D1614683

Musculoskeletal Ultrasound-Guided Regenerative Medicine

Yasser El Miedany
Editor

Musculoskeletal Ultrasound-Guided Regenerative Medicine

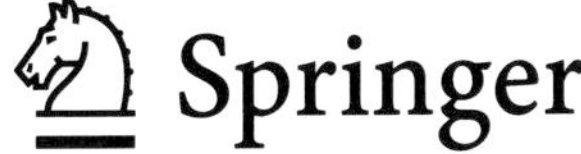

Editor
Yasser El Miedany
Institute of Medical Sciences
Canterbury Christ Church University
Canterbury, Kent, UK

ISBN 978-3-030-98255-3 ISBN 978-3-030-98256-0 (eBook)
https://doi.org/10.1007/978-3-030-98256-0

This Springer imprint is published by the registered company Springer Nature Switzerland AG
The registered company address is: Gewerbestrasse 11, 6330 Cham, Switzerland

To my friends
True friends are never apart, may be in distance, never in heart

Foreword

It is my pleasure to write this foreword for the textbook *Musculoskeletal Ultrasound and Interventional Regenerative Medicine*. Ultrasonography of the musculoskeletal system began over 50 years ago primarily focusing on the diagnosis of tendon pathology. Since then, we have seen significant advances in technology and now we are able to visualize structures as small as peripheral nerve branches. We have also subsequently advanced our ability to image musculoskeletal pathology. Subtle areas of tendinosis, partial tearing of small ligaments of the fingers, and peripheral nerve disorders are now readily identified. Color Doppler applications also allow us to identify neovascularity within tendinosis and inflammation in synovitis.

Paralleling these advancements in imaging of anatomy and pathology is our further understanding of pathology on a histologic and biochemical level. This information has allowed us to investigate novel treatments for musculoskeletal pathology. Musculoskeletal sonography now plays an important role where subtle pathology can be identified and then treatments can be directed to the area of concern using ultrasound guidance. Such treatments have progressed from routine anesthetics and corticosteroids to new regenerative medicine applications.

This textbook reviewing the current state of ultrasound guided regenerative medicine is a timely body of work. The authors have nicely reviewed essential topics to provide an overview of regenerative medicine. Subsequently, diagnostic and interventional musculoskeletal ultrasound techniques are reviewed specific to each joint and other applications. In addition to regenerative medicine treatments, other novel topics include spine applications and high frequency peripheral nerve ultrasonography. I commend the editor and authors of this textbook for providing an essential overview of an important topic that has the potential to alter how we think about the diagnosis and treatment of musculoskeletal disorders.

Professor of Radiology, University of Cincinnati Jon A. Jacobson
Cincinnati, OH, USA

Preface

Regenerative medicine is the branch of medicine that develops methods to repair, regrow, or replace damaged or diseased cells, organs or tissues. Broadly, it includes the generation and use of therapeutic stem cells, tissue engineering and the production of artificial organs. The year 2021 represents the dawn of a new era of regenerative medicine, as the field of regenerative medicine reached a remarkable milestone. By mid-2021, four women regained full sexual function after the successful implantation of lab-grown vaginas created from their own cells. In August 2021, the Alliance for Regenerative Medicine (ARM), in collaboration with GlobalData, published a new report highlighting that 2021 has already been a "year of firsts and records" for the regenerative medicine sector with significant clinical milestones, commercial progress and investment.

For the first time ever, CRISPR gene-editing technology was deployed in vivo in human patients — to treat ATTR amyloidosis — with extremely positive interim Phase 1 results. An ex vivo approach has shown compelling early-stage results in sickle cell and beta thalassemia patients. Regenerative medicine is on track to have the highest annual number of regulatory approvals of new gene therapy and gene-modified cell therapy products, with three already approved and an additional four to receive regulatory decisions across the USA and Europe in the remainder of 2021.

The rationale for this book is a gap that needs filling on the application of regenerative medicine in musculoskeletal diseases both in terms of concepts and management. So, this book has been written aiming at discussing the recent developments in regenerative medicine and its therapeutic potential, guided by musculoskeletal ultrasonography scanning. The book starts with an introductory section including three chapters on the principles of regenerative medicine and regenerative options for musculoskeletal disorders. Next is the section of diagnostic and interventional musculoskeletal ultrasound which includes eight chapters representing a clinician's guide to region-specific musculoskeletal ultrasonography and image optimization. The following section deals with regenerative medicine procedures carried out under ultrasound guidance This include six chapters discussing hydrodissection, high-frequency peripheral nerve ultrasound, prolotherapy, interventional physiatry and US-guided spinal procedures. The fourth section includes the role of regenerative therapies in sports medicine. The section comes in three chapters discussing US-guided exercises, musculoskeletal US in sports, and the use of US and regenerative therapies in sports injuries. The last section deals with the challenges, perspectives and future directions for regenerative medicine.

The main theme of this book is to deliver a very practical and reader-friendly guide. It delivers the science-based evidence and advanced knowledge of regenerative medicine. Further, it provides the most recent developments in this field together with examples of recent practical approaches which would be of value for the readers/researchers in their standard practice/clinical trials. With its 21 key chapters, this book is expected to fill an important void in the current literature. It represents what can be considered the best current thinking on regenerative medicine. Therefore, *Musculoskeletal Ultrasound Guided Regenerative Medicine* can serve as both an excellent introductory material and a very good reference as well as resource for implementation in standard clinical practice and future reading. Special thanks to my colleagues and friends for their support throughout the whole project which helped to make this book complete.

This book has been the outcome of cooperative effort of a large international cohort of leaders in regenerative medicine and musculoskeletal ultrasonography. They have done a superb job in producing authoritative chapters including vast amounts of scientific and clinical data to create state-of-the-art descriptions of regenerative medicine and its application in the variable musculoskeletal disorders. Special thanks to Jeimylo do Castro, Medical Director at SMARTMD, Philippines, for his support and collaboration throughout the whole project which helped to make this book complete. Personally, I feel privileged to have compiled this work and am enthusiastic about all that it offers our readers. I hope you too will find this edition a uniquely valuable educational resource.

Canterbury, UK Yasser El Miedany

London, UK
26 December 2021

Contents

Contributors

Paschenelle Celis Physical Medicine & Rehabilitation Department, Clinica OS Habitares, Quezon City, Philippines

Ke-Vin Chang Department of Physical Medicine and Rehabilitation, National Taiwan University Hospital, Bei-Hu Branch, Taipei, Taiwan

Angela N. Cortez Department of Physical Medicine & Rehabilitation, University of California at Davis, Sacramento, CA, USA

Jeimylo C. de Castro Chair, Physical Medicine and Rehabilitation Department, The Medical City-South Luzon, Sta. Rosa, Laguna, Philippines

Medical Director/CEO, SMARTMD Center for Non-Surgical Pain Interventions, Makati City, Philippines

Rhoel James Timothy O. Dejano Department of Internal Medicine, University of Cebu Medical Center, Cebu City, Philippines

Franklin San Pedro Domingo Department of Physical Medicine & Rehabilitation, Center for Regenerative Medicine, Pain Management Service, Makati Medical Center, Makati City, Philippines

Samia Elazab Galala University, Suez, Egypt

Faculty of Dentistry, Cairo University, Giza, Egypt

Yasser El Miedany Institute of Medical Sciences, Canterbury Christ Church University, Canterbury, Kent, UK

Tolga Ergönenç Akyazı Hospital Pain and Palliative Care, Sakarya, Turkey

Jeffrey D. Gross Stem Cell Whisperer, SPINE & ReCELLebrate, Henderson, NV, USA

Daniel Habbal Sydney Kimmel Medical College, Thomas Jefferson University, Philadelphia, PA, USA

Troy P. Henning Rehabilitation and Performance Medicine, Swedish Medical Group, Seattle, WA, USA

Kaitlin Jayendran McMaster University, Hamilton, ON, Canada

Jonathan Kirschner Department of Physiatry, Hospital for Special Surgery, New York, NY, USA

Department of Rehabilitation Medicine, UT Health San Antonio, TX, San Antonio, USA

King Hei Stanley Lam The Hong Kong Institute of Musculoskeletal Medicine, Kowloon, Hong Kong

Department of Family Medicine, The Faculty of Medicine, The Chinese University of Hong Kong, New Territory, Hong Kong

Department of Family Medicine, The Faculty of Medicine, The University of Hong Kong, Hong Kong, Hong Kong

Chih-Peng Lin Department of Anesthesiology, National Taiwan University Hospital and National Taiwan University College of Medicine, Taipei, Taiwan

Alexander R. Lloyd University of Pittsburgh Medical Center, Department of PM&R, Pittsburgh, PA, USA

Daniel R. Lueders University of Pittsburgh Medical Center, Pittsburgh, PA, USA

Nicola Maffulli Department of Musculoskeletal Disorders, University of Salerno School of Medicine and Dentistry, Salerno, Italy

Queen Mary University of London, Barts and the London School of Medicine and Dentistry Centre for Sports and Exercise Medicine, Mile End Hospital, London, UK

Gerard A. Malanga New Jersey Regenerative Institute LLC, Cedar Knolls, NJ, USA

Department of Physical Medicine and Rehabilitation, Rutgers University, New Jersey Medical School, Newark, NJ, USA

Liza Maniquis-Smigel Hilo, HI, USA

Robert Monaco Department of Sports Medicine, Atlantic Health System, Morristown, NJ, USA

William D. Murrell Plancher Orthopaedics and Sports Medicine, Fellowship Program, New York City, NY, USA

411th Hospital Center, Jacksonville Naval Airstation, Jacksonville, FL, USA

Michael Francis Obispo, MD, PTRP, RMSK Department of Physical and Rehabilitation Medicine, De La Salle Medical and Health Sciences Institute, Dasmariñas, Cavite, Philippines

Kentaro Onishi University of Pittsburgh Medical Center, Department of PM&R and Orthopedic Surgery, Pittsburgh, Pennsylvania, USA

Hector L. Osoria Department of Sports Medicine, Atlantic Health System, Morristown, NJ, USA

Levent Özçakar Hacettepe University Medical School, Department of Physical and Rehabilitation Medicine, Ankara, Turkey

Susan Plummer Faculty of Medicine, Health and Social Care, Canterbury Christ Church University, Canterbury, Kent, UK

Adam Pourcho Rehabilitation and Performance Medicine, Swedish Medical Group, Seattle, WA, USA

Piyaporn Pramuksun Department of Physical Medicine and Rehabilitation, Bhumibol Adulyadej hospital, Bangkok, Thailand

Joseph Purita The Institute of Regenerative Medicine, Boca Raton, FL, USA

Aditya Raghunandan Department of Physiatry, Hospital for Special Surgery, New York, NY, USA

Department of Rehabilitation Medicine, UT Health San Antonio, TX, San Antonio, USA

Dean Reeves Private Practice of Physical Medicine and Rehabilitation, Roeland Park, KS, USA

Kenneth Dean Reeves Private Practice of Physical Medicine and Rehabilitation, Roeland Park, KS, USA

Vincenzo Ricci Physical and Rehabilitation Medicine Unit, Luigi Sacco University Hospital, ASST Fatebenefratelli-Sacco, Milano, Italy

Allison N. Schroeder University of Pittsburgh Medical Center, Pittsburgh, PA, USA

Jeffrey Smith University of Pittsburgh Medical Center, Department of PM&R, Pittsburgh, Pennsylvania, USA

Jeffrey A. Strakowski Department of PM&R, The Ohio State University, OhioHealth Riverside Methodist Hospital, Columbus, OH, USA

Daniel Chiung-Jui Su Department of Physical Medicine and Rehabilitation, Chi-Mei Hospital, Tainan, Taiwan

Donald Tsung-Yung Tang Department of Pain Managemet, Taichung Tzu Chi Hospital, Taichung, Taiwan

Lauren Vernese Rehabilitation and Performance Medicine, Swedish Medical Group, Seattle, WA, USA

Nagib Atallah Yurdi Reem Hospital, Abu Dhabi, United Arab Emirates

Yung-Tsan Wu Department of Physical Medicine and Rehabilitation, Tri-Service General Hospital, School of Medicine, National Defense Medical Center, Taipei, Taiwan

Integrated Pain Management Center, Tri-Service General Hospital, School of Medicine, National Defense Medical Center, Taipei, Taiwan

Part I

Regenerative Medicine

1 Fundamentals and Applications of Regenerative Medicine

Yasser El Miedany

Introduction

Regenerative medicine (RM) is a new medical specialty that implements advances in the study of cells and tissue engineering to understand how the body repair/heals itself. The capability to successfully generate replacement cells, heal tissues, and repair ligaments has been one of the most fascinating and anticipated medical developments of the twenty-first century. Gradually, the concept of RM has expanded and become multifaceted, including cell therapy, tissue engineering, and gene therapy. Global attention to the field is growing at a rapid pace. A Nobel Prize winner in medicine (2012), Dr. Shinya Yamanaka, is a prime example of this recognition, for his discovery in converting a human skin cell to a stem cell [1]. This rapidly expanding science is expected to become a breakthrough solution through its potential impact across many therapeutic areas. This has been reflected by the level of investment in this science, as the global market is estimated to reach $50.5 billion by 2025 [2]. In real-life application, RM is anticipated to play a major transformative role in mainly in two therapeutic areas, cardiovascular and musculoskeletal diseases.

Y. El Miedany (✉)
Institute of Medical Sciences, Canterbury Christ Church University, Canterbury, Kent, UK

Applying the term "regenerative medicine," to musculoskeletal injuries, describes a rapidly growing new approach of musculoskeletal medicine, which employs evidence-based treatments that focus on augmenting the body's endogenous repair capabilities. This is not only limited to the specific injury site but also the region of injury. This has been made possible by the precise application of autologous, allogeneic, or proliferative agents. Musculoskeletal (MSK) diseases encompass more than 100 disorders characterized by injuries to joints and soft tissue [3]. Worldwide, the market for regenerative medicine is quite big. In December 2016, the US Congress passed the twenty-first Century Cures Act with the intent of further incentivizing pharmaceutical and medical device companies to pursue advancements in technology that aid patients who are in dire need of care. The Act was intended to create a comprehensive policy framework for RM, which allowed the US Food and Drug Administration (FDA) to more efficiently expedite its development and approval processes by building on already established approaches, including fast-track, breakthrough therapy designation, accelerated approval, and priority review [4]. In response, in November 2017, the FDA established a new framework called RM Advanced Therapy (RMAT) designation [5].

The chapter will expand to discuss phases of the regenerative medicine, existing and new cell sources, as well as its clinical applications,

Y. El Miedany (ed.), *Musculoskeletal Ultrasound-Guided Regenerative Medicine*,
https://doi.org/10.1007/978-3-030-98256-0_1

including both the potential regenerative medicine interventions for the treatment of major musculoskeletal diseases, their limitations, and the convergence of regenerative medicine and rehabilitation. The chapter will conclude with the potential for transforming healthcare through regenerative medicine, ethics in musculoskeletal regenerative medicine, the need for regenerative medicine curriculum particularly for next-generation physicians, and lastly a look forward toward achieving maturity of the regenerative medicine field.

Standard Forms of Therapy vs. Regenerative Medicine

To understand the innovative role of regenerative medicine, it would be very helpful to compare it to the standard management approaches. This was reviewed in a recent review article by Mulvaney et al. [6]. Standard treatment modalities, basically, act by stopping/minimizing the pain levels or reduction of the inflammatory process with the aim of facilitating the endogenous repair mechanisms. Management modalities vary to include pharmaceutical agents such as anti-inflammatory drugs [7, 8], destructive modalities (e.g., radio frequency ablation of nerves, botulinum toxin injections) [9], and surgical methods that permanently alter the functioning of a joint, including joint fusion, spine fixation, and partial or total arthroplasty.

Standard Pharmacotherapy

Anti-inflammatory therapy includes both nonsteroidal anti-inflammatory drugs (NSAIDs) and corticosteroid medications. These are widely recommended for acute and chronic painful musculoskeletal conditions. However, published Cochrane Database Systemic Reviews revealed that in the medical literature, there is poor justification to show that these anti-inflammatory medications are able to promote better long-term tissue healing [10, 11]). In fact, NSAIDs may interfere with tissue healing [2, 3]. A well-executed randomized controlled trial (RCT), published in 2017, compared intra-articular steroid injections to normal saline injections for the treatment of knee osteoarthritis over a 2-year follow-up period. Results did not show any association with improvement in pain. In addition, in the cohort treated with steroid injections into the knee joints, there was evidence of accelerated osteoarthritis as shown in MRI scans [12]. There is substantial evidence that the standard local steroid injections, which usually is combined with local anesthetic, have toxic effects on chondrocytes both in vivo and vitro. This negative impact on the cartilage has been attributed to the steroids therapy [13, 14]. Regarding the use of steroids in treating tendinopathy, a meta-analysis of 41 RCTs outcomes, published in 2010 by Coombes and colleagues, revealed that "at four weeks post-injection, the non-injection groups had better pain and function in comparison to the injected group" [15]. In addition, a randomized controlled trial, which compared local steroid injections to placebo (saline) injections, demonstrated worse outcomes in the corticosteroid injection group after 1 year [16].

The pathophysiologic basis for using anti-inflammatory therapy for the treatment of tendinopathies was a matter of debate, if not rebutted. In an early published study (1999) authored by Kraushaar and Nirschl, sections of human lateral epicondyle tendons from patients suffering from tendinitis of the extensor tendons were assessed using electron microscopy. Results revealed that there was a noticeable absence of cells associated with inflammation; hence, "tendinitis" can be a misnomer. They successfully demonstrated that, instead, the underlying pathology represented a chronic degenerative status referred to as "tendinosis" [17].

Considering local spinal injections, epidural steroid injections is considered one of the most common procedures in the setting of subacute and chronic lumbar pain. An updated Cochrane review, which evaluated the outcomes of 18 RCTs, concluded that "there is currently insufficient evidence to support the use of steroid injection therapy in subacute and chronic low-back pain" [18]. Many standard orthopedic surgeries, including arthroscopic surgery for the repair of knee meniscal tears in patients over the age of 40, have been shown in a recent meta-analysis of nine RCTs to be no better than sham surgery or conservative treatment; in fact, they accelerate the degeneration process in the affected knee joints [19, 20].

Lastly, opioid therapy has also long been a cornerstone in the management of chronic non-neoplastic musculoskeletal pain. However, chronic narcotic therapy has inadvertently contributed to a national epidemic of opioid-related deaths [21]. This is in addition to the well-known opioid-associated adverse effects. These include opioid-induced hyperalgesia, constipation, as well as tolerance or lack of long-term efficacy or improved quality of life [22].

Lastly, when compared to other allopathic options, including knee and hip arthroplasty with a 90-day mortality rate of 0.7% in the Western hemisphere [23], regenerative medicine treatment modalities have a lower incidence of adverse events with a growing body of statistically significant medical literature illustrating both their safety and efficacy [24].

Basics of Regenerative Medicine

Local Tissue Metabolic Changes

Studying the metabolic process in painful musculoskeletal conditions and the associated local tissue metabolic changes reveals a shift toward a catabolic state. Such catabolic, sub-optimal healing environment has been attributed to several factors including the following: exposure to toxins (including many pharmaceuticals), obesity, poor diet, lack of regular exercise, chronic systemic inflammation, chronic infection, poor sleep quality, hormonal disturbances, and chronic stress [25, 26].

In addition, with aging, the body moves toward senescence (a condition or process of deterioration with age or loss of a cell's power of division and growth) with a gradual shift from a balanced catabolic/anabolic status to one that slightly favors catabolic environment, consequently resulting in gradual tissue degeneration. At some point, this slow senescence becomes clinically manifested in the form of chronic injuries.

The net result of such metabolic changes is impairment of the body's ability to self-repair, which sometimes may reach a state of failure in the setting of chronic injury. Several reasons have been identified for such inadequate or failed self-repair process; these are shown in Table 1.1.

Table 1.1 Reasons for inadequate or failed self-repair process in musculoskeletal pain

1. The body fails to recognize an injury and consequently fails to initiate an effective healing response
2. The repair mechanism is overwhelmed by ongoing tissue insults such as chronic repetitive movements without adequate recovery, ligamentous laxity resulting in pathologic joint movement, and functional movement disorders resulting in pathologic movement
3. The repair mechanisms are inhibited by a suboptimal healing milieu

The Potential of Regenerative Medicine in Achieving Metabolic Balance

These data paved the way for healthcare professionals to consider alternative approaches for patients' management. The regenerative medicine treatment model represents an innovative treatment modality, where there is a shift in the balance from catabolism and tissue degeneration toward anabolism and tissue repair on a local and/or regional level. In fact, each of the reasons for failure to self-repair can be considered a potential target for regenerative medicine. One target of regenerative medicine treatment is to augment the anabolic environment through the stimulation of native and natural processes. Therefore, regenerative medicine offers solutions to repair, restore, or replace skeletal elements and associated tissues that are affected by acute injury, chronic degeneration, genetic dysfunction, or cancer-related defects [6]. The goal is to improve quality of life and outcomes for people with musculoskeletal injury or degradation.

The Induction of Self-Regeneration

Conceptually, although the term "regenerative medicine" includes the creation of artificial organs and their subsequent implantation; its most realistic definition refers to the set of processes used to repair or replace tissue or organ function by stimulating and inducing their own self-regeneration. Schematically, this discipline encompasses two therapeutic strategies: those based on the use of living cells or cell-based therapies and those based on tissue engineering using different scaffolds and matrices with biocompatible materials, alone or in combination, to provide support and facilitate the repair of tissue damage [27, 28]. Among cell therapies, one may differentiate two types of products based on mature cells, grafts or implants, and those using stem or progenitor cells.

The application of different regenerative techniques has enabled the development of different basic, preclinical and clinical studies with encouraging results for the treatment of various diseases, including those of musculoskeletal origin [29, 30]. The first set of strategies to repair damage to the bone or cartilage tissue consisted of transplantation or implantation of autografts to provide a supply of cells able to provide an influx of osteo- or chondro-inducting factors. However, these methods have limitations in their bioavailability and the size of the lesion to be repaired. Alternatives, such as allogeneic and/or xenogeneic transplants, need further analysis regarding the risk of rejection, disease transmission, and/or teratogenicity.

The therapeutic potential of each strategy depends on the nature of damage to repair. Its widespread application is still subject to the resolution of technical and biological aspects; however, advances in this field are growing rapidly, in particular those related to cellular therapies applied to musculoskeletal diseases, one of the most promising fields for medium-term treatments [31–33].

Phases of the Regenerative Medicine

Most of the techniques adopted in regenerative medicine interventions depend on precise injections of autologous, allogeneic, or proliferative agents, which initiate (or reinitiate) a productive healing cascade by stimulating a repair response. Often this is accomplished in three phases (Fig. 1.1): First comes *phase 1*: an acute inflammatory reaction is initiated in the target tissue. This focuses the body's ability to heal itself by providing "initial injury debridement" through the action of macrophages and subsequently paves the way for the proliferative phase of tissue repair, among many other key functions [34].

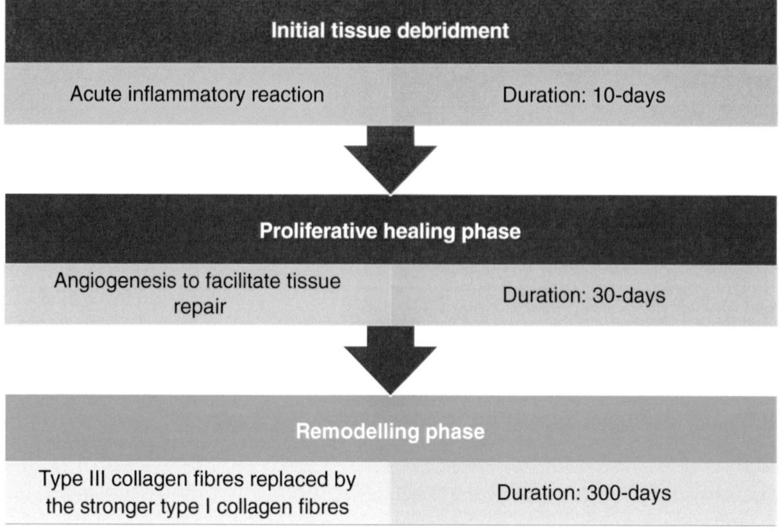

Fig. 1.1 Phases of regenerative medicine enhanced tissue healing

This inflammatory phase lasts for 10 days. This is followed by *phase 2*: the "proliferative healing phase" lasts for 30 days and involves chemical messengers released from the injury site, which recruit fibroblasts to the injury location and induce local angiogenesis at the site to facilitate tissue repair. Lastly, comes *Phase 3*: "the remodeling phase" is the final phase of tissue healing, during which the rapidly laid down type 3 collagen fibers are gradually replaced by stronger, more organized type 1 collagen fibers [35]. This remodeling takes up to 300 days to complete.

The Importance of Image Guidance

Successful regenerative medicine treatment relies not only on an accurate diagnosis but also on precise guidance of injections. Most of the injectates administered in regenerative medicine are costly to prepare or purchase; therefore, an ultrasound-guided application, along with detailed knowledge of sonographic anatomy, plays an important role in the success of the procedures [36]. It would be also nearly impossible to assess the effectiveness of therapies without knowing precisely where they were placed in or near the injured tissue. Hall [37] carried out a review of palpation-guided versus ultrasound-guided peripheral injections; he reported a remarkably low level of accuracy when injections are performed based on palpation-guided landmarks. Thus, it is highly recommended that soft tissue structures, such as ligaments, tendons, joint capsules, and muscles, should be injected using real-time ultrasound guidance. Many spine targets have reasonable medical literature supporting the use of ultrasound guidance [38, 39]. Fluoroscopic guidance is suitable for intervertebral disc and transforaminal epidural injections, as well as for subchondral and intraosseous injections.

Fundamentals of Cell Therapies

To understand the fundamentals and the potential of cell therapies in musculoskeletal diseases, analogies can be drawn with the composition of a classic drug. Not surprisingly, and to bridge gaps, cellular therapies are considered drugs and as such must meet all stages of drug development, including their adequate manufacturing practices and conditions (GMP). By definition, the principal component or "active ingredient" of cell therapy is the cell itself, while the "carrier" would be represented by growth factors and/or biomaterials that facilitate structural integration or differentiation of cells. The cell component may be composed of mature or undifferentiated cells. Thus, chondrocytes or cartilage explants developed for the treatment of chondral defects are an example of the first type. However, the use of differentiated cells has not satisfactorily met expectations. Currently, attention has focused on the progenitor cells with improved biological properties and superior plasticity to those already differentiated [40, 41].

A stem or progenitor cell is defined in terms of its ability to divide asymmetrically, i.e., self-renewing itself while maintaining its undifferentiated state, or divide and differentiate into other cell types. Broadly speaking, and depending on their origin, stem cells are grouped into two categories: embryonic stem cells (ESC) and adult stem cells (ASC). This classification carries other intrinsic differentiation potential. Thus, embryonic stem cells (ESC), deriving from the embryonic blastocyst can differentiate into cells belonging to any of the three embryonic layers: ectoderm, endoderm, and mesoderm (from which skeletal tissues originate) (Fig. 1.2).This totipotency (ability of developing into a complete organism or differentiating into any of its cells or tissues), however, can cause problems when undergoing therapeutic application, arising from their high proliferation capacity and the possibility of ectopic teratoma formation. Thus, the most reasonable approach, from the point of view of their therapeutic application, is to use cells with limited differentiation potential, specific to an embryonic single-layer lineage.

Experimentally, it is possible to induce reprogramming of adult cells to a pluripotent (capable of giving rise to several different cell types) immature state, called induced pluripotent stem cells (iPSC), but its application is still under investigation. While scientific advances to avoid the risk arising from the application of the previ-

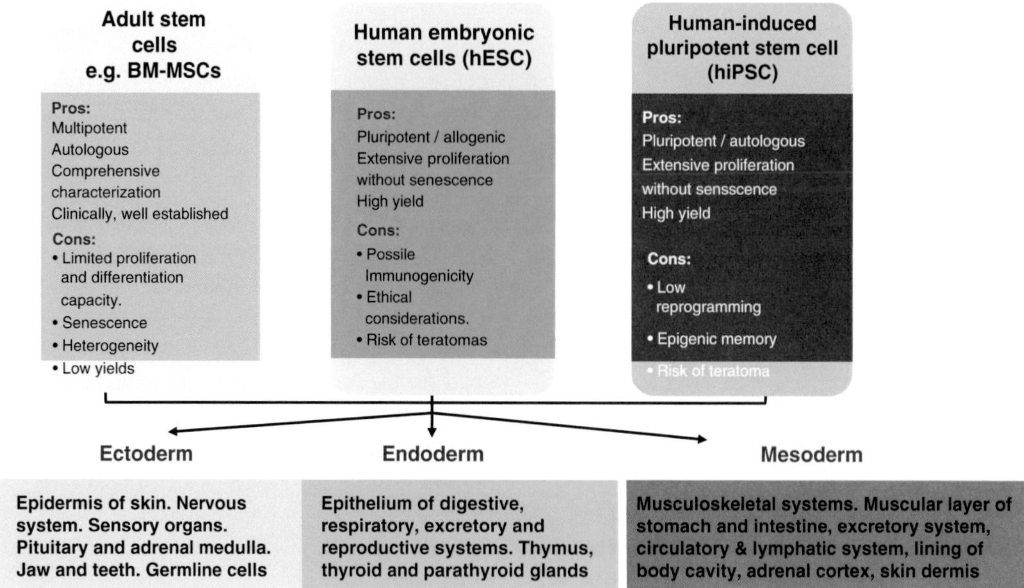

Fig. 1.2 Pros and cons of using adult stem cells and pluripotent stem cells for clinical applications. Comparison of the BM-MSCs, hESCs, and hiPSCs for application in regenerative medicine. Pluripotent stem cells derivation and subsequent tissue generation ability. hESCs can be derived from the inner cell mass of a blastocyst at the final stage of preimplantation development. hiPSCs can be obtained through reprogramming somatic cells using the forced expression of OCT4, SOX2, KLF4, and NANOG. These cells can subsequently be differentiated into any derivative of the three germ layers (ectoderm, endoderm, and mesoderm). BM-MSC bone marrow-derived mesenchymal stem cell, hESC human embryonic stem cell, hiPSC human-induced pluripotent stem cell

ous cell types have been made, the best current option is the use of natural skeletal progenitor cells, mesenchymal stem cells (MSC) [27].

The Mesodermal Embryonic Stem Cells

Mesenchymal stem cells (MSCs) are mesodermal embryonic stem cells from which adult connective tissues develop. Therefore, they constitute progenitor cells of other specialized cells, such as chondrocytes, osteoblasts, adipocytes, tenocytes, myoblasts, as well as others. They retain their self-renewal capacity, which facilitates their in vitro expansion [42, 43]. In addition to differentiating into different lineages, if subjected to an appropriate postimplantation stimulus in vitro or in vivo, they have immunomodulatory properties [44]. Originally, they were described in the bone marrow stroma. They are currently known to be virtually ubiquitous, although adipose tissue, along with bone marrow, is the most common source of MSC. However, the frequency of MSCs in tissues decreases with age [45], and more importantly, the tissue of origin seems to confer particular characteristics that can alter their immunomodulatory properties [46, 47]. This variability may be related to the fact that MSCs are actually a heterogeneous population of cells. In fact, due to the absence of a single common tag, the definition of an MSC is performed according to the performance of three minimum criteria: their ability to adhere to culture medium, the presence of various cell surface markers and the absence hematopoietic lineage markers, and, finally, their in vitro ability to commit to osteogenic, chondrogenic, and adipogenic lineages, generally determined by histochemical staining. Given the relative laxity of the selection criteria, one of the challenges lies in the unambiguous characterization of MSC as a single entity, a task that has not yet been achieved.

The immunomodulatory functions of MSC, one of the aspects of their therapeutic potential, are gaining more importance and have already been applied in different pathologies. The study of the immunomodulatory potential of MSCs was described originally by studying their effect on regulatory T cells, such as Ras initiation and mediators of transplant rejection. Numerous evidences have shown that under inflammatory conditions, MSC may inhibit T cell effector responses or increase Treg-mediated regulatory function. Furthermore, they can also exert various effects on other immune cells. Thus, MSC inhibit the maturation of dendritic cells, preventing their migration to the lymph nodes and their antigen-presenting function; they modulate macrophages and NK cells, and suppress the proliferation and terminal differentiation of B15 cells. The mechanisms through which they carry out these functions are both dependent on cell contact and through secretion of soluble factors [48, 49].

Stem Cell-Microenvironment Communication

Manipulation of the tissue microenvironment has become a promising method to enhance the regenerative abilities of stem cells/progenitors for musculoskeletal repair. The composition of the microenvironment is determined by the resident cells, extracellular matrix, cytokines, and chemokines as well as the biomechanical property and nutrient status. The microenvironment is altered by the homeostasis and degenerative stage of the native tissue. All the alterations of the surrounding host microenvironment will definitely change the biology of the implanted stem cells/progenitors. Thus, a thorough understanding of the stem cell-microenvironment communication would therefore accelerate the success of musculoskeletal repair [43].

The interaction between stem cells and local microenvironment goes in both directions. Not only the microenvironment can impose on the fate of stem cells but also stem cells can positively affect the local microenvironment of injured tissues. In Fang's study [50] using a rat peripheral nerve injury model, except from generating neurons, transplanted embryonic spinal cord cells were found to have a regulatory effect on local Schwann cells in the distal nerve and induced them to produce proximal axons to facilitate nerve regeneration.

Amyotrophic lateral sclerosis (ALS) is a progressive disease that affects nerve cells in the brain and spinal cord, causing loss of muscle control. Due to the low bioavailability and short half-life in vivo, in clinics, the expected outcomes of the intrathecal administration of neurotrophic factors alone were hard to achieve. Pawlukowska et al. [51] performed a clinical study using the autologous lineage negative (Lin^-) stem cells to treat ALS. The authors thought Lin^- stem cell-based therapy would be a reasonable and promising alternative for classic ALS treatments, because the Lin^- stem cells could produce the trophic support for the host's neurons, stimulate the secretion of neurotrophins (NTs), and differentiate into oligodendrocyte progenitor cells or neurons. The authors completed a clinical trial to assess the impact of intrathecal administration of bone marrow Lin^- stem cells in 32 patients suffering from ALS on articulation; it was demonstrated that 6 patients achieved the improvement of articulation after 28 days, 23 patients remained stable, and 3 deteriorated. Although some valuable findings were observed, several limitations should be acknowledged, such as the small number of patients, the lack of control group, and a short observation period.

During muscle regeneration, as reviewed by Dort et al. [52], the spatial recruitment of pro-inflammatory and anti-inflammatory macrophages was reported to be different and is related to their temporal recruitment, meaning that pro-inflammatory macrophages were found located close to proliferating satellite cells, while anti-inflammatory macrophages were found close to the regenerating area containing differentiated myoblasts. Depletion of pro-inflammatory macrophages resulted in impaired muscle regeneration in animal models. The suppression of the switch of macrophage from pro-inflammatory phenotype to anti-inflammatory phenotype reduced muscle fiber growth but did not affect the clearance of necrotic tissues. At the cellular level, pro-inflammatory macrophages promote myoblast proliferation and inhibit differentiation, while anti-inflammatory macrophages inhibit myoblast proliferation and stimulate their differentiation and myofiber growth. Direct coculture of macrophages also promoted proliferation and inhibited apoptosis of myogenic cells. Altogether, these findings suggest that different subsets of macrophages have complementary roles in the regulation of satellite cell/myoblast function, myogenesis progression, and optimal muscle regeneration.

Existing and New Cell Sources

Most regenerative medicine strategies rely on an ample cell source, but identifying and obtaining sufficient numbers of therapeutic cells is often a challenge. Stem, progenitor, and differentiated cells derived from both adult and embryonic tissues are widely being explored in regenerative medicine, although adult tissue-derived cells are the dominant cell type used clinically to date due to both their ready availability and perceived safety [53, 54]. All FDA-approved regenerative medicine therapies and the vast majority of strategies explored in the clinic use adult tissue-derived cells. There is great interest in obtaining greater numbers of stem cells from adult tissues and in identifying stem cell populations suitable for therapeutic use in tissues historically thought not to harbor stem cells [55].

Therefore, sources can be stratified into two main types of stem cells, embryonic and non-embryonic. Embryonic stem cells (ESC) are obtained from embryos, whereas non-embryonic stem cells (NESC) are derived from essentially any adult tissue, such as placenta, blood, the umbilical cord, and adipose tissue. As noted above, most of the treatments available or under evaluation are related to the non-embryonic stem cell treatment.

Platelet-rich plasma treatment or PRP is very popular, given its association with professional athletes. PRP is a patient's own blood that is spun down in a machine, which will allow for the blood to separate into its various components. The plasma, which contains growth factors and platelets, is drawn from the solution and injected into the tendons, ligaments, muscles, and joints due to its healing property. There have been several studies publishing the benefits of PRP treatment, and its presence helps increase treatment options for specific musculoskeletal ailments [56].

Stem cells obtained from adipose tissue represent a viable source. Adipose tissue stem cells are obtained via needle biopsy or liposuction. The sample must be minced profusely washed and chemically treated and then incubated for 30 minutes and neutralized. This process is similar for both bone marrow and placenta stem cells, which also have to be aspirate and harvested appropriately prior to usage [57].

Each option for stem cells has its own risks and benefits. For example, cells obtained from adipose tissue and bone marrow include more available stem cells compared to PRP, whereas the PRP has the advantage of being easier to obtain and utilize. The advantage of the stem cells, obtained from the amniotic tissue, is that is has been used for wound healing, while adipose stem cells have been utilized in surgeries to speed up tissue repair.

Studies aiming to understand the processes that control stem cell renewal are being leveraged for both purposes, with the prototypical example being studies with hematopoietic stem cells (HSCs) [58]. For example, exposure of HSCs in vitro to cytokines that are present in the HSC niche leads to significant HSC expansion, but this increase in number is accompanied by a loss of repopulation potential [59, 60]. Coculture of HSCs with cells implicated in the HSC niche and in microenvironments engineered to mimic native bone marrow may improve maintenance of HSC stemness during expansion, enhancing stem cell numbers for transplantation. For example, direct contact of HSCs with MSCs grown in a 3D environment induces greater CD34+ expansion than with MSCs grown on 2D substrate [61]. Another example is that culture of skeletal muscle stem cells on substrates with mechanical properties similar to normal muscle leads to greater stem cell expansion [62] and can even rescue impaired proliferative ability in stem cells from aged animals [63].

Standard Interventions for the Treatment of Major Musculoskeletal Diseases and Their Limitations

Osteoarthritis

Osteoarthritis (OA) is considered the most common joint disease mainly among older adults [64], with a high global prevalence [66]. As life expectancy is surging for both men and women worldwide, the years of life lived with disability is also expected to increase. This demonstrates the impact of increased life span without a corresponding improvement in health span. The underlying pathology of OA includes degradation of the hyaline articular cartilage and the abnormal remodeling of the joint tissues, which results in loss of joint function. Cartilage is avascular, has low cellularity, and, therefore, has a limited capacity for repair. Daily wear and tear or injury leads to the structural deterioration of articular cartilage at the joint surface. The early stages of OA are characterized by the formation of partial thickness chondral defects. If left untreated, the defects will extend into the marrow spaces of subchondral bone, giving access to bone marrow stem cells (BMSCs). The repair tissue formed by infiltrating BMSCs is typically fibrous rather than hyaline [65].

Effective treatments for OA are currently lacking [66]. Early-stage management includes glucosamine/chondroitin supplement therapy and hyaluronic acid injections. However, their efficacy has been highly debated [67, 68]. On the other hand, surgical management is mainly in the form of total joint replacement, which is widely used; however, surgeries are considered a late-stage treatment option and, as expected, carry significant risks, which gets higher with patient age [69, 70]. Other early-stage interventions are available and focus on initiating cell-based repair. Reparative techniques, such as abrasion arthroplasty [71], debridement [72], and microfracture [73], aim to encourage infiltration of stem cells from the marrow spaces of the underlying subchondral bone, to stimulate repair of the damaged tissue. Restorative techniques such as mosaicplasty [74] involve removing cartilage plugs from non-load-bearing regions of the joint and implanting them into the osteochondral defect zone. Another restorative surgical technique is autologous chondrocyte implantation (ACI) [75]; here, patient-derived autologous chondrocytes are harvested from the non-load-bearing region of the articular cartilage, expanded in monolayer culture, and implanted at the site of the defect underneath a periosteal flap. This technique often utilizes a collagen scaffold to support the implanted cells and is referred to as matrix-assisted ACI (MACI). Following recently published NICE guidelines (2017) [76], ACI is now a recommended treatment; however, patient selection criteria are restrictive. While ACI has been relatively successful compared to other techniques such as mosaicplasty [75], there are a number of drawbacks associated with the treatment (Table 1.2).

Osteoporosis

Osteoporosis is a disease characterized by low bone mass and structural deterioration of bone tissue, leading to bone fragility. Worldwide, it has high prevalence with an estimated 22 million women, and 5.5 million men being affected within the EU [77], and over 8.9 million fractures annually of osteoporotic fractures [78].

Osteoporosis is caused by an imbalance in bone turnover homeostasis, leading to accelerated trabecular bone loss that results in a more porous structure. When associated with falls, the incidence of osteoporotic fractures gets higher [79]. Osteoporosis predominantly affects the older adults, and in association with increased fracture risk, there is a corresponding increase in the likelihood of morbidity. Unlike OA, there are a number of effective pharmacological treatments available for osteoporosis. Treatment types can be divided into two categories: antiresorptive and anabolic agents. Antiresorptive treatments reduce bone turnover and preserve bone mineral density (BMD). Anabolic agents stimulate bone forma-

Table 1.2 Standard treatment options vs cell therapy for chronic musculoskeletal diseases

Musculoskeletal disease	Risk/incidence	Standard management	Challenges	Cell/tissue therapy	Challenges
Fracture healing	Worldwide incidence of osteoporotic fractures: 8.9 million fractures each year	Plate and screw	Nonunion	Mesenchymal stem cells (MSC) combined with/without calcium sulfate Allogenic bone graft containing stem cells G-CSF-mobilized Hemopoietic stem cells with collagen scaffold for nonunion fracture healing	Uncontrolled MSC cell differentiation Immunologic rejection
Osteoarthritis	Worldwide incidence of: Knee OA: 3.8% Hip OA: 0.85% Lifetime risk of developing symptomatic knee OA: Men: ~40% Women: ~47% Higher risk in obese people	*Moderate OA:* Glucosamine sulfate Hyaluronic acid injections *Severe*: Total joint replacement *Reparative techniques:* Abrasion arthroplasty Debridement Microfracture	Conflicting outcomes (some in favor, others not) Late-stage option Risk of infection Need for redoing Limited repair option Results, typically, in fibrocartilaginous tissue	Restorative techniques: Mosaicplasty Autologous chondrocyte implantation (ACI) Matrix-assisted ACI (MACI)	Expensive Invasive process to procure chondrocytes, Limited number of cells Dedifferentiation during monolayer expansion Recommended for patients with knee OA who did not receive any previous treatments Formation of fibrocartilaginous tissue
Osteoporosis	Incidence in EU: Women: 22 million Men: 5.5 million	Pharmacotherapy Antiresorptive: Bisphosphonates Denosumab Anabolic: Parathyroid hormone Combined: Romosozumab Others: Calcium and vitamin D	Poor adherence Concerns regarding long-term therapy-associated side effects Atypical femur fracture Osteonecrosis of the jaw Limited duration of therapy Expensive	Stem cell therapy: Introduction of exogenous mesenchymal stem cells Small molecules that recruit endogenous stem cells to osteoporotic sites Stem cell stimulation and transplantation have the ability to reverse bone demineralization	Uncertainty of stem cell fate and biodistribution following cell transplantation

Myopathy	Sarcopenia (*mean age 67 years*): Men: 4.6% Women: 7.9%	Resistive exercise	Difficulty to do without assistance due to frailty of the sufferers Limited success	Myogenic stem cells to improve regeneration of old muscles	Massive rapid death of transplanted donor cells Minimal cell dispersal that is required to supply all muscles throughout the body
	Duchenne muscular dystrophy: Males:1 in 3500–6000 Women: 1:50,000,000	Genetic intervention steroids	Need to target skeletal and heart muscles Side effects Masks/delays symptoms only	Autologous bone marrow mononuclear Autologous myoblasts Myoblasts	Only a small percentage of stem cells replaced the damaged muscles Often must administer stem cells from donors

tion, thereby increasing BMD. It has been shown that some forms of combination or sequential therapy may offer a synergistic effect on BMD [80, 81]. While these treatments have been suggested to slow the progression of osteoporosis, they fail to offer long-term effective solutions [77] and are associated with variable side effects [82, 83], particularly with longer duration of therapy.

Myopathies

Myopathies (muscular diseases) are a key group of diseases that affect a fair percentage of the population [84, 85]. A common form of myopathy is sarcopenia [86], which is age-related loss of muscle mass and strength. Sarcopenia is associated with frailty and is more prevalent in older adults. There are also numerous genetic diseases, such as muscular dystrophies [87], for example, Duchene muscular dystrophy (DMD), and limb girdle muscle dystrophy. So far, there are limited effective treatments to combat the progression of muscular degeneration. Muscle itself has a resident population of stem cells, known as satellite cells [88]. These cells are responsible for the regeneration of muscle fibers following exercise or injury. However, the satellite cell-mediated repair mechanism can become compromised. For example, Duchene muscle dystrophy is characterized by continuous rounds of degeneration and regeneration of muscle fibers that results in a depletion of the muscle stem cell pool [89], leading to a loss of skeletal muscle mass. Currently, there are no approved drugs that consistently result in an increase in both muscle mass and strength, making treatment for myopathies extremely limited [90].

The Convergence of Regenerative Medicine and Rehabilitation

Regenerative rehabilitation lies at the intersection of regenerative medicine and rehabilitation research. While regenerative medicine approaches provide unique opportunities to regenerate, repair, and/or replace various tissues and organs, these approaches often fall short in the long-term treatment of chronic, disabling conditions. Regenerative medicine or rehabilitation approaches provide a foundation for the restoration of tissue architecture, promotion of organ function, reduction of disability, or improvement of quality of life. However, it is the combination of both approaches working synergistically that can optimize or maximize the functional outcome of the individual (Fig. 1.3) [91].

Current approaches in regenerative medicine involve the use of cells and/or biologics with or without scaffolding materials with the goal of replacing injured or lost tissue resulting from trauma or disease. However, the medical care process does not stop after transplantation of the cell or tissue construct in the clinic. Using the principles of rehabilitation sciences to maximize the outcome in the treatment of disabling condi-

Regenerative medicine
*Cells and tissues
*Matrices / scaffolds
*Biologics
*Enabling technology
Rehabilitation
*External stimulation
*Assistive Technology
*Therapeutic Physical activity
Regenerative rehabilitation
*Enhance tissue / organ function
*Reduce disabilities
*Increase quality of life

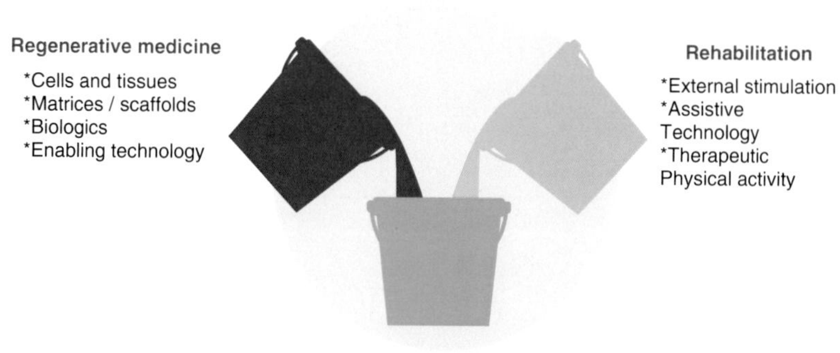

Fig. 1.3 Merging rehabilitation and regenerative medicine: the goals of the regenerative rehabilitation approach are to synergize regenerative medicine approaches with rehabilitation techniques to enhance the clinical outcomes for the patient

tions by regenerative medicine, impose the need to reconsider the standard management approaches, taking into account the role of post-transplantation rehabilitation. For example, the consequences of central nervous systems injuries illustrate the need for collaboration in clinical care and research in regenerative medicine and rehabilitation. Trauma to the central nervous system not only involves nerve cells but also the peripheral targets these cells innervate, including internal organs and the musculoskeletal system. Rehabilitation prior to regenerative therapies can set the stage for improved recovery by preconditioning the individual, while posttransplant physical activity may help cells to integrate and form appropriate connections with the host tissue. Activity-dependent performance of tasks not only shapes behaviors but also strengthens synapses and promotes neuronal plasticity [92, 93]. In general, the timing, dosing, and duration of rehabilitation strategies for neurologic or musculoskeletal injuries varies, and their optimal integration with regenerative therapies is an area in need of further study.

On the other hand, the inappropriate pairing of regenerative and rehabilitative approaches can have deleterious side effects (e.g., pain and spasticity following inappropriate peripheral inputs) and requires monitoring [94]. Thus, the foundation for regenerative rehabilitation can be laid by harnessing physical substrates to refine, direct, and mold components to the desired regenerative endpoint while monitoring for adverse effect to restore and improve the functionality of the individual [95]. As new regenerative medicine strategies enter human clinical trials, increased collaborations with rehabilitation clinicians will be important to optimize outcomes. It will also be important for rehabilitation clinicians to plan for potential changes in rehabilitation practice to accommodate regenerative medicine treatments.

Transforming Healthcare Through Regenerative Medicine

The expansion of regenerative medicine as a scientific discipline, with its core principles of rejuvenation, regeneration, and replacement (the 3R's), is shifting the paradigm in healthcare from symptomatic treatment in the twentieth century to curative treatment in the twenty-first century [96–98]. This is evidenced by the rapid increase in regenerative medicine clinical trials in each specialty [99, 100], which can be broadly classified as using either cell- or tissue-based products. The Food and Drug Administration in the US and the European Medicines Agency have more complex classification systems of regenerative medicine products, including cellular therapy, gene therapy, stimulators of endogenous repair, biologic-device combination products, and human tissue and xenotransplantation [101]. Broadly, the regulatory requirements can be based on the pillars of sterility, stability, and potency, and these need to be addressed prior to successful clinical translation in the future [102].

Cell-based therapies work either via stimulation of endogenous repair through extracellular factors or differentiation and functional replacement of endogenous cell types [100]; they include stem cell implantation or infusion to treat hematopoietic diseases, cardiac conditions, and Parkinson's disease. Most of the pioneering work has been performed using hematopoietic stem cells due to the early bone marrow transplant work, making them the most well-studied stem cell type [103]. In particular, adult mesenchymal stem cells have gained interest as they avoid the ethical concerns of using embryonic stem cells, which can be rapidly expanded in vitro and avoid immunogenicity. Studies have shown contradictory results on the efficacy of the transplanted cells, with patient variability with regard to response; further work is needed to elucidate cell identity and health to ensure patient safety (Fig. 1.4).

The tissue engineering strand of regenerative medicine incorporates cells with biodegradable scaffolds to engineer replacement tissues like dermis or cartilage [104] and whole organs such as trachea and bladder [105]. Limitations of synthetic polymer scaffolds, such as infection, extrusion, and degradation product toxicity, have encouraged interest in decellularized matrices as well biologics for use as scaffolds as one of the

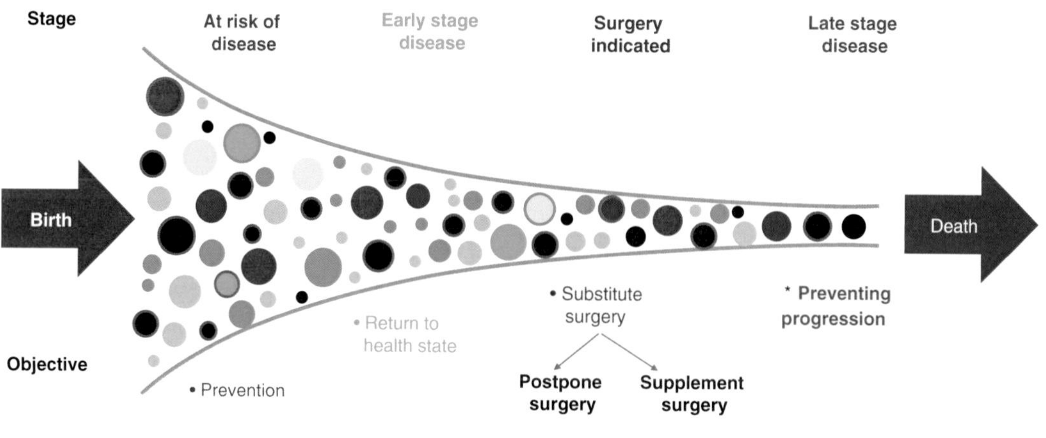

Fig. 1.4 Therapeutic objectives for the different stages of each musculoskeletal diseases

more effective ways of replicating native tissue anisotropy [106]. Decellularized matrices provide durability, enhanced integration, and biocompatibility while avoiding allosensitization [105]. This may explain why many of the significant breakthroughs and first-in-man studies have utilized this technique, combined with autologous cell seeding with some success [105–107], and even showed promise in vitro for more complex structures, such as pulmonary and aortic valves as well as whole organs such as heart and liver [108, 109].

Controversies in Regenerative Medicine

The regenerative medicine field has been shrouded in controversy. Significant potential gains have led to several high-profile allegations of research misconduct [110, 111]. There is also a growing stem cell tourism industry based on unproven treatments that aims to capitalize on stem cell hype [112, 113]. Desperate patients would rather approach private clinics offering experimental stem cell treatments, with unproven safety and efficacy profiles, than wait for outcomes of clinical trials [113]. Media coverage and direct advertising of stem cell therapies as well as the political, ethical, and religious controversies surrounding human embryonic stem cells can contribute not only to increased public awareness but also inflated expectations of regenerative medicine products, and there continues to be a significant gap between the perceived and realistic benefits [114]. A concerted effort from the scientific community as well as robust outcome data from clinical trials will be needed to temper unrealistic claims [99, 100].

Ethics in Musculoskeletal Regenerative Medicine

Recent challenges emerged between clinical scientists and research ethical committees (RECs) when choosing or evaluating the regenerative medicine clinical trials for a musculoskeletal disorder and choosing the appropriate regenerative medicine (RM) comparator. RM is an umbrella term for a variety of techniques, including cell-based interventions, biomaterial implantation, gene transfer, and tissue engineering1e4. Due to the characteristics of RM interventions, such as the invasive nature, the application of such technologies in early-stage disease, and the novelty and even hype of the field, a new light is shed on ethical challenges [115, 116]. Therefore, in regenerative medicine, ethical considerations go hand in hand with scientific questions.

Basically, the objectives of RM interventions are closely linked to the stage of the disease. The natural course of a disease over time can follow a staged pattern, progressing from mild to worse. In musculoskeletal disorders, four main stages can be identified: (1) at risk of the disease, (2) early-stage disease with minor symptoms, (3) intervention indicated, and (4) late-stage disease with severe symptoms (conservative measures only) (Fig. 1.4) [117]. Currently, musculoskeletal RM interventions are being developed for the full range of these different stages, and in all these stages, one or more objectives can be discerned. Accordingly, seven types of RM interventions can be defined based on disease stages. In the "at risk" stage of disease, the objective of the intervention is prevention, while in an early stage of disease, the objective is return to a healthy state or slow the progression of disease. RM can be aimed at substituting the surgical treatment, or at supplementing treatment. Other interventions are aimed at postponing surgery. RM in a late-stage disease, where an alternative is lacking, is aimed at slowing disease progression or restoration of function [116, 117].

The comparator in RM clinical trials Although conducting clinical trials for invasive interventions involve practical and ethical hurdles, the RCT is the default when the objective is to assess efficacy of an intervention [118–120]. The main types of comparators in RCTs are placebo, standard of care, or no intervention. Examples of standard of care include the following: a conventional surgical procedure, another RM intervention, pain management, and physiotherapy. As RM interventions are invasive interventions, a placebo that optimally blinds participants and investigators requires an invasive placebo, or a sham intervention. For symptomatic patients, delayed treatment or historical control groups can be considered and approved by the Food and Drug Administration (FDA). However, optimal comparability with historical and delayed treatment control groups should be ensured to limit bias. This can be achieved by proper demographic analysis and ensuring comparability in follow-up. However, though a sham procedure is demonstrated to be an ethically acceptable comparator in RM trials with certain objectives, it is less appropriate for musculoskeletal RM interventions that aim at preventing disease or substituting a surgical treatment. The latter may be compared to "standard of care." A placebo as a comparator can also be applied within an add-on design, which means that it is provided on top of standard treatment [121–123].

Informed Consent Another condition for determining the acceptability of sham is whether valid informed consent can be obtained by taking the elements of disclosure, competence, and voluntariness into account [124]. It has been suggested that the use of an invasive intervention, such as sham, could foster therapeutic misconception [125].

Here, the participant confuses care with research, which could compromise a valid consent. Therapeutic misconception may especially occur in the field of RM, where expectations of researchers and participants are high [126]. Therefore, in sham-controlled RM trials, one should take safeguards to decrease the chance of therapeutic misconception, for example, by prolonged reflection time, reevaluation of understanding prior to inclusion and during a trial, and avoiding confusing linguistics [127, 128]. In general, efforts should be made to enhance understanding, both through the content and the manner of providing the information in consent forms [129, 130]. Furthermore, one should be aware whether the potential participant is in an acute or chronic stage of disease: a participant with a recent onset disease might not fully understand the consequences of participating due to anxiety and stress, and also voluntariness might be impaired [131]. In participants with chronic disease, the competence and voluntariness is less expected to be compromised.

Regenerative Medicine Curriculum for Next-Generation Physicians

To ensure that regulated regenerative therapies are provided for patient care, educating a specialized workforce that can distinguish safe and valid regenerative options is warranted [132, 133]. Regenerative approaches, however, remain underemphasized in medical school education, including in the United States [134, 135]. As a result, there is a paucity of physicians adequately trained in regenerative principles and practices, necessitating earlier and systematic introduction to this transdisciplinary field that imposes a novel lexicon and new know-how [136, 137].

Curriculum development and its outcomes: Ongoing efforts aim to bridge curricular gaps and prepare the next generation physician. The regenerative medicine curriculum for medical students offers a comprehensive educational experience that encompasses discovery, development, and delivery of next-generation patient management modalities targeted to address root cause of disease [138]. Guiding principles for the introductory "Regenerative Medicine and Surgery Course" included the following: (i) early introduction of regenerative medicine concepts in medical education training; (ii) dynamic teaching methods, such as interactive, simulation, and laboratory experiences to maximize student engagement; (iii) multidisciplinary, patient-centric approach to comprehend bench-to-bedside translation and iterative optimization; (iv) all-inclusive group discussion involving patients and faculty along with students; and (v) online education modules and medical student presentations to ensure learning proficiency. Encompassing a patient-centric paradigm, the "Regenerative Medicine and Surgery Course" is a prototype dedicated to medical students and integrated within the medical school curriculum. Assessment of outcomes which includes completion of learning objectives is monitored by online tests, group teaching, and simulated clinical examinations, along with continuity across medical school training. Success is documented by increased awareness and proficiency in domain-relevant content, as well as specialty identification through practice exposure, research engagement, clinical acumen, and education-driven practice advancement [139] (Fig. 1.5).

Regenerative medicine shapes education: Regenerative therapies will permeate the future clinical landscape, in particular for diseases that have been proven intractable to current management strategies [140]. Yet, education in regenerative medicine is lagging behind scientific and clinical advances. This threatens to

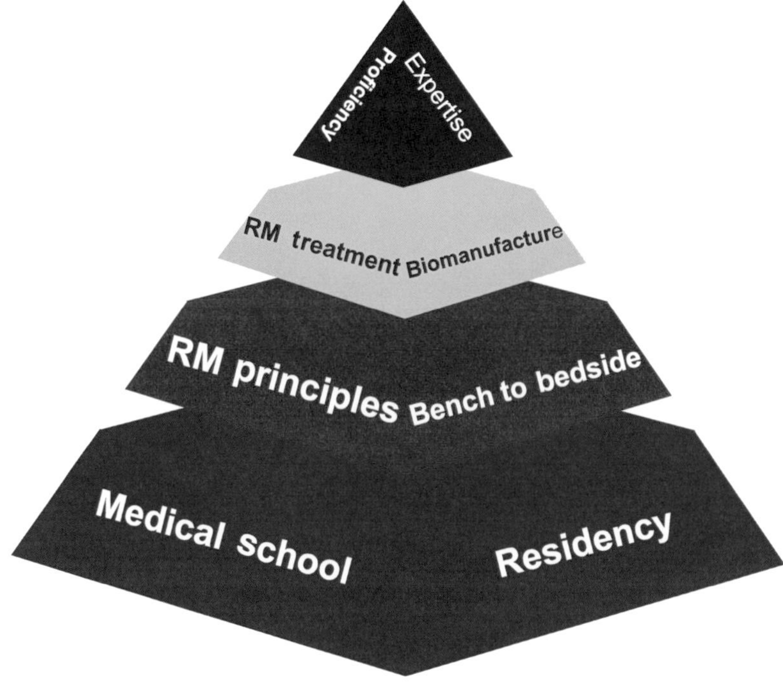

Fig. 1.5 Regenerative medicine and surgery curriculum. Fundamental principles of the "regenerative medicine and surgery course" curriculum are introduced early in medical school training and longitudinally expanded in residency and clinical fellowship, allowing for core proficiency to develop into advanced expertise of the next-generation specialized workforce

leave the physicians-in-training ill-equipped to address the changing needs in patient care [141]. A systematic review of medical school curricula included no reports of regenerative medicine courses dedicated for medical students [142]. In line with the projection that regenerative care will represent 10% of all healthcare in the next decade [143], a comprehensive, patient-centered course is needed to prepare healthcare providers.

Maturity of the Regenerative Medicine Field

The ultimate goal of regenerative medicine is to completely restore missing or damaged tissues to a level functionally and aesthetically indistinguishable from the pre-injury/diseased state. This entails not only regeneration of the specific tissues (such as nerve, muscle, bone, skin, and vasculature) but also integration of the tissues with each other and the healthy surrounding tissue. Apart from vascularized composite allotransplantation, reconstruction with like tissues through regeneration of autologous tissue is still a distant goal, and different tissues are at widely varying stages of maturity. Bone regeneration is most advanced, with several FDA-approved therapies currently in use clinically [144]. Numerous technologies for regenerating skin are available, although final outcomes are still suboptimal [145, 146]. Several technologies to regenerate large diameter arteries are in development or in clinical trials [147]. However, regeneration of peripheral nerves is limited to 5–7 cm [148], and reinnervation of end organs is not guaranteed. Moreover, the ability to integrate those individual tissues into a functioning whole is only in the early stages of development. Variables such as cell source and host species play critical roles in the successful integration of the graft with the host. In the case of spinal cord injury, human cells transplanted into rodent spinal cord take over 1 year to mature [149] and differentiate into glial cells and neurons, with functional recovery beginning more than 1 year after grafting [91].

In conclusion, regenerative technologies, aimed at restoring form and function, inform the prospect of transforming standard-of-care practices.1,2 The evolution from the traditional perspective of "fighting disease" to the increasingly actionable paradigm of "restoring health" begets a new skill set imperative for the developing healthcare practitioner.3 This lack of ethical standards creates difficulties for scientists and research ethical committees when designing or evaluating RM clinical trials. The quest for regenerative solutions has, however, exposed a major gap in current healthcare education. A call for evidence-based adoption has underscored the necessity to establish rigorous regenerative medicine educational programs early in training.

References

1. Hossain I, Milne C. Can regenerative medicine help close the gap between the medicine pipeline and public health burden of cardiovascular and musculoskeletal diseases? Clin Ther. 2018;40(7):1066–75.
2. Global regenerative medicines market—analysis and forecast (2017–2025) (Focus on therapy, applications, market share analysis, 22 country analysis, and competitive landscape). Market Research, Business Wire. Available at: www.reportlinker.com/p05292525/Global-Regenerative-Medicines-Market-Analysis-and-Forecast-Focus-on-Therapy-Applications-Market-Share-Analysis-22-Country-Analysis-and-Competitive-Landscape.html. Accessed 12 Oct 2020.
3. Musculoskeletal Disorder (MSD) Signs and Symptoms. Mohawk College. Available at: www.mohawkcollege.ca/employees/occupational-health-tolerability/ergonomics/musculoskeletal-disorder-msd-signs-and-symptoms. Accessed 12 Oct 2020.
4. US Food and Drug Administration, Office of the Commissioner. 21st Century Cures Act. Available at: www.fda.gov/RegulatoryInformation/LawsEnforcedbyFDA/SignificantAmendmentstotheFDCAct/21stCenturyCuresAct/default.htm. Accessed 12 Oct 2020.
5. US Food and Drug Administration, Center for Biologics Evaluation and Research. Cellular & gene therapy products—regenerative medicine advanced therapy designation. Available at: www.fda.gov/BiologicsBloodVaccines/CellularGeneTherapyProducts/ucm537670.htm. Accessed 12 Oct 2020.
6. Mulvaney S, Tortland P, Shiple B, Curtis K. Regenerative medicine options for chronic mus-

culoskeletal conditions: a review of the literature. Endurance and Sports Medicine; 2018;4:6–15.
7. Kaushal M, Kutty NG, Rao CM. Nitrooxyethylation reverses the healing-suppressant effect of Ibuprofen. Mediat Inflamm. 2006;4:24396.
8. Su WH, Cheng MH, Lee WL. Nonsteroidal anti-inflammatory drugs for wounds: pain relief or excessive scar formation? Mediat Inflamm. 2010;2010:413238.
9. Salari M, Sharma S, Jog MS. Botulinum toxin induced atrophy: an uncharted territory. Toxins. 2018;10(8):313.
10. Pattanittum P, Turner T, Green S, Buchbinder R. Non-steroidal anti-inflammatory drugs for treating lateral elbow pain in adults. Cochrane Database Syst Rev. 2013;31(5):CD003686.
11. McLauchlan GJ, Handoll HH. Interventions for treating acute and chronic Achilles tendinitis. Cochrane Database Syst Rev. 2001;2:CD00232.
12. McAlindon TE, LaValley MP, Harvey WF, et al. Effects of intraarticular triamcinolone vs saline on knee cartilage volume and pain in patients with knee osteoarthritis: a randomized clinical trial. JAMA. 2017;317(19):1967–75.
13. Farkas B, Kvell K, Czompoly T, Illes T, Bardos T. Increased chondrocyte death after steroid and local anesthetic combination. Clin Orthop Relat Res. 2010;468(11):3112–20.
14. Dragoo JL, Danial CM, Braun HJ, Pouliot MA, Kim HJ. The chondrotoxicity of single-dose corticosteroids. Knee Surg Sports Traumatol Arthrosc. 2012;20(9):1809–14.
15. Coombes BK, Bisset L, Vicenzino B. Efficacy and safety of corticosteroid injections and other injections for management of tendinopathy: a systematic review of randomized controlled trials. Lancet. 2010;376:1751–67.
16. Coombes BK, Bisset L, Brooks P, Khan A, Vicenzino B. Effect of corticosteroid injection, physiotherapy or both on clinical outcomes in patients with unilateral lateral epicondylalgia: a randomized controlled trial. JAMA. 2013;309(5):461–9.
17. Kraushaar BS, Nirschl RP. Tendinosis of the elbow (tennis elbow). Clinical features and findings of histological, immunohistochemical, and electron microscopy studies. J Bone Joint Surg Am. 1999;81(2):259–78.
18. Staal JB, de Bie RA, de Vet HC, Hildebrandt J, Nelemans P. Injection therapy for subacute and chronic low back pain: an updated Cochrane review. Spine (Phila Pa 1976). 2009;34(1):49–59.
19. Lee DY, Park YJ, Kim HJ, Nam DC, Park JS. Arthroscopic meniscal surgery versus conservative management in patients aged 40 years and older: a meta-analysis. Arch Ortho and Trauma Surg. 2018;138(12):1731–9.
20. Siemieniuk RAC, Harris IA, Agoritsas T, et al. Arthroscopic surgery for degenerative knee arthritis and meniscal tears: a clinical practice guideline. Brit J Sports Med. 2018;52:313.
21. Nuckols TK, Anderson L, Popescu I, Diamant AL, Doyle B, et al. Opioid prescribing: a systematic review and critical appraisal of guidelines for chronic pain. Ann Intern Med. 2014;160(1):38–47.
22. Chaparro LE, Furlan AD, Deshpande A, Mailis-Gagnon A, Atlas S, Turk DC. Opioids compared to placebo or other treatments for chronic low-back pain. Cochrane Database Syst Rev. 2013;8:CD004959.
23. Singh JA, Kundukulam BS, Riddle DL, Strand V, Tugwell P. Early postoperative mortality following joint arthroplasty: a systematic review. J Rheumatol. 2011;38(7):1507–13.
24. Hernigou P, Auregan JC, Dubory A, Flouzat-Lachaniette CH, Chevallier N, Rouard H. Subchondral stem cell therapy versus contralateral total knee arthroplasty for osteoarthritis following secondary osteonecrosis of the knee. Int Orthop. 2018;42(11):2563–71.
25. Anderson K, Hamm RL. Factors that impair wound healing. J Am Col Clin Wound Spec. 2014;4:84–91.
26. Gosling CM, Forbes AB, Gabbe BJ. Health professionals perceptions of musculoskeletal injury and injury risk factors in Australian triathletes: a factor analysis. Phys Ther Sport. 2013;14(4):207–12.
27. López J. Regenerative medicine applied to treatment of musculoskeletal diseases. Reumatol Clin. 2014;10(3):139–40.
28. Henson F, Getgood A. The use of scaffolds in musculoskeletal tissue engineering. Open Orthop J. 2011;5(Suppl. 2):261–6.
29. Giordano A, Galderisi U, Marino IR. From the laboratory bench to the patient's bedside: an update on clinical trials with mesenchymal stem cells. J Cell Physiol. 2007;211:27–35.
30. Tabar V, Studer L. Pluripotent stem cells in regenerative medicine: challenges and recent progress. Nat Rev Genet. 2014;15:82–92.
31. Antebi B, Pelled G, Gazit D. Stem cell therapy for osteoporosis. Curr Osteoporos Rep. 2014;12:41–7.
32. Huselstein C, Li Y, He X. Mesenchymal stem cells for cartilage engineering. Biomed Mater Eng. 2012;22:69–80.
33. Nie H, Lee CH, Tan J, Lu C, Mendelson A, Chen M, et al. Musculoskeletal tissue engineering by endogenous stem/progenitor cells. Cell Tissue Res. 2012;347:665–76.
34. Kharraz Y, Guerra J, Mann CJ, Serrano AL, Munoz-Canoves P. Macrophage plasticity and the role of inflammation in skeletal muscle repair. Mediat Inflamm. 2013;2013:491497.
35. Sasaki K, Yamamoto N, Kiyosawa T, Sekido M. The role of collagen arrangement change during tendon healing demonstrated by scanning electron microscopy. J Electron Microsc. 2012;61(5):327–34.
36. Sibbitt WL, Peisajovich A, Michael AA, Park KY, Sibbitt RR, et al. Does sonographic needle guidance affect the clinical outcome of intraarticular injections? J Rheumatol. 2009;36:1892–902.

37. Hall MD. The accuracy and efficacy of palpation versus image-guided peripheral injections in sports medicine. Curr Sports Med Rep. 2013;12(5):296–303.
38. Yun DH, Kim HS, Yoo SD, Kim DH, Chon JM, et al. Efficacy of ultrasound-guided injections in patients with facet syndrome of the low lumbar spine. Ann Rehab Med. 2012;36:66–71.
39. Galiano K, Obwegeser AA, Bodner G, Freund M, Maurer H, et al. Ultrasound guidance for facet joint injections in the lumbar spine: a computed tomography-controlled feasibility study. Anesth Analg. 2005;101:579–83.
40. Fuentes-Boquete IM, Arufe Gonda MC, Diaz Prado SM, Hermida Gomez T, de Toro Santos FJ, Blanco Garcia FJ. Treatment of joint cartilage lesions with cell therapy. Reumatol Clin. 2007;3:S63–9.
41. Ibarra C, Garciadiego D, Martinez V, Velasquillo C. Tissue engineering and osteoarthritis. Reumatol Clin. 2007;3:S19–22.
42. Richardson SM, Kalamegam G, Pushparaj PN, Matta C, Memic A, Khademhosseini A, Mobasheri R, Poletti FL, Hoyland JA, Mobasheri A. Mesenchymal stem cells in regenerative medicine: focus on articular cartilage and intervertebral disc regeneration. Methods. 2016;15(99):69–80.
43. Huang Y-C, Li Z, Li J, Lyu F-J. Interaction between stem cells and the microenvironment for musculoskeletal repair. Stem Cells Int. 2020;2020:3, Article ID 7587428. https://doi.org/10.1155/2020/7587428.
44. Mobasheri A, Csaki C, Clutterbuck AL, Rahmanzadeh M, Shakibaei M. Mesenchymal stem cells in connective tissue engineering and regenerative medicine: applications in cartilage repair and osteoarthritis therapy. Histol Histopathol. 2009;24(3):347–66.
45. Mobasheri A, Kalamegam G, Musumeci G, Batt ME. Maturitas. 2014;78:188–98.
46. World Health Organization, Office of Information. Population ageing: a public health challenge: by 2020 more than 1000 million people aged 60 years and older will be living in the world, more than 700 million of them in developing countries, rev. ed., World Health Organization, Geneva, 1998.
47. United Nations, Dept. of Economic and Social Affairs, Population Division. World population ageing: 1950–2050. New York: United Nations; 2002.
48. Orth P, Cucchiarini M, Kohn D, Madry H. Eur Cell Mater. 2013;25:299–316.
49. Orth P, Rey-Rico A, Venkatesan JK, Madry H, Cucchiarini M. Stem Cells Cloning. 2014;7:1–17.
50. Zeng X, Zhang L, Sun L, et al. Recovery from rat sciatic nerve injury in vivo through the use of differentiated MDSCs in vitro. Exp Ther Med. 2013;5(1):193–6.
51. Pawlukowska W, Baumert B, Gołąb-Janowska M, et al. Influence of lineage-negative stem cell therapy on articulatory functions in ALS patients. Stem Cells Int. 2019;2019:7213854.
52. Dort J, Fabre P, Molina T, Dumont NA. Macrophages are key regulators of stem cells during skeletal muscle regeneration and diseases. Stem Cells Int. 2019;2019:4761427.
53. Mao AS, Mooney DJ. Regenerative medicine: current therapies and future directions. Proc Natl Acad Sci U S A. 2015;112(47):14452–9.
54. Fisher MB, Mauck RL. Tissue engineering and regenerative medicine: recent innovations and the transition to translation. Tissue Eng Part B Rev. 2013;19(1):1–13.
55. Lane SW, Williams DA, Watt FM. Modulating the stem cell niche for tissue regeneration. Nat Biotechnol. 2014;32(8):795–803.
56. Kennedy MI, Whitney K, Evans T, LaPrade RF. Platelet-rich plasma and cartilage repair. Curr Rev Musculoskelet Med. 2018;11(4):573–82.
57. Chu DT, Nguyen Thi Phuong T, Tien NLB, et al. Adipose tissue stem cells for therapy: an update on the progress of isolation, culture, storage, and clinical application. J Clin Med. 2019;8(7):917.
58. Mendelson A, Frenette PS. Hematopoietic stem cell niche maintenance during homeostasis and regeneration. Nat Med. 2014;20(8):833–46.
59. Zhang CC, Lodish HF. Murine hematopoietic stem cells change their surface phenotype during ex vivo expansion. Blood. 2005;105(11):4314–20.
60. Walasek MA, van Os R, de Haan G. Hematopoietic stem cell expansion: challenges and opportunities. Ann N Y Acad Sci. 2012;1266:138–50.
61. Zhang Y, Chai C, Jiang XS, Teoh SH, Leong KW. Coculture of umbilical cord blood CD34+ cells with human mesenchymal stem cells. Tissue Eng. 2006;12(8):2161–70.
62. Kim BS, Mooney DJ. Scaffolds for engineering smooth muscle under cyclic mechanical strain conditions. J Biomech Eng. 2000;122(3):210–5.
63. Cosgrove BD, et al. Rejuvenation of the muscle stem cell population restores strength to injured aged muscles. Nat Med. 2014;20(3):255–64.
64. Centers for Disease Control and Prevention (CDC). Prevalence of doctor-diagnosed arthritis and arthritis-attributable activity limitation – United States, 2007–2009. Morb Mortal Week Rep. 2010;59(39):1261.
65. Cross M, Smith E, Hoy D, et al. The global burden of hip and knee osteoarthritis: estimates from the global burden of disease 2010 study. Ann Rheum Dis. 2014;73(7):1323–30.
66. Jevons LA, Houghton FD, Tare RS. Augmentation of musculoskeletal regeneration: role for pluripotent stem cells. Regen Med. 2018;13(2):189–206.
67. Aggarwal A, Sempowski IP. Hyaluronic acid injections for knee osteoarthritis. Systematic review of the literature. Can Fam Physician. 2004;50:249–56.
68. Ogata T, Ideno Y, Akai M, et al. Effects of glucosamine in patients with osteoarthritis of the knee: a systematic review and meta-analysis. Clin Rheumatol. 2018;37(9):2479–87.

69. Pritzker K, Gay S, Jimenez S, et al. Osteoarthritis cartilage histopathology: grading and staging. Osteoarthr Cartil. 2006;14(1):13–29.
70. D'apuzzo MR, Pao AW, Novicoff WM, Browne JA. Age as an independent risk factor for postoperative morbidity and mortality after total joint arthroplasty in patients 90 years of age or older. J Arthroplast. 2014;29(3):477–80.
71. Johnson LL. Arthroscopic abrasion arthroplasty: a review. Clin Orthop Relat Res. 2001;391:S306–17.
72. Insall J. The Pridie debridement operation for osteoarthritis of the knee. Clin Orthop Relat Res. 1974;101:61–7.
73. Mithoefer K, Williams RJ, Warren RF, et al. Chondral resurfacing of articular cartilage defects in the knee with the microfracture technique. J Bone Joint Surg Am. 2006;88(1 Suppl. 2):294–304.
74. Bentley G, Biant L, Vijayan S, Macmull S, Skinner J, Carrington R. Minimum ten-year results of a prospective randomised study of autologous chondrocyte implantation versus mosaicplasty for symptomatic articular cartilage lesions of the knee. J Bone Joint Surg Br. 2012;94(4):504–9.
75. Brittberg M, Lindahl A, Nilsson A, Ohlsson C, Isaksson O, Peterson L. Treatment of deep cartilage defects in the knee with autologous chondrocyte transplantation. N Engl J Med. 1994;331(14):889–95.
76. NICE guidelines: autologous chondrocyte implantation for treating symptomatic articular cartilage defects of the knee. https://www.nice.org.uk/guidance/ta477. Accessed 12 Oct 2020.
77. Hernlund E, Svedbom A, Ivergård M, et al. Osteoporosis in the European Union: medical management, epidemiology and economic burden. Arch Osteoporos. 2013;8(1–2):1–115.
78. Johnell O, Kanis J. An estimate of the worldwide prevalence and disability associated with osteoporotic fractures. Osteoporosis Int. 2006;17(12):1726–33.
79. Dargent-Molina P, Favier F, Grandjean H, et al. Fall-related factors and risk of hip fracture: the EPIDOS prospective study. Lancet. 1996;348(9021):145–9.
80. Kanis JA. Assessment of fracture risk and its application to screening for postmenopausal osteoporosis: synopsis of a WHO report. Osteoporosis Int. 1994;4(6):368–81.
81. Tsai JN, Uihlein AV, Lee H, et al. Teriparatide and denosumab, alone or combined, in women with postmenopausal osteoporosis: the DATA study randomised trial. Lancet. 2013;382(9886):50–6.
82. Khan AA, Sandor GK, Dore E, et al. Bisphosphonate associated osteonecrosis of the jaw. J Rheumatol. 2009;36(3):478–90.
83. Nieves JW, Cosman F. Atypical subtrochanteric and femoral shaft fractures and possible association with bisphosphonates. Curr Osteoporos Rep. 2010;8(1):34–9.
84. Nedergaard A, Henriksen K, Karsdal MA, Christiansen C. Musculoskeletal ageing and primary prevention. Best Pract Res Clin Obstetr Gynaecol. 2013;27(5):673–88.
85. Woolf AD, Pfleger B. Burden of major musculoskeletal conditions. Bull WHO. 2003;81(9):646–56.
86. Patel HP, Syddall HE, Jameson K, et al. Prevalence of sarcopenia in community-dwelling older people in the UK using the European Working Group on Sarcopenia in Older People (EWGSOP) definition: findings from the Hertfordshire Cohort Study (HCS). Age Ageing. 2013;42(3):378–84.
87. Emery AE. The muscular dystrophies. Lancet. 2002;359(9307):687–95.
88. Mauro A. Satellite cell of skeletal muscle fibers. J Biophys Biochem Cytol. 1961;9(2):493–5.
89. Webster C, Blau HM. Accelerated age-related decline in replicative life-span of Duchenne muscular dystrophy myoblasts: implications for cell and gene therapy. Somat Cell Mol Genet. 1990;16(6):557–65.
90. Meriggioli MN, Roubenoff R. Prospect for pharmacological therapies to treat skeletal muscle dysfunction. Calcif Tissue Int. 2015;96(3):234–42.
91. Rose LF, Wolf EJ, Brindle T, et al. The convergence of regenerative medicine and rehabilitation: federal perspectives. npj Regen Med. 2018;3(19):1–7.
92. Nash MS, et al. Cardiometabolic syndrome in people with spinal cord injury/disease: guideline-derived and nonguideline risk components in a pooled sample. Arch Phys Med Rehabil. 2016;97:1696–705.
93. Budde H, Wegner M, Soya H, Voelcker-Rehage C, McMorris T. Neuroscience of exercise: neuroplasticity and its behavioral consequences. Neural Plast. 2016;2016:3643879.
94. Wang L, Conner JM, Nagahara AH, Tuszynski MH. Rehabilitation drives enhancement of neuronal structure in functionally relevant neuronal subsets. Proc Natl Acad Sci U S A. 2016;113:2750–5.
95. Ambrosio F, et al. The emerging relationship between regenerative medicine and physical therapeutics. Phys Ther. 2010;90:1807–14.
96. Nelson TJ, Behfar A, Terzic A. Strategies for therapeutic repair: the "R3" regenerative medicine paradigm. Clin Transl Sci. 2008;1:168–71.
97. World regenerative medicines market – opportunities and forecasts, 2013–2020. Allied Market Research report. 2014. https://www.alliedmarketresearch.com/regenerative-medicines-market. Accessed 12 Oct 2020.
98. Remarks of President Barack Obama. The White House. 2009. https://www.whitehouse.gov/the-press-office/remarks-president-prepared-deliverysigning-stem-cell-executive-order-and-scientifi. Accessed 12 Oct 2020.
99. Trounson A. New perspectives in human stem cell therapeutic research. BMC Med. 2009;7:29.
100. Trounson A, Thakar RG, Lomax G, Gibbons D. Clinical trials for stem cell therapies. BMC Med. 2011;9:52.
101. Lee MH, Arcidiacono JA, Bilek AM, Wille JJ, Hamill CA, Wonnacott KM, Wells MA, Oh SS. Considerations for tissue-engineered and regenerative medicine product development prior to clini-

cal trials in the United States. Tissue Eng Part B Rev. 2010;16(1):41–54.
102. Jessop ZM, Al-Sabah A, Francis WR, et al. Transforming healthcare through regenerative medicine. BMC Med. 2016;14:115.
103. Ford CE, Hamerton JL, Barnes DW, Loutit JF. Cytological identification of radiation-chimaeras. Nature. 1956;177:452–4.
104. Cao Y, Vacanti JP, Paige KT, Upton J, Vacanti CA. Transplantation of chondrocytes utilizing a polymer-cell construct to produce tissue engineered cartilage in the shape of a human ear. Plast Reconstr Surg. 1997;100:297–304.
105. Macchiarini P, Jungebluth P, Go T, Asnaghi MA, Rees LE, Cogan TA, Dodson A, Martorell J, Bellini S, Parnigotto PP, Dickinson SC, Hollander AP, Mantero S, Conconi MT, Birchall MA. Clinical transplantation of a tissue-engineered airway. Lancet. 2008;372:2023–30.
106. Atala A, Bauer SB, Soker S, Yoo JJ, Retic AB. Tissue-engineered autologous bladders for patients needing cystoplasty. Lancet. 2006;367:1241–6.
107. Gonfiotti A, Jaus MO, Barale D, Baiguera S, Comin C, Lavorini F, Fontana G, Sibila O, Rombolà G, Jungebluth P, Macchiarini P. The first tissue-engineered airway transplantation: 5-year follow-up results. Lancet. 2014;383(9913):238–44.
108. Ott HC, Matthiesen TS, Goh SK, Black LD, Kren SM, Netoff TI. Perfusion decellularized matrix: using nature's platform to engineer a bioartificial heart. Nat Med. 2008;14(2):213–21.
109. Soto-Gutierrez A, Zhang L, Medberry C, Fukumitsu K, Faulk D, Jiang H. A whole-organ regenerative medicine approach for liver replacement. Tissue Eng Part C Methods. 2011;17(6):677–86.
110. Cyranoski D. Acid bath offers easy path to stem cells. Nat News. 2014. http://www.nature.com/news/acid-bath-offers-easy-path-to-stem-cells-1.14600. Accessed 12 Oct 2020.
111. Vogel G. Regenerative medicine. Report finds misconduct by surgeon. Science. 2015; 348(6238):954–5.
112. Alta CR. On the road (to a cure?) — stem-cell tourism and lessons for gene editing. N Engl J Med. 2016;374:901–3.
113. Matthews KR, Iltis AS. Unproven stem cell-based interventions and achieving a compromise policy among the multiple stakeholders. BMC Med Ethics. 2015;16:75.
114. Bubela T, Li MD, Hafez M, Bieber M, Atkins H. Is belief larger than fact: expectations, optimism and reality for translational stem cell research. BMC Med. 2012;10:133.
115. Niemansburg SL, van Delden JJ, Dhert WJ, Bredenoord AL. Regenerative medicine interventions for orthopedic disorders: ethical issues in the translation into patients. Regen Med. 2013;8(1):65e73.
116. Niemansburg SL, Teraa M, Hesam H, van Delden JJ, Verhaar MC, Bredenoord AL. Stem cell trials for vascular medicine: ethical rationale. Tissue Eng A. 2014;20(19–20):2567–74.
117. de Windt TS, Niemansburg SL, Vonk LA, van Delden JM, Roes KCB, Dhert WJA, Bredenoord AL. Ethics in musculoskeletal regenerative medicine; guidance in choosing the appropriate comparator in clinical trials. Osteoarthr Cartil. 2019;27(1):34–40.
118. Koudstaal S, Niemansburg SL, Dib N, Wallet J, Doevendans PA, Bredenoord AL, et al. Placebo in autologous cell-based interventions: hard pill to swallow? J Am Coll Cardiol. 2014;63(25 Pt A):2877–9.
119. Schulz KF, Grimes DA. Blinding in randomised trials: hiding who got what. Lancet. 2002; 359:696–700.
120. Horng S, Miller FG. Ethical framework for the use of sham procedures in clinical trials. Crit Care Med. 2003;31:S126–30.
121. Ergina PL, Cook JA, Blazeby JM, Boutron I, Clavien PA, Reeves BC, et al. Challenges in evaluating surgical innovation. Lancet. 2009;374(9695):1097–104.
122. Cook JA. The challenges faced in the design, conduct and analysis of surgical randomised controlled trials. Trials. 2009;10:9.
123. Farrokhyar F, Karanicolas PJ, Thoma A, Simunovic M, Bhandari M, Devereaux PJ, et al. Randomized controlled trials of surgical interventions. Ann Surg. 2010;251(3):409–16.
124. Brock DW. Philosophical justifications of informed consent in research. In: Emanuel EJ, Grady C, Crouch RA, editors. The Oxford textbook of clinical research ethics. Oxford: Oxford University Press; 2008. p. 606–12.
125. Gillett GR. Unnecessary holes in the head. IRB. 2001;23(6):1–6.
126. Cho Mildred K, David M. Therapeutic misconception and stem cell research. Nat Rep Stem Cell. 2013; https://doi.org/10.1038/stemcells.2007.88. (online pub).
127. Lidz CW, Appelbaum PS. The therapeutic misconception: problems and solutions. Med Care. 2002;40(9 Suppl):V55–63.
128. Horng S, Grady C. Misunderstanding in clinical research: distinguishing therapeutic misconception, therapeutic misestimation, and therapeutic optimism. IRB. 2003;25(1):11–6.
129. Flory J, Emanuel E. Interventions to improve research participants' understanding in informed consent for research: a systematic review. JAMA. 2004;292(13):1593–601.
130. Nishimura A, Carey J, Erwin PJ, Tilburt JC, Murad MH, McCormick JB. Improving understanding in the research informed consent process: a systematic review of 54 interventions tested in randomized control trials. BMC Med Ethics. 2013;14:28.
131. Gammelgaard A, Rossel P, Mortensen OS. Patients' perceptions of informed consent in acute myocardial

infarction research: a Danish study. Soc Sci Med. 2004;58(11):2313–24.
132. Marks P, Gottlieb S. Balancing safety and innovation for cell-based regenerative medicine. N Engl J Med. 2018;378:954–9.
133. Badylak S, Rosenthal N. Regenerative medicine: are we there yet? NPJ Regen Med. 2017;2:2.
134. Knoepfler PS. Call for fellowship programs in stem cell-based regenerative and cellular medicine: new stem cell training is essential for physicians. Regen Med. 2013;8:223–5.
135. Bussel II, Stupple A, Moody KJ, Lefkowitz DM. Call to action: medical students for regenerative medicine. Rejuvenation Res. 2010;13:1–2.
136. Webster A. Regenerative medicine and responsible research and innovation: proposals for a responsible acceleration to the clinic. Regen Med. 2017;12:853–64.
137. Griffith L, Swartz M, Tranquillo R. Education for careers in tissue engineering and regenerative medicine. Ann Biomed Eng. 2006;34:265–9.
138. Waldman SA, Terzic A. Managing innovation to maximize value along the discovery–translation–application continuum. Clin Pharmacol Ther. 2017;101:8–12.
139. Wyles SP, Hayden RE, Meyer FB, et al. Regenerative medicine curriculum for next-generation physicians. npj Regen Med. 2019;4:3.
140. Tolar J. Regenerative solutions for inherited diseases. Clin Pharmacol Ther. 2018;103:763–6.
141. Terzic A, Pfenning MA, Gores GJ, Harper CM Jr. Regenerative medicine build-out. Stem Cells Transl Med. 2015;4:1373–9.
142. Agarwal A, Wong S, Sarfaty S, Devaiah A, Hirsch AE. Elective courses for medical students during the preclinical curriculum: a systematic review and evaluation. Med Educ Online. 2015;20:26615.
143. Terzic A, Folmes CD, Martinez-Fernandez A, Behfar A. Regenerative medicine: on the vanguard of health care. Mayo Clin Proc. 2011;86:600–2.
144. Ong JL, editor. Translating biomaterials for bone graft: bench-top to clinical applications. New York: CRC Press; 2016.
145. Chaudhari AA, et al. Future prospects for scaffolding methods and biomaterials in skin tissue engineering: a review. Int J Mol Sci. 2016;17(12):1974.
146. Chua AW, et al. Skin tissue engineering advances in severe burns: review and therapeutic applications. Burns Trauma. 2016;19(4):3.
147. Laschke MW, Menger MD. Bioengineered vascular grafts off the shelf. Lancet. 2016;387:1976–8.
148. Daly W, Yao L, Zeugolis D, Windebank A, Pandit A. A biomaterials approach to peripheral nerve regeneration: bridging the peripheral nerve gap and enhancing functional recovery. J R Soc Interface. 2012;9:202–21.
149. Lu P, et al. Prolonged human neural stem cell maturation supports recovery in injured rodent CNS. J Clin Invest. 2017;127:3287–99.

2 Regenerative Options for Musculoskeletal Disorders

Daniel Habbal, Kaitlin Jayendran, Nagib Atallah Yurdi, William D. Murrell, Nicola Maffulli, and Gerard A. Malanga

Introduction

Given the aging US population, and increasing prevalence of obesity, the prevalence of osteoarthritis (OA) can be expected to increase in the coming decades. It has been projected that by the year 2040, one in four adults aged 18 years and older will have doctor-diagnosed arthritis [1]. OA significantly diminishes quality of life through pain and loss of joint function and can present a significant economic burden. In 2013, the national arthritis-attributable medical costs totaled to $140 billion, which is equivalent to $2,117 of additional medical costs per adult with arthritis [2]. Current treatments for early OA include conservative approaches such as weight loss, physical therapy, utilization of nonsteroidal anti-inflammatory drugs (NSAIDs), topical anti-inflammatory gels, and intra-articular corticosteroid injections. These approaches aim to provide symptom relief and improve quality of life but are shown to only be effective in the short term [3]. Conservative approaches have not been proven to significantly modify disease progression or successfully prevent final joint replacement in the advanced disease stage [4]. In cases of more advanced OA, operative approaches include high tibial osteotomy, unilateral joint arthroplasty, and partial and total joint arthroplasty. Unfortunately, these procedures can fail due to implant loosening, infection, persistent pain, and instability indicating a more complex revision procedure [5]. Implant durability presents a particular challenge for younger patients. The lifetime risk of revision in younger patients, under the age of 70 years, has shown to reach up

D. Habbal
Sydney Kimmel Medical College, Thomas Jefferson University, Philadelphia, PA, USA
e-mail: Daniel.Habbal@students.jefferson.edu

K. Jayendran
McMaster University, Hamilton, ON, Canada
e-mail: jayendrk@mcmaster.ca

N. A. Yurdi
Reem Hospital, Abu Dhabi, United Arab Emirates

W. D. Murrell (✉)
Plancher Orthopaedics and Sports Medicine Fellowship Program, New York City, NY, USA

411th Hospital Center, Jacksonville Naval Airstation, Jacksonville, FL, USA

N. Maffulli
Department of Musculoskeletal Disorders, University of Salerno School of Medicine and Dentistry, Salerno, Italy

Queen Mary University of London, Barts and the London School of Medicine and Dentistry Centre for Sports and Exercise Medicine, Mile End Hospital, London, UK
e-mail: n.maffulli@qmul.ac.uk

G. A. Malanga
New Jersey Regenerative Institute LLC, Cedar Knolls, NJ, USA

Department of Physical Medicine and Rehabilitation, Rutgers University, New Jersey Medical School, Newark, NJ, USA

Y. El Miedany (ed.), *Musculoskeletal Ultrasound-Guided Regenerative Medicine*,
https://doi.org/10.1007/978-3-030-98256-0_2

to 35% [6]. In order to reduce medical costs and risks to patients, improved strategies for early disease management and treatment of OA are needed. Orthobiologics may be an option to prevent patient OA progression prior to an advanced disease state.

Basic Science of Orthobiologics

Regenerative treatment methods are the new frontier of surgical intervention – the use of orthobiologic therapies holds the potential to transform medical and surgical practices significantly and is already heralded as the most modern method of healing and therapeutics in current medicine [7]. The term orthobiologics refers to biologically augmented substances, derived from naturally occurring biomaterials, used to heal musculoskeletal injuries. Orthobiologics are used to improve the healing of ligaments, bones, and muscles, as well as accelerate the biological processes of regeneration and repair in response to injury [8].

Primary studies conducted by orthopedic surgeon John Connolly and others inspired the modern use of bone marrow in surgical treatments [7], as it was concluded that bone marrow, upon transplantation, could act as versatile osteogenic reconstructors at the site of injury [9]. It was discovered that bone marrow contained mixed connective tissue progenitors – more commonly known as "mesenchymal stem cells (MSC)" as coined by Arnold Caplan, the researcher credited for providing their most common name [7]. As described by Caplan, MSCs are "infinitely divisible progenitor cells whose progeny may possibly give rise to skeletal tissues, such as bone, cartilage, marrow stroma, adipocyte, muscle, tendon, ligaments, [and] connective tissue." However today, we know that this is not the case and that most likely the cells are more immunomodulating in nature [10, 11]. Current scientific evidence suggests that MSCs are derived from perivascular cells called pericytes [12], as both fetal and adult MSCs "expressed both pericyte mesenchymal stem cell markers in situ" and were both found to be "clonally multipotent in culture" [13]. It is hypothesized that blood vessel walls harbor reserves of these progenitor cells, which activate and detach at the site of breakage and inflammation [7]. These MSCs are considered to have immunomodulatory, anti-inflammatory, and trophic properties; they provide bioactive molecules to the site of inflammation or injury that locally inhibit immune response and apoptosis, as well as accelerate the process of regenerative repair [7].

Orthobiologic medicine harnesses the immunomodulatory capacity of MSCs to provide therapeutic effects against a variety of clinical pathologies and injuries [7]. As we further our understanding of MSCs, we in turn further our understanding of the regenerative capacity of individuals. Current research clearly demonstrates that every bodily tissue has ubiquitous, intrinsic regenerative abilities due the presence of tissue-specific progenitor cells [11]. Careful manipulation of this regenerative ability could produce enhanced clinical outcomes, ranging from accelerating healing to scar-less regeneration [10]; therein lies the basis of orthobiologics in modern medicine. The most common orthobiologic therapy is platelet-rich plasma (PRP) – which is composed of platelets, which are nonnucleated cells with vesicles containing bioactive factors that regulate wound healing [7] and plasma containing both bioactive molecules and chemokines that assist in the detachment of MSCs from their perivascular origins, as well as mitogens, which stimulate MSC replication [14]. The introduction of PRP results in signaling an increased presence of MSCs at the site of injury and is expected to enhance regeneration and healing. The working concentration of PRP is typically 1,000,000 platelets/μl in 5 ml of plasma, and this composition has been associated with improved clinical outcomes [15].

The ability to biologically engineer MSC-mediated immunomodulatory activity is the fundamental principle behind a large spectrum of clinical trials using orthobiologic therapies. The modern challenges we face involve delivery of such therapies, in the right amounts, in the right places, and at the right time. It is important to acknowledge that MSCs harvested from differing anatomical locations, and from a variety of donors, are expected to have differing intrinsic biochemistries. However, recent clinical trials have reported that such differences do not significantly impact the efficacy of isolated autologous or culturally expanded allogeneic MSCs [7].

Selected Orthobiologics to Treat Primary MSK Conditions

Rotator Cuff Tendinopathy

PRP – It was found to be incredibly effective in treating rotator cuff tendinopathies, as seen in a random-effects meta-analysis by Hamid et al. that reviewed eight RCTs. Four studies compared PRP injection with normal saline, and four RCTs used rehabilitation programs and dry needling as control interventions. The meta-analysis showed that PRP injection was a safe and effective treatment for long-term pain control and shoulder function in patients with rotator cuff tendinopathies [16].

BMAC ± PRP – One systematic review by Di Matteo et al. looked at the available clinical evidence on the application of cell-based therapies for the management of rotator cuff tears. All the papers included suggested an improvement of rotator cuff tendinopathies with cell-based approaches with a satisfactory safety profile. The study also highlights a lack of high-level evidence and the presence of controversial issues with the standardization of these biologic approaches, specifically in regards to inter-product variability and application strategies [17].

MFAT – In addition, Robinson et al. studied the safety and clinical outcomes of patients treated with micro-fragmented adipose tissue for shoulder pain secondary to rotator cuff pathology. Significant improvements in VAS scores and pain disability index scores with no major adverse events were observed at 6 months [18].

Lateral Epicondylitis

PRP – A systematic review and meta-analysis of nine RCTs by Huang et al. compared PRP to corticosteroid (CS) in the management of lateral epicondylitis [19]. Short-term data analysis showed a statistically significant improvement with CS over PRP for pain relief with medium effect size, while the improvement in pain scores reversed long term with PRP providing significantly better pain relief with a very large effect size [19].

BMAC – Singh et al. studied the treatment of tennis elbow patients with a single injection of BMA and showed a significant improvement in short- to medium-term follow-up [20].

ASC – Khoury et al. studied the effect of adipose-derived stromal cell (ASC) injection as a therapeutic procedure on the common extensor tendinopathy. Eighteen tennis players with chronic, recalcitrant lateral epicondylitis (LE) underwent clinical evaluation and MRI before intervention. Tennis players with recalcitrant LE showed significant clinical improvement and structural repair at the origin of the common tendon origin after injection of autologous ASCs [21].

KOA

PRP – Orthobiologics have been increasingly used to treat musculoskeletal conditions such as OA and tendinopathies. Belk et al. performed a meta-analysis on 18 studies that compared the efficacy and safety of PRP with hyaluronic acid (HA) in the treatment of knee OA (KOA). The meta-analysis showed a benefit of using PRP over hyaluronic acid in treating OA with six out of 11 studies showing significantly better VAS scores at latest follow-up, and three out of six studies showing significant improvement in subjective IKDC outcome scores. Additionally, the meta-analysis showed that leukocyte-poor PRP may be a superior line of treatment for KOA over leukocyte-rich PRP [22].

BMAC – Bone marrow aspirate and concentrate are a heterogeneous mixture of mixed connective tissue progenitors that have been found to accelerate bone regenerative repair and have the ability to be immunomodulatory [23]. One systematic review by Keeling et al. used eight studies to evaluate the efficacy of isolated BMAC injection in the treatment of OA of the knee joint. Patients demonstrated significant improvement from baseline to latest follow-up across 34 of 36 patient-reported outcomes, and the authors concluded that BMAC injection is effective in improving pain and patient-reported outcomes in patients with KOA at short- to midterm follow-up. However, BMAC did not demonstrate superiority in relation to other biologic therapies commonly used in the treatment of OA, including PRP and MFAT [24].

MFAT – Gobbi et al. performed a multicentric, international, open-label study to assess the use of micronized adipose tissue (MFAT) in elderly patients with 2-year follow-up. Patients were followed up to 24 months with Knee Injury and Osteoarthritis Outcome Score (KOOS). Statistical models were used to assess KOOS subscores and the probability of exceeding the minimally clinically important difference (MCID) or patient acceptable symptom state (PASS) and to assess the effect of the treatment variables on KOOS – pain. Seventy-five patients with 120 primary treatments, mean age of 69.6 years (95%CI 68.3–70.9), BMI of 28.4 (95%CI 27.3–29.6), and KL grade of 2–4 KOA were treated with a single MFAT injection. Patients with KL grade 2 disease had the best results in KOOS – pain ($P = 0.001$), at 6, 12, and 24 months. Fourteen treatments (11.7%, 9 patients) failed prior to the study endpoint and underwent knee arthroplasty. This study demonstrated that a single-dose MFAT injection can lead to clinical, functional, and quality of life improvement at 2 years in elderly patients, in KL grades 2–4 of KOA. These findings provide evidence that this treatment modality could be a safe and cost-effective option to other commonly available treatments in carefully selected patients [25].

CAS – The use of conditioned autologous serum has been assessed for treating KOA by Schneider and co-workers in their recent publication a novel technique of preconditioning autologous blood with gold particles (GOLDIC®) and injection in patients. This prospective observational study that was retrospectively assessed was performed on 64 patients, with 89 knees (mean age: 64.8 years; 89 knees) treated with gold-induced cytokines (GOLDIC) with moderate to severe KOA with radiographically proven KOA. All participants received four ultrasound-guided intra-articular knee injections of GOLDIC® at 3–6 day intervals. Western Ontario and McMaster Universities Osteoarthritis Index (WOMAC) and Knee Injury and Osteoarthritis Outcome Score (KOOS) were evaluated at baseline; 1, 3, and 6 months; and 1, 2, and 4 years (T1–T6). The incidence of treatment-related severe adverse events (SAEs) was recorded. Intra-articular gelsolin level in patients with effusion was determined. KOOS and WOMAC scores improved for the full duration of the study ($P < 0.05$), and minimal clinically important difference (MCID) was observed at all time points in all KOOS subscores, with no reported SAEs. No statistically significant evidence of an association between patient demographics and outcome were identified. Nine patients failed treatment, with 32 months mean time to failure, and underwent total knee arthroplasty. This study demonstrated that GOLDIC is good for conservative management of moderate to severe KOA. The CAS produces rapid and sustained improvements in all indices after treatment, with no SAEs [26].

SVF – There is also a growing body of research supporting the use of adipose-derived mesenchymal stem cells to treat orthopedic conditions. Autologous stromal vascular fraction (SVF) has recently been used as an efficient medium for the administration of adipose-derived mesenchymal stem cells. A systematic review of 11 studies by Shanmugasundaram et al. evaluated the safety and efficacy of SVF injection for the treatment of KOA. The majority of patients reported improvement in pain, range of motion (ROM), and functional outcome scores. The authors concluded SVF injection is a safe and effective technique for the management of KOA and could serve as an interim option for patients who failed other conservative and arthroscopic options [27].

In the future, stem cell-based injection therapy can possibly be used as an alternative conservative treatment. Before mainstream adoption, additional evidence, especially for cost-effectiveness, long-term safety, and additional adverse event reporting, needs to be demonstrated for treatment in several MSK conditions. This is particularly true for those who have failed nonoperative treatment before surgical repair is taken.

Orthobiologics to Augment Current Orthopedic Surgical Procedures

Rotator Cuff Tears

Rotator cuff tear, both partial and full thickness, can be a debilitating source of pain and can cause significant shoulder dysfunction. As surgical repair has become the gold standard, one would assume that all repairs heal. However, some literature shows that the failure rate of rotator cuff repair exceeds 50%. Higher repair rates could be achieved by adding orthobiologics to help reattachment to the bone [7].

PRP – It has been shown to stimulate tendon stem cells to differentiate into tenocytes and facilitate collagen extracellular matrix production [28]. One systematic review and meta-analysis by Ryan et al. investigated the clinical and imaging outcomes of 4 types of PRP therapies in rotator cuff repairs and found significant reductions in retear rates [29].

BMAC – Another study by Cole et al. compared the clinical outcome of arthroscopic rotator cuff repair with and without augmentation using BMAC to identify persistent structural defects following surgery [30]. MSCs injected into the shoulder at the time of surgical repair showed improved tendon quality on postoperative MRI at 1-year postop [30]. The longest-term study with a 10-year follow-up was carried out by Hernigou et al., which compared 45 patients who received BMAC during a rotator cuff repair to a matched control group of 45 patients who did not receive MSCs. Nearly 100% of repairs with MSC augmentation had healed by 6 months versus 67% of repairs without MSC treatment. The study also showed a substantial improvement in the level of tendon integrity at the 10-year follow-up visit for patients treated with BMAC [31]. Further investigation is needed into these new and evolving treatments; however, they show promise for improving rotator cuff repair healing and functional outcome.

ACL Tears

Regenerative therapies have the potential to improve current surgical interventions in the area of ligament repair via improved graft incorporation and strengthening, trophic induction, and microenvironment facilitation [7]. Andriolo et al. performed a systematic review of all the preclinical and clinical papers dealing with the application of PRP as a biological enhancer during ACL reconstructive surgery [32]. The majority of papers did not show beneficial effects in terms of graft integration; however, there was some evidence that PRP administration could positively contribute to graft maturation over time [32].

Meniscal Tears

Biomechanical and clinical data by Baratz et al. have demonstrated the importance of the meniscus and of meniscal preservation for protection of the articular cartilage, distribution of forces, and as a secondary stabilizer [33]. Given the limited blood supply, there has been an increasing interest in biologic augmentation of these repairs to enhance healing [7]. Kaminski et al. performed an RCT to study the effect of PRP augmentation for meniscus repair and found improvements in both meniscus healing and functional outcome [34]. Another study by Massey et al. reviewed the results of meniscus repairs with and without bone marrow aspiration concentrate [35]. Both the control group and BMAC meniscus repair group had improved outcomes at 1-year postoperatively with respect to VAS, Lysholm, and IKDC. Authors found that meniscus repair outcomes were improved at 6 weeks and 3 months postoperatively when BMAC was used in the repair [35]. On the other hand, the use of ASCs for meniscal repair is largely unexplored [36]. One recent study by Sasaki et al. studied the effects of ASC-seeded hydrogels on the repair of a meniscal transplant model and found that ASC-seeded hydrogels preloaded enhanced healing of radial meniscal tears [36]. More studies are needed to properly assess the use of this biologic in the treatment of meniscal pathologies.

Cartilage Repairs

Cartilage repair has long been an area of difficulty within orthopedics. There have been many recent studies that have been published studying the effects of biologics on the treatment of cartilage pathology.

PRP – Campbell et al. reported on the quality of three meta-analyses that evaluated PRP injection therapy for cartilage degenerative conditions. Authors found that IKDC scores improved at 6-month follow-up, and WOMAC and VAS improved at 3- and 6-month follow-ups compared to hyaluronic acid (HA) [37].

BMAC – Another study by Cotter et al. demonstrated that BMAC may also help stimulate hyaline cartilage repair. Results showed robust tissue response with cartilage restoration procedures at various defined time points after surgery [38].

PBPC – Peripheral blood progenitor cells use in cartilage repair was studied in an RCT by Saw et al., with 50 patients randomized to control (HA) and intervention (PBSC + HA) groups [39]. Histologic and MRI evaluation showed that injections of autologous PBSC in combination with HA resulted in an improvement of the quality of articular cartilage repair over isolated HA injections [39]. Although results are promising, the use of orthobiologics in cartilage repair continues to require additional evidence to support clinical use.

Quantifying Outcomes of Orthobiologics

The use of orthobiologics is growing rapidly in both research, translation, and clinical applications. However, there has been a scarcity of real-world patient outcome data for the vast majority of orthobiologic treatments. This includes quality measures, characterization of injectate, cost, adverse events, and long-term follow-up [40]. Therefore, there has been a great effort to increase available evidence, based on clinical outcomes, to provide a potential road map on delivering quality for facilities providing orthobiologic therapies [41]. To provide feedback on the safety and efficacy of these treatments, observational practice registries have emerged in clinical environments throughout the world [42]. A clinical outcomes registry is an organized system for collecting patient outcomes as data points relevant to the effect of treatment on pathology or injury. A key benefit of this type of registry is its agility; the registry can quickly identify underperforming treatments by linking the treatment to patient-reported outcome measures (PROs) and adverse events (AEs). For the field of orthobiologics, this is critical, as data and information about the efficacy of treatments is growing, but not fully known [43, 44].

One recent outcome registry, by Drs. Rogers, Malanga, and Bowen, provides comprehensive coverage of a broad array of regenerative medicine treatments. This includes PRP, hyaluronic acid, bone marrow, adipose-derived mesenchymal cells, and a variety of other regenerative medicine treatments. The most common orthobiologic treatment employed in the registry was PRP (64%), followed by adipose (17%), and then by BMAC (12%). Although still in its early stages, registries will allow physicians to begin patient-reported outcome data collection and contribute to reporting outcomes of the successes and failures of biologic therapy. The future holds many potential avenues of progression for this tracking system, with one potential next-gen application being a data biologics software that will streamline the collection and reporting of these important outcome data.

Future of Orthobiologics

The overall field of orthobiologics is at a critical junction in time. Scientists, translation clinicians, and practitioners jointly have to collaborate to ensure that the necessary evidence needed for further legitimizing the use of orthobiologics is established and accepted by regulating bodies and professional organizations. Recently, there has been increased regulatory action of the use of orthobiologics clinically, and overall this has been positive as many bad actors have been brought to light [45]. What is missing from most published investigations are the quality measures, characterization of injectate, cost, adverse events, and long-term follow-up [40]. To advance the clinical practice forward either providers will depend on industry to provide injectates (most likely allogenic), create their own labs (expensive and difficult to run), or the creation of central labs that collect, process, perform quality assurance, and delivery may become a reality in more of the world as is being currently seen in some part of Europe at very reasonable costs [46].

The other critical area of growth requires more expansive use of registries by clinical orthobiologic practitioners that are both easy to use by patients and providers alike, to allow for very nimble adjustments to patient protocols and products used [47, 48].

Bibliography

1. Hootman JM, Helmick CG, Barbour KE, Theis KA, Boring MA. Updated projected prevalence of self-reported doctor-diagnosed arthritis and arthritis-attributable activity limitation among US adults, 2015-2040. Arthritis Rheumatol. 2016;68(7):1582–7. https://doi.org/10.1002/art.39692.
2. Murphy LB, Cisternas MG, Pasta DJ, Helmick CG, Yelin EH. Medical expenditures and earnings losses among US adults with arthritis in 2013. Arthritis Care Res (Hoboken). 2018;70(6):869–76. https://doi.org/10.1002/acr.23425. Epub 2018 Apr 16.
3. Crawford DC, Miller LE, Block JE. Conservative management of symptomatic knee osteoarthritis: a flawed strategy? Orthop Rev (Pavia). 2013;5(1):e2. https://doi.org/10.4081/or.2013.e2. PMID: 23705060; PMCID: PMC3662262.
4. Grässel S, Muschter D. Recent advances in the treatment of osteoarthritis. F1000Res. 2020;9:F1000 Faculty Rev-325. https://doi.org/10.12688/f1000research.22115.1. PMID: 32419923; PMCID: PMC7199286.
5. Evans JT, Walker RW, Evans JP, Blom AW, Sayers A, Whitehouse MR. How long does a knee replacement last? A systematic review and meta-analysis of case series and national registry reports with more than 15 years of follow-up. Lancet. 2019;393(10172):655–63. https://doi.org/10.1016/S0140-6736(18)32531-5. Epub 2019 Feb 14. Erratum in: Lancet. 2019 Feb 20;: PMID: 30782341; PMCID: PMC6381229.
6. Bayliss LE, Culliford D, Monk AP, Glyn-Jones S, Prieto-Alhambra D, Judge A, Cooper C, Carr AJ, Arden NK, Beard DJ, Price AJ. The effect of patient age at intervention on risk of implant revision after total replacement of the hip or knee: a population-based cohort study. Lancet. 2017;389(10077):1424–30. https://doi.org/10.1016/S0140-6736(17)30059-4. Epub 2017 Feb 14. Erratum in: Lancet. 2017 Apr 8;389(10077):1398. PMID: 28209371; PMCID: PMC5522532.
7. Murrell WD, Anz AW, Badsha H, Bennett WF, Boykin RE, Caplan AI. Regenerative treatments to enhance orthopedic surgical outcome. PM R. 2015;7(4 Suppl):S41–52. https://doi.org/10.1016/j.pmrj.2015.01.015.
8. Dhillon MS, Behera P, Patel S, Shetty V. Orthobiologics and platelet rich plasma. Indian J Orthop. 2014;48(1):1–9. https://doi.org/10.4103/0019-5413.125477. PMID: 24600055; PMCID: PMC3931137.
9. Connolly JF. Clinical use of marrow osteoprogenitor cells to stimulate osteogenesis. Clin Orthop Relat Res. 1998;355:Suppl):S257-66. https://doi.org/10.1097/00003086-199810001-00026.
10. Caplan AI. Mesenchymal stem cells. J Orthop Res. 1991;9(5):641–50. https://doi.org/10.1002/jor.1100090504.
11. Caplan AI. Mesenchymal stem cells: time to change the name! Stem Cells Transl Med. 2017;6(6):1445–51. https://doi.org/10.1002/sctm.17-0051. Epub 2017 Apr 28. PMID: 28452204; PMCID: PMC5689741.
12. Murphy MB, Moncivais K, Caplan AI. Mesenchymal stem cells: environmentally responsive therapeutics for regenerative medicine. Exp Mol Med. 2013;45(11):e54. https://doi.org/10.1038/emm.2013.94. PMID: 24232253; PMCID: PMC3849579.
13. Caplan AI. All MSCs are pericytes? Cell Stem Cell. 2008;3(3):229–30. https://doi.org/10.1016/j.stem.2008.08.008.
14. Haynesworth SE, Goldberg VM, Caplan AI. Diminution of the number of mesenchymal stem cells as a cause for skeletal aging. In: Musculoskeletal soft-tissue aging: impact on mobility, section 1, chapter 7, Eds. JA Buckwalter, VM Goldberg, and SL-Y Woo, American Academy of Orthopaedic Surgeons, Publishers; 1994, 79–87.
15. Marx RE. Platelet-rich plasma (PRP): what is PRP and what is not PRP? Implant Dent. 2001;10(4):225–8. https://doi.org/10.1097/00008505-200110000-00002.
16. A Hamid MS, Sazlina SG. Platelet-rich plasma for rotator cuff tendinopathy: a systematic review and meta-analysis. PLoS One. 2021;16(5):e0251111.

https://doi.org/10.1371/journal.pone.0251111. PMID: 33970936; PMCID: PMC8109792.
17. Di Matteo B, Ranieri R, Manca A, Cappato S, Marcacci M, Kon E, Castagna A. Cell-based therapies for the treatment of shoulder and elbow tendinopathies: a scoping review. Stem Cells Int. 2021;24(2021):5558040. https://doi.org/10.1155/2021/5558040. PMID: 33995531; PMCID: PMC8096562.
18. Robinson DM, Eng C, Mitchkash M, Tenforde A, Borg-Stein J. Outcomes after micronized fat adipose transfer for glenohumeral joint arthritis and rotator cuff pathology: a case series of 18 shoulders. Muscle Ligaments Tendons J. 2020;10(393) https://doi.org/10.32098/mltj.03.2020.06.
19. Huang K, Giddins G, Wu LD. Platelet-rich plasma versus corticosteroid injections in the management of elbow epicondylitis and plantar fasciitis: an updated systematic review and meta-analysis. Am J Sports Med. 2020;48(10):2572–85. https://doi.org/10.1177/0363546519888450. Epub 2019 Dec 10.
20. Singh A, Gangwar DS, Singh S. Bone marrow injection: a novel treatment for tennis elbow. J Nat Sci Biol Med. 2014;5(2):389–91. https://doi.org/10.4103/0976-9668.136198. PMID: 25097421; PMCID: PMC4121921.
21. Khoury M, Tabben M, Rolón AU, Levi L, Chamari K, D'Hooghe P. Promising improvement of chronic lateral elbow tendinopathy by using adipose derived mesenchymal stromal cells: a pilot study. J Exp Orthop. 2021;8(1):6. https://doi.org/10.1186/s40634-020-00320-z. PMID: 33501619; PMCID: PMC7838228.
22. Belk JW, Kraeutler MJ, Houck DA, Goodrich JA, Dragoo JL, McCarty EC. Platelet-rich plasma versus hyaluronic acid for knee osteoarthritis: a systematic review and meta-analysis of randomized controlled trials. Am J Sports Med. 2021;49(1):249–60. https://doi.org/10.1177/0363546520909397. Epub 2020 Apr 17.
23. Kim GB, Seo MS, Park WT, Lee GW. Bone marrow aspirate concentrate: its uses in osteoarthritis. Int J Mol Sci. 2020;21(9):3224. https://doi.org/10.3390/ijms21093224. PMID: 32370163; PMCID: PMC7247342.
24. Keeling LE, Belk JW, Kraeutler MJ, Kallner AC, Lindsay A, EC MC, Postma WF. Bone marrow aspirate concentrate for the treatment of knee osteoarthritis: a systematic review. Am J Sports Med. 2021:3635465211018837. https://doi.org/10.1177/03635465211018837. Epub ahead of print.
25. Gobbi A, Dallo I, Rogers C, Striano RD, Mautner K, Bowers R, Rozak M, Bilbool N, Murrell WD. Two-year clinical outcomes of autologous microfragmented adipose tissue in elderly patients with knee osteoarthritis: a multi-centric, international study. Int Orthop. 2021;45(5):1179–88. https://doi.org/10.1007/s00264-021-04947-0. Epub 2021 Mar 2.
26. Schneider U, Kumar A, Murrell W, Ezekwesili A, Yurdi NA, Maffulli N. Intra-articular gold induced cytokine (GOLDIC®) injection therapy in patients with osteoarthritis of knee joint: a clinical study. Int Orthop. 2021;45(2):497–507. https://doi.org/10.1007/s00264-020-04870-w. Epub 2021 Jan 6.
27. Shanmugasundaram S, Vaish A, Chavada V, Murrell WD, Vaishya R. Assessment of safety and efficacy of intra-articular injection of stromal vascular fraction for the treatment of knee osteoarthritis-a systematic review. Int Orthop 2021;45(3):615–625. doi: https://doi.org/10.1007/s00264-020-04926-x. Epub 2021 Jan 12.
28. Wang JH, Nirmala X. Application of tendon stem/progenitor cells and platelet-rich plasma to treat tendon injuries. Oper Tech Orthop. 2016;26(2):68–72. https://doi.org/10.1053/j.oto.2015.12.008. PMID: 27574378; PMCID: PMC5000850.
29. Ryan J, Imbergamo C, Sudah S, Kirchner G, Greenberg P, Monica J, Gatt C. Platelet-rich product supplementation in rotator cuff repair reduces retear rates and improves clinical outcomes: a meta-analysis of randomized controlled trials. Arthroscopy. 2021;37(8):2608–24. https://doi.org/10.1016/j.arthro.2021.03.010. Epub 2021 Mar 17. PMID: 33744318; PMCID: PMC8349828.
30. Cole BJ, Verma NN, Yanke AB, Bach BR, Otte RS, Chubinskaya S, Romeo AA, Southworth TM, Naveen NB. Prospective randomized trial of biologic augmentation with mesenchymal stem cells in patients undergoing arthroscopic rotator cuff repair. Orthop J Sports Med. 2019;7(7 suppl 5):2325967119S00275. https://doi.org/10.1177/2325967119S00275. PMCID: PMC6667873.
31. Hernigou P, Flouzat Lachaniette CH, Delambre J, Zilber S, Duffiet P, Chevallier N, Rouard H. Biologic augmentation of rotator cuff repair with mesenchymal stem cells during arthroscopy improves healing and prevents further tears: a case-controlled study. Int Orthop. 2014;38(9):1811–8. https://doi.org/10.1007/s00264-014-2391-1. Epub 2014 Jun 7.
32. Andriolo L, Di Matteo B, Kon E, Filardo G, Venieri G, Marcacci M. PRP augmentation for ACL reconstruction. Biomed Res Int. 2015;2015:371746. https://doi.org/10.1155/2015/371746. Epub 2015 May 5. PMID: 26064903; PMCID: PMC4430629.
33. Baratz ME, Fu FH, Mengato R. Meniscal tears: the effect of meniscectomy and of repair on intraarticular contact areas and stress in the human knee. A preliminary report. Am J Sports Med. 1986;14(4):270–5. https://doi.org/10.1177/036354658601400405.
34. Kaminski R, Kulinski K, Kozar-Kaminska K, Wielgus M, Langner M, Wasko MK, Kowalczewski J, Pomianowski S. A prospective, randomized, double-blind, parallel-group, placebo-controlled study evaluating meniscal healing, clinical outcomes, and safety in patients undergoing meniscal repair of unstable, complete vertical meniscal tears (bucket handle) augmented with platelet-rich plasma.

Biomed Res Int. 2018;11(2018):9315815. https://doi.org/10.1155/2018/9315815. PMID: 29713647; PMCID: PMC5866900.
35. Massey PA, Zhang A, Stairs CB, Hoge S, Carroll T, Hamby AM. Meniscus repair outcomes with and without bone marrow aspiration concentrate. Orthop J Sports Med. 2019;7(7 suppl 5):2325967119S00283. https://doi.org/10.1177/2325967119S00283. PMCID: PMC6668001.
36. Sasaki H, Rothrauff BB, Alexander PG, Lin H, Gottardi R, Fu FH, Tuan RS. In vitro repair of meniscal radial tear with hydrogels seeded with adipose stem cells and TGF-β3. Am J Sports Med. 2018;46(10):2402–13. https://doi.org/10.1177/0363546518782973. Epub 2018 Jul 12.
37. Campbell KA, Saltzman BM, Mascarenhas R, Khair MM, Verma NN, Bach BR Jr, Cole BJ. Does intra-articular platelet-rich plasma injection provide clinically superior outcomes compared with other therapies in the treatment of knee osteoarthritis? A systematic review of overlapping meta-analyses. Arthroscopy. 2015;31(11):2213–21. https://doi.org/10.1016/j.arthro.2015.03.041. Epub 2015 May 29.
38. Cotter EJ, Wang KC, Yanke AB, Chubinskaya S. Bone marrow aspirate concentrate for cartilage defects of the knee: from bench to bedside evidence. Cartilage. 2018;9(2):161–70. https://doi.org/10.1177/1947603517741169. Epub 2017 Nov 10. PMID: 29126349; PMCID: PMC5871125.
39. Saw KY, Anz A, Siew-Yoke Jee C, Merican S, Ching-Soong Ng R, Roohi SA, Ragavanaidu K. Articular cartilage regeneration with autologous peripheral blood stem cells versus hyaluronic acid: a randomized controlled trial. Arthroscopy. 2013;29(4):684–94. https://doi.org/10.1016/j.arthro.2012.12.008. Epub 2013 Feb 4.
40. Marenah M, Li J, Kumar A, Murrell W. Quality assurance and adverse event management in regenerative medicine for knee osteoarthritis: current concepts. J Clin Orthop Trauma. 2019;10(1):53–8. https://doi.org/10.1016/j.jcot.2018.09.005. Epub 2018 Sep 18. PMID: 30705533; PMCID: PMC6349654.
41. Chiauzzi E, Rodarte C, DasMahapatra P. Patient-centered activity monitoring in the self-management of chronic health conditions. BMC Med. 2015;13:77.
42. Bai Y, Welk GJ, Nam YH, Lee JA, Lee JM, Kim Y, Meier NF, Dixon PM. Comparison of consumer and research monitors under semistructured settings. Med Sci Sports Exerc. 2016 Jan;48(1):151–8. https://doi.org/10.1249/MSS.0000000000000727.
43. Centeno CJ, Al-Sayegh H, Freeman MD, Smith J, Murrell WD, Bubnov R. A multi-center analysis of adverse events among two thousand, three hundred and seventy-two adult patients undergoing adult autologous stem cell therapy for orthopaedic conditions. Int Orthop. 2016;40:1755–65.
44. Gagnier JJ. Patient reported outcomes in orthopaedics. J Orthop Res 2017;35:2098-2108. El-Daly I, Ibraheim H, Rajakulendran K, Culpan P, Bates P. Are patient-reported outcome measures in orthopaedics easily read by patients? Clin Orthop Relat Res. 2016;474:246–55.
45. FDA Extends Enforcement Discretion Policy for Certain Regenerative Medicine Products. https://www.fda.gov/news-events/press-announcements/fda-extends-enforcement-discretion-policy-certain-regenerative-medicine-products. U.S. Food and Drug Administration. 01 Nov 2021.
46. Lucas S, Tencerova M, von der Weid B, Andersen TL, Attané C, Behler-Janbeck F, Cawthorn WP, Ivaska KK, Naveiras O, Podgorski I, Reagan MR, van der Eerden BCJ. Guidelines for biobanking of bone marrow adipose tissue and related cell types: report of the biobanking working group of the International Bone Marrow Adiposity Society. Front Endocrinol (Lausanne). 2021;12:744527. https://doi.org/10.3389/fendo.2021.744527. PMID: 34646237; PMCID: PMC8503265.
47. Yurdi NA, Tulpule S, Malanga G, Rogers C, Murrell WD. Chapter 42. Measuring outcomes in orthobiologics – registry. In: Dhillon M, editor. Orthobiologics. Salubris; 2021.
48. Jenio FZ, Scholes C, Marenah M, Li J, Cowley M, Ebrahimi M, Harrison-Brown M, Murrell WD. Quality in practice: implementation of a clinical outcomes registry in regenerative medicine. Ann Transl Med. 2019;7(7):130. https://doi.org/10.21037/atm.2019.02.38. PMID: 31157251; PMCID: PMC6511570.

The Nuts and Bolts of Regenerative Medicine as It Pertains to the Joint

3

Joseph Purita

Regenerative medicine has dramatically changed the approaches of treating degenerative conditions in a joint. Typically, when we are discussing joints, there are a few major aspects that we need to address. Rather than deal with the esoteric, the focus of this chapter is on the more common afflictions of joints and how regenerative medicine may effectively treat them. These conditions can be divided into three major aspects. Those affecting the articular cartilage, those affecting the soft tissue aspects of the joint, and finally those conditions affecting joint circulation. The soft tissue aspects deal with the ligaments, tendons, and muscles that contribute to the integrity of the knee. We must keep in mind that typically these conditions are many times interrelated to each other. One condition may predispose the joint to other problems and combine with other problems. The main emphasis of this chapter is on conditions of the articular cartilage. A word of caution should be given. Some of the recommendations in this chapter may not be allowed in your country. We urge that you check with the appropriate authorities in your country if you have questions on certain procedures.

J. Purita (✉)
The Institute of Regenerative Medicine,
Boca Raton, FL, USA

Articular Cartilage

Joints are unique in that they are subjected to decades of wear and tear. Articular cartilage is hyaline cartilage and is 2–4 mm thick [1]. Unlike most tissues, articular cartilage does not have blood vessels, nerves, or lymphatics. It is composed of a dense extracellular matrix (ECM) with a sparse distribution of highly specialized cells called chondrocytes. The ECM is principally composed of water, collagen, and proteoglycans, with other non-collagenous proteins. The glycoproteins present in lesser amounts. Together, these components help to retain water within the ECM, which is critical to maintain its' unique mechanical properties. The articular cartilage is divided into four main sections.

The superficial zone has Type II collagen with an orientation that is parallel to joint. The superficial zone protects the deeper layers from shear stresses and makes up approximately 10–20% of articular cartilage thickness. It has flattened chondrocytes, condensed collagen fibres, and sparse proteoglycans sparse proteoglycans. It is the only zone where articular cartilage progenitor cells have been found. The integrity of this layer is imperative in the protection and maintenance of deeper layers. Of significance in this layer is a compound called lubricin. Lubricin was originally identified as a lubricating glycoprotein present in the synovial fluid (SF). It is specifically synthesized and expressed by articular

Y. El Miedany (ed.), *Musculoskeletal Ultrasound-Guided Regenerative Medicine*,
https://doi.org/10.1007/978-3-030-98256-0_3

chondrocytes of the superficial zone. It is recognized to have a major protective role in preventing cartilage wear, helps in synovial cell adhesion and proliferation, and reduces the coefficient of friction of the articular cartilage surface.

The intermediate layer has Type II collagen, having an oblique or random organization. It is the thickest layer with round chondrocytes and abundant proteoglycan content. The intermediate layer represents 40% to 60% of the total cartilage volume. Functionally, the intermediate layer is the first line of resistance to compressive forces.

The deep zone is responsible for providing the greatest resistance to compressive forces, given that collagen fibrils are arranged perpendicular to the articular surface. The deep zone contains the largest diameter collagen fibrils in a radial disposition, the highest proteoglycan content, and the lowest water concentration. The rounded chondrocytes are typically arranged in columnar orientation, parallel to the collagen fibres, and perpendicular to the joint line. The deep zone represents approximately 30% of articular cartilage volume.

The last zone is called the tidemark. The tidemark divides the superficial, uncalcified cartilage from the deeper calcified cartilage division. The tidemark is found only in joints.

When we are dealing with regenerative procedures in the joint, we are most interested in the chondrocytes [2]. Chondrocytes are metabolically active cells that synthesize and turnover a large volume of extracellular matrix (ECM) components, such as collagen, glycoproteins, proteoglycans, and hyaluronan. They do, however, respond to a variety of stimuli, including growth factors, mechanical loads, piezoelectric forces, and hydrostatic pressures. The metabolic activities of chondrocytes are altered by many factors that are present within their chemical and mechanical environment. Most important among these factors are the pro- and anti-inflammatory cytokines and growth factors that have anabolic and catabolic effects. In essence, regenerative medicine is attempting to manipulate these cytokines to lead to repair and decreased inflammation.

Ligaments and Tendons and Their Effects on Joint Problems

Ligaments and tendons are intimately related to the joint. A malfunction in one or both of these entities can result in a disaster for the joint. The treatment of ligamentous and tendon injuries is similar yet different from that of the joint. These structures are similar in composition, but there are some significant differences. In the tendon, the collagen fibrils are aligned parallel to each other and to the long axis of the tendon, whereas in the ligament, the fibrils are not as uniformly orientated to allow for multiaxial loading patterns. The treatment of these injuries is similar to articular cartilage injuries.

Platelet-Rich Plasma (PRP)

In regenerative medicine procedures, a good concept to consider is that one is planting a garden. Any garden has three main components. It consists of soil or in this case a scaffold, seeds which in our case are regenerative cells including stem cells, and fertilizer which in our case are growth factors derived from among other things platelets. Platelet-rich plasma is derived from the patient's own blood; therefore, it is an autologous product. Platelets are composed of three main components. The three main components are lysosomes, the dense granules, and the alpha granules. The alpha granules contain the most important factors controlling regeneration. The following diagram illustrates these facts (Fig. 3.1). It gives an excellent breakdown of each entity and its various subparts. As we can see, a platelet is a complicated structure.

The growth factors are one of the most important aspects of the platelets for our purposes. However, we cannot minimize the importance of other aspects such as dense granules and lysosomes. The question as to what the most important growth factors from the platelets are is like asking what the most important instruments in a symphony orchestra are. They all have importance. For discussion purposes, we will centre on a hand full of these factors. Numerous protein

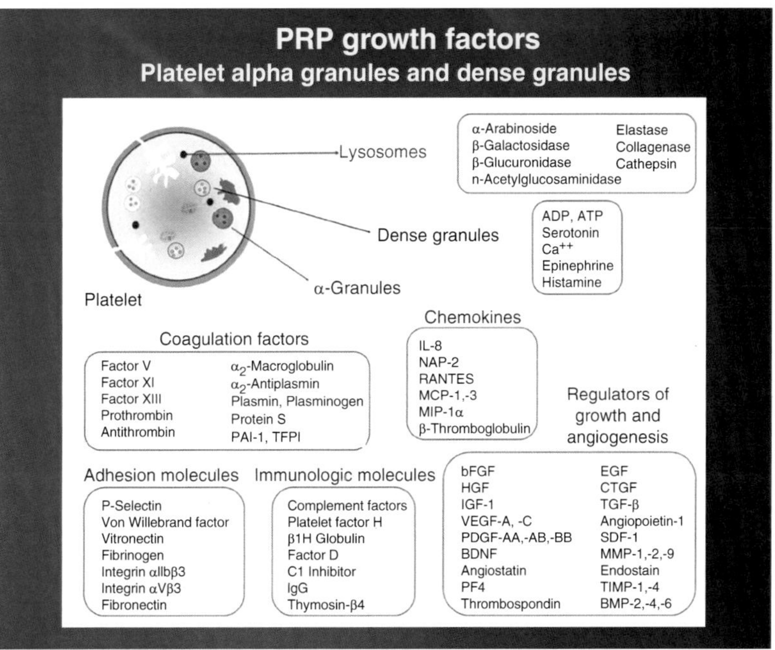

Fig. 3.1 PRP growth factors

growth factors are contained in the alpha granules of platelets: platelet-derived growth factor (PDGF), transforming growth factor (TGF), platelet factor interleukins (IL), platelet-derived angiogenesis factor (PDAF), vascular endothelial growth factor (VEGF), epidermal growth factor (EGF), insulin-like growth factor IGF, fibronectin, and a host of others. When we are dealing with the different growth factors, we need to realize they typically consist of a family [3]. For instance, there are a few types of IGF. Most growth factors have more than one type, some such as FGF can have 22 different types (realize that some of these forms can have significantly different effects). Both age and gender account for variations in specific GFs present in PRP. This may partially explain some of the inconsistent results of PRP clinical trials. It is well known that the biological half-lives of most growth factor peptides are very short, and this may limit the effectiveness of the current intra-articular injection therapies [4]. Combining a growth factor with hyaluronic acid (HA), for example, allows for a more prolonged delivery of the growth factor, potentially enhancing this widely used clinical treatment for cartilage degeneration and joint pain. HA gels have been prepared as injectable carrier vehicles for growth factors and bioactivity assays demonstrate that sustained release is achieved over periods as long as 10–15 days. HA itself can have many different properties, including acting as a signalling molecule [5].

Realize that growth factors from platelets represent only one source of growth factors. The other major source comes from various types of stem cells, cells of the immune system, and other regenerative cells. Many studies have shown that the growth factor release from platelets lasts about 7 days. A few years back, it was very popular to activate the platelets ahead of their injection. This was typically done by adding thrombin to the platelet mixture. However, there were some potential problems with the thrombin, such as an allergic reaction by the patient. That being said, we must realize that when platelets come into contact with collagen, they become activated. Essentially, most all tissue contains collagen. Also, when there are some RBCs in the platelet product, they will contribute some thrombin and further activate the platelets. There are some conditions which may require the use of only the platelet growth factors without the platelets. When we are only using the platelet growth factors, this is called platelet lysate. There are no platelets in a lysate. A lysate may be used in some intravenous applications. A good method of producing a lysate is by using an ultrasonic cleaner and using it to lysis the platelets.

When we are looking at a PRP product, we must realize that a PRP is more than platelets. The following diagram (Fig. 3.2) shows the various components of a PRP product [6]. An effective PRP preparation has many different components. Where we get into problems when dealing with a PRP preparation is what type of preparation are we dealing with. In other words, how was it made? What does it consist of?

The problem we have discovered is that there is no consistent classification of PRP products. This may be one the reasons why there is a discrepancy in results that are reported. A good attempt to classify PRP products was made by Mirsha et al. They classified PRP according to platelet content, WBC content, and platelet activation. There were four main classifications. Type 1 had increased amounts of WBCs and no platelet activation with either 5× or more of platelet concentration from baseline (Type 1A) or less than 5× concentration from baseline (Type 1B). Type 2 is similar with the difference being activated platelets and 5× more (Type 2A) or 5× less (Type 2B) concentration of platelets from the baseline. Type 3 had minimal or no WBCs with no platelet activation and either 5× more (Type 3A) or 5× less (Type 3B) platelet concentration than baseline. Type 4 had little or no WBCs with platelet activation and either 5× more platelet concentration from baseline (Type 4A) or less than 5× platelet concentration from baseline (Type 4B). This is a very good attempt in trying to compare "apples to apples" when we are looking at clinical studies. It gives us some indication as to what the PRP was composed of.

Another paper by Lana and Purita et al. further classifies PRP [6]. In their paper, they expanded the classification to include other perimeters. These perimeters included method made, presence of red blood cells, the number of spins used to produce the PRP product, and finally light activation. We are now realizing the that light activation is becoming more and more important in the field of regenerative medicine. There is more to follow later in the chapter concerning photo modulation. A synopsis of classification of Lana et al. can be found below (Table. 3.1). It is called the MARSPILL PRP classification.

The ultimate question becomes the following: Which form of PRP works best? Should different forms of PRP be used for different clinical conditions? Is a leucocyte poor (LP) PRP product (sometimes called a pure PRP) more effective in the joint than a leucocyte-rich (LR) PRP product? Unfortunately, there are no easy answers here. However, when we sift thru science, some important trends emerge.

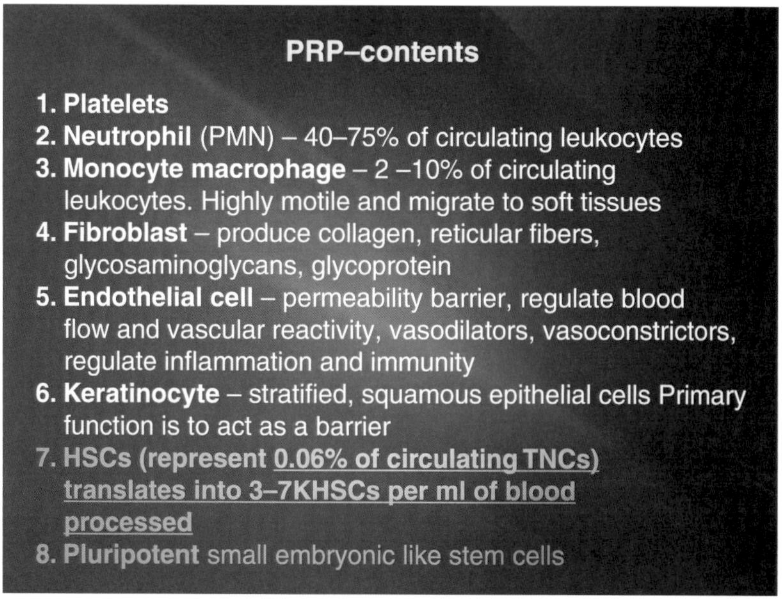

Fig. 3.2 PRP contents

Table 3.1 MARSPILL PRP classification

Marspill PRP classification

Table 2. Marspill classification

Letter	Relates to	Type
M	Method	Handmade (H) Machine (M)
A	Activation	Activated (A+) Not activated (A–)
R	Red blood cells	Rich (RBC-R) Poor (RBC-P)
S	Spin	One spin (Sp1) Two spins (Sp2)
P	Platelet number (folds basal)	PL 2–3 PL 6–8 PL 4–6 PL 8–10
I	Image guided	Guided (G+) Not guided (G–)
L	Leukocyte concentration	Rich (Lc-R) Poor (Lc-P)
L	Light activation	Actived (A+) Not activated (A–)

Lc: Leukocyte concentration; PL: Platelet concentration; RBC: Red blood cell.

There are some misconceptions in the field of PRP that I call "Urban Legends of PRP". It seems that many times companies are using their marketing ploys and trying to represent them as clinical science. There are very few papers showing clinical evidence that (LP) PRP is more effective than (LR) PRP in the joint. However, there is ample systemic review and meta-analysis showing that (LR) is more effective. Dr. William Parrish [7] has presented a number of peer-reviewed articles on these concepts. There are some huge takeaways that we obtain from the various Parrish articles. Realize these concepts are not just those of Dr. Parrish but are prevailing scientific attitudes. As Dr. Parrish mentions "growth factors represent only a single aspect of the bioactivity of platelets. Furthermore, platelets represent only one aspect of the potential bioactivity of PRP".

Let us take a better look at some of these ideas. We can start with red blood cells (RBCs). Granted we do want diminished numbers of RBCs. But there is a prevailing attitude that RBCs cause inflammation. There is no literature supporting this. On the contrary, there are good clinical examples that RBCs do not cause inflammation. When a patient tears an ACL ligament, he or she typically develops a bloody effusion. The patient may have discomfort from the effusion, but they typically do not develop an inflammatory response from the blood. Another good example concerns the use of a blood patch for a spinal leak. If something (in this case whole blood) were inflammatory, would we want to put it on the dura? What other purpose might RBCs serve. They are a source of thrombin, which is of the upmost importance for helping platelet activation. Furthermore, the RBCs help in the growth factor release from the platelets. In addition, RBCs also release nitric oxide and glutathione, both of which can have beneficial effects on the cellular matrix and environment.

Another misconception is the presence of neutrophils. In many circles, neutrophils are vilified as one of the major causes of inflammation. Again, as Dr. Parrish explains, only under certain conditions are neutrophils actually bad as far as regeneration is concerned [8]. The following diagram is from one of Parrish's papers. As is pointed out, neutrophils cause inflammation when they are activated. We see that they will secrete those cytokines, which cause inflammation. This is the classical injury-induced inflammation. This is what will hopefully get a bacterial infection under control. Remember, neutrophils are powerful antibacterial agents. In their destruction of bacteria, they will cause some collateral damage to the surrounding tissue. When the neutrophils are primed but not activated, some interesting things happen. The neutrophils actually secrete anti-inflammatory growth factors, which can lead to repair. The following diagram is an excellent summation of this concept put forth by Parrish (Fig. 3.3). As we can see in the diagram, the neutrophils actually produce IL-10 and IL-1 antagonist which are potent master anti-inflammatory cytokines. They also produce TGF-b. These three cytokines can be instrumental in tissue repair. They also give a stop signal to turn off an inflammatory cycle.

We know that we can manipulate the neutrophils a bit with photo modulation. Photo modulation, as evidenced by Morgan et al. [9], has an effect on neutrophils. Studies indicates that phototherapy can have a significant impact on neutrophils, the effect of which varies according to the specific type of phototherapy. We have utilized photo modulation for years in our clinic.

While photo modulation may help the neutrophils produce some anti-inflammatory growth factors, there are other aspects of neutrophils to consider.

Macrophages: A Secret Weapon in a PRP

Another important cell group found in a proper PRP product involves monocytes, which become macrophages. The concept that macrophages should be part of PRP product is steadily becoming more accepted. The macrophage is at the centre of the "immune solar system". They have profound effects on various immune cells. Our

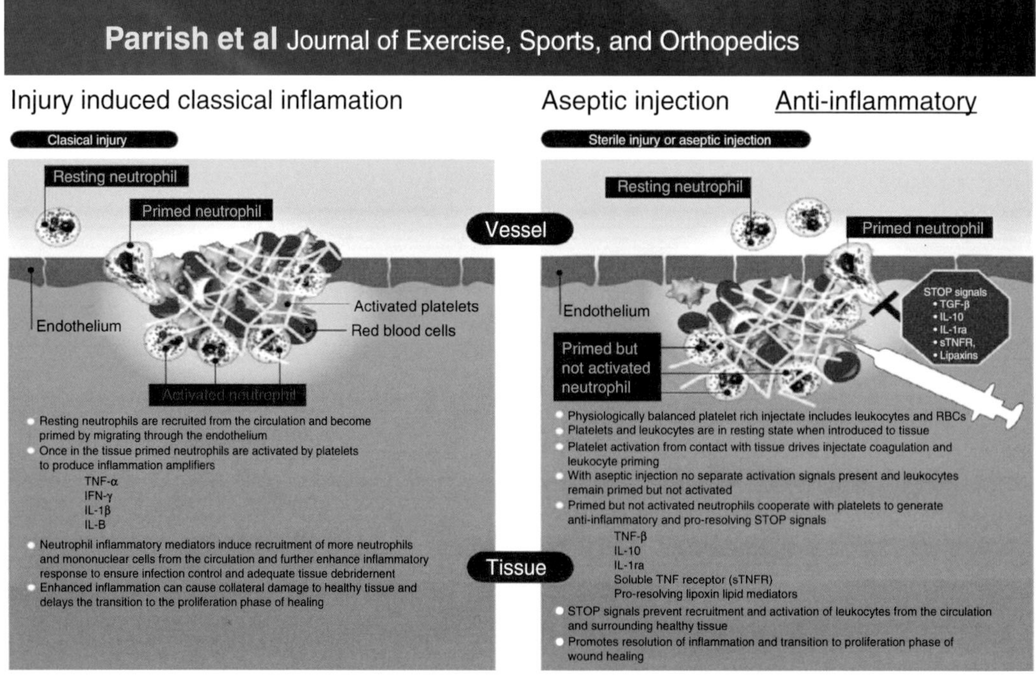

Fig. 3.3 Parrish et al. Journal of Exercise, Sports, and Orthopedics. (Used with the permission of DR. W. Parrish)

immune system and stem cell therapy are intimately related. There are two types of macrophages in the immune system. Macrophages have prominent plasticity and are classified into activated M-1 or activated M-2 macrophages [10]. The macrophage type depends on the specific micro-environment they are found in. These two types have significantly different actions not only in the immune system but also in general repair. M-1 macrophages are pro-inflammatory and possess remarkable antimicrobial abilities via the secretion of various inflammatory cytokines and chemokines. M-2 macrophages are immunomodulatory by releasing IL-10 (interleukin 10) and trophic factors to promote tissue repair and resolve inflammation. Put in simple terms, M1-type macrophages release cytokines that inhibit the proliferation of surrounding cells and damage contiguous tissue, and M2-type macrophages release cytokines that promote the proliferation of contiguous cells and encourage tissue repair. The clinical impact of M-1/kill and M-2/repair responses is immense, playing pivotal roles in curing (or causing) many diseases, including infections, cancer, autoimmunity, and atherosclerosis. Realize that mesenchymal stem cells and their secretory patterns have a profound effect on the polarization of macrophages.

In the field of regenerative medicine, we are more concerned with the M-2 macrophage. The M-2 macrophage conversion is influenced by its environment. This is where mesenchymal stem cells can be of great importance. By secreting certain growth factors, such as IL-3 and IL-4, they are able to influence the polarization of the macrophages to move towards the M-2 category. IL-4-induced macrophages stimulate arginase activity by converting arginine to polyamines and collagen precursors that are crucial for tissue modelling and wound healing. Macrophages were shown to be responsible for regeneration by actively metabolizing arginine with arginase into ornithine and urea. This is of upmost importance, since ornithine is required for many repair processes. It is a precursor of the polyamines required for cell proliferation and collagen synthesis for extracellular matrix construction. Collagen synthesis is critical for articular cartilage formation, ligamentous and tendon healing, and the list goes on and on.

In summation, we can see that a proper PRP product is required for the best chance of success in regenerative medicine. As Dr. Parrish's has pointed out, we want to use the full complements of the whole blood. We certainly need to concentrate the platelets but at the same time need other components of the whole blood to complement platelet action. A PRP works like a symphony orchestra. All components contribute to the whole. Platelets, RBCs, and leucocytes work synergistically to accomplish repair. They help to control the magnitude and duration of the repair process. There is no doubt that a "pure" PRP (LP-PRP) product will typically cause less of an inflammatory response. The reason for this is typically the LP- PRP product may be an inferior one. I base this on my clinical experience over the last dozen years or so and thousands of cases.

We utilize PRP treatments in the less severe conditions. This includes disorders of the shoulder, including bursitis and rotator cuff tears. Also included in this grouping, we find tendonitis of a variety of tendons, including tennis elbow, Achilles tendonitis, and plantar fasciitis. PRP typically works well with muscle tears, sprains, trigger points, and meniscus tears of the knee. We have had good success with mild to moderate degenerative arthritis of various joints and disorders of the spine especially facet joints. Most of the time, in our primary treatments PRP will be combined with a free fat graft. Experience has taught us that many articular cartilage problems require bone marrow aspirate combined with PRP and a fat graft. There are platelets found in a bone marrow aspirate; however, their numbers are not like those found in the peripheral blood. We typically perform an additional PRP (processed from the blood) when using bone marrow aspirate. There are many different commercial preparations for a bedside PRP. It is probably wise when one is starting out to use one of these kits. As more experience is obtained, then one can manufacture their own PRP. Some final thoughts concerning PRP preparations. It has been described in the literature (2018) that subjecting a PRP preparation to four degrees centigrade for approximately 20 minutes and at the same time reducing the amount of plasma in the total volume to no more than 25% will enhance the release of the growth factors from the alpha granules [11].

One final thought on PRP products. A new concept concerning PRP products is called platelet microparticles. Platelet-derived microparticles (PMP) are the small plasma membrane vesicles (0.05–1 μm) shed from platelets upon their activation, constituting the major pool of microparticles circulating in the blood, and are considered a communication mediator between cells, triggering responses such as inflammation and angiogenesis. P-EVs might be not only a next-generation alternative to PRP but also a potential vehicle for the administration of drugs and other molecules, including mRNA, miRNA, and lncRNA. They are likely to provide a better option than exosomes, which are derived from expensive stem cells or progenitor cells, to modulate cell activity in treating many disorders.

Matrix Metalloproteases (MMP) A2M

Before moving on to stem cells, matrix metalloproteases (MMP) need to be addressed. At neutral pH, only specialized MMPs can degrade across the triple helix of the extracellular matrix. Degradation of cell attachment substrates induces a special form of apoptosis in ECM-dependent mesenchymal cells (anoikis). MMPs can also release suppressive effects and stimulate cellular proliferation and differentiation. MMPs can also exert various anti-inflammatory and pro-healing effects. MMPs can destroy old or excessive matrix to provide room for cells. Protease cleavage plays a role in inactivation of inflammatory cytokines and is imperative for activation of anabolic growth factors. One of the best-known clinical compounds in the MP world is called A2M. A2M is also known as alpha 2-macroglobulin. It is produced in the liver and in macrophages. It is a broad-spectrum multipurpose protease inhibitor having a high concentration in blood (up to 6 mg/ml). It inhibits MMPs and ADAMTS degradation proteases while binding and helping regulate cytokines and grow factors. There are a number of commercially available kits that can concentrate the A2M. This may help in the overall repair process. It does not seem to be a game changer.

Stem Cells: The Drivers of Regeneration

Some Generalities

Getting back to the gardening concept, the stem cells represent the seeds in the regenerative medicine garden. We must realize that we are lucky if a few percent of the stem cells survive. We need to be cognizant of the fact that we would live about 2 days without stem cells. The major sources of stem cells in the regenerative medicine field are those derived from typically the bone marrow as an aspirate or those found in adipose tissue. There are a limited number of stem cells found in the circulating blood. The two main types of stem cells we are dealing with include mesenchymal stem cells and hemopoietic stem cells. We shall discuss both. Before discussing the various aspect of different stem cell types, we should present some of their basic science.

When we are discussing a cell, we will typically give it a specific name rather than calling it a mesenchymal cell etc. The specific name will typically begin with the initials CD. CD stands for cluster of differentiation. The CD designation represents the cell surface molecules, which are used to identify the stem cells and the stage of a stem cell. Stem cell identification can be made by having a particular CD marker (CD+) or not having it (CD-). Some examples include the following: mesenchymal stem cells (MSC) (CD 70+, CD90+, CD105+, CD34-) and hematopoietic stem cells (HSC) (CD34+, CD59+, CD90+, CD133). Adult stem cells are found in many tissues. The primary role of stem cells is to maintain and repair the tissue in which they are found.

Most adult stem cells are multipotent, not pluripotent. The vast majority of procedures will involve multipotent cells. However, there is one type of cell called a very small embryonic-like stem cell that is pluripotent. More will be discussed about this cell later in the chapter.

There are distinct differences between stem cells and progenitor cells. Stem cells are typically self-renewing, they are long lived, and they have a low regenerative capacity. On the other hand, progenitor cells (often referred to as transit-amplifying cells) are non-renewing, they are short lived, and they have a high proliferative capacity.

Stem Cell Niche

When discussing stem cells, we need to discuss their environment. This is called the stem cell niche [1]. The niche is composed of many moving parts. The first part of the niche consists of various cellular components: such as tissue specific cells such as mesenchymal cells and other cells and tissues such as blood vessels. The second component deals with secreted factors. These include chemokines and their receptors, growth factors, and their receptors, hormones, etc. The third component deals with inflammation and scarring. This component works closely with macrophages, T-cells, and the immune system. The fourth component deals with the extracellular matrix. This component has fibronectin and collagen in addition to the basement membrane. The fifth component involves physical forces, such as elasticity, stiffness, and shear forces. The sixth and last component deals with hypoxia and metabolism and its various ramifications. Realize that all these components are interacting with cell surface of the stem cell. The cell surface should be considered the eyes and ears of the cell. Unfortunately, bad omega-6 fatty acid tends to accumulate in this area. To combat the omega-6s, we try to give the patient omega-3s and omega-9 to displace the omega-6s. Diet and supplements contribute to the niche health. This is one of the reasons why diet and supplements are so important.

What Are the Major Stem Cells

Embryonic Stem Cells

There are many different types of stem cells, but we basically deal with a handful. The first cell to discuss is the embryonic cell. This is a cell that is draped in controversy. Putting ethical issues aside, why do we not want to use these cells? There are two concerning facts about these cells. First, they are unpredictable. They could potentially form a tumour in the host patient. This is sometimes referred to as a teratoma. Secondly, they act as a foreign tissue. When they are recognized by the body, there could be an allergic reaction triggering what is called a graft vs. host disease. This can be a life-threating problem of which there is not typically an easy solution. With our present technology, these cells seem destined to be used for disease modelling. They have great potential but not with our present technology. One fact to mention about these cells is that they have what are called Yamanaka factors. These are four proteins called SOX2, OCT4, KLF4, and c-myc. These factors are the four master genes that allow cells to be rejuvenated and reprogrammed. These genes wind back the developmental clock. They are typically found in pluripotent cells. If one sees these factors in a cell, then that cell typically will have some pluripotent qualities. This seems to be a common thread in cells, which seem to have great regenerative potential.

Induced Pluripotent Stem Cells (IPS CELLS)

Induced pluripotent stem cells (IPS) are another type of stem cell. They are produced when adult cells have been genetically reprogrammed to an embryonic stem cell-like state. This practice involes expressing genes and factors important for maintaining the defining properties of embryonic stem cells. This reprogramming is typically done by means of a viral vector or by enzymatic means. Clinically, these cells are still not ready for widespread use. But iPS cells have made their mark in a different way. They have become an important tool for modelling and investigating human diseases, as well as for screening drugs. Time will tell where these cells will lead us to. One potential problem with these cells is that although they may act as a pluripotent cell, their DNA is old and may reflect upon the functioning of the cell. Telomere degradation is a problem not just with these cells but most stem cells in general. If we can reverse some telomere damage, we might make a more efficient stem cell. Nevertheless, IPS cells seem to hold great regenerative potential.

Multilineage-Differentiating Stress-Enduring Cells (Muse Cells)

A Muse cell is found in adipose or bone marrow tissue. They are typically isolated in fat using severe cellular stress conditions, including long-term exposure to the proteolytic enzyme collagenase, serum deprivation, low temperatures, and hypoxia. Under these conditions, a highly purified population of Muse-AT cells is isolated without the utilization of cell sorting methods. These cells are probably pluripotent, not multipotent like other adult stem cells. These cells have a very high survival rate upon transplantation into other parts of the body. Unlike embryonic cells, they do not seem to form tumours! They are highly resistance to the following: hypoxia, acidosis, change of temperatures, toxic environment, etc. These cells may take on more importance as time goes on. They seem well suited to the joint due to their ability to survive harsh conditions, such as those found in the joint. At present, it seems that we will have more success in harvesting these cells from adipose tissue. Their harvesting is relatively simple, and typically the harvest will produce adequate numbers.

Very Small Embryonic-Like Stem Cells (V Cells)

Very small embryonic-like stem cells (V Cells) are slowly gaining acceptance in the scientific world. They were first described in 2006 by Ratajczak et al. [12] They were discovered in bone marrow aspirate. They have some unique properties. They have pluripotent markers SSEA-1, Oct-4, Nanog, and Rex-1. V cells have an open chromatin with a high nucleus/cytoplasm ratio. They also have large amounts of telomerase telling us that their DNA should be fairly well preserved. V cells are about one third the size of regular cells. Typically, the V cells circulate in the blood in an inactive form. They are "awakened" by a physiological stress. In a clinical setting, these cells are kept at four degrees centigrade in a hypoxic setting for approximately 12 hours. This temperature and hypoxic stress will activate the cells. There are a number of methods which are utilized to increase the release of these cells into the circulation from the bone marrow. Vitamin A or intravenous CoQ-10 are known stimulators of these cells. They are used in both an intravenous and intra-articular fashion. They also have a specific marker on their cell membrane for parathyroid hormone (PTH). We use parathyroid hormone not only on V cell procedures but also on all of our stem cell procedures. It is pointed out in the literature that PTH is chondro-regenerative [13]. PTH seems to increase stem cell output from the marrow. The PTH is delivered via a patch (should be available in early 2019) with penetrating molecules and also in an oral homeopathic form. One very important aspect of these cells is that in clinical studies, they seem to cause lengthening of the telomeres of the immune system when they are given intravenously. Typically, we are as healthy as our immune system. These cells will certainly become more widely accepted as time goes on. What role they will play in joint regeneration remains to be seen, but I suspect they will eventually play a significant role. Typically, approximately 200 CCs of blood will produce about 30 CCs of the final product. Most of the time, the V cell solution is given intravenously. Many times, five or so CCs will be given as an intra-articular injection. We are still in the process of evaluating the V cells as a viable option of articular problems.

Mesenchymal Stem Cells

Mesenchymal stem cells have a long and storied history. For quite some time, they were thought to be the omnipotent cells of the stem cell field. This concept has changed somewhat due to the input of Dr. Arnold Caplan of Case Western Reserve. Dr. Caplan coined the term *mesenchymal stem cell* in 1987; in 2011, he coined the term *medicinal signalling cell* and declared it was outside of the stem cell category [14]. Dr. Caplan has now given us the concept that the mesenchymal stem cell is more of an immune modulator rather than an actual driver of tissue regeneration. This concept is still not universally accepted but is steadily gaining acceptance. Some general characteristics of the MSCs are as follows. They have plastic adherence. They are positive for the following CD markers 73, 90, and 105. They are negative for hematopoietic CD markers 45, 34, 14 or 11b, 10 or 79α, and HLA-DR. They are multipotent in nature. They seem to possess both immunomodulatory and tropic properties.

We need to have the realization that this class of cells can be isolated from almost every tissue in the human body. The central connecting aspect to explain this fact is that all of these tissues are vascularized and that every blood vessel in the body has mesenchymal cells in abluminal locations. These perivascular cells can be summarily called pericytes. Eventually, when an injury occurs, these pericytes become activated MSCs.

MSCs are being used therapeutically because they undergo homing to the sites of inflammation or tissue injury and they secrete massive levels of bioactive agents [12]. The injury response will make the MSC become immunomodulatory. This immune modulation has some profound effects on the immune system, such as T-cells, Treg cells, and dendritic cells. At the same time, MSCs have some trophic effects, including angiogenic, mitotic, antiapoptotic, chemoattractive, and regenerative. Perhaps a good way to look at MSCs is to consider them as the body's Navy Seals. They get injected into a hostile area. Chances are they will not survive. But they will secure the area so that the rest of the other cells can do their job. One other aspect of MSCs is their antibacterial properties. They produce a compound called LL-37 or human cathelicidin antimicrobial peptide [15]. This will help prevent infections in joints when MSCs are utilized. The LL-37 is responsible for preventing women from developing sepsis during their menstrual periods due to the high number of MSCs in the menstrual blood. Like macrophages, MSCs can polarize into two different types. The inflammatory milieu determines the path the MSCs take [13]. Following an injury, the inflammatory milieu is typically high. The high level of inflammatory products results in a type II MSC. The type II MSC results in immune modulation, increases Treg cell production while suppressing T-cell responsiveness. They also produce a number of valuable growth factors, such as TGF, FGF, IGF, IL-10, and CXCL-12. These are all important in regeneration. The type I MSC results in the activation of M-1 macrophages and T-cells, which among other things contributes to autoimmune diseases. In regenerative medicine, we are more interested in the type II MSC. As can be seen, regenerative medicine is intimately tied in to the immune system. They can profoundly affect each other. It is imperative to understand their symbiosis.

MSCs Sources

MSCs are found in many different tissue types. From a clinical point of view, there are two main sources of these cells. They are found in the bone marrow aspirate, but typically as the age of the patient increases, the number of MSCs diminishes in the bone marrow. When we start out as a newborn, one out of every 10,000 cells in our marrow is an MSC; by the time we reach age 80, one out of every two million cells is an MSC. Herein lies the problem; as we age, do we have enough MSCs from the bone marrow alone? No one knows the answer to this question. I feel that the MSCs from the marrow need to be supplemented. One very good solution to this problem is the use of adipose tissue. Adipose tissue is a rich source of MSCs [15]. The supply stays relatively constant and does not vary much with age. Adipose tissue is rich in many different cell types, MSCs being one of them. A potential problem with the MSCs in adipose is to release them. Free fat grafts work well as a supply of MSCs and Muse cells. However, when we want to increase the number of stem cells per volume, then it will be necessary to break down the adipose tissue to release the MSCs. The method of harvesting the cells is a simple liposuction technique similar to that employed by a plastic surgeon. When doing the liposuction, it is performed with tumescent fluid consisting of a mixture of 30 CCs of 2% lidocaine and one ampule of epinephrine in 500 CCs of normal saline. Typically, the harvesting is performed from the abdominal region around the waist line, where the cell concentration is greatest. One caveat to keep in mind, not all fat is the same. There are more cells for CC in a lean person when compared to an obese person. Also, the cell profile in a lean person is different from that of an obese person. The lean person will have a cell profile which is more conducive to regeneration. The lean person will have more regenerative cells. The profile can be changed somewhat when pretreating the patient with certain cytokine growth factors.

There are many methods of breaking down the adipose tissue into its component parts. These methods involve both enzymatic breakdown of the fat. There are machines which utilize mechanical methods of breaking down the adipose tissue to its component parts. The automated machines are fairly expensive as are the processing kits that come with them. For most people in the field, a more cost-effective choice involves a simple kit, which includes either collagenase or lecithin. This is a step-by-step process that is easily reproducible and produces a fairly reliable SVF product. The automated kits offer a timesaving but a great cost of money.

The product produced when fat is broken down is called stromal vascular fraction (SVF) [16]. One of the main components of the SVF is the mesenchymal stem cells. There are a number of other cell types in the SVF. Some of these cells include adipocytes and attached progenitor cells, Treg cells and macrophages, endothelial cells, and fibroblasts. The hemopoietic stem cells appear to be short lived and not as effective as those in the bone marrow. Are there any drawbacks to SVF? As was stated earlier in the chapter, one needs to check the regulatory issues in the country they are practicing as it pertains to the legality of SVF. From a scientific point of view, there are some concerns when using SVF. The question is when creating SVF if we are throwing away some important cells such as Muse cells. Furthermore, the structural niche of the adipose tissue might be damaged, which dramatically reduces the viability of the cells [16]. Nevertheless, SVF is a good choice in the treatment of joint afflictions in the field of regenerative medicine. Typically, when SVF is employed, it is given as both an intra-articular injection and intravenously. Some studies indicate that the cells get trapped in the lungs when given intravenously. This may very well be the case, but they will nevertheless release their growth factors having a systemic effect on the body. There now seems to be an explanation for the long-term effects of stem cells yet their short survivability. It is felt that monocytes phagocytize MSCs and ultimately produce Treg cells, which have rather long-lasting effects [17]. Is adipose tissue alone the best treatment for a joint? There is no clear-cut answer, and this I suspect will continue to be an ongoing controversy. My opinion is to use both adipose tissue and marrow aspirate. We like a free fat graft in most of our initial procedures. The amount of graft used depends on the joint size. It can be from 4 to 8 CCs of free fat graft. Also, the use of a free fat graft seems to potentiate the effect of the SVF.

Hematopoietic Stem Cells

MSCs are very important in the field of regenerative medicine. They are the ultimate immune modulators and at the same time cause some trophic regeneration of tissue. They are the body's Navy Seals. However, the cells which truly drive regeneration are the hematopoietic stem cells (HSCs). By far, the largest concentration of HSCs in the body is found in the bone marrow. The primary engine of new bone and cartilage formation in vivo is through the recruitment and differentiation of cells classically defined as hematopoietic in origin.

Numerous scientific articles have pointed out that the HSCs are the true drivers of regeneration [18]. The classical marker of human HSC is CD34. HSCs are thought to possess a good deal of plasticity. Plasticity refers to the capacity of cells (stem or differentiated) to adopt the biological properties (gene expression profile, phenotype, etc.) of other differentiated types of cells (that may belong to the same or different lineages). If MSCs are considered Navy Seals, then HSCs can be considered the regular army. Although HSCs are found in many different tissues, they are found in the biggest concentration in the bone marrow. When we are discussing bone marrow, the best source is in the region of the posterior superior spine near the S.I. joint. It is not recommended to obtain marrow aspirate from a long bone due to the diminished numbers of stem cells.

Techniques for Obtaining HSCs From Bone Marrow

Bone marrow should be harvested from the posterior ilium. Bone marrow aspiration is very technique driven. Drs. Muschler and Hernigou have given us some excellent techniques when drawing bone marrow aspirate [19]. Dr. Hernigou et al. concluded that the optimal syringe size was 10 mL combined with a rapid pull of the plunger optimizing the negative pressure [20]. This may cause more pain, but cell numbers will be much higher! Dr. Muschler has shown that the best aspirations result when there is not a large aspirate from one area. It is the recommendation of the author that bone marrow aspirations be performed with multiple 10 CC syringes. In each syringe, harvest approximately 3–4 CCs of marrow aspirate (each syringe should have approximately 1 CC of heparin). At the same time, each aspiration must be performed from a different geographic area. Initially, a few years ago, all bone marrow aspirates underwent centrifugation. The reason for this was that the bone marrow aspirate was taken for one geographic area, resulting in whole blood "contamination". Many physicians would aspirate 60 CCs for one location. This was an easy technique, but it typically results in low numbers of regenerative cells. It did result in a large amount of whole blood being aspirated. In order to get rid of the whole blood, it was necessary to perform centrifugation. This is a very simplistic approach. There may now be some better alternatives.

Centrifugation does concentrate the various stem cells found in the marrow, giving us higher numbers on a CC per CC basis. For years, this was considered the gold standard of bone marrow aspiration. Now some changes are in the wind. There are now a number of physicians who are recommending a non-centrifuged bone marrow aspirate. There are some important concepts that non-centrifuged marrow brings forth. One question to ask is what cells are discarded when marrow aspirate is centrifuged. An excellent paper by Bhartiya et al. [21] discussed the fact that among other cells, the V cells seem to be discarded with centrifugation. Further evaluation of centrifugation shows both good and bad aspects. Some aspects attributed to centrifugation include the fact that it can change the shape of the cells and interfere with their secretory pattern. The stress of centrifugation can increase growth factor release. Centrifugation can decrease the "respiratory burst" from neutrophils diminishing oxygen availability to cells diminishing cell viability. Decreased "respiratory burst" may point macrophages more towards an M-1 inflammatory macrophage. Thus, we see both the good and bad of centrifugation. A hybrid product may provide the best of both worlds. You make sure that you have the pluripotent cells and non-disturbed cells from the initial non-centrifuged marrow aspirate. Centrifuge another portion of marrow aspirate to increase the cell numbers of multipotent cells and growth factor release. This is the perfect marriage of multipotent and pluripotent cells. It straddles both schools of thought. We call this the Hybrid Purebred™ technique.

We must remember that bone marrow aspirate is much more than just HSCs. There are a whole plethora of different cell types, including MSCs,

RBCs, WBCs, platelets, V cells, and many other different cell types. One fact to keep in mind is that typically bone marrow aspirate is much richer in cytokine growth factors than a PRP. For example, there is approximately 23 times more interleukin 1 antagonist in bone marrow aspirate versus PRP [22]. This is one of the reasons bone marrow always tromps PRP as a better alternative. However, sometimes bone marrow aspirate may be an overkill for a minor problem.

I typically use a Jamshidi needle for bone marrow harvesting. We will harvest from several different depths and different locals. Only local anaesthesia (10 CCs lidocaine) is used on the periosteum. Also, avoid a drill which will burn the bone. A hammer works much better and gives the operator more control. Another pearl to pass along. Depending upon the joint, we will utilize approximately 12 CCs of uncentrifuged marrow and 30 CCs of marrow aspirate to produce 5CCs of concentrated marrow aspirate. If you have a patient who is a difficult blood draw, then you can obtain the blood from the bone marrow stick after harvesting the marrow aspirate. Just aspirate from one area.

What Cell Combinations Seem to Work Best for the Joint?

When we are dealing with a degenerative arthritis of a joint, a protocol that has worked well for us involves bone marrow, PRP, and a free fat graft. At the initial procedure, we are utilizing all of these components. The amount of material injected depends upon the joint. For a knee, there is typically no problem with the amount of material injected. This may include 8 CCs of a PRP product, 6–8 CCs of a free fat graft, and 10–17 CCs of a combination bone marrow product (both centrifuged and non-centrifuged). For a hip or ankle, the amounts will be less typically about one half the amount put into the knee. For shoulders, the amounts injected would be similar to the knee. If one wants the best possible combination of cells, then I would add SVF. I have done these combinations many times at my clinics outside the United States. Depending upon the amount of SVF produced, some would be injected into the joint, while the rest would be given intravenously. We must remember that bone marrow supplies large numbers of HSCs while fat, especially SVF, supplies large numbers of MSCs. This is the combination we strive for. Once the initial injections are performed, we will usually have the patient get three additional PRP injections spaced about 1 month apart. We also utilize growth factor patches on every patient. Many of the patients are also utilizing oral cytokine formulas.

Avascular Necrosis and Ligamentous Problems

We will mention these problems in passing. In avascular necrosis (AVN), there is a problem with the circulation in a portion of the bone of the joint. The causes are varied in nature. We have had good success in treating these problems similarly to an osteoarthritis of the joint. There is some new research that suggests injecting the affected bone directly with the cell combination. Time will tell if this is a better treatment method of this problem. Most extra-articular ligamentous problems can usually be handled with a PRP injection, possibly enhanced with a free fat graft. When one is dealing with an injury to a ligament that is intra-articular such as an ACL injury, then there appears to be better results utilizing the same method as an osteoarthritis. In another words, a combination of bone marrow, PRP, and fat would be utilized while at the same time utilizing some type of imaging.

Why Does There Seem to Be Differences in Success Between Different Joints?

Many experienced regenerative medicine physicians will mention the fact that there is a difference in success between different joints in the body. For instance, knees and ankles seem to be more successful than hips when discussing treatment outcomes. What is the reason for this? There was recently an article published [23], which gives a good explanation on the reason for the discrepancy. Apparently, we can generate new proteins in joint cartilage, and this ability is more pronounced in joints farther from the centre of the body, such as the ankles, than in those nearer, such as the hips. The researchers found that the prevalence of younger proteins was tied to the abundance of a microRNA that blocks the action of a messenger RNA that inhibits the production of new collagen proteins. This may be an explanation as to why typically there is more success in ankle and knee treatments than in hips.

What Else Is Used to the Stem Cell Procedures for Better Efficiency?

There is quite a bit of interest in products that are derived from cord blood, amniotic, and placenta tissue. These products have many desirable components, including, in some cases, actual stem cells. However, for instance, in the United States, these products contain growth factors but typically not stem cells that are metabolically active. Having metabolically active stem cells is not allowed under current FDA guidelines. Nevertheless, these products have their place as an adjunct when using autogenous stem cells especially in an older patient. One needs to keep aware of the shifting rules of various regulatory bodies concerning these products.

Extracorporeal Shock Wave Therapy (ESWT)

ESWT is a high-power sound wave that causes mechanical stimulation of cells, resulting in increased expression of cytokines and growth factors [24]. ESWT applied to an area of chronic inflammation may enable acute inflammatory mediators to be released, facilitating an appropriate progression of healing. It will allow stem cells to hom to the area. There are other physiological changes, including changes to the cell membrane and its permeability, release of neurotransmitters, and antibacterial effects. ESWT also includes induction of vessel growth, stem cell migration, and differentiation. Finally, ESWT therapy includes release of NO (nitric oxide) and various other growth factors. Extracorporeal shock waves significantly promoted the proliferation and self-renewal of MSCs in vitro and accelerated the cartilage repair process in vivo, indicating favourable clinical outcomes. The scientific studies indicated that there was an increase in mitochondria size and activity in the stem cells. There are various EWST machines on the market. We consider them a valuable adjunct in our treatment protocols.

Hyperbaric Oxygen Therapy

A number of studies suggest that hyperbaric oxygen will mobilize stem cells in the body, making them available for repair. A study by S. Thom et al. (Univ of Penn) showed that hyperbaric oxygen will cause rapid mobilization of stem/progenitor cells in humans [25]. The mobilization is thought to be caused by a nitric oxide (NO)-dependent mechanism [25]. Stem cell activation occurs via release of stem cell active cytokine C-kit ligand (SCF). Over a course of 20 treatments, the marrow stem cell output increased eightfold. It is this increase in stem cells that seems to be responsible for the clinical results obtained from hyperbaric oxygen. The practical drawbacks with hyperbaric oxygen are that it is expensive and time-consuming. What we have used as a substitute is a nitric oxide generator.

As we age, we find that the amounts of NO in our bodies diminishes. Most of the time, instead of hyperbaric oxygen, we will utilize a NO generator to hopefully increase the levels. We have found that an excellent source of NO is a product called Neo-40. Neo-40 is a product that was developed by the Univ. of Texas. It is taken orally and produced from a beet derivative. We will typically have the patients take two to three tablets a day. There is one very important fact to remember. NO actions depend upon the neighbourhood it is found in. In some circumstances, it can act as an inflammatory agent and not contribute towards regeneration. These actions are dependent on which enzyme produces NO. This enzyme is called nitric oxide synthase. There are three forms of synthase called inducible, neuronal, and endothelial. Inducible is actually inflammatory, and the NO it produces works to destroy bacteria and others; unfortunately, it will also destroy cells as a collateral damage. The endothelial is the one which affects the bone marrow and will have a direct effect on the release of stem cells from the bone marrow. Also, it helps to increase circulation. As one reads the literature, one will discover that NO is a very important signalling molecule. It can have very profound effects on the body.

Photoactivation of PRP and Stem Cells

Photoactivation is thought to act at least in part by modulating the pro- and anti-inflammatory properties of leucocytes. However, it appears to have effects on all cells [23]. Photo biomodulation (PBM), also known as low level light therapy, is the use of red, near-infrared, and other colours of light to stimulate healing, relieve pain, and reduce inflammation [26]. The primary chromophores have been identified as cytochrome c oxidase in mitochondria and calcium ion channels (possibly mediated by light absorption by opsins). Secondary effects of photon absorption include increases in ATP, a brief burst of reactive oxygen species, an increase in nitric oxide, and modulation of calcium levels. Tertiary effects include activation of a wide range of transcription factors leading to improved cell survival, increased proliferation and migration, and new protein synthesis [24]. In my experience, I have utilized the AdiLight for many years with excellent success. The AdiLight works on a few different levels. When white blood cells (WBC) from the peripheral blood are photoactivated under AdiLight for 10 minutes, pro-inflammatory cytokines (IL1, IL2, IL6, and TNF alpha) are inhibited and anti-inflammatory cytokines (IL1Ra and IL10) are induced as well as the observation of beta endorphin release. This is a highly desired response when pathophysiological conditions, resulting from chronic inflammation states and irritation, are considered. When adipose and bone marrow-derived stem cells are extracted from an individual, the cells are in a semi-dormant state, due to lack of physiological activation. In the body, stem cells and progenitor cells are activated by a detailed and complex physiological cascade repair system. This involves the release of growth factors and chemokines from platelets. Moreover, when the adipose-derived or bone marrow stem cells are photoactivated for 20 minutes with the AdiLight device, they show increased release of signalling factors, such as integrins, vascular endothelial growth factor, thymosin beta 4, and interleukin 1 receptor antagonist.

When we are discussing photo modulation, we would be amiss if we did not discuss low-level light therapy (LLLT), more commonly known as laser therapy. Molecular and cellular mechanisms of LLLT are becoming better understood. Mitochondria are principal photoreceptors, while ATP, cAMP, NO, and ROS are primary mediators. Certain transcription factors, such as NF-kB, AP-1, etc., are activated. Transcription factors are proteins involved in the process of converting or transcribing DNA into RNA; they help turn genes on and off at the right time. Laser therapy is pro-survival, antiapoptotic, anti-inflammatory, pro-angiogenic, and pro-proliferation. Whatever cells are designed to do will be improved by LLLT. Cells with lots of mitochondria respond well to LLLT [27]. Also, pain relief is significant and inflammation is reduced.

Prolotherapy

The author of this chapter does not have first-hand knowledge of the use of prolotherapy in treating joint problems. Prolotherapy is a procedure where a natural irritant is injected into the soft tissue of an injured joint. The irritant kick-starts the body's healing response. The irritant used can include high-concentration dextrose. Some of the newer thinking now is that a PRP is a prolotherapy treatment. Prolotherapy works by causing a temporary, low-grade inflammation at the injection site, activating fibroblasts to the area, which, in turn, synthesize precursors to produce mature collagen and thus reinforce connective tissue. This is essentially the mechanism of action of PRP, etc. Many prolotherapists recommend injection's both intra-articular and extra-articular.

Ozone Therapy

Ozone therapy pulls from a few different fields. It is postulated that ozone has analgesic, anti-inflammatory, immunomodulatory, and trophic properties Typically, ozone (O3) is injected into the joint. The cost of a medical grade ozone generator is 500 dollars and up. A series of injections are given usually about once a week for about 6 or 7 weeks. The injection will consist of 10–20 CCs of ozone injected into the joint. Some physicians recommend the additional injections of some homeopathic compounds called Traumeel and Zeel. The concentration of ozone is variable according to various studies. We have used a concentration of 10–40 μg/ml. Some recommendations are to start with a lower dose and then give higher doses. Ozone has a number of effects on the joint, including PGE2 inhibition, NO synthesis, inhibition of pro-inflammatory cytokines (IL-1, TNF, IFN), stimulation of anti-inflammatory cytokines (IL-4, IL-10, IL-13), and growth factors, such as TGF beta and IGF-1. There seems to be some promise to ozone therapy, and further clinical trials are underway. It seems to be a good adjunct in regenerative therapies. One other important aspect of ozone therapy is the ability it has on affecting the NAD/NADH ratio, which is so important in the production of cellular energy in the form of ATP.

Allogenic Cell Products

Most of the cell products, we are utilizing come from the patient himself. However, there are a number of products that are allogenic in that they come from another person. One must be aware of the regulations of the country in which they are practicing. For instance, in the United States, there is much interest in various products from placenta, cord blood, and amniotic tissue. Typically, these products are registered with the US FDA as a 361-tissue product. A 361-tissue product contains tissue but does not contain live cells that have a metabolic purpose. The tissue is rich in a variety of growth factors, etc. However, if these products contain live cells with a metabolic profile, then they become a 351 with the FDA, which requires an Investigational New Drug (IND) application, clinical testing, and several years of analysis. The bottom line is that these products essentially only contain growth factors and not live active cells. They can be used as an adjunct to PRP and other procedures. If indeed there are live cells in these products, then this is probably a violation of FDA regulations. However, this is beyond the scope of this chapter. One other word of caution, many of these products are said to be immune privileged. This is probably not an accurate statement. A better term to describe these cells is to say that they are "immune evasive". This means that the immune system of the body will ultimately attack these cells. There is always a possibility that these cells can cause an immune response, especially if given intravenously.

Cytokine Therapy

Cytokines are proteins that are secreted by a wide variety of cells. They have a specific effect on the interactions of the cells. Cytokines are various growth factors that act as signalling molecules telling cells what to do. Cytokines can be compared to the body's cell phone system. This is how cells communicate with each other. These forms of communication are called the "crines" of communication. One type of communication is autocrine, in which the cell acts upon itself. Another type is juxtacrine, in which the cell requires close contact with a neighbouring cell. The third type of communication is paracrine, in which one cell targets a neighbouring cell. Lastly, the final form of cellular communication is endocrine. This is where one cell will communicate with a distant cell. There are many different subclasses of cytokines. Most all problems in medicine are a result of an imbalance of cytokines. Many conditions have either too much or too little of certain cytokines. We must realize that the different cells we inject into a patient typically do not survive very long in a hostile area such as the joint. Their important mission is to release various growth factors, which cause a variety of reactions such as stem cell homing to the area and telling various cells what to do. The stem cells found in the body are what ultimately achieve repair.

When we are discussing cytokines, it boils down to about six major cytokines. There are three master inflammatory cytokines and three master anti-inflammatory cytokines. The master inflammatory cytokines are IL-1, TNF, and IL-6. These cytokines typically cause most of the symptoms associated with the symptoms of degenerative arthritis of the joint. The master anti-inflammatory cytokines are IL-1 antagonist, IL-10, and IGF-1. The anti-inflammatory cytokines are found in PRP and bone marrow aspirate in varying concentrations. We have found that as we age, the concentrations of different anti-inflammatory cytokines diminish. We have used supplemental cytokines for a number of years with good clinical success. We have used these cytokines in various methods. Currently, we utilize a formula consisting of a blend of various cytokines that are mixed with penetrating molecules. They are placed on a Tegaderm patch, and the growth factors penetrate down into the joint. They should be commercially ready for sale towards the last quarter of 2018. We have also found that an oral cytokine mixture that is absorbed sublingually also seems to benefit the patients. There are two sources of these oral cytokines. They are Guna from Italy and Viatrexx from Canada. There are a number of combinations which seem to work well. A word of caution is to probably avoid the oral growth factors on patients who have a history of a cancer other than the common skin cancers.

Perhaps, the newest and most exciting aspect of cytokine therapy is from a company in Switzerland called Contrad. They have designed a GMP FDA registered growth factors transdermal patches. The technology is called SIGMOLECS. SIGMOLECS molecules induce signals to key amino acid sensors that govern gene expression of amino acid metabolism that then trigger specific physiological and metabolic activity. These SIGMOLECS molecules are structured according to these key amino acid sensors to trigger specific regenerative tasks.

Stem Cell Ageing Pathways May Be the Key to Regenerative Success

There is an old adage, namely, how stem cells age is how we age. There are a number of different pathways; however, we will address the major pathways. Perhaps one of the most important pathways concerns what are called the sirtuins. There are seven major sirtuin proteins. Sirtuins are a family of proteins that regulate cellular health. Sirtuins play a key role in regulating cellular homeostasis. Homeostasis involves keeping the cell in balance. The sirtuins have critical importance in the health of the mitochondria and subsequent production of ATP. Stem cells produce energy by glycolysis, which has low energy demands; however, when stem cells begin differentiating, then more ATP is needed and energy production switches to oxidative phosphorylation. NAD and its substrates are of critical importance of proper functioning of the sirtuins.

Another very important pathway is called the AMPK pathway. AMPK stands for adenosine monophosphate-activated protein kinase. One of the central regulators of cellular and organismal metabolism in eukaryotes is AMP-activated protein kinase (AMPK), which is activated when intracellular ATP production decreases. AMPK has critical roles in regulating growth and reprogramming metabolism. AMPK acts as a master switch to regulate cell functions, such as uptake of glucose, burning of fats, and formation of new mitochondria. If the AMPK pathway is under control, then there is a better chance of regenerative medicine success. Some compounds that will stimulate this pathway include metformin and a supplement called berberine.

The FOXO family of forkhead transcription factors plays an important role in longevity and tumour suppression, by upregulating target genes involved in stress resistance, metabolism, cell cycle arrest, and apoptosis.

FOXO proteins activate genes that maintain healthy joints and bone structure. People with osteoarthritis have significantly lower FOXO proteins. FOXO transcription factors modulate autophagy, which promotes cellular turnover, and maintenance FOXO factors are important for stem cell production and DNA repair. FOXO1 and FOXO3 promote mitophagy, which is mitochondrial autophagy. FOXO proteins suppress tumorigenesis in cancer. FOXO factors increase the antioxidant capacity of cells, and reactive oxygen species and oxidative stress activate FOXO pathway to adapt to the stress. Inactivity of FOXO factors accelerates atherosclerosis and compromises stem cell proliferation. FOXO proteins inhibit adipogenesis or the differentiation of adipocytes. Thus, they promote fat burning and prevent fat gain. FOXO3 activity protects against Parkinson's disease and promotes neuronal survival. FOXO transcription factors play an important role in determining ageing and longevity.

The Nrf2 pathway has been referred to as the "master regulator of antioxidant, detoxification and cell defense gene expression". The Nrf2 pathway modulates numerous genes responsible for inflammatory response, rebuilding tissue, immune system response, inhibiting cancer production, and preventing its spread, cognitive processes. It regulates production of crucial antioxidants, such as glutathione and superoxide dismutase, or SOD.

One must remember that there are other important pathways that can have a direct effect on stem cells and their environment.

Senescent Cells

One topic that is often overlooked is that of senescent cells. Although senescent cells can no longer replicate, they remain metabolically active and commonly adopt an immunogenic phenotype, consisting of a pro-inflammatory secretome (cytokines). These cells are capable of doing damage on a molecular level. They will accumulate growth factors, proteases, and inflammatory factors that disrupt normal tissue function. Senescent cells have long been implicated in ageing and decreased success in stem cell procedures. There now exist agents to eliminate these cells. These agents are called senolytic agents. There is now much research into senolytic agents, which will destroy senescent cells in the hope of reversing osteoarthritis. Typically, people accumulate significant senescent cell burdens around age 60. It seems that the use of senolytic agents may become the standard treatment as time goes on. There are a number of supplements such as quercetin, fisetin, and black tea. We have had fairly good use with the senolytic agents in our office.

Supplements to Increase Success

Supplements have a place in the field of regenerative medicine. We have utilized a number of supplements. To go to the specifics of each supplement is beyond the scope of this chapter. I will touch upon a few of the important ones. I am very high on a product called Neo-40. This is a supplement that is taken orally. It seems to increase the amount of nitric oxide (NO) in the body. Hopefully, this in turn will have a similar effect as hyperbaric oxygen. We know that hyperbaric oxygen works on a principle of increasing NO, which will increase stem cell output. Another product high on the list is UltraCur. This is a product which utilizes a very potent form of curcumin. It is potent in that it has much higher bioavailability than the typical curcumin product. This will hopefully reduce inflammation in the extracellular matrix. It seems to help block interleukin 1 actions. The third product is called StemXCell. This product seems to increase stem cell output from the bone marrow. Tests in the lab show it to be similar to GCSF. The last product we use is called CH-Alpha. This appears to be a product that has a number of clinical studies, which show that it appears to be a good source of collagen to help accomplish repair. Of course, a good multivitamin and hormonal balance also is needed for higher success.

Citations

1. Sophia Fox AJ, Bedi A, Rodeo SA. The basic science of articular cartilage. Sports Health. 2009;1(6):461–8.
2. Akkiraju H, Nohe A. Role of chondrocytes in cartilage formation, progression of osteoarthritis and cartilage regeneration. J Dev Biol. 2015;3(4):177–92. Epub 2015 Dec 18.
3. Bafico A, Aaronson SA. Classification of growth factors and their receptors. In Holland-Frei cancer medicine. 6th edition. B C Decker: Hamilton; 2003.
4. Cole BJ, Seroyer ST, Filardo G, Bajaj S, Fortier LA. Platelet-rich plasma: where are we now and where are we going? Sports Health. 2010;2(3):203–10.
5. Litwiniuk M, Krejner A. Hyaluronic acid in inflammation and tissue regeneration. Wounds. 2016;28(3):78–88.
6. Lana JFSD, Purita J. Contributions for classification of platelet rich plasma – proposal of a new classification: MARSPILL. Regen Med. 2017;12(5):565–74.
7. Parrish WR, Roides B, Hwang J, Mafilios M, Story B, Bhattacharyya S. Normal platelet function in platelet concentrates requires non-platelet cells: a comparative in vitro evaluation of leucocyte-rich (type 1a) and leucocyte-poor (type 3b) platelet concentrates. BMJ Open Sport Exerc Med. 2016;2(1):e000071. collection 2016.
8. Parrish W, et al. Physiology of blood components in wound healing: an appreciation of cellular cooperativity in platelet rich plasma action. J Exerc Sports Orthop. 2017;4(2):1–14.
9. Morgan MC, Rashid RM. The effects of phototherapy on neutrophils. Int Immunopharmacol. 2009;9(4):383–.
10. Martinez FO, Gordon S. The M1 and M2 paradigm of macrophage activation: time for reassessment. F1000Prime Rep. 2014;6:13. https://doi.org/10.12703/P6-13. E Collection 2014.
11. Etulian J, et al. An optimized protocol for platelet-rich plasma preparation to improve its angiogenic and regenerative properties. Sci Rep. 2018;8:Article number: 1513.
12. Chacón-Martínez CA, Koester J, Wickström SA. Signaling in the stem cell niche: regulating cell fate, function and plasticity. Development. 2018;145:dev165399. https://doi.org/10.1242/dev.165399. Published 1 August 2018.
13. Sampson ER, Hilton MJ, Tian Y, Chen D, Schwarz EM, Mooney RA, Bukata SV, O'Keefe RJ, Awad H, Puzas JE, Rosier RN, Zuscik MJ. Teriparatide as a chondro regenerative therapy for injury-induced osteoarthritis. Sci Transl Med. 2011;3(101):101ra93. https://doi.org/10.1126/scitranslmed.3002214.
14. Kaplan A. Mesenchymal stem cells: time to change the name! Stem Cells Transl Med. 2017;6(6):1445–51.
15. Krasnodembskaya A, Song Y, Fang X, Gupta N, Serikov V, Lee J-W, Matthay MA. Antibacterial effect of human mesenchymal stem cells is mediated in part from secretion of the antimicrobial peptide LL-37. Stem Cells. 2010;28(12):2229–38. https://doi.org/10.1002/stem.544.
16. Alexander RW. Understanding adipose-derived stromal vascular fraction (AD-SVF) cell biology and use on the basis of cellular, chemical, structural and paracrine components: a concise review. J Prolother. 2012;855–69
17. de Witte S. Immunomodulation by therapeutic mesenchymal stromal cells (MSC) is triggered through phagocytosis of MSC by monocytic cells. Stem Cells. 2018;36(4):602–15.
18. Grcevic, et al. In vivo mapping identifies mesenchymal progenitor cells. Stem Cells. 2012;30:187–96.
19. Muschler G, et al. Aspiration to obtain osteoblast progenitor cells from human bone marrow: the influence of aspiration volume. J Bone Joint Surg. 1997;79-A(11):1699–709, Cleveland Clinic.
20. Hernigou P, et al. Benefits of small volume and small syringe for bone marrow aspirations of mesenchymal stem cells. Int Orthop. 2013;37(11):2279–87.
21. Bhartiya D, Shaikh A, Nagvenkar P, Kasiviswanathan S, Pethe P, Pawani H, Mohanty S, Rao SG, Zaveri K, Hinduja I. Very small embryonic-like stem cells with maximum regenerative potential get discarded during cord blood banking and bone marrow processing for autologous stem cell therapy. Stem Cell Dev. 2012;21(1):1–6.
22. Cassano JM, Kennedy JG, Ross KA, Fraser E, Goodale MB, Fortier LA. Bone marrow concentrate and platelet-rich plasma differ in cell distribution and interleukin 1 receptor antagonist protein concentration. Knee Surg Sports Traumatol Arthrosc. 2018;26(1):333–42.
23. Hsueh M-F, Önnerfjord P, Bolognesi MP, Easley ME, Kraus VB. Analysis of "old" proteins unmasks dynamic gradient of cartilage turnover in human limbs. Sci Adv. 2019;5(10):eaax3203. https://doi.org/10.1126/sciadv.aax3203.
24. Zhang L, Fu XB, Chen S, Zhao ZB, Schmitz C, Weng CS. Efficacy and safety of extracorporeal shock wave therapy for acute and chronic soft tissue wounds: a systematic review and meta-analysis. Int Wound J. 2018;15(4):590–9. https://doi.org/10.1111/iwj.12902. Epub 2018 Apr 19
25. Thom SR. Hyperbaric oxygen – its mechanisms and efficiency. Plast Reconstr Surg. 2011;127:131s–41s.
26. Giannelli M, Chellini F, Sassoli C, Francini F. Photoactivation of bone marrow mesenchymal stromal cells with diode laser: effects and mechanisms of action. J Cell Physiol. 2013;228(1):172–81.
27. Michael R. Hamblin. Photo biomodulation or low-level laser therapy. J Biophotonics. 2016;9(11–12):1122–4.

Suggested Reading

Alexander RW. Understanding adipose-derived stromal vascular fraction (AD-SVF) cell biology and use on the basis of cellular, chemical, structural and paracrine components: a concise review. J Prolother. 2012;4

Bhartiya D, et al. Very small embryonic-like stem cells with maximum regenerative potential get discarded during cord blood banking and bone marrow processing for autologous stem cell therapy. Stem Cells Dev. 2012;21(1):1–6.

Caplan AI. Mesenchymal stem cells: time to change the name! Stem Cells Transl Med. 2017;6:1445–51.

Domen J, Wagers A, Weissman I. Bone marrow (Hematopoietic) stem cells. N.I.H. Stem Cell Information; n.d.

Hernigou P, et al. Benefits of small volume and small syringe for bone marrow aspirations of mesenchymal stem cells. Int Orthop. 2013;37(11):2279–87.

Parrish WR, Roides B. Platelet rich plasma: more than a growth factor therapy. Musculoskelet Regen. 2017;3:e1518.

Parrish W, et al. Physiology of blood components in wound healing: an appreciation of cellular co-operativity in platelet rich plasma action. J Exerc Sports Orthop. 2017;4(2):1–14.

Ratajczak MZ, et al. Very small embryonic/epiblast-like stem cells (VSELs) and their potential role in aging and organ rejuvenation--an update and comparison primitive small stem cells isolated from adult tissues. Aging (Albany NY). 2012;4(4):235–46.

Thom SR. Hyperbaric oxygen – its mechanisms and efficacy. Plast Reconstr Surg. 2011;127:131s–41s.

Zhang H, et al. Radial shockwave treatment promotes human mesenchymal stem cell self-renewal and enhances cartilage healing. Stem Cell Res Ther. 2018;9:54.

Part II

Diagnostic and Interventional MSK Ultrasound

Image Optimization

4

Franklin San Pedro Domingo

Desiderius Erasmus once said that, "in the kingdom of the blind, the one-eyed man is king". And, in the world of ultrasound, the transducer is the one eye that has to be optimized.

How an Ultrasound Image Is Generated

Physics defines sound as a form of mechanical energy transmitted by pressure waves in a material medium. Humans are capable of hearing sound in the frequency of 20–20,000 Hz. Ultrasound is anything above the range of the capability of human beings to hear sound. This is above the range of 20,000 Hz [1]. Diagnostic ultrasound is usually in the range of 3–17 MHz, which is well above the upper limit of hearing [2]. Novel systems using ultrahigh-frequency ultrasound use frequencies up to 70 MHz. This may allow better assessment of ultrastructural changes of very superficial peripheral nerves and other thin structures, such as pulleys, retinacula, and tendons [3].

The Piezoelectric Effect

Most ultrasound probes are fitted with piezoelectric crystals. And when electrical energy is applied to these crystals, it induces the crystals to vibrate, producing sound waves that are transmitted to the tissues under the ultrasound probe. Some of these sound waves are reflected back into the probe. The piezoelectric crystals can be said to be listening to these returning sound waves. These echoes that are going back to the probe then cause the crystals to vibrate. These vibrations are then converted back into electrical energy [4]. These electrical signals are then processed by the ultrasound machine and are displayed as dots or pixels on the screen. The stronger the returning echo received, the brighter the dot on the screen. Many ultrasound machines make use of 256 shades of grey to allow for good resolution on the generated image [5]. The process of sending, receiving and processing sound waves happens numerous times in just 1 second. There are newer systems that replace the piezoelectric crystal with a silicon chip. In development are submicrometre silicon-on-insulator resonator for ultrasound detection with the potential for imaging at a resolution comparable to that achieved with optical microscopy [6].

F. S. P. Domingo (✉)
Department of Physical Medicine & Rehabilitation, Center for Regenerative Medicine, Pain Management Service, Makati Medical Center, Makati City, Philippines

Y. El Miedany (ed.), *Musculoskeletal Ultrasound-Guided Regenerative Medicine*,
https://doi.org/10.1007/978-3-030-98256-0_4

Transducers

There are different kinds of transducers. And, they are described in the way that the transducer crystals are arranged in the head of the probe. The two most common types of transducers are the linear and the curvilinear (Fig. 4.1). The linear array is arranged in a straight line of crystals, giving it the ability to focus on the area directly below it. The image generated by this probe is rectangular or trapezoidal [7]. The thickness or slice of the ultrasound beam generated is very thin. This means that the needle has to be within this thin area when doing an ultrasound-guided procedure with the orientation of the needle being parallel to the probe. A curvilinear array is arranged in an arc. This generates a fanlike image on the screen. This gives it the advantage of having a wider field of view.

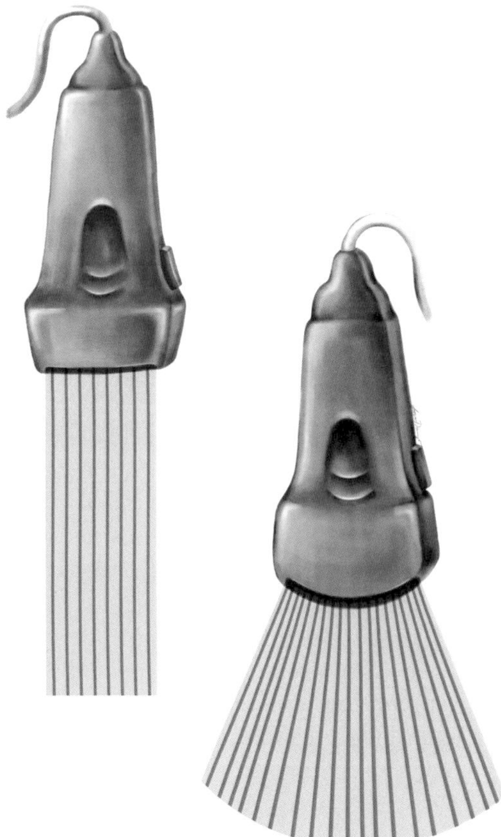

Fig. 4.1 A linear array on the left, generating a rectangular scan field. And, a curvilinear array on the right, generating an arc shaped scan field. (Illustration credits to Anna Melissa Domingo)

The Effect of Frequency, Gain and Focus on the Character of the Ultrasound Image

Frequency

The ultrasound machine has the capability to alter its transmitted frequency. The higher the frequency, the better the resolution. This comes at the expense of having less penetration. This is because higher frequencies are more attenuated or absorbed as they go thru tissue. These frequency settings can be used for targeted structures that are shallow. Lower frequency settings give the advantage of better penetration. This allows for the appreciation of deeper structures. However, this comes at the price of a poorer resolution [8]. Lower frequencies are best used for targeted structures that are deeper such as the hip.

Depth

Adjusting depth allows for the optimization of the size of the target tissue relative to the image seen on the monitor of the ultrasound machine [2] (Fig. 4.2). A good guide would be to keep the

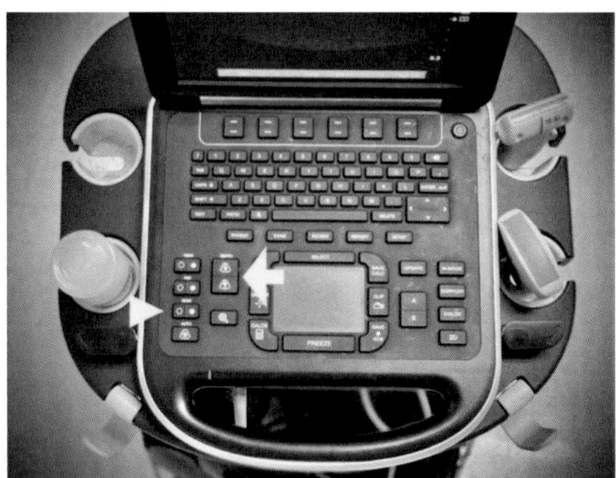

Fig. 4.2 Depth setting on arrow. And, gain setting on arrowhead. (Photo credits to Maria Olivia Domingo)

area of interest in the middle third of the screen by adjusting the depth accordingly. A too shallow depth setting may prevent the visualization of deeper relevant structures. And a too deep setting may take up the majority of the size of the screen. This leads to a smaller area on the screen to visualize the target structure.

When blood vessels or lung tissue are very close to the target area, proper depth adjustment is necessary. Satisfactory visualization of the said structures during the preliminary scan is needed to improve patient safety. There is usually a numerical guide on one side of the screen that can be used to approximate the depth of the target. This is also needed in planning the angle of approach and the length of the needle to be used during a procedure.

Gain

The gain setting enables the ultrasound machine to listen harder for the returning echo sent by the piezoelectric crystal. And the higher the gain, the more it can listen to the returning echoes. This would then lead to a brighter image on the screen. Gain setting can be calibrated for the far field, near field or the whole field. There can be problems with too much or too little gain. Too much gain can give a very bright washed-out appearance. And too little gain may give a very dark image. Too much or too little gain would prevent the appreciation of important surrounding structures. The proper adjustment for gain will not be evident until the probe is applied on the skin [2].

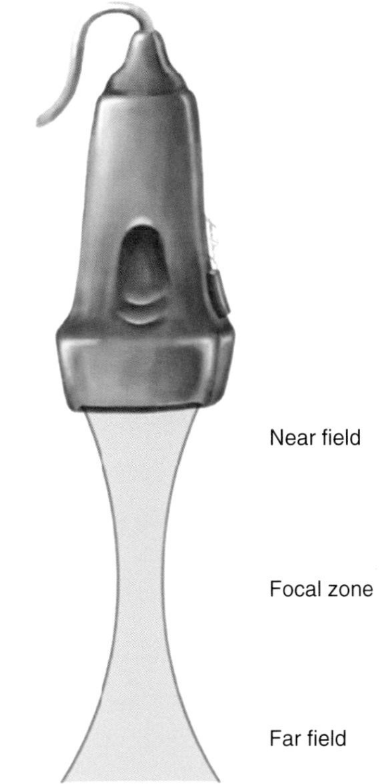

Fig. 4.3 Focus of an ultrasound beam. (Illustration credits to Anna Melissa Domingo)

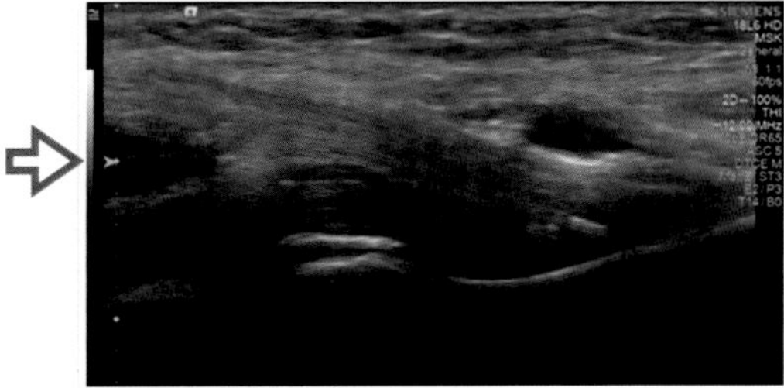

Fig. 4.4 An ultrasound scan of the distal biceps tendon. The open arrow is showing the focus indicator on the monitor. Note that the area of interest is at the middle third of the screen

Focal Zone

Proper adjustment of the beam focus is necessary for image clarity. The right focal zone setting allows for the improvement of the lateral resolution at the area of interest (Fig. 4.3). Lateral resolution refers to the ability of the transducer to discriminate between two objects positioned side by side. This is achieved by adjusting the depth at which the ultrasound beam is at its narrowest and most dense. Some machines do this automatically by assuming that the area of interest is at the middle third of the screen. Other ultrasound machines allow for the adjustment of the focal zone independent of the depth [2] (Fig. 4.4).

Doppler and Its Utility in Identifying Vascular Structures

The use of the Doppler function is important in identifying vascular flow. Proper identification of these structures will help to avoid inadvertently puncturing them during a procedure. Doppler can also be useful in helping to distinguish between nerves and vessels. Arteries can be distinguished by their more pulsatile flow and non-compressible nature [9].

Orientation Marker

Every transducer has a marker or notch on one side (Fig. 4.5). This enables the user to orient the probe properly in relation to what is being scanned under the probe. This is important in doing ultrasound-guided procedures in order to be able to determine on what side of the monitor the incoming needle will be displayed. On most machines, the orientation marker usually corresponds to the left side of the screen.

Some ultrasound probes have markers on their broader side that correspond to the middle or centreline of the screen. These machines may also have an option that allows the display to have a guideline running down the centre of the screen. This guides the interventionist when doing an out-of-plane injection.

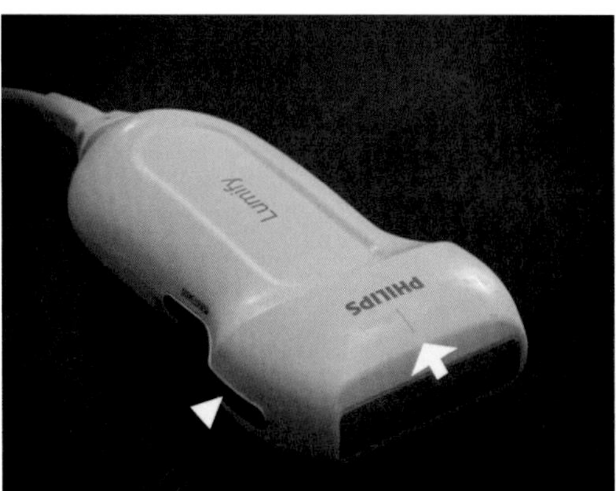

Fig. 4.5 Probe orientation marker on the arrowhead. Centreline indicator on the broader side of the transducer on the arrow. (Photo credits to Jose Franco Domingo, Sofia Victoria Domingo)

Techniques to Improve Needle Visualization

Probe Manipulation

The ultrasound probe allows for the visualization of the target structure in two dimensions. And, proper manipulation of the transducer can facilitate the formation of a mental picture of the scanned area in three dimensions.

Correct transducer handling allows for the proper acquisition of the target structure on the screen. The American Institute of Ultrasound in Medicine has defined these five transducer planes of manipulation [10]:

- Sliding glides the probe along the short or long axis of the structure (Figs. 4.6 and 4.7). This is done without rocking or tilting the probe.
- Rocking the probe refers to doing a heel-toe manoeuvre (Fig. 4.8). This can be used to

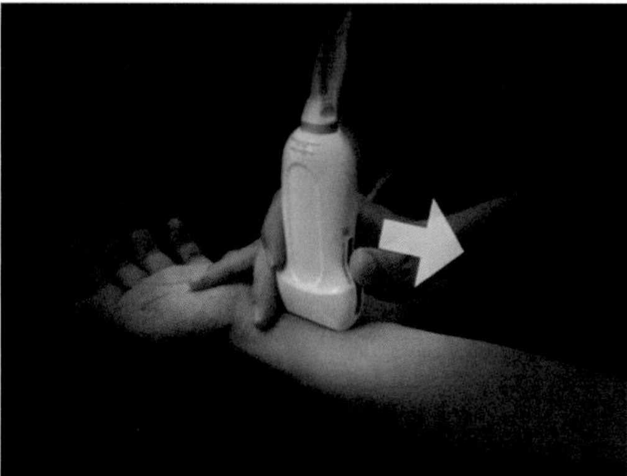

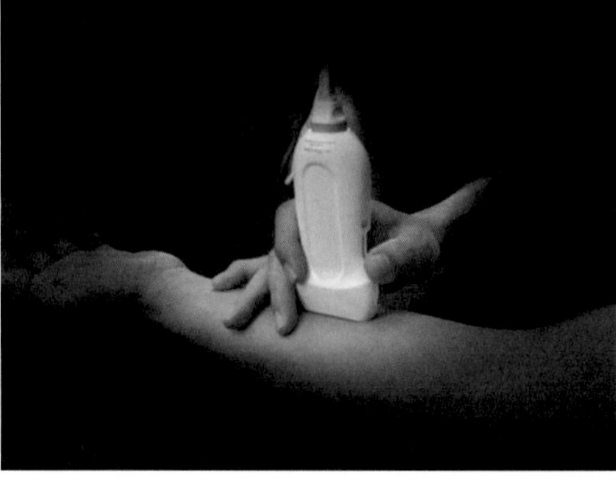

Fig. 4.6 Long-axis linear slide. (Photo credits to Maria Olivia Domingo, Jose Franco Domingo and Sofia Victoria Domingo)

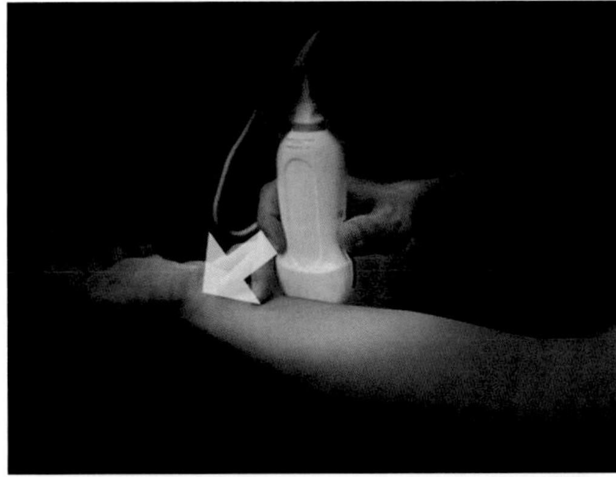

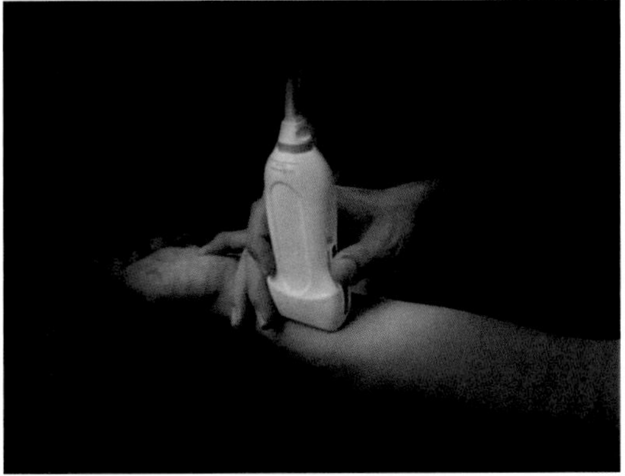

Fig. 4.7 Short-axis linear slide. (Photo credits to Maria Olivia Domingo, Jose Franco Domingo and Sofia Victoria Domingo)

decrease anisotropy when scanning in the long axis. This can also be used to improve the field of view. This manoeuvre can be done to facilitate better visualization of the needle during the injection of deeper structures. This can be done by doing a heel-toe manoeuvre to angle the transducer to be more parallel in relation to the needle in long axis. If one side of the probe loses contact with the skin during this manoeuvre, more gel can be added to the area. This is sometimes called a gel standoff technique.

- Tilting, wagging or toggling the probe can be done by doing a side-to-side motion (Fig. 4.9). This is done without moving the base or sliding. This changes the angle of incidence of the sound waves on the tissue.
- Rotating the transducer turns the probe in a clockwise or counterclockwise manner (Fig. 4.10). During an intervention, this manoeuvre helps in the visualization of the needle tip on its way to the target area.

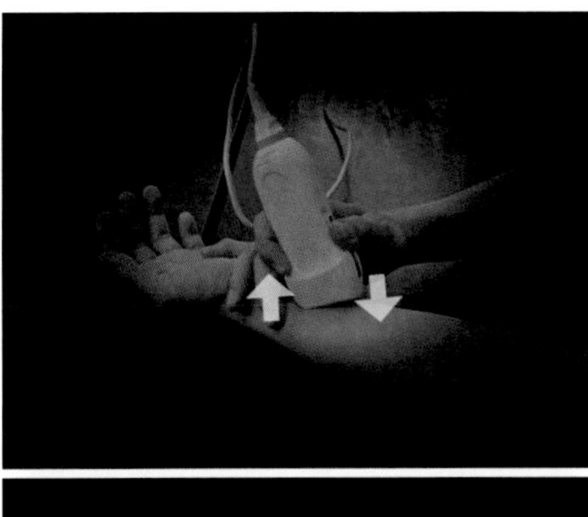

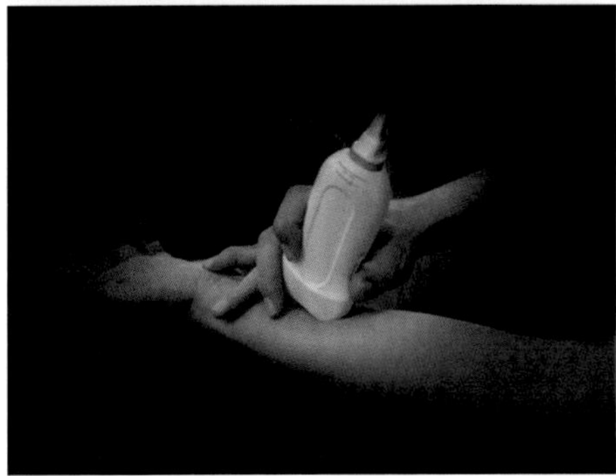

Fig. 4.8 Heel-toe manoeuvre. (Photo credits to Maria Olivia Domingo, Jose Franco Domingo and Sofia Victoria Domingo)

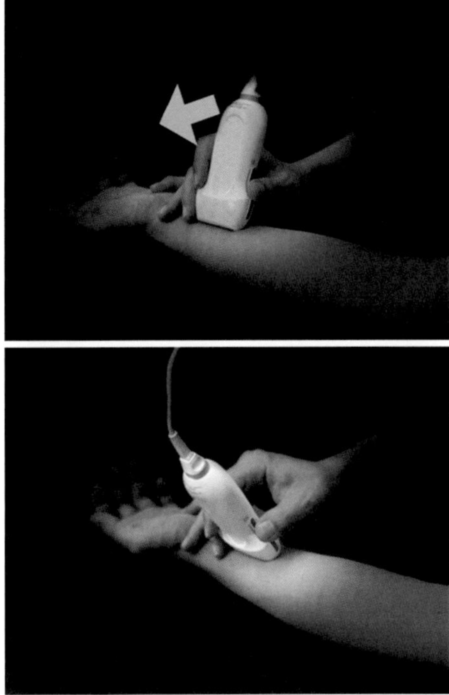

Fig. 4.9 Tilting the transducer. (Photo credits to Maria Olivia Domingo, Jose Franco Domingo and Sofia Victoria Domingo)

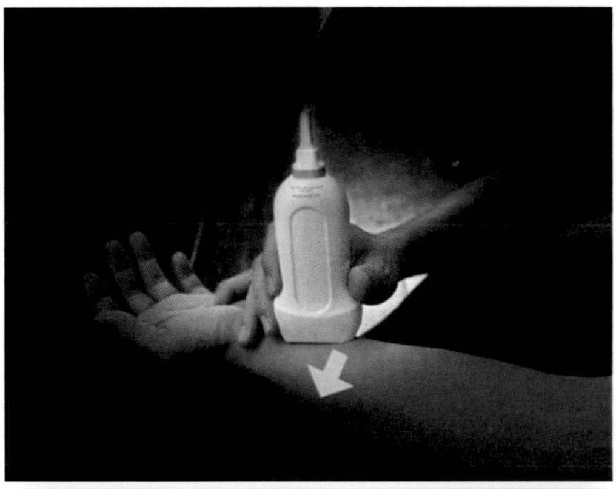

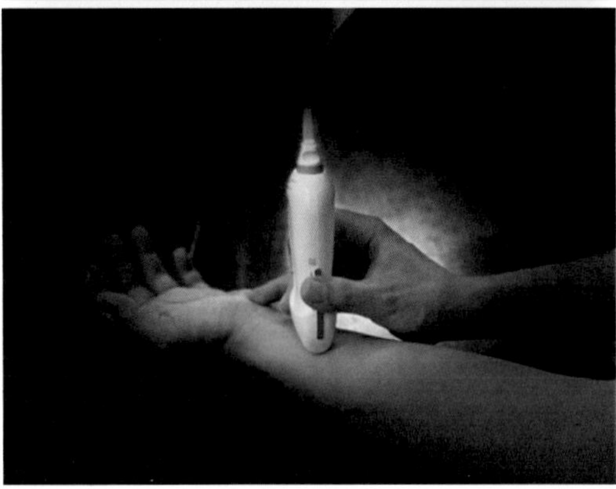

Fig. 4.10 Rotating the transducer. (Photo credits to Maria Olivia Domingo, Jose Franco Domingo and Sofia Victoria Domingo)

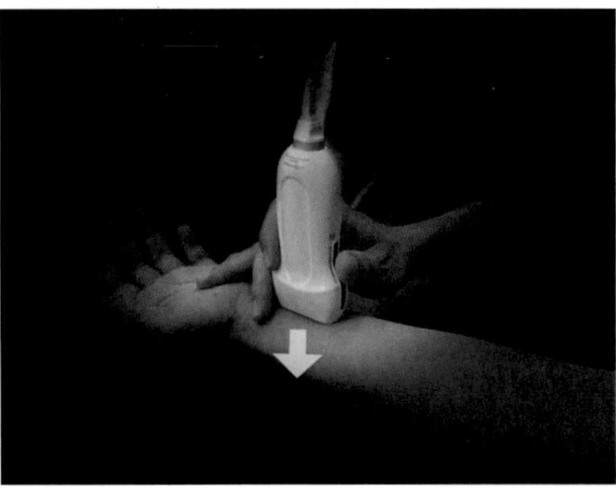

Fig. 4.11 Compression manoeuvre. (Photo credits to Maria Olivia Domingo, Jose Franco Domingo and Sofia Victoria Domingo)

- Compression involves pressing down on the transducer (Fig. 4.11). Too much compression may cause veins to collapse and cause subcutaneous tissue to appear thinner. This manoeuvre may be used for the visualization of deeper structures.

Ergonomics

Proper positioning of the patient and interventionist can be critical to the success of the procedure. Not only does this improves patient comfort and safety, but it also reduces the incidence of developing a repetitive stress injury [1].

Clinical Pearls

- Do an initial scan to survey the area and to confirm the diagnosis while looking out for structures to avoid.
- Visualize the target structure in three dimensions based on the two-dimensional ultrasound images.
- Plan for a shallow angle of approach to maximize needle visibility if feasible.
- Consider using the curvilinear probe for deeper structures.
- Practice good ergonomics to improve hand-eye coordination and needle to beam alignment.
- Apply a relaxed and even grip on the transducer while holding it at the base using the first three digits of the hand (Fig. 4.12).
- Stabilize the transducer by anchoring the fourth and fifth digit along with the heel of the palm on the patient.
- Do not add more than necessary compression on the patient's body with the transducer.

For beginners, it is best to start with an easy procedure they are comfortable with. The patient should be lying between the interventionist and the monitor. Position the patient in order for the physician to be able to align his eye with the nee-

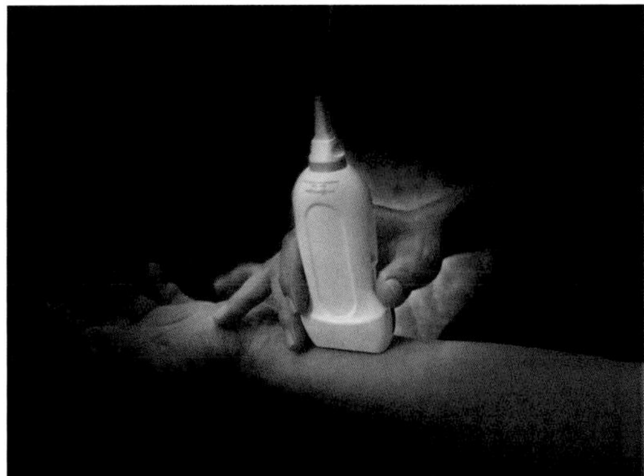

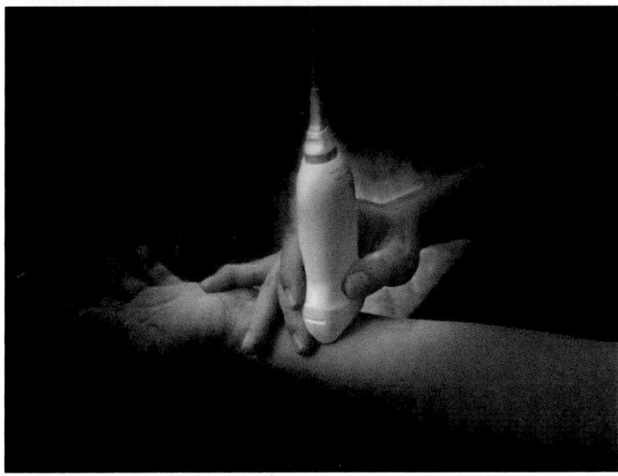

Fig. 4.12 How to hold the probe properly. (Photo credits to Maria Olivia Domingo, Jose Franco Domingo and Sofia Victoria Domingo)

dle, the transducer and the monitor all in one line of sight (Fig. 4.13). It is preferable for the patient to be in a supine or prone position to prevent a vasovagal reaction.

In summary, preparation is crucial to performing ultrasound-guided interventional procedures. It starts with a good knowledge of anatomy combined with a firm grasp on how to best optimize the imaging of the targeted structure. The fusion of image optimization, proper needle visualization, correct ergonomics and adequate preprocedural planning is needed to be able to guide the needle to the right place at the right time (Figs. 4.14 and 4.15)

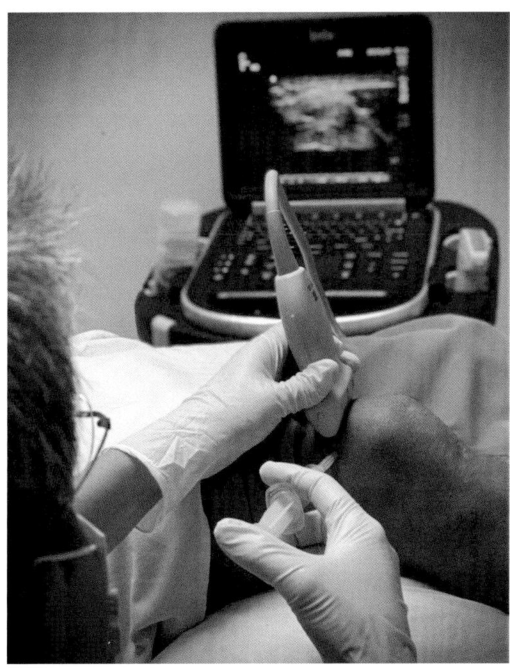

Fig. 4.13 Proper positioning of the patient allowing for a single line of sight from the interventionist, to the needle, the probe and the monitor. Note that the physician is comfortably seated with the right forearm resting on the bed for support. The linear probe can be seen to have the orientation marker that is used as a visual reference to improve the alignment of the slice of the ultrasound beam relative to the needle. (Photo credits to Michael Francis Obispo)

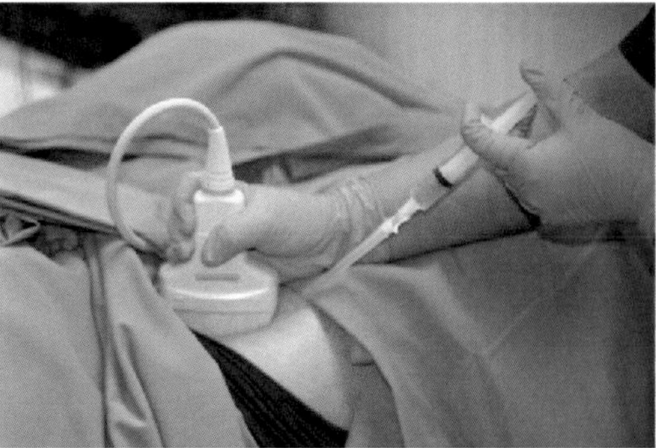

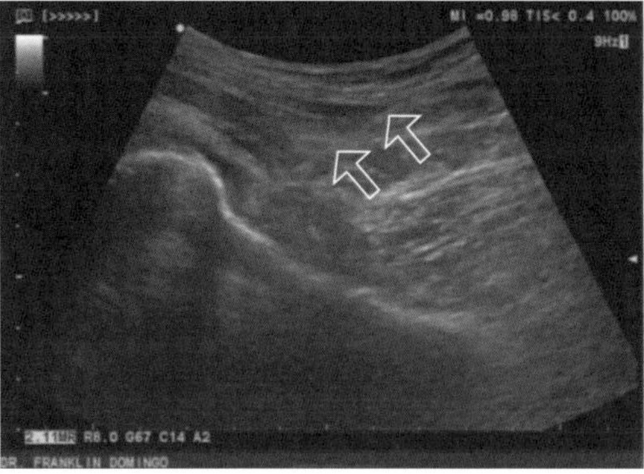

Fig. 4.14 In-plane approach for a hip procedure. The open arrows are pointing to the needle. The use of a curvilinear transducer allows for better needle visualization. A needle with a larger bore size is also easier to visualize. (Photo credits to Maria Olivia Domingo)

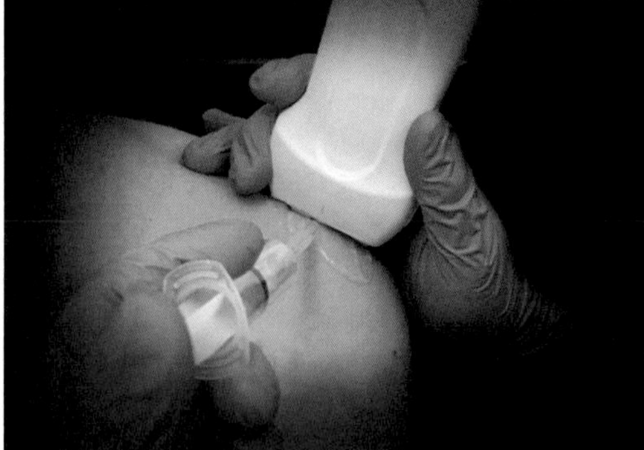

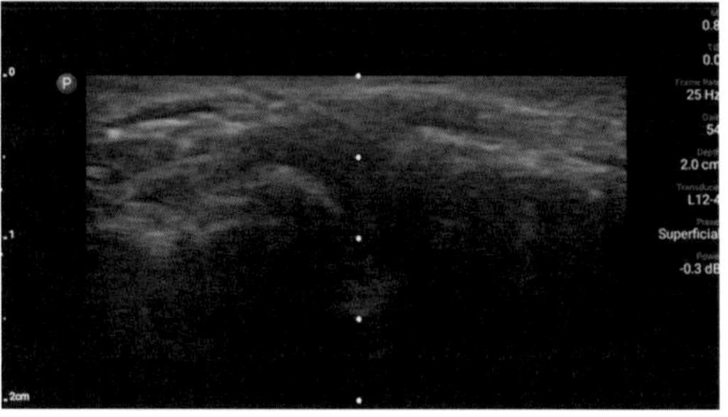

Fig. 4.15 Out-of-plane approach for an acromioclavicular joint injection. Note the centreline dots at the middle of the screen. This corresponds to the trajectory of the needle using the walk down technique. To do this technique, the needle is initially inserted superficially. Then, when the needle tip becomes visible, the needle is withdrawn and inserted at a deeper trajectory. This is done repeatedly at a steeper angle until the target is acquired. Note that in the picture, the non-dominant left hand is used to hold the needle. Practicing with the non-dominant hand can be helpful for more advanced procedures that require more dexterity. In addition, the depth of the target structure can be measured using the guide on the left side of the monitor to plan the pathway of the needle to the target. (Photo credits to Maria Olivia Domingo)

Clinical Pearls

- When injecting, hand movements should be very minimal, smooth and gradual.
- Use mainly the short axis linear slide manoeuvre to guide the needle. And, only use the tilt manoeuvre when necessary.
- Move only the probe or the needle. Do not move both at the same time.
- Ensure that what is being visualized primarily is the needle tip and not what looks like a partially visible short-appearing shaft.
- Do not move the needle if it is not visible.
- Keep the bevel of the needle facing up to allow for better visibility.
- To improve needle tip visibility, use a very minimal in and out or jiggling manoeuvre. A minimal side-to-side lateral movement can also be used.
- A small amount of saline solution can also be injected to confirm needle tip position.

Acknowledgements Photo credits to Maria Olivia Domingo, Jose Franco Domingo, Sofia Victoria Domingo and Michael Francis Obispo.

Illustration credits to Anna Melissa Domingo.

References

1. Strakowski JA. Introduction to musculoskeletal ultrasound: getting started. New York: Demos Medical Publishing; 2016.
2. Smith J, Finnoff JT. Diagnostic and interventional musculoskeletal ultrasound: part 1. Fundamentals. PM R. 2009;1(1):64–75.
3. Albano D, Aringhieri G, Messina C, De Flaviis L, Sconfienza LM. High-frequency and ultra-high frequency ultrasound: musculoskeletal imaging up to 70 MHz. Semin Musculoskelet Radiol. 2020;24(2):125–34.
4. Schwantes J, Byerly DW. Biceps Tendon Sheath Injection. 2021 Aug 15. In: StatPearls [internet]. Treasure Island: StatPearls Publishing; 2021.
5. Bruno MA. 256 Shades of gray: uncertainty and diagnostic error in radiology. Diagnosi. 2017;4(3):149–57.
6. Shnaiderman R, Wissmeyer G, Ülgen O, Mustafa Q, Chmyrov A, Ntziachristos V. A submicrometre silicon-on-insulator resonator for ultrasound detection. Nature. 2020;585(7825):372–8.
7. Bianchi S, Martinoli C. Ultrasound of the musculoskeletal system. Berlin: Springer; 2007. p. 12.
8. Bowness J, Taylor A. Ultrasound-guided regional Anaesthesia: Visualising the nerve and needle. Exp Med Biol. 2020;1235:21.
9. Smith J, Finnoff JT. Diagnostic and interventional musculoskeletal ultrasound: part 2. Clinical applications. PM R. 2009;1(2):162–77.
10. AIUM technical bulletin. Transducer manipulation. American Institute of Ultrasound in Medicine. J Ultrasound Med. 1999;18(2):169–75.

Shoulder

5

Daniel R. Lueders, Alexander R. Lloyd, and Allison N. Schroeder

Long Head of the Biceps Brachii

Anatomy and Ultrasound Evaluation

The biceps brachii has two heads – short and long – which act together to flex the shoulder and elbow and assist with forearm supination. The long head of the biceps brachii (LHBB) originates on the supraglenoid tubercle, rim of the glenoid, superior glenoid, and the joint capsule. The short head of the biceps brachii (SHBB) originates at the coracoid process of the scapula. These heads merge at the level of the pectoralis major and insert on the radial tubercle and as the lacertus fibrosus onto the deep fascia of the forearm. The LHBB follows a curvilinear course from its origin and passes through the rotator interval formed by the superior border subscapularis inferiorly, anterior border of the supraspinatus superiorly, and the base of the coracoid process medially. The coracohumeral ligament and the glenohumeral ligament also overlie the LHBB within this interval and restrain medial movement. The LHBB is encased in a synovial sheath that communicates with the glenohumeral joint.

D. R. Lueders (✉) · A. N. Schroeder
University of Pittsburgh Medical Center, Pittsburgh, PA, USA
e-mail: luedersdr2@upmc.edu; aschroe1@alumni.nd.edu

A. R. Lloyd
University of Pittsburgh Medical Center, Department of PM&R, Pittsburgh, PA, USA

For ultrasound evaluation of the LHBB, the patient should rest their arm adducted to the side and in neutral to slight external rotation. This brings the tendon anteriorly and allows the sonographer to trace the biceps tendon from its distal point at the pectoralis major to its proximal portion within the rotator interval. Failing to do this and leaving the patient internally rotated can hinder initial localization of the tendon and can prevent comfortable positioning of the probe to allow for optimal visualization of the tendon. The LHBB is generally superficial even in obese patients, making a high-frequency linear probe the best choice for exam. Decreasing both depth and focal zone to evaluate the proximal position of the tendon can improve visualization. The probe should be carefully adjusted to achieve a perpendicular view of the tendon and to eliminate artifact from anisotropy. This may be challenging, given the curvilinear path of the tendon, and requires constant reorientation of the probe. Maintaining a discrete visualization of the cortex of the humerus as a well-defined, hyperechoic structure underlying the biceps tendon indicates the probe is perpendicular to the contour of the bone and can assist with proper probe alignment.

The scan begins with the transducer in the transverse plane on the anterior aspect of the proximal shoulder. The LHBB tendon is identified in short axis within the bicipital groove of the humerus. (Fig. 5.1) The tendon should be scanned

Y. El Miedany (ed.), *Musculoskeletal Ultrasound-Guided Regenerative Medicine*, https://doi.org/10.1007/978-3-030-98256-0_5

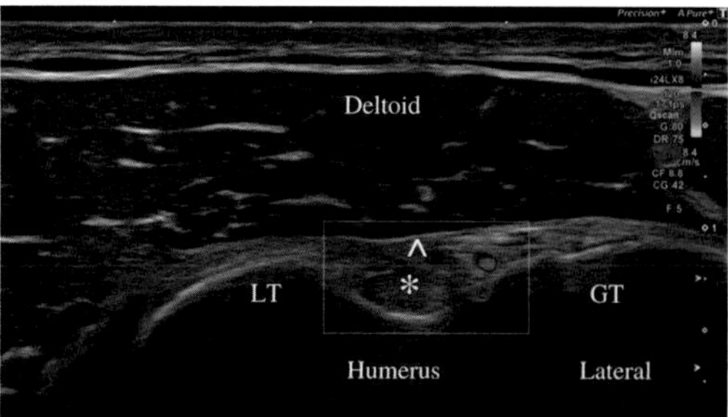

Fig. 5.1 Transverse view of the biceps brachii long head tendon in the intertubercular groove, or biceps tunnel. The biceps tendon (*) is seen as a dense, homogenous hyperechoic ovoid structure sitting between the humeral lesser tuberosity (LT) and greater tuberosity (GT). The hyperechoic fibrillar-appearing transverse humeral ligament (^) sits superficial to the biceps long head tendon and secures it within the biceps tunnel superior to the epiphyseal line

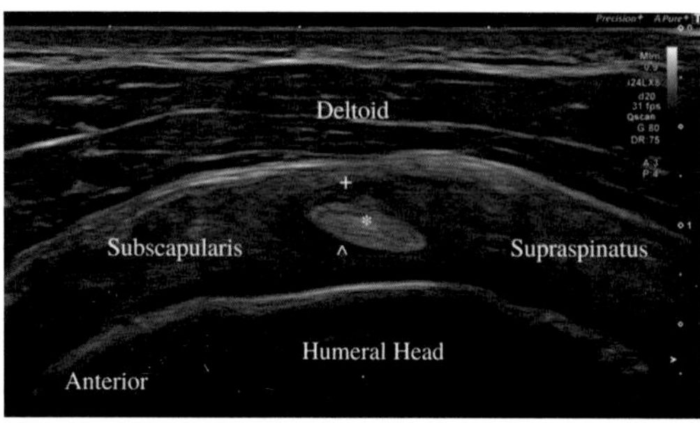

Fig. 5.2 Transverse view of the biceps brachii long head tendon at the rotator interval. The biceps tendon (star) is seen as a dense, homogenous hyperechoic ovoid structure sitting on the humeral head and deep to deltoid. The anterior, or leading edge, of supraspinatus forms the posterior margin of the rotator interval, while the cephalad-most fibers of subscapularis form the anterior margin of the rotator interval. The superficial rotator interval is comprised of the coracohumeral ligament (+), and the deep rotator interval is bordered by the superior glenohumeral ligament (^)

proximally through the rotator interval as this is a common site of pathology. (Fig. 5.2) The LHBB tendon has an oval shape proximal to the bicipital groove and migrates medially toward the glenoid at this point. This should not be confused for tendon subluxation. The tendon generally cannot be followed all the way to its origin on the supraglenoid tubercle because of the overlying bony anatomy. Some fibers may be seen blending with the surrounding tissues at this level as they move to their origin on the capsule and labrum.

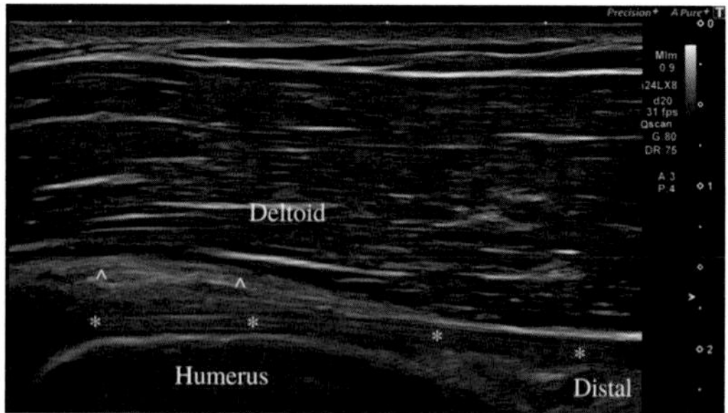

Fig. 5.3 Longitudinal view of the biceps brachii long head tendon in the intertubercular groove, or biceps tunnel. The biceps (*) courses adjacent to the humerus at the biceps tunnel, and the transverse humeral ligament (^) can be seen superficial to the tendon securing it in place

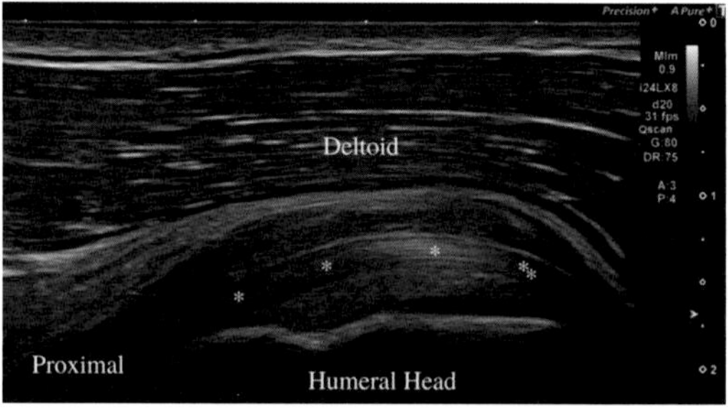

Fig. 5.4 Longitudinal view of the biceps brachii long head tendon (*) adjacent to the humeral head and deep to deltoid

The tendon should then be followed inferiorly to the level of its myotendinous junction just caudad from the traversing pectoralis major tendon, which is visualized emerging in long axis medial to the biceps long head tendon and subsequently traversing superficial to biceps tendon to insert on the lateral aspect of the humerus. Doppler evaluation should also be performed to identify an ascending branch of the anterior circumflex artery, which courses lateral to the LHBB tendon in the bicipital groove. Also of note, the transverse humeral ligament overlies the bicipital groove and appears as a thin, hyperechoic band superficial to LHBB tendon. The tendon should then be evaluated in a long axis view (Fig. 5.3). Maintaining this view over the entire course of the tendon can be challenging, particularly as the tendon curves into the rotator interval (Fig. 5.4). Increased pressure on the distal end of the transducer may assist with bringing the tendon paral-

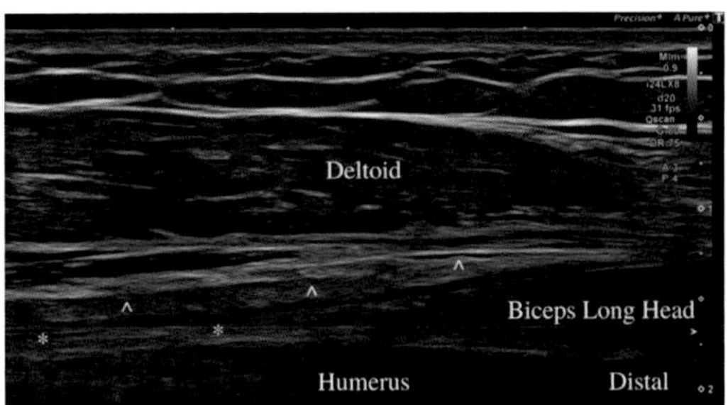

Fig. 5.5 Longitudinal view of the biceps brachii long head tendon (*) at its myotendinous junction distally. The broad, flat tendon of pectoralis major (^) is visualized superficial to the biceps tendon just proximal from the biceps myotendinous junction

lel to the plane of the transducer. The tendon should again be scanned from proximal to distal to evaluate for pathology at the myotendinous junction (Fig. 5.5).

Pathology

LHBB tendon pathology is seen most commonly within the first 3.5 cm from the tendon origin and within, or close to, the rotator interval [1]. Chronic degenerative injury to the LHBB may result in tendinosis. This phenomenon represents the noninflammatory mucoid degeneration and chondroid metaplasia of chronically injured tendons [2]. Tendinosis manifests as hypoechoic defects with changes to the fibrillar architecture of the tendon that give it an ill-defined heterogenous appearance [3]. Concomitant thickening of the tendon and Doppler flow may also be seen in the abnormal areas [3].

Anechoic clefts or irregularities in the superficial contour of the biceps tendon may indicate partial-thickness tearing [4]. Full-thickness tearing results in the complete absence tendon in the bicipital groove due to its retraction distally into the arm. The full extent of the bicipital groove should be evaluated distally to locate the retracted stump of the tendon. Of note, the collapsed bicipital tendon sheath may appear as a hyperechoic fascial structure within the bicipital groove and should not be mistaken for the biceps tendon [5]. Reactive effusion and debris can also fill the vacancy of the ruptured tendon and mimic an abnormal tendon [6].

The tendon sheath of the LHBB usually contains minimal to no fluid. However, because of the tendon sheath that communicates with the glenohumeral joint space, a glenohumeral joint effusion greater than 5 mL can result in peritendinous extravasation of the effusion down the tendon sheath to the level of the bicipital groove [7]. As a result, effusion within the LHBB sheath may indicate both LHBB tendon and glenohumeral joint pathology. Fluid resulting from glenohumeral effusion is usually evenly distributed circumferentially around and along the LHBB tendon and is not focally tender. This is in comparison to focal tenosynovitis, which is often painful with sonopalpation and demonstrates focal fluid deposition. Areas of tenosynovitis may also demonstrate hyperemia that can be seen with Doppler imaging. The presence of the anterior circumflex artery lateral to the tendon should not be confused with hyperemia. Fluid in the tendon sheath may finally be associated with rotator cuff tear. This is particularly the case when an effusion of the subacromial/subdeltoid bursa is also present [7, 8].

Subluxation or dislocation of the LHBB tendon occurs in the medial direction and generally results from disruption of the coracohumeral ligament. Suspicion for subluxation or complete dislocation of the tendon should arise when the tendon is not seen in the bicipital groove. During subluxation, the tendon can be observed subluxating medially out of the bicipital groove with external rotation and relocating back into the bicipital groove with internal rotation. When dislocation has occurred, the tendon has permanently migrated medially and may be difficult to visualize. LHBB subluxation or dislocation should not be confused with a complete tear of the tendon, which may similarly show an empty bicipital groove. To differentiate between the two, examiners must scan distally to visualize the most proximal portion of the tendon that can be visualized. This should then be followed more proximally. An abnormal tendon course that courses medial to the humerus indicates subluxation or dislocation, while discontinuity indicates rupture of the tendon.

While LHBB tendon pathology may be focal and isolated, it can be an indicator of glenohumeral joint or rotator cuff pathology [7–9]. Even damage to the LHBB tendon itself may reflect abnormal biomechanics within the shoulder triggered by pathology elsewhere in the rotator cuff [9].

Interventional Procedures

Limited evidence exists for dedicated regenerative procedures performed at the LHBB tendon. Prolotherapy protocols involving injection of the proximal biceps tendon almost always do so as part of a larger protocol for rotator cuff disease with multiple other tendons injected [10, 11]. It's difficult to make definitive conclusions as a result, because improvements in pain or function may have been related to effects at other locations. No studies have been performed with prolotherapy on isolated biceps tendon pathology.

With reference to PRP, a single pilot study evaluated the effect of PRP injections to the LHBB tendon in eight spinal cord injured patients with good overall outcomes [12]. Beyond this, no data was found about PRP injections for isolated proximal biceps tendon pathology. As previously mentioned, the biceps tendon may be affected by significant pathology of the supraspinatus and subscapularis tendons through disruption of the rotator interval and rotator pulley that may lead to tendon dysfunction [13]. Additionally, there is likely some bursal communication between the subacromial-subdeltoid bursa and the biceps tendon sheath when significant rotator cuff tearing is present [7]. However, use based on this evidence is largely speculative.

No systematic studies have been performed examining the effects of mesenchymal stem cells or hyaluronic acid on the biceps tendon.

Injection Approach #1

- Patient positioning – Supine.
- Transducer selection – High-frequency linear array transducer (>10MHz)
- Transducer position – Short axis to the long head of the biceps tendon at the intertubercular groove
- Needle selection – 25–27-gauge 1.5–2.5-inch needle, depending on body habitus
- Injectate selection – Anesthetize with local anesthetic. Inject with 5mL or less of volume including steroid, prolotherapy, or orthobiologic therapy. Volumes of 5mL or more commonly enter the glenohumeral joint and may be used for adhesive capsulitis [7].
- Needle trajectory and target – In-plane, lateral to medial, target is just superficial to the tendon within the sheath to ensure the safety of the ascending artery from the anterior humoral circumflex artery.
- Accuracy – Ultrasound-guided injections of the biceps tendon sheath are significantly more accurate than palpation-guided injections. Many practitioners struggle to accurately identify the correct location of the biceps tendon with palpation, leading to frequent needle placement error [14]. Recent comparative studies have found ultrasound-guided injections to be between 85% and 100% accurate with superior effectiveness [15–17]. Palpation-guided injections range in accuracy from 26% to 68% (Hashiuchi et al. [16]; Yiannakopoulos et al. [17]).
- Pearls/Pitfalls
  - The lesser tuberosity can be used as a backstop for the needle trajectory to facilitate proper placement
  - Injectate should flow easily and disseminate within the tendon sheath. Focal collection of the fluid indicates the needle is either outside of the sheath or within the tendon.
  - The anterior circumflex humeral artery, which typically lies lateral to the tendon, should always be visualized with Doppler prior to the injection and avoided during the procedure.

Injection approach #2

- Patient positioning – Supine
- Transducer selection – High-frequency linear array transducer (>10MHz)
- Transducer position – Long axis to the long head of the biceps tendon at the intertubercular groove

- Needle selection – 25–2-gauge 1.5–2.5-inch needle depending on body habitus
- Injectate selection – Same as above
- Needle trajectory and target – In-plane, inferior to superior, target is just superficial to the tendon within the sheath
- Accuracy – As above
- Pearls/Pitfalls
  - This approach provides another option in the event that approach #1 is not possible.
  - While this approach allows for a longer tendon target, it lacks simultaneous visualization of the anterior circumflex humeral artery and lacks a bony backstop if the injector misjudges the needle depth.

Supraspinatus Tendon

Anatomy and Ultrasound Evaluation

The supraspinatus tendon originates from the supraspinous fossa of the scapula. It courses superolaterally to pass under the acromion and over the superior aspect of the glenohumeral joint before inserting on the middle and superior facet of the greater tuberosity. The supraspinatus muscle has a complex architecture that permits it to provide significant stability to the humeral head during rotation and abduction at a variety of angles. This includes a ventral or anterior portion that inserts more anteriorly on the greater tuberosity and acts as an internal rotator, as well as a posterior portion that inserts posteriorly on the greater tuberosity and serves to abduct the shoulder [18, 19]. Each of these portions is subdivided into superficial, middle, and deep portions, each with its own insertion [18]. This complex architecture with resulting complex movement is thought to contribute to its susceptibility to injury [18]. The supraspinatus musculature and tendon are separated from surrounding musculature and bony prominences by the subacromial-subdeltoid (SASD) bursa, which functions to facilitate movement of the tendon. The SASD bursa is described separately. As the supraspinatus courses laterally toward its insertion, the supraspinatus forms the posterosuperior border of the rotator interval, which surrounds the proximal portion of the LHBB.

Ultrasound evaluation of the medial, proximal supraspinatus tendon is obscured by the bony acromion at rest in a neutral position. Placing the patient in a Crass position (hand behind the back with shoulder extension and internal rotation) or modified-Crass position (hand on the hip with shoulder in extension) angles the greater tuberosity anteriorly, pulling a larger portion of the supraspinatus out from underneath the acromion. The Crass position may obscure the rotator interval because of the internal rotation and be painful for patients with pathology [5]. The modified Crass is more commonly used as a result, but it should be noted that this position may overestimate the size of tendon tears [20]. It should be noted that part of the tendon will always be obscured by the coracoacromial arch and the supraspinatus should be evaluated to the maximal extent possible posterior and anterior to the acromial arch, recognizing the inherent limitations presented by the overlying bony architecture.

The supraspinatus tendon is superficial and can generally be imaged with a high-frequency linear probe within a few centimeters of the skin surface. The probe is placed over the superior and anterior aspect of the shoulder in a coronal oblique plane with the medial end of the transducer pointed towards the patient's ear. This will show the supraspinatus tendon in a long axis view (Fig. 5.6). The insertion of the supraspinatus tendon classically has a convex "bird's beak"

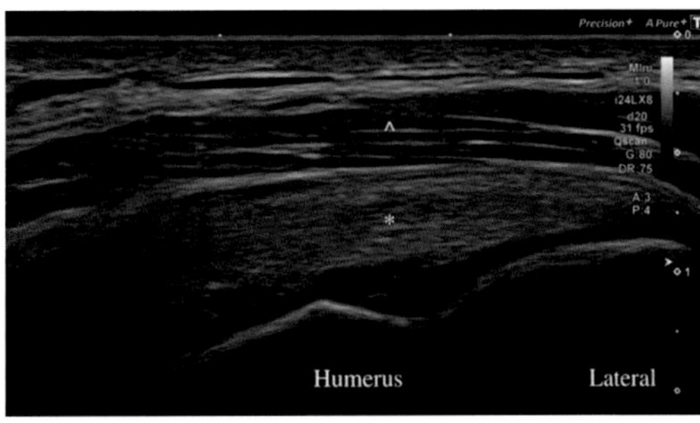

Fig. 5.6 Longitudinal view of the insertional supraspinatus (*) onto humerus. Deltoid (^) is superficial to supraspinatus

appearance as it inserts on the greater tuberosity. In this view, the greater tuberosity, bursal, and articular surfaces of the tendon can be evaluated for pathology. The tendon will appear fibrillar and hyperechoic with fibrocartilage often seen deep to the tendon over the facets. Hypoechoic articular cartilage may also be seen over the humeral head. Heel-toe of the transducer should be used over the insertion of the supraspinatus to eliminate anisotropy caused by the downward curve of the tendon at the insertion on the humerus.

The footprint of the supraspinatus covers approximately 25 mm of the greater tuberosity, and the entire footprint should be scanned [21]. The boundaries of the supraspinatus can be identified by scanning anteriorly until the biceps tendon is seen within the rotator interval and posteriorly until the infraspinatus comes into oblique view. The tendon should then be scanned superiorly in long axis until the acromion is encountered. The SASD bursa may be seen as a thin, hypoechoic line overlying the supraspinatus tendon, although it is collapsed in those without pathology and may be difficult to visualize.

Once long-axis evaluation has been completed, the transducer should be rotated 90° to evaluate the tendon in short axis (Fig. 5.7). Scanning should be started at the level of the humeral head with the proximal tendon in view over underlying articular cartilage. The tendon thickness generally measures 5–6 mm in thickness 1–2 cm from the insertion and may vary by approximately 0.5 mm between men and women

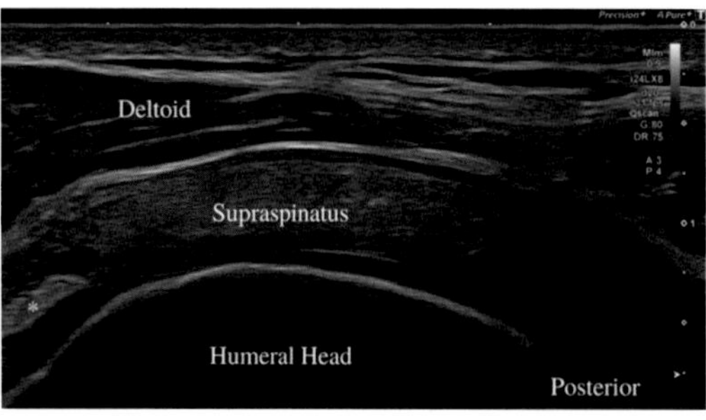

Fig. 5.7 Transverse view of the supraspinatus insertion onto humerus. The long head biceps brachii tendon (*) is visualized at the rotator interval and leading anterior edge of supraspinatus

[22–24]. As the tendon is scanned distally, it will thin as the articular portion of the humerus gives way to the more angulated facets of the greater tuberosity. The supraspinatus will insert on the superior and superior half of the middle facet. The infraspinatus will also be seen inserting onto the middle facet at this level and the fibers of both tendons often mingle at this level, making a definitive differentiation difficult. As with the long-axis portion of the scan, the transducer should be translated anteriorly until the biceps tendon is visualized within the rotator interval and posteriorly until the infraspinatus is viewed to ensure the entire footprint has been evaluated.

Dynamic evaluation is then performed to evaluate for any visible signs of subacromial impingement. With the supraspinatus footprint and the acromion in view, the patient should slowly abduct and adduct the shoulder. The supraspinatus will be observed passing underneath the acromion. The sonographer should observe for bunching of bursal tissue against the acromion, collecting fluid at the edge of the acromion representing an effusion in the bursa, or correspondence of pain with this movement.

The musculature of the supraspinatus can be visualized posteriorly for echotexture changes that may suggest muscle pathology such as denervation or disuse. Short-axis panoramic views of the muscle can allow comparison to the infraspinatus and teres minor for reference. The musculature should have a "starry sky" appearance with a largely hypoechoic echotexture interspersed with hyperechoic connective tissue. Increased hyperechogenicity should raise concern for underlying fatty or fibrous infiltration. The musculature can be traced into the tendon up until its passage under the acromion.

The deltoid musculature is also commonly viewed during diagnostic scans in this area, although dedicated diagnostic scanning is far less common than imaging of the rotator cuff. This is largely based on the low levels of pathology seen in the deltoid relative to the muscles of the rotator cuff. The muscle originates on the lateral third of the clavicle, the acromion, and on the spine of scapula. It inserts onto the anterolateral surface of the humerus. Because of its broad origins, the deltoid muscle assists with a variety of actions around the shoulder, including flexion, extension, internal rotation, external rotation, and abduction, although abduction is its main action. It is supplied by the axillary nerve and may show signs of denervation – atrophy, fibrosis, or fatty infiltration – in cases of axillary nerve injury The muscle may also be injured by direct blow resulting in contusion or muscle injury, which can also be visualized under ultrasound.

Pathology

The supraspinatus tendon is the most commonly torn tendon in the rotator cuff [25]. Ultrasound has been shown in several meta-analyses to be at least 90% specific and as good as MRI and potentially MR arthrogram in evaluating tearing of the tendon [26, 27]. Degenerative tears are frequently seen posterior to the biceps tendon near the junction of the supraspinatus and infraspinatus tendons [28]. The anterior supraspinatus tendon at the articular-sided footprint is also commonly affected, and concomitant cortical irregularity representing chronic injury may be seen [25]. Acute tears tend to occur more proximally and often lack the cortical irregularity seen in degenerative tears [5].

Tears are hypoechoic or anechoic areas within the substance of the tendon. Tears are described as partial- or full-thickness involving part of or the entire thickness of the tendon. Full-thickness tears appear as well-defined, hypoechoic, or anechoic disruptions in the fibrillar architecture of the tendon and may only affect part of the width of the tendon. Smaller tears may not change the overall shape of the tendon, while larger tears can lead to tendon volume loss, which flattens the typical convex appearance of the tendon [5]. Mixed hypoechoic and hyperechoic components can occur when a portion of the torn residual tendon is surrounded by fluid within the tear [29]. A complete tear is described as a full-width, full-thickness tear. Some partial-thickness tears may be difficult to evaluate based on their location or orientation, and secondary signs can be used to deduce underlying pathology. These signs include cortical irregularity at the footprint, effusion seen in the SASD bursa, a glenohumeral joint effusion, or a cartilage interface sign (hyperechoic line over the surface of the articular cartilage under the contour of the supraspinatus tendon) [3].

The location of a partial-thickness tear should also be defined as intrasubstance, bursal-sided, or articular-sided. An intrasubstance tear occurs within the tendon and does not extend to a surface of the tendon. Bursal-sided tears lead to loss of superficial fibers on the surface of the tendon, causing thinning of the tendon. The surrounding deltoid muscle and SASD bursa may then dip into this defect, causing loss of the typical convex appearance of the tendon. This is less common in articular-sided tears, because the cortical and articular surfaces underlying the tendon preserve the convex appearance of the tendon.

Chronic degeneration of the supraspinatus can result in tendinosis, which appears as a hypoechoic lesion within the tendon as described in more detail previously. Tendinosis should always be carefully differentiated from anisotropy. In particular, the convexity of the insertional footprint of the supraspinatus tendon may mislead sonographers into believing that tendinosis or tearing is present in the areas of hypoechogenicity, when this actually represents anisotropic tendon fibers. Tears in the supraspinatus may also involve other tendons of the rotator cuff. This is particularly the case for the infraspinatus, which intermingles fibers of its insertion toward the lateral edge of the supraspinatus tendon insertion on the middle facet. Tearing of the supraspinatus that extends posterior to the middle facet indicates likely involvement of the infraspinatus tendon. Tearing can also extend anteriorly into the rotator interval, coinciding with pathology of the subscapularis and biceps tendon.

The supraspinatus tendon is the most common rotator cuff tendon affected by calcific disease [30, 31]. The precise pathogenesis of tendon calcifications is unclear, and multiple different etiologies have been proposed [30–32]. Calcific lesions follow a predictable progression, resulting in the deposition of hydroxyapatite crystals within the tendon [32]. This involves a precalcific stage, where fibrocartilaginous metaplasia occurs within the tendon, followed by the painful formation of hydroxyapatite crystals on these metaplastic tissues that then calcify [32]. This is followed by resorption of the calcific lesion, which may also be painful secondary to increased edema and intratendinous pressure [30]. The pain in both of these stages may be related to ingrowth of neovessels and neonerves [33]. The area of previous calcification is eventually replaced by granulation tissue that is gradually remodeled into normal tendon [30].

On ultrasound, the appearance of these lesions can vary, and several classification systems have been devised to describe them as noted below [34]. While many lesions are hyperechoic with posterior acoustic shadowing, they may also be amorphous in appearance without significant posterior shadowing [34]. They may also take on several different appearances, including arc-shaped, fragmented with multiple components, nodular without shadowing, or cystic with an anechoic center [34]. The consistency of calcifications can also vary from hard, soft, or nearly liquid [35]. Soft or liquid calcifications may be isodense on ultrasound and absent on radiographs, making identification challenging. In these cases, the calcification can be identified as an amorphous echotexture within the tendon that will not become anisotropic with movement of the ultrasound probe [5]. As mentioned earlier, these lesions may also show color and power Doppler signal as a result of closely associated neovessels.

Calcific Disease Classification Systems	
Gärtner and Heyer Classification [36]	
Type I	Dense, well-circumscribed calcification
Type II	Soft contour/dense or sharp/transparent
Type III	Translucent/cloudy, not clearly circumscribed
Molé et al. Classification [37]	
Type A	Sharp contour, dense, homogenous
Type B	Sharp contour, dense, segmented
Type C	Soft contour, heterogeneous
Type D	Dystrophic calcification at the tendon insertion

Interventional Procedures

While corticosteroids are commonly used for shoulder pain, their utility for treatment of tendon injury has been increasingly questioned, given the non-inflammatory etiology of most chronic tendon abnormalities and the potentially harmful impact steroid has on tendon healing [2, 38] Attention has turned to alternative modes of treatment as a result, including platelet-rich plasma (PRP), prolotherapy, and mesenchymal stem cells.

Precise data on treatment of the supraspinatus tendon is muddied by the frequent use of the imprecise term "rotator cuff" in the literature, rather than specifying the tendons being treated. This makes it difficult to evaluate exactly what was targeted in many of these studies and to determine whether one or multiple tendons were addressed with the intervention. Additionally, much of the research has been done within the orthopedic community using platelet-rich plasma as an adjunct to surgical intervention as a way to augment healing outcomes. Several high-quality studies in these cases found borderline effects or failed to show an effect of PRP in these cases [39–43]. Some studies have reported faster healing, decreased retear rates, and lower rates of surgical failure or incomplete healing, but this may be more reliably the case for small to medium tears rather than large or massive tears [41, 44, 45]. The degree to which this reflects an improvement in functional outcomes is also questionable [44, 46]. A Cochrane review found similar findings to this effect [47].

Variable results have been reported for PRP injections as a nonoperative option for treatment of supraspinatus pathology. An RCT comparing PRP to saline injections into interstitial supraspinatus tears found no difference between PRP and saline [48]. At least one study comparing the effectiveness of dry needling with PRP to the supraspinatus tendon found a beneficial effect on pain and disability when PRP was injected into the lesion under ultrasound guidance [49]. Another study by Kesikburun et al. found no difference between PRP and saline, but the injections were placed in the subacromial space rather than in the tendon [50]. A recent meta-analysis by Lin et al. comparing PRP to steroid and prolotherapy found some indication that PRP improved long-term function more than other therapies and that prolotherapy improved long-term pain more than other therapies [51]. They also noted significant heterogeneity in their data [51]. In particular, the included studies contained a mix of diagnoses including supraspinatus tendinitis, clinically diagnosed subacromial impingement, and chronic tendinosis with 19 studies performing a subacromial injection and only two performing a supraspinatus tendon injection [51]. The effect of PRP composition on effectiveness is an additional consideration that likely influences outcome [52]. This was demonstrated in a 2019 study by Kim et al. that found improved response to PRP injection for degenerative rotator cuff tendinopathy when the injectate had higher levels of IL-1β or TGF-β1 [53]. This level of detail is often not obtained or reported in most PRP studies.

As mentioned above, prolotherapy has been considered for treatment of rotator cuff pathology, both alone and as an adjuvant to other regenerative therapies. However, prolotherapy has received significantly less research attention than PRP. A 2019 meta-analysis of prolotherapy trials for rotator cuff disease found only five randomized-controlled trials and three additional non-randomized trials [10]. While their synthesis of the data showed potential for effectiveness in pain reduction, range of motion improvement, and functional improvement, they also noted significant risk of bias and highly variable findings [10]. This was related to the heterogeneous and often small populations studied, variable sites and methods of injection, differing controls, and differing protocols used. While several studies found positive short-term results with intratendinous injection, long-term follow-up did not show significant differences compared to controls [54–56]. Definitive conclusions about the effectiveness of prolotherapy cannot be made at this time.

Hyaluronic acid has also been proposed as a treatment for rotator cuff tendinopathy, but results of trials to this effect are difficult to interpret, given the variable location of injection. A meta-analysis done by Osti et al. showed effectiveness of hyaluronic acid in treatment of shoulder pain in shoulders with rotator cuff tears; however, the studies included also reported a mix of intra-articular and subacromial locations for injection [57]. A 2019 study by Cai et al. found increased effectiveness of PRP injections when combined with hyaluronic acid injections, when injections were performed in the subacromial space [58]. Of note, research done by Wu et al. examining the effect of intratendinous injections of hyaluronic acid into the Achilles tendon showed a persistent inflammatory response lasting approximately 42 days with a significant increase in neovascularization [59]. These findings led them to recommend against intratendinous injection of hyaluronic acid [59].

While significant enthusiasm has surrounded the use of mesenchymal stem cells (MSC), either derived from adipose tissue or bone marrow, few studies have been performed on the effectiveness of these interventions on tendon pathology of the rotator cuff. Kim et al. evaluated the use of BMAC for rotator cuff pathology compared to an exercise program [60]. They found marginal improvement in pain and function scores at 3 months compared to exercise alone [60]. Jo et al. recently reported an unblinded, uncontrolled case series of adipose-derived MSC injection into rotator cuff tears, although which tendons of the rotator cuff were targeted was not clarified in the study [61]. Those in the high-dose treatment group ($1\text{x}10^8$ cells injected) improved in shoulder pain and disability index (SPADI) and visual analogue scale (VAS) with other tested parameters largely nonsignificant (Jo et al. [61]). These studies have yet to be replicated, and caution should be exercised in extrapolating their findings.

Injection Technique

- Patient positioning – Lateral decubitus with affected side facing up
- Transducer selection – High-frequency linear array transducer (>10MHz)
- Transducer position – Long axis to the supraspinatus tendon

- Needle selection – 25–27-gauge 1.5–2.5-inch needle, depending on body habitus and depth of target.
- Injectate selection – Anesthetize with local anesthetic. Inject with ~3 mL of volume including steroid, prolotherapy, or orthobiologic therapy.
- Needle trajectory and target – In-plane, lateral to medial. Target area of tendon pathology.
- Accuracy – Specific studies have not been performed on injections into the supraspinatus, although targeting specific lesions within the tendon without guidance would be extremely challenging. Many studies noted above use injection into the subacromial space with accuracy for these injections reported in the section on the SASD bursa.
- Pearls/Pitfalls
  - It is common to see apparent extension of the lesion under ultrasound guidance as the injectate expands collapsed areas of tearing with the injectate filling these potential spaces.
  - The overall space within an area of pathology may be very limited. Significant pressure should not be exerted during the procedure. Once significant resistance is met, the needle can be withdrawn and redirected to another area of pathology.
  - Some practitioners perform needle tenotomy during injection of PRP to further stimulate inflammation and healing in the area. [62].

Percutaneous needle barbotage/lavage of intratendinous calcific lesions has been found to be a safe and effective means of treating these lesions [63]. However, while short-term results after this procedure appear promising, one long-term follow-up study done by de Witte et al. found no difference in pain, function, or radiographic findings between those who had undergone barbotage and those who had an isolated subacromial corticosteroid injection [64, 65]. They theorize that this may be related to the natural course of calcific lesions, which often resolve on their own [30, 32, 64].

One-Needle Technique

- Patient positioning: Supine with several pillows under the affected shoulder to elevate it
- Transducer selection – High-frequency linear array transducer (>10MHz)
- Transducer position – Long axis to the supraspinatus tendon with the calcification in view
- Needle selection – 16–25-gauge needles have been used, but 18-gauge 2.5-inch needle is recommended
- Injectate selection – Anesthetize down to the lesion. 10mL syringe with 3 mL of 2% lidocaine and 3 mL normal saline attached to the first 10 mL syringe to aid with anesthetizing the lesion. Subsequent syringes can be filled with 6 mL of normal saline.
- Needle trajectory and target – In-plane, lateral to medial. Target calcification.
- Description – Puncture the calcification at a single location if possible. Once the needle is within the calcification, the plunger of the syringe should be gently pumped using back pressure to extract the calcific debris. Calcific debris should be seen returning into the syringe when pressure is released. Once the syringe becomes cloudy, it should be switched for another syringe. This procedure should be repeated until no further calcific debris returns.
- Pearls/pitfalls
  - The needle and syringe should be held in a dependent positioning, so that gravity carries debris away from the needle inlet to avoid reinjection of calcific debris.
  - A single-entry point should be used for best effect. If multiple puncture sites are made, it may not be possible to generate the intralesional back pressure that facilitates the removal of calcific debris.
  - Ensure multiple syringes with normal saline are readily available prior to beginning the procedure, since multiple are commonly required before all calcific debris is removed.
  - If the needle becomes clogged during the procedure, the needle can be withdrawn into the surrounding tissue and then threaded with a 25-gauge needle to clear the blockage.

Two-Needle Technique

- Patient positioning: Same position as above
- Transducer selection – High-frequency linear array transducer (>10MHz)
- Transducer position – Long axis to the supraspinatus tendon with the calcification in view
- Needle selection – 16–25-gauge needles have been used, but 18-gauge 2.5-inch needle is recommended
- Injectate selection – Anesthetize down to the lesion. 6 mL NS attached to 10 mL syringe for calcific tendinosis
- Needle trajectory and target – In-plane, lateral to medial. Target calcification.
- Description – In this technique, two needles are placed within the calcification: one anteriorly that will serve as the injecting needle and one posteriorly in a dependent position that will serve as the draining needle. When both needles have been placed, the syringe is attached to the anterior needle, and the calcification is irrigated with normal saline, which is allowed to drain from the posterior needle. This is done until no further calcific debris drains from the needle.
- Pearls/pitfalls
  - This technique is ideal when back pressure is lost as a result of multiple punctures.
  - If desired, the anterior needle may be repositioned after the procedure to perform a SASD bursa injection.

Subscapularis Tendon

Anatomy and Ultrasound Evaluation

The subscapularis muscle originates in the subscapular fossa on the ventral side of the scapula. It then courses posteromedially to the humerus under the coracoid process to insert anteromedially on the lesser tuberosity of the humerus. The subscapularis lies medial to the biceps tendon over the anterior shoulder and inferior to it in the rotator interval. It serves to internally rotate the shoulder.

The subscapularis is often evaluated after the biceps tendon because of its close proximity. The distal end of the subscapularis tendon is seen in long axis medial to the biceps tendon during short-axis evaluation of the proximal biceps tendon (Fig. 5.2). Positioning the patient in adduction and external rotation brings more the distal tendon into view and allows for Fig. optimization to better evaluate for pathology (Fig. 5.8). Heel-toe movements of the transducer eliminate anisotropy at the footprint of the tendon as it wraps around the humeral head. Full evaluation of the more proximal tendon is limited because of its depth and surrounding bony anatomy. The transducer should be translated superiorly and inferiorly at the lesser tuberosity to ensure that the entirety of the subscapularis tendon is evaluated in long axis.

The transducer is then rotated 90° to evaluate the tendon in short axis. The subscapularis contains several hypoechoic divisions within the tendon in this plane, which represent different tendon bundles and should not be interpreted as partial- or full-thickness tearing of the tendon (Fig. 5.9).

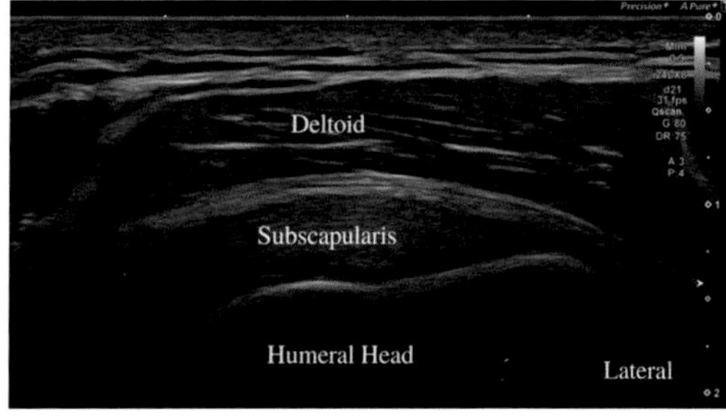

Fig. 5.8 Longitudinal view of the insertional subscapularis onto humerus

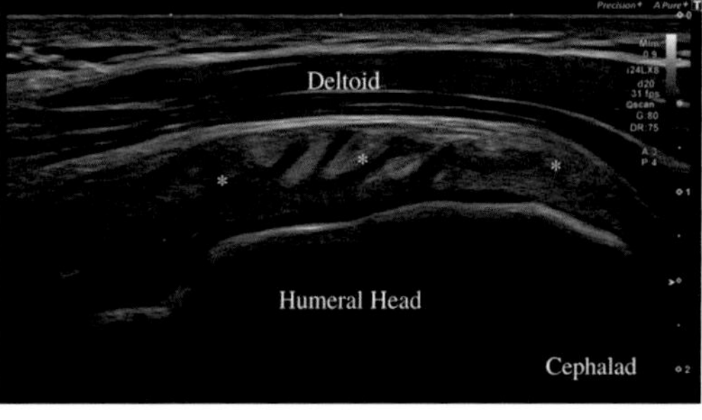

Fig. 5.9 Transverse view of the insertional subscapularis onto humerus. The subscapularis tendon has a unique multipennate appearance

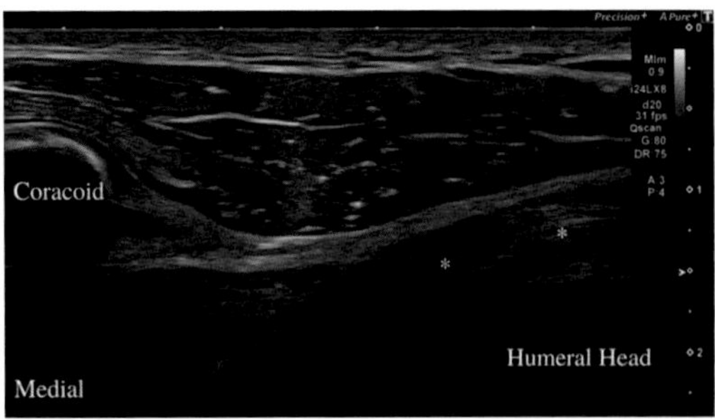

Fig. 5.10 Longitudinal view of subscapularis (*) medially deep to coracoid

Dynamic evaluation is performed to evaluate for subcoracoid impingement medially and bursal fluid that may become more prominent with shoulder internal and external rotation (Fig. 5.10). The subscapularis tendon is visualized in its long axis with the coracoid process visible medially and the humeral head visible laterally. The shoulder is then both passively and actively internally and externally rotated while visualizing the tendon passing under the coracoid process. Any dyskinetic bunching of tissue at the coracoid process, collection of fluid, or pain with this maneuver suggests an underlying pathology.

Pathology

Subscapularis tendon tears commonly occur as a result of acute trauma with the arm abducted and externally rotated and have a similar sonographic appearance as described in the section on the supraspinatus. Isolated subscapularis tears are uncommon and should prompt more thorough evaluation of the rotator cuff [66]. Partial-thickness subscapularis tears can be bursal-sided, interstitial, or articular-sided. The cephalad portion of the tendon is more commonly torn than the caudad portion and is commonly associated with a supraspinatus tear [6, 66].

Full-thickness subscapularis tears can be seen as a discontinuity in the tendon structure or outright retraction if the tear is large or complete. Tears of this nature are most common at the lesser tuberosity and can be seen more clearly in external rotation [5]. Avulsion tears will often demonstrate posterior acoustic shadowing behind the hyperechoic fragment.

It is important to recognize that subscapularis tears are often associated with biceps long head tendon instability, particularly in tearing of the cephalad subscapularis, because of the subscapularis contribution to the rotator interval and stabilizing ligaments that overlie the biceps tendon and constrain medial movement [13].

Subcoracoid impingement occurs as the subscapularis passes deep to the coracoid process. This impingement occurs with internal rotation and shoulder flexion, when the lesser tuberosity of the humerus comes into closest proximity with the coracoid, and can contribute to tendon degeneration, further exacerbating the impingement and increasing tendon thickness [67]. Subcoracoid impingement is much less common than subacromial impingement but may be seen in the settings of postoperative and post-traumatic lesser tuberosity abnormalities [67].

The subcoracoid bursa is located deep to the conjoined tendon of the short head of the biceps and coracobrachialis. It is an extension of the subacromial subdeltoid bursa and does not communicate with the glenohumeral joint. It is commonly enlarged in the setting of anterior rotator cuff pathology [6]. External rotation can draw the bursa out from underneath the coracoid and improve visualization [5]. It should be differentiated from the nearby subscapularis recess. This recess (sometimes known as the subscapularis bursa) is a recess of the glenohumeral joint and overlies the portion of the subscapularis tendon closest to the scapular neck. The recess is typically not visible during routine scanning but may be visible in the setting of an intra-articular effusion. If present, it lies in close proximity to the subscapularis tendon just caudal to the coracoid process [6].

Several studies have attempted to establish defined normal and abnormal coracohumeral distances, but multiple studies have shown mixed results regarding the predictive value of coracohumeral distance [68]. While distance is unlikely to be indicative in and of itself, abnormal sonographic appearance of the subscapularis tendon combined with abnormal contact under the coracoid in the setting of corresponding anterior shoulder pain is strongly suggestive of impingement.

Interventional Procedures

Data regarding the effectiveness of PRP for treatment of subscapularis pathology suffers from the same lack of specificity in language, target site, intervention protocols, and choice of outcome measures as the supraspinatus literature. In spite of the differences between pathology affecting the subscapularis and supraspinatus, both are often grouped together as rotator cuff pathology with most injections taking place within the subacromial space. As a result, specific data on subscapularis pathology and the effectiveness of PRP, prolotherapy, MSC, or hyaluronic acid is lacking at this time.

- Patient positioning – Supine with arm externally rotated
- Transducer selection – High-frequency linear array transducer (>10 MHz)
- Transducer position – Long axis to the subscapularis tendon
- Needle selection – 25–27-gauge 1.5–2.5-inch needle, depending on body habitus and depth of target. A longer needle is often needed for the subscapularis due to depth of the targeted structures.
- Injectate selection – Anesthetize with local anesthetic. Inject with ~3 mL of volume including steroid, prolotherapy, or orthobiologic therapy.
- Needle trajectory and target – In-plane, lateral to medial. Target area of tendon pathology.
- Accuracy – Studies to have not been performed evaluating the accuracy of these kinds of injections beyond general accuracy of injections into the subacromial space mentioned elsewhere.
- Pearls/pitfalls – None

Infraspinatus

Anatomy and Ultrasound Evaluation

The infraspinatus originates within the scapular infraspinous and courses laterally over the posterior glenohumeral joint to insert on the middle facet of the humoral greater tuberosity. The patient can be examined either seated or side-lying with the shoulder neutrally positioned. The lateral inserting tendon is superficial and should require minimal depth with a superficial focal zone for evaluation. A high-frequency linear probe is usually the best choice for this evaluation. Examination of the medial infraspinatus muscle belly requires greater depth to visualize the entirety of the muscle belly. This should be possible with a linear probe in most individuals but may require a lower frequency curvilinear probe in more muscular or obese individuals.

To identify the infraspinatus, the transducer is aligned in an axial oblique plane inferior to the spine of the scapula. The hyperechoic central tendon can be followed from medial to the lateral insertion of the tendon on the middle facet of the humeral greater tuberosity (Fig. 5.11). The full width of the tendon should be scanned in cephalad to caudad manner, with the most superior aspect of the tendon demarcated by the supraspinatus tendon inserting on the superior and middle facets. It's important not to confuse anisotropy from oblique supraspinatus fibers for infraspinatus pathology.

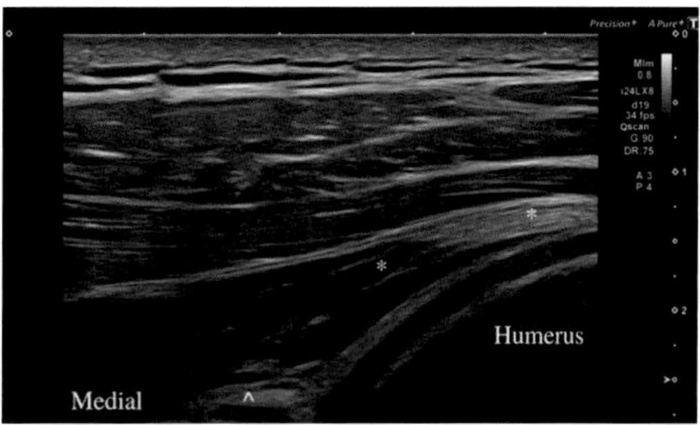

Fig. 5.11 Longitudinal view of infraspinatus (*) overlying the posterior glenohumeral joint. Deep to infraspinatus, the glenoid (^) and humeral head are visualized

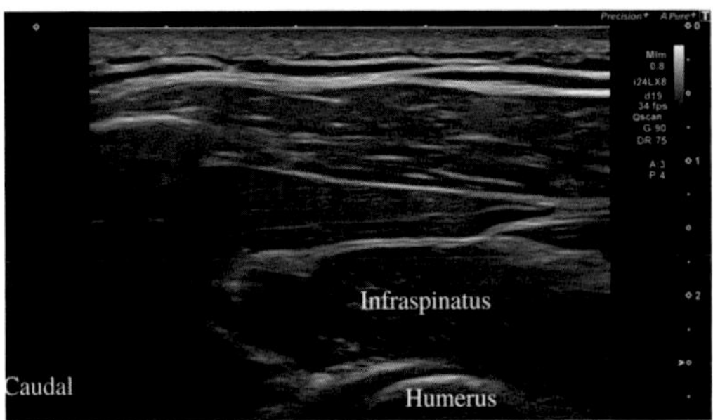

Fig. 5.12 Transverse view of infraspinatus overlying the scapula

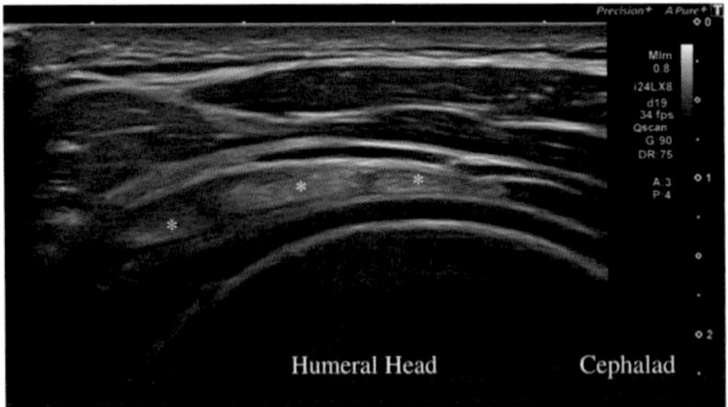

Fig. 5.13 Transverse view of infraspinatus (*) overlying the humeral head near its insertion

Toggling or rotating the probe should eliminate these areas of hypoechogenicity.

The infraspinatus should also be evaluated in short axis. The transducer is placed in a sagittal orientation just caudal from the spine of the scapula overlying the infraspinatus in short axis (Fig. 5.12). The musculature and punctate hyperechoic central tendon can be traced from medial to the lateral humeral insertion (Fig. 5.13). The appearance of the muscle belly of the infraspinatus should be compared to the appearance of the supraspinatus teres minor, since changes in muscle echotexture may reflect underlying fatty infiltration from chronic disuse, tearing, or denervation. The use of the panoramic scanning feature can facilitate visualization of the supraspinatus, infraspinatus, and teres minor in one image across the scapula to compare muscle bulk and echotextures.

Pathology

Isolated infraspinatus injury is rare, and tearing often coincides with supraspinatus pathology. Infraspinatus tearing appears similar to supraspinatus tearing as described previously. Full-thickness tears usually indicate concomitant supraspinatus tearing and rarely occur in isolation [5]. Chronic tendon injury can lead to tendinopathy and calcific disease in the infraspinatus through a similar process to that seen in the supraspinatus, although this pathology is less commonly seen [69].

Articular surface tearing of the infraspinatus tendon may also be seen in shoulder internal impingement. This occurs in a position abduction and external rotation of the shoulder [70, 71]. Such tearing is particularly common close to the infraspinatus-supraspinatus junction and may also been seen in conjunction with SLAP tears [70]. These injuries are commonly seen in throwing athletes, and the same torsion forces, shearing, and peel-back forces that result in a SLAP tear are also responsible for articular-sided infraspinatus tears [70]. Chronic microtrauma to the posterior capsule leads to thickening, fibrosis, and subsequent malpositioning of the humerus during abduction and external rotation [70]. Identification of an articular-sided infraspinatus tear should prompt supraspinatus evaluation and a shoulder MRI to assess the labrum.

Interventional Procedures

The evidence for regenerative treatment of the infraspinatus is limited. The vast majority of existing evidence has been done for generic rotator cuff pathology with injection into the subacromial space as described in the section on the supraspinatus. At time of writing, no systematic studies exist examining treatment specifically of the infraspinatus tendon with regenerative therapies. However, given the previously mentioned data on effective treatment regimens for the supraspinatus and rotator cuff, outcomes of similar treatment in the infraspinatus may be similar.

- Patient positioning – Lateral decubitus with affected side facing up
- Transducer selection – High-frequency linear array transducer (>10 MHz) or low-frequency curvilinear transducer (<10 MHz) may be

used for deep targets or to facilitate needle placement

- Transducer position – Long axis to the infraspinatus tendon
- Needle selection – 27-gauge 1.5-inch or 27-gauge 2.5-inch needle, depending on body habitus and depth of target.
- Injectate selection – Anesthetize with local anesthetic. Inject with ~3 mL of volume including steroid, prolotherapy, or orthobiologic therapy.
- Needle trajectory and target – In-plane, lateral to medial. Target area of tendon pathology.
- Accuracy – Studies to have not been performed evaluating the accuracy of these kinds of injections beyond general accuracy of injections into the subacromial space.
- Pearls/pitfalls: None

Teres Minor

Anatomy and Ultrasound Evaluation

The teres minor muscle primarily originates from the axillary border of the scapula caudal to the infraspinatus but also has two aponeurotic laminae that arise from the infraspinatus and teres major muscles. The muscle courses superolaterally to insert onto the humeral greater tuberosity inferior facet and directly on the shaft of the humerus. The teres minor externally rotates and adducts the humerus. It is important to note that the fusion of the infraspinatus and teres minor muscles is a normal variant that may be seen. In this case, the paired muscle bellies share a common aponeurosis that inserts broadly on the greater tuberosity [6].

For ultrasound examination, the patient can be maintained in the same neutral position as the infraspinatus evaluation. The teres minor muscle is identified just caudal from the infraspinatus muscle and has a more rounded appearance in short axis compared to the elongated appearance of the infraspinatus. A subtle ridge in the infraspinatus fossa may also be seen in short axis separating the muscle bellies of each muscle. In long axis, the tendon of the teres minor is very short relative to the infraspinatus and is obliquely oriented relative to the humerus because of its superolateral direction of insertion (Fig. 5.14). The muscle and tendon should be evaluated in short axis from the origin on the scapula to the insertion on the greater tuberosity (Fig. 5.15). While the infraspinatus and teres minor can be differentiated over the scapula, some examiners may find it easier to visualize the tendons over the humerus and trace the tendons back into the musculature to ensure the correct structure is evaluated. In these cases, the teres minor will be the smaller and more inferior tendon seen inserting on the inferior facet.

As previously mentioned, the thickness and echotexture of the teres minor should be evaluated relative to the musculature of the other rotator cuff muscles in the dorsal plane of the scapula. This comparison can be easily achieved for the infraspinatus given the proximity of the muscle

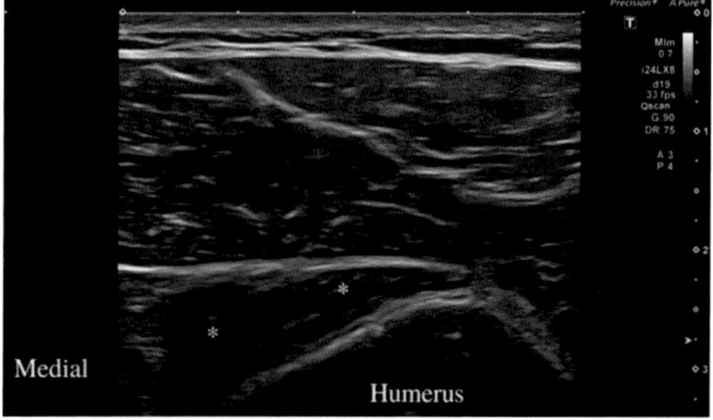

Fig. 5.14 Longitudinal view of teres minor (*) at its humeral insertion

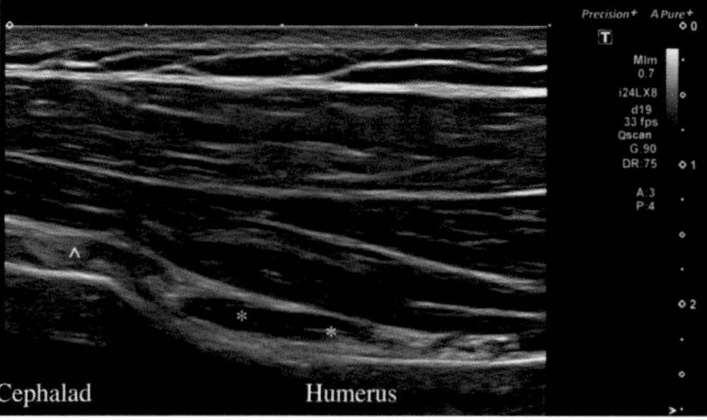

Fig. 5.15 Transverse view of the teres minor (*) at its humeral insertion. Infraspinatus (^) is visualized cephalad/proximal on the humerus from the teres minor

bellies. Comparison between all three muscles requires panoramic evaluation. Since the teres minor is the smallest of the rotator cuff muscles and is rarely injured, it often serves as a helpful reference point for pathology of the supraspinatus and infraspinatus.

Pathology

Teres minor pathology is rare relative to the other muscles of the rotator cuff. Teres minor tendon injury is usually related to acute trauma directly affecting the area. Extension of tears from the infraspinatus tendon into the teres minor tendon is also rare [5]. Signs of denervation may be observed in the teres minor and are commonly caused by impingement of the axillary nerve in the quadrilateral space as discussed elsewhere in this chapter. While the deltoid may be involved, isolated teres minor atrophy can also occur, depending on the exact location where the innervating nerve is entrapped [72]. The innervation of the teres minor has been found to be variable, likely explaining how the teres minor might be selectively affected over other muscles innervated by the axillary nerve [72]. The bundles within the teres minor may even be selectively affected, as noted in a 2019 study by Kang et al. [73].

Interventional Procedures

No systematic studies of regenerative treatment for the teres minor tendon pathology have been performed, likely because the rarity of teres minor pathology, so recommendations beyond those made for the general rotator cuff as discussed in the section on the supraspinatus cannot be made. If quadrilateral space pathology is suspected as a possible cause of denervation of the teres minor, evaluation and injection for this space is discussed in the section on the quadrilateral space. Injections into the teres minor and muscle are rare but follow the same procedural guidelines as those for the infraspinatus.

Subacromial/Subdeltoid Bursa (SASD Bursa)

Anatomy and Ultrasound Evaluation

The SASD bursa is located deep to the acromion, deltoid, and subdeltoid fascia [74] and superficial to the supraspinatus tendon [75, 76]. It averages 55.6 mm medial to lateral length and 55.7 mm in anterior to posterior width. It is a potential space and is very thin when not inflamed, scarred, or distended with fluid [75]. It may extend as far anterior as the acromioclavicular (AC) joint [75]. The SASD bursa does not communicate with the glenohumeral (GH) joint [76], unless a full-thickness rotator cuff tear exists. As it passes around the proximal humerus, the axillary nerve courses about 1.0 cm caudal to the posterolateral boarder of the SASD bursa (range 0.0–1.4 cm) [74, 77].

On ultrasound evaluation of the SASD bursa, the patient's arm in held in adduction and neutral rotation. The probe is oriented in long axis to the supraspinatus tendon in the coronal or coronal-oblique plane with the acromion in view (image of probe placement). A high-frequency linear array transducer is optimal and will be utilized in even the most muscular or obese patients, given the relatively superficial location of the bursa. The SASD is a thin potential space in normal states, appearing as a thin hypoechoic plane overlying the rotator cuff tendons (Fig. 5.16). When acutely or chronically inflamed, the bursa appears as a 2 mm or thicker complex comprised of an

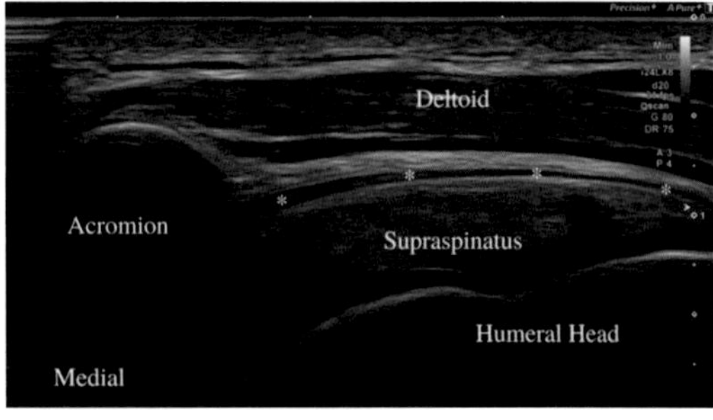

Fig. 5.16 The subacromial-subdeltoid bursa (*) in normal states is visualized as a thin, hypoechoic stripe superficial to the longitudinal supraspinatus and the hyperechoic peribursal fat deep to the overlying deltoid

inner layer of hypoechoic fluid between two layers of hyperechoic peribursal fat [78]. In cases of subtle bursal effusion, fluid accumulates in the most distal and dependent aspect of the bursa and may be visualized several centimeters distal to the insertion of the rotator cuff by sliding the probe laterally [8, 78]. Care should be taken to apply minimal pressure with the probe over the bursa so as to not artifactually displace a bursal effusion.

Pathology

Inflammation of the SASD bursa and pathology involving underlying rotator cuff tendons can lead to bursitis, and subacromial impingement occurs as the enlarged or distended bursa is mechanically traumatized between the rotator cuff tendons and the acromion. Pain related to SASD bursitis or impingement occurs with shoulder abduction, flexion, and internal rotation. SASD bursitis and subacromial impingement are associated with supraspinatus tendon thickening (0.6 mm thicker, $p = 0.048$) that occupation of a greater percentage of the subacromial interval between the acromion and humerus (7.5%, $p = 0.014$) when measured on ultrasound [79]. Dynamic ultrasound can identify dynamic subacromial impingement by passively or actively abducting the arm and evaluating for dyskinetic obstruction of the normal gliding of the SASD bursa under the acromion and pooling of fluid in the distal and lateral SASD bursa [78, 80]. Treatment of SASD bursitis and subacromial impingement consist of physical therapy to improve rotator cuff the glenohumeral stability, relative rest from provoking or exacerbating activities, oral or transdermal non-steroidal anti-inflammatory drugs (NSAIDs), physical modalities (therapeutic ultrasound, manual therapy), interventional procedures (injections), and surgery [81, 82].

Interventional Procedures

SASD bursa corticosteroid injections can successfully palliate symptoms [83]. Only two studies have reported on the injection of orthobiologics into the SASD bursa [84, 85]. Nejati et al. compared two ultrasound-guided injections of leukocyte-rich platelet-rich plasma (PRP) into the SASD bursa and about the rotator cuff tendons (RTC) to a course of physical therapy that progressed from passive range of motion exercises (ROM) to strengthening of the scapular stabilizers. Both interventions effectively reduced pain and disability with the physical therapy cohort showing greater improvement [84]. One study has compared a palpation-guided leukocyte-poor PRP injection to corticosteroid injection and showed that the corticosteroid injection significantly improved pain and function compared to the PRP injection [85]. These studies show that PRP can improve pain, function, and ROM but remain inferior to the more established corticosteroid injections and physical therapy [86].

The accuracy of US-guided SASD bursa injections is 65–100% [87, 88], as compared to 29–100% accuracy of palpation-guided injections [87, 89–92]. A systematic review and meta-analysis comparing US-guided versus palpation-guided SASD bursa corticosteroid injections showed statistically significant differences in pain ($p = 0.003$), function ($p < 0.001$), and range of motion ($p < 0.001$) [83] favoring US guidance.

Procedural protocol:

- Patient position – Lateral decubitus on the contralateral, unaffected side. The arm of the affected side should be adducted, slightly extended, and in slight internal rotation.
- Transducer selection – High-frequency, linear array transducer (>10 MHz).
- Transducer position – Long axis to supraspinatus tendon toward its humeral insertion with the acromion in view. The SASD bursa is identified superficial to the supraspinatus tendon and deep to the deltoid.
- Needle selection – 30-gauge, 1-inch; 27-gauge, 1.5-inch; or 25-gauge, 2-inch (depending on body habitus).
- Injectate selection – Anesthetize with lidocaine or Marcaine. Inject steroid or orthobio-

logic (most commonly PRP). Typically inject 3–5 mL of fluid.

- Needle trajectory and target structure – In-plane, lateral to medial approach to the SASD bursa.
- Pearls/pitfalls
  - Given the convexity of the shoulder, an entry point distal and lateral to the transducer should be chosen to ensure that the needle trajectory is perpendicular to the ultrasound beam.
  - The SASD bursa exists between the deltoid and rotator cuff tendons, which demonstrate differential motion in shoulder internal and external rotation movements and shoulder abduction. Slight movement in those planes can produce differential motion on ultrasound and aid in confirmation of the exact tissue plane of the SASD bursa.
  - A non-distended bursa can be a relatively non-distinct tissue plane, which can make confident identification and accurate injection challenging. Care must be taken to ensure intrabursal flow and not intratendinous or intramuscular deltoid deposition. Accurate intrabursal deposition may accomplish transient retro- or anterograde bursal distension and resolution as the injectate disperses throughout the bursa. Accumulation of fluid in one location without dispersion suggests extrabursal placement [83] and should prompt repositioning of the needle tip.

Acromioclavicular Joint

Anatomy and Ultrasound Evaluation:

The acromioclavicular (AC) joint is a diarthrodial articulation of the acromion and clavicle in the anterolateral shoulder that acts as a strut to anchor the complex movements of the scapula and arm to the thorax [93]. The articular surfaces of the acromion and clavicle are covered with hyaline cartilage. A meniscus-like fibrocartilaginous disc separates those surfaces but has a negligible contribution to joint function [93].

Static stabilizers of the AC joint include the superior, inferior, anterior, and posterior acromioclavicular ligaments, the coracoclavicular ligaments, and the coracoacromial ligaments. The coracoclavicular ligaments reinforce the inferior aspect of the AC joint and prevent superior displacement. Dynamic reinforcement of the joint is provided by the fascia of the overlying deltoid and trapezius muscles.

Ultrasound evolution of the AC joint can be performed with the patient seated or supine. The arm is adducted to the side and shoulder held in neutral rotation. The AC joint is superficial and best evaluated with a high-frequency linear array transducer. Localization of the joint can be facilitated and confirmed by multiple approaches. One reproducible means is to initially place the transducer in an anatomic sagittal plane transversely over the mid-clavicle. The clavicle then appears as a hyperechoic convexity of bone. The transducer is then carefully translated laterally toward the acromion, maintaining the clavicle in this transverse view, until the convex diaphysis of the clavicle flattens and broadens at its epiphysis before falling off into the hypoechoic joint space. The transducer is then maintained at this same position and rotated 90 degrees to longitudinal view of the distal clavicle at its articulation with the acromion (Fig. 5.17).

Normal AC joint space width has been reported in radiographic studies as 1–3 mm at the superior margin of the joint [94]. However, there can be significant variability in joint space measurement because of individual anatomic variations and US probe location. If concern for joint

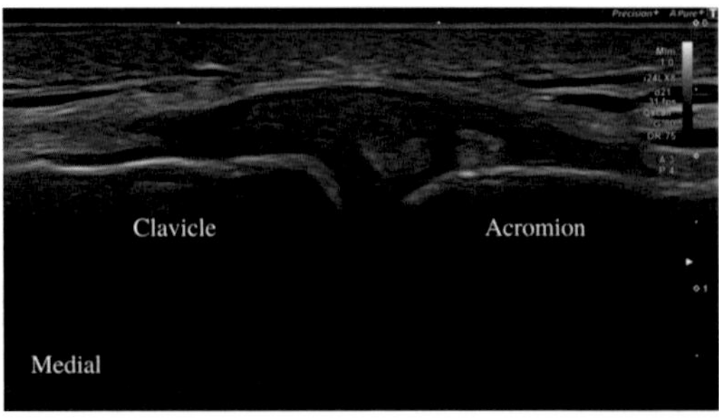

Fig. 5.17 Longitudinal view of the acromioclavicular joint

separation or widening exists, the contralateral AC joint width should be measured and assessed for symmetry. Dynamic evaluation for sonographic widening or narrowing and corresponding pain can be performed by having the patient cross-body adduct their ipsilateral hand to the contralateral shoulder. The acromioclavicular ligament is seen overlying the joint capsule. Other ligamentous stabilizers of the AC joint are obscured from sonographic visualization by surrounding bony anatomy.

The joint can also be evaluated in a long-axis and anatomic sagittal view by scanning along the clavicle in a sagittal oblique plane until the hyperechoic contour of the clavicle rises up superficially before dropping off into the hypoechoic joint space, which contains the hypoechoic fibrocartilaginous disc. This view is rarely used for diagnostic purposes but can be used for in-plane visualization of a needle during an AC joint injection, as described below. The supraspinatus tendon is deep to the AC joint, and a small extent of the tendon can often be visualized through to the joint space.

Pathology

The most common AC joint pathologies are osteoarthritis and ligamentous injury resulting in AC joint separation. AC joint osteoarthritis is characterized by joint space narrowing and cortical irregularities of the clavicle and/or acromion. AC joint degeneration can occur due to age-related degeneration, post-traumatic arthropathy, and, less commonly, distal clavicle osteolysis, inflammatory arthropathy, septic arthritis, and joint instability [95], each of which can contribute to fraying or tearing of the intra-articular disk and maceration of the chondral surface of the diarthrodial joint [96]. Patients with AC joint arthritis will have tenderness with palpation directly over the AC joint and pain with cross-body shoulder adduction [97]. AC joint arthritis is treated conservatively with physical therapy focused on ROM and strengthening of the pericapsular musculature (which is often ineffective), activity modification, NSAIDs, and intra-articular joint injection [95].

Acromioclavicular joint separation can occur secondary to a traumatic ligamentous sprain or chronic, attritional ligamentous disruption of one or several of the static stabilizers of the joint. The Rockwood classification system is the most commonly used system to classify injuries but is based on radiographic findings from bilateral anterior-to-posterior, axillary, and Zanca views. US correlates to the Rockwood classification are described in Table 5.1. Joint widening, superior clavicular displacement, and increased joint mobility can be identified by ultrasound evaluation; however, many ligaments that stabilize the AC joint cannot be directly visualized with ultrasound, and US measurements of displacement can be inconsistent, both of which can limit its diagnostic sensitivity in the context of suspected separation. AC joint effusion is identified as a hypoechoic, compressible fluid collection that superiorly distends in the joint space greater than 3 mm, and may result from acute injury, chronic degenerative changes, or communicating from the glenohumeral joint in the context of a full-thickness supraspinatus tear [98]. Treatment of AC joint separation depends on the type; anesthetic injections can be performed for pain control.

An os acromiale results from incomplete fusion of the anterior epiphysis of the acromion and is present in about 8% of the population and is present bilaterally in about one third of that population [100]. The os acromiale can relate to the lateral acromion by means of a separate articulation, a fibrocartilaginous union, or nearly complete fusion [100]. Pain can result from anterosuperior impingement of the underlying subscapularis tendon by a mobile os body or by secondary osteophytes. This synchondrosis should not be mistaken for a fracture or for the true AC joint. The acromion's articulation with the os acromiale can be differentiated from the true acromioclavicular joint by its orientation, which is approximately perpendicular to the plane of the acromioclavicular joint [6, 101].

Table 5.1 AC joint separation Rockwood classification with ultrasound correlation

Type	Definition AC ligament	CC ligament	Radiographs	US description
1	Sprain	Normal	Normal	Asymmetric joint space widening. Irregular-appearing capsular fibers. Hypoechogenic edema within the joint space. No step off between the clavicle and acromion
2	Torn	Sprain	Superiorly displaced lateral clavicle. Increased coracoclavicular distance <25%	Visible step off between the (medial) clavicle and (lateral) acromion. Joint space widening and increased clavicle mobility when stressed
3	Torn	Torn	Superiorly displaced lateral clavicle. Increased coracoclavicular distance 25–100%	More prominent step off between the clavicle and acromion. Joint space widening and increased clavicle mobility when stressed
4	Torn	Torn	Posteriorly displaced lateral clavicle	Horizontal instability with dynamic maneuvers with posterior clavicular displacement [99]
5	Torn	Torn	Superiorly displaced lateral clavicle. Increased coracoclavicular distance >100%	Acromioclavicular step off greater than 100%. Joint space widening when stressed
6	Torn	Torn	Inferiorly displaced lateral clavicle	There is a larger step off between the acromion and clavicle with the clavicle displaced inferiorly

An AC joint cyst results from glenohumeral joint fluid tracking into the acromioclavicular joint because of a massive rotator cuff tear, leading to significant distension of the superior joint capsule. On coronal evaluation of the AC joint, this can appear as hypoechoic fluid emerging from the underlying narrow joint space and termed a "geyser sign." This finding should prompt a full evaluation of the rotator cuff.

Interventional Procedures

AC joint anesthetic injection can be performed for diagnostic purposes in the context of AC joint arthritis or cysts to assist the clinic decision-making [102–104] and for analgesia in the setting of AC joint separation [105]. AC joint corticosteroid injections have been reported to have poor efficacy in symptom palliation and to achieve only short-term benefit [103, 106]. Definitive management can include surgical resection of the distal clavicle, but this can result in postoperative joint instability [95, 103, 106, 107]. Orthobiologics can be used to treat AC joint pathology, but only one study on prolotherapy has been reported. That study describes the use of ultrasound-guided injection of 15% dextrose prolotherapy into the AC joint (one or two injections 1 month apart) or near the distal acromion and showed substantial pain reduction with average visual analog scale (VAS) reduction of 4.3 points ($p < 0.01$) [108].

Despite the superficial location of the AC joint, accuracy of palpation-guided AC joint injections is very low (36.5–72%) [91, 109–112]. Ultrasound-guided injections of various approaches have accuracies of 90–100% but have not been directly compared [109, 110].

Procedural protocol: AC joint injection, anterior to posterior

- Patient position – Supine or seated. The ipsilateral shoulder and arm are held at the side in comfortable, neutral anatomic positions.
- Transducer selection – High-frequency, small-footprint linear array transducer (>10MHz). The small footprint aids in maneuverability of the probe and needle.
- Needle selection – 30-gauge, 1-inch; or 27-gauge, 1.5-inch.
- Injectate selection – Local anesthesia is often not used since the joint is so superficial. Inject anesthetic (for diagnostic purposes), steroid,

orthobiologic (PRP or prolotherapy). Typically inject <1 mL of fluid.

- Technique #1.
  - Transducer position – Short axis to clavicle over joint with no bony structures in view. Anatomic sagittal plane. The hypoechoic AC joint space is identified between the hypoechoic margins of the clavicle and acromion.
  - Needle trajectory and target – In-plane, anterior to posterior into AC joint.
  - Pearls/pitfalls

    The AC joint is very small; therefore, only the smallest volume as needed should be injected, usually about 1 mL.

    The location of the needle insertion site at the skin should take into account the convexity of the anterior shoulder and the depth of the joint space from the skin and the joint capsule to facilitate a near-parallel trajectory to the joint for optimal needle visualization.

    The transducer can be rotated 90 degrees to confirm that the needle tip is in the joint in an out-of-plane visualization between the clavicle and acromion.
- Technique #2
  - Transducer position – Long axis to clavicle and acromion with those bony contributions to the joint completely visualized. Anatomic axial plane. The hypoechoic AC joint space is identified between the hyperechoic convex margins of the clavicle and acromion.
  - Needle trajectory and target – Out-of-plane, anterior to posterior into the AC joint.
  - In an out-of-plane approach, the needle is visualized as a hyperechoic, punctate dot. The ultrasound transducer should be translated anteriorly (toward the sternum) to meet the needle tip shortly after it is inserted into the skin to identify its location and to estimate it's trajectory. Small-caliber translations anteriorly and posteriorly will aid in the triangulation of the superficial/deep and medial/lateral trajectory of the needle to inform whether withdrawal and redirection is necessary to ensure its continued accurate trajectory and its final location within the joint space.

    Pearls/pitfalls
    - Utilizing the walk-down technique is helpful in executing the injection.
    - The AC joint is very small; therefore, a small amount of fluid should be injected.
    - The transducer can be rotated 90 degrees to determine the anterior-posterior location of the needle tip within the joint.
- Technique #3: Lateral to medial AC joint injection
  - Patient position – Supine or seated. The ipsilateral shoulder and arm are held at the side in comfortable, neutral anatomic positions.
  - Transducer selection – High-frequency, small-footprint linear array transducer (>10 MHz).
  - Transducer position – Long axis to clavicle and acromion with those bony contributions to the joint completely visualized. Anatomic axial plane. The hypoechoic AC joint space is identified between the hyperechoic convex margins of the clavicle and acromion.
  - Needle selection – 30-gauge, 1-inch; or 27-gauge, 1.5-inch.
  - Injectate selection – Injection of local anesthesia with lidocaine or Marcaine, as the subcutaneous needle course is slightly longer than anterior-to-posterior approaches. Inject anesthetic (for diagnostic purposes), steroid, or orthobiologic (PRP or prolotherapy) to the joint. Typically inject about 1 mL of fluid.
  - Needle trajectory and target – In-plane, lateral to medial into AC joint.

    A generous gel standoff at the lateral aspect of the transducer overlying the acromion will facilitate an improved needle visualization, as there is often only a small amount of tissue overlying the acromion and AC joint. A gel standoff permits needle visualization and redirection before skin entry to optimize the approach to the joint and improve ultimate accuracy of needle placement. A skin entry that is too far lateral may dictate an approach trajectory that is too far media or lateral and can make entry into the joint unnecessarily challenging or impossible.

Sternoclavicular (SC) Joint

Anatomy and Ultrasound Evaluation

The SC joint is a saddle-shaped joint between the manubrium of the sternum and first rib medially and the medial end of the clavicle laterally [113]. It is the only articulation between the thorax and the upper limb. The SC joint is stabilized by the anterior and posterior sternoclavicular ligaments, the interclavicular ligaments, and the costoclavicular ligaments [113, 114]. A fibrocartilaginous disk separates the joint into clavicular and sternal compartments. Age-related degeneration can result in communication between these compartments [114, 115].

The sternoclavicular joint is visualized sonogramphically with the probe in a coronal or axial plane spanning the joint, with the clavicle visualized in long axis, and the sternum visualized medially (Fig. 5.18). A small-footprint linear array transducer is most commonly used and should be scanned in a cephalad to caudad maneuver to evaluate the entire joint.

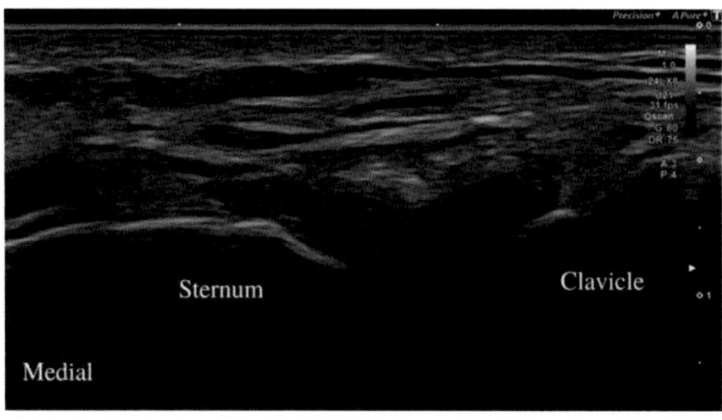

Fig. 5.18 Longitudinal view of the sternoclavicular joint

Pathology

Injuries of the SC joint are uncommon, but acute injuries can be severe to life-threatening. Ultrasound can identify subluxation or dislocation of the SC joint as an excessive, asymmetric step off between the sternum and clavicle. Comparison to the contralateral side is helpful. US can also identify atraumatic pathology, most commonly arthritis. SC joint arthritis occurs most commonly in patients with rheumatoid arthritis; is characterized by narrowing of the joint space, osteophytes, and para-articular cysts; and is amenable to corticosteroid injections. Septic arthritis is associated with increased joint fluid of mixed echogenicity and often requires aspiration and analysis of joint fluid or surgical washout [116].

Interventional Procedures

Description of the use of orthobiologics to treat the SC joint is scarce in the literature. One case reports the use of orthobiologics in the treatment of SC joint instability and describes the use of six injections of prolotherapy (a mixture of 22% dextrose and procaine was used for some injections and "more traditional" prolotherapy for others) and one leukocyte-poor PRP injection, followed by seven additional prolotherapy injections (22% dextrose and 1 mL of sodium morrhuate and procaine) into the bilateral SC joint capsular and ligamentous tissue that resulted in resolution of pain and popping symptoms [117].

The SC joint is not commonly injected, and different methods of guidance have been reported. Palpation-guided injections of the SC joint have a reported accuracy of 78%. Computed tomography (67% accuracy) [118, 119] and fluoroscopy [120] have been successfully used for needle guidance into the SC joint. Sonographic guidance is reported to have a 100% accuracy for injection of the SC joint [121].

Procedural protocol:

- Patient position – Supine or seated. The arm of the affected side is in neutral anatomic position.

- Transducer selection – High-frequency, small-footprint linear array transducer (>10 MHz).
- Transducer position – Spanning the SC joint with the clavicle in long axis.
- Needle selection – 30-gauge 1-inch; or 27-gauge 1.5-inch.
- Injectate selection – Can anesthetize with lidocaine or Marcaine. Inject anesthetic (for diagnostic purposes), steroid, or orthobiologic (PRP or prolotherapy). Typically inject <1 mL of fluid.
- Needle trajectory and target – Out-of-plane, anterior to posterior into the SC joint.
- Pearls/pitfalls.
  - A hyperechoic intra-articular disk may be visualized within the joint.
  - Take caution to avoid advancement of the needle beyond the SCJ where it can injure neurovasculature.
  - The transducer can be rotated 90 degrees to confirm that the needle tip is in the joint.

This injection can also be performed with the same setup using an in-plane, lateral to medial technique with gel standoff. This involves a lateral gel standoff and toe-ing in the medial side of the transducer. The smaller footprint and greater maneuverability of a small-footprint linear array transducer makes this easier. Such an approach, standoff, and small-footprint transducer improve the ease of injection, given the minimal subcutaneous tissue in this area through which to guide or redirect a needle to ensure placement within the joint space.

Glenohumeral (GH) Joint and Rotator Interval

Anatomy and Ultrasound Evaluation

The GH joint is a shallow ball and socket joint comprised of the articulation between the pear-shaped glenoid fossa of the scapula and the spheroidal humeral head. The shallow nature of this articulation affords the most range of motion of any joint in the body. The glenoid labrum is a fibrocartilaginous tissue that encircles the glenoid to extend the depth of the glenoid socket by 50%. The lax and redundant glenohumeral joint capsule allows for a wide range of motion and extends from the margins of the glenoid rim and labrum to the anatomic neck of the humerus. The capsule has several recesses in which fluid can accumulate in the setting of effusion (dependent axillary pouch, posterior and anterior recesses, subscapularis recess, sheath of the long head of the biceps tendon).

The joint is stabilized by both static and dynamic stabilizers. The glenohumeral ligaments provide static stability to the joint (Table 5.2). The glenoid labrum is composed of a fibrocartilaginous tissue and additionally contributes to

Table 5.2 Static stabilizers of the glenohumeral joint

Ligament	Biomechanics
Superior glenohumeral Ligament	Restraint to anteroinferior translation of long head of biceps (biceps pulley) and inferior translation at 0 degrees of abduction
Middle glenohumeral Ligament	Resists anterior and posterior translation in the midrange of abduction (~45 degrees of external rotation)
Inferior glenohumeral Ligament (Posterior Band)	Most important restraint to posterior subluxation at 90 degrees of flexion and internal rotation Tightness is linked to SLAP lesions
Inferior glenohumeral Ligament (Anterior Band)	Primary restraint to anterior/inferior translation 90 degrees abduction and maximal external rotation Weak link predisposing to Bankart lesions
Inferior glenohumeral Ligament (superior band)	Most important stabilizer of the joint
Coracohumeral ligament	From coracoid to rotator cable Limits posterior translation with should in flexion, adduction, and internal rotation Limits inferior translation in external rotation and adducted position Thickened in adhesive capsulitis

SGHL superior glenohumeral ligament, *MGHL* middle glenohumeral ligament, *IGHL* inferior glenohumeral ligament, *SLAP* superior labrum from anterior to posterior static stability by helping to create 50% of the glenoid socket depth. The anterior labrum anchors the inferior glenohumeral ligament, and the superior labrum anchors the biceps tendon. Several normal variants of the glenoid labrum occur and must not be mistaken for pathology, including a cord-like middle glenohumeral ligament (MGHL), sublabral foramen, sublabral foramen plus cord-like MGHL, and a Buford complex, which consists of an absent anterosuperior labrum and cord-like MGHL. Dynamic stabilizers consist of the periscapular muscles, biceps tendon, rotator interval, and rotator cuff muscles (supraspinatus, infraspinatus, teres minor, subscapularis). The rotator cuff muscles provide dynamic stability by compressing the humeral head against the glenoid.

At the rotator interval, the capsule is reinforced externally by the coracohumeral ligament (CHL) and internally by the superior glenohumeral ligament (SGHL) and traversed by the intra-articular portion of the long head of the biceps tendon [13]. The interval lies between the anterior margin of the supraspinatus and superior margin of the subscapularis tendon [13]. The intra-articular portion of the biceps tendon and the biceps pulley system lie within the rotator interval [13].

On ultrasound evaluation, the posterior GH joint is evaluated using a liner array transducer with the patient seated and the shoulder in neutral rotation. A lower frequency curvilinear array transducer may be necessary in patients with a large or more muscular body habitus. The transducer is placed in an oblique axial plane with the lateral end of the probe angled superiorly toward the humeral head just inferior to the scapular spine. The GH joint is visualized deep to the central tendon of the infraspinatus (Fig. 5.19). The articulation between the humeral head and glenoid should be evaluated from proximally under the acromion to distally to the humeral surgical neck. The posterior glenoid labrum can also be visualized and can be made more conspicuous with shoulder internal and external rotation.

The anterior GH joint and rotator interval are evaluated with the patient in a modified Crass position and the transducer in short axis to the

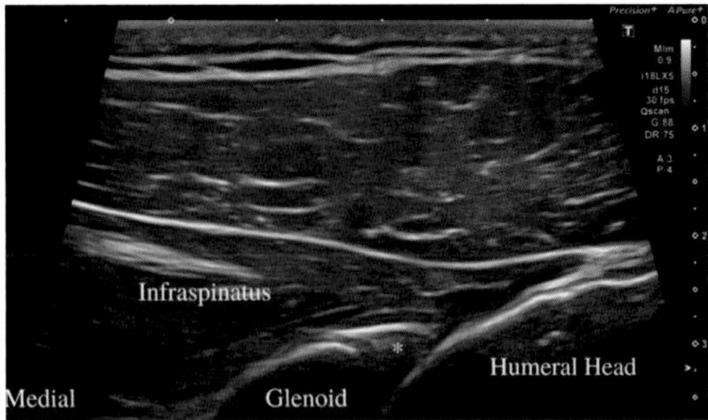

Fig. 5.19 Posterior glenohumeral joint. The posterior articulation the humeral head laterally with the glenoid, medially. The infraspinatus is visualized superficial to the joint space, and the glenoid labrum (*) is visualized as a hyperechoic triangular-appearing structure contiguous with the glenoid

proximal long head of the biceps tendon. The SGHL is located at the subscapularis side of the biceps brachii tendon with fibers merging with the CHL that lies superficial to the biceps tendon. The supraspinatus tendon lies posterolateral to the biceps tendon at the rotator interval, and the hypoechoic ligament, which separates them, should not be misinterpreted as a tendon tear [122]. (Fig. 5.2).

Pathology

A glenoid labral tear can occur secondary to trauma or repetitive microtrauma of overhead activities (SLAP). A labral tear is described by its location and can occur concomitantly with internal impingement, glenohumeral internal rotation deficit (GIRD), rotator cuff tears, and scapular dyskinesis. Ultrasound can be a highly specific tool to identify a posterior labral tear (98%), although it is not highly sensitive (63%) [123]. There is a substantial agreement between sonoarthrography and MR arthrography for the diagnosis of posterior labral tears [124]. Glenohumeral joint injection can be both diagnostic (using anesthetic) and therapeutic for labral injuries [125].

Ultrasound can be applied to accurately evaluate the shoulder after an acute dislocation or subluxation and has been shown to have 100% accuracy in several studies in identifying the characteristic hypoechoic or anechoic interval between the humeral head and the glenoid [126, 127]. Ultrasound can also identify a Hill-Sachs lesion and dynamically visualize engagement of the humeral lesion within the glenoid rim, an indication for surgical evaluation [128].

GH joint arthritis affects up to 32.8% of those over 60 years old and can develop after shoulder trauma, in the setting of rotator cuff degeneration, or secondary to rheumatoid arthritis [129]. Findings on ultrasound can include marginal osteophyte formation and joint space narrowing. Nonsurgical management of GH osteoarthritis includes activity moderation and modification, NSAIDs, injection therapies, and physical therapy (PT) focused on periscapular strengthening and stretching [130, 131] (1, 12. Surgical interventions can consist of debridement and capsular release, or a type of shoulder replacement) [131–133].

Adhesive capsulitis is characterized by limited range of motion (ROM) followed by shoulder pain. Shoulder external rotation is most commonly affected. It can be idiopathic or can be associated with diabetes mellitus, trauma, and immobilization. It is characterized by three clinical stages (Table 5.3). The most sensitive and specific ultrasound finding reported is a diminished sliding movement of the supraspinatus tendon beneath the acromion with shoulder abduction, which has a 91% sensitivity, 100% specificity, and 92% accuracy for detecting adhesive capsulitis [134]. Abnormal hypoechogenicity and hyperemia at the rotator interval have been demonstrated in up to 86% of patients with adhesive capsulitis [135]. Thickening of the coracohumeral ligament (3 mm vs 1.39 mm in controls) is also seen [136].

Table 5.3 Clinical stages of adhesive capsulitis

Clinical stage	Description
Freezing/Painful	Gradual onset of diffuse pain (6 weeks–9 months)
Frozen/Stiff	Decreased ROM affecting activities of daily living (4–9 months or more)
Thawing	Gradual return of motion (5–26 months)

Nonsurgical management of GH adhesive capsulitis can include PT, extracorporeal shock wave therapy, corticosteroid injections, and capsular hydrodistension. Most patients will see complete resolution of pain and full return of glenohumeral motion after conservative treatment and time [137–142]. Manipulation under anesthesia or arthroscopic capsular release can be considered in refractory cases [137].

Interventional Procedures

In patients with GH joint arthritis, injection of HA has had shown mixed outcomes. Several small retrospective case series [143–147] and one retrospective case-control study [148] reported a significant reduction in pain and improvement in function in patients with GH arthritis treated with HA, but two large randomized controlled trial did not show superiority of HA to placebo [149, 150]. The majority of the studies utilized palpation guidance for the injections, which may confound the results [144, 146–150]. Only one study reports the injection of PRP into the GH joint, and this was in the context of GH adhesive capsulitis. Cell-based therapies have limited evidence in treating patients with GH joint arthritis. One case series of 115 patients with GH joint arthritis with or without RTC tear showed improved pain and physical function for up to 2 years following bone marrow aspirate concentrate (BMAC) injection, but the study was limited by heterogeneity in the patient population and lack of a control group [151]. A case series of the use of microfragmented adipose tissue (MFAT) to treat 20 patients with GH arthritis and concomitant rotator cuff tear resulted in improvements in pain and function at 12 months [152].

Although orthobiologic injections into the GH joint are sometimes implemented to treat glenoid labral pathology, there are no PubMed indexed studies describing or supporting PRP injections to treat labral pathologies [153].

Ultrasound-guided interventional procedures are commonly performed to treat GH adhesive capsulitis. Corticosteroid injections are generally accepted as a mainstay of treatment with short-term efficacy, although a high degree of variance is seen in the dose of corticosteroid administered, location of injection, and performance of concomitant procedures at the time of steroid injection [154–159]. Several studies have compared the clinical efficacy of anterior (rotator interval) to posterior GH joint injections in patients with frozen shoulder with two studies showing no clinical difference [160, 161] and one showing faster and more significant improvement with steroid injection into the rotator interval [162]. Hydrodistension of the joint capsule with a high volume of injectate is commonly used to treat adhesive capsulitis, but one meta-analysis of 12 studies reported that it had only a small, clinically insignificant effect [140]. The use of orthobiologics to treat adhesive capsulitis is emerging, with one study demonstrating that injection of a single dose of intra-articular PRP was more effective than intra-articular corticosteroid injection on improving pain, function, and ROM [163] and was more effective than procaine on pain and function [164]. Some advocate for the use of orthobiologics rather than corticosteroids to treat adhesive capsulitis in diabetics to minimize blood sugar elevation, but this has not been specifically reported in the literature.

The use of ultrasound guidance greatly improves the accuracy of GH joint injections relative to palpation-guided injections. Palpation-guided anterior GH joint injections are 26–95.7% accurate [165, 166] and posterior GH joint injections 42–96% accurate [92, 167–169]. Ultrasound guidance of injections to the GH joint improves accuracy to 92% with an anterior approach (rotator interval) [170] and to 92.5–100% with a posterior approach [168, 170–173].

Procedural protocol: Posterior approach to GH joint

- Patient position – Lateral decubitus with the affected side up. The arm should be in neutral or slight internal rotation.
- Transducer selection – Low-frequency, curvilinear (>10 MHz), or midrange linear array transducer
- Transducer position – Short axis to the joint in the oblique axial plane. The transducer should be placed just lateral to the inferior scapular spine.
- Needle selection – 25-gauge, 2.5-inch (or longer if larger body habitus)
- Injectate selection – Anesthetize with lidocaine or Marcaine. Inject steroid or orthobiologic (most commonly PRP). Typically inject 3–5 mL of fluid or > 10 mL if treating adhesive capsulitis.
- Needle trajectory and target structure – In-plane, lateral to medial approach into to the GH joint. Needle will traverse through the infraspinatus musculotendinous unit. Greater glenohumeral internal rotation and cross-body adduction will pull the infraspinatus tendon anteriorly, ensuring that the needle traverses more through musculature than tendon. Ensure that the needle tip is deep to the infraspinatus and glenoid labrum, adjacent to the hypoechoic articular cartilage of the humeral head
- Pearls/pitfalls
  - Take care to identify to not to injure the glenoid labrum.
  - The injectate should flow readily into the large, accommodating GH joint. Visible accumulation of injectate in one area suggests extraarticular placement and should prompt redirection of the needle tip.
  - Placement of the needle superficial and medial to the GH joint poses risk of injury to neurovascular structures in spinoglenoid notch.

Procedural protocol: Anterior approach to GH joint at rotator interval

- Patient position – Supine. The arm adducted and in slight GH external rotation.
- Transducer selection – High-frequency linear array transducer (>10MHz)
- Transducer position – Anatomic axial plane over the rotator interval with the long head of the biceps tendon in short axis.
- Needle selection – 27-gauge 1.5-inch; or 25-gauge 2.5-inch
- Injectate selection – Anesthetic with lidocaine or Marcaine. Inject steroid or orthobiologic.

Volume of about 5 mL, or > 10 mL if treating adhesive capsulitis.
- Needle trajectory and target – In-plane, lateral to medial approach into the space deep to the coracohumeral ligament and superficial to the LHBT.
- Pearls/pitfalls.
  - Slight external rotation of the arm improves visualization of the long head of the biceps tendon and structures of the rotator interval.

Spinoglenoid Notch

Anatomy and Ultrasound Evaluation

The spinoglenoid notch is formed between the lateral side of the scapular spine and the posterior part of the glenoid, and the spinoglenoid ligament spans these two bony structures of the scapula [174]. The suprascapular nerve traverses the spinoglenoid notch before innervating infraspinatus. The suprascapular artery and vein course lateral to the suprascapular nerve in the spinoglenoid notch and occupy 68.5% of the suprascapular notch [175].

During sonographic evaluation, the spinoglenoid notch is localized medial to the posterior GH joint by translating the transducer medial and from the joint and rotating the medial end of the transducer slightly cephalad (Fig. 5.20). Color doppler should be applied to identify the vascular structures within the spinoglenoid notch. Dynamic engorgement of the vein when the arm is in external rotation should not be mistaken for a spinoglenoid notch cyst.

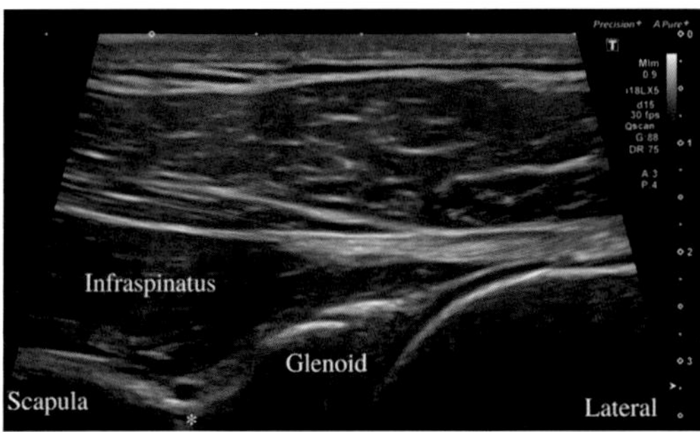

Fig. 5.20 The spinoglenoid notch (*) is visualized between the scapular spine medially and the glenoid laterally. The suprascapular nerve lies within the spinoglenoid notch and infraspinatus superficial to that nerve

Pathology

Compression of the suprascapular nerve in the spinoglenoid notch results in infraspinatus denervation. Neural injury can be secondary to a spinoglenoid notch ganglion cyst [176, 177], GH paralabral cyst secondary to posteroinferior glenoid labral tear (most common) [178, 179], or traction injury, as seen in volleyball players [180]. Cysts can be difficult to visualize on ultrasound due to their deep location. Placing the ipsilateral hand on the contralateral shoulder may make spinoglenoid notch more superficial and improve diagnostic assessment. Paralabral cysts are most commonly visualized in the superficial region of the spinoglenoid notch. If denervation has occurred, the infraspinatus muscle will appear atrophied and hyperechoic relative to the ipsilateral supraspinatus and to the contralateral infraspinatus. The volume of a paralabral cyst has been shown to directly correlate with the degree of infraspinatus atrophy [179]. Infraspinatus denervation can be confirmed with electrodiagnostic studies. Varicosities and enlarged spinoglenoid notch veins are also seen at the spinoglenoid notch. Veins are not stationary and will dynamically vary in size with different shoulder movements. Color Doppler should be used to rule out the presence of blood flow in any cystic-appearing structure.

Interventional Procedures

A sonographically lateral-to-medial spinoglenoid notch paralabral cyst aspiration can have up to an 86% success rate for pain reduction [181]. The use of orthobiologics to treat pathology of the spinoglenoid notch region has not been reported.

Procedural protocol: Spinoglenoid notch injection or cyst aspiration

- Patient position – Lateral decubitus with the affected side up. The arm should be in neutral or slight internal rotation.
- Transducer selection – Low-frequency, curvilinear (>10 MHz)
- Transducer position – Just inferior and parallel to the lateral edge of the spine of the scapula. The medial end of the transducer should be rotated slightly cephalad to optimize visualization of the spinoglenoid notch.
- Needle selection – 27-gauge, 1.5-inch; 25-gauge, 2.5-inch (or longer if larger body habitus) needle can be used for local anesthetic. An 18-gauge 2.5- or 3.5-inch needle should be used for aspiration of a cyst.
- Injectate selection – Anesthetize with lidocaine or Marcaine. Inject steroid or orthobiologic (most commonly PRP). Typically inject 3–5 mL.
- Needle trajectory and target structure – In-plane, medial to lateral approach to the spinoglenoid notch cyst.
- Pearls/pitfalls
  - Color Doppler should be used to rule out the presence of blood flow in any cystic-appearing structure to ensure that the targeted structure is not vasculature.
  - If one wishes to both aspirate/inject in the spinoglenoid notch and to inject into the posterior GH joint, the same needle entry point can be used by slightly withdrawing the needle from the spinoglenoid notch and redirecting the needle more steeply to the more lateral GH joint.

Suprascapular Notch

Anatomy and Ultrasound Evaluation

The suprascapular notch is a U- or V-shaped notch in the lateral body scapula within the supraspinous fossa, which is located just medial to the base of the coracoid and about 3 cm medial from the supraglenoid tubercle [182]. Table 5.4 details the six different anatomical classifications of the notch character [183]. The superior transverse scapular ligament traverses superficial to the notch and forms a roof to a foramen through which through suprascapular nerve travels. The suprascapular artery travels superficial to the ligament [183].

Table 5.4 Suprascapular notch anatomy

Type	Rate of occurrence	Description
1	6–22%	Notch is absent. The superior border forms a wide depression from the medial angle to the coracoid process
2	8–31%	Notch is a blunted V-shaped occupying the middle third of the superior boarder
3	29–60%	Notch is U-shaped with nearly parallel margins
4	3–13%	Notch is V-shaped and very small
5	6–18%	Notch is minimal and U-shaped with a partially ossified ligament
6	2–6%	Notch is a foramen since the ligament is completely ossified

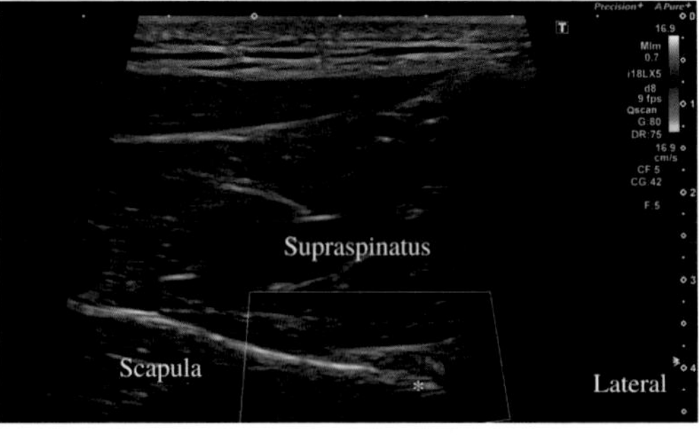

Fig. 5.21 Longitudinal view of the suprascapular notch (*)

Ultrasound evaluation of the suprascapular notch is performed using a curvilinear array transducer with the patient in the seated position. The transducer is placed in long axis to the supraspinatus tendon within the supraspinous fossa just cephalad to the scapular spine. The transducer is angled in a caudad direction and oriented almost directly in a coronal plane, which facilitates visualization of the notch (Fig. 5.21). Depth and focus should be adjusted to optimize the image of the deep suprascapular notch as the muscular bulk of lateral trapezius and supraspinatus can vary greatly between individuals [184].

Pathology

Compression of the suprascapular nerve at the suprascapular notch can occur secondary to a glenohumeral paralabral cyst, a space-occupying lesion, or a massive supraspinatus tear or from repetitive traction related to overhead sports [185]. The notch type (V-shaped is more commonly associated with pathology) and distance from the glenoid may be correlated with injury risk [186, 187]. Pathologic compression can result in infraspinatus atrophy and possibly supraspinatus atrophy, and patients may complain of shoulder pain, demonstrate arm abduction and external rotation weakness, and maintain intact sensation. Ultrasound evaluation should assess for supraspinatus and infraspinatus atrophy, manifested as muscular hyperechogenicity relative to adjacent or superficial musculature and loss of muscular bulk. A paralabral cyst or other space-occupying lesion may be visualized within or adjacent to the suprascapular notch as a rounded or oval hypoechoic lesion with well-defined margins that remains relatively fixed with dynamic shoulder movements [184].

Interventional Procedures

The suprascapular nerve provides sensation to the posterior GH joint and can be blocked prior to surgical procedures or in the setting of severe GH joint pathology not amenable to surgery. The accuracy of ultrasound-guided suprascapular notch injections for suprascapular neural blockade has been reported to be 100% in one cadaveric study [188]. However, another study utilizing EMG current intensity reported that only 18.5% of suprascapular nerve injections were believed to be close enough to the nerve; however, it could be reasonably postulated that the spread of anesthetic injectate or other medication could still result in a sufficient neural blockade [189]. Other studies have shown no difference between ultrasound-guided and landmark-guided suprascapular nerve blocks [190, 191]. There are no reports of the injection of orthobiologics agents near the suprascapular notch.

Procedural protocol: Suprascapular nerve block at the suprascapular notch

- Patient position – Seated with ipsilateral hand placed on contralateral shoulder.
- Transducer selection – Low-frequency, curvilinear (<10 MHz)
- Transducer position – Parallel to the spine of the scapula over the supraspinatus fossa with US beam angled caudally to visualize the suprascapular notch.
- Needle selection – 25-gauge, 3.5-inch needle
- Injectate selection – Anesthetize with lidocaine or Marcaine. Inject anesthetic or steroid. Typically inject 3–5 mL.
- Needle trajectory and target – In-plane, medial to lateral (preferred) adjacent to the suprascapular nerve within the suprascapular notch and deep to the superior transverse scapular ligament. Injection can also be performed lateral to medial; however, this requires a much steeper angle of injection, which decrease clarity of needle visualization and makes needle tracking more challenging.
- Pearls/pitfalls
  - Toe-ing in of the lateral end of the transducer or application of a beam-steering mode will improve needle visualization.
  - Color Doppler should be applied to identify the suprascapular artery above the superior transverse scapular ligament and to plan an injection course that ensures its safety.

Quadrilateral Space

Anatomy and Ultrasound Evaluation

The axillary nerve and posterior circumflex humeral artery course from the axilla anteriorly to the posterior shoulder through the quadrilateral space, which is bordered superiorly by the teres minor, inferiorly by the teres major, medially by the long head of triceps, and laterally by the humeral surgical neck. Beyond the quadrilateral space, the axillary nerve innervates the deltoid and teres minor and provides sensation from the lateral arm.

A linear transducer is used to evaluate the quadrilateral space with the patient in a prone or sitting position and the arm internally rotated. A posterior longitudinal view of the humeral head and surgical neck is obtained with the teres minor visualized transversely. The posterior circumflex humeral artery and axillary nerve can be visualized in short axis at the inferior boarder of the teres minor at the humerus. Tracing those neurovascular structures more proximally along their course and medially, the humerus falls off and then the true quadrilateral space is visualized (Fig. 5.22). Translating more laterally, the posterior humeral circumflex artery and axillary nerve are distinctly visualized adjacent to humerus (Fig. 5.23). The transducer can then be rotated 90 degrees to evaluate the neurovascular structures in long axis.

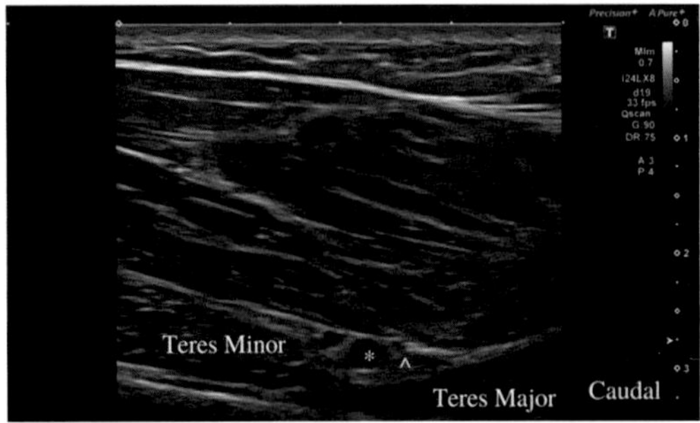

Fig. 5.22 The posterior humeral circumflex artery (*) and axillary nerve (^) are visualized coursing between the teres minor and teres major within the quadrilateral space

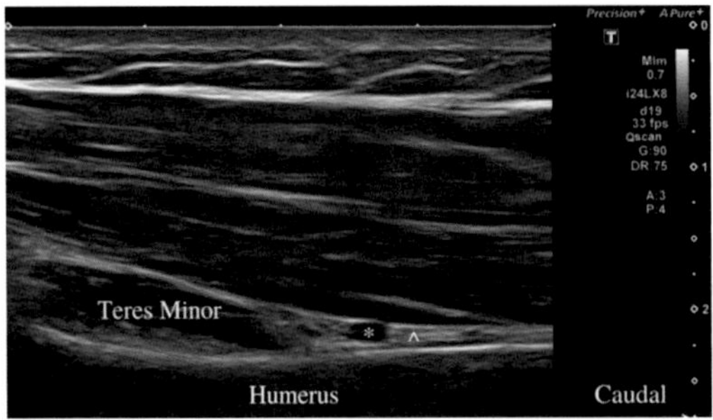

Fig. 5.23 The posterior humeral circumflex artery (*) and axillary nerve (^) are visualized adjacent to the posterior humerus, caudal from the teres minor

Pathology

Quadrilateral space syndrome (QSS) results from compression or traction of the axillary nerve (neurogenic), the posterior circumflex humeral artery (PCHA) (vascular), or both structures as they traverse the quadrilateral space. QSS is most common in volleyball [192–195], baseball [137, 196–198] (17, 18, 20, 21, 22), and swimming athletes, who perform repetitive overhead movements of abduction and external rotation [199]. Additional etiologies include mechanical compression secondary to improper crutch use or cast application, fibrous bands [200], and paralabral cysts [179], or iatrogenic injury during shoulder arthroscopy [201]. QSS with involvement of the axillary nerve will result in selective atrophy of the teres minor and sparing of deltoid, as axillary innervation to deltoid occurs proximal from the quadrilateral space. Isolated teres minor weakness and shoulder external rotation can be difficult to diagnose clinically. Ultrasound can identify isolated teres minor atrophy with an intact distal tendon, manifested as relative loss of bulk and muscular hyperechogenicity compared to the adjacent infraspinatus [184]. Ultrasound can also be used to dynamically evaluate the quadrilateral space compressive lesions or masses.

Interventional Procedures

Diagnostic axillary neural blockade within the quadrilateral space is the most common intervention at this location [202]. There are no studies to date describing the injection of an orthobiologic agent in the management of quadrilateral space syndrome. The accuracy of injection into the quadrilateral space has not been described.

Procedural protocol: Quadrilateral space/axillary perineural injection

- Patient position – Lateral decubitus on contralateral side. The affected side should be up and the affected arm fully abducted with the patient's hand resting on the back of their head.

- Transducer selection – High-frequency, linear (>10 MHz)
- Transducer position – In the axial plane, and mid-humerus. Find the long head of the triceps at the spiral groove and follow the triceps proximally into the axilla to the humeral head. Visualize the axillary nerve anterior to the inferior joint capsule.
- Needle selection – 25-gauge 2-inch needle (or larger depending on body habitus)
- Injectate selection – Anesthetize with lidocaine or Marcaine. Inject anesthetic or steroid. Typically inject 3–5 mL.
- Needle trajectory and target – In-plane, posterolateral to anteromedial through the triceps long head and targeting the axillary nerve and a perineural injection.
- Pearls/pitfalls:
  - The patient can be positioned prone, and a needle trajectory through the teres major can be taken, rather than a lateral decubitus position and approach through the long head of the triceps.

Pectoralis Major

Anatomy and Ultrasound Evaluation

The pectoralis major is a broad muscle in the anterior chest and shoulder that functions as a strong adductor and internal rotator of the shoulder. It has three heads of origin and a lateral insertion to the lateral lip of the humeral bicipital groove. The clavicular head originates from the anteromedial two thirds of the clavicle and superior sternum. The sternal head originates from the inferior sternum and costal cartilage of the medial first through fifth ribs. The abdominal head originates from the fifth and sixth ribs. Each head forms a lamina, and those laminae fuse to form a trilaminar distal tendon that twists 90 degrees just before it's insertion on the lateral lip of the bicipital groove, such that the clavicular head inserts more distally and the sternal and abdominal heads more proximally on the humerus [203]. The tendon measures about 5 cm in medial to lateral length and 4 cm in craniocaudal width [204]. The tendon of the pectoralis major has a unique U shape with the anterior fibers coming from the clavicular head and superior sternal segments and the posterior fibers coming from the inferior sternal and abdominal segments [204].

Ultrasound examination of the pectoralis major tendon at its insertion is most commonly carried out using a linear transducer with the arm abducted and externally rotated while the patient is supine. The transducer is placed in the anatomic axial plane over the bicipital groove with the bicep tendon in short axis. The transducer is then moved distally, and the pectoralis major will come into view as it courses from medial to lateral. It can be visualized in long axis coursing superficial to the coracobrachialis and biceps on its way to insert on the lateral edge of the bicipital groove (Fig. 5.24). The integrity of the tendon and the entire craniocaudal and mediolateral course should be evaluated. The tendon should have a fibrillar pattern and the superficial clavicular/sternal head and the deeper sternal/abdominal heads can be evaluated [205] (Fig. 5.25). The transducer can be moved medially to evaluate the muscle bulk as well. The muscle can be followed all the way to its origin on the clavicle, sternum, and ribs, but this is less commonly performed.

Pathology

Traumatic rupture of the pectoralis major is an uncommon sports injury that typically occurs while performing a bench press during maximal

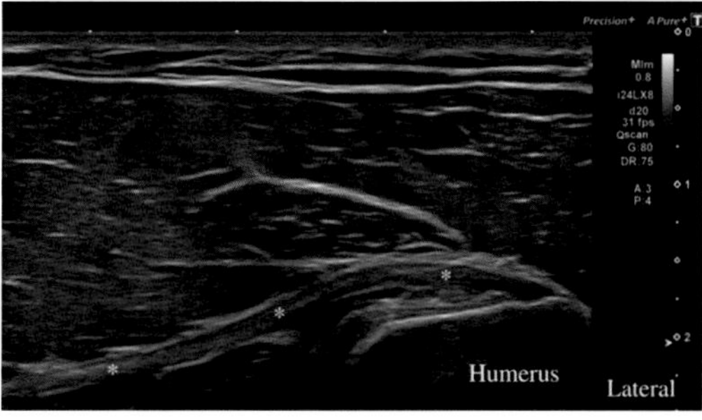

Fig. 5.24 Longitudinal view of the distal pectoralis major tendon (*) inserting onto humerus

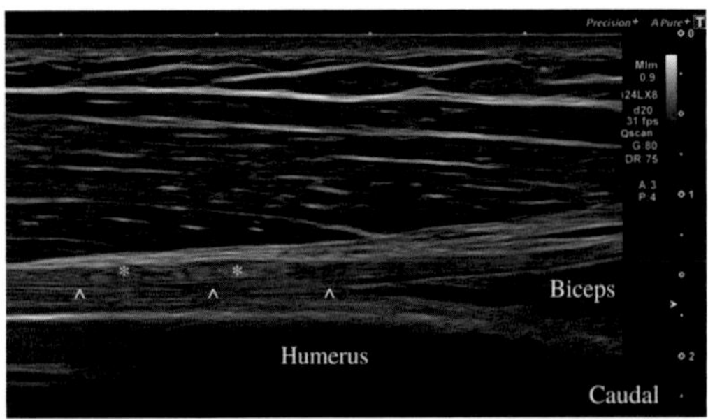

Fig. 5.25 Transverse view of the distal pectoralis major tendon (*). The long head biceps brachii tendon (^) is visualized deep to the pectoralis major tendon

Table 5.5 Anatomic classification of pectoralis major tears [209]

Type	Injury Pattern
I	Contusion or sprain
II	Partial tear
III	Complete tear
III-A	at muscle origin
III-B	at muscle belly
III-C	at myotendinous junction
III-D	at tendinous insertion

eccentric contraction with the arm in forced external rotation with extension and abduction of the humerus [206, 207]. Tear occur most commonly in active men between the ages of 20–40 [208]. Tears have historically been classified by the system described by Tietjen in 1980 (Table 5.5) [209]. Rupture most commonly occurs at the distal insertion of the inferior fibers of the sternocostal head, followed by the superior fibers of the sternocostal head or the myotendinous junction [206]. In cases of rupture, the tendon will either have a wavy appearance (if tear occurs in the muscle or near the myotendinous junction) or will not be visualized (distal tear), and edema or fluid can be seen anterior to the coracobrachialis muscle. The tendon of the pectoralis major is a stabilizer to the long head of the biceps, so when it is ruptured, the biceps tendon will be elevated off of the humerus [184]. With time, adhesions may form a pseudotendon between the retracted muscle and stump of the actual tendon [210]. Anatomic surgical repair results in better outcomes than conservative treatment alone [211].

Procedural protocol: Pectoralis major

Technique #1

- Patient position – Supine, shoulder held at side and externally rotated
- Transducer selection – High-frequency, linear (>10 MHz)
- Transducer position – In the axial plane just distal to the deltopectoral interval. Find the biceps brachii long head in its transverse plane, and track it to its myotendinous junction. Just cephalad to biceps long head myotendinous junction, the pectoralis major tendon is visualized as a laminar-appearing tendon in its longitudinal axis to its humeral insertion.
- Needle selection – 25-gauge 2-inch needle (or larger depending on body habitus and muscularity)
- Injectate selection – Anesthetize with lidocaine or Marcaine. Inject anesthetic or steroid. Typically inject 3–5 mL.
- Needle trajectory and target – In-plane, lateral to medial in plane with the tendon at its humeral insertion to perform a peritendinous injection.

Technique #

- Patient position – Supine, shoulder held at side and externally rotated
- Transducer selection – High-frequency, linear (>10 MHz)
- Transducer position – In the anatomic sagittal plane just distal to the deltopectoral interval. Find the biceps brachii long head in its longitudinal plane, and track it to its myotendinous junction. It is here the it sits deep to the tendon of pectoralis major. This plane can be translated medially to identify and to target a pectoralis major myotendinous injury.
- Needle selection – 25-gauge 2-inch needle (or larger depending on body habitus and muscularity)
- Injectate selection – Anesthetize with lidocaine or Marcaine. Inject anesthetic or steroid. Typically inject 3–5 mL.
- Needle trajectory and target – Cephalad to caudad, in an anatomic sagittal plane transverse to the pectoralis major.

References

1. Buck FM, et al. Degeneration of the long biceps tendon: comparison of MRI with gross anatomy and histology. AJR Am J Roentgenol. 2009;193(5):1367–75.
2. Buck FM, et al. Magnetic resonance histologic correlation in rotator cuff tendons. J Magn Reson Imaging. 2010;32(1):165–72.
3. Jacobson JA, et al. Full-thickness and partial-thickness supraspinatus tendon tears: value of US signs in diagnosis. Radiology. 2004;230(1):234–42.
4. Skendzel JG, et al. Long head of biceps brachii tendon evaluation: accuracy of preoperative ultrasound. AJR Am J Roentgenol. 2011;197(4):942–8.
5. Jacobson J. Fundamentals of musculoskeletal ultrasound. 3rd ed. Philadelphia: Elsevier, Inc.; 2018.
6. Bianchi S, Martinoli C. Ultrasound of the musculoskeletal system. Berlin: Springer Science & Business Media; 2007.
7. Nwawka OK, et al. Volume and movement affecting flow of Injectate between the biceps tendon sheath and Glenohumeral joint: a cadaveric study. AJR Am J Roentgenol. 2016;206(2):373–7.
8. Hollister MS, et al. Association of sonographically detected subacromial/subdeltoid bursal effusion and intraarticular fluid with rotator cuff tear. AJR Am J Roentgenol. 1995;165(3):605–8.
9. Beall DP, et al. Association of biceps tendon tears with rotator cuff abnormalities: degree of correlation with tears of the anterior and superior portions of the rotator cuff. AJR Am J Roentgenol. 2003;180(3):633–9.
10. Catapano M, et al. Effectiveness of dextrose Prolotherapy for rotator cuff tendinopathy: a systematic review. PM R. 2020;12(3):288–300.
11. Seven MM, et al. Effectiveness of prolotherapy in the treatment of chronic rotator cuff lesions. Orthop Traumatol Surg Res. 2017;103(3):427–33.
12. Ibrahim VM, et al. Use of platelet rich plasma for the treatment of bicipital tendinopathy in spinal cord injury:: a pilot study. Top Spinal Cord Inj Rehabil. 2012;18(1):77–8.
13. Petchprapa CN, et al. The rotator interval: a review of anatomy, function, and normal and abnormal MRI appearance. AJR Am J Roentgenol. 2010;195(3):567–76.
14. Gazzillo GP, et al. Accuracy of palpating the long head of the biceps tendon: an ultrasonographic study. PM R. 2011;3(11):1035–40.
15. Aly AR, Rajasekaran S, Ashworth N. Ultrasound-guided shoulder girdle injections are more accurate and more effective than landmark-guided injections: a systematic review and meta-analysis. Br J Sports Med. 2015;49(16):1042–9.
16. Hashiuchi T, et al. Accuracy of the biceps tendon sheath injection: ultrasound-guided or unguided injection? A randomized controlled trial. J Shoulder Elb Surg. 2011;20(7):1069–73.
17. Yiannakopoulos CK, et al. Ultrasound-guided versus palpation-guided corticosteroid injections for tendinosis of the long head of the biceps: a randomized comparative study. Skelet Radiol. 2020;49(4):585–91.
18. Kim SY, et al. Three-dimensional study of the musculotendinous architecture of supraspinatus and its functional correlations. Clin Anat. 2007;20(6):648–55.
19. Vahlensieck M, Haack K a, Schmidt HM. Two portions of the supraspinatus muscle: a new finding about the muscles macroscopy by dissection and magnetic resonance imaging. Surg Radiol Anat. 1994;16(1):101–4.
20. Ferri M, et al. Sonography of full-thickness supraspinatus tears: comparison of patient positioning technique with surgical correlation. AJR Am J Roentgenol. 2005;184(1):180–4.
21. Ruotolo C, Fow JE, Nottage WM. The supraspinatus footprint: an anatomic study of the supraspinatus insertion. Arthroscopy. 2004;20(3):246–9.
22. Bretzke CA, et al. Ultrasonography of the rotator cuff. Normal and pathologic anatomy. Investig Radiol. 1985;20(3):311–5.
23. Karthikeyan S, et al. Ultrasound dimensions of the rotator cuff in young healthy adults. J Shoulder Elb Surg. 2014;23(8):1107–12.
24. Kim K, et al. Ultrasound dimensions of the rotator cuff and other associated structures in Korean healthy adults. J Korean Med Sci. 2016;31(9):1472–8.
25. Schaeffeler C, et al. Tears at the rotator cuff footprint: prevalence and imaging characteristics in 305 MR arthrograms of the shoulder. Eur Radiol. 2011;21(7):1477–84.
26. de Jesus JO, et al. Accuracy of MRI, MR arthrography, and ultrasound in the diagnosis of rotator cuff tears: a meta-analysis. AJR Am J Roentgenol. 2009;192(6):1701–7.
27. Roy JS, et al. Diagnostic accuracy of ultrasonography, MRI and MR arthrography in the characterisation of rotator cuff disorders: a systematic review and meta-analysis. Br J Sports Med. 2015;49(20):1316–28.
28. Kim HM, et al. Location and initiation of degenerative rotator cuff tears: an analysis of three hundred and sixty shoulders. J Bone Joint Surg Am. 2010;92(5):1088–96.
29. van Holsbeeck MT, et al. US depiction of partial-thickness tear of the rotator cuff. Radiology. 1995;197(2):443–6.
30. Chianca V, et al. Rotator cuff calcific tendinopathy: from diagnosis to treatment. Acta Biomed. 2018;89(1-s):186–96.
31. Sansone V, et al. Calcific tendinopathy of the shoulder: clinical perspectives into the mechanisms, pathogenesis, and treatment. Orthop Res Rev. 2018;10:63–72.
32. Uhthoff HK, Loehr JW. Calcific tendinopathy of the rotator cuff: pathogenesis, diagnosis, and management. J Am Acad Orthop Surg. 1997;5(4):183–91.

33. Hackett L, et al. Are the symptoms of calcific tendinitis due to Neoinnervation and/or neovascularization? J Bone Joint Surg Am. 2016;98(3):186–92.
34. Chiou HJ, et al. The role of high-resolution ultrasonography in management of calcific tendonitis of the rotator cuff. Ultrasound Med Biol. 2001;27(6):735–43.
35. Farin PU. Consistency of rotator-cuff calcifications. Observations on plain radiography, sonography, computed tomography, and at needle treatment. Investig Radiol. 1996;31(5):300–4.
36. Gärtner J, Heyer A. Calcific tendinitis of the shoulder. Orthopade. 1995;24(3):284–302.
37. Molé D, et al. Results of endoscopic treatment of non-broken tendinopathies of the rotator cuff. 2. Calcifications of the rotator cuff. Rev Chir Orthop Reparatrice Appar Mot. 1993;79(7):532–41.
38. Dean BJ, et al. The risks and benefits of glucocorticoid treatment for tendinopathy: a systematic review of the effects of local glucocorticoid on tendon. Semin Arthritis Rheum. 2014;43(4):570–6.
39. Castricini R, et al. Platelet-rich plasma augmentation for arthroscopic rotator cuff repair: a randomized controlled trial. Am J Sports Med. 2011;39(2):258–65.
40. Flury M, et al. Does pure platelet-rich plasma affect postoperative clinical outcomes after arthroscopic rotator cuff repair? A randomized controlled trial. Am J Sports Med. 2016;44(8):2136–46.
41. Jo CH, et al. Does platelet-rich plasma accelerate recovery after rotator cuff repair? A prospective cohort study. Am J Sports Med. 2011;39(10):2082–90.
42. Malavolta EA, et al. Platelet-rich plasma in rotator cuff repair: a prospective randomized study. Am J Sports Med. 2014;42(10):2446–54.
43. Randelli P, et al. Platelet rich plasma in arthroscopic rotator cuff repair: a prospective RCT study, 2-year follow-up. J Shoulder Elb Surg. 2011;20(4):518–28.
44. Carr JB 2nd, Rodeo SA. The role of biologic agents in the management of common shoulder pathologies: current state and future directions. J Shoulder Elb Surg. 2019;28(11):2041–52.
45. Zhang Q, et al. Are platelet-rich products necessary during the arthroscopic repair of full-thickness rotator cuff tears: a meta-analysis. PLoS One. 2013;8(7):e69731.
46. Wang A, et al. Do postoperative platelet-rich plasma injections accelerate early tendon healing and functional recovery after arthroscopic supraspinatus repair? A randomized controlled trial. Am J Sports Med. 2015;43(6):1430–7.
47. Moraes VY, et al. Platelet-rich therapies for musculoskeletal soft tissue injuries. Cochrane Database Syst Rev. 2013;12:Cd010071.
48. Schwitzguebel AJ, et al. Efficacy of platelet-rich plasma for the treatment of interstitial supraspinatus tears: a double-blinded, randomized controlled trial. Am J Sports Med. 2019;47(8):1885–92.
49. Rha DW, et al. Comparison of the therapeutic effects of ultrasound-guided platelet-rich plasma injection and dry needling in rotator cuff disease: a randomized controlled trial. Clin Rehabil. 2013;27(2):113–22.
50. Kesikburun S, et al. Platelet-rich plasma injections in the treatment of chronic rotator cuff tendinopathy: a randomized controlled trial with 1-year follow-up. Am J Sports Med. 2013;41(11):2609–16.
51. Lin MT, et al. Comparative effectiveness of injection therapies in rotator cuff tendinopathy: a systematic review, pairwise and network meta-analysis of randomized controlled trials. Arch Phys Med Rehabil. 2019;100(2):336–349.e15.
52. Mautner K, et al. A call for a standard classification system for future biologic research: the rationale for new PRP nomenclature. PM R. 2015;7(4 Suppl):S53–s59.
53. Kim SJ, et al. Effect of platelet-rich plasma on the degenerative rotator cuff tendinopathy according to the compositions. J Orthop Surg Res. 2019;14(1):408.
54. Cole B, et al. Ultrasound-guided injections for supraspinatus tendinopathy: corticosteroid versus glucose prolotherapy - a randomized controlled clinical trial. Shoulder Elbow. 2018;10(3):170–8.
55. George J, et al. Comparative effectiveness of ultrasound-guided Intratendinous Prolotherapy injection with conventional treatment to treat focal supraspinatus tendinosis. Scientifica (Cairo). 2018;2018:4384159.
56. Lin CL, Huang CC, Huang SW. Effects of hypertonic dextrose injection in chronic supraspinatus tendinopathy of the shoulder: a randomized placebo-controlled trial. Eur J Phys Rehabil Med. 2019;55(4):480–7.
57. Osti L, et al. Clinical evidence in the treatment of rotator cuff tears with hyaluronic acid. Muscles Ligaments Tendons J. 2015;5(4):270–5.
58. Cai YU, et al. Sodium hyaluronate and platelet-rich plasma for partial-thickness rotator cuff tears. Med Sci Sports Exerc. 2019;51(2):227–33.
59. Wu PT, et al. Intratendinous injection of hyaluronate induces acute inflammation: a possible detrimental effect. PLoS One. 2016;11(5):e0155424.
60. Kim SJ, et al. Effects of bone marrow aspirate concentrate and platelet-rich plasma on patients with partial tear of the rotator cuff tendon. J Orthop Surg Res. 2018;13(1):1.
61. Jo CH, et al. Intratendinous injection of autologous adipose tissue-derived mesenchymal stem cells for the treatment of rotator cuff disease: a first-in-human trial. Stem Cells. 2018;36(9):1441–50.
62. Finnoff JT, et al. Treatment of chronic tendinopathy with ultrasound-guided needle tenotomy and platelet-rich plasma injection. PM R. 2011;3(10):900–11.
63. Gatt DL, Charalambous CP. Ultrasound-guided barbotage for calcific tendonitis of the shoulder: a systematic review including 908 patients. Arthroscopy. 2014;30(9):1166–72.
64. de Witte PB, et al. Rotator cuff calcific tendinitis: ultrasound-guided needling and lavage versus subacromial corticosteroids: five-year outcomes of

a randomized controlled trial. Am J Sports Med. 2017;45(14):3305–14.
65. de Witte PB, et al. Calcific tendinitis of the rotator cuff: a randomized controlled trial of ultrasound-guided needling and lavage versus subacromial corticosteroids. Am J Sports Med. 2013;41(7):1665–73.
66. Morag Y, et al. The subscapularis: anatomy, injury, and imaging. Skelet Radiol. 2011;40(3):255–69.
67. Radas CB, Pieper HG. The coracoid impingement of the subscapularis tendon: a cadaver study. J Shoulder Elb Surg. 2004;13(2):154–9.
68. Navarro-Ledesma S, et al. Is coracohumeral distance associated with pain-function, and shoulder range of movement, in chronic anterior shoulder pain? BMC Musculoskelet Disord. 2017;18(1):136.
69. Sansone V, et al. Calcific tendinopathy of the rotator cuff: the correlation between pain and imaging features in symptomatic and asymptomatic female shoulders. Skelet Radiol. 2016;45(1):49–55.
70. Fessa CK, et al. Posterosuperior glenoid internal impingement of the shoulder in the overhead athlete: pathogenesis, clinical features and MR imaging findings. J Med Imaging Radiat Oncol. 2015;59(2):182–7.
71. Tirman PF, et al. Posterosuperior glenoid impingement of the shoulder: findings at MR imaging and MR arthrography with arthroscopic correlation. Radiology. 1994;193(2):431–6.
72. Friend J, et al. Teres minor innervation in the context of isolated muscle atrophy. Surg Radiol Anat. 2010;32(3):243–9.
73. Kang Y, et al. The pattern of idiopathic isolated teres minor atrophy with regard to its two-bundle anatomy. Skelet Radiol. 2019;48(3):363–74.
74. Beals TC, Harryman DT 2nd, Lazarus MD. Useful boundaries of the subacromial bursa. Arthroscopy. 1998;14(5):465–70.
75. Birnbaum K, Lierse W. Anatomy and function of the bursa subacromialis. Acta Anat (Basel). 1992;145(4):354–63.
76. Kennedy MS, Nicholson HD, Woodley SJ. Clinical anatomy of the subacromial and related shoulder bursae: a review of the literature. Clin Anat. 2017;30(2):213–26.
77. Duranthon LD, Gagey OJ. Anatomy and function of the subdeltoid bursa. Surg Radiol Anat. 2001;23(1):23–5.
78. van Holsbeeck M, Strouse PJ. Sonography of the shoulder: evaluation of the subacromial-subdeltoid bursa. AJR Am J Roentgenol. 1993;160(3):561–4.
79. Michener LA, et al. Supraspinatus tendon and subacromial space parameters measured on ultrasonographic imaging in subacromial impingement syndrome. Knee Surg Sports Traumatol Arthrosc. 2015;23(2):363–9.
80. Bureau NJ, et al. Dynamic sonography evaluation of shoulder impingement syndrome. AJR Am J Roentgenol. 2006;187(1):216–20.
81. Beard DJ, et al. Arthroscopic subacromial decompression for subacromial shoulder pain (CSAW): a multicentre, pragmatic, parallel group, placebo-controlled, three-group, randomised surgical trial. Lancet. 2018;391(10118):329–38.
82. Haahr JP, et al. Exercises versus arthroscopic decompression in patients with subacromial impingement: a randomised, controlled study in 90 cases with a one year follow up. Ann Rheum Dis. 2005;64(5):760–4.
83. Wu T, et al. Ultrasound-guided versus blind subacromial-subdeltoid bursa injection in adults with shoulder pain: a systematic review and meta-analysis. Semin Arthritis Rheum. 2015;45(3):374–8.
84. Nejati P, et al. Treatment of subacromial impingement syndrome: platelet-rich plasma or exercise therapy? A randomized controlled trial. Orthop J Sports Med. 2017;5(5):2325967117702366.
85. Say F, Gurler D, Bulbul M. Platelet-rich plasma versus steroid injection for subacromial impingement syndrome. J Orthop Surg (Hong Kong). 2016;24(1):62–6.
86. Schneider A, et al. Platelet-rich plasma and the shoulder: clinical indications and outcomes. Curr Rev Musculoskelet Med. 2018;11(4):593–7.
87. Rutten MJ, et al. Injection of the subacromial-subdeltoid bursa: blind or ultrasound-guided? Acta Orthop. 2007;78(2):254–7.
88. Dogu B, et al. Blind or ultrasound-guided corticosteroid injections and short-term response in subacromial impingement syndrome: a randomized, double-blind, prospective study. Am J Phys Med Rehabil. 2012;91(8):658–65.
89. Ahn KS, et al. Ultrasound elastography of lateral epicondylosis: clinical feasibility of quantitative elastographic measurements. AJR Am J Roentgenol. 2014;202(5):1094–9.
90. Mathews PV, Glousman RE. Accuracy of subacromial injection: anterolateral versus posterior approach. J Shoulder Elb Surg. 2005;14(2):145–8.
91. Partington PF, Broome GH. Diagnostic injection around the shoulder: hit and miss? A cadaveric study of injection accuracy. J Shoulder Elb Surg. 1998;7(2):147–50.
92. Eustace JA, et al. Comparison of the accuracy of steroid placement with clinical outcome in patients with shoulder symptoms. Ann Rheum Dis. 1997;56(1):59–63.
93. Mazzocca AD, Arciero RA, Bicos J. Evaluation and treatment of acromioclavicular joint injuries. Am J Sports Med. 2007;35(2):316–29.
94. Petersson CJ, Redlund-Johnell I. Radiographic joint space in normal acromioclavicular joints. Acta Orthop Scand. 1983;54(3):431–3.
95. Mall NA, et al. Degenerative joint disease of the acromioclavicular joint: a review. Am J Sports Med. 2013;41(11):2684–92.
96. Saccomanno MF, Ieso CDE, Milano G. Acromioclavicular joint instability: anatomy, biomechanics and evaluation. Joints. 2014;2(2):87–92.
97. Chronopoulos E, et al. Diagnostic value of physical tests for isolated chronic acromioclavicular lesions. Am J Sports Med. 2004;32(3):655–61.

98. Jacobson JA. Fundamentals of musculoskeletal ultrasound E-book. Philadelphia: Elsevier Health Sciences; 2017.
99. Hobusch GM, et al. Ultrasound of horizontal instability of the acromioclavicular joint : a simple and reliable test based on a cadaveric study. Wien Klin Wochenschr. 2019;131(3-4):81–6.
100. Sammarco VJ. Os acromiale: frequency, anatomy, and clinical implications. J Bone Joint Surg Am. 2000;82(3):394–400.
101. Boehm TD, et al. Ultrasonographic appearance of os acromiale. Ultraschall Med. 2003;24(3):180–3.
102. Armstrong A. Evaluation and management of adult shoulder pain: a focus on rotator cuff disorders, acromioclavicular joint arthritis, and glenohumeral arthritis. Med Clin North Am. 2014;98(4):755–75. xii
103. Jacob AK, Sallay PI. Therapeutic efficacy of corticosteroid injections in the acromioclavicular joint. Biomed Sci Instrum. 1997;34:380–5.
104. Chang Chien GC, et al. Ultrasonography leads to accurate diagnosis and management of painful acromioclavicular joint cyst. Pain Pract. 2015;15(7):E72–5.
105. Mikell C, Gelber J, Nagdev A. Ultrasound-guided analgesic injection for acromioclavicular joint separation in the emergency department. Am J Emerg Med. 2020;38(1):162.e3–5.
106. van Riet RP, Goehre T, Bell SN. The long term effect of an intra-articular injection of corticosteroids in the acromioclavicular joint. J Shoulder Elb Surg. 2012;21(3):376–9.
107. Gokkus K, et al. Limited distal clavicle excision of acromioclavicular joint osteoarthritis. Orthop Traumatol Surg Res. 2016;102(3):311–8.
108. Hsieh PC, et al. Ultrasound-guided Prolotherapy for acromial Enthesopathy and acromioclavicular joint Arthropathy: a single-arm prospective study. J Ultrasound Med. 2019;38(3):605–12.
109. Borbas P, et al. The influence of ultrasound guidance in the rate of success of acromioclavicular joint injection: an experimental study on human cadavers. J Shoulder Elb Surg. 2012;21(12):1694–7.
110. Sabeti-Aschraf M, et al. Ultrasound guidance improves the accuracy of the acromioclavicular joint infiltration: a prospective randomized study. Knee Surg Sports Traumatol Arthrosc. 2011;19(2):292–5.
111. Scillia A, et al. Accuracy of in vivo palpation-guided acromioclavicular joint injection assessed with contrast material and fluoroscopic evaluations. Skelet Radiol. 2015;44(8):1135–9.
112. Wasserman BR, et al. Accuracy of acromioclavicular joint injections. Am J Sports Med. 2013;41(1):149–52.
113. van Tongel A, et al. A cadaveric study of the structural anatomy of the sternoclavicular joint. Clin Anat. 2012;25(7):903–10.
114. Bearn JG. Direct observations on the function of the capsule of the sternoclavicular joint in clavicular support. J Anat. 1967;101(Pt 1):159–70.
115. Brossmann J, et al. Sternoclavicular joint: MR imaging—anatomic correlation. Radiology. 1996;198(1):193–8.
116. Yood RA, Goldenberg DL. Sternoclavicular joint arthritis. Arthritis Rheum. 1980;23(2):232–9.
117. Stein A, McAleer S, Hinz M. Microperforation prolotherapy: a novel method for successful nonsurgical treatment of atraumatic spontaneous anterior sternoclavicular subluxation, with an illustrative case. Open Access J Sports Med. 2011;2:47–52.
118. Peterson CK, et al. CT-guided sternoclavicular joint injections: description of the procedure, reliability of imaging diagnosis, and short-term patient responses. AJR Am J Roentgenol. 2010;195(6):W435–9.
119. Taneja AK, et al. Diagnostic yield of CT-guided sampling in suspected sternoclavicular joint infection. Skelet Radiol. 2013;42(4):479–85.
120. Galla R, et al. Sternoclavicular steroid injection for treatment of pain in a patient with osteitis condensans of the clavicle. Pain Physician. 2009;12(6):987–90.
121. Pourcho AM, Sellon JL, Smith J. Sonographically guided sternoclavicular joint injection: description of technique and validation. J Ultrasound Med. 2015;34(2):325–31.
122. Middleton WD, et al. Pitfalls of rotator cuff sonography. AJR Am J Roentgenol. 1986;146(3):555–60.
123. Taljanovic MS, et al. Sonography of the glenoid labrum: a cadaveric study with arthroscopic correlation. AJR Am J Roentgenol. 2000;174(6):1717–22.
124. Ogul H, et al. Sonoarthrographic examination of posterior labrocapsular structures of the shoulder joint. Br J Radiol. 2020;93(1106):20190886.
125. Park D. Evaluation of Posterosuperior labral tear with shoulder sonography after intra-articular injection: a case series. Am J Phys Med Rehabil. 2017;96(3):e48–51.
126. Boswell B, et al. Emergency medicine resident-driven point of care ultrasound for suspected shoulder dislocation. South Med J. 2019;112(12):605–9.
127. Abbasi S, et al. Diagnostic accuracy of ultrasonographic examination in the management of shoulder dislocation in the emergency department. Ann Emerg Med. 2013;62(2):170–5.
128. Khoury V, Van Lancker HP, Martineau PA. Sonography as a tool for identifying engaging hill-Sachs lesions: preliminary experience. J Ultrasound Med. 2013;32(9):1653–7.
129. Kerr R, et al. Osteoarthritis of the glenohumeral joint: a radiologic-pathologic study. AJR Am J Roentgenol. 1985;144(5):967–72.
130. Crowell MS, Tragord BS. Orthopaedic manual physical therapy for shoulder pain and impaired movement in a patient with glenohumeral joint osteoarthritis: a case report. J Orthop Sports Phys Ther. 2015;45(6):453–61. a1-3
131. Saltzman BM, et al. Glenohumeral osteoarthritis in the young patient. J Am Acad Orthop Surg. 2018;26(17):e361–70.
132. van der Meijden OA, Gaskill TR, Millett PJ. Glenohumeral joint preservation: a review of

management options for young, active patients with osteoarthritis. Adv Orthop. 2012;2012:160923.
133. Sayegh ET, et al. Surgical treatment options for Glenohumeral arthritis in young patients: a systematic review and meta-analysis. Arthroscopy. 2015;31(6):1156–1166.e8.
134. Ryu KN, et al. Adhesive capsulitis of the shoulder joint: usefulness of dynamic sonography. J Ultrasound Med. 1993;12(8):445–9.
135. Lee JC, et al. Adhesive capsulitis: sonographic changes in the rotator cuff interval with arthroscopic correlation. Skelet Radiol. 2005;34(9):522–7.
136. Homsi C, et al. Ultrasound in adhesive capsulitis of the shoulder: is assessment of the coracohumeral ligament a valuable diagnostic tool? Skelet Radiol. 2006;35(9):673–8.
137. Redler LH, Dennis ER. Treatment of adhesive capsulitis of the shoulder. J Am Acad Orthop Surg. 2019;27(12):e544–54.
138. Struyf F, Meeus M. Current evidence on physical therapy in patients with adhesive capsulitis: what are we missing? Clin Rheumatol. 2014;33(5):593–600.
139. Lee S, et al. The effects of extracorporeal shock wave therapy on pain and range of motion in patients with adhesive capsulitis. J Phys Ther Sci. 2017;29(11):1907–9.
140. Saltychev M, et al. Effectiveness of Hydrodilatation in adhesive capsulitis of shoulder: a systematic review and meta-analysis. Scand J Surg. 2018;107(4):285–93.
141. Griesser MJ, et al. Adhesive capsulitis of the shoulder: a systematic review of the effectiveness of intra-articular corticosteroid injections. J Bone Joint Surg Am. 2011;93(18):1727–33.
142. Jain TK, Sharma NK. The effectiveness of physiotherapeutic interventions in treatment of frozen shoulder/adhesive capsulitis: a systematic review. J Back Musculoskelet Rehabil. 2014;27(3):247–73.
143. Porcellini G, et al. Intra-articular glenohumeral injections of HYADD(R)4-G for the treatment of painful shoulder osteoarthritis: a prospective multicenter, open-label trial. Joints. 2015;3(3):116–21.
144. Silverstein E, Leger R, Shea KP. The use of intra-articular hylan G-F 20 in the treatment of symptomatic osteoarthritis of the shoulder: a preliminary study. Am J Sports Med. 2007;35(6):979–85.
145. Noel E, et al. Efficacy and safety of Hylan G-F 20 in shoulder osteoarthritis with an intact rotator cuff. Open-label prospective multicenter study. Joint Bone Spine. 2009;76(6):670–3.
146. Di Giacomo G, de Gasperis N. Hyaluronic acid intra-articular injections in patients affected by moderate to severe Glenohumeral osteoarthritis: a prospective randomized study. Joints. 2017;5(3):138–42.
147. McKee MD, et al. NASHA hyaluronic acid for the treatment of shoulder osteoarthritis: a prospective, single-arm clinical trial. Med Devices (Auckl). 2019;12:227–34.
148. Merolla G, et al. Efficacy of Hylan G-F 20 versus 6-methylprednisolone acetate in painful shoulder osteoarthritis: a retrospective controlled trial. Musculoskelet Surg. 2011;95(3):215–24.
149. Kwon YW, Eisenberg G, Zuckerman JD. Sodium hyaluronate for the treatment of chronic shoulder pain associated with glenohumeral osteoarthritis: a multicenter, randomized, double-blind, placebo-controlled trial. J Shoulder Elb Surg. 2013;22(5):584–94.
150. Blaine T, et al. Treatment of persistent shoulder pain with sodium hyaluronate: a randomized, controlled trial. A multicenter study. J Bone Joint Surg Am. 2008;90(5):970–9.
151. Centeno CJ, et al. A prospective multi-site registry study of a specific protocol of autologous bone marrow concentrate for the treatment of shoulder rotator cuff tears and osteoarthritis. J Pain Res. 2015;8:269–76.
152. Striano RD, et al. Refractory shoulder pain with osteoarthritis, and rotator cuff tear, treated with micro-fragmented adipose tissue. J Orthop Spine Sports Med. 2018;2(1):014.
153. Jong BY, Goel DP. Biologic options for Glenohumeral arthritis. Clin Sports Med. 2018;37(4):537–48.
154. Wang W, et al. Effectiveness of corticosteroid injections in adhesive capsulitis of shoulder: a meta-analysis. Medicine (Baltimore). 2017;96(28):e7529.
155. Xiao RC, et al. Corticosteroid injections for adhesive capsulitis: a review. Clin J Sport Med. 2017;27(3):308–20.
156. Paruthikunnan SM, et al. Intra-articular steroid for adhesive capsulitis: does hydrodilatation give any additional benefit? A randomized control trial. Skelet Radiol. 2019.
157. Yoon SH, et al. Optimal dose of intra-articular corticosteroids for adhesive capsulitis: a randomized, triple-blind, placebo-controlled trial. Am J Sports Med. 2013;41(5):1133–9.
158. Shang X, et al. Intra-articular versus subacromial corticosteroid injection for the treatment of adhesive capsulitis: a meta-analysis and systematic review. Biomed Res Int. 2019;2019:1274790.
159. Kim YS, et al. Comparison of high- and low-dose intra-articular triamcinolone acetonide injection for treatment of primary shoulder stiffness: a prospective randomized trial. J Shoulder Elb Surg. 2017;26(2):209–15.
160. Prestgaard T, et al. Ultrasound-guided intra-articular and rotator interval corticosteroid injections in adhesive capsulitis of the shoulder: a double-blind, sham-controlled randomized study. Pain. 2015;156(9):1683–91.
161. Ogul H, et al. Ultrasound-guided shoulder MR arthrography: comparison of rotator interval and posterior approach. Clin Imaging. 2014;38(1):11–7.
162. Sun Y, et al. The effect of corticosteroid injection into rotator interval for early frozen shoulder: a randomized controlled trial. Am J Sports Med. 2018;46(3):663–70.
163. Barman A, et al. Single intra-articular platelet-rich plasma versus corticosteroid injections in the treat-

ment of adhesive capsulitis of the shoulder: a cohort study. Am J Phys Med Rehabil. 2019;98(7):549–57.
164. Lin J. Platelet-rich plasma injection in the treatment of frozen shoulder: a randomized controlled trial with 6-month follow-up. Int J Clin Pharmacol Ther. 2018;56(8):366–71.
165. Sethi PM, Kingston S, Elattrache N. Accuracy of anterior intra-articular injection of the glenohumeral joint. Arthroscopy. 2005;21(1):77–80.
166. Shao X, et al. Transcoracoacromial ligament Glenohumeral injection technique: accuracy of 116 injections in idiopathic adhesive capsulitis. Arthroscopy. 2018;34(8):2337–44.
167. Catalano OA, et al. MR arthrography of the glenohumeral joint: modified posterior approach without imaging guidance. Radiology. 2007;242(2):550–4.
168. Patel DN, et al. Comparison of ultrasound-guided versus blind glenohumeral injections: a cadaveric study. J Shoulder Elb Surg. 2012;21(12):1664–8.
169. Esenyel CZ, et al. Accuracy of anterior glenohumeral injections: a cadaver study. Arch Orthop Trauma Surg. 2010;130(3):297–300.
170. Souza PM, et al. Arthrography of the shoulder: a modified ultrasound guided technique of joint injection at the rotator interval. Eur J Radiol. 2010;74(3):e29–32.
171. Choudur HN, Ellins ML. Ultrasound-guided gadolinium joint injections for magnetic resonance arthrography. J Clin Ultrasound. 2011;39(1):6–11.
172. Gokalp G, Dusak A, Yazici Z. Efficacy of ultrasonography-guided shoulder MR arthrography using a posterior approach. Skelet Radiol. 2010;39(6):575–9.
173. Ogul H, et al. Magnetic resonance arthrography of the glenohumeral joint: ultrasonography-guided technique using a posterior approach. Eurasian J Med. 2012;44(2):73–8.
174. Plancher KD, et al. The spinoglenoid ligament. Anatomy, morphology, and histological findings. J Bone Joint Surg Am. 2005;87(2):361–5.
175. Aktekin M, et al. The significance of the neurovascular structures passing through the spinoglenoid notch. Neurosciences (Riyadh). 2003;8(4):222–4.
176. Lichtenberg S, Magosch P, Habermeyer P. Compression of the suprascapular nerve by a ganglion cyst of the spinoglenoid notch: the arthroscopic solution. Knee Surg Sports Traumatol Arthrosc. 2004;12(1):72–9.
177. Steinwachs MR, et al. A ganglion of the spinoglenoid notch. J Shoulder Elb Surg. 1998;7(5):550–4.
178. Phillips CJ, Field AC, Field LD. Transcapsular decompression of shoulder ganglion cysts. Arthrosc Tech. 2018;7(12):e1263–7.
179. Tung GA, et al. MR imaging and MR arthrography of paraglenoid labral cysts. AJR Am J Roentgenol. 2000;174(6):1707–15.
180. Ferretti A, De Carli A, Fontana M. Injury of the suprascapular nerve at the spinoglenoid notch. The natural history of infraspinatus atrophy in volleyball players. Am J Sports Med. 1998;26(6):759–63.
181. Chiou HJ, et al. Alternative and effective treatment of shoulder ganglion cyst: ultrasonographically guided aspiration. J Ultrasound Med. 1999;18(8):531–5.
182. Sangam MR, et al. A study on the morphology of the suprascapular notch and its distance from the glenoid cavity. J Clin Diagn Res. 2013;7(2):189–92.
183. Rengachary SS, et al. Suprascapular entrapment neuropathy: a clinical, anatomical, and comparative study. Part 2: anatomical study. Neurosurgery. 1979;5(4):447–51.
184. Martinoli C, et al. US of the shoulder: non-rotator cuff disorders. Radiographics. 2003;23(2):381–401. quiz 534
185. Boykin RE, et al. Suprascapular neuropathy. J Bone Joint Surg Am. 2010;92(13):2348–64.
186. Urguden M, et al. Is there any effect of suprascapular notch type in iatrogenic suprascapular nerve lesions? An anatomical study. Knee Surg Sports Traumatol Arthrosc. 2004;12(3):241–5.
187. Bayramoglu A, et al. Variations in anatomy at the suprascapular notch possibly causing suprascapular nerve entrapment: an anatomical study. Knee Surg Sports Traumatol Arthrosc. 2003;11(6):393–8.
188. Blasco L, et al. Ultrasound-guided proximal and distal suprascapular nerve blocks: a comparative cadaveric study. Pain Med. 2019;21(6):1240–7.
189. Taskaynatan MA, et al. Accuracy of ultrasound-guided suprascapular nerve block measured with neurostimulation. Rheumatol Int. 2012;32(7):2125–8.
190. Laumonerie P, et al. Ultrasound-guided versus landmark-based approach to the distal suprascapular nerve block: a comparative cadaveric study. Arthroscopy. 2019;35(8):2274–81.
191. Laumonerie P, et al. Distal suprascapular nerve block-do it yourself: cadaveric feasibility study. J Shoulder Elb Surg. 2019;28(7):1291–7.
192. van de Pol D, et al. High prevalence of self-reported symptoms of digital ischemia in elite male volleyball players in the Netherlands: a cross-sectional national survey. Am J Sports Med. 2012;40(10):2296–302.
193. Vlychou M, et al. Embolisation of a traumatic aneurysm of the posterior circumflex humeral artery in a volleyball player. Br J Sports Med. 2001;35(2):136–7.
194. Atema JJ, et al. Posterior circumflex humeral artery injury with distal embolisation in professional volleyball players: a discussion of three cases. Eur J Vasc Endovasc Surg. 2012;44(2):195–8.
195. Reekers JA, et al. Traumatic aneurysm of the posterior circumflex humeral artery: a volleyball player's disease? J Vasc Interv Radiol. 1993;4(3):405–8.
196. Ligh CA, Schulman BL, Safran MR. Case reports: unusual cause of shoulder pain in a collegiate baseball player. Clin Orthop Relat Res. 2009;467(10):2744–8.
197. Kee ST, et al. Ischemia of the throwing hand in major league baseball pitchers: embolic occlusion from aneurysms of axillary artery branches. J Vasc Interv Radiol. 1995;6(6):979–82.

198. Nuber GW, et al. Arterial abnormalities of the shoulder in athletes. Am J Sports Med. 1990;18(5):514–9.
199. McClelland D, Hoy G. A case of quadrilateral space syndrome with involvement of the long head of the triceps. Am J Sports Med. 2008;36(8):1615–7.
200. Perlmutter GS. Axillary nerve injury. Clin Orthop Relat Res. 1999;368:28–36.
201. Lo IK, Burkhart SS, Parten PM. Surgery about the coracoid: neurovascular structures at risk. Arthroscopy. 2004;20(6):591–5.
202. Chen H, Narvaez VR. Ultrasound-guided quadrilateral space block for the diagnosis of quadrilateral syndrome. Case Rep Orthop. 2015;2015:378627.
203. Wolfe SW, Wickiewicz TL, Cavanaugh JT. Ruptures of the pectoralis major muscle. An anatomic and clinical analysis. Am J Sports Med. 1992;20(5):587–93.
204. Fung L, et al. Three-dimensional study of pectoralis major muscle and tendon architecture. Clin Anat. 2009;22(4):500–8.
205. Lee YK, et al. US and MR imaging of pectoralis major injuries. Radiographics. 2017;37(1):176–89.
206. Chiavaras MM, et al. Pectoralis major tears: anatomy, classification, and diagnosis with ultrasound and MR imaging. Skelet Radiol. 2015;44(2):157–64.
207. Provencher MT, et al. Injuries to the pectoralis major muscle: diagnosis and management. Am J Sports Med. 2010;38(8):1693–705.
208. ElMaraghy AW, Devereaux MW. A systematic review and comprehensive classification of pectoralis major tears. J Shoulder Elb Surg. 2012;21(3):412–22.
209. Tietjen R. Closed injuries of the pectoralis major muscle. J Trauma. 1980;20(3):262–4.
210. Rehman A, Robinson P. Sonographic evaluation of injuries to the pectoralis muscles. AJR Am J Roentgenol. 2005;184(4):1205–11.
211. Kircher J, et al. Surgical and nonsurgical treatment of total rupture of the pectoralis major muscle in athletes: update and critical appraisal. Open Access J Sports Med. 2010;1:201–5.

6 Ultrasound-Guided Elbow Injection Techniques

Tolga Ergönenç

Ultrasound-Guided Elbow Injection Techniques

This chapter describes the injection techniques that are most commonly used around the elbow joint. The objective is to precisely define the position and alignment of the transducer and needle to ensure accurate tissue placement. This section also includes short clinical descriptions of each condition with anatomical details. The drugs, doses, and volumes mentioned are those used in clinical practice by the author. This section includes the following injection techniques commonly used in the elbow:

1. Elbow joint injection
2. Common extensor tendon injection (tennis elbow)
3. Common flexor tendon injection (golfer's elbow)
4. Olecranon bursa injection
5. Ulnar collateral ligament (UCL)
6. Ulnar nerve at the elbow
7. Deep branch of radial nerve at the elbow (posterior interosseous nerve syndrome)

Each procedure includes the following subheadings:

(a) Brief anatomy
(b) Common cause
(c) Injection indications
(d) Equipment needed
(e) Injection technique
    (i) Patient position
    (ii) Transducer position
    (iii) Needle direction and approach
    (iv) Target

Elbow Joint Injection

(a) Brief Anatomy

The distal humerus, proximal radius, and proximal ulna comprise the elbow joint, which is a complicated and compound joint produced by the articulations of three bones. The humeral/ulnar joint functions similarly to a hinge joint, allowing elbow flexion and extension. Forearm rotation is possible, thanks to the proximal radioulnar joint and the radiohumeral joint. The joint capsule encases the entire elbow joint.

The posterolateral approach is the safest and most straightforward method which accessing the elbow joint.

T. Ergönenç (✉)
Akyazı Hospital Pain and Palliative Care, Sakarya, Turkey
e-mail: ergonenc@ultrasoundmsk.org

Y. El Miedany (ed.), *Musculoskeletal Ultrasound-Guided Regenerative Medicine*,
https://doi.org/10.1007/978-3-030-98256-0_6

(b) Common Cause

Elbow intra-articular injections can be used to treat a variety of pathologic conditions.

Symptoms of a painful elbow joint may be caused by either an intrinsic process, such as infection or osteoarthritis, or an extrinsic process, such as a fracture or dislocation. Repetitive stress and overuse can also cause injury and pain in the joint.

(c) Injection Indications

The etiology of a painful and swollen joint can be determined by ultrasound-guided diagnostic aspiration of joint fluid to evaluate if the accumulation is due to inflammatory or noninflammatory arthritis, infection, or crystal-induced arthropathy.

Steroids, hyaluronic acid, local anesthetic, Platelet Rich Plasma (PRP), and ozone can be injected into the joint in various situations.

(d) Equipment Needed
- 25-gauge needle.
- One syringe (5 ml).
- High-frequency linear array transducer/small hockey stick.
- Injectate: 1.0 mL of local anesthetic and 1 mL of injectable corticosteroids (2–3 mL ozone 15–25 mcg/ml).

(e) Injection Technique

(i) Patient Position
- Prone, propped up on a cushion with elbows overhead (lateral elbow joint) or elbow over the edge of the examination table with arm drooping over the edge of the table (posterior elbow joint injection) (Figs. 6.1 and 6.2).
- Sitting, the arm resting on a table with the elbow in slight flexion, the forearm pronated.

(ii) Transducer Position
- The radial head and capitellum are easily identified when the transducer is placed in the long axis of the radius above the posterior portion of the radiohumeral joint (Fig. 6.3).

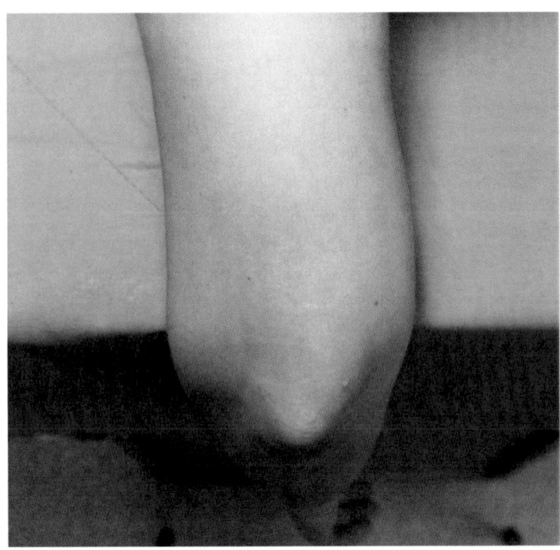

Fig. 6.1 The patient's position of the posterior elbow joint injection. The elbow joint flexes to 90 degrees, and the arm droops over the table's edge

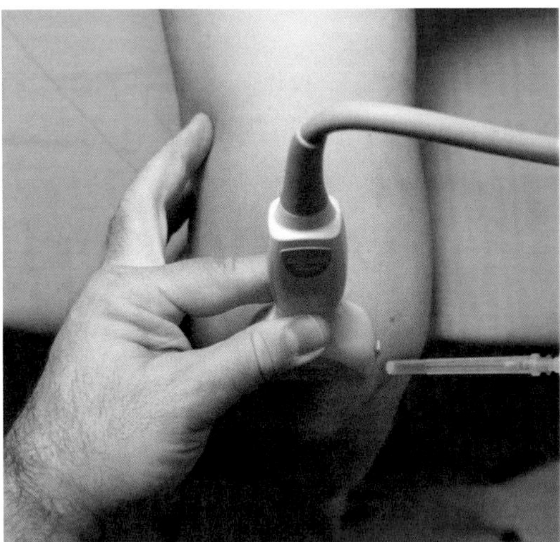

Fig. 6.2 The patient and transducer position of the posterior elbow joint injection with an in-plane approach

(iii) Needle Direction and Approach
- Out-of-plane approach, posterior to anterior direction (Fig. 6.4a, b).
- In-plane approach, distal to proximal direction (Fig. 6.5).

(iv) Target
- Radiocapitellar joint (Figs. 6.6, 6.7, and 6.8).

Common Extensor Tendon Injection (Tennis Elbow)

(a) Brief Anatomy

The extensor carpi radialis brevis tendon, the extensor digitorum communis tendon, the extensor digiti minimi tendon, and the extensor carpi ulnaris tendon are the four major components of the common extensor tendon (CET) anatomically which are origin on the anterior facet of the lateral epicondyle of the humerus. Wrist extension and radial/ulnar deviation are the functions of the CET.

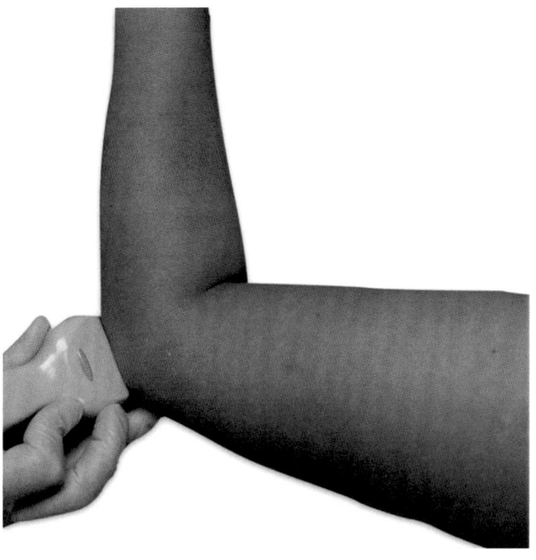

Fig. 6.3 The transducer position of the elbow joint injection. The elbow in slight flexion, the forearm pronated. Move the transducer over the posterior aspect of the radiohumeral joint to identify the gap between the radial head and capitellum of the humerus

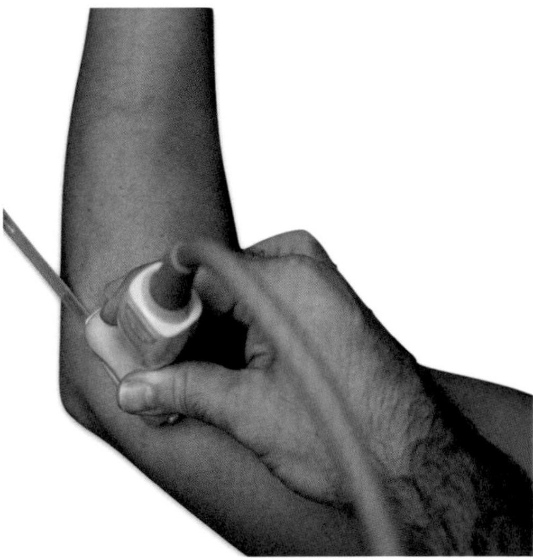

Fig. 6.5 In-plane approach, the needle is inserted at 45 degrees to the transducer in a distal to proximal direction

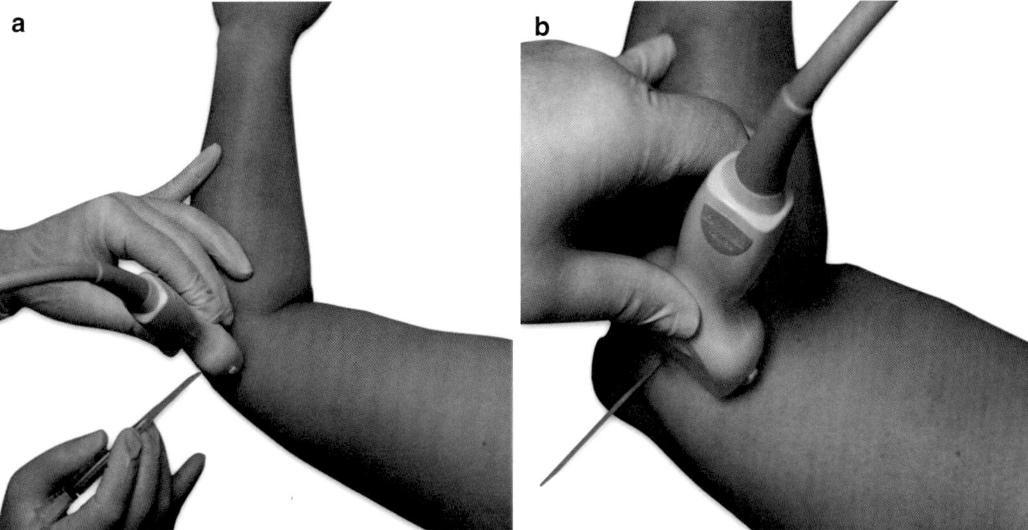

Fig. 6.4 (**a**) For best visualization of the radiohumeral joint, tilt the transducer. (**b**) Out-of-plane approach, the needle is inserted at 45 degrees to the transducer in a lateral to medial direction

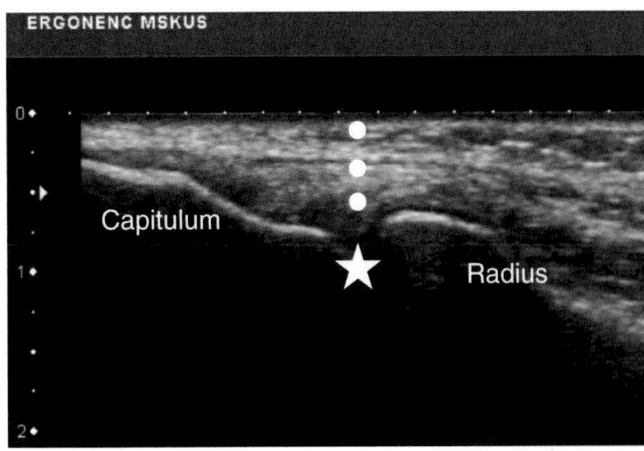

Fig. 6.6 Long-axis sonogram of the radiocapitellar joint (*). Out-of-plane walk-down approach. White circle needle tip

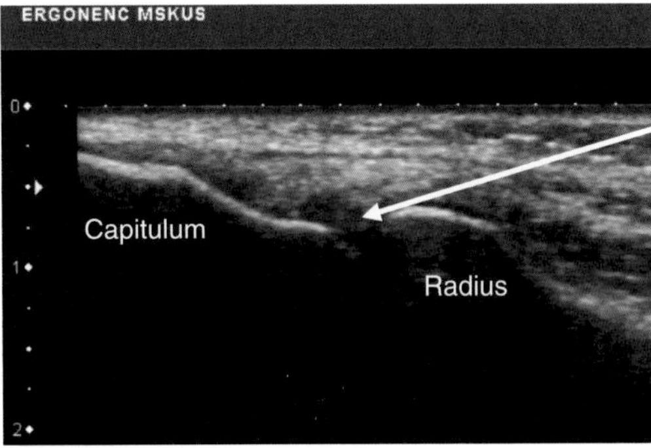

Fig. 6.7 Long-axis sonogram of the radiocapitellar joint. In-plane approach

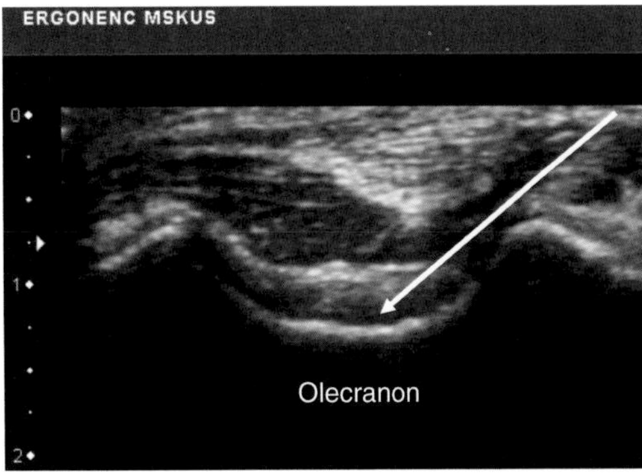

Fig. 6.8 Sonogram of the posterior elbow joint injection with an in-plane approach

(b) Common Cause

Extensor tendinopathy (tennis elbow) is a condition caused by repetitive stress/overuse injuries and microtrauma. Occupational disorders and physically demanding activities such as sport are implicated in the etiology.

(c) Injection Indications

CET injection can be performed on patients with persistent pain despite that conservative treatment. Steroids, local anesthetic, PRP, and ozone can be injected for extensor tendinopathy.

(d) Equipment Needed
- 25-gauge needle.
- One syringe (5 ml).
- High-frequency linear array transducer.
- Injectate: 1.0 mL of local anesthetic and 1 mL of injectable corticosteroids (1–2 mL ozone 15–25 mcg/ml).

(e) Injection Technique
(i) Patient Position
- Supine or sitting, the arm resting on a table with the elbow at approximately 90 degrees of flexion.

(ii) Transducer Position
- The common extensor tendon is easily identified when the transducer is placed in the long axis to the CET at its origin on the lateral epicondyle (Fig. 6.9).

(iii) Needle Direction and Approach
- The needle is inserted distal to proximal into the transducer at a 45-degree angle, passing through the extensor tendon to reach the epicondyle's anterolateral facet.
- In-plane (Fig. 6.9).

(iv) Target
- CET/lateral epicondyle anterolateral facet (Fig. 6.10).

Common Flexor Tendon Injection (Golfer's Elbow)

(a) Brief Anatomy

The anterior aspect of the medial epicondyle is the origin of the common flexor tendon (CFT) at the elbow. The CFT comprises four superficial group muscles of the forearm's flexor (pronator

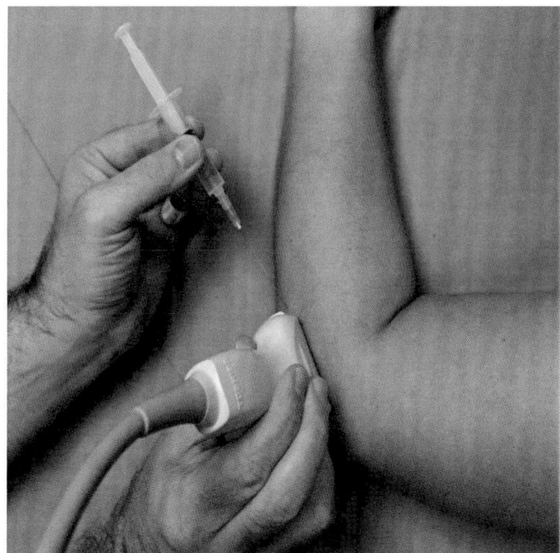

Fig. 6.9 The patient and transducer position of the common extensor tendon injection with an in-plane approach. The transducer is placed long axis over the lateral elbow joint. The needle is inserted distal to proximal into the transducer at a 45-degree angle, passing through the extensor tendon to reach the epicondyle's anterolateral facet

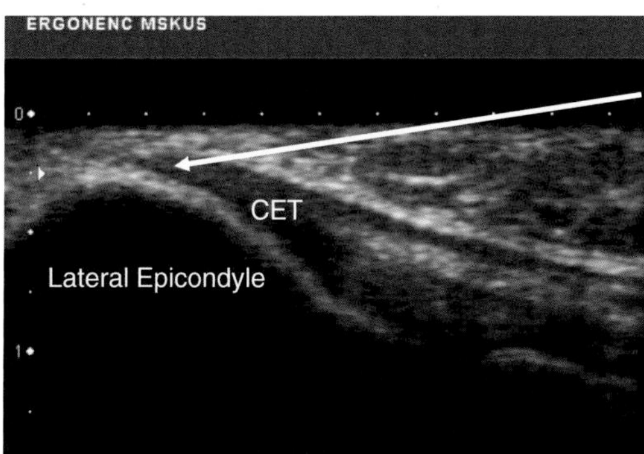

Fig. 6.10 Long-axis sonogram of the common extensor tendon and radiocapitellar joint. Injection for the tennis elbow with an in-plane approach

teres, palmaris longus, flexor carpi radialis, flexor carpi ulnaris). Forearm pronation, wrist flexion, and wrist flexion-adduction are all functions of the CFT muscles.

(b) Common Cause

Flexor tendinopathy (golfer's elbow) is a condition caused by repetitive stress/overuse injuries and microtrauma. Another consideration is that there are many occupations where repetition and excessive grasping are necessary that can cause inflammation and degeneration of the medial epicondyle.

(c) Injection Indications

CFT injection can be performed on patients with persistent pain despite that conservative treatment. Steroids, local anesthetic, PRP, and ozone can be injected for flexor tendinopathy.

(d) Equipment Needed
  - 25-gauge needle.
  - One syringe (5 ml).
  - High-frequency linear array transducer.
  - Injectate: 1.0 mL of local anesthetic and 1 mL of injectable corticosteroids (1–2 mL ozone 15–25 mcg/ml).

(e) Injection Technique
  (i) Patient Position
    - Supine or sitting, the arm resting on a table with the wrist in supine and medial compartment facing the interventionist (Fig. 6.11).

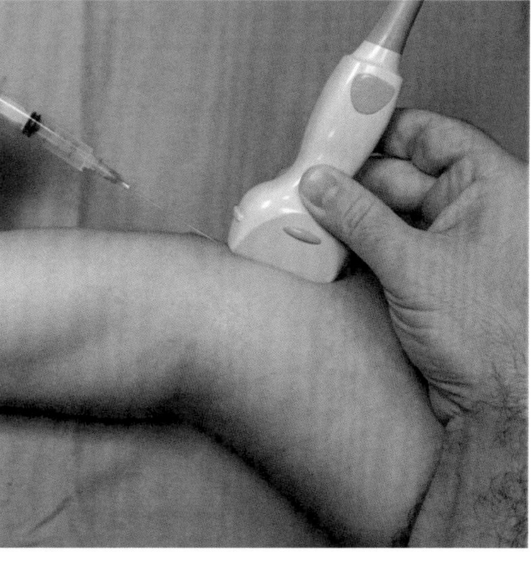

Fig. 6.11 The patient and transducer position of the common flexor tendon injection with an in-plane approach. The transducer is placed long axis over the medial elbow. The needle is inserted distal to proximal into the transducer at a 45-degree angle, passing through the flexor tendon to reach the medial epicondyle's interface

(ii) Transducer Position
- The common flexor tendon is easily identified when the transducer is placed in the long axis to the CFT at its origin on the medial epicondyle (Fig. 6.11).

(iii) Needle Direction and Approach
- The needle is inserted distal to proximal into the transducer at a 45-degree angle, passing through the flexor tendon to reach the medial epicondyle's interface.
- In-plane.

(iv) Target
- CFT/anterior facet of the medial epicondyle. Injection should not be performed to the medial collateral ligament (Fig. 6.12).

Olecranon Bursa Injection

(a) Brief Anatomy

The olecranon bursa is located between the skin of the extensor surface of the elbow and the olecranon process of the ulna, and it aids in the reduction of friction between two adjacent surfaces. It contains very little fluid in its normal state and is not visible with ultrasound. It has no communication with the joint.

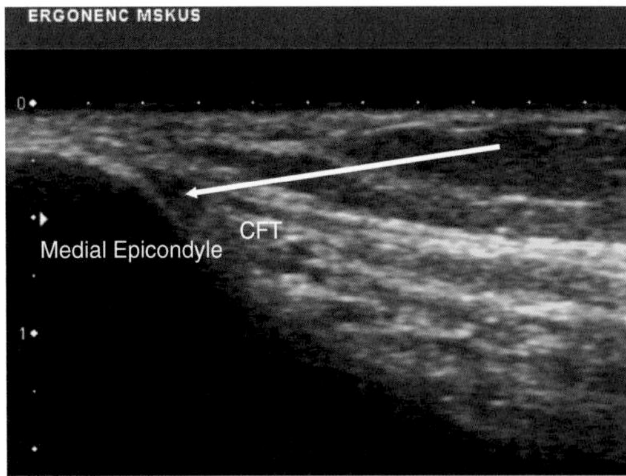

Fig. 6.12 Long-axis sonogram of the common flexor tendon and medial epicondyle. Injection for the golfer's elbow with an in-plane approach

(b) Common Cause

Olecranon bursitis can be caused by various factors, including direct trauma such as a fall or blow to the olecranon, infection such as septic bursitis, and inflammatory conditions such as rheumatoid arthritis and gout.

(c) Injection Indications

Chronic or recurring bursitis that has not responded to conservative treatment can be treated with aspiration of the olecranon bursa. In the case of septic bursitis, corticosteroids should not be injected.

(d) Equipment Needed
- 18-gauge needle.
- One syringe for aspiration (10–20 ml).
- One syringe for injectate (5 ml).
- High-frequency linear array transducer.
- Injectate: 1.0 mL of local anesthetic and 1 mL of injectable corticosteroids.

(e) Injection Technique

(i) Patient Position

Supine, prone, or sitting.
- Supine: the shoulder is internally rotated and with about 30 degrees flexion.
- Sitting: with the arm resting on a table in front and the elbow flexed at the edge of the examination table, with the shoulder partially abducted, and the elbow flexed, the distal arm hangs off the side, to approximately 90 degrees.
- Prone: the shoulder partially abducted and the elbow flexed at the edge of the examination table, allowing for the distal arm to hang off of the side.

(ii) Transducer Position
- Supine, prone, or sitting: the transducer is positioned long axis or short axis over the bursa of the olecranon.

(iii) Needle Direction and Approach
- The needle punctures the skin at a 45-degree angle with an in-plane

approach, that directly visualizes the bursa is allowed (Figs. 6.13 and 6.14).

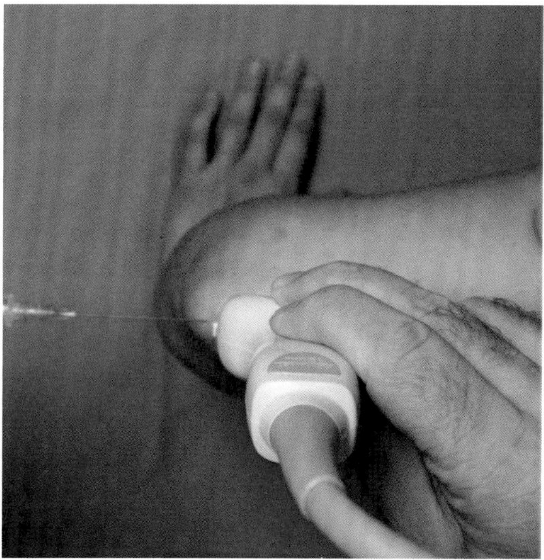

Fig. 6.13 The patient and transducer position of the olecranon bursa injection with an in-plane approach. The transducer is placed long axis over the olecranon bursa. The needle is inserted parallel into the transducer, lateral to medial. The olecranon bursa is not visible in its usual state

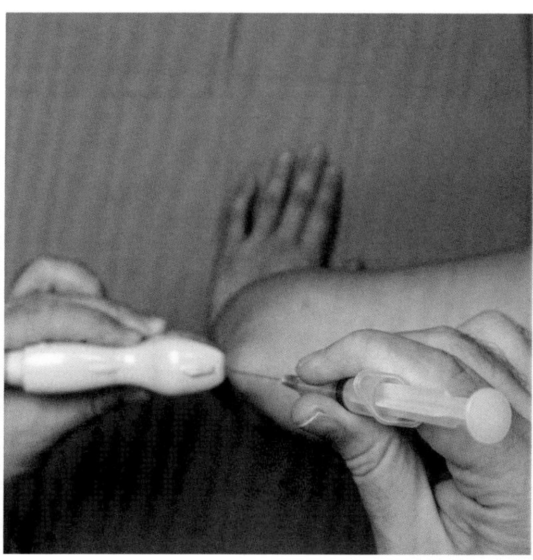

Fig. 6.14 The patient and transducer position of the olecranon bursa injection with an in-plane approach. The transducer is placed long axis over the olecranon bursa. The needle is inserted parallel into the transducer, proximal to distal. The olecranon bursa is not visible in its usual state

(iv) Target
  - Center of the olecranon bursa.

Ulnar Collateral Ligament (UCL)

(a) Brief Anatomy

The medial stabilizer of the elbow is the ulnar collateral ligament (UCL) that consists of three portions as an anterior, posterior, and transverse segment.

(b) Common Cause

The anterior segment of the UCL is responsible for the primary stabilization of the medial elbow, and this segment is critical during joint valgus stress.

During the overhead throwing, a tremendous amount of valgus stress is applied to the elbow in many cases. Repetitive microtrauma or single-throw injury can occur in sports activities.

(c) Injection Indications

Injection of regenerative solutions or only needle tenotomy can be performed on patients with persistent pain despite that conservative treatment.

(d) Equipment Needed
  - 25-gauge needle.
  - One syringe (5 ml).
  - High-frequency linear array transducer.
  - Injectate: 1.0 mL of local anesthetic and 1 mL of injectable corticosteroids.

(e) Injection Technique
  (i) Patient Position
    - Supine or sitting, elbow flexion with 30 degrees and the shoulder externally rotated, and the arm abducted at least 45 degrees.

  (ii) Transducer Position
    - On the medial elbow, a slight oblique plane exists. To the CFT, the UCL appears to be quite deep (Fig. 6.15).

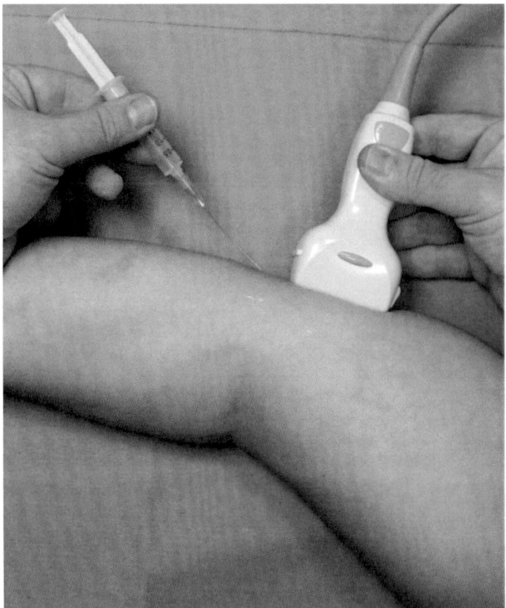

Fig. 6.15 The patient and transducer position of the ulnar collateral ligament injection with an in-plane approach. Elbow flexion with 30 degrees and the shoulder externally rotated, and the arm abducted at least 45 degrees

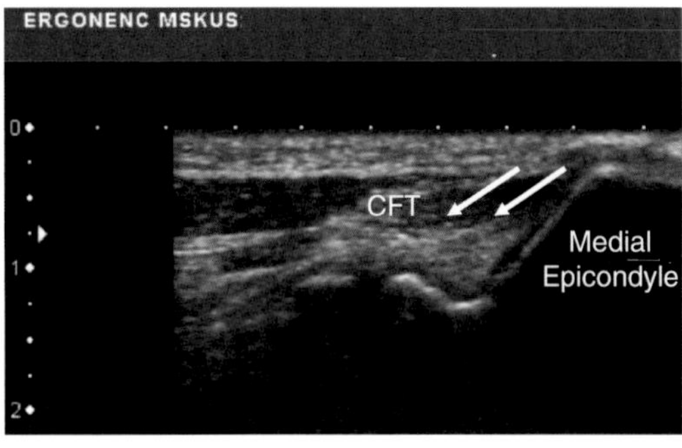

Fig. 6.16 Long-axis sonogram of the common flexor tendon and medial epicondyle and ulnar collateral ligament (white arrows). The needle should be inserted distal to proximal with an in-plane approach to the transducer

(iii) Needle Direction and Approach
- The needle should be inserted distal to proximal with an in-plane approach to the transducer.

(iv) Target
- Hypoechoic area of the pathologic ligament (Fig. 6.16).
- Take care to locate the ulnar nerve and avoid injecting too posteriorly, where the ulnar nerve may be located.

Ulnar Nerve at the Elbow

(a) Brief Anatomy

The ulnar nerve arises from the C8 and T1 nerve roots. It travels through the cubital tunnel before entering the flexor compartment of the forearm, where it is found between the two heads of the flexor carpi ulnaris muscle. About 5 cm proximal to the wrist, the ulnar nerve splits into dorsal and palmar branches.

(b) Common Cause

Numerous mechanisms can result in the entrapment or injury of the ulnar nerve at the elbow (cubital tunnel) or wrist (Guyon's canal). Dynamically evaluating the ulnar nerve at the elbow is beneficial in detecting ulnar subluxation, one of the most common causes of neuropathy.

(c) Injection Indications

Patients who have prolonged pain owing to ulnar nerve entrapment despite conservative treatment may benefit from the ulnar perineural injection. It could also be utilized for diagnostic purposes.

(d) Equipment Needed
- 25-gauge needle.
- One syringe (5 ml).
- High-frequency linear array transducer.
- Injectate: 1.0 mL of local anesthetic and 1–2 mL of injectable corticosteroids.
- For hydrodissection of the nerve up to 10–15 mL total volume (0.9% NaCl, local anesthetic, ± dextrose solution).

(e) Injection Technique

(i) Patient Position
- Supine, the shoulder abducted 90 degrees and the elbow flexed approximately 90 degrees.
- Sitting, the elbow flexed 90 degrees with the hand on the table.

(ii) Transducer Position
- At the elbow, place the transducer transverse position to the ulnar nerve.

(iii) Needle Direction and Approach
- The needle should be inserted medial to lateral with an in-plane approach (Fig. 6.17).
- The needle should be inserted distal to proximal with an out-of-plane approach (Fig. 6.18).

(iv) Target
- Spread medication around the circumference of the ulnar nerve. Create a "target sign" of injectate around the nerve (Fig. 6.19).

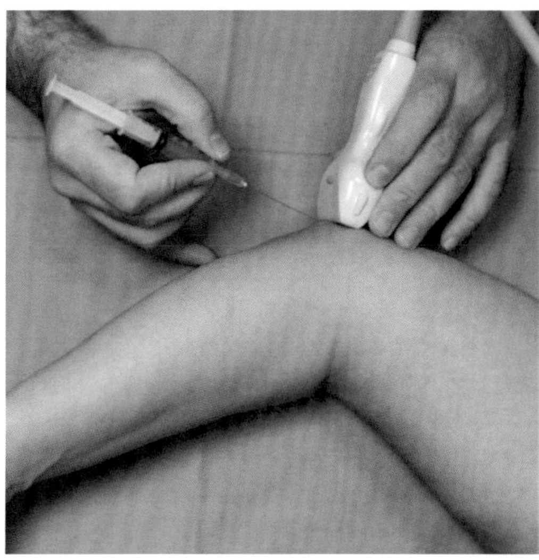

Fig. 6.18 The patient and transducer position of the ulnar perineural injection with an out-of-plane approach. The elbow flexed 90 degrees with the hand on the table

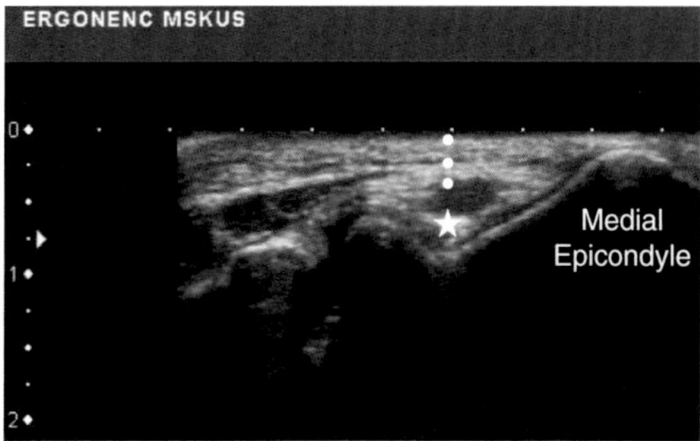

Fig. 6.19 Axial view of the ulnar nerve (*) at the cubital tunnel level. Out-of-plane walk-down approach. White circle needle tip

Deep Branch of Radial Nerve at the Elbow (Posterior Interosseous Nerve Syndrome)

(a) Brief Anatomy

The posterior interosseous nerve (PIN) is the terminal motor branch of the radial nerve.

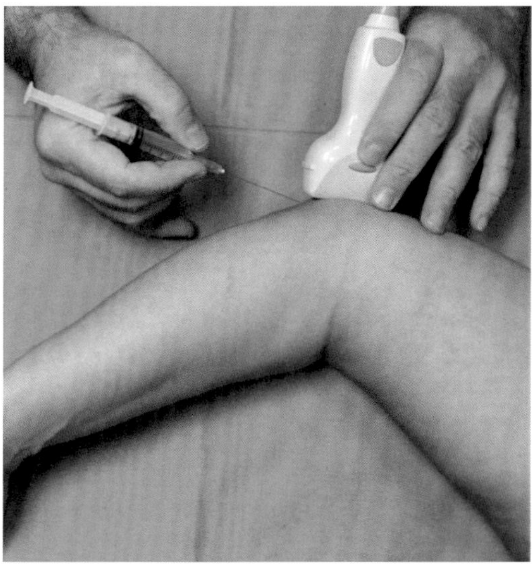

Fig. 6.17 The patient and transducer position of the ulnar perineural injection with an in-plane approach. The elbow flexed 90 degrees with the hand on the table

(b) Common Cause

Numerous mechanisms can result in the entrapment or injury of the median nerve PIN near or below the supinator muscle. Hypertrophy of the supinator muscle, fibrous bands, soft-tissue masses, radial head, and neck fractures may cause and compress the PIN.

(c) Injection Indications

Patients who have prolonged clinical signs due to PIN syndrome despite conservative treatment may benefit from this injection.

(d) Equipment Needed
- 25-gauge needle.
- One syringe (5 ml).
- High-frequency linear array transducer.
- Injectate: 1.0 mL of local anesthetic and 1–2 mL of injectable corticosteroids.
- For hydrodissection of the nerve up to 15–20 mL total volume (0.9% NaCl, local anesthetic, ± dextrose solution).

(e) Injection Technique
  (i) Patient Position
  - Sitting, the elbow flexed 90 degrees with the hand on the table and the forearm neutral or pronated (Fig. 6.20).

  (ii) Transducer Position
  - Place the transducer in a transverse position at the level of the distal humerus, find the radial nerve, and follow it distally until it splits into the superficial sensory branch and PIN.

  (iii) Needle Direction and Approach
  - The needle should be inserted lateral to medial with an in-plane approach (Fig. 6.20).

  (iv) Target
  - Spread medication around the circumference of the PIN. Create a "target sign" of injectate around the nerve (Fig. 6.21).

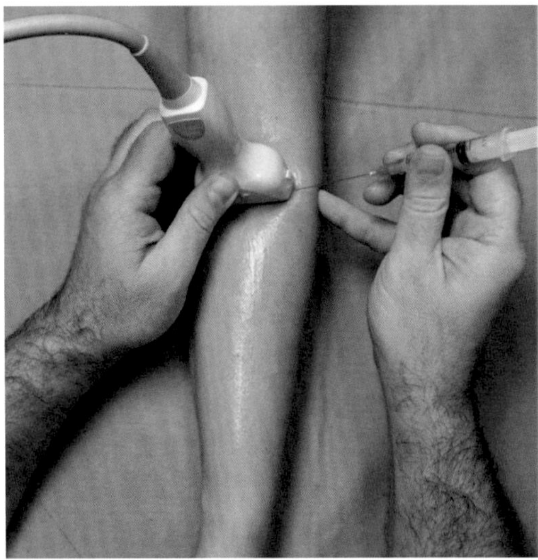

Fig. 6.20 The patient and transducer position of the PIN injection with a short-axis in-plane approach

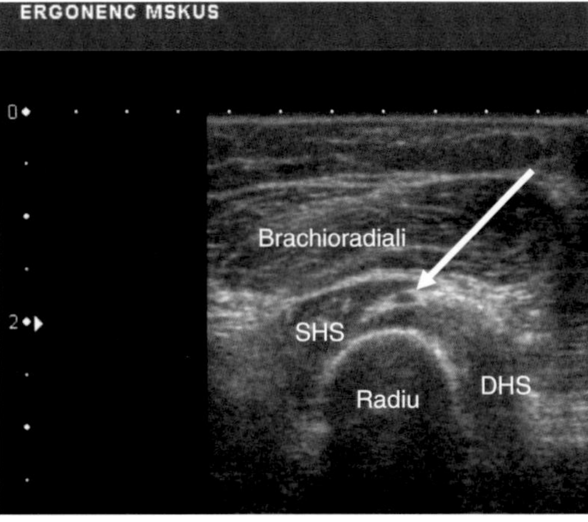

Fig. 6.21 Sonogram of the deep branch of the radial nerve (white arrow), PIN injection with a short-axis in-plane approach. Deep head of supinator (DHS). Superficial head of supinator (SHS)

7 Wrist and Hand

Vincenzo Ricci and Levent Özçakar

Introduction

In clinical practice, disorders of the wrist and hand are commonplace and may result in significant functional limitations in daily activities. Owing to the superficial localization of most of the anatomical structures in this region, ultrasound (US) imaging is widely considered a suitable modality for diagnostic and therapeutic procedures [1, 2]. Tendons, joints, ligaments, nerves, and other peculiar soft tissues of the wrist and hand are all potential pain generators, and if clearly visualized, they are all "reachable" under US guidance for prompt interventions [1–4].

The aim of this chapter is to provide a practical guide as to how US imaging and guidance can be used to correctly plan for regenerative interventions of this anatomical region. The authors will try to illustrate how relevant anatomical structures (commonly involved in hand/wrist pathologies) can be thoroughly scanned and safely accessed [5].

V. Ricci (✉)
Physical and Rehabilitation Medicine Unit, Luigi Sacco University Hospital, ASST Fatebenefratelli-Sacco, Milano, Italy

L. Özçakar
Hacettepe University Medical School, Department of Physical and Rehabilitation Medicine, Ankara, Turkey

Wrist – Sonoanatomy and Interventional Techniques

Due to the high anatomical complexity of the wrist and the small sizes of the structures, US examination of this region can be "planned" with standardized positions of the patient, the sonographer, and the probe. Herewith, during the examination, they need to be dynamically modified depending on the anatomical structure and/or the clinical question [2–4].

Starting with the patient in sitting position (face-to-face with the physician) and the forearm pronated over the examination bed, a dorsal longitudinal scan can be used as the initial window to explore joint fluid [2]. Axial scan can be performed for prompt "sonographic navigation" as regards the six extensor compartments [2]. Using Lister's tubercle as a bony landmark, the probe can be shifted from ulnar to radial and vice versa (with a fan-like movement). Immediately on the radial side of the tubercle, it is possible to visualize the extensor carpi radialis brevis and longus tendons (2nd compartment) and the extensor pollicis brevis and abductor pollicis longus tendons (1st compartment) more radially. Immediately on the ulnar side of the tubercle, it is possible to visualize the extensor pollicis longus tendon (3rd compartment). Moving further ulnar, the extensor indicis proprius and extensor digitorum communis tendons (4th compartment), the extensor digiti minimi tendon (5th compartment), and the

Y. El Miedany (ed.), *Musculoskeletal Ultrasound-Guided Regenerative Medicine*,
https://doi.org/10.1007/978-3-030-98256-0_7

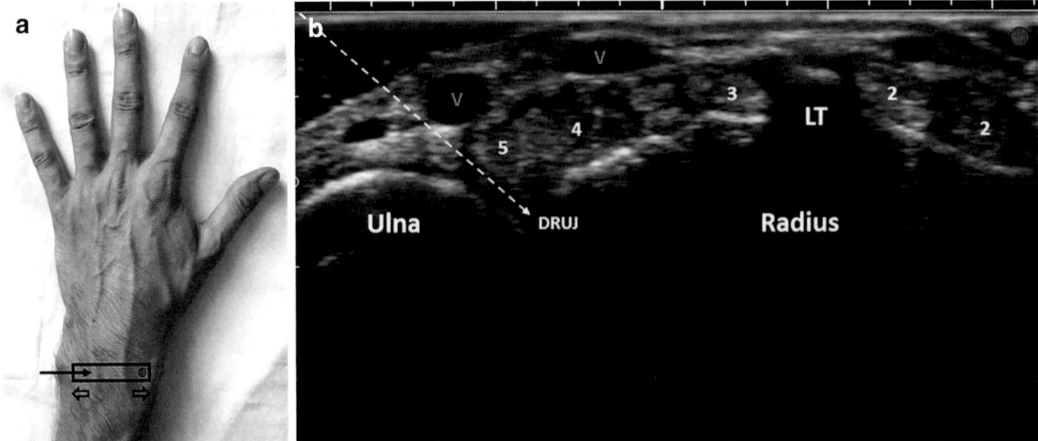

Fig. 7.1 Positioning the probe (*black rectangle*) in a transverse plane over the dorsal aspect of the wrist (**a**), Lister's tubercle (*LT*) and the extensor tendons can be visualized in the short-axis view (**b**). Using the in-plane technique, the needle (*black arrow*) (**a**) can be advanced from ulnar to radial direction in order to perform an intra-articular injection of the distal radioulnar joint (*DRUJ*) (**b**). Void arrows fan-like movement of the probe, V vein, 2, 2nd extensor compartment, 3, 3rd extensor compartment, 4, 4th extensor compartment, 5, 5th extensor compartment, dotted arrow needle's pathway

extensor carpi ulnaris tendon (6th compartment) can be imaged as well [2]. As the probe is shifted distally/proximally, tendons of the 1st and 3rd compartments will be seen as crossing over the 2nd compartment as the proximal and distal intersections, respectively [6]. In this position, an US-guided injection of the distal radioulnar joint (DRUJ) can also be performed using an in-plane technique and ulnar to radial approach (Fig. 7.1). The needle tip must be advanced deep to the extensor digiti minimi tendon, overcoming the joint capsule, in order to release the drug inside the articular space between the two bony surfaces [7].

Once identified in the short-axis view, each and every extensor tendon can be scanned in the long-axis view throughout their courses, i.e., from the proximal myotendinous junction until the distal attachment. Of note, the extensor digiti minimi tendon is usually located just superficial to the distal radioulnar joint [8], and through a slightest tilt/shift of the probe, the dorsal radioulnar ligament can be clearly visualized immediately below this tendon (Fig. 7.2). This ligament normally presents a "sloped" course due to the different alignment of the distal ends of radius and ulna [9]. Using this sonographic acoustic window, US-guided (regenerative) injection for this small ligament can readily be performed using an out-of-plane technique and dorsal to volar approach (Fig. 7.2).

To better evaluate the 1st extensor compartment, we can ask the patient to move the forearm in a neutral position over the examination bed, with a supportive object in the palm to stabilize the hand (Fig. 7.3) [4]. In this particular position, US-guided injections for the synovial sheaths of the tendons (and/or hydrodissection of the interface between the tendons and the extensor retinaculum) can be performed with an in-plane technique and dorsal to volar approach – also avoiding the radial artery (Fig. 7.3) [10]. Rotating the probe 90 degrees, US-guided needling of the dorsal retinaculum (e.g., in case of chronic thickening/fibrosis) can be performed using an in-plane technique and distal to proximal approach (Fig. 7.3). For sure, both short- and long-axis views of the 1st extensor compartment (Fig. 7.3) can be used for intra-tendinous injections (e.g., with orthobiologic agents) if clinically indicated. In the same position, dynamic sonotracking of the 1st extensor compartment (i.e., elevator technique) in a distal direction allows to visualize the crossing between the tendons and the radial

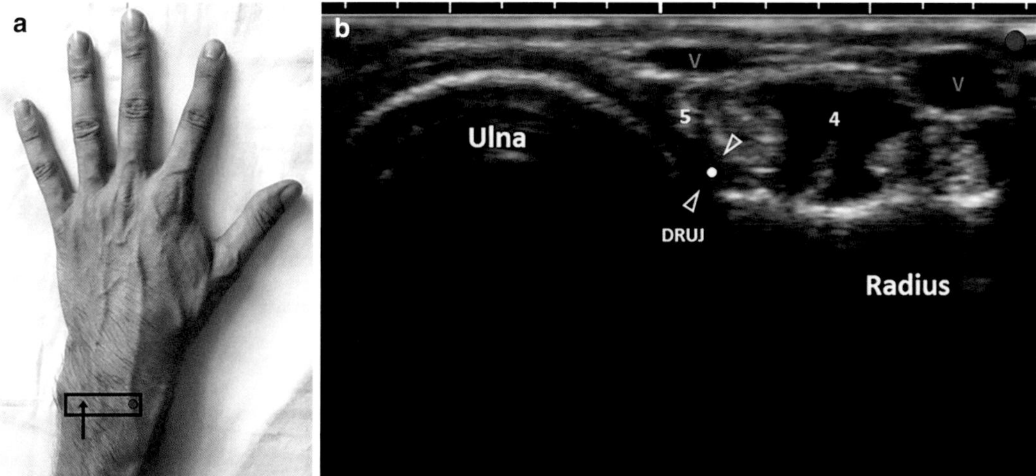

Fig. 7.2 Positioning the probe (*black rectangle*) in a transverse plane over the dorsal aspect of the wrist (**a**), the dorsal radioulnar ligament (*void arrowheads*) can be visualized in the long-axis view just below the extensor digiti minimi tendon (*5*) (**b**). Using the out-of-plane technique, the needle (*black arrow*) (**a**) can be advanced from cranial to caudal direction in order to target the ligament (**b**). V vein, DRUJ distal radioulnar joint, 4, 4th extensor tendon compartment, white dot, needle in the short-axis view

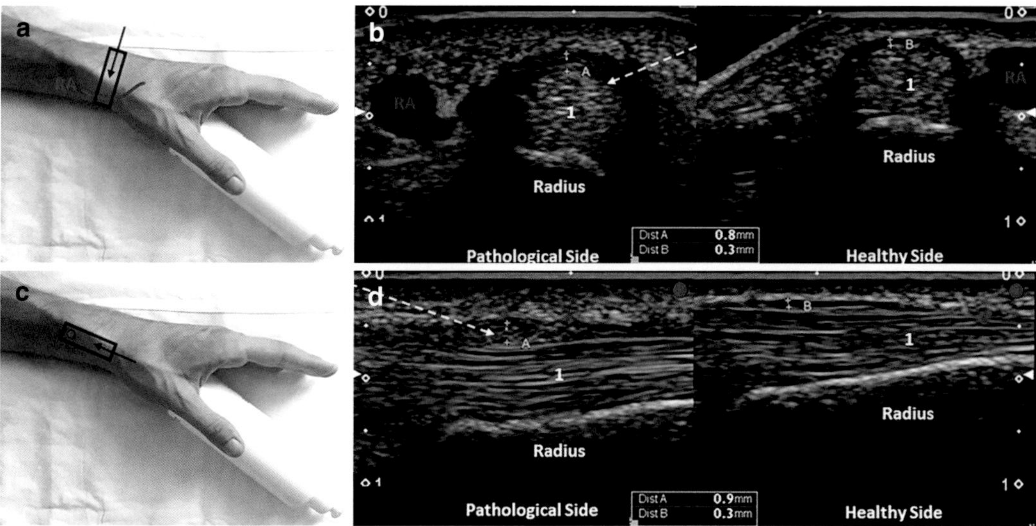

Fig. 7.3 Positioning the probe (*black rectangle*) in a transverse plane over the radial aspect of the wrist (**a**), the 1st extensor compartment (*1*) can be visualized in the short-axis view between the cortical bone of the radius and the retinaculum (*calipers*) (**b**). Using the in-plane technique, the needle (*black arrow*) (**a**) can be advanced from dorsal to volar direction in order to perform intra-sheath injection and/or hydrodissection of the interface between the retinaculum and the tendons (**b**). Rotating the probe (*black rectangle*) 90 degrees (**c**), the needle (*black arrow*) can be advanced for a distal to proximal direction to perform the needling of a thickened retinaculum (*calipers*) (**d**). RA radial artery, dotted arrow, needle's pathway

artery at the level of the carpal bones and in a proximal direction allows to identify the anatomical intersection between the 1st and 2nd compartments (Fig. 7.4). Of note, the intersection sites are considered as potential pain generators in the wrist due to excessive friction with inflam-

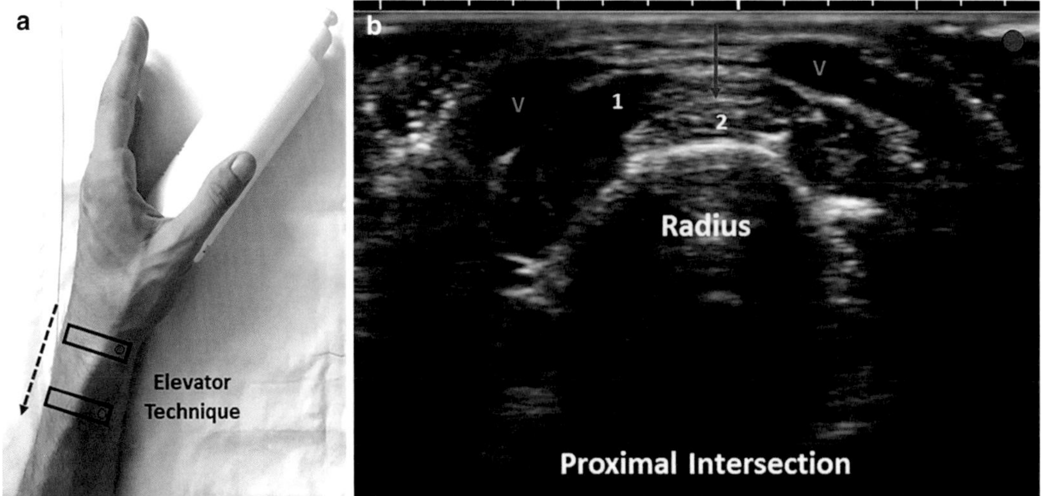

Fig. 7.4 Positioning the probe (*black rectangle*) in a transverse plane over the radial aspect of the wrist and using the "elevator technique" in a distal to proximal direction (**a**), the intersection between the 1st (*1*) and the 2nd (*2*) extensor compartments is clearly visible (**b**). Of note, the tendinous and muscular components of the extensor units are both present at this level. V vein, red arrow, tendon-tendon interface

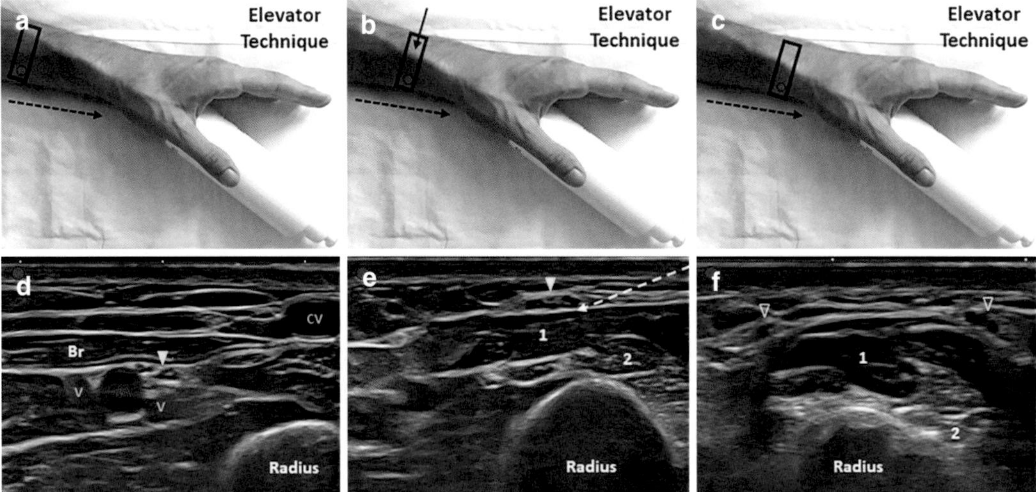

Fig. 7.5 Positioning the probe (*black rectangle*) in a transverse plane over the radial aspect of the wrist and using the "elevator technique" in a proximal to distal direction (**a**–**c**), the superficial branch of the radial nerve (*yellow arrowhead*) (**d**) can be seen piercing the superficial fascia of the forearm (**e**) and diverging in different ending branches (*void yellow arrowheads*) distally (**f**). Using the in-plane technique, the needle (*black arrow*) (**b**) can be advanced from dorsal to volar direction in order to perform hydrodissection of the nerve from the nearby soft tissues (**e**). CV cephalic vein, Br brachioradialis muscle, RA radial artery, V vein, 1, 1st extensor compartment, 2, 2nd extensor compartment, dotted arrow, needle's pathway

matory phenomena and overuse tendinopathies. Indisputably, US-guided interventions can easily be planned at any specific level for any specific target alike [11]. Without changing the position of the patient (as in Fig. 7.3), a proximal to distal sonotracking for the superficial branch of the radial nerve (SBRN) is possible (Fig. 7.5) [12] whereby it pierces the antebrachial fascia and splits into its terminal branches [13]. Using this acoustic window, US-guided hydrodissection of this sensory nerve from the surrounding soft tissues can be performed using an in-plane technique and dorsal to volar approach (Fig. 7.5). This procedure might be clinically indicated in patients with proximal intersection syndrome or chronic De Quervain syndrome coupled with neural irritation (i.e., neuritis) or after surgical release of the 1st extensor compartment with local adhesions that impair physiological gliding of the SBRN [14, 15].

As previously underlined, continuous repositioning of the forearm may be necessary to "follow" a specific structure and/or correctly visualize a small/curved target. Indeed, asking the patient to grip an object with the fingers, it is possible to "raise" the wrist from the examination bed in order to easily scan the extensor carpi ulnaris (ECU) tendon at the level of the ulnar groove and over the ulnocarpal joint (Fig. 7.6) [3, 4]. Likewise, an US-guided injection of the synovial sheath of the ECU tendon or hydrodissection of the interface between the tendon and the retinaculum can be performed using an in-plane technique and dorsal to volar approach (Fig. 7.6). Rotating the probe 90 degrees (longitudinal plane), the triangular fibrocartilage complex (TFCC) would be scanned in the ulnocarpal space deep to the ECU tendon (Fig. 7.7). An active radial deviation of the wrist is paramount to increase the size of the ulnocarpal space in order to better visualize the deep tissues [16]. Using the same position, an US-guided injection of the TFCC/ulnocarpal space can be readily performed with an out-of-plane technique and dorsal to volar approach in regenerative medicine (Fig. 7.7) [17]. It is noteworthy that the TFCC is crucial for the stabilization of the distal radial-ulnar and ulnocarpal joints. It is composed of an articular disk, meniscus homolog, ulnocarpal ligament, dorsal and volar radioulnar ligaments, and ECU tendon sheath. Of note, the prestyloid recess is a synovial space between the articular disk and the meniscus homolog that may be filled with minimal fluid in a normal condition [18]. Following the ECU tendon in the long-axis view, its distal attachment to the base of the 5th metacarpal bone can also be visualized (Fig. 7.8).

While the dorsal transverse approach is useful to promptly evaluate the extensor tendon compartments of the wrist, the dorsal longitudinal scan is paramount to correctly differentiate the carpal bones and the articular surfaces [2, 3]. Positioning the probe "bridged" between the distal end of the radius and the 2nd metacarpal bone, scaphoid and trapezoid can be seen. Herein, a portion of the dorsal radiocarpal recess is located superficial to the scaphoid cortex (Fig. 7.9). Progressively shifting the probe towards the ulnar side, the scaphoid and capitate bones can be seen at the level of Lister's tubercle (Fig. 7.10). More laterally, scaphoid is replaced by lunate and the dorsal radiolunotriquetral (RLT) ligament is

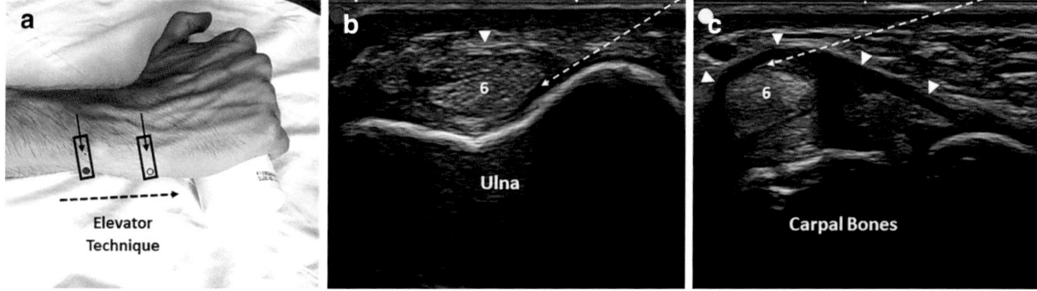

Fig. 7.6 Positioning the probe (*black rectangle*) in a transverse plane over the ulnar aspect of the wrist and using the "elevator technique" (**a**), the 6th extensor compartment (*6*) can be visualized in the short-axis view in the ulnar groove (**b**) and over the carpal bones (**c**). Using the in-plane technique, the needle (*black arrow*) (**a**) can be advanced from dorsal to volar direction in order to perform an intra-sheath injection of the extensor carpi ulnaris tendon (**b**) or hydrodissection of the interface between the tendon and the retinaculum (**c**). White arrowhead, retinaculum, dotted arrow, needle's pathway

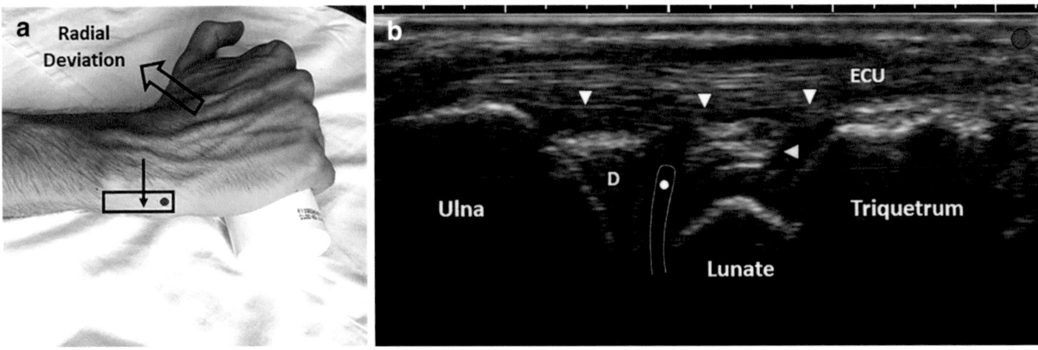

Fig. 7.7 Positioning the probe (*black rectangle*) in a longitudinal plane over the ulnar aspect of the wrist under active radial deviation (**a**), the articular disk (*D*), the homologous meniscus (*yellow arrowhead*), and the prestyloid recess (*white dotted line*) can all be visualized under the extensor carpi ulnaris (*ECU*) tendon and ulnar collateral ligament (*white arrowheads*), between the distal end of the ulna and the carpal bones (**b**). Using the out-of-plane technique, the needle (*black arrow*) (**a**) can be advanced from dorsal to volar direction in order to reach the ulnocarpal space and target the TFCC. White dot, needle in the short-axis view located inside the prestyloid recess

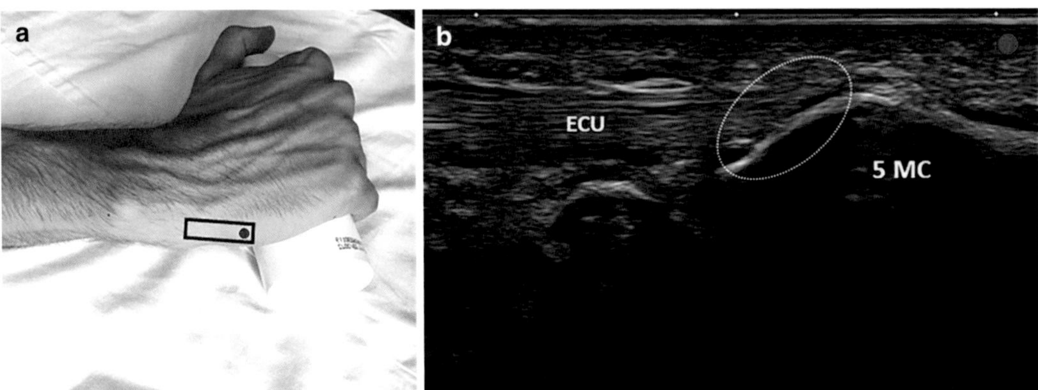

Fig. 7.8 Positioning the probe (*black rectangle*) in a longitudinal plane over the ulnar aspect of the wrist/hand (**a**), the distal attachment of the extensor carpi ulnaris (*ECU*) tendon to the base of the 5th metacarpal bone (*5MC*) can be easily visualized and targeted (**b**). White dotted circle, enthesis of the extensor carpi ulnaris tendon

clearly visible in the short-axis view (Fig. 7.11). Using this position, an US-guided injection of the dorsal recess of the radiocarpal joint (e.g., for synovitis) can be performed with an out-of-plane technique and dorsal to volar approach [10, 19].

Rotating the probe in a transverse oblique plane, the dorsal RLT ligament can be depicted in the long-axis view [8, 9] whereby an US-guided injection (in-plane, radial to ulnar approach) can be performed (Fig. 7.12).

The longitudinal dorsal approach of the wrist allows a panoramic evaluation of the dorsal radiocarpal and midcarpal recesses to be checked for effusion and/or synovitis [2, 3]. Shifting the probe more laterally (ulnar), the ulnocarpal space is seen with the TFCC interposed between the distal end of ulna and the carpal bones (Fig. 7.13). Using this acoustic window, an US-guided injection of the ulnocarpal space/TFCC can be performed with an out-of-plane technique and dorsal to volar approach [17].

Starting from the basic scan at the level of Lister's tubercle in a transverse plane (Fig. 7.1), it is possible to slowly shift the probe more distally until the dorsal scapholunate ligament is clearly visualized in its long-axis view (Fig. 7.14) [8, 9].

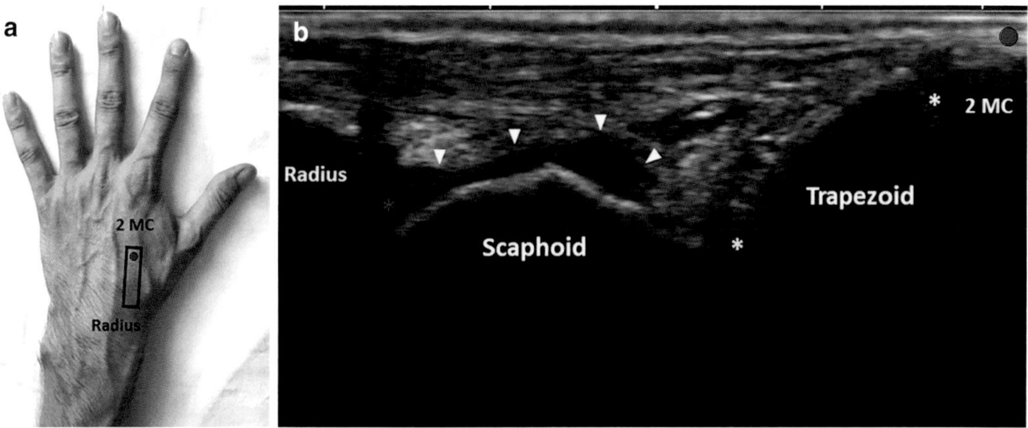

Fig. 7.9 Positioning the probe (*black rectangle*) in a longitudinal plane over the dorsal aspect of the wrist between the distal end of the radius and the 2nd metacarpal bone (*2MC*) (**a**), scaphoid and trapezoid are visible (**b**). Red asterisk, radiocarpal joint, yellow asterisk, midcarpal joint, white asterisk, carpometacarpal joint, white arrowheads, dorsal radiocarpal recess

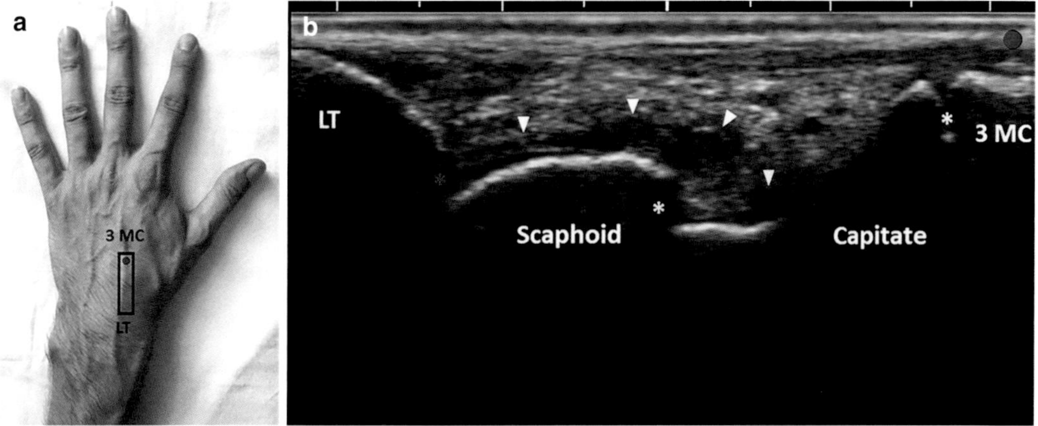

Fig. 7.10 Positioning the probe (*black rectangle*) in a longitudinal plane over the dorsal aspect of the wrist between Lister's tubercle (*LT*) and the 3rd metacarpal bone (*3MC*) (**a**), scaphoid and capitate are visible (**b**). Red asterisk, radiocarpal joint, yellow asterisk, midcarpal joint, white asterisk, carpometacarpal joint, white arrowheads, dorsal radiocarpal recess, yellow asterisk, dorsal midcarpal recess

Especially after wrist trauma, sonographic evaluation of this ligament is paramount because an eventual partial/complete tear may be associated with acute/chronic instability of the carpal bones [20]. In addition to the direct signs of ligament injury (i.e., focal/complete defect of the echostructure), the indirect ultrasonographic sign (enlargement of the scapholunate space as compared to the contralateral side) and dynamic imaging (separation of the bones during active radial/ulnar deviation) would, for sure, be useful to precisely evaluate this anatomical structure in routine daily clinical practice [21].

In patients with synovitis of the radiocarpal joint, this sonographic window can be used to perform an US-guided injection of the dorsal recess (overlying the dorsal scapholunate ligament) with an in-plane technique and ulnar to radial approach (Fig. 7.14). With the same technique, the needle tip can be advanced until/inside the injured ligament (in the space between the bones) for an injection [19].

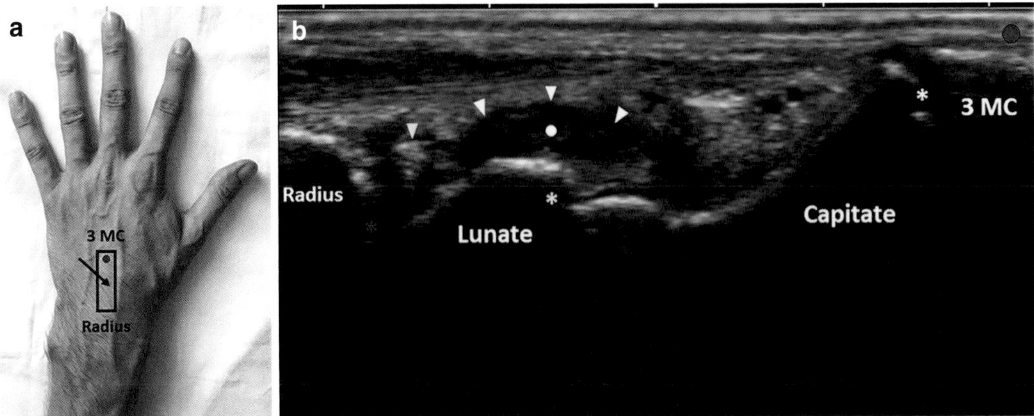

Fig. 7.11 Positioning the probe (*black rectangle*) in a longitudinal plane over the dorsal aspect of the wrist between the distal end of the radius and the 3rd metacarpal bone (*3MC*) (**a**), lunate and capitate are visible (**b**). Using the out-of-plane technique, the needle (*black arrow*) (**a**) can be advanced from dorsal to volar direction in order to visualize it in the short-axis view (*white dot*) inside the dorsal radiocarpal recess (*white arrowheads*) (**b**). Red asterisk, radiocarpal joint, yellow asterisk, midcarpal joint, white asterisk, carpometacarpal joint, yellow arrowhead, dorsal radiolunotriquetral ligament (short-axis view)

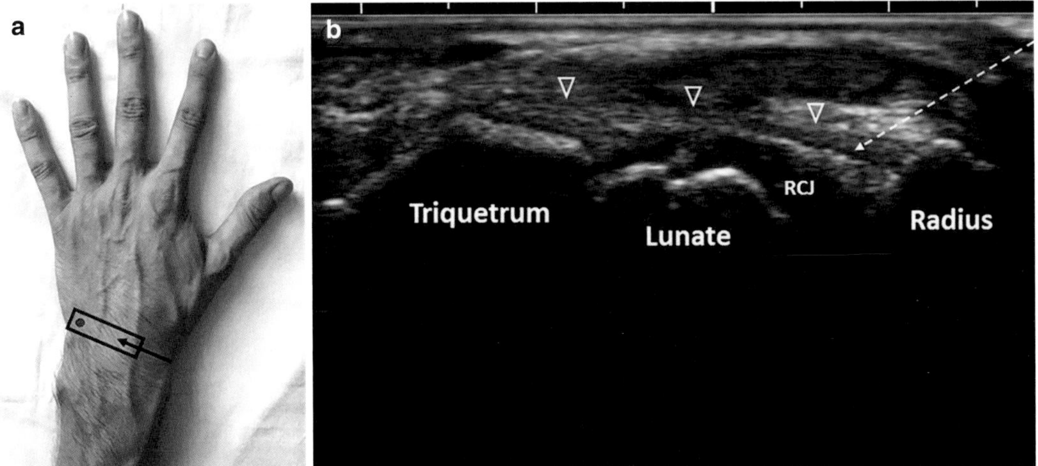

Fig. 7.12 Positioning the probe (*black rectangle*) in a transverse oblique plane over the dorsal aspect of the wrist (**a**), the dorsal radiolunotriquetral ligament (*void arrowheads*) is visible in the long-axis view (**b**). Using the in-plane technique, the needle (*black arrow*) (**a**) can be advanced from radial to ulnar direction to target the ligament (**b**). Void arrow, needle's pathway, RCJ radiocarpal joint

Another basic scan of the wrist is the transverse (palmar) approach at the level of the distal third of the forearm. Radius, ulna, and the overlying pronator quadratus muscle can be easily recognized to "orientate" the sonographic evaluation (Fig. 7.15). Of note, unlike the dorsal view, radius and ulna present a regular alignment on the same horizontal plane in the volar view. Progressively moving the probe towards the fingers, the proximal and distal segments of the carpal tunnel can be depicted using specific bony landmarks, i.e., scaphoid and pisiform for the proximal carpal tunnel (Fig. 7.16) and trapezium and hamate for the distal carpal tunnel (Fig. 7.17) [2, 22, 23]. Herein, complete sonotracking of the median nerve, from proximal to distal, is necessarily per-

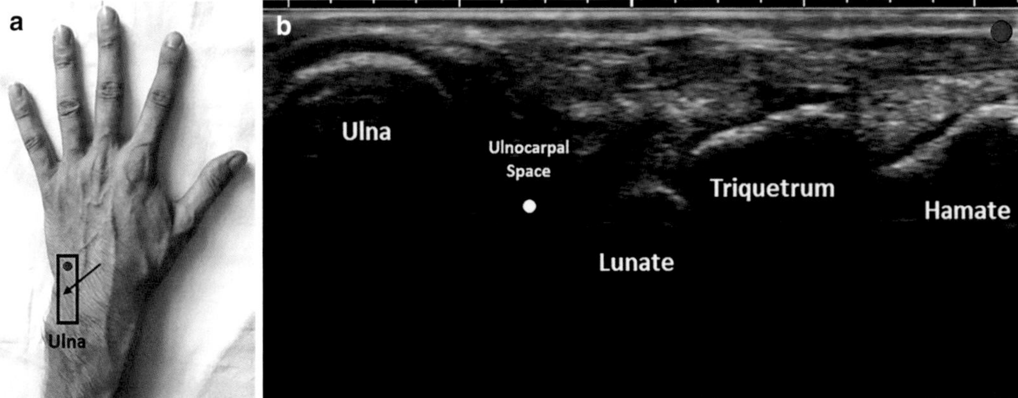

Fig. 7.13 Positioning the probe (*black rectangle*) in a longitudinal plane over the dorsal aspect of the wrist (**a**), the ulnocarpal space is clearly visible between the distal end of the ulna and the carpal bones (**b**). Using the out-of-plane technique, the needle (*black arrow*) (**a**) can be advanced from dorsal to volar direction until it is visualized in the short-axis view (*white dot*) in the "target space" before the injection (**b**). Of note, using the dorsal approach is more difficult to clearly distinguish the different components of the TFCC as compared with the ulnar approach shown in Fig. 7.7. As such, this acoustic window would be useful if the ulnocarpal space (but not a specific smaller structure) is the target of the injection

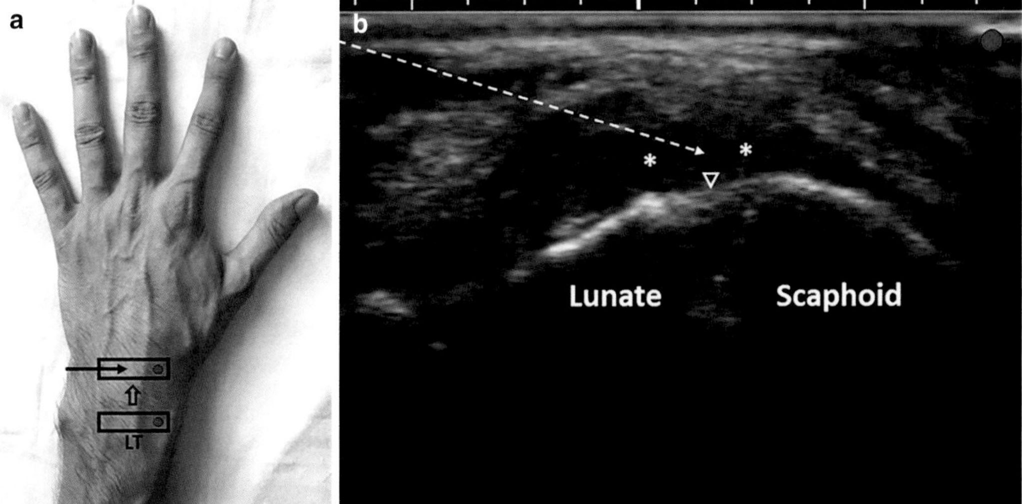

Fig. 7.14 Positioning the probe (*black rectangle*) in a transverse plane over Lister's tubercle (*LT*) and gradually moving the probe distally (**a**), the dorsal scapholunate ligament (*void arrowhead*) is visible in its long-axis view (**b**). Using the in-plane technique, the needle (*black arrow*) (**a**) can be advanced from ulnar to radial direction to inject the dorsal radiocarpal recess, overlying the ligament (*white asterisks*) (**b**). Of note, with the same technique, the dorsal scapholunate ligament can be targeted. Void arrow, needle's pathway

formed in the transverse view (elevator technique) exploring the sonoanatomy of different sections of the tunnel. Again, US-guided perineural injections can easily be performed in the short-axis view using the in-plane technique and radial to ulnar (or ulnar to radial) approach for several purposes (perineural corticosteroid injection, nerve hydrodissection using dextrose, etc.) (Fig. 7.16) [24, 25]. Additionally, the ulnar nerve can also be sonotracked proximally (starting

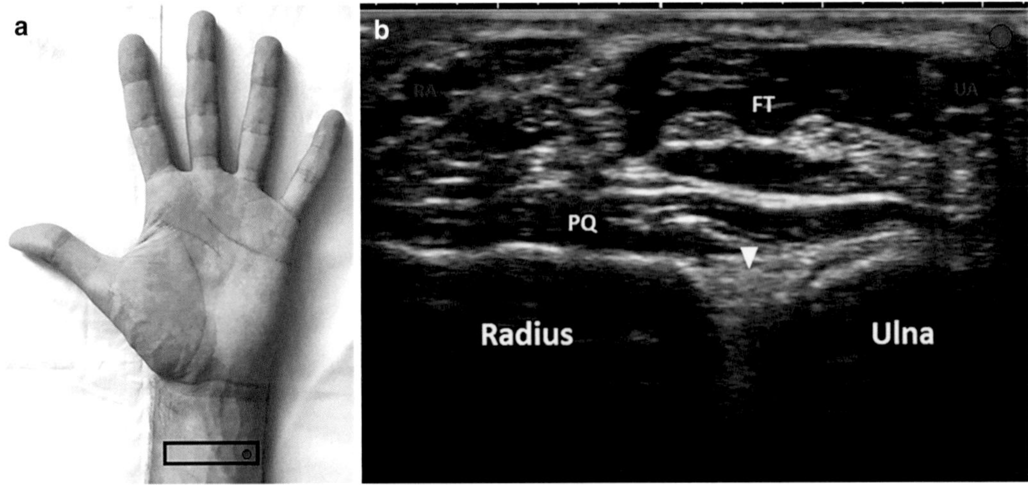

Fig. 7.15 Positioning the probe (*black rectangle*) in a transverse plane over the volar aspect of the distal third of the forearm (**a**), the pronator quadratus (*PQ*) muscle can be used as an anatomical landmark (**b**). RA radial artery, UA ulnar artery, FT flexor tendons, white arrowhead, interosseous membrane

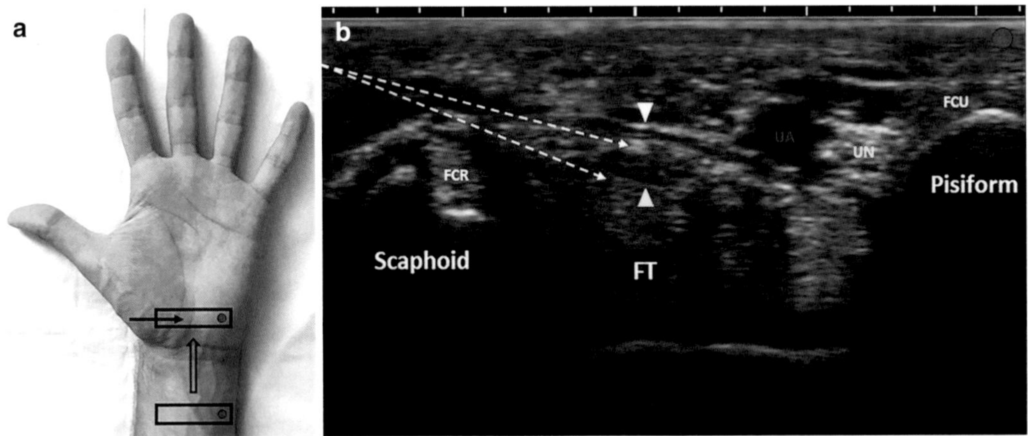

Fig. 7.16 Positioning the probe (*black rectangle*) in a transverse plane over the pronator quadratus muscle and gradually moving the probe distally (**a**), the proximal section of the carpal tunnel is clearly visible (**b**). Using the in-plane technique, the needle (*black arrow*) (**a**) can be advanced from radial to ulnar direction to hydrodissect the interfaces between the median nerve (*yellow arrowhead*), flexor tendons (*FT*), and the transverse carpal ligament (*white arrowhead*) (**b**). Of note, with the same technique, a perineural injection can also be performed. FCR flexor carpi radialis tendon, FCU flexor carpi ulnaris tendon, UA ulnar artery, UN ulnar nerve, dotted arrows, needle's pathways

from Guyon's canal) in order to visualize the origin of the dorsal cutaneous branch in the anatomical space located between the flexor carpi ulnaris and pronator quadratus muscles (Fig. 7.18) [12]. At this level, both nerves can be targeted under US guidance with an in-plane technique and ulnar to radial approach.

Rotating the probe 90 degrees, the median nerve can be visualized in its long-axis view (Fig. 7.19), particularly useful to confirm its compression while passing under the transverse carpal ligament (i.e., hourglass sign) [26]. Keeping the probe in a longitudinal plane, it is possible to shift it in an ulnar direction to visual-

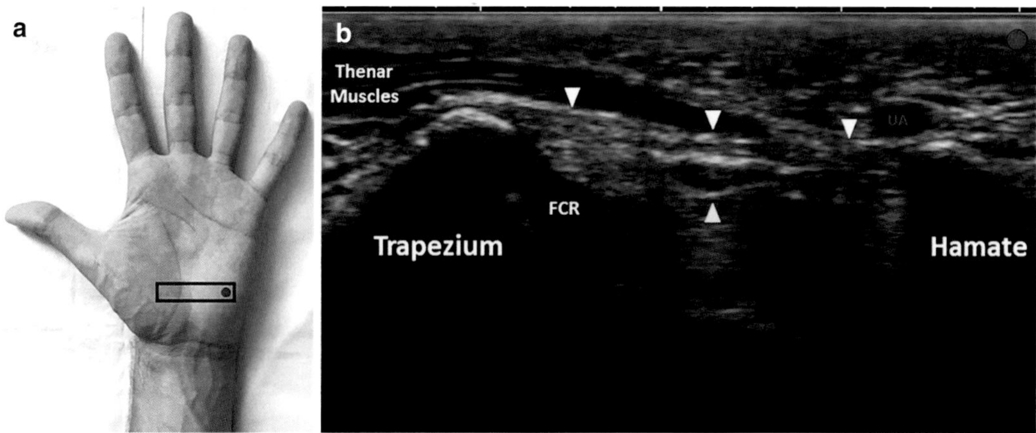

Fig. 7.17 Positioning the probe (*black rectangle*) in a transverse plane over the palmar aspect of the hand (**a**), the distal section of the carpal tunnel can be evaluated (**b**). At this level, the transverse carpal ligament (*white arrowheads*) appears thicker compared to its proximal segment. Also note the anisotropy pertaining to the flexor carpi radialis (*FCR*) tendon. Yellow arrowhead, median nerve, UA ulnar artery

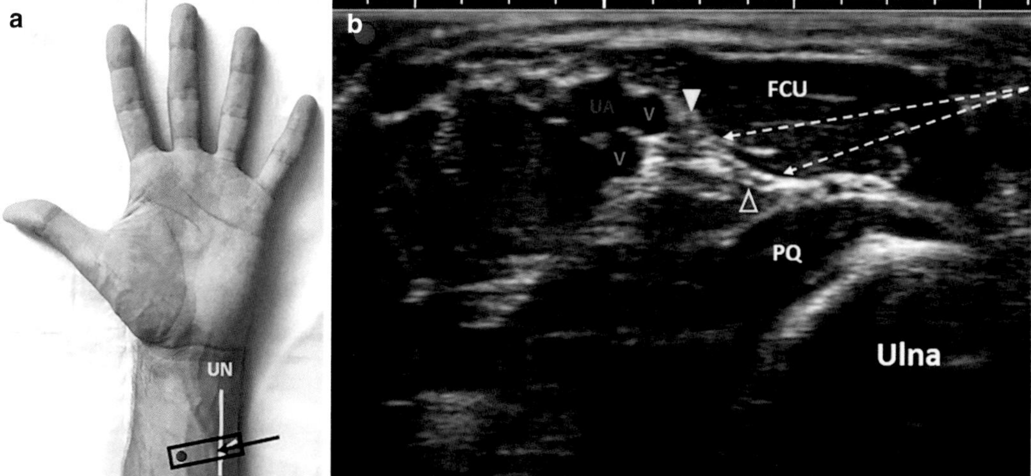

Fig. 7.18 Positioning the probe (*black rectangle*) in an oblique transverse plane over the volar aspect of the distal third of the forearm (**a**), the dorsal cutaneous branch (*void yellow arrowhead*) of the ulnar nerve (*yellow arrowhead*) can be visualized in the anatomical space between the flexor carpi ulnaris (*FCU*) and pronator quadratus (*PQ*) muscles (**b**). Using the in-plane technique, the needle (*black arrow*) (**a**) can be advanced from ulnar to radial direction to target the neural structures (**b**). UN ulnar nerve, UA ulnar artery, V vein, dotted arrows, needle's pathways

ize the attachment of the flexor carpi ulnaris tendon to pisiform (anatomical location of a small insertional bursa) (Fig. 7.20). Similarly, shifting the probe in a radial direction, the flexor carpi radialis tendon is visualized passing over scaphoid and attaching to the base of the 2nd metacarpal bone (Fig. 7.20) [27, 28].

Hand – Sonoanatomy and Interventional Techniques

With the patient in sitting position (face-to-face with the physician) and the forearm supinated (resting on the examination bed or a pillow), a volar approach can be considered as the simplest

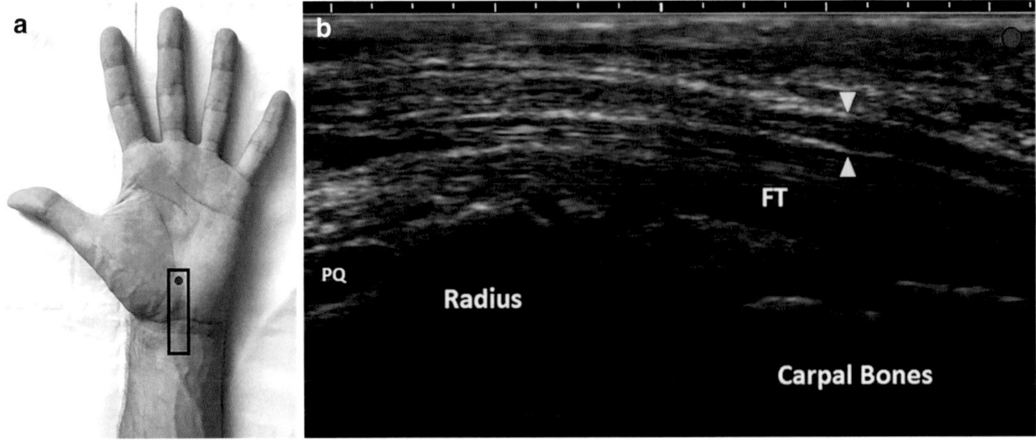

Fig. 7.19 Positioning the probe (*black rectangle*) in a longitudinal plane over the volar aspect of the wrist (**a**), the median nerve (*yellow arrowheads*) in the long-axis view can be seen superficial to the flexor tendons (*FT*) (**b**). During active flexion/extension of the fingers, the nerve can be visualized to glide but less than the tendons. PQ pronator quadratus muscle

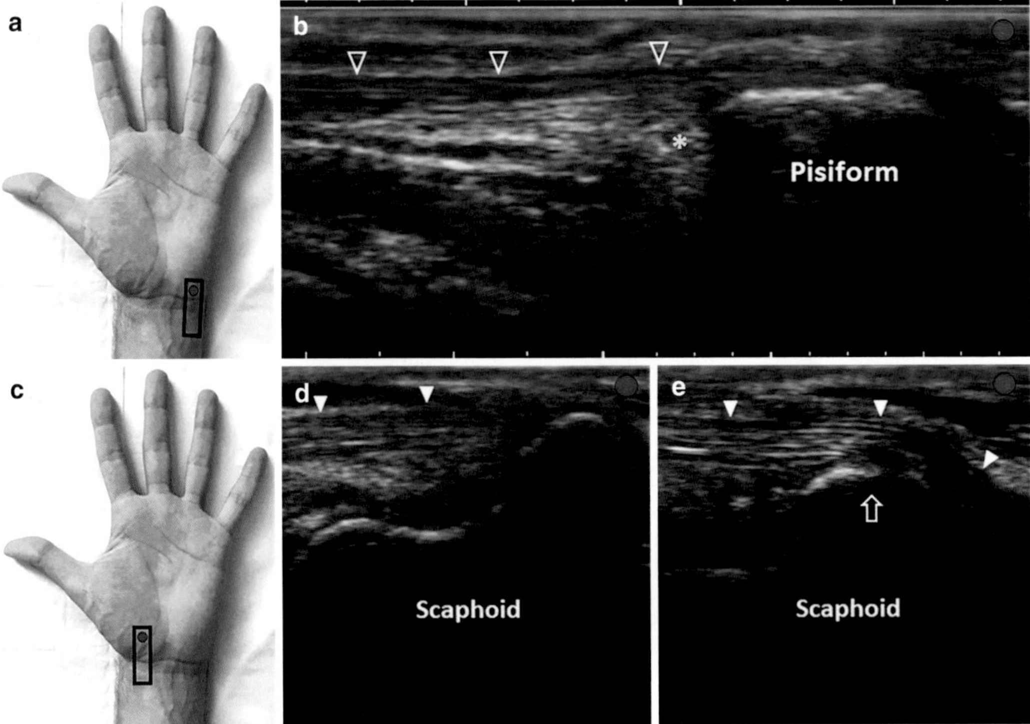

Fig. 7.20 Positioning the probe (*black rectangle*) in a longitudinal plane over the volar and ulnar aspect of the wrist (**a**), the attachment site of the flexor carpi ulnaris tendon (*void arrowheads*) over the pisiform bone is well visualized (**b**). Of note, in some patients, a synovial bursa can be located in the tendon-bone interface (*yellow asterisk*). On the other hand, shifting the probe (*black rectangle*) at the radial side of the wrist (**c**), the peculiar shape of the volar surface of the scaphoid bone can be used as an anatomical landmark to promptly recognize the overlying flexor carpi radialis tendon (*white arrowheads*) (**d**). At this level, gently tilting the probe, the anatomical course of the tendon over the distal pole of the scaphoid (*void arrow*) is better depicted (**e**). This is a critical point where excessive friction can lead to tenosynovitis and/or tendinopathies

way to start with [2]. Positioning the probe in a longitudinal plane over the metacarpophalangeal (MCP) joint, flexor tendons overlying the volar plate are easily recognized (Fig. 7.21). In addition to static imaging, tendons' gliding can be thoroughly assessed during active and passive flexion/extension [29]. Of note, the dynamic part of the examination is paramount if mechanical impingement between the tendons and the surrounding tissues (e.g., hypertrophic pulley, stenosing tenosynovitis, postsurgical adhesions, local osteophytes, cortical irregularities after a trauma, subluxation of the small joints of the fingers) is clinically suspected [3, 4, 29]. In the same plane, the attachment site of the flexor digitorum profundus tendon on the base of the distal phalanx can be visualized distally (Fig. 7.21). Using either the long- or short-axis views, an US-guided injection of the synovial sheath of the tendons (and/or of the interface pulley-tendon) can easily be performed using an in-plane technique (Fig. 7.22) [19, 30]. Herewith, to reduce the procedure-related pain, an interdigital approach avoiding the puncture of the highly innervated palmar skin of the hand has also been described [19, 31].

The long-axis view of flexor tendons can be considered as a useful sonographic approach also for diagnosis and interventions of pathologies related with the palmar aponeurosis (i.e., tiny

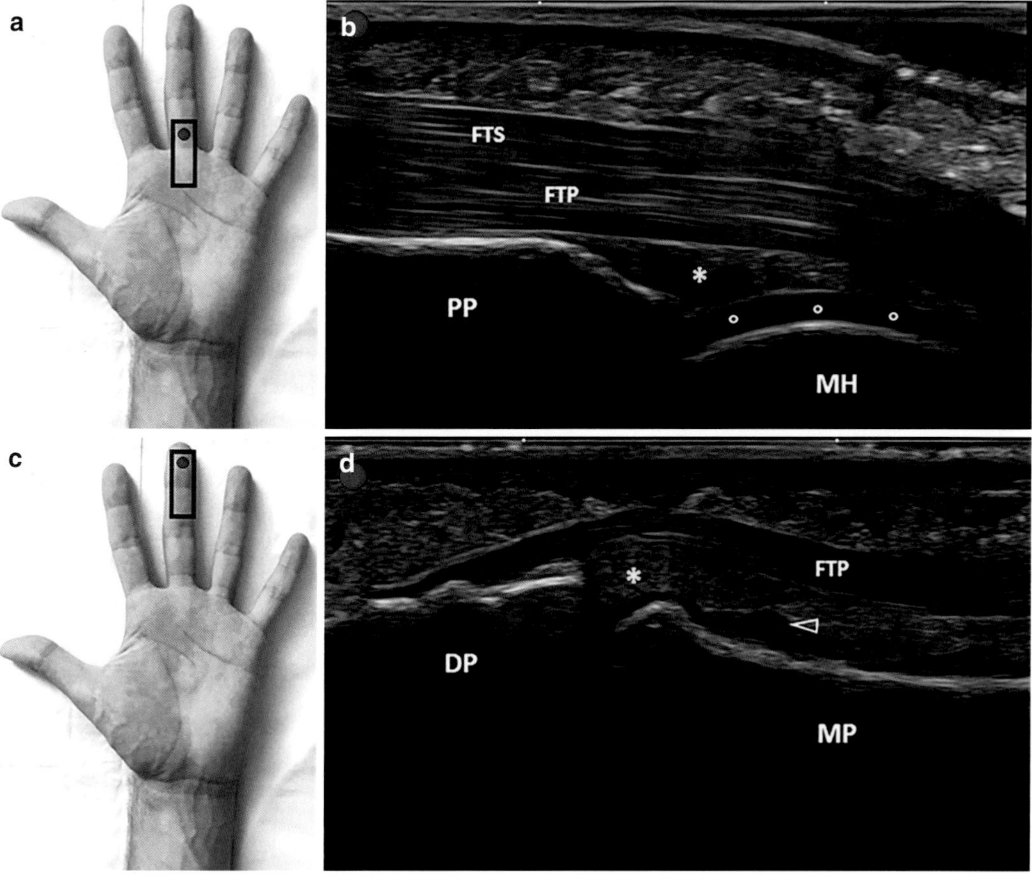

Fig. 7.21 Positioning the probe (*black rectangle*) in a longitudinal plane over the volar aspect of the finger at the level of the metacarpophalangeal joint (**a**), the superficial (*FTS*) and deep (*FTD*) flexor tendons are easily recognizable just over the volar plate (*yellow asterisk*) (**b**). Gradually shifting the probe (*black rectangle*) in a distal direction (**c**), the attachment site of the deep flexor tendon (*FTD*) to the base of the distal phalanx (*DP*) can be depicted (**d**). MH metacarpal head, PP proximal phalanx, white dots, cartilage, MP, middle phalanx, void arrowhead, articular recess

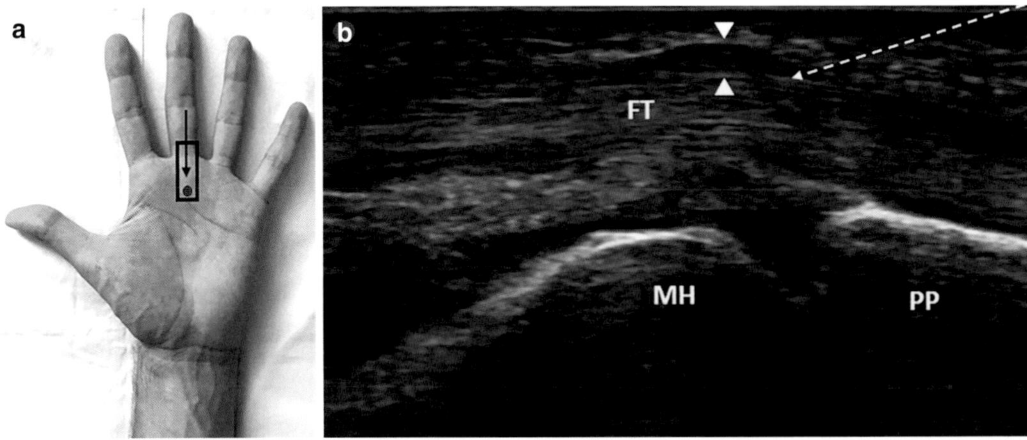

Fig. 7.22 Positioning the probe (*black rectangle*) in a longitudinal plane over the volar aspect of the finger (**a**), an intervention can be planned in patients with pathologies of the flexor tendons (*FT*) (e.g., tenosynovitis, trigger finger). Using the in-plane technique, the needle (*black arrow*) can be advanced from a distal to proximal direction (**a**) to inject the synovial sheath of the tendons and/or to hydrodissect the interface between the tendons and the pulley (*white arrowheads*) (**b**). MH metacarpal head, PP proximal phalanx, dotted arrow, needle's pathway

anatomical structure located superficial to the flexor tendons) (Fig. 7.23) [32]. For instance, fibrous nodules originating from the palmar fascia of the hand (i.e., Dupuytren's disease) are common in clinical practice whereby dynamic assessment of the tendons allows the physician to promptly evaluate the presence of local adhesions [29, 32]. This dynamic/precise evaluation is paramount to correctly plan for the details of the US-guided procedure, e.g., injection inside the nodule and/or hydrodissection of the tendons and the palmar aponeurosis [4, 19].

Rotating the probe 90 degrees, the short-axis view of the flexor tendons (Fig. 7.24) will allow full evaluation using the "elevator technique" and dynamic scanning to observe the tendon motions from a different perspective. As mentioned above, this acoustic window can also serve as a convenient/safe way for guided injections of the interface between pulley and flexor tendons (and/or their sheath) with an in-plane ulnar to radial (or radial to ulnar) approach [19, 30].

Keeping the forearm supinated, it is possible to put the probe in a longitudinal oblique plane over the volar aspect of the thenar eminence to visualize the trapezio-scaphoid and trapezio-metacarpal joints (Fig. 7.25). Using this positioning, both joints can also be targeted using an out-of-plane technique and radial to ulnar approach [33]. At this level, another important anatomical structure, potentially involved in thumb pain, is the flexor pollicis longus tendon. It courses between the superficial and deep heads of the flexor pollicis brevis muscle (Fig. 7.26) [34]. Following this tendon in the short-/long-axis view from proximal to distal, its relationship with the (radial and ulnar) sesamoid bones of the thumb at the level of the 1st metacarpophalangeal joint is well depicted [35].

Using a large amount of gel and gentle compression of the probe, the dorsal aspect of the MCP joint can be clearly visualized, i.e., recognizing the cartilage of the metacarpal head, the dorsal plate, and the capsule interface (Fig. 7.27) [2]. This sonographic window can be used to perform an US-guided injection of the MCP joint with an out-of-plane technique and radial to ulnar (or vice versa) approach [1, 19]. Of note, with the same technique, the proximal and distal interphalangeal joints can be injected under US guidance as well. Likewise, it is again possible to visualize/target the extensor tendons of the fingers using different techniques, i.e., static and dynamic, short- and long-axis views (Figs. 7.28 and 7.29) [4, 36].

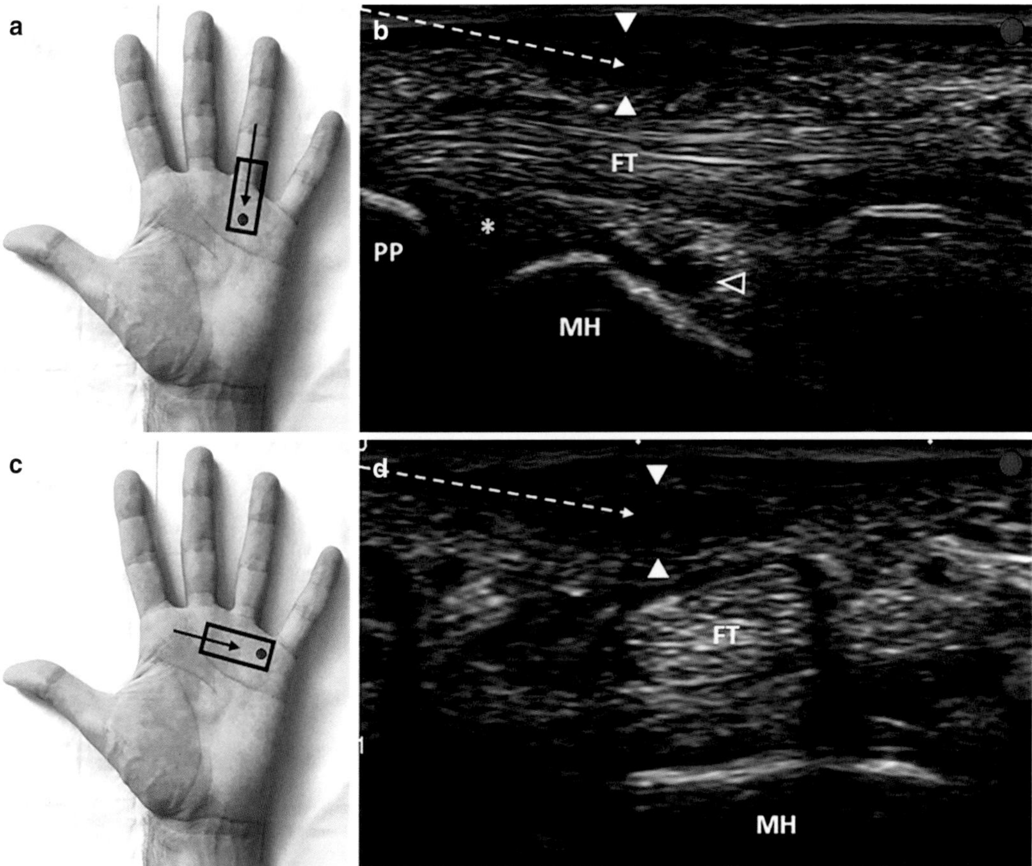

Fig. 7.23 Positioning the probe (*black rectangle*) in a longitudinal plane over the volar aspect of the hand (**a**), the needle (*black arrow*) can be advanced from a distal to proximal direction (**a**) to inject a focal thickening (*white arrowheads*) of the palmar aponeurosis in Dupuytren's contracture (**b**). On the other hand, positioning the probe (*black rectangle*) in a transverse plane (**c**), the same procedure can be performed with the in-plane technique and radial to ulnar (or ulnar to radial) approach (**d**). Void arrow, needle's pathway, FT flexor tendons, MH metacarpal head, PP proximal phalanx, yellow asterisk, volar plate, void arrowhead, articular recess

Asking the patient to grip an object within the fingers, it would be possible to "tension" the sagittal bands and identify them as curved hypoechoic structures originating from the dorsal interossei muscles – incapsulating the extensor tendons (Fig. 7.30) [36]. These sagittal bands (i.e., the main component of the extensor hood) are thin structures made of connective tissue, and they act as passive stabilizers (the "cuff") of the extensor tendons in the dorsal aspect of the MCP joints during finger flexion/extension [37]. Like elsewhere, seeing under US also means access to any structure; therefore, when necessary, US-guided injections of the sagittal bands can be performed using this acoustic window (Fig. 7.30).

Last but not least, another important ligament of the thumb, frequently involved in traumatic injuries and thus a possible target for regenerative interventions, is the ulnar collateral ligament [38]. Asking the patient to lie the thumb over an object while the forearm is partially pronated, this ligament can be visualized statically or dynamically – during movements of the interphalangeal joint of the thumb (helping to distinguish the ligament from the overlying adductor pollicis

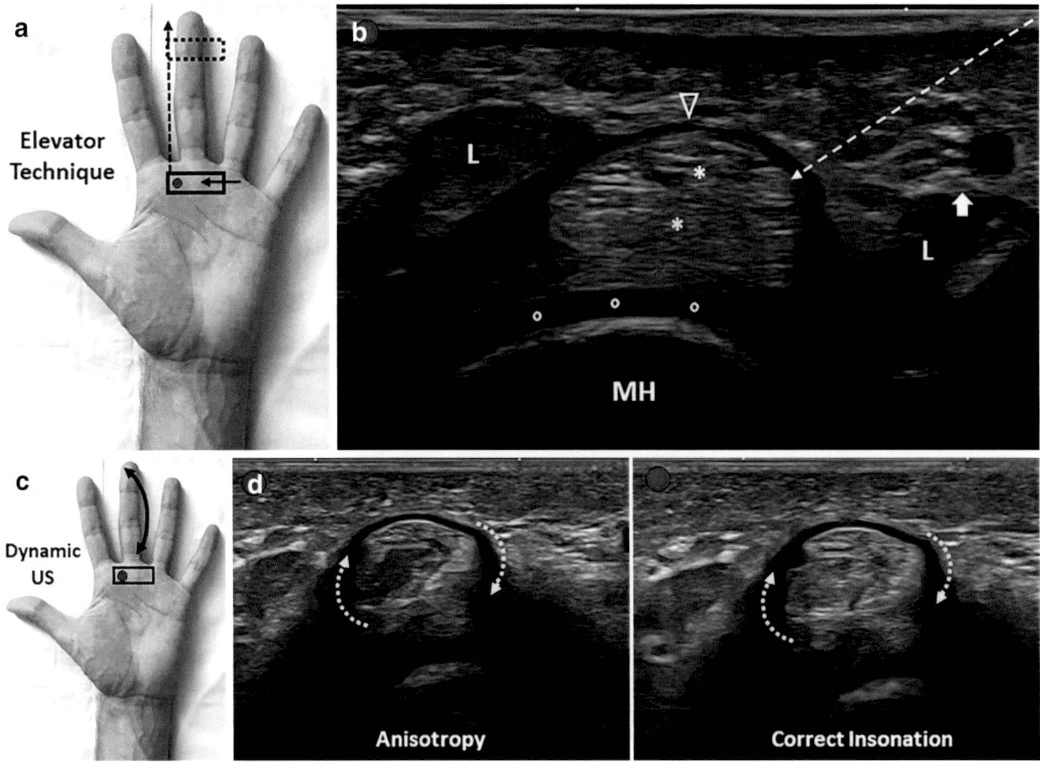

Fig. 7.24 Positioning the probe (*black rectangle*) in a transverse plane over the volar aspect of the finger and using the "elevator technique" (**a**), the superficial (*white asterisk*) and deep (*yellow asterisk*) flexor tendons can be completely evaluated (**b**). Using the in-plane technique, the needle (*black arrow*) can be advanced from ulnar to radial (or radial to ulnar) direction (**a**) to inject the synovial sheath of the tendons and/or to hydrodissect the interface between the pulley (*void arrowhead*) and the tendons, avoiding the neurovascular bundle (*white arrow*) (**b**). During active flexion/extension of the finger (*double black arrow*) (**c**), axial twisting (*yellow dotted arrows*) of the superficial and deep flexor tendons can be promptly evaluated, also paying attention to the anisotropy (**d**). L lumbricals, white dotted arrow, needle's pathway, red asterisk, volar plate, white dots, cartilage, MH metacarpal head

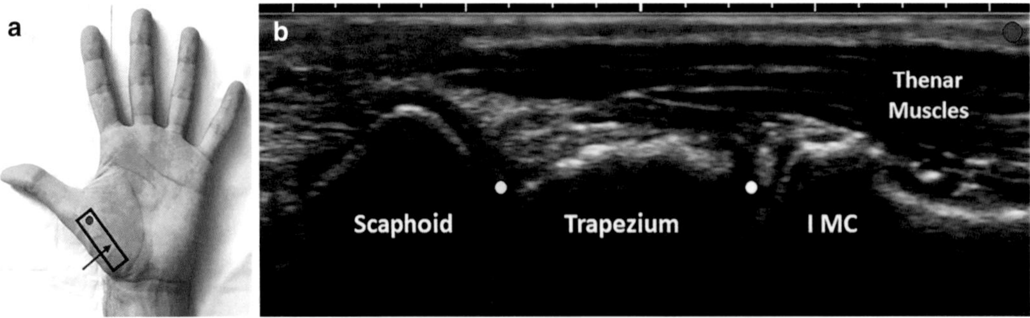

Fig. 7.25 Positioning the probe (*black rectangle*) in a longitudinal oblique plane over the volar aspect of the thenar eminence (**a**), trapezio-scaphoid (*yellow dot*) and trapezio-metacarpal (*white dot*) joints can be depicted (**b**). Using the out-of-plane technique, the needle (*black arrow*) can be advanced from radial to ulnar direction (**a**) to target one or both of the articular surfaces (**b**). On the other hand, keeping the probe in the same position and using the in-plane technique, the needle (*black arrow*) can be advanced from a distal to proximal direction (**c**) to inject the trapezio-metacarpal joint with hypertrophic synovitis (*yellow asterisk*) and bulging of the capsule (*white arrowhead*) (**d**). I MC, 1st metacarpal bone, void arrow, needle's pathway

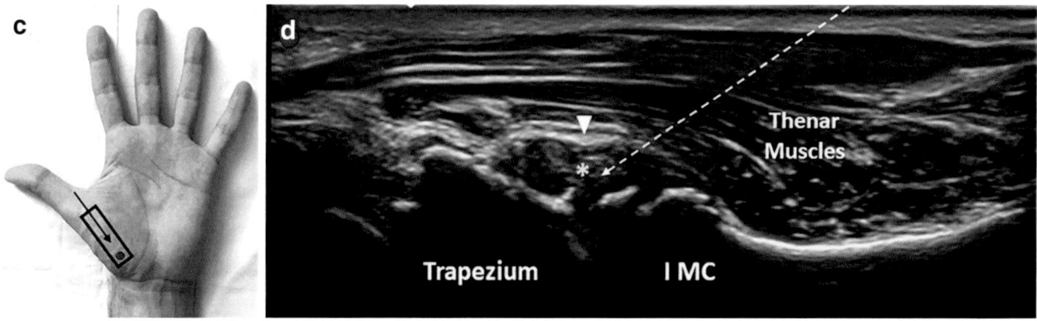

Fig. 7.25 (continued)

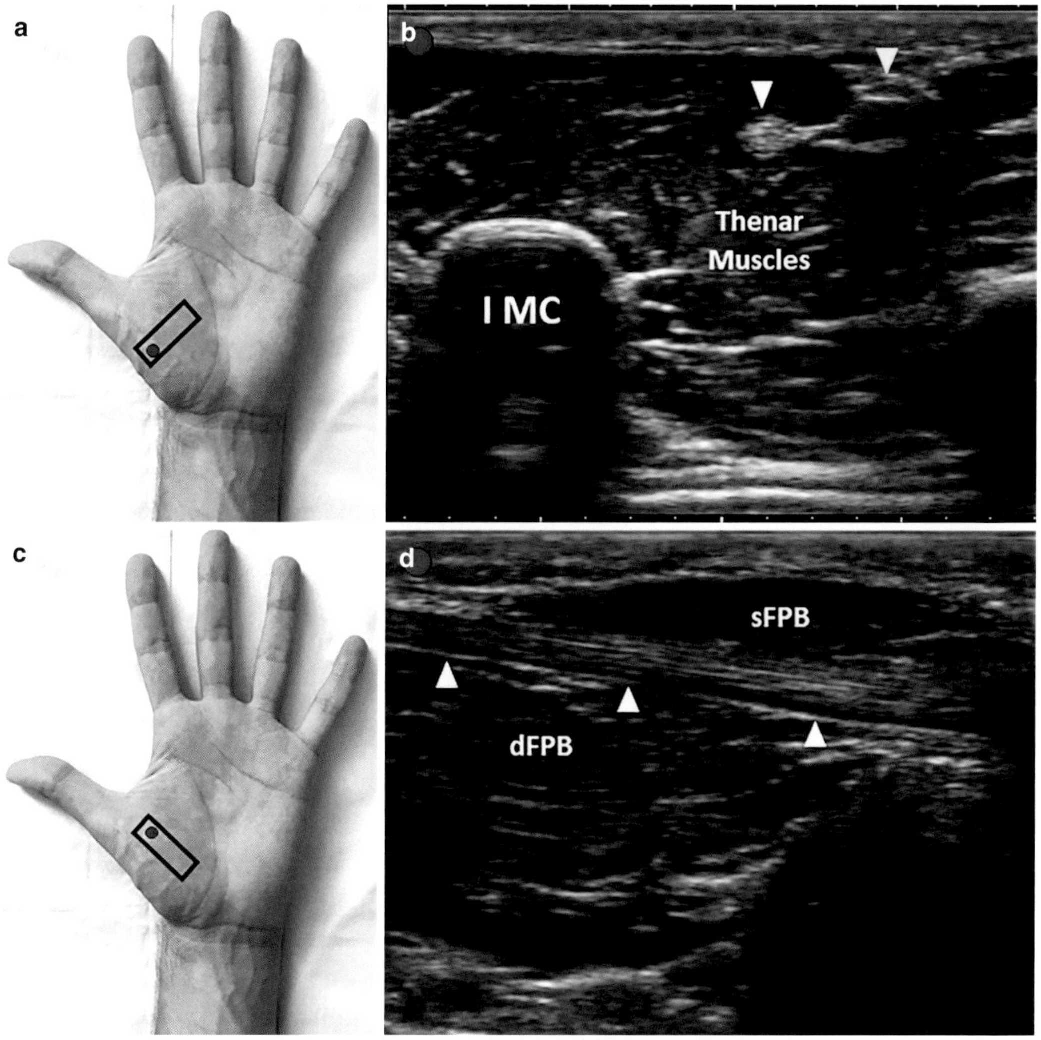

Fig. 7.26 Positioning the probe (*black rectangle*) in a transverse oblique plane over the volar aspect of the thenar eminence (**a**), the flexor pollicis longus tendon (*white arrowhead*) is visualized in the short-axis view (**b**). The close spatial relationship between the tendon and the digital nerve of the thumb (*yellow arrowhead*) is noteworthy if an intervention must be performed at this level (**b**). Rotating the probe (*black rectangle*) 90 degrees (**c**), the same tendon (*white arrowheads*) can be evaluated, in the long-axis view, encircled by the superficial (*sFPB*) and deep (*dFPB*) components of the flexor pollicis brevis muscle (**d**). I MC, 1st metacarpal bone

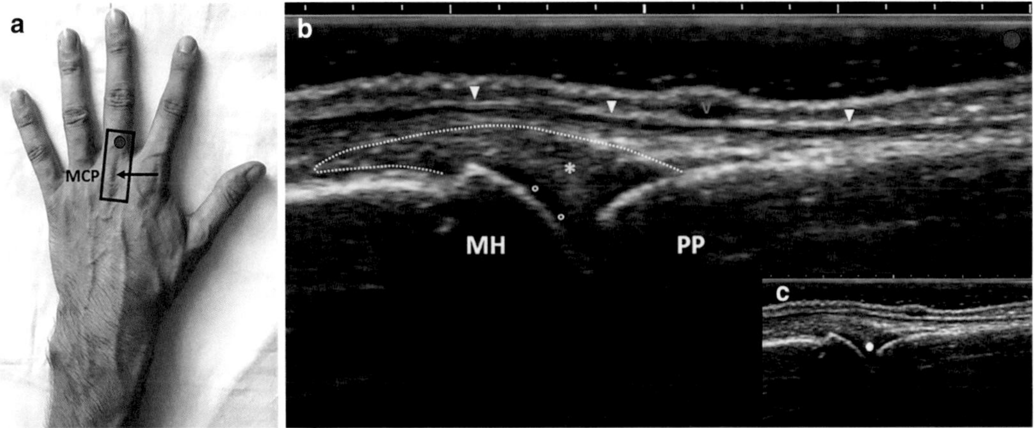

Fig. 7.27 Positioning the probe (*black rectangle*) in a longitudinal plane over the dorsal aspect of the metacarpophalangeal (*MCP*) joint (**a**), the articular surface interposed between the metacarpal head (*MH*) and the proximal phalanx (*PP*) can be clearly visualized (**b**). The cartilage surface of the metacarpal bone (*white dots*), dorsal plate (*yellow asterisk*), joint capsule (*white dotted line*), and the extensor tendon (*white arrowheads*) are all imaged using enough gel and gentle compression of the probe (**b**). Using the out-of-plane technique, the needle (*black arrow*) can be advanced from radial to ulnar (or ulnar to radial) direction (**a**) to target/inject the joint space (*white dot*) between the two bones (**c**). V vein

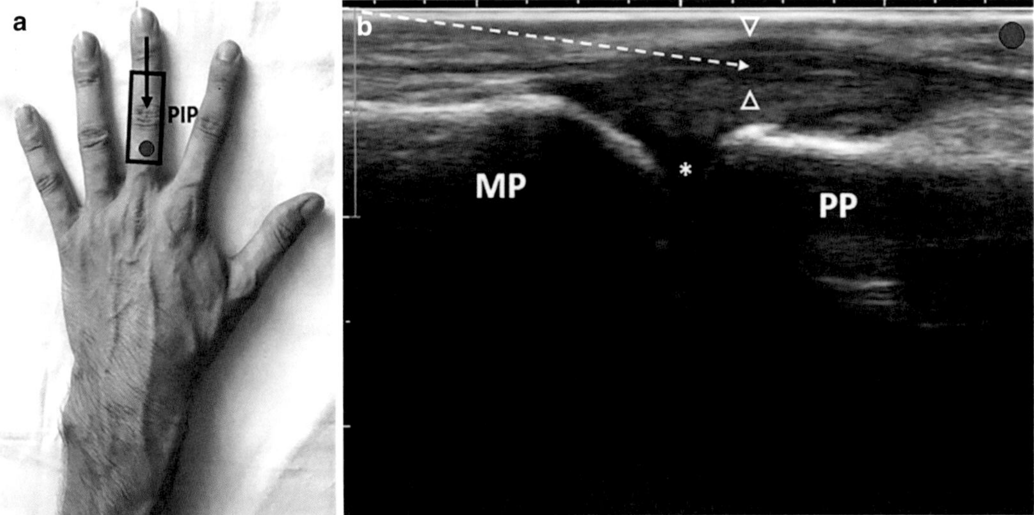

Fig. 7.28 Positioning the probe (*black rectangle*) in longitudinal plane over the dorsal aspect of the proximal interphalangeal (*PIP*) joint (**a**), a focal and hypoechoic thickening of the extensor tendon (*void arrowheads*) is depicted in a patient with hand trauma (**b**). Using the in-plane technique, the needle (*black arrow*) can be advanced from distal to proximal direction (**a**) to target the tendon (**b**). MP; middle phalanx, PP; proximal phalanx, dotted arrow; needle's pathway, white asterisk; joint effusion

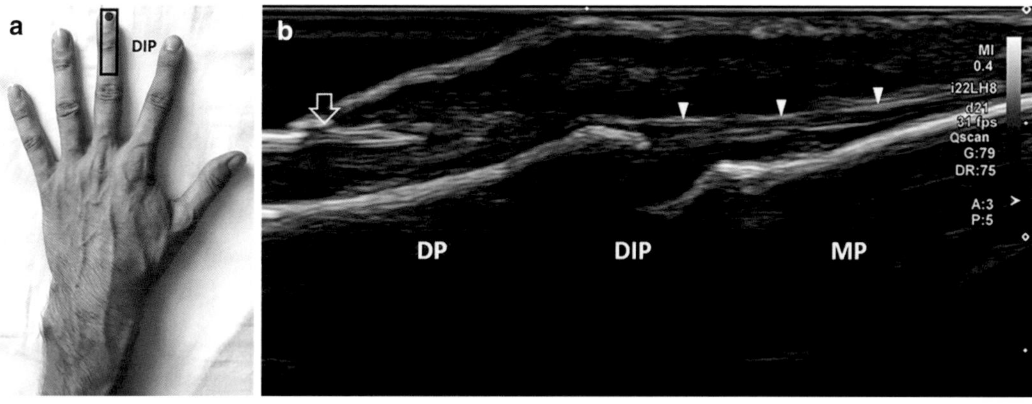

Fig. 7.29 Positioning the probe (*black rectangle*) in a longitudinal plane over the dorsal aspect of the distal interphalangeal (*DIP*) joint (**a**), the attachment site of the extensor tendon (*white arrowheads*) over the base of the distal phalanx (*DP*) can be visualized (**b**). Void arrow, nail, MP middle phalanx

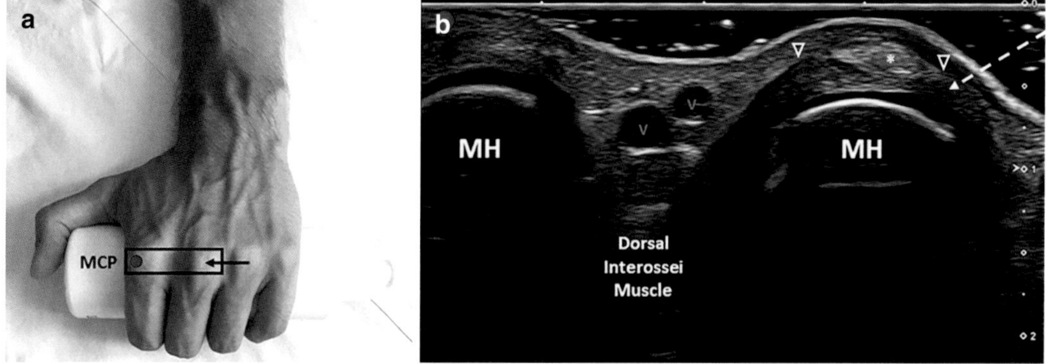

Fig. 7.30 Positioning the probe (*black rectangle*) in a transverse plane over the dorsal aspect of the metacarpophalangeal (*MCP*) joints (while the patient is gripping the gel tube) (**a**), the anatomical complex composed of the extensor tendon (*yellow asterisk*) and the sagittal bands (*void arrowheads*) can be depicted in a state of "mechanical tension" over the metacarpal heads (*MH*) (**b**). Using the in-plane technique, the needle (*black arrow*) can be advanced from ulnar to radial (or radial to ulnar) direction (**a**) to target the (injured) sagittal bands (**b**). V vein, void arrow, needle's pathway

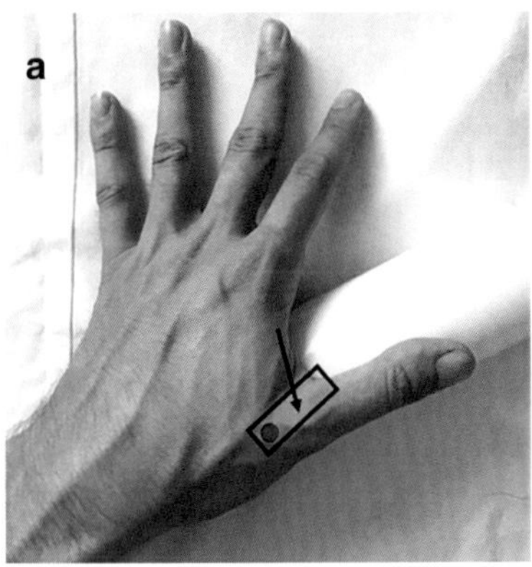

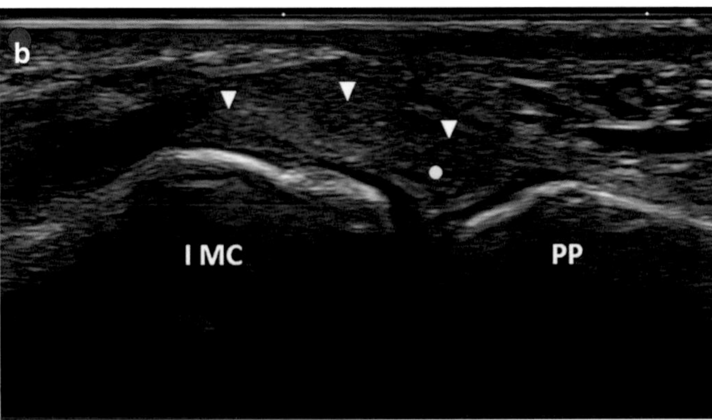

Fig. 7.31 Positioning the probe (*black rectangle*) in a longitudinal oblique plane over the ulnar aspect of the base of the thumb (**a**), the ulnar collateral ligament (*white arrowheads*) is seen between the 1st metacarpal (*I MC*) bone and the proximal phalanx (*PP*) of the thumb (**b**). Using the out-of-plane technique, the needle (*black arrow*) can be advanced from cranial to caudal direction (**a**) to target the ligament (*yellow dot*) (**b**)

aponeurosis). The out-of-plane technique with a cranial to caudal approach can simply be used to target the ulnar collateral ligament (Fig. 7.31).

References

1. Colio SW, Smith J, Pourcho AM. Ultrasound-guided interventional procedures of the wrist and hand: anatomy, indications, and techniques. Phys Med Rehabil Clin N Am. 2016;27(3):589–605.
2. Özçakar L, Kara M, Chang KV, et al. EURO-MUSCULUS/USPRM basic scanning protocols for wrist and hand. Eur J Phys Rehabil Med. 2015;51(4):479–84.
3. Bianchi S, Martinoli C. Ultrasound of the musculoskeletal system. Berlin: Springer; 2007. p. 425–95.
4. Ricci V, Özçakar L. From "Ultrasound imaging" to "ultrasound examination": a needful upgrade in musculoskeletal medicine. Pain Med. 2019. https://doi.org/10.1093/pm/pnz231. [published online ahead of print].
5. Ricci V, Özçakar L. Life after ultrasound: are we speaking the same (or a new) language in physical and rehabilitation medicine? J Rehabil Med. 2019;51(3):234–5.
6. Draghi F, Bortolotto C. Intersection syndrome: ultrasound imaging. Skeletal Radiol. 2014;43(3):283–7.
7. Smith J, Rizzo M, Sayeed YA, Finnoff JT. Sonographically guided distal radioulnar joint injection: technique and validation in a cadaveric model. J Ultrasound Med. 2011;30(11):1587–92.
8. Gitto S, Draghi F. Normal sonographic anatomy of the wrist with emphasis on assessment of tendons, nerves, and ligaments. J Ultrasound Med. 2016;35(5):1081–95.
9. Gitto S, Messina C, Mauri G, et al. Dynamic high-resolution ultrasound of intrinsic and extrinsic ligaments of the wrist: how to make it simple. Eur J Radiol. 2017;87:20–35.
10. Orlandi D, Corazza A, Silvestri E, et al. Ultrasound-guided procedures around the wrist and hand: how to do. Eur J Radiol. 2014;83(7):1231–8.
11. Sekizkardeş M, Özdemir S, Aydin G, et al. Intersection syndrome revised: let's talk much more about it using ultrasound. Am J Phys Med Rehabil. 2018;97(9):e89.
12. Chang KV, Mezian K, Naňka O, et al. Ultrasound imaging for the cutaneous nerves of the extremities and relevant entrapment syndromes: from anatomy to clinical implications. J Clin Med. 2018;7(11):457.
13. Meng S, Tinhofer I, Weninger WJ, et al. Anatomical and ultrasound correlation of the superficial branch of the radial nerve. Muscle Nerve. 2014;50(6):939–42.
14. Bianchi S, Becciolini M, Urigo C. Ultrasound imaging of disorders of small nerves of the extremities: less recognized locations. J Ultrasound Med. 2019;38(11):2821–42.
15. Chang KV, Hung CY, Özçakar L. Snapping thumb and superficial radial nerve entrapment in De Quervain disease: ultrasound imaging/guidance revisited. Pain Med. 2015;16(11):2214–5.
16. Hung CY, Chang KV, Özçakar L. Dynamic and Doppler ultrasound imaging for the diagnosis of triangular fibrocartilage complex and ulnocarpal wrist instability. Am J Phys Med Rehabil. 2016;95(7):e111–2.
17. Wu WT, Chang KV, Mezian K, et al. Ulnar wrist pain revisited: ultrasound diagnosis and guided injection for triangular fibrocartilage complex injuries. J Clin Med. 2019;8(10):1540.
18. Pesquer L, Scepi M, Bihan M, et al. Normal ultrasound anatomy of the triangular fibrocartilage of the wrist: a study on cadaver and on healthy subjects. J Clin Ultrasound. 2009;37(4):194–8.

19. Hsiao MY, Wang TG. Intraarticular injections – upper limb. In: Özçakar L, editor. Ultrasound imaging & guidance for musculoskeletal interventions in physical and rehabilitation medicine. Edi.Ermes: Milan; 2019.
20. Padmore CE, Stoesser H, Langohr GDG, et al. Carpal kinematics following sequential scapholunate ligament sectioning. J Wrist Surg. 2019;8(2):124–31.
21. Rodriguez RM, Ernat JJ. Ultrasonography for dorsal-sided wrist pain in a combat environment: technique, pearls, and a case report of dynamic evaluation of the scapholunate ligament. Mil Med. 2019. https://doi.org/10.1093/milmed/usz157. [published online ahead of print].
22. Chen IJ, Chang KV, Lou YM, et al. Can ultrasound imaging be used for the diagnosis of carpal tunnel syndrome in diabetic patients? A systemic review and network meta-analysis. J Neurol. 2019. https://doi.org/10.1007/s00415-019-09254-8. [published online ahead of print].
23. Kaymak B, Özçakar L, Cetin A, et al. A comparison of the benefits of sonography and electrophysiologic measurements as predictors of symptom severity and functional status in patients with carpal tunnel syndrome. Arch Phys Med Rehabil. 2008;89(4):743–8.
24. Güven SC, Özçakar L, Kaymak B, et al. Short-term effectiveness of platelet-rich plasma in carpal tunnel syndrome: a controlled study. J Tissue Eng Regen Med. 2019;13(5):709–14.
25. Wu YT, Chen SR, Li TY, et al. Nerve hydrodissection for carpal tunnel syndrome: a prospective, randomized, double-blind, controlled trial. Muscle Nerve. 2019;59(2):174–80.
26. Wu CH, Chang KV, Özçakar L, et al. Sonographic tracking of the upper limb peripheral nerves: a pictorial essay and video demonstration. Am J Phys Med Rehabil. 2015;94(9):740–7.
27. Luong DH, Smith J, Bianchi S. Flexor carpi radialis tendon ultrasound pictorial essay. Skeletal Radiol. 2014;43(6):745–60.
28. Draghi F, Gregoli B, Bortolotto C. Pisiform bursitis: a forgotten pathology. J Clin Ultrasound. 2014;42(9):560–1.
29. Bianchi S, Martinoli C, de Gautard R, et al. Ultrasound of the digital flexor system: normal and pathological findings. J Ultrasound. 2007;10(2):85–92.
30. Bianchi S, Gitto S, Draghi F. Ultrasound features of trigger finger: review of the literature. J Ultrasound Med. 2019;38(12):3141–54.
31. Abdulsalam AJ, Mezian K, Ricci V, et al. Interdigital approach to trigger finger injection using ultrasound guidance. Pain Med. 2019;20(12):2607–10.
32. Morris G, Jacobson JA, Kalume Brigido M, et al. Ultrasound features of palmar fibromatosis or Dupuytren contracture. J Ultrasound Med. 2019;38(2):387–92.
33. Smith J, Brault JS, Rizzo M, et al. Accuracy of sonographically guided and palpation guided scaphotrapeziotrapezoid joint injections. J Ultrasound Med. 2011;30(11):1509–15.
34. Rawat U, Pierce JL, Evans S, et al. High-resolution MR imaging and US anatomy of the thumb. Radiographics. 2016;36(6):1701–16.
35. Bianchi S, Becciolini M. Ultrasound evaluation of sesamoid fractures of the hand: retrospective report of 13 patients. J Ultrasound Med. 2019;38(7):1913–20.
36. Lee SA, Kim BH, Kim SJ, et al. Current status of ultrasonography of the finger. Ultrasonography. 2016;35(2):110–23.
37. Clavero JA, Alomar X, Monill JM, et al. MR imaging of ligament and tendon injuries of the fingers. Radiographics. 2002;22(2):237–56.
38. Draghi F, Gitto S, Bianchi S. Injuries to the collateral ligaments of the metacarpophalangeal and interphalangeal joints: sonographic appearance. J Ultrasound Med. 2018;37(9):2117–33.

Ultrasound of the Hip/Thigh: Regenerative Medicine Focus

8

Robert Monaco, Hector L. Osoria, and Piyaporn Pramuksun

Introduction

Injuries to the hip and thigh are some of the most common in all of musculoskeletal medicine. Hip injuries represent at least 6% of all sports injuries affecting adults and are even more prevalent among older individuals. The thigh is the most commonly injured muscle group in the body. The hip joint is often affected by arthritis, and many tendons around the hip region can be involved in pathology. Secondary to the wide length and depth of the region and its structures, it is best to break down the hip into selective regions. These include the following with the key structures listed in each area.

Regions of the Hip

Anterior: Hip joint, acetabular labrum, iliopsoas complex, rectus femoris, lateral femoral cutaneous nerve

Medial: Adductor tendons, pubic symphysis, inguinal region, femoral neurovasculature

Lateral: Greater trochanter, gluteal tendons, iliotibial tract

Posterior: Piriformis/external rotators, sciatic nerve, hamstring origin

Thigh: Anterior quadriceps complex, posterior hamstring complex

There is broad overlap of structures and pain referral patterns in these regions requiring clinicians to have extensive anatomic knowledge and a broad differential diagnosis. Radiographs are the initial assessment for all types of pathology in the region and may help the clinician narrow down differential diagnosis. Ultrasound is limited in its ability to assess deep intra-articular injuries affecting the osteoarticular surface in the hip and groin. Examples include articular cartilage injuries, subtle fractures or bone stress injuries, and small labral tears. These are better evaluated using MRI or MRI arthrography. The role of ultrasound is growing rapidly for diagnosis and interventional procedures. Ultrasound can help assess both intra- and extra-articular collections of fluid including joint, bursal, or synovial pathology. It is extremely useful for the assessment of muscles and tendon pathologies. It is the test of choice for the evaluation of snapping in the region due to its ability to perform dynamic maneuvers. Ultrasound is readily available, relatively low in cost, has short exam times, and can be done at the point of care. These attributes make it an excellent choice to start the process of hip pain evaluation and for guided injections.

R. Monaco (✉) · H. L. Osoria
Department of Sports Medicine, Atlantic Health System, Morristown, NJ, USA

P. Pramuksun
Department of Physical Medicine and Rehabilitation, Bhumibol Adulyadej Hospital, Bangkok, Thailand

Y. El Miedany (ed.), *Musculoskeletal Ultrasound-Guided Regenerative Medicine*, https://doi.org/10.1007/978-3-030-98256-0_8

Common clinical indications for sonography of the region are:

1. Evaluation for effusion/synovitis and to guide aspiration or injection
2. Evaluation for bursal or fluid collection in the region for aspiration/injection (bursitis, seroma, labral cyst, etc.)
3. Evaluation for athletic hip pain, especially of the groin
4. Evaluation for muscle, tendon, bursal, or hernia pathology
5. Evaluation for snapping in the region

Other indications include the postoperative hip replacement patient with continued pain, which is beyond the scope of this regenerative text chapter.

A variety of ultrasound frequencies are used, in general to scan the wide regions of the hip and thigh. This will depend on the anatomy of the patient and the depth of the structure being evaluated. A curvilinear probe at 2–6 MHZ is ideal for many of the deeper structures, particularly in the posterior hip region. High-frequency linear probes are used for the evaluation of the superficial tendons. A focused exam protocol of each region should be followed. The hip joint should be evaluated in all regions as it may refer pain to all these areas.

We will review the common sonoanatomy of the regions and discuss common clinical pathologies with specific focus on those where regenerative ultrasound-guided procedures can assist in diagnosis and treatment options.

Anterior Hip Region

Sonoanatomy

A common framework for assessing the anterior hip is to divide it into intra-articular and extra-articular structures. The following structures should be evaluated when performing an ultrasound of the anterior hip:

Checklist:

Intra-articular:

1. Hip joint and capsule
2. Femoral head bone anatomy
3. Articular cartilage
4. Hip labrum

Extra-articular:

1. Rectus femoris tendons (direct and indirect)
2. Sartorius
3. Iliopsoas complex
4. Femoral neurovascular structures
5. Lateral femoral cutaneous nerve (if clinical history warrants)

The hip joint is a synovial ball-and-socket joint between the femoral head and the pelvic acetabulum. The joint capsule surrounds the joint and is reinforced by three ligaments – the iliofemoral (Y ligament of Bigelow), ischiofemoral, and pubofemoral ligaments. The femoral head should be, in general, egg shaped but may have abnormalities such as cam or other developmental deformities. The capsule inserts anteriorly at the intertrochanteric line; however, it reflects redundantly back to the femoral head-neck junction; these layers are 2–3 mm each and therefore about 4–6 mm when viewed under ultrasound at the level of the femoral head-neck junction. The femoral head is covered by hyaline cartilage, whereas the acetabulum is lined by hyaline cartilage in an inverted U shape with a fibrocartilage labrum attached to the acetabular rim [60, 75]. The acetabulum of the pelvis is a deep socket, providing more inherent stability in conjunction with the acetabular labrum and ligamentous structures, compared to the shoulder. However, despite the greater stability of the joint, there is still a great degree of mobility in all planes – sagittal, transverse, and frontal [46]. In addition to functionally increasing the surface area of the acetabulum, the labrum also provides a suction-seal mechanism to help maintain the femoral head positioned in the acetabulum. Under ultrasound, the fibrocartilage of the labrum should be hyperechoic and appear triangular in shape [44, 46]. Ultrasonography of the anterior hip joint is best accomplished with a curvilinear probe due to the depth of the hip joint. One can use the bony landmarks to orient the probe quickly over the joint. Placing it at the mid distance between the anterior superior iliac spine and the pubic tuber-

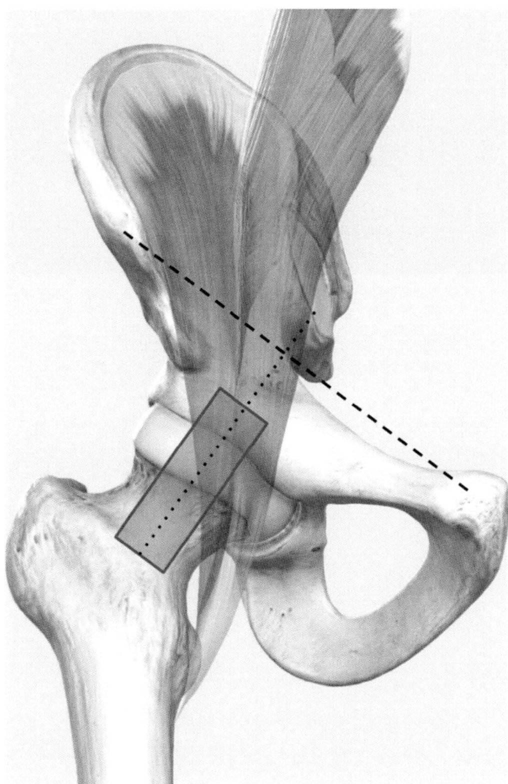

Fig. 8.1 Schematic of probe placement (blue box) for the assessment of the anterior hip joint in-plane with the femoral head-neck junction, bisecting the plane between the ASIS and the pubic tubercle

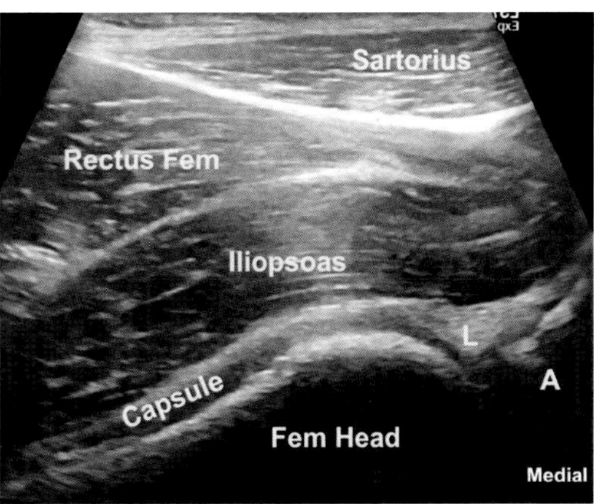

Fig. 8.2 Anterior longitudinal sonographic view of the hip joint. (A) Acetabulum, (L) acetabular labrum

cle at a 30-degree angle will line up with the joint (Fig. 8.1). One can also find the joint by placing the probe transversely on the thigh to visualize the hyperechoic outline of the femur and pivot 30 degrees to line up parallel with the femoral head and neck. Normal sonoanatomy of the hip joint is noted in Fig. 8.2. With further medial translation, one may also identify the femoral neurovascular bundle. These are best visualized in the transverse plane.

The bony anatomy of the hip and pelvis provides attachment points for various muscular structures that cross the hip joint and provide movement about the hip (Fig. 8.3).

The iliopsoas tendon is formed by the continuation of the iliacus muscle combined with the psoas muscle to form this common tendon which crosses the anterior-medial aspect of the hip joint (Fig. 8.3b). It courses deep and slightly laterally to insert into the lesser trochanter. The Iliopsoas bursa, the largest in the body, lies between the iliopsoas muscle complex and the surfaces of the pelvis and proximal femur [3, 17]. Visualization of the iliopsoas tendon can be achieved with the transducer first in the transverse plane over the femoral head (Fig. 8.3c); then the lateral edge of the transducer is angled superiorly to align the probe in parallel with the inguinal ligament until the AIIS is visualized in this view. The hyperechoic iliopsoas tendon will be seen here in the short axis just superficial to the bony contour of the ilium, distal to the AIIS, with hypoechoic iliacus muscle still partially surrounding the tendon more proximally. This is also where the iliopsoas bursa would be visualized for abnormal fluid volume. The iliopsoas tendon should be evaluated along its length in both long and short axes.

The rectus femoris is primarily a knee extensor; however, it is also a weaker hip flexor relative to the iliopsoas complex. The rectus has two main heads and is really a muscle within a muscle. The direct head of the rectus femoris originates at the anterior inferior iliac spine, whereas the indirect head attaches at the superior-posterior aspect of the acetabulum [17]. The origin of the direct head of the rectus can be easily identified just proximal and medial to the joint space at its attachment into the anterior inferior iliac spine. It is easy in longitudinal views to see its attachment and muscle tendon junction (Fig. 8.4a). With the

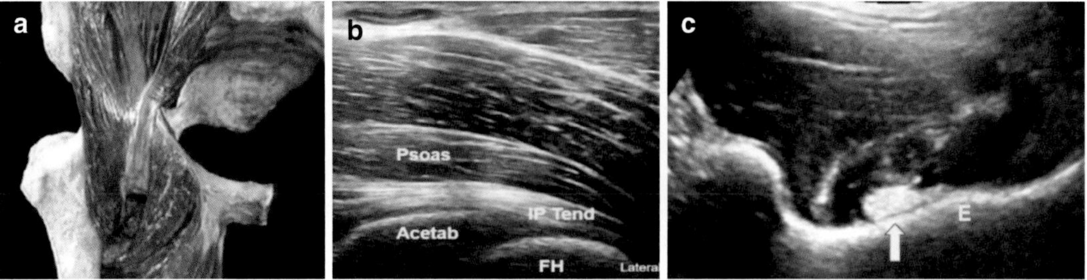

Fig. 8.3 (**a**) Cadaveric iliopsoas complex, tendon over the eminence. (**b**) Note the iliopsoas tendon in the long axis over the acetabulum and femoral head, (**c**) transverse view of the iliopsoas tendon (yellow arrow) the iliopectineal eminence (E)

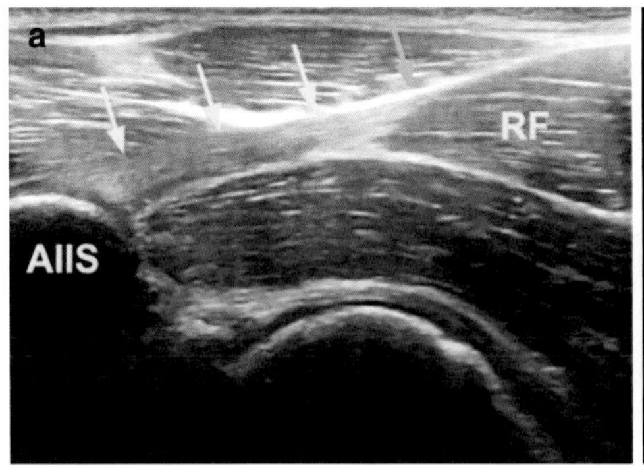

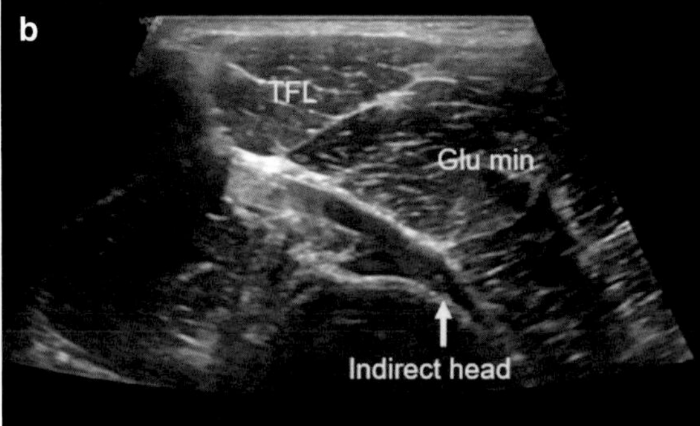

Fig. 8.4 (**a**) Longitudinal view of the rectus femoris (RF) with its tendon (yellow arrows) seen attaching to the anterior inferior iliac spine (AIIS); myotendinous junction (green arrow). (**b**) Longitudinal view of the indirect head of the rectus femoris (arrow)

direct head in a transverse plane axis, one can translate the probe laterally to partially reveal the indirect head traveling proximally and deep, though it will be anisotropic at this angle (Fig. 8.4b). Pivot 30 degrees cranially to line up on the tendon attachment to the posterior acetabulum [44].

More cephalad originating at the anterior superior iliac spine are the sartorius and the tensor fasciae latae muscles. A tensor fasciae latae does not cross the hip anteriorly but courses laterally and inserts into the iliotibial band.

The lateral femoral cutaneous nerve exits to the pelvis under the inguinal ligament and provides sensation to the lateral thigh [17] (Fig. 8.5). The nerve can be traced in the tissue plane very superficial to the sartorius muscle and medial to the ASIS, and it should be followed proximally to the level of the inguinal ligament to assess for nerve entrapment [44, 86]. Sonopalpation can be used to help identify nerve pathology and a contralateral comparison to help determine irregularities. There are natural variants in the location of the nerve which include posterior to and across the ASIS; anterior to the ASIS but within the substance of the inguinal ligament; through the tendinous origin of the sartorius muscle; between the sartorius tendon and thick fascia of the iliopsoas muscle; and deep to the inguinal ligament, overlying the thin fascia of the iliopsoas muscle [5].

Pathologies Common pathologies in the region with potential regenerative procedural options are noted below. It is important to distinguish between intra-articular and extra-articular processes, but these may overlap.

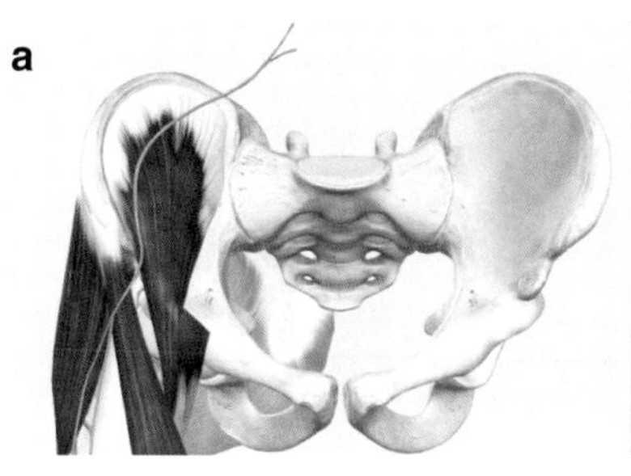

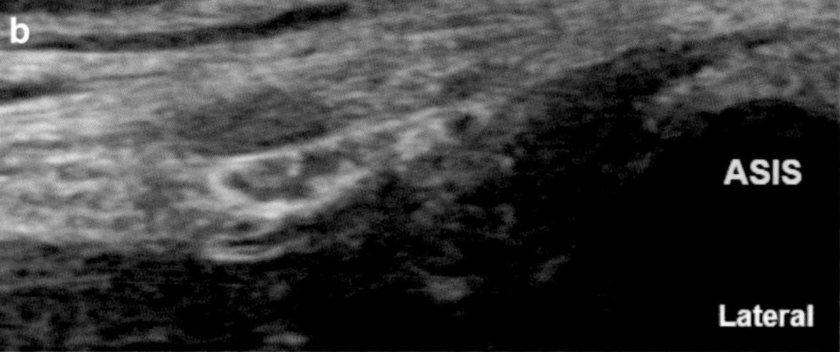

Fig. 8.5 (**a**) Schematic of typical path of the lateral femoral cutaneous nerve. (**b**) Transverse view of the LFCN (green outline)

Intra-articular Hip effusion/joint (mechanical vs. inflammatory), labral pathology.

The clinician should first try to determine if the source of pain is from an intra-articular and/or an extra-articular source. Evidence of a hip effusion is strongly suggestive of an intra-articular process. Fluid in the joint can be secondary to multiple etiologies, and ultrasound cannot distinguish this directly. These include, but are not limited to, mechanical joint irritation, synovitis, systemic inflammatory conditions, tumors (pigmented villonodular synovitis), and infections. The clinician needs to clinically correlate to determine the appropriate evaluation and treatment steps. When indicated, aspiration or diagnostic injection may provide further information.

The most common source of an intra-articular hip effusion and pain in adults is hip osteoarthritis. It is the second most common form of arthritis. It usually presents unilaterally with pain–usually felt in the groin or thigh, stiffness, and restricted range of motion of which internal rotation is often the earliest to be limited. Pain from hip arthritis is typically exacerbated by both active and passive movement and alleviated by rest [2]. Inflammatory conditions which can manifest in the hip and present similarly to hip osteoarthritis include, but are not limited to, rheumatoid arthritis, psoriatic arthritis, and reactive arthritis. These would typically also present with systemic or other extra-articular exam findings associated with these conditions. Many pathologies in the joint can cause an effusion, specifically injuries to the labrum and hyaline cartilage. Under ultrasound, an effusion is diagnosed when there is 7 mm or great capsular distension as measured from the femoral neck surface to the outer edge of the joint capsule or when there is a greater than 1 mm side-to-side difference compared to the non-affected side [44] (Fig. 8.6).

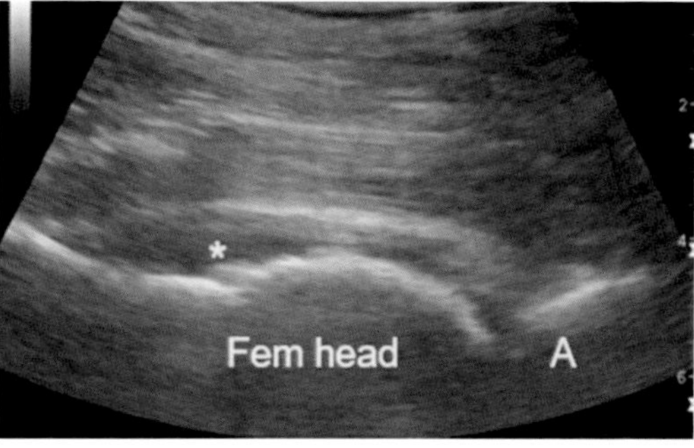

Fig. 8.6 Hip effusion: hypoechoic effusion (*) which does not follow the femoral head contour

The hip labrum can be visualized under ultrasound but only a small portion. For the diagnosis of labral tears, it has a sensitivity of 81% and a specificity of 49% [85]. However, the visualized part is the most commonly injured section. Dynamic testing can help evaluate labral detachment. Criteria for labral tears are displacement or absence of labrum, hypoechoic cleft through the base of the labrum causing detachment with or without displacement, intrasubstance hypoechoic linear clefts (Fig. 8.7a), and cystic (Fig. 8.7b) or irregular formations. Mixed echogenicity without definite tearing and irregular margins are interpreted as degenerative changes [88]. Linear probes with high frequency are recommended. However, MR arthrogram is a gold standard for

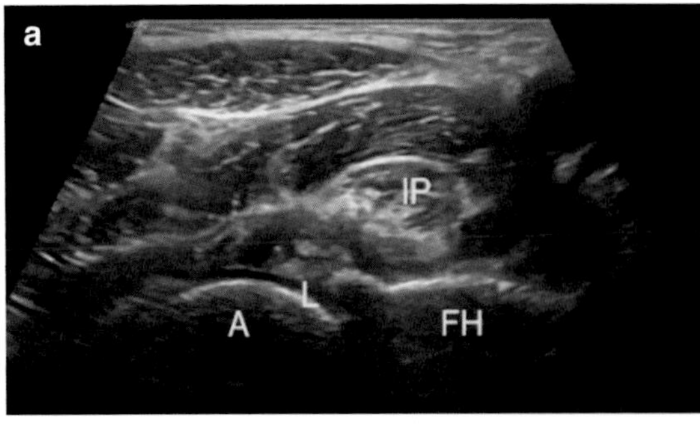

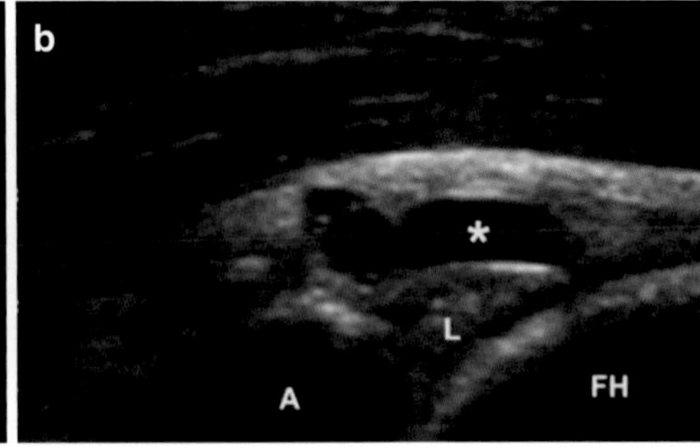

Fig. 8.7 (**a**) Transverse view of the hip joint showing intrasubstance hypoechoic cleft suggesting labral tear with cyst formation. (**b**) Longitudinal view showing paralabral cyst (*): well-defined cyst near the labrum of the hip joint. Acetabulum (A), labrum (L), iliopsoas (IP), femoral head (FH)

the diagnosis of labral tears. Femoral acetabular impingement (FAI) is a condition in which the shape of the femoral head and acetabular sockets are not compatible due to inappropriate bony overgrowth of the femoral head, acetabulum, and/or both and can be a cause of labral pathology. The location of the overgrowth determines the type of FAI: pincer type involves overgrowth of the acetabulum, cam impingement occurs with overgrowth of the femoral head, and combined type involves both. The clinical presentation of FAI typically involves pain with hip flexion, internal rotation, and/or adduction. Often, the bony deformity leads to damage to the cartilage of the acetabular labrum or the femoral head. Physical examination of these patients typically reveals limited internal rotation of the hip and reproduction of pain with the hip flexed at 90°, internal rotation, and adduction. Although ultrasonography can assist with identification of the femoral head morphology, MRI may still be needed to better evaluate for a chondral injury or labral pathology.

Extra-articular Hip

"Snapping hip" is a common name for the symptoms of audible or palpable and often painful snapping of the iliopsoas tendon during movement. The original pathophysiology was described as the iliopsoas tendon translating taughtly translating over the iliopectineal eminence of the pelvis [66]. While this is one mechanism, more recent dynamic ultrasound imaging studies have actually demonstrated that the more frequent cause of the snap is an internal rapid torsion of a flipped psoas tendon within the iliacus muscle when the hip goes from the FABER position to extension and neutral [3, 29, 40]. Sonographic assessment for this form of medial or "internal" snapping hip is performed by assessing the iliopsoas tendon in transverse axis and having the patient ask to reproduce the snapping sensation, usually by bringing the hip into flexion, abduction, and external rotation, then straightening the leg. If the patient has a snapping hip caused by the psoas major tendon, there will be an abrupt snapping of the psoas major tendon from internally over the accessory tendon or occasionally over the superior pubic ramus [40]. The abnormal movement of the psoas tendon during the snap has been associated with irritation of the tendon leading to iliopsoas bursitis and tendonitis. The patient may also have lateral or "external" snapping hip, which is usually caused by snapping of the gluteus maximus tendon or iliotibial band over the greater trochanter [21].

Often, the irregular snapping of the iliopsoas tendon can cause tendon irritation and inflammation leading to an iliopsoas tendinopathy or tendinitis. Another potential cause of this tendinopathy is an overly tight iliopsoas unit which rubs against the underlying acetabular labrum and may also cause labrum pathology. Direct overuse in athletes will also cause tendonitis. This iliopsoas pathology may cause hip bursitis in the adjacent iliopsoas bursa [3]. Iliopsoas bursitis, the largest bursa in the body, can mimic hip effusion (Fig. 8.8). However, bursitis is outside the joint capsule; thus, it will not distend

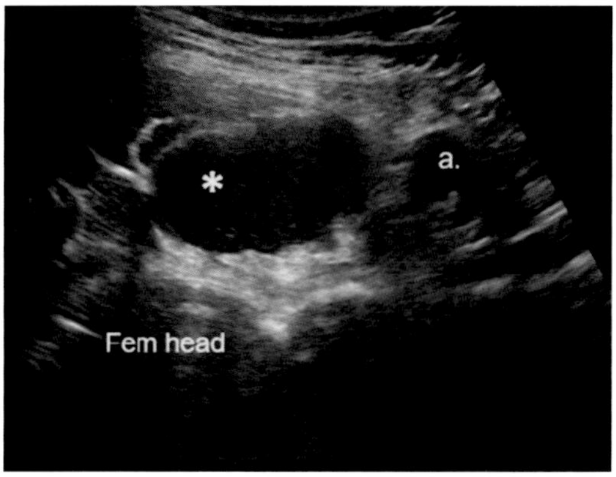

Fig. 8.8 Well-defined thin-walled hypoechoic fluid collection (*) along the line of the iliopsoas tendon in a short-axis view with the femoral artery (a) seen medially

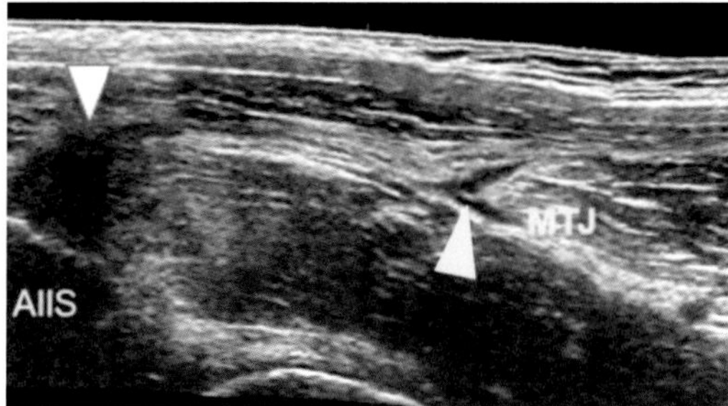

Fig. 8.9 Longitudinal views of the rectus femoris direct head show a myotendinous junction hypoechoic tear (yellow arrowhead) and insertional AIIS attachment hypoechoic defect (white arrowhead) of the rectus femoris

the joint. Fifteen percent of iliopsoas bursitis can communicate with the joint. Iliopsoas bursitis can extend all the way up into the pelvis. Like any fluid collection, it can have multiple etiologies including mechanical irritation and infection. The use of Doppler may help assist in categorizing the type of fluid, but aspiration and analysis and/or injection may be indicated to definitively diagnose and treat the condition.

The rectus femoris tendon may also experience various pathologies that can be assessed via ultrasound. These include tendinosis, calcifications, and partial or full thickness tears (Fig. 8.9). Common changes seen in tendinopathies include sonographic appearance of hypoechoic tendon with loss of fibrillar pattern, tendon thickening with or without partial tearing, and positivity to power Doppler signal. The tendon is more often strained or tendinopathic than completely avulsed off the AIIS [17]. One should also assess for a rectus tendon tear or bony avulsion of the AIIS in adolescents or growing athletes.

The indirect head injury is more common in kicking sports and dancers and may be missed clinically. The common presentation is chronic hip pain which may mimic labral or other hip joint pathology and are more commonly seen as overuse injuries as opposed to acute traumatic injuries. Rectus femoris indirect head pathology may be more common than direct head [13]. Pathology can also progress to direct head.

Lateral femoral cutaneous nerve (LFCN): Entrapment or neuroma of this nerve can cause meralgia paresthetica. This condition usually results from chronic compression of the LFCN. The patient may present with numbness, paresthesia, hyperesthesia, or neuropathic pain in the anterior lateral thigh which is innervated by the LFCN [39].

Procedures

Ultrasound injections around the hip joint may be extremely valuable for both diagnostic and therapeutic purposes. Injections can help diagnose or narrow down the pain generator, help manage painful conditions, and/or serve as a bridge to delay surgery. Percutaneous procedures around the hip joint are an excellent alternative to more invasive procedures. Ultrasound is the ideal modality for this secondary to its real-time guidance, low cost, portability, lack of ionizing radiation, and additional diagnostic information obtained. Due to the complexity of the region including its neurovascular structures, with rare exception, all hip procedures should be ultrasound guided.

The most common procedures in the anterior hip region are the following:

1. Hip joint/labral complex injection/aspiration
2. Iliopsoas injection/bursal aspiration
3. Lateral femoral cutaneous nerve hydrodissection

Hip Joint/Labrum Injection/Aspiration

Ultrasound-guided hip joint procedures can be performed in the office setting with no risk of radiation exposure with an excellent accuracy of around 97–100% [26]. There are multiple techniques to inject the hip joint (Table 8.1).

The anterior approach is the most common where the needle is directed in-plane down to the femoral head-neck junction. The patient should lie in a supine position with the leg extended. Rolling the leg into internal rotation can help increase joint fluid which gives better visualization of the joint space. Align the probe along the long axis of the femoral neck. Before injection, use Doppler to evaluate the femoral neurovascular structures. They reside a good 2.5 cm from the joint. One also wants to avoid the femoral circumflex vessels anterior using Doppler. The needle path should be planned aiming at the femoral head-neck junction using a lateral to media, distal to proximal approach (Fig. 8.10). A long needle, usually a 22 gauge 3 inch or longer, is needed depending on body habitus. In obese patients, coated needle or beam steer mode will assist and improve needle

Table 8.1 Hip joint injection approaches

Technique	Anterior approach (in plane) (Fig. 8.10)	Transverse approach (in plane) (Fig. 8.11)	Lateral approach (out of plane) (Fig. 8.12)
Patient position	Supine position with the leg in neutral or internal position		Side-lying position
Probe positioning	Halfway between ASIS and pubic symphysis (not tubercle), the hip joint will be at 2.5 cm medial	Probe oriented axially over the femoral head and acetabular rim in view	Transversely on the trochanter with the acetabulum in view
Target	Femoral head-neck junction	Pierce the thick joint capsule into the joint	
Needle size	25 g 1.5 inch for local anesthesia; 18–22 g 3–4 inch for injection		
Probe	Low frequency curvilinear or high frequency linear for transverse	Curvilinear frequency	
Injected agents	Corticosteroids (40–80 mg) Hyaluronic acid (vary by product/prefer single dose) Platelet Rich Plasma/bone marrow aspirate/microfat 3–6 ml 25% dextrose with 0.5% lidocaine 4–8 ml		

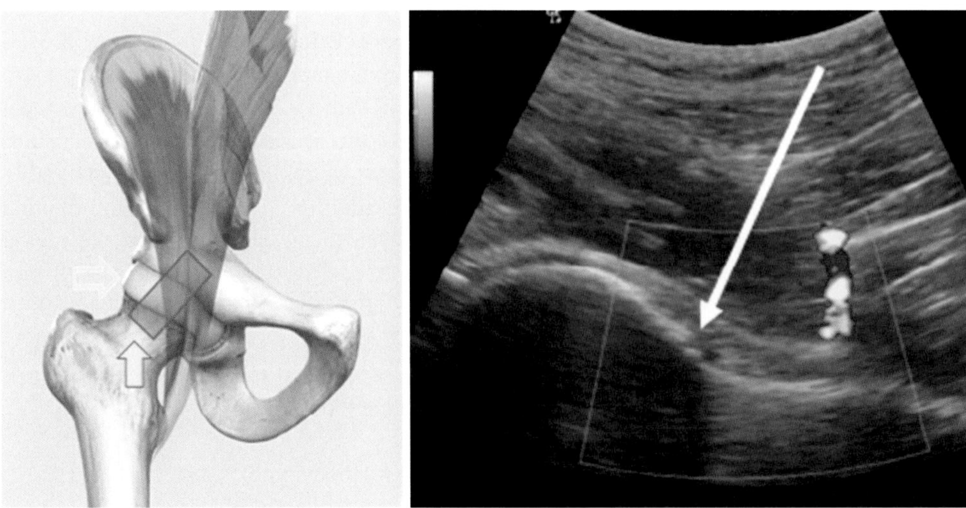

Fig. 8.10 Anterior approach targeted at the femoral head-neck junction (arrow). Note and avoid femoral circumflex vessels

visualization if available on the machine. A curvilinear low-frequency probe is often used. The needle position should be confirmed in both longitudinal and transverse planes before injection. Injection should be under sterile technique, while watching the flow into the joint or use power Doppler to see flow in the joint to confirm position. One can also aspirate if an effusion is present or to confirm intra-articular position.

Another technique is a transverse approach. This approach has shorter skin to target distance which may be suitable for larger patients. The patient is supine and the probe is placed transversely on the femoral head with the acetabulum in view. The needle is introduced lateral to medial, targeted toward femoral cartilage, psoas, or labrum (Fig. 8.11). A third approach is the longitudinal anterior approach. With this approach, one can also target the gluteal tendons as well as the joint with one injection approach (Fig. 8.12).

The most common injection in the hip region is diagnostic lidocaine with or without steroid. Diagnostic anesthetic intra-articular hip injections help differentiate between intra- and extra-articular pathology and help predict a response of total hip arthroplasty [28]. Studies to date have shown short-term benefit of steroid injections into the hip joint for osteoarthritic-type inflammatory conditions. Steer et al. showed a significant response up to 8 weeks after injection; however, there was no significant change in any imaging finding of effusion-synovitis [84].

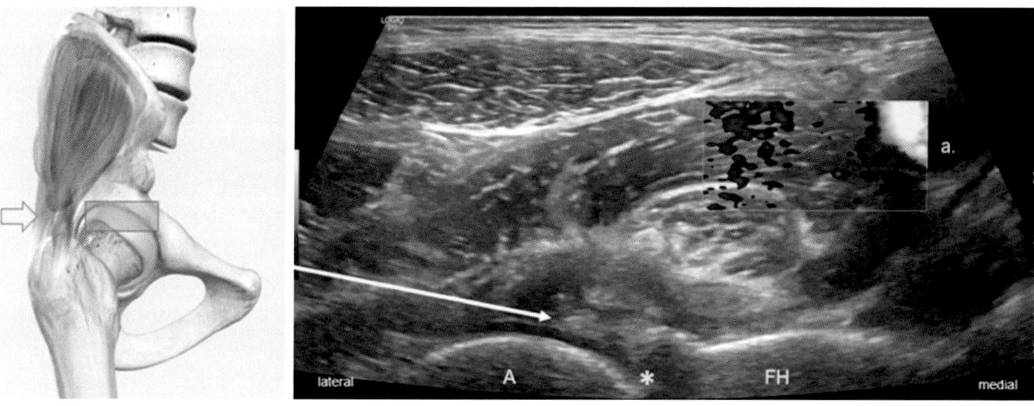

Fig. 8.11 Transverse approach: anterior supine position, lateral to medial approach to inject the joint at the labral complex. Note femoral vessels medial

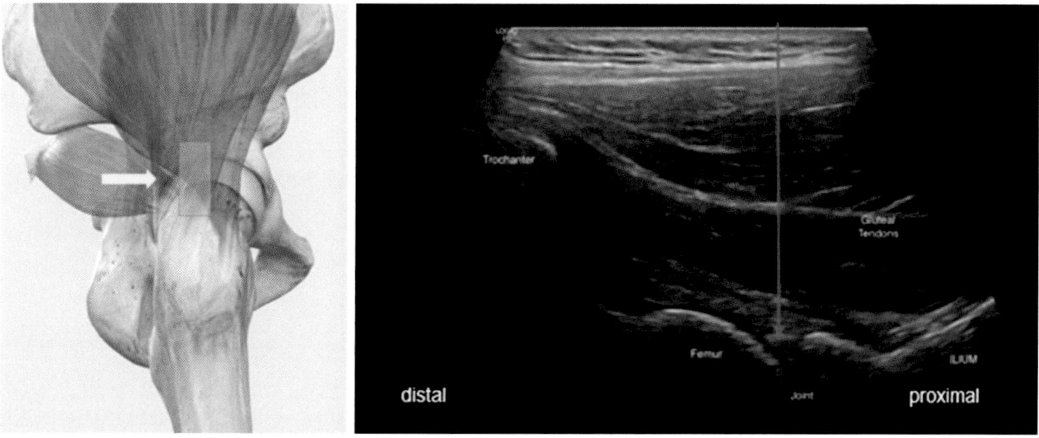

Fig. 8.12 Side-lying position, posterior to anterior approach, longitudinal view, out-of-plane technique. Acetabulum (A), femoral head (FH), needle target (asterisk)

Effusion does not seem to be helpful in determining who will respond. Recent studies also showed some potential adverse joint findings, accelerated OA progression, subchondral insufficiency fracture, complication of osteonecrosis, and rapid joint destruction, including bone loss after intra-articular corticosteroid injection in some patients [52]. Patient involvement in decision making on using steroid injections in this joint is advised.

Hyaluronic acid may be another choice for inflammatory hip conditions. There are limited studies compared to the knee with older studies suggesting a reduced effectiveness. More recent work indicates that intra-articular injections for mild-moderate hip OA may help in reducing pain and improving function [56]. With the ease of office-based ultrasound injections, this is now a reasonable option in the treatment paradigm; however, cost is an issue as it is usually not covered by many insurance plans.

Orthobiologics have an increasing role in hip pathology, including arthritis. Platelet-rich plasma (PRP) has shown promising outcomes in osteoarthritis condition, particularly of the knee. Multiple randomized controlled studies have shown both improvements of pain and increased function as compared to placebo or hyaluronic acid. Studies to date have been mixed on PRP in the hip, as studies have suffered from multiple issues, such as lack of classification of the PRP products and other methodological weaknesses. One randomized controlled study showed that PRP had statistically significant reduction in VAS at 6 months in hip OA patients when compared with hyaluronic injection [24], while three other RCTs showed no statistically significant changes [10, 30, 31]. PRP may have more efficacy in early osteoarthritis of the hip. Unfortunately, most hip osteoarthritis is picked up later in the process. PRP appears to be safe with limited to no side effects. Further research needs to be done in the area.

Recently, mesenchymal stem cells/medicinal signaling cells (MSCs) have been used more frequently in treating patients with osteoarthritis. Bone marrow and adipose tissue contain mesenchymal stem cells, which have chondrogenic properties and anti-inflammatory and regenerative effects [88]. Currently, there is no level 1 RCT on treating hip OA. However, early limited studies show very good potential for good clinical outcomes. Mardones et al. [59] studied ten patients with three doses weekly of intra-articular hip autologous BM-MSC injection. They showed an improvement in pain, function, and range of motion with no safety issues after the follow-up period of 16–40 months. Another preliminary results from six patients using autologous adipose-derived MSC also showed a positive outcome with no reported adverse effect after intra-articular hip injections [23].

Labrum Injection

One may occasionally inject in or around the labrum in specific cases. These include distinct labral tears or large labral cysts or calcifications in the region causing pain. Positioning is similar in the supine position with the needle being directed to the labral pathology (Fig. 8.13). Intra-articular injections can also be used in cases as it will bathe the labrum with the injectate. Hip labrum mainly consists of fibrocartilage and dense connective tissue which is thought to be avascular; therefore, like other fibrocartilage, it may be difficult to heal [57]. PRP has been used

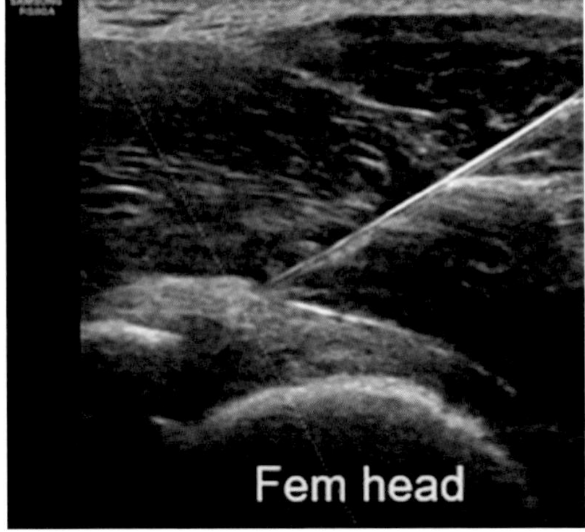

Fig. 8.13 Longitudinal view of the labrum with needle above the anterior hip labrum

to help augment cartilage tissue healing through the natural healing process [89]. According to a recent pilot study by De Luigi et al., the use of leukocyte-rich PRP injection has shown promising outcome in improving function and reducing pain in eight labral tear patients [27].

Iliopsoas Bursal Injection

The iliopsoas tendon/bursal complex can be injected and/or aspirated for a variety of conditions (Table 8.2), most commonly bursal collections, snapping tendon, and iliopsoas tendinosis/tendinitis.

Iliopsoas bursitis injections are commonly performed in the supine position with the leg extended in neutral. The ultrasound probe should start in the transverse plane over the femur then translated superiorly towards the femoral neck; when the elongation of the femoral neck is noted, the medial portion of the probe should be rotated superiorly to angle in parallel with the inguinal ligament and femoral neck. Long-axis views should be used for confirmation. The femoral neurovascular structures should be identified medially. The needle is inserted in a lateral to medial approach targeting the hypoechoic fluid collection.

For snapping hips, the same approach is used. If bursal/tendon fluid is not well visualized, the needle tip should be placed between the iliopsoas and the ilium (Fig. 8.14). Watch the flow of fluid to lift off the iliopsoas tendon from the acetabular brim of the ilium and halo the tendon. This helps confirm the appropriate needle tip placement. This should be the area consistent with pathology on the dynamic ultrasound exam. Diagnostic maneuvers postinjection are needed to help assess if this is the source of pain.

In cases of tendon pathology, the long-axis approach on tendon can be easier for tenotomy or peritendinous injection as a greater length of tendon is accessible with one approach. See Fig. 8.3b for longitudinal views.

Anesthetics, cortisone, and orthobiologics are the primary substances injected. Results of a study performed by Blankenbaker et al. [12]

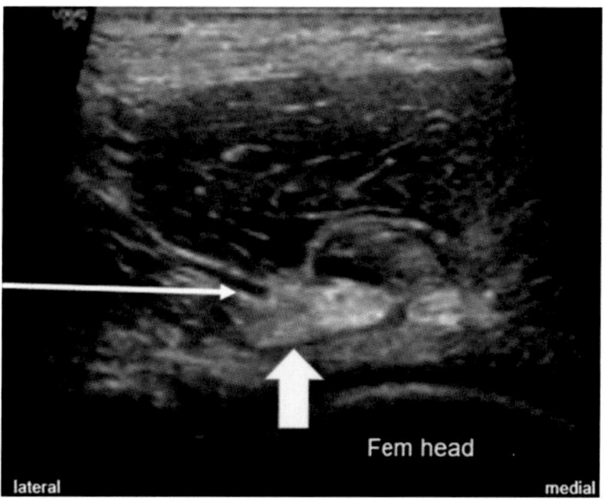

Fig. 8.14 Iliopsoas tendon complex. Transverse view of needle path using a lateral to medial approach. Note the two heads iliopsoas tendon at the level of the acetabular rim

Table 8.2 Iliopsoas tendon/bursa injection approaches

Pathology	Iliopsoas bursitis	Snapping hip	Iliopsoas tendinopathy
Patient position	Supine position with the leg in neutral or internal position		
Probe positioning	Transversely over the femoral head, then shifted superiorly and angled parallel to the inguinal ligament		Consider switch to the long axis for better needle positioning
Target	The hypoechoic fluid collection (Fig. 8.20) or between the iliopsoas and the ilium (unclear bursa)	Iliopsoas tendon at the area of pain and snapping	Pathologic tendon
Needle size	25 g 1.5 inch for local anesthesia; 18–22 g 1.5–3 inch for injection		
Probe	Medium to high frequency linear		
Injected agents	Corticosteroids (40–80 mg) Platelet- Rich Plasma/bone marrow aspirate/microfat 3–6 ml 25% dextrose with 0.5% lidocaine 4–8 ml Tenotomy		

showed that US-guided corticosteroid injection in the iliopsoas bursa has diagnostic and therapeutic benefits for patients with groin pain and clinically suspected snapping iliopsoas tendon, even if the snapping cannot be demonstrated sonographically. A positive response to corticosteroid injection is a predictor of a good surgical outcome if surgical release of the iliopsoas tendon is needed. High-volume injection may be tried, but no clinical outcome studies are available. Orthobiologic injection as well as tenotomy may play a role in case of tendinosis, tendinitis, or partial tear. Although limited study has been done, orthobiologic studies with PRP have shown good efficacy in treating tendon pathology in similar tendons, particularly for tendinosis. Further research is needed.

Hydrodissection on Lateral Femoral Cutaneous Nerve

The lateral femoral cutaneous nerve, when well visualized, is amenable to high-volume injection (Table 8.3). Ultrasound with clinical palpation is required to identify and reproduce symptoms in the patient. In a supine position, the ultrasound probe is placed to locate the nerve as previously described. It is best found transversely near the ASIS and between the sartorius and the tensor fasciae latae. The needle is introduced in a lateral to medial approach, targeting just below the LFCN in the fascial plane. The needle bevel should be turned facing the nerve to avoid nerve damage. Inject the fluid and watch fluid flow around the nerve. Inject until the entire nerve is haloed; oftentimes, 20 cc or more of fluid may be needed.

Table 8.3 Lateral femoral cutaneous nerve injection approach

Patient position	Supine position with the leg in neutral or internal position
Probe positioning	Over the nerve where abnormality is noted or pain/Tinel's sign on sonopalpation
Target	LFCN in the fascial plane between the sartorius and the tensor fasciae latae
Needle size	25 g 1.5 inch for anesthesia and injection
Probe	Highest frequency linear
Injected agents	Normal saline Corticosteroids (40 mg) 25% dextrose with 0.5% lidocaine Leukocyte-poor PRP 5–20 cc around the nerve – enough to dissect tissue and halo the nerve

Hydrodissection with normal saline, 25% dextrose or leukocyte-poor PRP or PPP has been used in treating nerve entrapment. Although, there have been limited studies showing efficacy on treating meralgia paresthetica, case reports and the authors clinical experience have shown immediate, long-term relief of numbness associated with severe, chronic MP after hydrodissection [64].

Medial Hip Region

Introduction

The medial hip region is an anatomically complex region for which pathology often presents as groin pain. Groin pain is very common, especially in certain sports that involve repetitive cutting, planting, and pivoting. The close proximity of the inguinal structures in males makes the evaluation of this region very challenging. Discussion of inguinal-related pain including hernias is not reviewed in this chapter but should strongly be considered in the differential. The primary musculoskeletal structures involved in medial hip pathology are the adductor tendons, the rectus abdominis insertion, and the pubic symphysis. Fortunately, unlike the posterior hip, many of the structures are superficial. Many terms are used interchangeably in the literature to describe groin pain. Athletic pubalgia, sports hernia, sportsman's hernia, Gilmore groin, adductor dysfunction or tendinopathy, and osteitis pubis are various terms used to describe entities that are either in the same spectrum of disease or share similar mechanisms of injury and clinical manifestation [18]. Clinicians should clearly define pathologic structures. While ultrasound is very useful in evaluating this region, MRI is often additionally needed to fully assess the entire region including the osseous structures.

Sonoanatomy

The following structures should be visualized as part of the medial hip checklist:

1. Symphysis pubis
2. Rectus abdominis
3. Adductor tendons
4. Pectineus muscle
5. Inguinal structures and hernia evaluation are beyond the scope of this chapter

The medial hip and thigh are highlighted by the adductor muscle group – the adductor longus (AL), adductor magnus (AM), and adductor brevis (AB), the gracilis and pectineus muscles [17, 46]. The primary proximal attachment of the adductor muscles is the AL on the inferior aspect of the pubis. The tendon has approximately 40% anterior tendon attachment and 60% posterior direct muscular attachment. It makes an aponeurosis with the tendon of the rectus abdominis. The AL is the most superficial of the three prime adductors with the AB and AM respectively deeper and have near complete muscular attachments at the pubis just lateral to that of the AL. The gracilis is the most medial of the adductor group and attaches inferior to the AB and AL on the anterior-medial border of the pubis. Ultrasonography of the adductor groups is best accomplished when the patient is positioned supine with the hip in flexion and abduction with a linear transducer in the longitudinal axis to the adductor muscles. To identify the AL, AB, and AM layered from superficial to deep, follow them proximally to their insertion at the pubis – attachments at the pubis from superficial to deep should proceed as follows: AL tendon, AL muscle, AB muscle, AM muscle [70, 76] (Fig. 8.15).

Rectus Abdominus

Superficially overlying the pubis, there is a continuous aponeurosis connecting the AL tendon and the rectus abdominis. This aponeurosis also blends with the fibrocartilage disc and capsule of the pubic symphysis. Notably, fibers of the aponeurosis both remain ipsilateral and cross to the contralateral side of the rectus abdominis. Sonographic evaluation of the distal rectus insertion is accomplished by continuing to scan in the cranial direction from the adductor insertion and rotating the probe slightly to the true sagittal plane in line with the rectus abdominis. The rectus tendon should be scanned across its width and proximally to the myotendinous junction. Additionally, the probe should be rotated 90 degrees and the tendon should be scanned in short access [44, 70].

Pubic Symphysis

The pubic symphysis is a nonsynovial joint containing a fibrocartilaginous disc covered by a thin layer of hyaline cartilage. It unites the superior rami of the pubic bones bilaterally connecting the anterior aspect of the pelvic ring [1]. The pubic symphysis can be accessed with ultrasound by

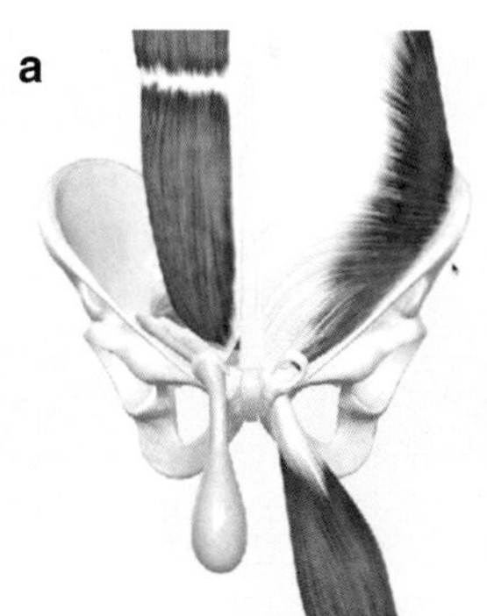

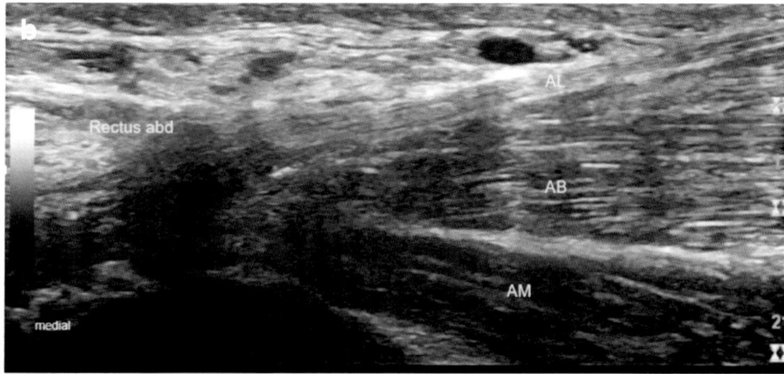

Fig. 8.15 (**a**) Overview of anatomy. Note rectus, adductor, obliques, and proximity of structures of inguinal canal in men. (**b**) Longitudinal view of layers of the adductor longus (AL), adductor brevis (AB), and adductor magnus (AM) attached to the pubic symphysis (P)

placing the probe with the midline of the synthesis in the transverse plane. From this view, a side-to-side comparison of the rectus-adductor aponeurosis over the pubic bones can also be made.

Pathology

Adductor/Rectus Aponeurosis

Groin pain is a symptom of many possible pathologies, with adductor/rectus injury at the pubis being the most common. Adductor attachment injuries may result from overuse microtears or acute injuries. This is a common and difficult problem to manage particularly in athletes in sports involving frequent twisting and cutting movements. The adductor longus attachment is most typically the involved site; however, the distal rectus attachment at the pubis and rectus-adductor aponeurosis may also be implicated [58, 61, 62, 77]. Pathologies of the adductor tendon insertion can include tendinopathic thickening greater than the normal 3–4 mm, full or partial tendon tears, or calcific tendinopathy (Fig. 8.16). Full thickness AL tendon tears are rare, but if present, there may be tendon retraction and hematoma noted in these cases [44, 70] (Fig. 8.17). Alternatively, if the pathology is located at the rectus aponeurosis attachment to the pubis, one may see a hypoechoic fluid layer in between the rectus-adductor aponeurosis and the pubic bone or thickening of the aponeurosis; this is more easily assessed with a simultaneous side-to-side comparison of both aponeuroses over the pubic symphysis in the transverse plane if there is not bilateral pathology. MRI is more useful than ultrasound in evaluating these subtle defects and can also evaluate for bone edema in the region. Ultrasound is useful for dynamic study as well.

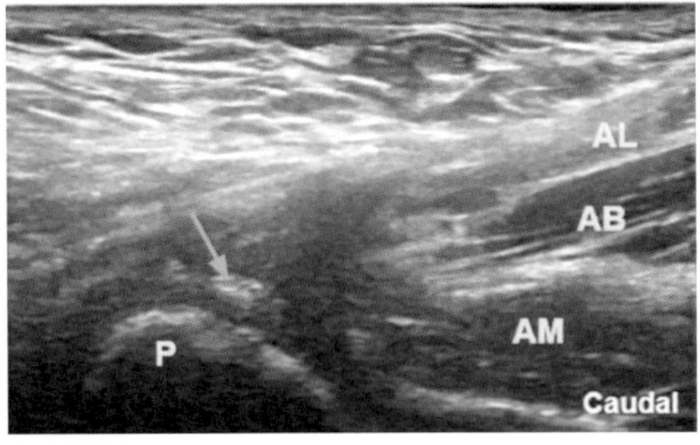

Fig. 8.16 Longitudinal view of adductor showing calcific tendinopathy (green arrow) at the pubic symphysis (P)

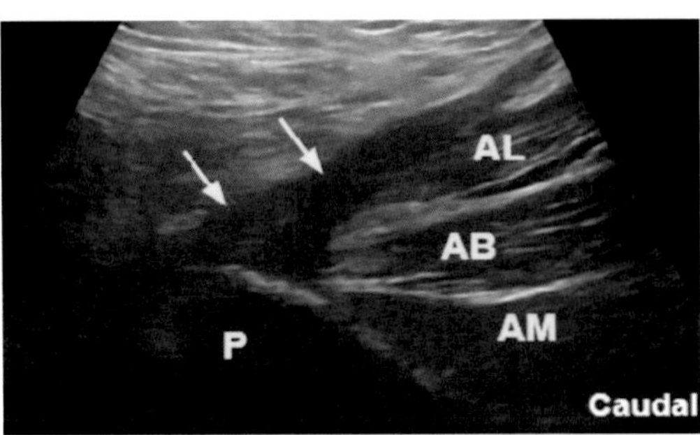

Fig. 8.17 Longitudinal full thickness adductor longus tendon tear

Osteitis Pubis

Osteitis pubis is a degenerative condition associated with various possible factors including trauma, overuse, inflammatory conditions, and infections. Studies in athletes have demonstrated biomechanical factors associated with osteitis pubis including decreased hip range of motion and muscle imbalances and environmental factors such as participation in sports with frequent kicking, twisting, and cutting [4, 72]. Ultrasound findings of osteitis pubis are cortical irregularity along the borders of the pubic bone, capsular thickening, and increased fluid in the pubic symphysis [1] (Fig. 8.18b). Dynamic ultrasound may show joint instability; however, MRI is more sensitive than ultrasound for the evaluation of the bone in this region.

Procedures

In patients with groin pain who fail to improve with conservative treatment, local injection can be useful for diagnostic purposes as well as therapeutic treatment. There are two common injections: the adductor/rectus aponeurosis and osteitis pubis (Table 8.4). For injections of the adductor origin, the patient is positioned supine with the leg slightly abducted and externally

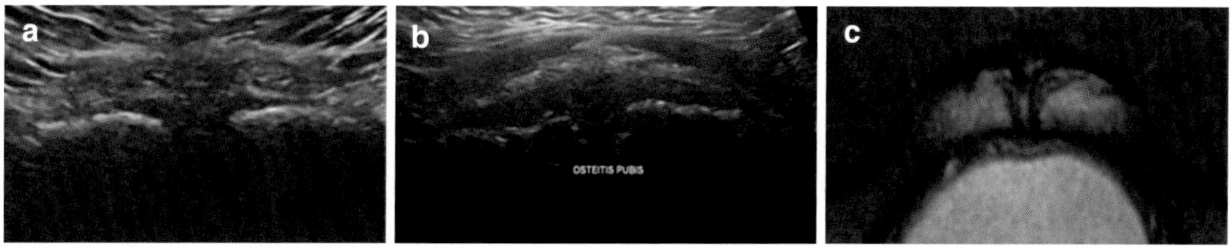

Fig. 8.18 (**a**) Transverse view demonstrating a normal pubic symphysis, (**b**) cortical irregularities and edema which can be seen in osteitis pubis, (**c**) MRI coronal plane showed intense marrow edema both sides of the symphysis pubis with subchondral sclerosis

Table 8.4 Adductor and pubic symphysis injection techniques

Procedure	Adductor injection	Osteitis pubis
Patient position	Supine with the leg slightly abducted and externally rotated	Supine with frog leg position
Probe positioning	At adductor tendon	Above pubic symphysis (Fig. 8.18)
Target	Pathologic tendon	Irregularity of the joint or into joint capsule
Needle size	25 g 1.5 inch for anesthesia and injection	
Probe	Medium to high frequency linear	
Injected agents	Corticosteroids (40 mg) PRP 4–6 ml Tenotomy	Corticosteroids (40 mg) PRP 2 ml 25% dextrose with 0.5% lidocaine

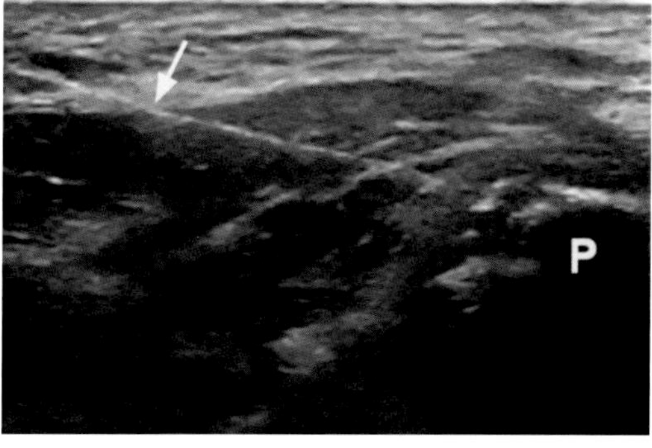

Fig. 8.19 Longitudinal view of needle placement for adductor calcification at the pubis (P)

rotated at the hip. Place the probe longitudinally at the adductor longus tendon (Fig. 8.15), and use transverse planes to confirm the three tendons. Injection is usually performed with a 25 g 1.5 inch needle in the long axis, approaching distal to proximal. Because of the superficial nature of the tendon and tight position, a small hockey stick probe can help facilitate the injection. A gel standoff pad is often required secondary to the sharp angle of the tendon anteriorly. Alternate between long and short axes during the injection to help better identify needle position and span the pathologic area.

Adductor tendon pathology can be effectively treated with corticosteroid injection. The study showed injection of local anesthetic and steroid into the adductor enthesis may help in pain relief for up to 1 year [79]. Like in other tendinopathies, PRP injection also has promising outcomes after intratendinous injection. According to a retrospective case series of 408 consecutive patients treated by a single ultrasound-guided PRP injection for tendinopathy in various sites, adductor longus tendinopathy demonstrated significantly improved functional outcome [25]. If a tear of the adductor is associated with spread up the aponeurosis (sports hernia) and particularly to the opposite side, surgical fixation is most likely warranted. Percutaneous tenotomy or barbotage using a needle (Fig. 8.19) or Tenex™ may also be considered for severe calcifications. New research is being done on ultrasound-guided tendon release as well. No data is available on the use of microfat or bone marrow cells in this tendon.

For osteitis pubis injections, patients lay supine. The joint can be injected in a variety of manners. The most common is in-plane with a standoff gel pad used to facilitate needle visualization. Alternatively, the clinician can use an out-of-plane technique with a walk-down technique with probe placed over the anterior aspect of the pubic symphysis. Neurovascular structure should be identified. A 25 g 1.5 inch needle should be introduced anterosuperior to posteroinferior approach aiming at pathology of irregularity of the pubic symphysis or direct into the joint capsule the pubic symphysis has a very tight joint space, so only 1–2 ml can be injected.

Local steroid injections are most commonly used for osteitis pubis treatment. Various studies report short-term pain relief. There is a high rate of nonresponder [20]. The underlying condition causing the joint irritation needs to be addressed for successful long-term treatment. This is usually the hip adductor myotendinous junction or adductor tendon-rectus sheath aponeurosis. Orthobiologic injections have limited studies in this pathology with only some case reports or small pilot studies. One study showed that monthly injection for two consecutive treatments of prolotherapy showed efficacy in athletes with groin pain [87]. Another case report found that combining PRP with needle tenotomy effectively improved the symptoms [80]. Further research is needed.

Lateral Hip Region

Introduction

Lateral hip pain is an extremely common problem requiring evaluation. Pain in this region is most commonly associated with tendon and bursa abnormalities at the greater trochanter. Pain can also be referred to this area from other structures, most commonly the hip joint. Evaluation starts with a thorough history and physical exam focusing the evaluation of the entire hip complex. A kinetic chain approach to movement deficits is helpful in addressing the underlying origin of pain. Ultrasound is critical to providing information on the diagnosis of pathology and in guiding interventions.

Sonoanatomy

The lateral hip is defined by the greater trochanter, an essential landmark with prominent muscular attachments, and a large bursa protecting the area. The trochanter is easily palpable and consists of four facets (Fig. 8.20), of which the lateral facet is palpable [71].

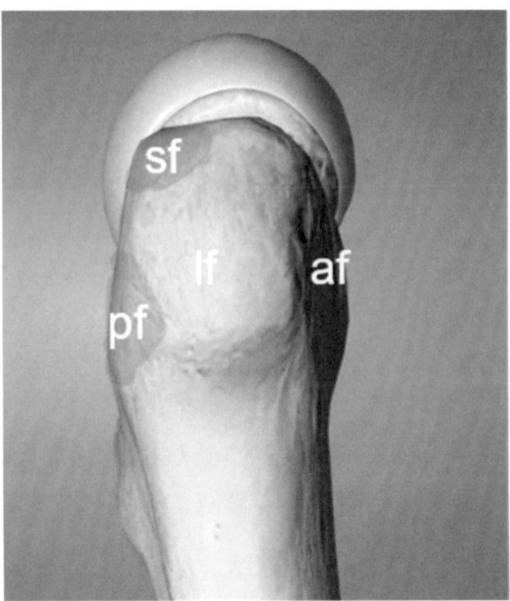

Fig. 8.20 sf superior-posterior facet, af anterior facet, lf lateral facet, pf posterior facet

The tendons originate on the ilium, with the gluteus minimus being the deepest structure. The gluteus minimus attaches to the anterior facet and runs deep to the gluteus medius on the ilium. The gluteus medius is bipennate and has two muscular attachments, the main one into the superior-lateral facet while its thick posterior band inserts into the superior aspect of the posterior facet [42] (Fig. 8.2). The maximus muscle does not attach to the trochanter; instead, it runs superficially sending fibers to insert onto the linea aspera of the femur and posterior hooks into the iliotibial band (ITB). Underneath the maximus lies the trochanteric bursa covering the posterior facet and parts of the lateral facet above the medius. The small bursa also sits between the attachment of the medius and minimus at the respective facets.

The tensor fasciae latae and iliotibial band (ITB) originate at the superior ilium and anterior superior iliac spine (ASIS), just posterior to the iliac tubercle. The ITB begins in the posterior lateral aspect forming from the fascia of the tensor fascia lata (TFL). There is a coalescence of these fibers from the TFL, ITB, and gluteal aponeurosis over the trochanter before they disperse distally to multiple sites. The ITB is involved in lateral hip and lateral knee stabilization. These are best seen in a longitudinal plane.

The gluteal muscles are the main external rotators and abductor muscles of the hip and assist in hip extension and stabilization. They are active during standing and walking motion.

Ultrasound Technique

The following structures should be visualized as part of the lateral hip checklist:

1. Trochanter facets (anterior, superficial posterior lateral, lateral, posterior)
2. Gluteus minimus tendon and muscle
3. Gluteus medius bipennate muscle with attachments
4. Trochanteric bursa
5. Iliotibial band
6. Tensor fasciae latae
7. Gluteus maximus muscle

Start the evaluation by positioning the patient in the lateral decubitus position, preferably with the hip slightly flexed to a fetal position. Place the probe transversely over the trochanter (Fig. 8.21) and identify the facets. The apex of the greater trochanter demarcates the division between the anterior and lateral facets. Assessment of the gluteus minimus attachment at the anterior facet is done by rotating the probe and translating anteriorly to have the anterior facet centered in the transverse plane, then rotating 90° to assess the tendon in the longitudinal axis (Fig. 8.22). The same

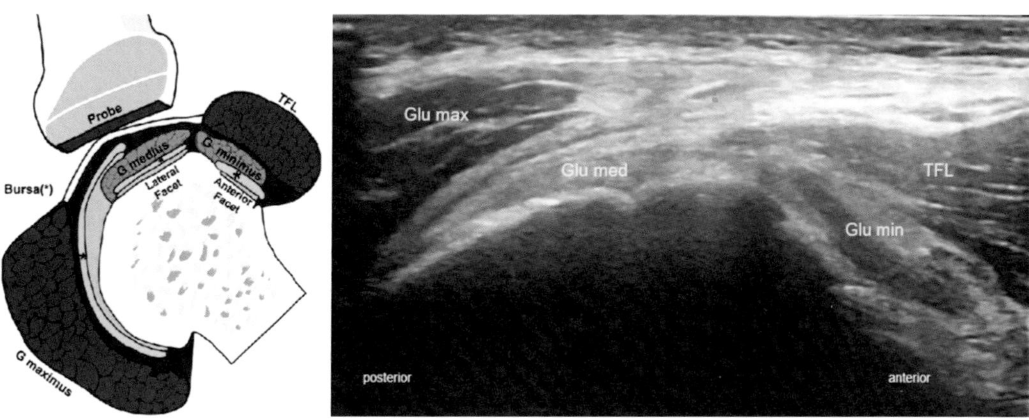

Fig. 8.21 Schematic and corresponding transverse view over the greater trochanter demonstrating gluteal muscle attachments

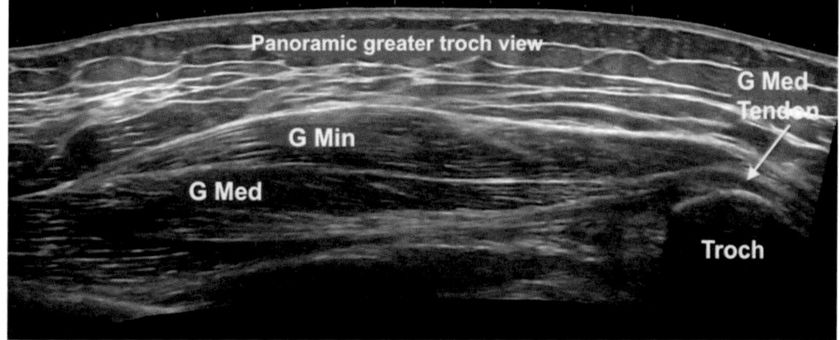

Fig. 8.22 The picture showed a bipennate gluteus medius, one band attached to the superior-posterior and lateral facets

technique should be used over the lateral and superoposterior facets for the assessment of the two gluteus medius attachments. Returning to the apex of the greater trochanter and translating slightly posteriorly to the lateral facet will allow for best visualization of the trochanteric bursa [45].

Evaluate the tendons for pathology in both longitudinal and transverse planes. As in many tendons, anisotropy may be encountered, mimicking a tear. Evaluate the posterior zone for fluid in the bursa and in the small bursal area at each tendon-bone interface. Characterize any bursal fluid. If there is pain or it is clinically, evaluate the TFL at its origin and ITB. The TFL tendon is on average about 2 mm thick and should have no significant side-to-side difference; look for any tendinopathy or partial tear.

If the patient has snapping, perform dynamic maneuvers for subluxation of the ITB and gluteus maximus over the greater trochanter. Ultrasound with its dynamic capabilities is the test of choice. Perform with the probe transverse over the trochanter. Move the hip into flexion and extension and evaluate for tissue movement and sonopalpation of reproducible snap. The ITB/gluteal aponeurosis may snap over the anterior trochanter with flexion and extension of the hip. It may also be seen with adduction and internal rotation of the hip with flexion/extension of the leg and flexed knee. Evaluation with light probe pressure or in the standing position may be required to reproduce symptoms.

Pathology

Pain at the lateral hip is usually referred to as greater trochanteric syndrome. It is most commonly seen in females in the 50s and 60s. It is best to describe the actual pathology using ultrasound. It has a reported prevalence of around 18% [81]. The etiology of greater trochanteric pain is often multifactorial, with symptoms arising from a variety of structures including gluteal tendinopathy, bursopathy, intra-articular hip disorders, posterior external rotator structures, and the sacroiliac or spine/lumbar complex. At the trochanter, the gluteus medius is the most common anatomic pathologic injured structure followed by the minimus. Isolated bursopathy is uncommon among symptomatic patients. Ultrasound compares favorably to MRI for the evaluation of these tendons with a sensitivity of 90% and a specificity of 95% [91] and may exceed it for specific tendon disease secondary to its dynamic component and high spatial resolution. The tendons have a similar spectrum of pathology to other tendons (partial tear, complete, tendinosis, calcifications, etc.). Tendons may fail in the anterior aspect initially and then proceed posteriorly similar to the rotator cuff [42]. Look for diffuse thickening and hypoechoic signal as the hallmarks of tendinosis (Fig. 8.23b).

Enthesopathic changes in the tendon are not uncommon and may not correlate with pain and should be clinically correlated. Abnormal

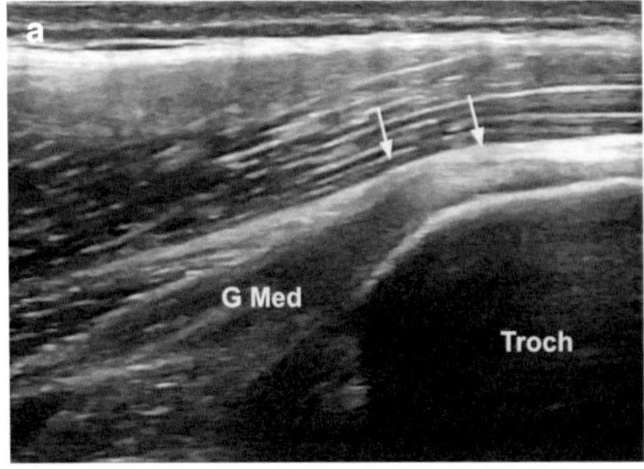

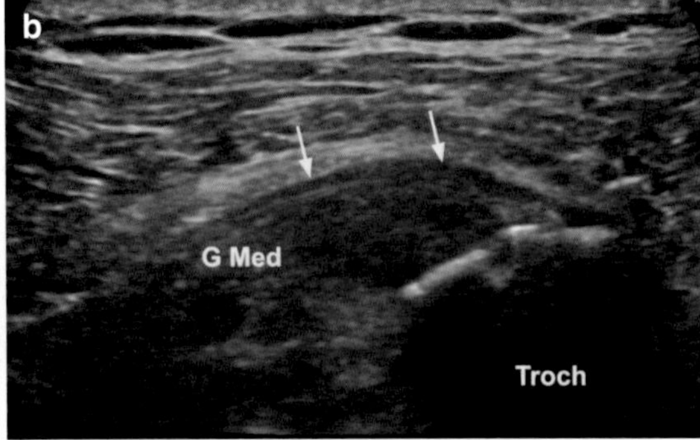

Fig. 8.23 (**a**) Ultrasound view showed a normal gluteal tendon (yellow arrows). (**b**) Gluteus medius severe tendinosis demonstrating significantly thickened tendon (yellow arrows) with small cortical irregularity at the greater trochanter

Doppler tendon vascularity is less conspicuous in these tendons than others. Muscle disorders of the gluteal tendons are less common. One may see some changes associated with tendon pathology such as atrophy and retraction. Complete tears may appear similar to the rotator cuff with a "bald" facet. Calcific deposits are often associated with tendinopathy, but like in the shoulder may be benign findings. A variety of presentations can occur from small lesions at the enthesis to large deposits causing significant bursal pain. Hydroxyapatite deposition and varying stages of calcific tendon pathology may be present [53]. Clinical correlation is critical.

Trochanteric bursal swelling is infrequent unless direct trauma is present (Fig. 8.24). Direct trauma may cause significant large swelling. Like all bursitis and fluid collections, the differential should also include systemic inflammatory disorders and rarely infection. Most trochanteric bursal swelling is secondary to tendon pathology, especially of the medius. Again, isolated bursal swelling is uncommon.

Gluteus Medius Bursitis

Chronic tendon pathology likely leads to an impingement-type phenomenon and chronic bursal issues similar to the shoulder. Abnormal hip mechanics secondary to intra-articular pathology likely plays a large role. Pain can also be referred to this area from the hip joint and other areas as previously noted.

Pain proximal to the trochanter at the ilium should be evaluated for tendinosis of the ITB or TFL (Fig. 8.25). In TFL tendon pathology, it is commonly seen as a repetitive overuse injury in

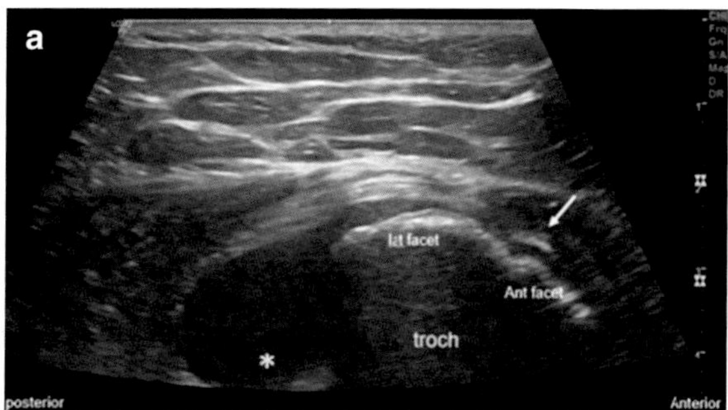

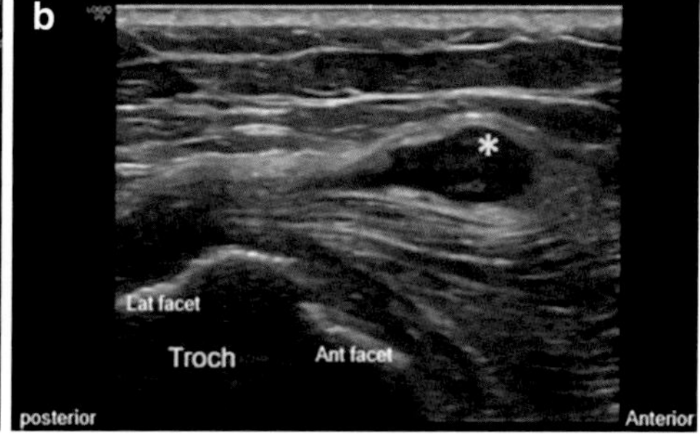

Fig. 8.24 (**a**) Trochanteric bursitis (asterisk) with anterior calcification (white arrow) at the gluteus minimus tendon. (**b**) Ultrasonography showed hypoechoic area of fluid collection (asterisk) with gluteus medius and gluteus minimus partial tear

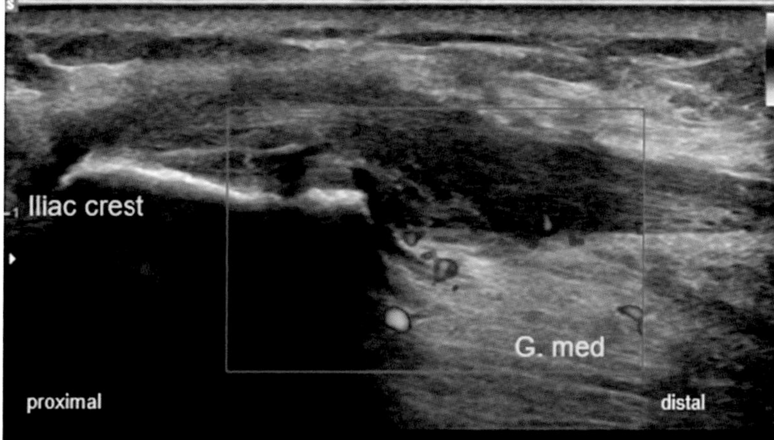

Fig. 8.25 Sonographic longitudinal view of TFL partial tear (long axis)

runners/cross trainers. It is more common in females and presents as local pain. Full thickness tears are rare.

Snapping can occur as previously noted and is associated with ITB/gluteal aponeurosis thickening.

Procedures

The common procedures to the lateral hip revolve around the gluteal tendons (Table 8.5). A variety of substances can be injected, each with varying pros and cons. These include corticosteroid, dextrose, saline, and biologics such as PRP, MFAT, and BMAC.

The procedures in the region are noted below.

Tendon: tenotomy, barbotage, orthobiologics, high-volume injection

Bursa: injection and aspiration

Table 8.5 Lateral hip injection techniques

Pathology	Trochanteric bursitis	Gluteal tendinopathy
Patient position	Placed in the side-lying fetal (lateral decubitus) position	
Probe positioning	Placed transversely to identify the facets and/or the tendon/bursal pathology	
Target	Trochanteric bursa	Pathologic tendon
Needle size	25 g 1.5 inch for anesthesia and 22 g 3 inch for injection Consider larger needles (18 g) for tenotomy or use specialized equipment with Tenex™	
Probe	Medium to high frequency linear	
Injected agents	Corticosteroids (40–80 mg) Platelet Rich Plasma/bone marrow aspirate/microfat 3–6 ml Tenotomy (6–9 needle passes)	

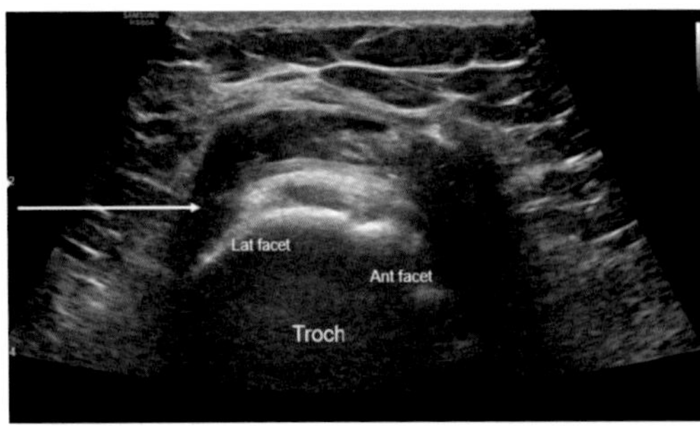

Fig. 8.26 Transverse view of the trochanteric bursa demonstrating the needle trajectory (arrow) for a lateral to medial approach

The patient is placed in the side-lying (lateral decubitus) fetal position. The probe is placed transversely to identify the facets and/or the tendon/bursal pathology. A 25 g or above needle is used for local soft tissue anesthesia. Then a 22 g 3 inch needle is used to advance in plane with the transducer from posterior to anterior. The target is primarily the trochanteric bursa (Fig. 8.26), but depending on diagnosis may be the tendon for regenerative procedures. Long-axis views of the tendon can also be used. It is best to determine this on an individual case basis.

Corticosteroids with anesthetics can play a role in acute inflammation control. This can allow pain reduction facilitating physical therapy. Labrosse et al. noted on average a 55% reduction in pain [54]. These injections are best done ultrasound guided through the same technique described above. These injections should be limited secondary to long-term potential risk of corticosteroids on tendons. The clinician should inject the bursa directly and avoid the tendon using steroids. Cortisone should not be used in high-grade partial or full thickness tears secondary to rupture possibilities. As previously noted, since most bursal issues are secondary to tendon pathology, treating the tendon is critical. For tendinopathy, a recent high-quality study by Fitzpatrick showed excellent results of single-dose leukocyte-rich PRP injection under ultrasound guidance in patients with chronic gluteal tendinopathy >4 months when compared with corticosteroid injection with sustained improvement for 2 years [36]. There was also a promising outcome in treating gluteus medius tendinopathy from combining LR-PRP injection with needle tenotomy [55]. A systematic review study also showed a clinical improvement of PRP injection in recalcitrant greater trochanteric pain syndrome when compared with surgery [90]. Moreover, a study comparing LP-PRP injection with corticosteroid injection in 24 patients with greater trochanteric pain syndrome revealed that PRP injection helps decrease pain up to 24 weeks, significantly longer than cortisone [11]. Platelet-rich plasma may also have indications for tendon pathology at the origin of the ITB and TFL in cases of pathology not responsive to standardized treatments. High-volume dissection was also shown to be effective in greater trochanteric pain. A case series study showed short to medium pain relief after high-volume dissection with 10 ml 0.5% Marcaine and 50 mg hydrocortisone into the area of greatest pain over the greater trochanter followed by structured rehabilitation [64].

The use of MSCs in the gluteal tendon still has limited study. One case report reported a significant improvement in pain and function after pure bone marrow injection in a gluteus medius tendon with calcific tendinopathy [41]. Tendon calcifications can be treated with barbotage/aspiration or needle tenotomy. Tenotomy has been studied by Jacobson with good results [45]. A large needle is passed through the tendon to facilitate controlled tendon injury and stimulate tendon recovery; the number of tendon passes is often based on feel with return to normal tissue characteristics. Sonographic guidance is critical. Recovery usually takes 3 months [45]. Instrumented procedures such as Tenex™ can also be used for large calcifications or tendinosis. A recent case series on percutaneous ultrasonic tenotomy in gluteal tendinopathy with a 22-month follow-up showed an improvement in VAS, functional score with no reported complication, and good patient satisfaction [7].

Posterior Hip Region

Introduction

The posterior hip is one of the most challenging areas for evaluation. It may best be referred to as the sub- or deep gluteal space. The area has multiple structures and deep layers of tissue, making physical exam, sonographic imaging, and interventions challenging. Pain can be from the tendons of the external rotators, as well as the extensive neurological structure in the area, particularly the sciatic nerve. Multiple pathologies in this area have been incorporated into the all-inclusive "piriformis syndrome," which lacks diagnostic precision.

Deep gluteal syndrome is perhaps a better term to encompass pain in this region [68]. Pain in the region is commonly referred to from the spine as well. Evaluation starts with a thorough history and physical exam, including the spine and kinetic chain movement pattern analysis. A kinetic chain approach to movement deficits is helpful in addressing the underlying origin of pain. Ultrasound with sonopalpation is critical to provide information on the diagnosis of pathology and guide interventions. Guided diagnostic injections can also be helpful to differentiate the pain generator for further treatment options.

Sonoanatomy

The posterior hip/subgluteal space encompasses the region. The area encompasses the following key structures to be scanned.

Posterior hip checklist:

Deep external rotators:

1. Piriformis
2. Obturator internus
3. Gemelli
4. Quadratus femoris
5. Sciatic nerve
6. Ischial tuberosity/bursa – hamstring origin

Its boundaries are posteriorly, the gluteus maximus; anteriorly, the posterior acetabulum, hip joint capsule, and proximal femur; laterally, the gluteal tuberosity; medially, the sacrotuberous ligament; superiorly, the inferior margin of the sciatic notch; and inferiorly, the proximal origin of the hamstrings at the ischial tuberosity. The superior and inferior gluteal, sciatic, posterior femoral cutaneous, and pudendal nerves traverse the deep gluteal space (Fig. 8.27).

The sciatic nerve is a key structure in the region. It runs out the sciatic notch with the superior gluteal artery and neve. It runs posterior to the piriformis though six variations are noted in the literature. Limited research suggests these variations do not appear to be associated with increased pain [4]. The nerve then heads laterally to the thigh and exits the space over the quadratus femoris muscle between the ischium and the trochanter. It is about 1.2 cm from the ischial tuberosity with close association to the hamstring origin. Fibrous bands may be located along the course of the nerve causing tethering and in some cases pain and sciatica-like symptoms [16].

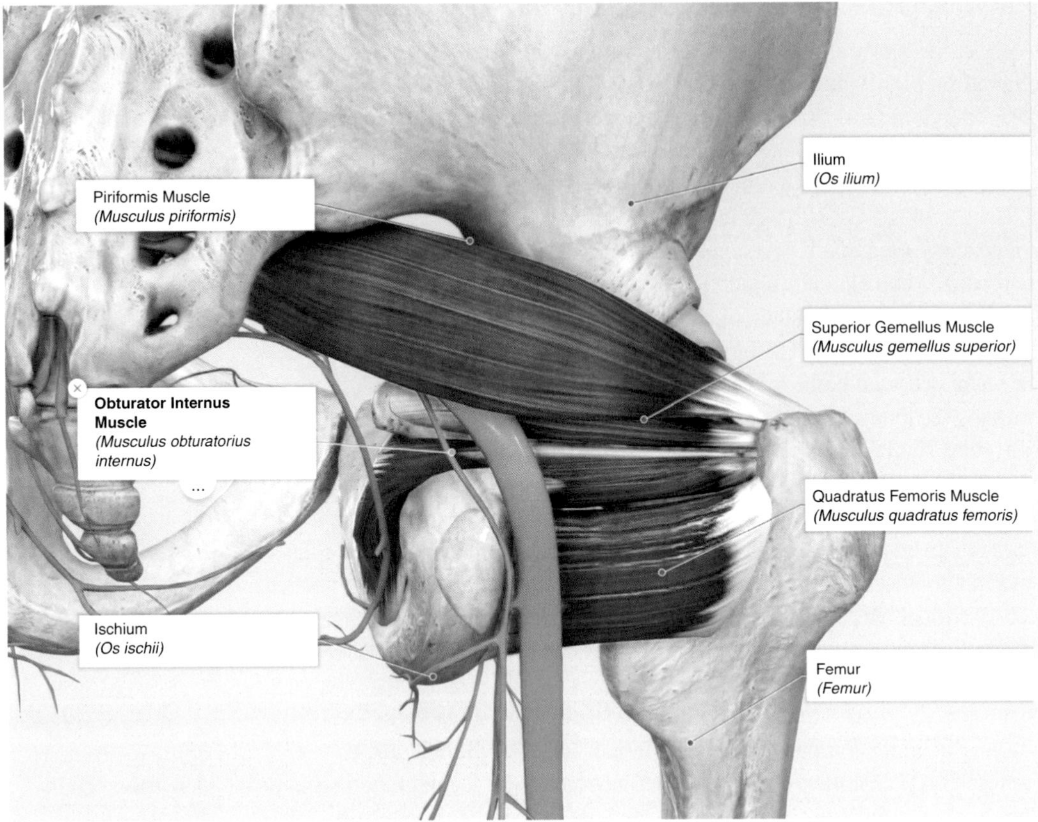

Fig. 8.27 Anatomy of the deep posterior hip musculature in relation to the sciatic nerve

The muscle tendon units in the space include from superior to inferior the piriformis, superior gemellus, obturator internus, inferior gemellus, and quadratus femoris (Fig. 8.27). The piriformis occupies a key position and runs laterally through the greater sciatic foramen, becomes tendinous, and inserts in the medial aspect of the trochanter. Its attachment is often not distinct from the conjoint tendons of the obturator internus and superior and inferior gemelli. The piriformis is a key external rotator and is stretched with hip flexion, adduction, and internal rotation. The most important of the conjoint tendons is the obturator internus, which makes a 90-degree turn to the anterior pelvis. These tendons also work to stabilize the hip and externally rotate. The quadratus femoris is a quadrilateral-type muscle that sits between the trochanter and the ischium. It can be involved in ischiofemoral impingement of the muscle and sciatic nerve which sits directly in this space.

Just distal and medial to the quadratus sits the ischial tuberosity and the attachment of the hamstring tendon. The hamstrings originate from the ischial tuberosity, except for the short head of the biceps femoris; the semimembranosus tendon is attached to the superolateral facet of the ischial tuberosity and the conjoint tendon of the biceps femoris, and the semitendinosus is attached to the inferomedial facet. The sciatic nerve lies approximately 1.2 cm lateral to the ischial tuberosity or the outer border of the semimembranosus tendon. Thus, the proximal part of this muscle complex is close to the sciatic nerve. The position of the tendon attachments of the conjoint tendon and semimembranosus is noted in Fig. 8.28.

Ultrasound

Sonographic evaluation in this region is done with the patient prone and a pillow placed under

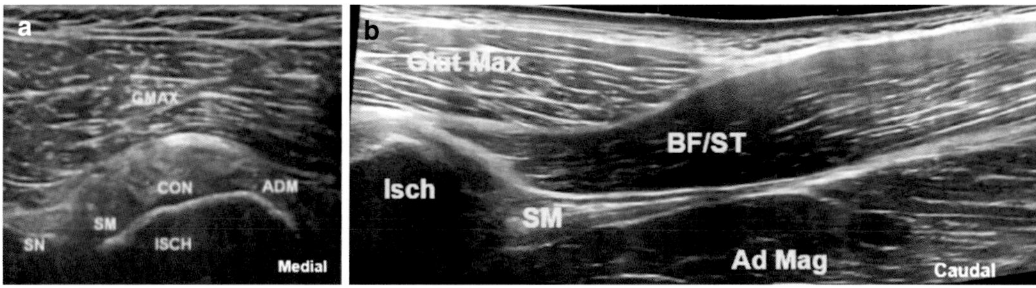

Fig. 8.28 (**a**) Transverse image of hamstring origin. Note the conjoint tendon (CON) attachment at the ischium (ISCH), the adductor magnus (ADM) medially, semimembranosus (SM), sciatic nerve (SN) laterally, and gluteus maximus (GMAX) superficially. (**b**) Longitudinal image of hamstring origin (BF biceps femoris long head, ST semitendinosus)

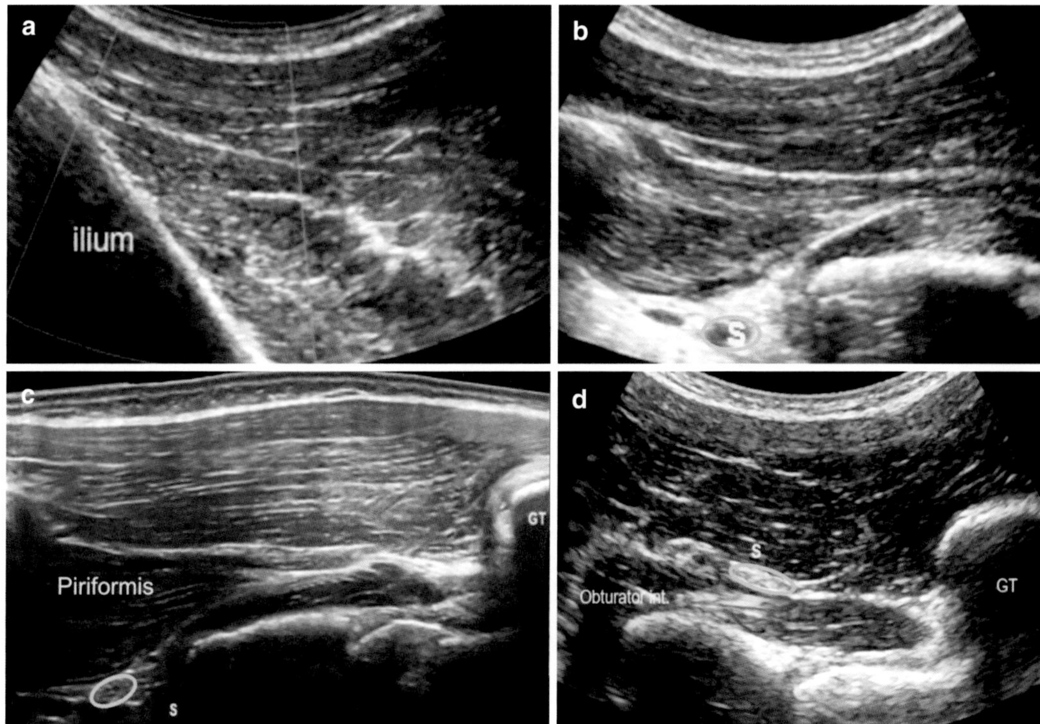

Fig. 8.29 Scanning sequence of the posterior hip from cranial to caudal. (**a**) The hyperechoic ilium is first noted in the lateral posterior region. (**b**) At the notch the piriformis is well visualized with the sciatic nerve (S, green outline). (**c**) The piriformis is seen attaching to the superior-posterior border of the greater trochanter (GT). (**d**) Caudal to the piriformis the characteristic right-angle appearance of the obturator internus hooking around the superior border of the obturator fossa and attaching to the greater trochanter

the pelvis. A curvilinear probe is required to best see these structures. The effective use of sonopalpation and dynamic maneuvers may assist in the evaluation of the pain generators.

Scanning of the posterior hip should be done sequentially beginning with the hyperechoic ilium first noted in the medial posterior region (Fig. 8.29a). Move distally until the sciatic notch is apparent. The use of Doppler may help localize the superior gluteal artery that runs with the sciatic nerve (Fig. 8.29b). An attempt to find the sciatic nerve at this level can be done but is challenging in obese patients. Evaluate the piriformis – which runs at a 30-degree angle through the notch – in the long axis by pivoting the probe toward the trochanter (Fig. 8.29c). Dynamic maneuvers of hip external and internal rotation help identify the muscle. Take note of the muscle complex thickness as it may be associated with piriformis syndrome and comparison to the opposite side may be needed. Transverse views of the posterior gluteal region may provide further diagnostic information, however are more challenging and take extensive practice. Recent literature suggests ultrasound may be of value in diagnosing piriformis syndrome, but more work needs to be done [92]. Moving the probe more distally, one will note the obturator internus running into the pelvis and the conjoint tendon (Fig. 8.29d). Again, dynamic maneuvers are very helpful for localization.

The quadratus muscle is seen easily between the ischium and the posterior trochanter. Note the sciatic nerve sitting in the fossa (Fig. 8.30). Use extreme internal/external rotation to evaluate ischiofemoral impingement. Dynamic maneuvers may help illicit pain and help evaluate for potential ischiofemoral impingement.

Pathology

Pathology in this region is difficult to note on imaging tests and may be multifactorial. It is best to use the term subgluteal/deep gluteal syndrome which can include pathology to multiple structures vs. piriformis syndrome. Four main entities will be reviewed.

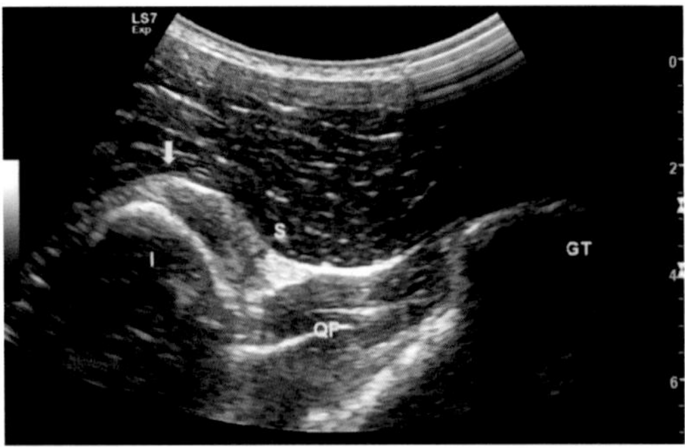

Fig. 8.30 Transverse view of posterior pelvis over the quadratus femoris muscle between greater trochanter and ischial tuberosity with sciatic nerve superficially. Note hamstring origin (arrow) (I ischium, S sciatic nerve, GT greater troch, QF quadratus femoris)

Piriformis Pain Syndrome Piriformis syndrome is a subgroup of deep gluteal syndrome, but not all deep gluteal syndrome is piriformis. Potential pain in the piriformis complex can occur from multiple sources including hypertrophy of the muscle, spasm, possibly anomalous course of sciatic, or anomalous fibrous attachments and lastly postsurgical fibrosis [16, 51, 68].

Gemelli-Obturator Internus Syndrome The gemelli-obturator is often painful to palpation. The sciatic runs under the piriformis and over the complex and may be affected by a scissor-like effect between the two muscles causing entrapment. The obturator is often more painful to clinical exams than the piriformis [48]. The nerve is attached to the gemelli-obturator internus complex by connective tissue, which can lead to sciatic entrapment [8]. Muscular spasm or myofascial pain syndrome, acute strain, hematoma, abscess/pyomyositis, tendinitis, and bursitis of the obturator internus can cause posterior hip pain as well [51]. Ultrasound and MRI exams are often negative or show subtle changes, but pain is noted over the tendon suggestive of mechanical wear.

Quadriceps Femoris and Ischiofemoral Impingement Ischiofemoral impingement (IFI) is a hip pain related to narrowing of the space between the ischial tuberosity and lesser trochanter of the femur (Fig. 8.30). This leads to muscle tendon and neurological changes. The space typically measures about 23 mm and can be considered narrowed if less than 17 mm. Most measurements are based on static MR images [74]. The condition can be related to repetitive overuse or inflammation in the area entrapping the muscle and/or sciatic nerve. Patients usually present with pain for prolonged sitting and with a long stride. Injection can be helpful both diagnostically and therapeutically. It is mainly seen in middle-aged to elderly women but can also be identified in pediatric patients [69].

Fibrous/Fibrovascular Bands Fibrous-type bands are not uncommon in the region and can compromise the sciatic nerve and result in entrapment-like syndromes. Symptoms present similar to sciatica but no back pain. These bands are often found in cases during arthroscopy Three types of bands occur, starting at the sciatic notch, then obturator-gemelli complex, and lastly in the area of the ischial tunnel [16].

Hamstring Conditions affecting the proximal origin of the hamstring may also be a source of pain. A full spectrum of pathology at the hamstring – tear, acute, chronic partial, tendinosis, calcifications (Fig. 8.31), apophyseal injuries – can occur. These can cause chronic inflammatory changes and adhesion causing fibrous scar and effect the sciatic nerve in the ischial tunnel. Patients often have pain with sitting and pain on firing of the hamstring muscles. It is often seen in runners and may not respond well to therapy.

Procedures

Clinicians can perform diagnostic and therapeutic injections (Table 8.6) in the region to assist in evaluation and treatment. Most injections will use a curvilinear probe at lower frequencies. The

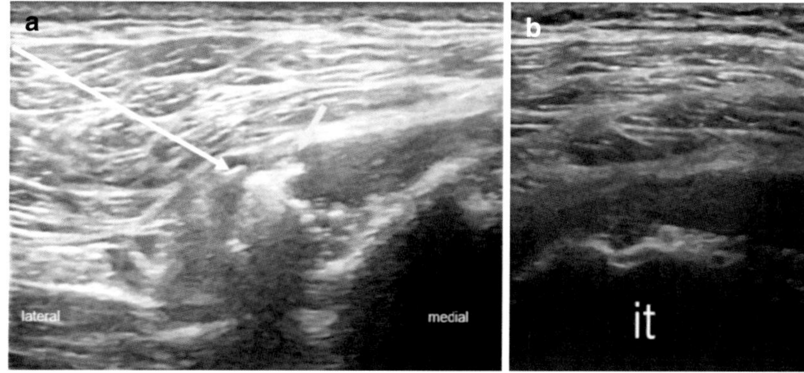

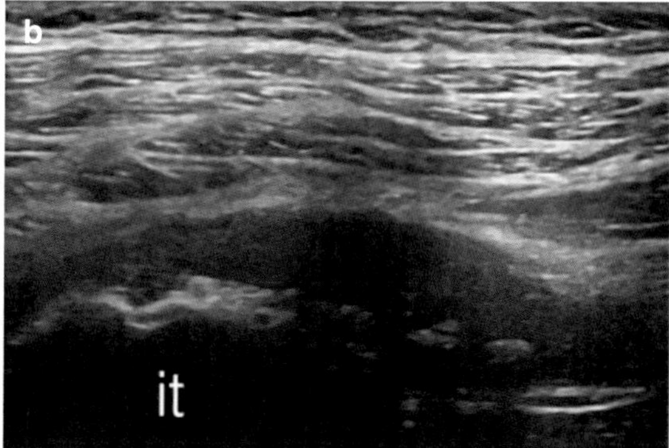

Fig. 8.31 (**a**) Transverse and (**b**) short-axis view of a calcific and tendinopathic hamstring origin with needle path shown in A

Table 8.6 Posterior hip injection techniques

Procedure	Piriformis injection	Peri-sciatic hydrodissection	Ischiofemoral space	Hamstring origin
Patient position	Placed in prone position (place a rolled pillow under the pelvis)			
Probe positioning	Placed transversely over the piriformis and confirmation is done with ext/int rotation		Transversely transverse on sciatic, long view on quadratus femoris	Transverse over the origin
Target	Superior to the piriformis or piriformis muscle belly	Peri-sciatic area	Quadrangle shape of the quad femoris with the sciatic nerve above it	Pathologic tendon of hamstring origin
Needle size	25 g 1.5 inch for anesthesia and 22 g 3 inch for injection			
Probe	Low frequency curvilinear			Medium to high frequency linear
Injected agents	Corticosteroids (40 mg) 25% dextrose with 0.5% lidocaine Normal saline PRP (consider LP-PRP or PPP on peri-sciatic area) 5–20 cc around the nerve – enough to dissect tissue and halo the nerve			Corticosteroids (40 mg) PRP Tenotomy

target of the injection should be based on history, physical exam, and imaging findings, including sonopalpation.

The piriformis muscle may be a source of pain and can be easily targeted. Injections can be helpful diagnostically and potentially therapeutic. The setup for this injection is as follows: The patient is placed in the prone position – it may be helpful to place a rolled pillow under the pelvis to allow for an easier sonographic window with less probe tilting. The probe is placed transversely over the piriformis and confirmation is done with external/internal rotation. Identify the location of the sciatic nerve, in most cases deep (anterior) and medial to the piriformis. Use Doppler to confirm neurovascular structures to avoid. One enters in-plane from a lateral to medial approach, though a medial to lateral approach can also be used. At first, a 25/27 gauge needle is used for superficial anesthesia, then followed by a 22 gauge approximately 3 inch needle. There is debate on the location of the injectate in the literature. We perform the following when this is the possible pain source: first, fluid is placed in the fascia superior to the piriformis, particularly if it appears more hyperechoic and enlarged versus the opposite side; then do a hydrodissection with saline of this fascia; next, the muscle belly of the piriformis may be targeted with an injection by moving the needle slightly anterior into the muscle.

If pain is in the obturator-gemelli complex or abnormality is noted, the same technique should be used to inject it. Carefully track the sciatic nerve to avoid iatrogenic injury. A medial to lateral approach may be easier in some cases to avoid the sciatic. Hydrodissection of this area may be beneficial if no pathology is visualized as accessory bands may play a role in pain of the sciatic. The accuracy of US-guided piriformis injections has been validated in cadaver studies, with an accuracy of 95% in a 2008 study by Finnoff et al. [34] In a study of 57 patients, US-guided anesthetic-only injection into the piriformis was shown to have a significant benefit in pain reduction. Corticosteroid may not provide additional benefit over lidocaine alone [63].

Ischiofemoral Space/Peri-sciatic Hydrodissection

Pain may be isolated more closely to the ischiofemoral space requiring a diagnostic and/or therapeutic injection. Differential in this area includes sciatic nerve entrapment, ischiofemoral impingement, hamstring tendinosis, and ischial bursitis. The injection will be done in the prone position with a pillow placed under the pelvis to reduce probe angle and facilitate better needle visualization. The space is found as described prior between the ischium and the trochanter. The quadrangle shape of the quadriceps femoris is easily recognized with the sciatic nerve sitting above it. Again, dynamic maneuvers of internal/external rotation will help facilitate its vision. The probe will be placed transversely to see a transverse view of the sciatic and long view of the quadratus. The approach will be from a lateral to medial aspect. Depending on the pathology, one can position the needle in multiple positions. For a diagnostic evaluation, one can target the area in the quadratus that shows pain or changes on MRI which is usually deep and lateral to the sciatic nerve. For those having sciatic-type symptoms, a peri-sciatic hydrodissection can be done of the sciatic nerve [15]. This may help alleviate symptoms, especially if fascial bands are present along the sciatic. The sciatic will need to be targeted at different regions but usually is affected from the obturator complex down through the quadratus femoris space. In cases of prior hamstring injury, the sciatic may also be encompassed in hyperechoic fibrous scar tissue and cause symptoms mimicking hamstring pain or sciatic-type pain. Regardless of the site of sciatic pathology, the technique will remain the same. Locate the sciatic again using a transverse ultrasound scan. A lateral to medial approach will be used. After anesthesia, a 22 g 3 inch needle can be used to place copious saline around the nerve to halo the nerve and hydrodissect the region. Typical volumes are around 10–20 cc. Pure (leukocyte-poor) PRP or PPP may be used or saline with dextrose. Depending on the length of symptoms, one may need to do multiple areas.

Hamstring Origin

The hamstring origin is often a source of pain in the posterior gluteal region and may be associated with ischiogluteal bursitis. Injection can be of value in this area for diagnostic and therapeutic purposes. The patient is again placed in the prone positions with pillows to prop up the pelvis. Placing the leg off the table in slight flexion can also assist in the evaluation of the tendon insertion. The approach will be with the probe transverse over the origin from a lateral to medial approach. The sciatic will sit more anterior and lateral to the tendon. The position is similar to the ischiofemoral space injection but slightly more distal on the body. Usually a needle between 1.5 and 3 inches will suffice depending on body habitus. Use Doppler and note the sciatic nerve position. The target in these injections is usually the tendinopathic origin of the hamstring, usually the conjoint tendon of the semitendinosus and biceps femoris. Oftentimes, calcifications and enthesopathic changes are the target. Occasionally, there is an isolated ischiogluteal bursitis that is isolated and can be injected. However, more commonly tendon pathology is the source of bursal swelling. Corticosteroids are targeted toward the bursa, while orthobiologic preparations would be targeted toward the tendon.

Piriformis cortisone injections under ultrasound guided have shown an improvement in half of the subjects, as noted by Jeong et al. [47]. Using a physiotherapy protocol combined with triamcinolone injections, Fishman et al. [35] found that 279 (79%) of 353 patients with piriformis syndrome had at least 50% improvement. The use of orthobiologic in this area still has limited study to date; however, the outcome might be promising like treating tendon pathology in other areas of the body. More research is needed.

Deep gluteal pain or piriformis pain may be associated with sciatic pathology. If sciatic entrapment is considered, a high-volume injection of the nerve can be done. Burke et al. reported 50% had extended relief [15]; however diagnosis was not subsetted making it difficult to determine responders and the underlying diagnosis. High-volume dissection may also help in recalcitrant cases to hopefully decrease fascial adhesions.

In ischiofemoral impingement patients, corticosteroid injection under ultrasound guidance at the quadratus femoris muscle has shown promising outcome in 2 weeks' follow-up [6]. An injection of 8 mL of 0.25% lidocaine at the quadratus femoris in lower buttock pain patients also showed to help decrease pain with good patient satisfaction [49]. Orthobiologic studies are limited in this area. One case report showed a good outcome after five injections of prolotherapy with polydeoxyribonucleotide sodium [50].

Hamstring Origin

The effects of corticosteroid peritendinous injection at proximal hamstring tendinopathy were good in various studies. Zissen et al. stated that corticosteroid injection under effective technique is safe with intermediate- to long-term clinical improvement [93]. Because of cortisone effects on tendons, this should be done in a limited amount of times and avoided in high-grade injuries.

The use of PRP injection in this area is also common with studies showing promising outcomes. A retrospective study concluded that PRP injection helped improve clinical outcome in the majority of the patients in the study [33]. A double-blind randomized controlled trial in 19 hips showed outcomes improvement in both PRP and whole blood intratendinous injection [9]. Tenotomy with PRP injection demonstrated a good clinical outcome as well as improvement of tendon echogenicity and intratendinous calcified resolution [34]. Adipose tissue combined with high-density platelet-rich plasma (HD-PRP) has been reported in one case report which showed clinical improvement after injection [67].

Conclusion

The posterior hip is a challenging area to diagnose and treat. The anatomy is complex, and pain may be multifactorial and referred. Ultrasound can be helpful in making an accurate diagnosis and developing a treatment plan and is critical to guided injections in the region.

Thigh

Introduction

The thigh muscles are the most commonly injured in the body. Muscle trauma mainly results from sporting activities and accounts for 15–50% of sports injuries. Muscle injuries are the most common injuries in sports, with hamstring injuries accounting for 29% of all injuries in athletes. Muscle contusion is one of the most common causes of morbidity from sports-related injuries, together with sprains and strains. The region is broken down into the anterior thigh focusing on the quadriceps and the posterior hamstrings. Our discussion is limited to the proximal aspects around the hip. Sonography can provide valuable information to the clinician at the point of care. This section will focus on high-grade muscle injuries, hematoma evacuation, Morel-Lavallée injuries, and review regenerative procedures.

Sonoanatomy

The anterior thigh is made up of the quadriceps muscles. With a transducer in the transverse plane over the mid-thigh, the most superficial structure is the rectus femoris muscle which is overlying the vastus intermedius, and the two are separated by a fascial plane. Deep to the vastus intermedius is the femur. Medially adjacent to the rectus femoris and vastus intermedius lies the vastus medialis and laterally the vastus lateralis. Evaluation is best in the transverse plane with confirmation in the longitudinal plane for pathology (Fig. 8.32).

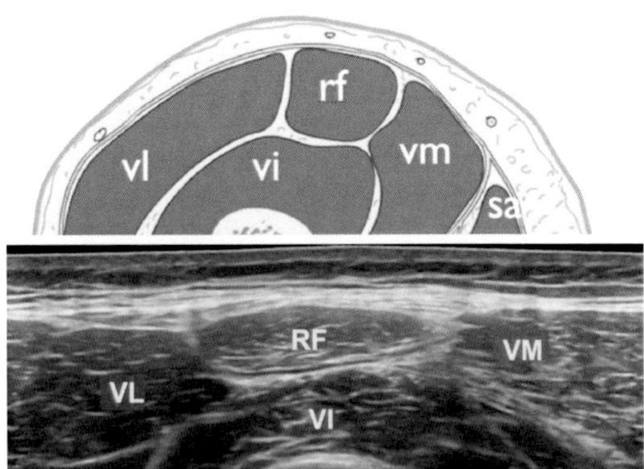

Fig. 8.32 Schematic and corresponding transverse view of quadriceps muscles at the proximal third of the thigh. Vastus lateralis (VL), rectus femoris (RF), vastus intermedius (VI), vastus medialis (VM)

Evaluation of the posterior thigh involves the assessment of the muscles of the hamstring – the semimembranosus, semitendinosus, and biceps femoris long and short heads – and the sciatic nerve. The orientation of the muscles from lateral to medial are biceps femoris, semitendinosus, then semimembranosus; these should be identified in the short axis at the mid-thigh. The short head of the biceps femoris lies deep to the long head and adjacent to the shaft of the femur. It is not commonly involved in proximal hamstring injuries. At the proximal hamstring, the semimembranosus is primarily a tadpole-like peripheral tendon and the semitendinosus is very muscular. Within the semitendinosus muscle, there is a notable hyperechoic raphe [44]. The semitendinosus and biceps long head come together to form the conjoint tendon to attach at the ischial tuberosity. The sciatic runs under the biceps/semitendinosus muscle and above the adductor magnus (Fig. 8.33).

Pathology

Muscle Injuries

Injuries to the muscles of the thigh can involve partial or complete muscle tears. These are the most commonly injured muscles in the body. There are various grading systems of muscle injuries based on both clinical and imaging criteria [18, 38]. It is best to describe the pathology on ultrasound in its entirety including length and cross-sectional area of injury, involvement of tendon pathology, proximity to sciatic nerve, amount

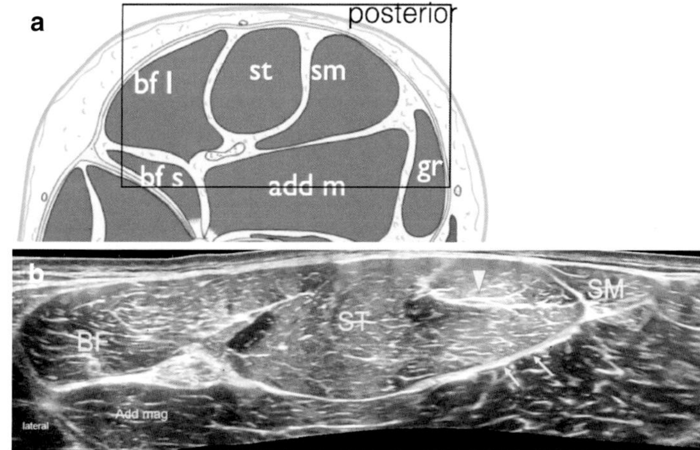

Fig. 8.33 (**a**) Cross section schematic of the posterior proximal thigh (**b**). Transverse view of the proximal third of the hamstring. Biceps femoris (BF), sciatic nerve (S), semitendinosus (ST), semimembranosus (SM). Note the peripheral semimembranosus tendon (arrow) and the raphe (arrowhead) through the semitendinosus

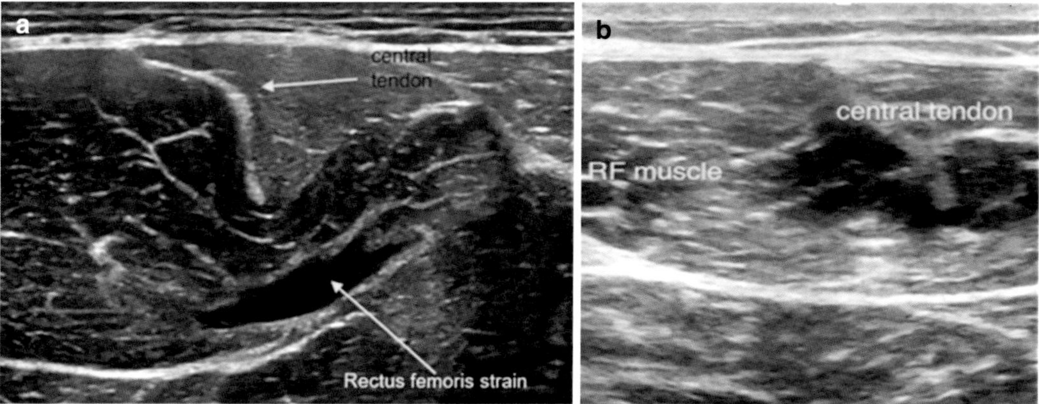

Fig. 8.34 (**a**) Transverse view of rectus femoris strain with normal central tendon and (**b**) with central tendon involvement

of hematoma, retraction of tendon, calcifications, and Doppler activity, to name a few. In general, you find the following: grade 1 injuries subtle, focal changes in echogenicity with no architectural distortion; grade 2 injuries may demonstrate some discontinuous muscle fibers with localized hypervascularity and altered echogenicity resulting from hematoma; and grade 3 injuries demonstrate complete discontinuity of muscle fibers, hematoma, and muscle fiber retraction [38].

The most commonly injured muscle in the anterior thigh is the rectus femoris. Most injuries to the rectus femoris are at the proximal myotendinous junction. Injuries in the proximal third can be to the muscle. More significant injuries may demonstrate altered echogenicity on ultrasonography with fluid around the central tendon or an ill-defined central tendon [32] (Fig. 8.34).

In the hamstring, the biceps is the most common injured muscle (Fig. 8.35b). Injuries to the conjoint tendon will have a worse and longer prognosis for recovery.

Hematoma

Hematomas can be identified as hypoechoic fluid collections (Fig. 8.36). There are two main types – those caused by direct trauma and indirect from muscle tears. Hematomas form in the intermuscular and/or intramuscular compartments. Sometimes, mixed hematomas can occur. Ultrasound is useful

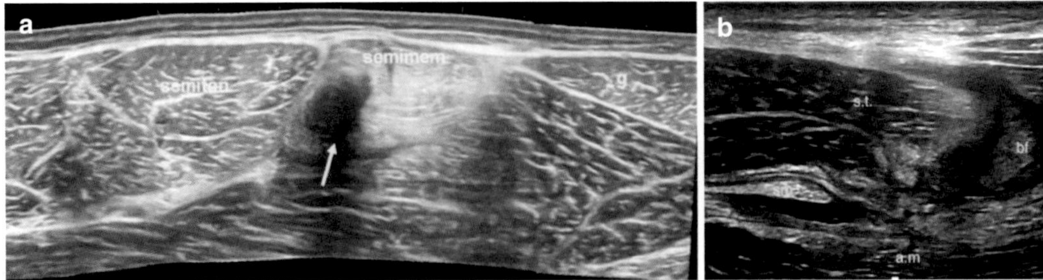

Fig. 8.35 (**a**) Transverse view through the proximal thigh showing a partial tear (yellow arrow) of semimembranosus muscle. (**b**) Note hypoechoic fluid around the semimembranosus (sm), as well as a tear of the biceps femoris (bf). At the conjoint tendon consistent with a high-grade sprain (g gracilis muscle)

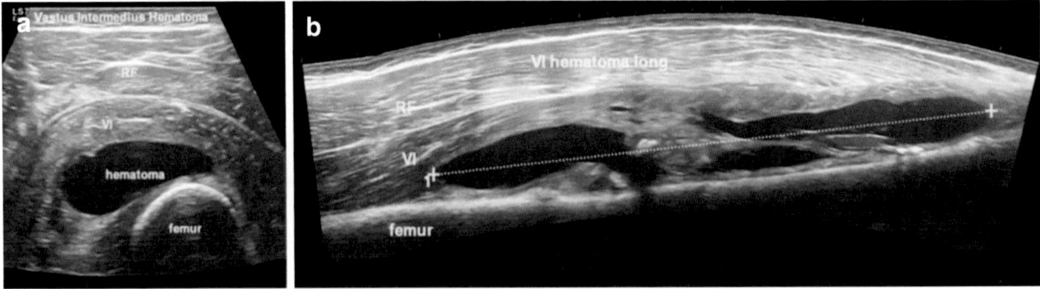

Fig. 8.36 (**a**) Short-axis view of vastus intermedius (VI) muscle hematoma seen deep to the rectus femoris (RF). (**b**) Longitudinal view of vastus intermedius hematoma

for the evaluation of muscle hematoma, to characterize the type of fluid, its extent, and its volume. A hematoma may be underappreciated on physical exams, especially in large athletes. Acutely the fluid is hypoechoic, but will turn to mixed echogenicity in time as the heme products settle and are metabolized. The best time to evaluate for a hematoma is usually about 48–72 hours from injury. The hematoma's length may play a greater role in recovery than width. Evacuation of large hematomas using ultrasound may help accelerate recovery from injury [73].

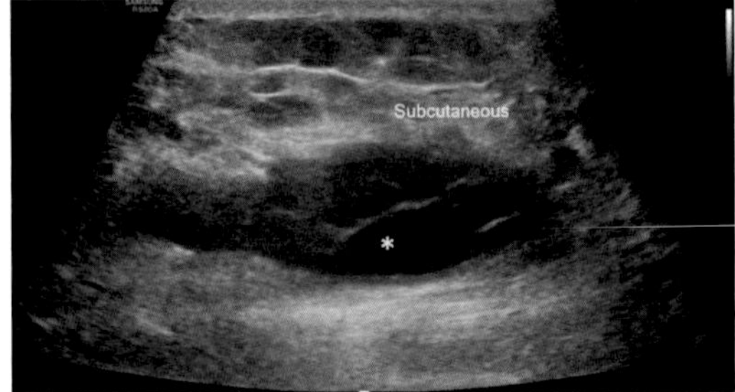

Fig. 8.37 Longitudinal view of the thigh showed a hypoechoic fluid collection (asterisk) between subcutaneous tissue and muscle consistent with a Morel-Lavallée lesion

Morel-Lavallée Lesions/Seroma

A post-traumatic condition which can be readily diagnosed with ultrasound as a fluid collection between the subcutaneous tissue and the underlying thigh fascia is known as a Morel-Lavallée lesion (Fig. 8.37). A traumatic injury to the thigh results in a collection of blood, lymph, fat, plasma, and/or debris in this potential space. These lesions tend to be well defined and smoothly marginated, especially as they age. In early stages of less than 1 month, they tend to be more heterogeneous with more irregular margins [65]. There are six subtypes of these injuries, and they have a high rate of recurrence. Ultrasound can easily identify this pathology, which often can be missed if the clinician does not have a high level of suspicion.

Procedures

Hematoma/Seroma Aspiration

The most common procedure in the thigh revolves around aspiration of hematomas or seromas. Hematomas or seromas, if large (greater than 5–10 ml), should be considered to be evacuated, particularly in the active athlete requiring an accelerated return to play. The approach to the hematoma will be dependent on the location. Most will require large needles usually in the range of 14–18 g depending on the echogenicity and age of the hematoma/seroma [43]. In chronic situations, one may need to irrigate the hematoma. Hematomas and seromas have high rates of recurrence and should be compressed post aspiration and followed closely with ultrasound, usually every few days until resolved.

There is really no data to help determine if injection of medications post aspiration is helpful. Some things to consider would be chronicity, where with chronic hematomas it may make sense to add a corticosteroid to assist in the process of emulsifying older fibrous tissue and blood products. In cases of recurrent hematomas, it may make some sense to use platelet-rich fibrin or platelet-poor plasma, but no data is available. Anecdotal evidence and basic science suggests avoiding corticosteroids in the acute traumatic hematoma. In regard to seromas, for recurrence, one of the options to consider is the use of sclerosing agents such as doxycycline; platelet-rich fibrin can alternatively be considered, but this has not been adequately studied to date [9, 83].

Muscle Injections

Muscle tears of the thigh may be treated with regenerative approaches, particularly after hematoma aspiration. Most treatments will be of grade two injuries and higher, as minor injuries as minor injuries will require no regenerative treatments. PRP may play a role in hamstring injuries, but the data to date has been mixed. Animal studies suggest that platelet-poor plasma (PPP) may be a much better choice to stimulate myocytes [19]. At this time, high-dose platelet/leukocyte-rich PRP should likely be avoided. Data seems more optimistic on leukocyte-poor/low-platelet-dose PRP or platelet-poor plasma (PPP) in these injuries. Bradley et al. showed an improvement in return times of one game in NFL players treated with ACP/leukocyte-poor/low-platelet PRP products [14]. Rossi showed that a single injection of autologous PRP with a rehabilitation program significantly shortened time to return to sports after an acute grade 2 muscle injury when compared with the control group; however, the rate of recurrence was not significant between the two groups [78]. Grassi et al. in a systematic review and meta-analysis concluded there was no evidence for an improvement in return to sport or reduction in future injury in PRP-treated cases [37]. The studies were limited by methodological matters as there were tremendous heterogeneities regarding the injectant preparation, optimum platelet concentration, presence of leukocytes, and volume of PRP which should be administered as well as the number of and timing of treatments. Sheth concluded PRP may help in grade 1–2 muscle strains but not in the hamstring [82]. Further research is needed on this, in particular potential doses, volume, and timing issues. The use of microfat/adipose may be of value in grade 3 tears requiring scaffolding, but no research is available to guide treatment decisions at this time.

Percutaneous injection treatments may also play a role in chronic injuries that have developed fibrosis, particularly around the sciatic nerve (Fig. 8.38). As previously discussed, high-volume hydrodissection around the sciatic nerve may be of value in fibrosis (Fig. 8.38b). Similar techniques can also be used around chronically fibrosed muscle tears with poor healing. Further research is needed as cases are limited to case reports [22].

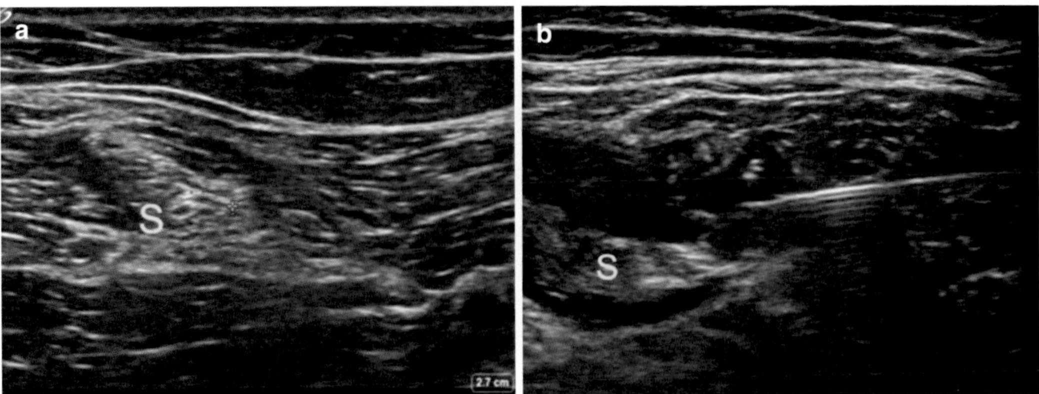

Fig. 8.38 (**a**) Cross-sectional view demonstrating fibrosis around the sciatic nerve (S); (**b**) needle placement during peri-sciatic nerve hydrodissection

Conclusion

The hip region is probably the most complex musculoskeletal area for sonography. Multiple layers in this broad region, deep structures, referred pain, and the wide scope of pathology make physical exam, diagnostic tests, and interventional procedures challenging. The chapter has provided an overview of the critical sono-anatomy of the region, focusing on each specific compartment: anterior, medial (groin), lateral, posterior, and the thigh. We have reviewed common pathologies that are amenable to intervention with a focus on key regenerative procedures. In summary, ultrasound provides a powerful tool at the point of care allowing the clinician to do a cost-effective targeted assessment of pathology/pain and when indicated targeted regenerative procedures.

References

1. Allen GM, Wilson DJ. Symphysis pubis in ultrasound guided musculoskeletal injections (Ch. 44). Philadelphia: Elsevier; 2018. p. 212–4.
2. Altman R, Alarcon G, Appelrouth D, Bloch D, Borenstein D, Brandt K, et al. The American College of Rheumatology criteria for the classification and reporting of osteoarthritis of the hip. Arthritis Rheum. 1991;34(5):505–14.
3. Anderson CN. Iliopsoas Pathology. DeLee, Drez, & Miller's orthopaedic sports medicine. 5th ed. Philadelphia: Elsevier; 2020. p. 979–89.
4. Angoules AG. Osteitis pubis in elite athletes: diagnostic and therapeutic approach. World J Orthop. 2015;6(9):672–9.
5. Aszmann OC, Dellon ES, Dellon AL. Anatomical course of the lateral femoral cutaneous nerve and its susceptibility to compression and injury. Plast Reconstr Surg. 1997;100(3):600–4.
6. Backer MW, Lee KS, Blankenbaker DG, Kijowski R, Keene JS. Correlation of ultrasound-guided corticosteroid injection of the quadratus femoris with MRI findings of ischiofemoral impingement. AJR Am J Roentgenol. 2014;203(3):589–93. https://doi.org/10.2214/AJR.13.12304.
7. Baker CL, Mahoney JR. Ultrasound-guided percutaneous tenotomy for gluteal tendinopathy. Orthop J Sports Med. 2020;8(3):2325967120907868.
8. Balius R, Susín A, Morros C, et al. Gemelli-obturator complex in the deep gluteal space: an anatomic and dynamic study. Skeletal Radiol. 2018;47(6):763–70. Leigh RE. Obturator internus spasm as a cause of pelvic and sciatic distress. J Lancet. 1952;72(6):286–287.
9. Bansal A, Bhatia N, Singh A, Singh A. Doxycycline sclerodesis as a treatment option for persistent Morel-Lavallée lesions. Injury. 2013;44(1):66–9.
10. Battaglia M, Guaraldi F, Vannini F, Rossi G, Timoncini A, Buda R, et al. Efficacy of ultrasound-guided intra-articular injections of platelet-rich plasma versus hyaluronic acid for hip osteoarthritis. Orthopedics. 2013;36(12):e1501–8.
11. Begkas D, Chatzopoulos S, Touzopoulos P, Balanika A, Pastroudis A. Ultrasound-guided platelet-rich plasma application versus corticosteroid injections for the treatment of greater trochanteric pain syndrome: a prospective controlled randomized comparative clinical study. Cureus. 2020;12(1):e6583.
12. Blankenbaker DG, De Smet AA, Keene JS. Sonography of the iliopsoas tendon and injection of the iliopsoas bursa for diagnosis and manage-

ment of the painful snapping hip. Skeletal Radiol. 2006;35(8):565–71.
13. Bordalo-Rodrigues M, Rosenberg ZS. MR imaging of the proximal rectus femoris musculotendinous unit. Magn Reson Imaging Clin N Am. 2005;13(4):717–25.
14. Bradley J, Lawyer TJ, Ruef S, Towers JD, Arner JW. Platelet-rich plasma shortens return to play in national football league players with acute hamstring injuries. Orthop J Sports Med. 2020;8(4):2325967120911731. Published online 2020 Apr 17. https://doi.org/10.1177/2325967120911731.
15. Burke CJ, Walter WR, Adler RS. Targeted ultrasound-guided perineural hydrodissection of the sciatic nerve for the treatment of piriformis syndrome. Arthroscopy. 2020;36(5):1465–7.
16. Carro LP, Hernando MF, Cerezal L, Navarro L, Saenz I, Fernandez AA, Castillo AO, Ortiz A. Deep gluteal space problems: piriformis syndrome, ischiofemoral impingement and sciatic nerve release. Muscles Ligaments Tendons J. 2016;6(3):384–96.
17. Chahla J, Kraeutler MJ, Pascual-Garrido C. pelvis, hip, and thigh injuries, in netter's sports medicine. 2nd ed. Philadelphia: Elsevier; 2018. p. 425–433.e1.
18. Chan O, DelBuono A, Best TM, Maffulli N. Acute muscle strain injuries: a proposed new classification system. Knee Surg Sports Traumatol Arthrosc. 20:2356–62.
19. Chellini F, et al. Review: influence of platelet rich and platelet poor plasma on endogenous mechanisms of skeletal muscle repair/regeneration. Int J Mol Sci. 2019 Feb;20(3):683. https://doi.org/10.3390/ijms20030683.
20. Choi H, McCartney M, Best TM. Treatment of osteitis pubis and osteomyelitis of the pubic symphysis in athletes: a systematic review. Br J Sports Med. 2011;45:57–64.
21. Choi YS, Lee SM, Song BY, Paik SH, Yoon YK. Dynamic sonography of external snapping hip syndrome. J Ultrasound Med. 2002;21(7):753–8.
22. Courseault J, Kessler E, Moran A, Labbe A. Fascial hydrodissection for chronic hamstring injury. Curr Sports Med Rep. 2019;18(11):416–20.
23. Dall'Oca C, Breda S, Elena N, Valentini R, Samaila EM, Magnan B. Mesenchymal Stem Cells injection in hip osteoarthritis: preliminary results. Acta Biomed. 2019;90(1-S):75–80.
24. Dallari D, Stagni C, Rani N, Sabbioni G, Pelotti P, Torricelli P, et al. Ultrasound-guided injection of platelet-rich plasma and hyaluronic acid, separately and in combination, for hip osteoarthritis: a randomized controlled study. Am J Sports Med. 2016;44(3):664–71.
25. Dallaudière B, Lempicki M, Pesquer L, Louedec L, et al. Efficacy of intra-tendinous injection of platelet-rich plasma in treating tendinosis: comprehensive assessment of a rat model. Eur Radiol. 2013;23(10):2830–7.
26. Daniels EW, Cole D, Jacobs B, Phillips SF. Existing evidence on ultrasound-guided injections in sports medicine. Orthop J Sports Med. 2018;6(2):2325967118756576.
27. De Luigi AJ, Blatz D, Karam C, Gustin Z, Gordon AH. Use of platelet-rich plasma for the treatment of acetabular labral tear of the hip: a pilot study. Am J Phys Med Rehabil. 2019;98(11):1010–7.
28. Deshmukh AJ, Thakur RR, Goyal A, Klein DA, Ranawat AS, Rodriguez JA. Accuracy of diagnostic injection in differentiating source of atypical hip pain. J Arthroplasty. 2010;25(6 Suppl):129–33.
29. Deslandes M, Guillin R, Cardinal E, Hobden R, Bureau NJ. The snapping iliopsoas tendon: new mechanisms using dynamic sonography. AJR Am J Roentgenol. 2008;190(3):576–81.
30. Di Sante L, Villani C, Santilli V, Valeo M, Bologna E, Imparato L, et al. Intra-articular hyaluronic acid vs platelet-rich plasma in the treatment of hip osteoarthritis. Med Ultrason. 2016;18(4):463–8.
31. Doria C, Mosele GR, Caggiari G, Puddu L, Ciurlia E. Treatment of early hip osteoarthritis: ultrasound-guided platelet rich plasma versus hyaluronic acid injections in a randomized clinical trial. Joints. 2017;5(3):152–5.
32. Douis H, Gillett M, James SLJ. Imaging in the Diagnosis, Prognostication, and Management of Lower Limb Muscle Injury. Semin Musculoskelet Radiol. 2011;15(1):27–41.
33. Fader RR, Mitchell JJ, Traub S, Nichols R, Roper M, Dan OM, EC MC. Platelet-rich plasma treatment improves outcomes for chronic proximal hamstring injuries in an athletic population. Muscles Ligaments Tendons J. 2015;4(4):461–6.
34. Finnoff J, Fowler SP, Lai JK, Santrach PJ, Willis EA, Sayeed YA, Smith J. Treatment of chronic tendinopathy with ultrasound-guided needle tenotomy and platelet-rich plasma injection. PM R. 2011;3:900–11.
35. Fishman LM, Dombi GW, Michaelsen C, Ringel S, Rozbruch J, Rosner B, Weber C. Piriformis syndrome: diagnosis, treatment, and outcome--a 10-year study. Arch Phys Med Rehabil. 2002;83(3):295–301. https://doi.org/10.1053/apmr.2002.30622.
36. Fitzpatrick J, Bulsara MK, O'Donnell J, McCrory PR, Zheng MH. The effectiveness of platelet-rich plasma injections in gluteal tendinopathy: a randomized, double-blind controlled trial comparing a single platelet-rich plasma injection with a single corticosteroid injection. Am J Sports Med. 2018;46(4):933–9. https://doi.org/10.1177/0363546517745525. Epub 2018 Jan 2
37. Grassi A, Napoli F, Romandini I, Samuelsson K, Zaffagnini S, Candrian C, Filardo G. Is platelet-rich plasma (PRP) effective in the treatment of acute muscle injuries? a systematic review and meta-analysis. Sports Med. 2018;48(4):971–89.
38. Grassi A, Quaglia A, Cantana GL, Zaffagnini S. An update on the grading of muscle injuries: a narra-

tive review from clinical to comprehensive systems. Joints. 2016;4(1):39–46.
39. Grossman MG, Ducey SA, Nadler SS, Levy AS. Meralgia paresthetica: diagnosis and treatment. J Am Acad Orthop Surg. 2001;9(5):336–44.
40. Guillin R, Cardinal E, Bureau NJ. Sonographic anatomy and dynamic study of the normal iliopsoas musculotendinous junction. Eur Radiol. 2009;19(4):995–1001.
41. Henderson RG, Colberg RE. Pure bone marrow aspirate injection for chronic greater trochanteric pain syndrome: a case report. Pain Manag. 2018;8(4):271.
42. Hoffman DJ, Smith J. Sonoanatomy and pathology of the posterior band of the gluteus medius tendon. J Ultrasound Med. 2017;36:389–99.
43. Isaacson AJ, Stavas JM. Image-guided drainage and sclerodesis of a Morel-Lavallee lesion. J Vasc Interv Radiol. 2013;24(4):605–6.
44. Hip JJ, Anatomy T. Fundamentals of musculoskeletal ultrasound. 2nd. ed. Philadelphia: Elsevier; 2013. p. 162–213.
45. Jacobson JA, Yablon CM, Troy Henning P, et al. Greater trochanteric pain syndrome. Percutaneous tendon fenestration versus platelet-rich plasma injection for treatment of gluteal tendinosis. J Ultrasound Med. 2016;35:2413–20.
46. Javidan P. The hip. In: Silman A, Smolen Jm Weixman M, Hochlberg M, Gravallese E, editors. Rheumatology. 7th ed. Philadelphia: Elsevier; 2019. p. 681–9.
47. Jeong HK, Lee GY, Lee EG, Joe EG, Lee JW, Kang HS. Long-term assessment of clinical outcomes of ultrasound-guided steroid injections in patients with piriformis syndrome. Ultrasonography. 2015;34(3):206–10. https://doi.org/10.14366/usg.14039. Epub 2015 Jan 23
48. Khodaee M, Jones D, Spittler J. Obturator internus and obturator externus strain in a high school quarterback. Asian J Sports Med. 2015;6(3):e23481.
49. Kim D, Yoon D, Yoon K. Ultrasound-guided quadratus femoris muscle injection in patients with lower buttock pain: novel ultrasound-guided approach and clinical effectiveness. Pain Physician. 2016;19:E863–70.
50. Kim W, Shin H, Koo G, Park H, Ha Y, Hee Y. Ultrasound-guided prolotherapy with polydeoxyribonucleotide sodium in ischiofemoral impingement syndrome. Pain Pract. 2014;14(7):649–55. https://doi.org/10.1111/papr.12215.
51. Kizaki K, Uchida S, Shanmugaraj A, Aquino CC, Duong A, Simunovic N, Martin HA, Ayeni OR. Deep gluteal syndrome is defined as a non-discogenic sciatic nerve disorder with entrapment in the deep gluteal space: a systematic review. Knee Surg Sports Traumatol Arthrosc. https://doi.org/10.1007/s00167-020-05966-x.
52. Kompel AJ, Roemer FW, Murakami AM, Diaz LE, Crema MD, Guermazi A. Intra-articular corticosteroid Injections in the hip and knee: perhaps not as safe as we thought? Radiology. 2019;293(3):656–63.
53. Kong A, Van der Vliet A, Zadow S. MRI and US of gluteal tendinopathy in greater trochanteric pain syndrome. Eur Radiol. 2007;17(7):1772–83. https://doi.org/10.1007/s00330-006-0485-x.
54. Labrosse JM, Cardinal E, Leduc BE, Duranceau J, Rémillard J, Bureau NJ, Belblidia A, Brassard P. Effectiveness of ultrasound-guided corticosteroid injection for the treatment of gluteus medius tendinopathy. AJR Am J Roentgenol. 2010;194(1):202–6. https://doi.org/10.2214/AJR.08.1215.
55. Lee JJ, Harrison JR, Boachie-Adjei K, Vargas E, Moley PJ. Platelet-rich plasma injections with needle tenotomy for gluteus medius tendinopathy: a registry study with prospective follow-up. Orthop J Sports Med. 2016;4(11):2325967116671692. eCollection 2016 Nov.
56. Letizia Mauro G, Scaturro D, Sanfilippo A, Benedetti MG. Intra-articular hyaluronic acid injections for hip osteoarthritis. J Biol Regul Homeost Agents. 2018;32(5):1303–9.
57. Lewis CL, Sahrmann SA. Acetabular labral tears. Phys Ther. 2006;86(1):110–21.
58. Major NM, et al. Hips and pelvis (Ch. 14). In: Musculoskeletal MRI. 3rd ed. Philadelphia: Elsevier; 2020. p. 47–375.
59. Mardones R, Jofre CM, Tobar L, Minguell JJ. Mesenchymal stem cell therapy in the treatment of hip osteoarthritis. J Hip Preserv Surg. 2017;4(2):159–63.
60. Martinoli C, Garello I, Marchetti A, Palmieri F, Altafini L, Valle M, et al. Hip ultrasound. Eur J Radiol. 2012;81(12):3824–31.
61. Martinoli C. Hip ultrasound. Eur J Radiol. 2012;81(12):3824–31.
62. Meyers WC, et al. Management of severe lower abdominal or inguinal pain in high-performance athletes. Am J Sports Med. 2000.; SAGE Publications Inc. STM;28(1):2–8.
63. Misirlioglu TO, Akgun K, Palamar D, Erden MG, Erbilir T. Piriformis syndrome: comparison of the effectiveness of local anesthetic and corticosteroid injections: a double-blinded, randomized controlled study. Pain Physician. 2015;18(2):163–71.
64. Morton S, Chan O, Price J, Pritchard M, Crisp T, Perry JD, Morrissey D. High volume image-guided injections and structured rehabilitation improve greater trochanter pain syndrome in the short and medium term: a combined retrospective and prospective case series. Muscles Ligaments Tendons J. 2015;5(2):73–87.
65. Neal C, Jacobson JA, Brandon C, Lalume-Brigido M, Morag Y, Gandikota G. Sonography of Morel-Lavallée Lesions. J Ultrasound Med. 2008;27(7):1077–81.
66. Nunziata A, Blumenfeld I. Snapping hip; note on a variety. Prensa Med Argent. 1951;38(32):1997–2001.
67. Onishi K, Alderman D, Alexander R. Autologous adipose-derived stromal/stem cells with platelet rich plasma as biocellular regenerative therapy in the treatment of chronic proximal hamstring tendon tear.

2013 Poster Presentation, Association of Academic Physiatry.
68. Park J, Lee Y, Lee Y, Shin S, Kang Y, Koo K. Deep gluteal syndrome as a cause of posterior hip pain and sciatica-like pain. Bone Joint J. 2020;102-B(5):556–67.
69. Patti JW, Ouellette H, Bredella MA, Torriani M. Impingement of lesser trochanter on ischium as a potential cause for hip pain. Skeletal Radiol. 2008;37(10):939–41.
70. Pesquer L, Reboul G, Silvestre A, Poussange N, Meyer P, Dallaudiere B. Imaging of adductor-related groin pain. Diagn Interv Imaging. 2015;96(9):861–9.
71. Pfirrmann CW, Chung CB, Theumann NH, Trudell DJ, Resnick D. Greater trochanter of the hip: attachment of the abductor mechanism and a complex of three bursae—MR imaging and MR bursography in cadavers and MR imaging in asymptomatic volunteers. Radiology. 2001;221(2):469–77. 28.
72. Prather H, Hunt D, Zierenberg A. Soft tissue pathology: bursal, tendon, and muscle diseases, in surgery of the hip. 2nd ed. Philadelphia: Elsevier; 2020. p. 450–67.
73. Quiñones PK, Hattori S, Yamada S, Kto Y, Ohuchi H. Ultrasonography-guided muscle hematoma evacuation. Arthrosc Tech. 2019;8(7):e721–5.
74. Rettig A, Meyers S, Bhadra A. Platelet-rich plasma in addition to rehabilitation for acute hamstring injuries in NFL players: clinical effects and time to return to play. OJS. 2013;1:1–5.
75. Robben SG, Lequin MH, Diepstraten AF, den Hollander JC, Entius CA, Meradji M. Anterior joint capsule of the normal hip and in children with transient synovitis: US study with anatomic and histologic correlation. Radiology. 1999;210(2):499–507.
76. Robertson BA, et al. The anatomy of the pubic region revisited. Sports Med. 2009;39(3):225–34.
77. Robinson P, Barron DA, Parson W, Grainger AJ, Schilders EMG, O'Connor PJ. Adductor-related groin pain in athletes: correlation of MR imaging with clinical findings. Skeletal Radiol. 2004;33(8):451–7.
78. Rossi LA, Romoli ARM, Altieri BAB, Flor JAB, Scordo WE, Elizondo CM. Does Platelet-rich plasma decrease time to return to sports in acute muscle tear? A randomized controlled trial. Knee Surg Sports Traumatol Arthrosc. 2017;25:3319–25.
79. Schilders E, Bismil Q, Robinson P, O'Connor PJ, Gibbon WW, Talbot JC. Adductor-related groin pain in recreational athletes: role of the adductor enthesis, magnetic resonance imaging, and entheseal pubic cleft injections. J Bone Joint Surg Am. 2009;91:2455–60.
80. Scholten PM, Massimi S, Dahmen N, Diamond J, Wyss J. Successful treatment of athletic pubalgia in a lacrosse player with ultrasound-guided needle tenotomy and platelet-rich plasma injection: a case report. PM R. 2015;7:79–83.
81. Segal NA, Felson DT, Torner JC, Zhy Y, Curtis JR, Niu J, Nevitt MC. Greater trochanteric pain syndrome: epidemiology and associated factors. Arch Phys Med Rehabil. 2007;88(8):988–92.
82. Sheth U, Dwyer T, Smith I, Wasserstein D, Theodoropoulos J, Takhar S, Chahal J. Does platelet-rich plasma lead to earlier return to sport when compared with conservative treatment in acute muscle injuries? a systematic review and meta-analysis. Arthroscopy. 2018;34(1):281–288.e1.
83. Singh R, Rymer B, Youssef B, Lim J. The Morel-Lavallée lesion and its management: A review of the literature. J Orthop. 2018;15:917.
84. Steer KJD, Bostick GP, Woodhouse LJ, Nguyen TT, Schankath A, Lambert RGW, et al. Can effusion-synovitis measured on ultrasound or MRI predict response to intra-articular steroid injection in hip osteoarthritis? Skeletal Radiol. 2019;48(2):227–37.
85. Stone TJ, Long N, Petchprapa CN, Adler RS. Sonoarthrography of the hip labrum: ultrasound evaluation of the anterosuperior acetabular labrum following joint distension with magnetic resonance arthrographic correlation. J Orth Rhe Sp Med. 2016;1(2):108.
86. Tagliafico A, Serafini G, Lacelli F, Perrone N, Valsania V, Martinoli C. Ultrasound-guided treatment of meralgia paresthetica (lateral femoral cutaneous neuropathy): technical description and results of treatment in 20 consecutive patients. J Ultrasound Med. 2011;30(10):1341–6.
87. Topol GA, Reeves KD, Hassanein KM. Efficacy of dextrose prolotherapy in elite male kicking-sport athletes with chronic groin pain. Arch Phys Med Rehabil. 2005;86:697–702.
88. Tremolada C, Colombo V, Ventura C. Adipose tissue and mesenchymal stem cells: state of the art and lipogems(R) technology development. Curr Stem Cell Rep. 2016;2:304–12.
89. Vora A, Borg-Stein J, Nguyen RT. Regenerative injection therapy for osteoarthritis: fundamental concepts and evidence-based review. PM R. 2012;4(5 Suppl):S104–9.
90. Walker-Santiago R, Wojnowski NM, Lall AC, Maldonado DR, Rabe SM, Domb BG. Platelet-rich plasma versus surgery for the management of recalcitrant greater trochanteric pain syndrome: a systematic review. Arthroscopy. 2020;36(3):875–88. https://doi.org/10.1016/j.arthro.2019.09.044. Epub 2019 Dec 25
91. Westacott DJ, Minns JL, Foguet P. The diagnostic accuracy of magnetic resonance imaging and ultrasonography in gluteal tendon tears--a systematic review. Hip Int. 2011;21(6):637–45. https://doi.org/10.5301/HIP.2011.8759.
92. Wu Y-Y, Guo X-Y, Chen K, He F-D, Quan J-R. The feasibility and reliability of an ultrasound examination to diagnose piriformis syndrome. World Neurosurg. 2019. https://doi.org/10.1016/j.wneu.2019.11.098.
93. Zissen M, Wallace G, Stevens K, Fredericson M, Beaulieu C. High hamstring tendinopathy: MRI and ultrasound imaging and therapeutic efficacy of percutaneous corticosteroid injection. AJR Am J Roentgenol. 2010;195:993–8.

Ultrasound Imaging of the Knee Joint

9

Daniel Chiung-Jui Su and Ke-Vin Chang

Introduction

Knee pain is one of the most common complaints that patients seek help for. When checking for knee problems, we have to see the whole lower limb as a unit and look for if there are other defects of biotensegrity existing in other joints, such as hips and ankles. Malalignment of the lower limb will cause serial problems and cannot be treated completely if the malalignment has not been identified and corrected.

Once we address the biotensegrity of the lower limb, we can specify our target into the knee joint, where we can divide the knee into the anterior region, medial region, posterior region, posterior medial corner, posterior lateral corner, and ligament-capsule-menisci complex.

Anterior Region

In the anterior region, the suprapatellar recess is used as the target for intra-articular injection of platelet rich plasma (PRP) or high concentration glucose. Effusion should be aspirated first before the injection to ensure that the concentration of the injectate is sufficient (Figs. 9.1 and 9.2).

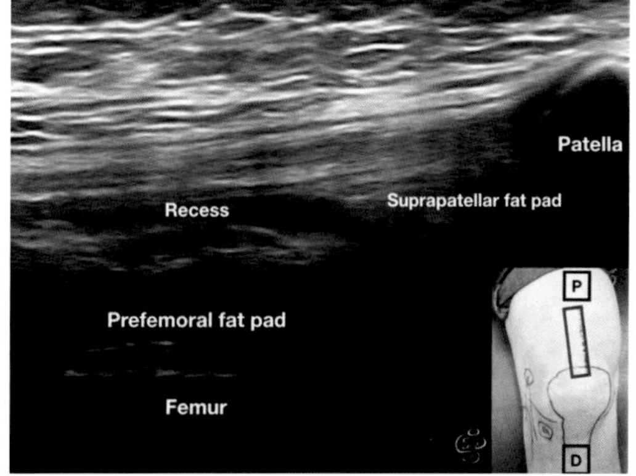

Fig. 9.1 By asking the patient to forcefully extend the knee, we can assess the effusion amount in the suprapatellar recess

The extension mechanism of the knee is maintained through the quadriceps tendon, patellar bone, patellar tendon, patellar retinacula, Hoffa's fat pad, and the prepatellar tissue [1]. Tendinopathy in this region, or increased blood flow under the power Doppler imaging, may imply failure of the extension mechanism. Therefore, we should always check for the integrity of the lower limb globally before we look into local injuries.

The anterior cruciate ligament (ACL) is the major stabilizer during anterior drawing of the tibia at all flexion angles and during internal rotation of the tibia at flexion angles less than 35

D. C.-J. Su
Department of Physical Medicine and Rehabilitation, Chi-Mei Hospital, Tainan, Taiwan

K.-V. Chang (✉)
Department of Physical Medicine and Rehabilitation, National Taiwan University Hospital, Bei-Hu Branch, Taipei, Taiwan

Y. El Miedany (ed.), *Musculoskeletal Ultrasound-Guided Regenerative Medicine*,
https://doi.org/10.1007/978-3-030-98256-0_9

degrees. Therefore, if the patient is presented with a positive anterior drawer test or Lachman test, we should further check the ACL under ultrasound or through magnetic resonance imaging. ACL insertion can be seen under the ultrasound with the maximal flexion of the knee.

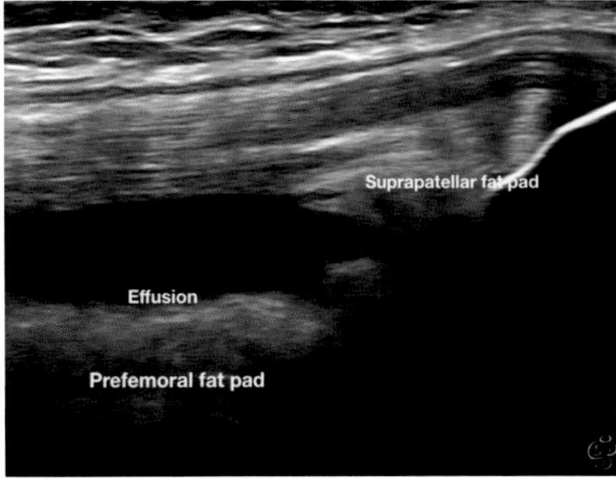

Fig. 9.2 Effusion may appear in the suprapatellar recess. If so, the effusion should be aspirated first before the injection to ensure that the concentration of the injectate (PRP or high concentration glucose) is sufficient

Three bony landmarks, including the anterior notch over the tibia plateau, intermeniscal ligament, and intercondylar eminence, can be used to identify the position of the ACL (Fig. 9.3). Insertion of the ACL is inside the anterior notch at the tibia plateau, and the fiber of the ACL should be in between the intermeniscal ligament and the intercondylar eminence (Fig. 9.4). By performing an anterior drawer test, we can assess the ACL more easily (Fig. 9.5). The anteromedial and posterolateral bundles can be differentiated by pivoting the probe (Fig. 9.6). The posterolateral bundle is more hyperechoic compared to the anteromedial bundle due to its course [2] (Fig. 9.7).

The coronary ligaments of the knee, also known as the meniscotibial ligaments, help to

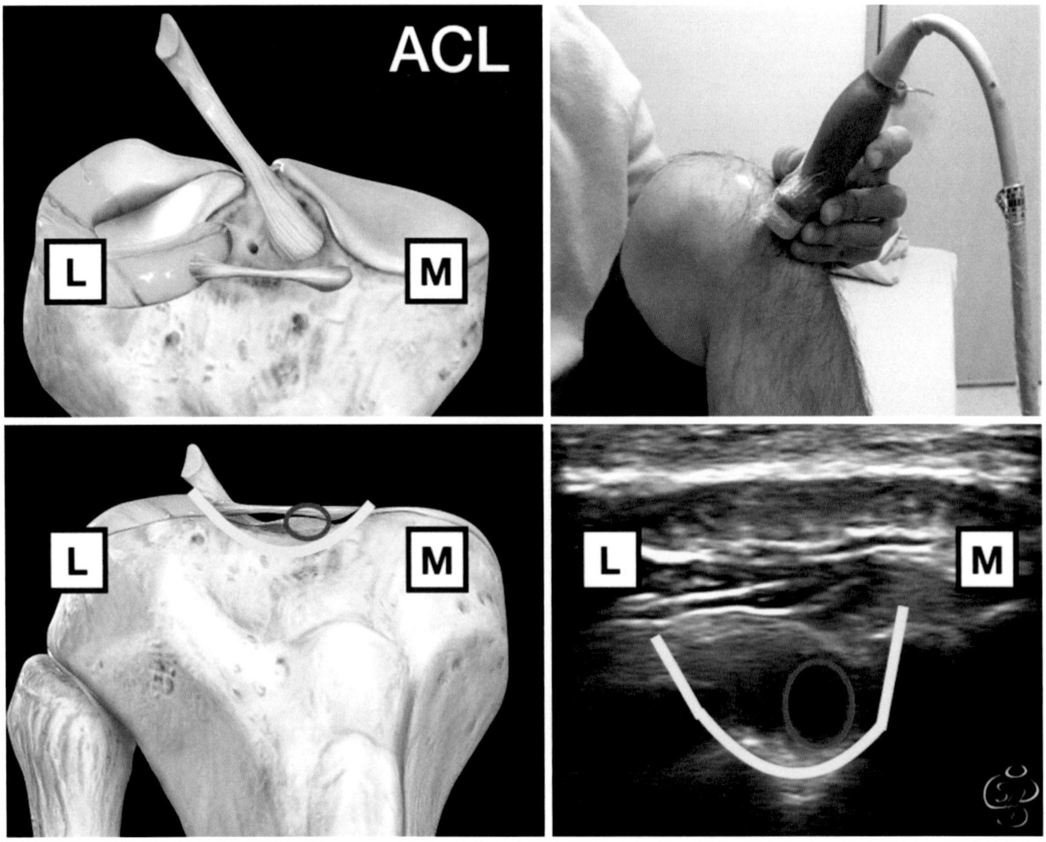

Fig. 9.3 Probe position of the ACL insertion in a transverse view. ACL is inserted at the medial corner of the anterior notch at the tibia plateau. The anterior notch at the tibia plateau is the first marker to identify the ACL position

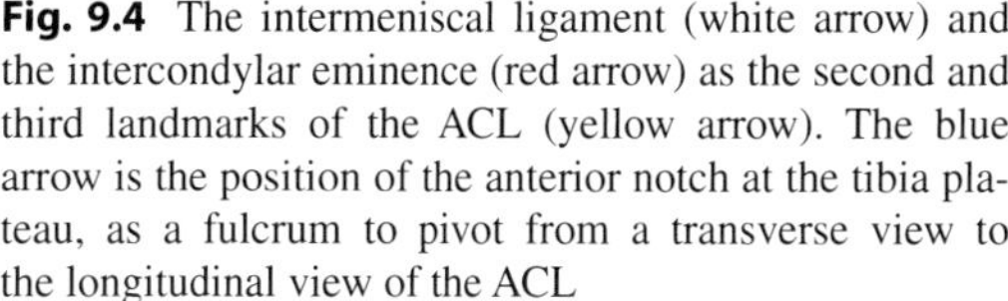

Fig. 9.4 The intermeniscal ligament (white arrow) and the intercondylar eminence (red arrow) as the second and third landmarks of the ACL (yellow arrow). The blue arrow is the position of the anterior notch at the tibia plateau, as a fulcrum to pivot from a transverse view to the longitudinal view of the ACL

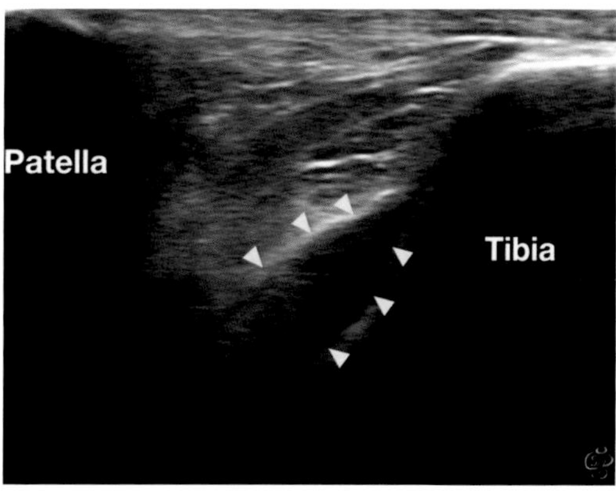

Fig. 9.5 Dynamic testing by performing an anterior drawer test can make the morphologic change of the ACL more easily seen. A swollen ACL is seen (yellow arrow)

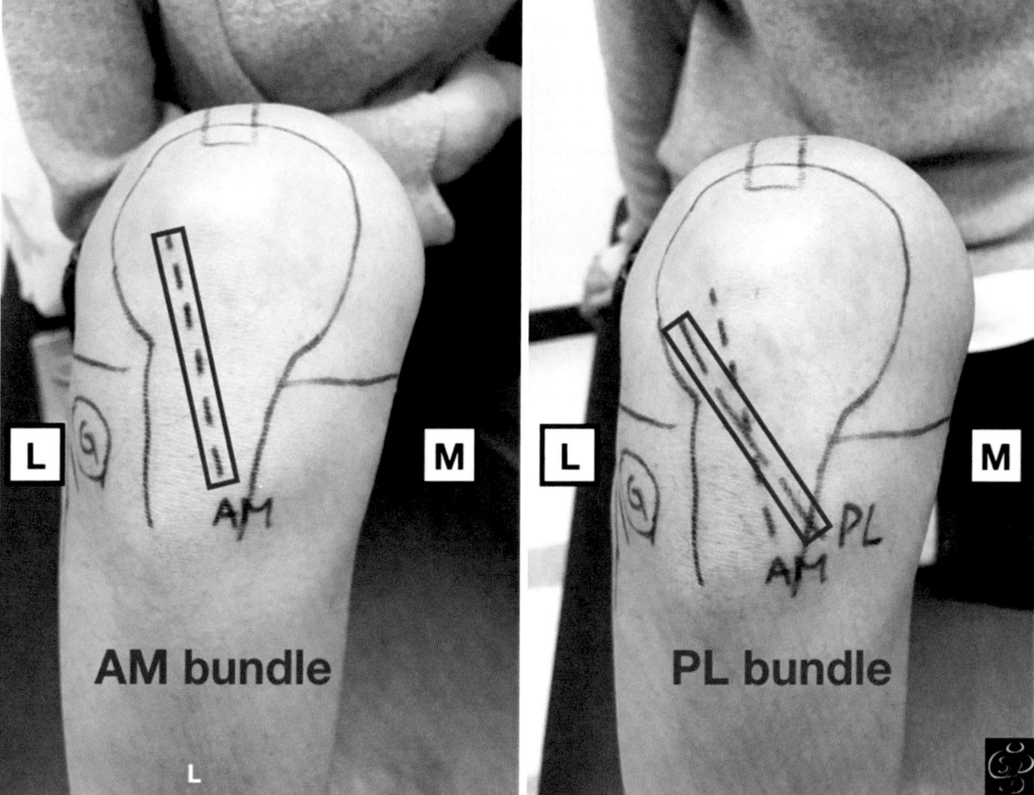

Fig. 9.6 Proper probe position to scan the anteromedial (AM) and posterolateral (PL) bundle of the ACL

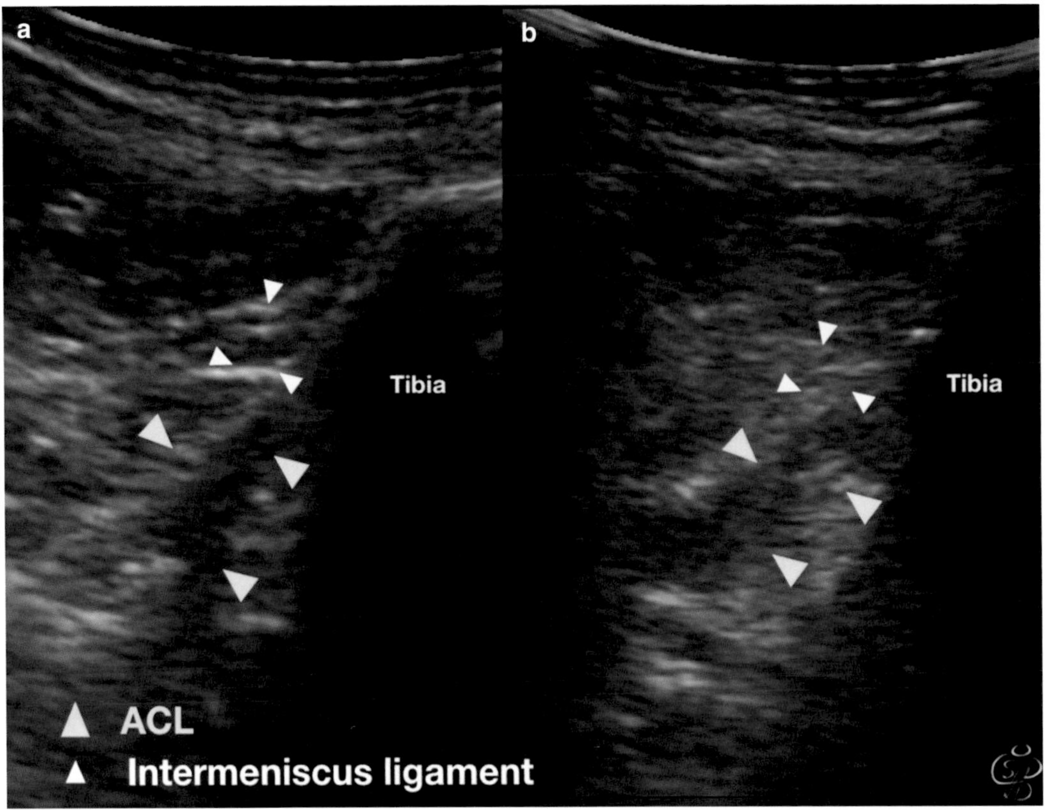

Fig. 9.7 The posterolateral bundle is more hyperechoic than the anteromedial bundle due to its course that is more parallel to the probe. (**a**) Anteromedial bundle. (**b**) Posterolateral bundle

stabilize the meniscus on the tibia plateau, by connecting the inferior edge of the menisci to the periphery of the tibial plateau. These ligaments are easily sprained or torn and can cause symptomatic discomfort. Ultrasound-guided regenerative injection in this ligament can help prevent hitting the genicular artery/vein accidently.

The anterolateral ligament (ALL) functions as a stabilizer for internal rotation of the tibia when the knee is flexed to more than 35 degrees. Proximally, ALL originates near the origin of the lateral collateral ligament (LCL), and distally, it attaches on the area between Gerdy's tubercle and the fibular head (Fig. 9.8). By flexing the knee to more than 35 degrees and internally rotating the tibia, lesions over the ALL (Fig. 9.9) will be more prominent [3–5].

By putting the probe between the Gerdy's tubercle and the fibular head, we can have a transverse view of the ALL. Injection through the short axis can cover all the structures including the Gerdy's tubercle, fibular head, and ALL if injured.

Medial Region

The medial side of the knee is a common area where painful symptoms exist. Several structures including the medial collateral ligament, medial coronary ligament, medial meniscus, medial plica, posterior oblique ligament, and pes anserinus bursa can all lead to tenderness. The muscle at the medial knee including semimembranosus, semitendinosus, sartorius, gracilis, and adductor muscles should be checked for potential tendinopathy.

With the probe turns to the coronal plane, we can obtain the longitudinal view of the medial

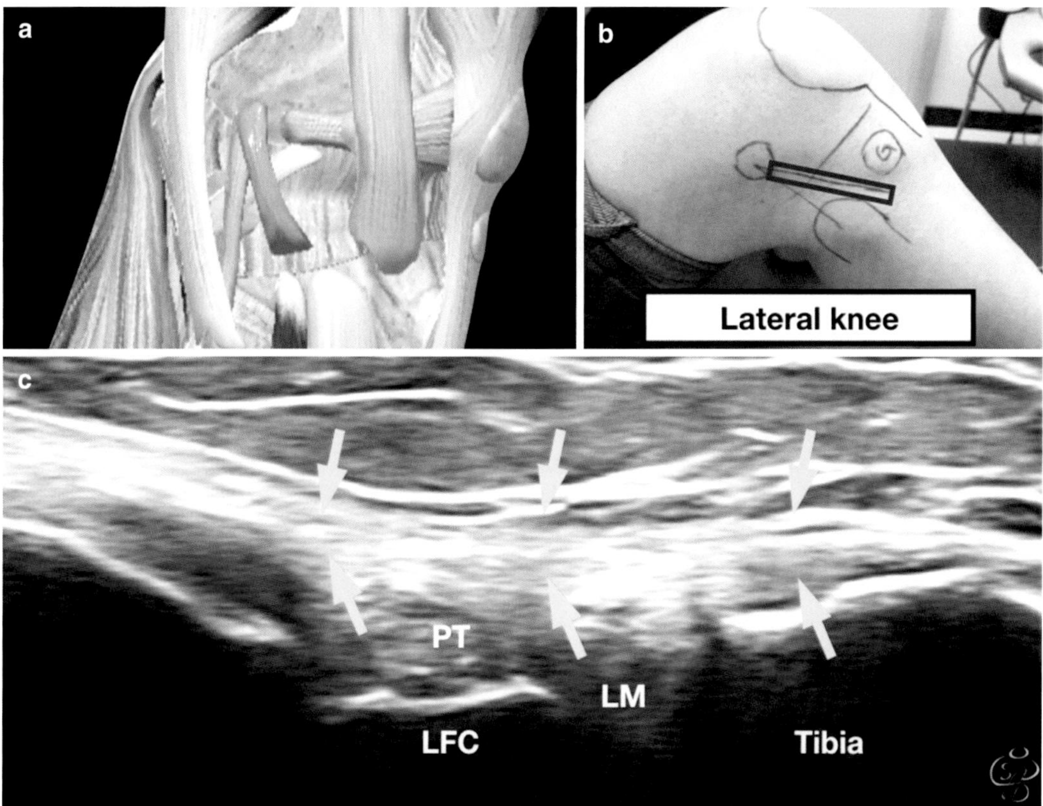

Fig. 9.8 Anterolateral ligament (ALL). (**a**) Anatomy of the ALL – the ALL has the common origin as the LCL and inserts in between the fibular head and Gerdy's tubercle. (**b**) Probe position of the ALL. (**c**) Sonogram of the longitudinal view of the ALL (yellow arrow). Popliteus tendon (PT), lateral femoral condyle (LFC), lateral meniscus (LM)

collateral ligament. The superficial and deep layers of the MCL can be identified. Swelling, partial tear, or even complete tear of the MCL can be seen with tenderness when compressed (Fig. 9.10). Coexisting injury of the MCL with ACL or PCL is common. We can use the Swain test to detect MCL complex injury. When the knee is flexed to 90 degrees, rotate the tibia externally to tighten the MCL and to test the tensegrity of the ligament complex. Pain along the medial side of the knee indicates injury to the MCL complex [6].

The pes anserinus is a conjoined tendon consisting of the sartorius, gracilis, and semitendinosus tendon. It is a highly tensioned area with infrapatellar branch of the saphenous nerve lying on top of it and inferomedial branch of the genicular nerve underneath it (Fig. 9.11). These nerves make it a sensitive area and susceptible to chronic pain when overuse or chronic friction due to malalignment and/or laxity [7]. Regenerative injection in this region can strengthen the area if there is tendinopathy, whereas biotensegrity of the lower extremity from the foot up to the hip has to be treated to truly eliminate the problem.

Posteromedial Corner

From the posterior border of the superficial MCL to the medial border of the PCL is the region called the posteromedial corner (PMC). In this area, the important structures include the posterior oblique ligament, three arms of

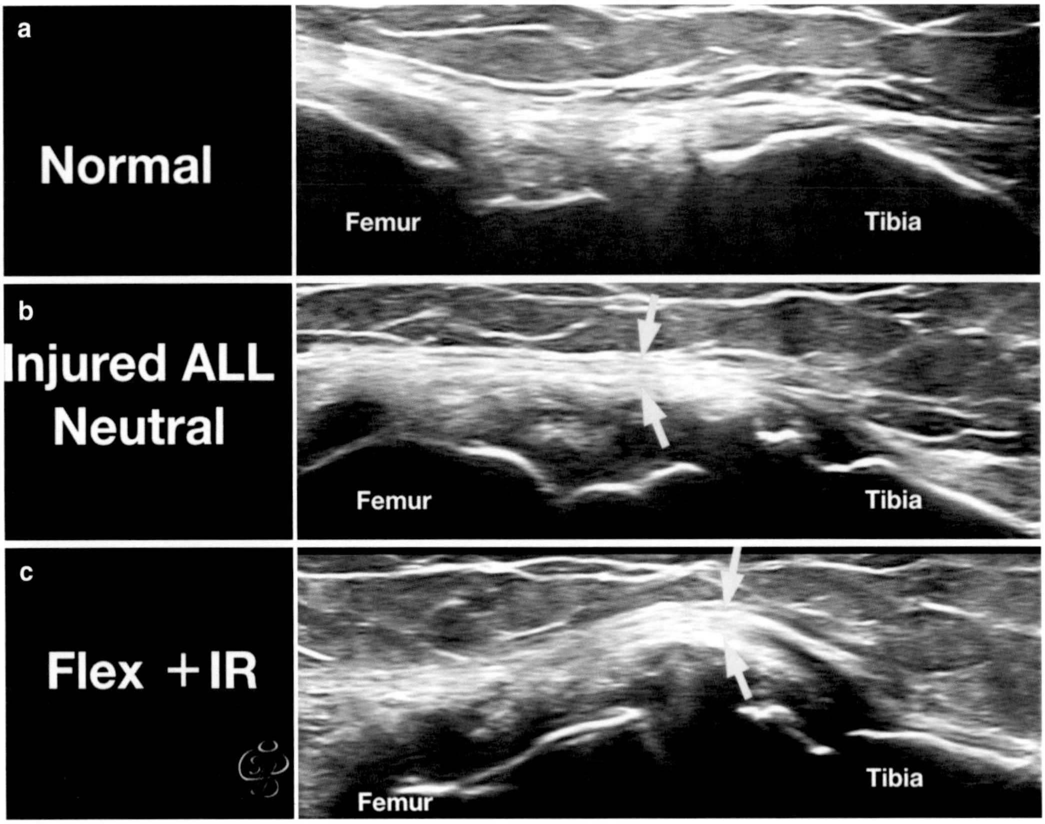

Fig. 9.9 Anterolateral ligament (ALL) helps to prevent the tibia from excessive internal rotation when the knee flex is more than 35 degrees. (**a**) Normal morphology of the ALL. (**b**) Injured ALL in knee neutral position. (**c**) By flexing the knee to more than 35 degrees and internally rotating the tibia, lesions over the ALL will be more prominent with an extruded lateral meniscus

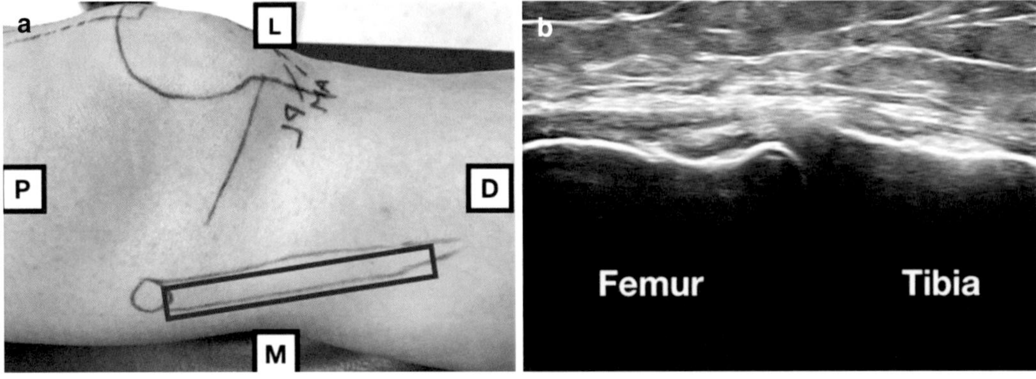

Fig. 9.10 Medial collateral ligament (MCL). (**a**) Probe position for scanning the MCL (**b**) Normal appearance of the MCL, consisting of superficial and deep layers. (**c**) Swelling and partial tears of both the superficial and deep layer of MCL

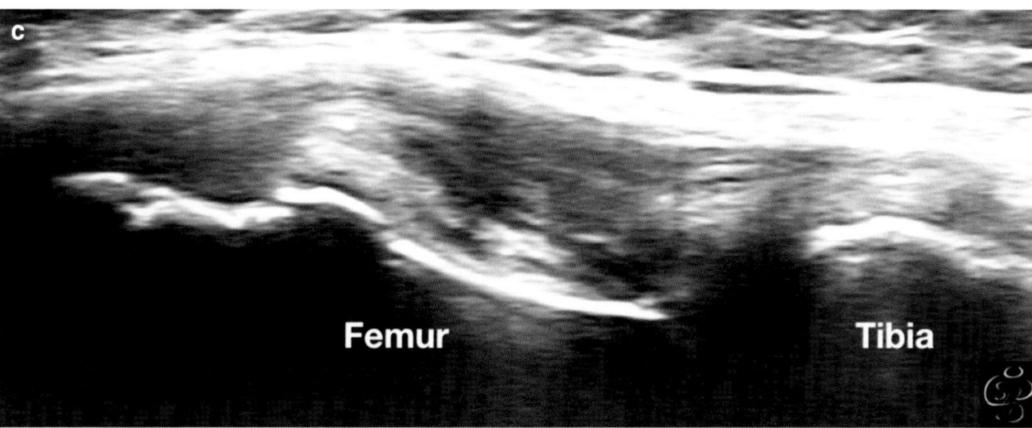

Fig. 9.10 (continued)

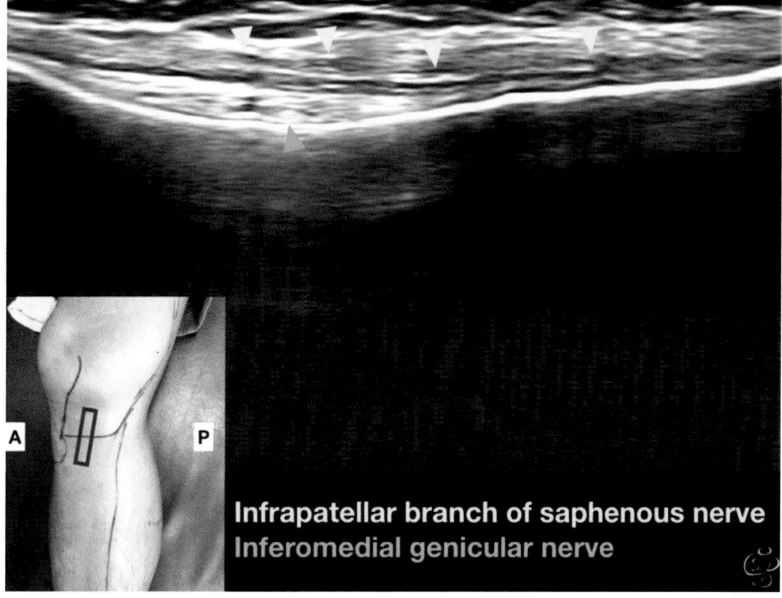

Fig. 9.11 Pes anserinus is in between the infrapatellar branch of saphenous nerve (yellow arrow) and inferomedial genicular nerve (green arrow)

the semimembranosus tendon, oblique popliteal ligament, and posterior horn of the medial meniscus [8].

The PMC is the primary stabilizer of the knee in extension during weight-bearing. It provides one-third of the restraint to valgus stress when the knee is in extension. Injury to this region will cause anteromedial rotatory instability (AMRI), which is defined as anterior translation and external rotation of the tibia relative to the femur. This area is likely to be injured together with the ACL and is therefore an important region for regenerative medicine [9].

When we move the probe posteriorly, the posterior oblique ligament (POL) can be seen (Fig. 9.12). Unlike the MCL, it only has one single layer. Its main function is to help stabilize the posterior tibial translation in knee extension and plays a crucial role in patients with posterior cruciate ligament laxity [8, 10, 11].

The semimembranosus muscle inserts on the posterior side of the tibia. It has several attach-

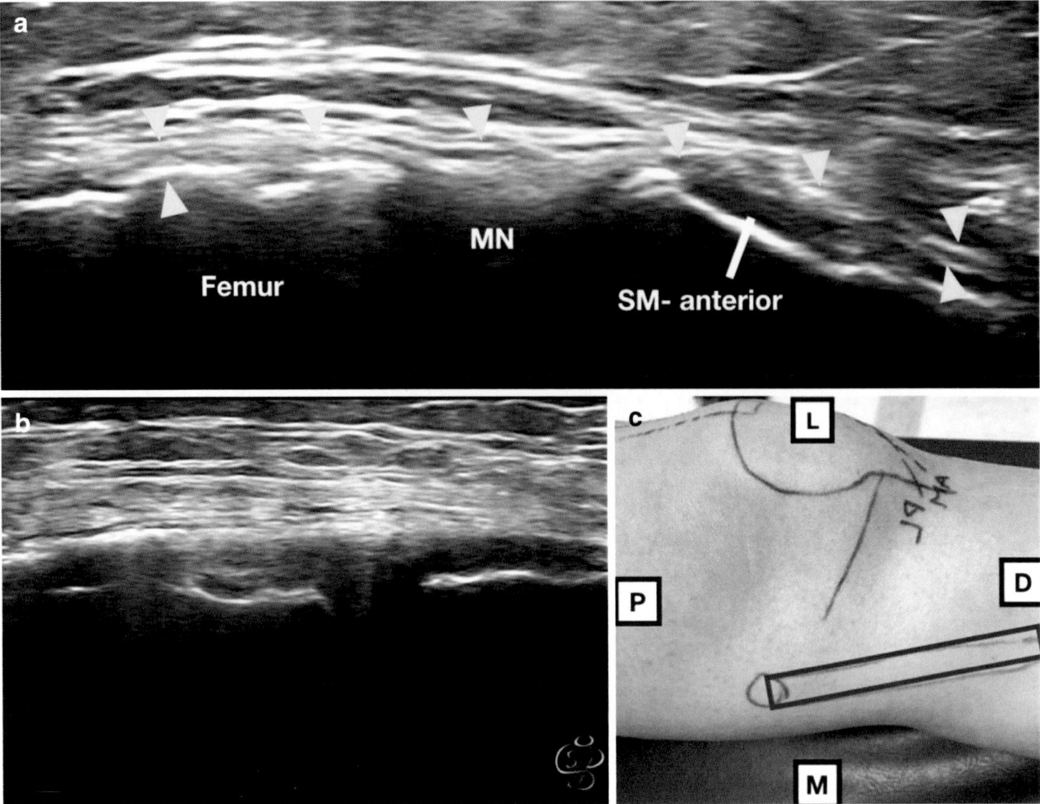

Fig. 9.12 Posterior oblique ligament. (**a**) Sonogram of a longitudinal view of the POL, which consists of one layer only. (**b**) Swelling of the POL. (**c**) Probe position of the POL, which is more posterior of the MCL

ments distal to the main common tendon, including the direct arm (Figs. 9.13 and 9.14), the anterior arm (Fig. 9.15) that circles to the front of the tibia, and the oblique popliteal arm (Fig. 9.16) that contributes to the oblique popliteal ligament.

Of the three arms, the oblique popliteal arm is found to be the primary ligamentous restraint to knee hyperextension. It expands from the semimembranosus tendon and courses superolaterally, then attaches to the fabella or the tendon of the lateral head of the gastrocnemius. There is also an aponeurotic fascia extending from the OPL to the medial gastrocnemius and plantaris, which helps dissipate stress concentration at the enthesis, thereby reducing tear.

In addition, the middle genicular neurovascular bundle passes through the midportion of the OPL and supplies the posterior knee capsule and PCL. This makes the midportion of the OPL a potential entrapment site [12–14].

Posterior Region

The popliteus muscle originates from the lateral condyle of the femur as a rounded tendon and inserts on the posterior surface of the tibia. It is an intra-articular and extra-synovial structure at the femoral origin and extra-articular at the muscular or myotendinous portion. The popliteus muscle, the popliteus tendon, and the popliteal fibular ligament make up the popliteus musculotendinous complex [15, 16]. It provides dynamic and static resistance to external rotation, assuming a major role with higher degrees of knee flexion.

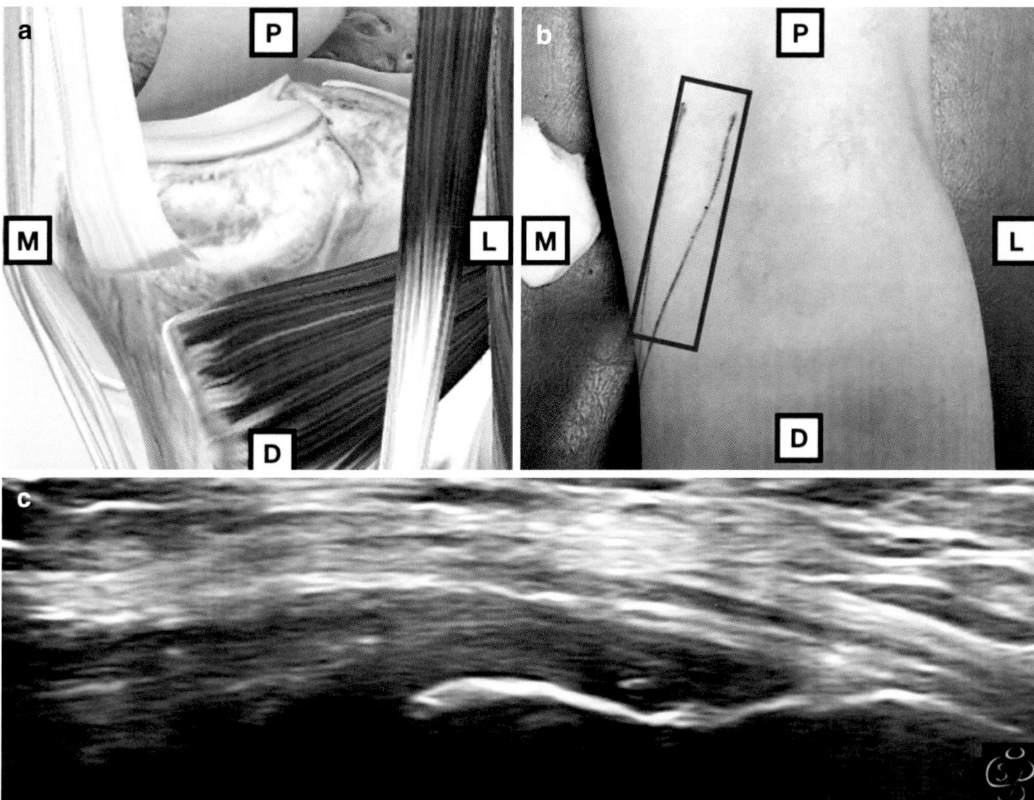

Fig. 9.13 Direct arm of the semimembranosus tendon. (**a**) Anatomy of the semimembranosus direct arm. (**b**) Proper probe position. (**c**) Normal sonographic appearance of the direct arm of the semimembranosus tendon in a longitudinal view

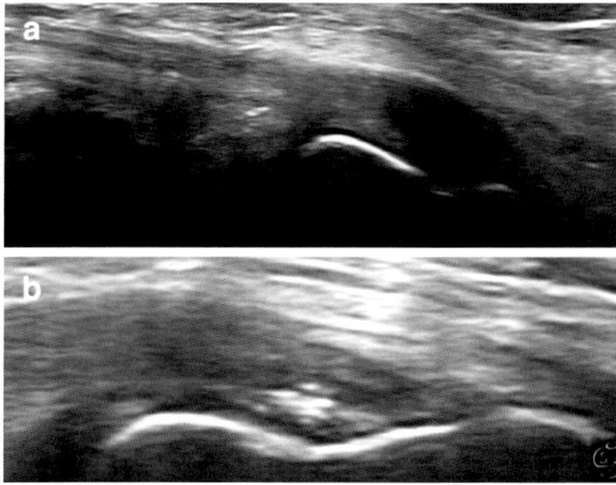

Fig. 9.14 Sonograms of the semimembranosus direct head. (**a**) Semimembranosus tendinopathy. (**b**) Calcification of the semimembranosus tendon

It helps create initial flexion from full extension, assists PCL when running downhill, and pulls on the lateral meniscus while bending the knee [17, 18].

It is often locked in a flexed shortened position after patients undergo knee surgery or experience severe trauma to the knee. Under ultrasound scanning, we should look for partial tear or sprain of the muscle or tendinopathy (Fig. 9.17). Regenerative injection could be done under ultrasound guidance to prevent injury of the popliteal vessels and tibial nerve.

The plantaris muscle originates from the inferior part of the lateral supracondylar ridge and inserts on the medial side of the calcaneus. Partial

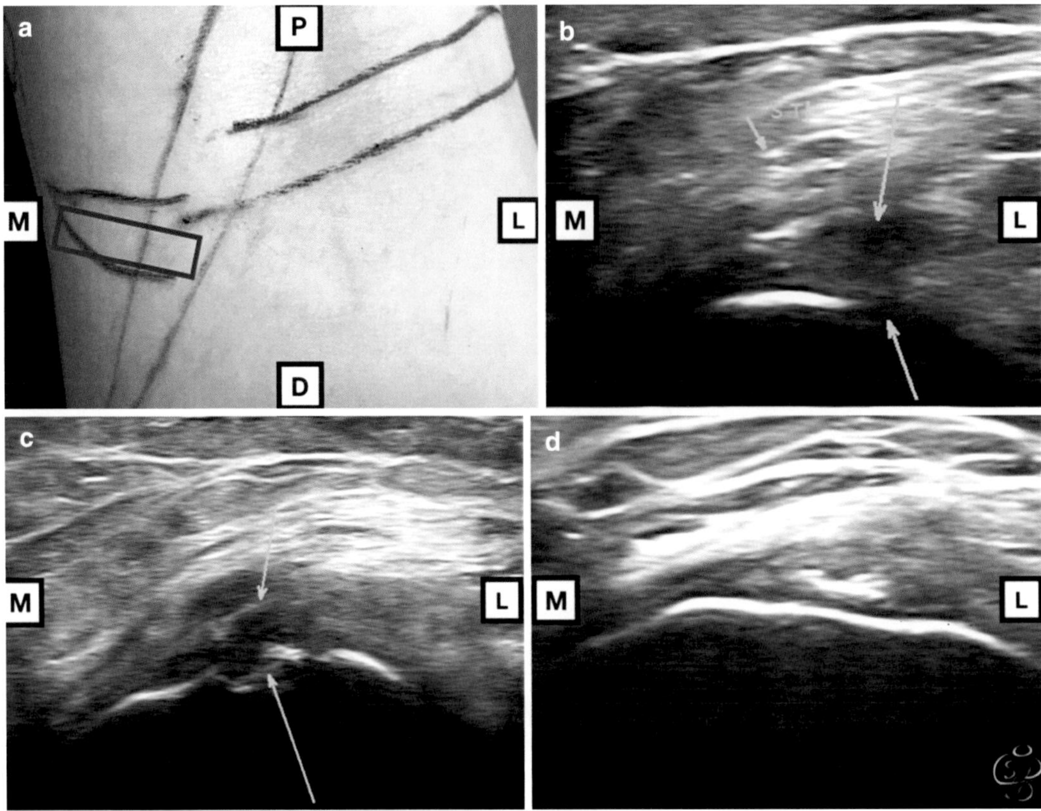

Fig. 9.15 Anterior arm of the semimembranosus tendon. (**a**) Probe position for the anterior arm of the semimembranosus tendon. (**b**) Tendinopathy of the anterior arm. (**c**) Avulsion of the anterior arm. (**d**) Calcification of the anterior arm

tear at the muscle combined with tendinopathy is not uncommon in athletes [19, 20] (Figs. 9.18 and 9.19).

The PCL serves as one of the main stabilizers of the knee and helps resist excessive posterior translation of the tibia relative to the femur. Therefore, chronic laxity of the PCL causes shear force to the anterior knee ligaments combining with an increased pressure over the patellofemoral joint and leads to anterior knee pain. Regenerating a torn PCL (Figs. 9.20 and 9.21) can help stabilize the knee and restore the tensegrity [21–23].

The fabella is a sesamoid bone and is more prevalent in Asian population. It serves as the common origin of the OPL, the arcuate ligament, and the FFL, as well as part of the plantaris muscle. It also has a close relationship with the peroneal nerve [24]. Dynamic ultrasound scanning can identify if there is peroneal nerve snapping/entrapment related to the fabella and can be treated by ultrasound-guided hydrodissection.

Posterolateral Corner

The posterolateral corner (PLC) is the most important restraint to varus stress, and it also acts as a secondary restraint to posterior tibial translation. Three major structures have been described as the primary stabilizers of the PLC: the lateral collateral ligament, the popliteal fibular ligament, and the popliteus tendon. Besides the three major structures, the fabellofibular ligament and arcuate

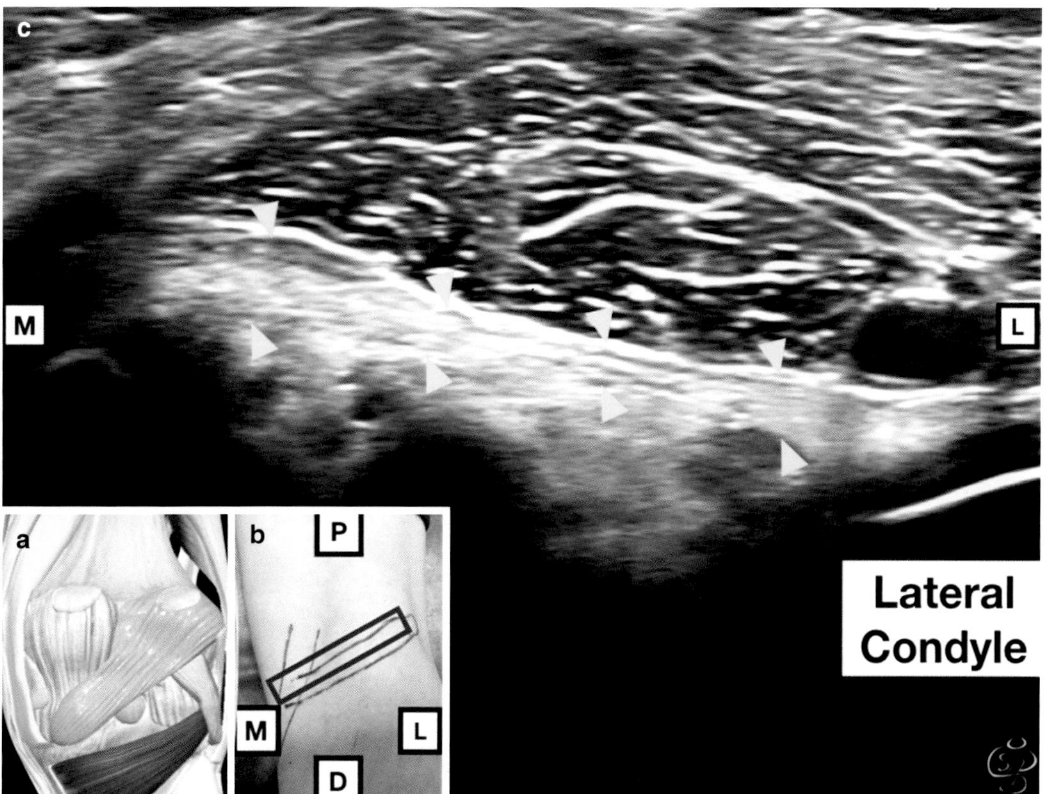

Fig. 9.16 Oblique popliteal ligament (OPL). (**a**) Anatomy of the OPL. (**b**) Probe position of the OPL. (**c**) Sonogram of the longitudinal view of the OPL (yellow arrow), expanding from the semimembranosus tendon to the lateral femoral condyle

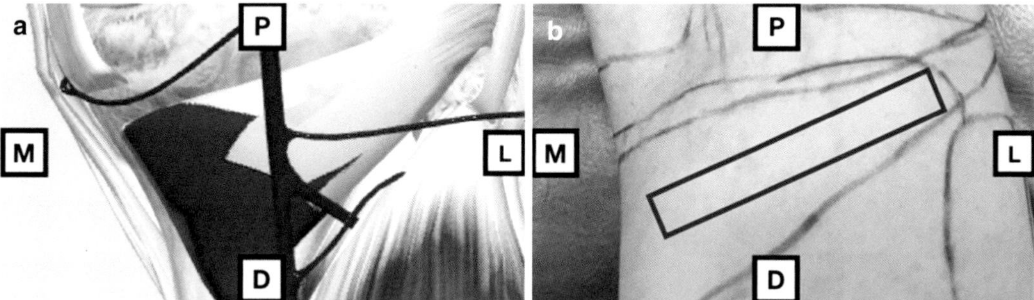

Fig. 9.17 Popliteus muscle and tendon. (**a**) Anatomy of the popliteus muscle, which is underneath the popliteal artery (red arrowhead). (**b**) Probe position of the longitudinal view of the popliteus muscle. (**c**) Normal popliteus muscle (yellow arrowhead) in a longitudinal view. (**d**) Near complete tear of the popliteus muscle (green arrowhead)

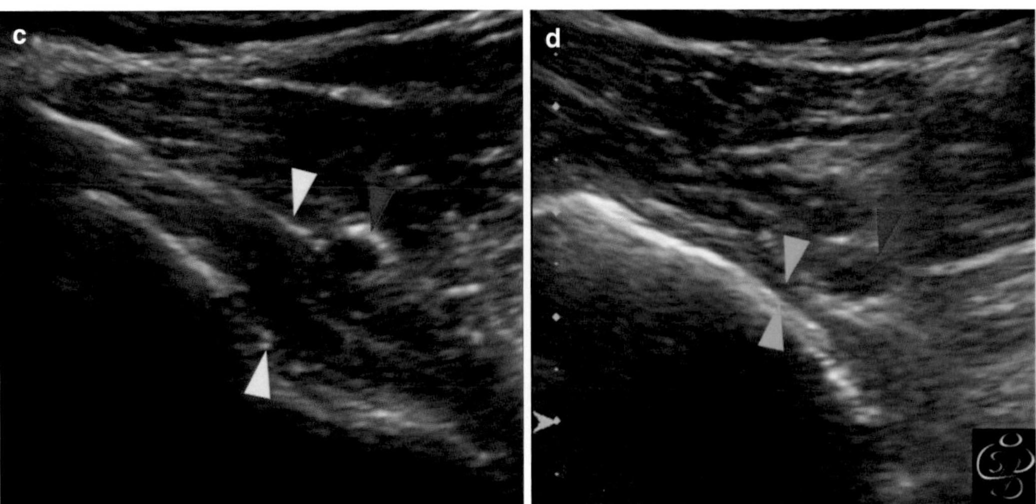

Fig. 9.17 (continued)

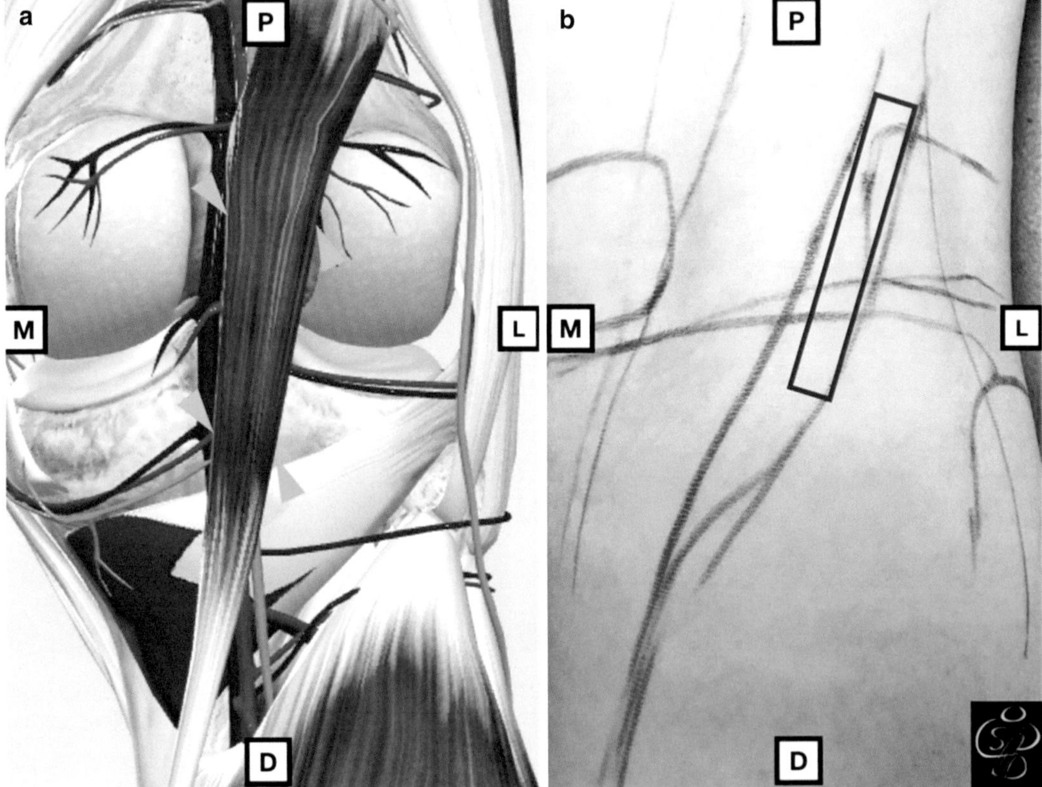

Fig. 9.18 Plantaris muscle. (**a**) Anatomy of the plantaris muscle (yellow arrowhead). (**b**) Probe position of the plantaris muscle

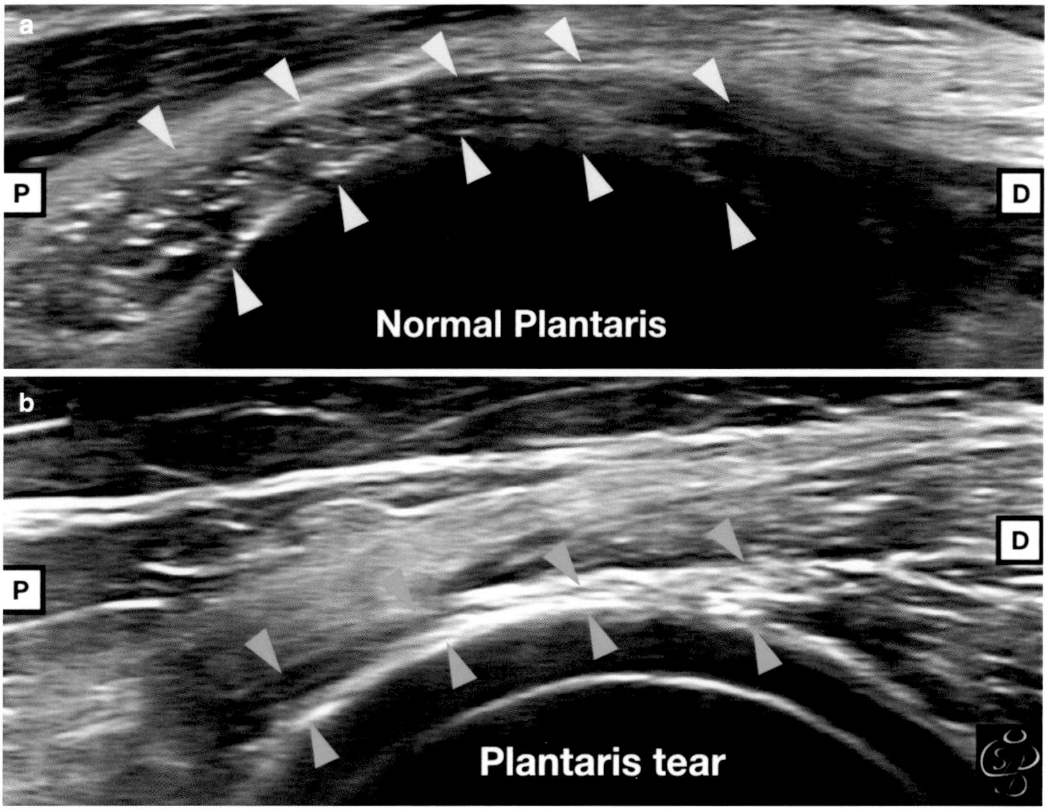

Fig. 9.19 Plantaris muscle. (**a**) Longitudinal view of the normal plantaris muscle. (**b**) Longitudinal view of a near complete tear of the plantaris muscle

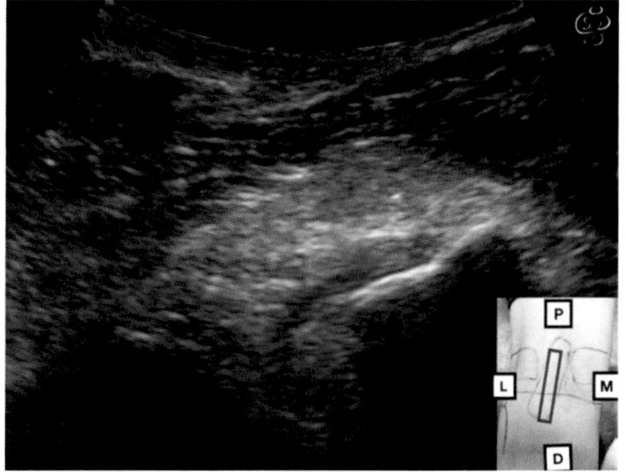

Fig. 9.20 Sonogram of the normal posterior cruciate ligament in the longitudinal view

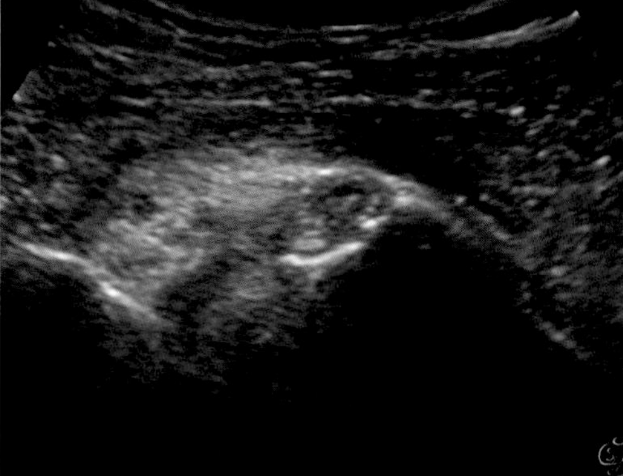

Fig. 9.21 Sonogram of the torn posterior cruciate ligament in the longitudinal view

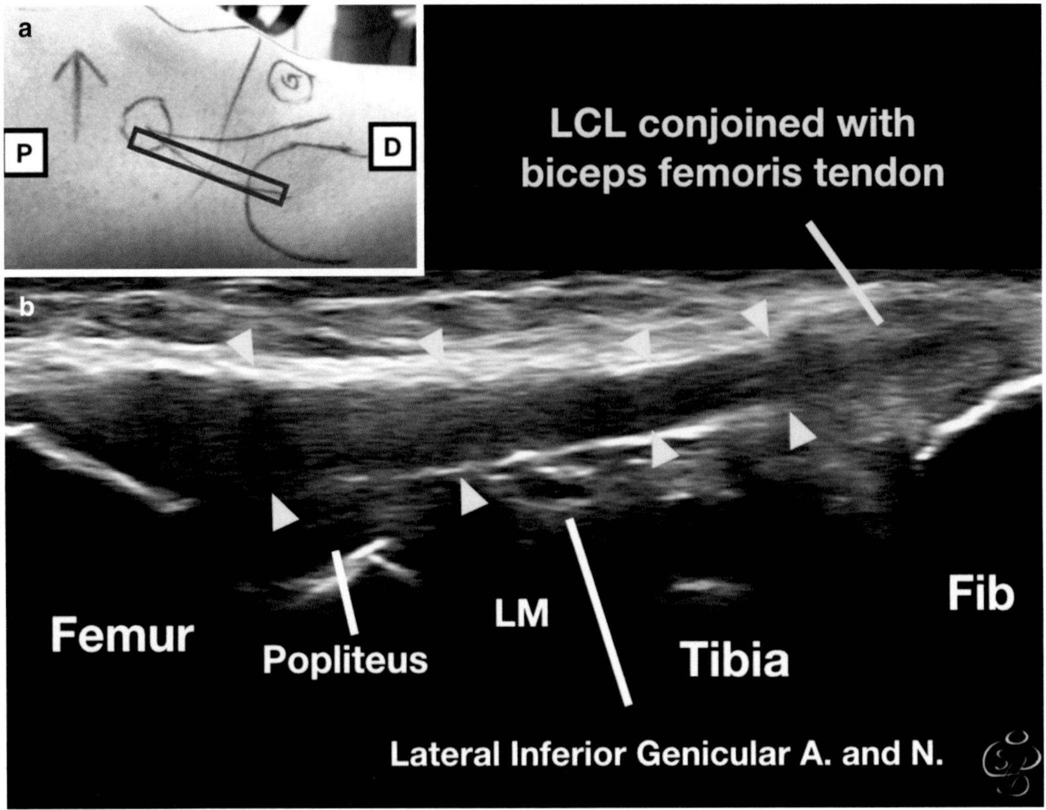

Fig. 9.22 Lateral collateral ligament. (**a**) Probe position of the LCL. (**b**) Sonogram of the longitudinal view of the LCL (yellow arrowhead). The lateral inferior genicular artery and nerve are underneath the LCL and lying right above the lateral meniscus (LM). Note that the LCL joins the insertion of the biceps femoris at the fibular head and should not be misdiagnosed as ligament injury

ligament are crucial for the tensegrity of this region [25].

The dial test is used in detecting isolated or concomitant PCL injury. The test is used to test the integrity of the posterior and posterolateral corner of the knee, when performing regenerative injection.

The test is performed in two steps. First, put the patient in a prone position with both knees flexed to 30 degrees and externally rotate the tibia simultaneously. If more than 10 degrees of external rotation is noted comparing to the other one, PLC injury is likely. Second, flex the knee to 90 degrees and perform external rotation again. If there is still increased external rotation in the previous problematic leg, then a combined PLC and PCL injury is indicated because the PCL is responsible for rotational stability when the knee flexion is at 90 degrees [17].

The lateral collateral ligament (LCL) is the primary varus stabilizer of the knee. It also limits external rotation and posterior displacement of the tibia. It has a broad insertion (Fig. 9.22) and covers 38% of the fibular head [26].

The popliteal fibular ligament (PFL) is a tendinous band and acts as a major stabilizer of the PLC. It originates from the popliteus tendon proximal to the myotendinous junction and inserts on the fibular styloid process. Using the posterior fibular head as the fulcrum, the probe is

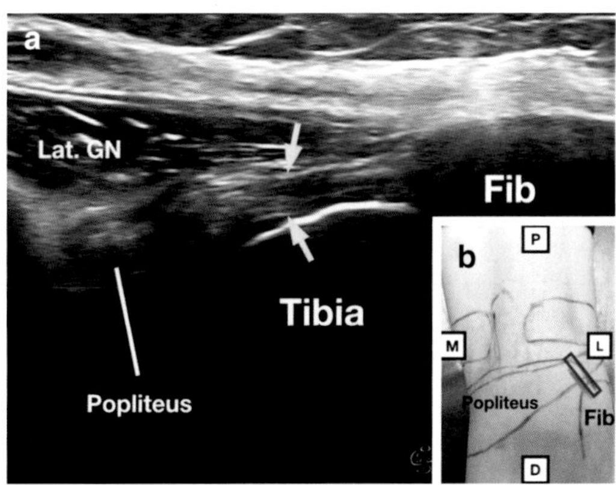

Fig. 9.23 Popliteal fibular ligament (PFL). (**a**) Longitudinal view of the PFL (yellow arrow). (**b**) Probe position of the PFL

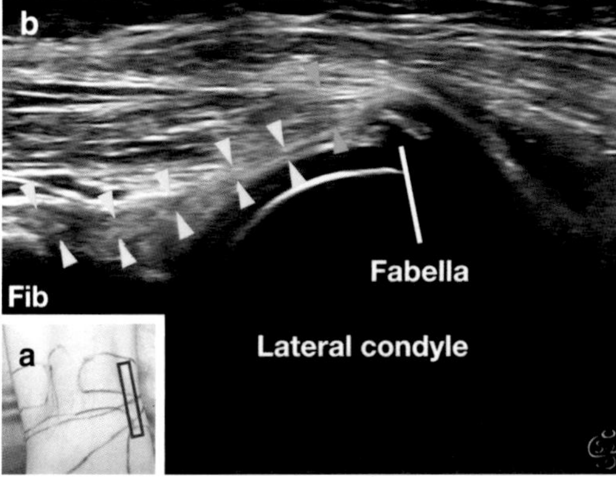

Fig. 9.24 Fabellofibular ligament (FFL). (**a**) Probe position of the FFL. (**b**) Sonogram of the longitudinal view of the FFL (yellow arrowhead). The tendon of the gastrocnemius muscle (green arrow) can be identified surrounding the fabella and embedding it

pivoted 45 degrees toward the center of the knee. A hypoechoic ligament will be seen as a ligament connecting the popliteus tendon and fibular head (Fig. 9.23). The fibular end of the ligament is posterior to the insertion of the lateral collateral ligament [16, 18].

The fabellofibular ligament (FFL) serves as a static stabilizer of the knee, which tenses in full extension. It runs from the base of the fabella to the styloid process of the fibular head (Fig. 9.24).

The arcuate ligament is inversely related to the FFL (Fig. 9.25). It extends from the femur condyle to the tip of the fibular head, which is hard to differentiate with the posterior capsule sometimes [16].

Both the FFL and arcuate ligament, together with PFL and LCL, help guard the tensegrity of the PLC.

When injecting PLC for regeneration, the peroneal nerve and popliteal vessels should be marked after ultrasound scanning, to prevent iatrogenic injury to the nerve.

Ligament-Capsule-Menisci Complex

The menisci are crescent-shaped wedges of the fibrocartilage situated on the medial and lateral aspect of the knee. Menisci are stabilized through a ligament-capsule-menisci complex. The loss of the complex integrity leads to a significant increased amount of extrusive displacement of the menisci.

When there is chronic instability of the knee due to ligament laxity or tear, menisci will be damaged eventually. Therefore, when there is a meniscus tear, we must not treat the meniscus only, but also have to treat the ligament-capsule-menisci complex and all the stabilizing ligaments which are compromised.

Meniscus tear can be divided into four grades (0–3) based on the MRI findings according to Reicher et al. [27]. Studies have shown that intrameniscal injections of PRP have the ability to achieve pain relief and halt progression on MRI over 6 months in patients with grade 2 meniscal lesions [28].

The posterior meniscofemoral ligament (PMFL), or the ligament of Wrisberg, helps stabilize the lateral meniscus. The PMFL originates from the lateral meniscus and crosses superiorly behind the PCL and inserts on the medial condyle of the femur. Using the curve probe, find the posterior medial border of the lateral meniscus first and pivot it to align the other end of the probe to the lateral border of the medial condyle.

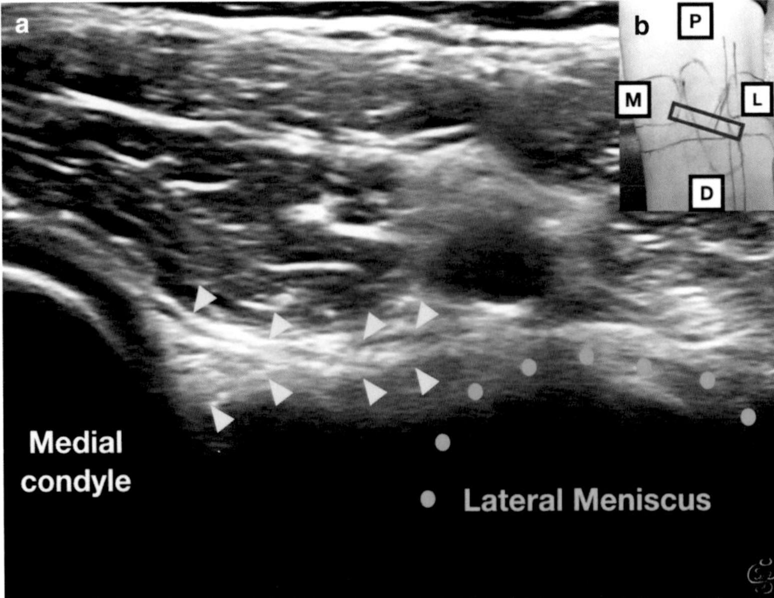

Fig. 9.26 Posterior meniscofemoral ligament (PMFL). (**a**) Sonogram of the longitudinal view of the PMFL (yellow arrow). The green dots indicate the posterior edge of the lateral meniscus. (**b**) Probe position of the PMFL

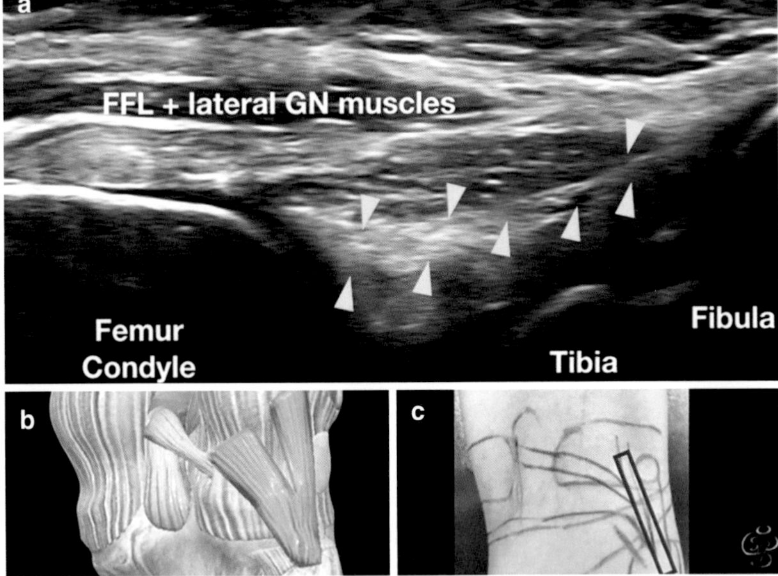

Fig. 9.25 Arcuate ligament (AL). (**a**) Anatomy of the AL. (**b**) Probe position of the AL. (**c**) Sonogram of the longitudinal view of the AL (yellow arrow). The size of the AL is inversely related to FFL. We can see marked AL with relatively thin and FFL blended together with the tendon of the gastrocnemius muscle in this patient without fabella

This will result in a clear view of the PMFL (Fig. 9.26).

Other than the aforementioned coronary ligaments and PMFL, there is another structure worth noting: the anterior intermeniscal ligament (AIML). It connects the anterior horn of the medial and lateral menisci. Matthieu et al. revealed that resection of the AIML leads to substantial changes in knee biomechanics [29]. Regenerative injection of the supporting structures helps stabilize the menisci.

Under ultrasound, once we localized the ACL by a previously described method, the AIML is seen as a hyperechoic, dot-like structure lying above the ACL. After localizing the dot, we can pivot the probe 90 degrees to have a longitudinal view of the AIML and have an in-plane injection.

References

1. Astur DC, Oliveira SG, Badra R, Arliani GG, Kaleka CC, Jalikjian W, et al. Updating of the anatomy of the extensor mechanism of the knee using a three-dimensional viewing technique. Rev Bras Ortop. 2011;46(5):490–4.
2. Hsiao MY, Chang KV, Ozcakar L. Ultrasonography of the anterior cruciate ligament: not an easy structure in knee joint imaging. Am J Phys Med Rehabil. 2016;95(9):e145–6.
3. Claes S, Vereecke E, Maes M, Victor J, Verdonk P, Bellemans J. Anatomy of the anterolateral ligament of the knee. J Anat. 2013;223(4):321–8.
4. Parsons EM, Gee AO, Spiekerman C, Cavanagh PR. The biomechanical function of the anterolateral ligament of the knee. Am J Sports Med. 2015;43(3):669–74.
5. Stijak L, Bumbasirevic M, Radonjic V, Kadija M, Puskas L, Milovanovic D, et al. Anatomic description of the anterolateral ligament of the knee. Knee Surg Sports Traumatol Arthrosc. 2016;24(7):2083–8.
6. Marchant MH Jr, Tibor LM, Sekiya JK, Hardaker WT Jr, Garrett WE Jr, Taylor DC. Management of medial-sided knee injuries, part 1: medial collateral ligament. Am J Sports Med. 2011;39(5):1102–13.
7. Lee JH, Kim KJ, Jeong YG, Lee NS, Han SY, Lee CG, et al. Pes anserinus and anserine bursa: anatomical study. Anat Cell Biol. 2014;47(2):127–31.
8. Dold AP, Swensen S, Strauss E, Alaia M. The posteromedial corner of the knee: anatomy, pathology, and management strategies. J Am Acad Orthop Surg. 2017;25(11):752–61.
9. Geiger D, Chang E, Pathria M, Chung CB. Posterolateral and posteromedial corner injuries of the knee. Radiol Clin N Am. 2013;51(3):413–32.
10. Tibor LM, Marchant MH Jr, Taylor DC, Hardaker WT Jr, Garrett WE Jr, Sekiya JK. Management of medial-sided knee injuries, part 2: posteromedial corner. Am J Sports Med. 2011;39(6):1332–40.
11. De Maeseneer M, Marcelis S, Boulet C, Kichouh M, Shahabpour M, de Mey J, et al. Ultrasound of the knee with emphasis on the detailed anatomy of anterior, medial, and lateral structures. Skelet Radiol. 2014;43(8):1025–39.
12. Fam LPD, Fruheling VM, Pupim B, Ramos CH, de Moura MFA, Namba M, et al. Oblique popliteal ligament - an anatomical study. Rev Bras Ortop. 2013;48(5):402–5.
13. Hedderwick M, Stringer MD, McRedmond L, Meikle GR, Woodley SJ. The oblique popliteal ligament: an anatomic and MRI investigation. Surg Radiol Anat. 2017;39(9):1017–27.
14. Morgan PM, LaPrade RF, Wentorf FA, Cook JW, Bianco A. The role of the oblique popliteal ligament and other structures in preventing knee hyperextension. Am J Sports Med. 2010;38(3):550–7.
15. Barker RP, Lee JC, Healy JC. Normal sonographic anatomy of the posterolateral corner of the knee. AJR Am J Roentgenol. 2009;192(1):73–9.
16. Chahla J, Moatshe G, Dean CS, LaPrade RF. Posterolateral corner of the knee: current concepts. Arch Bone Joint Surg. 2016;4(2):97–103.
17. Petrillo S, Volpi P, Papalia R, Maffulli N, Denaro V. Management of combined injuries of the posterior cruciate ligament and posterolateral corner of the knee: a systematic review. Br Med Bull. 2017;123(1):47–57.
18. Shon OJ, Park JW, Kim BJ. Current concepts of posterolateral corner injuries of the knee. Knee Surg Relat Res. 2017;29(4):256–68.
19. Bianchi S, Sailly M, Molini L. Isolated tear of the plantaris tendon: ultrasound and MRI appearance. Skelet Radiol. 2011;40(7):891–5.
20. Chang KV, Wu WT, Ozcakar L. Ultrasonography imaging for the diagnosis and guided injection of Plantaris tendon strain in a patient with tennis leg. Am J Phys Med Rehabil. 2018;97(6):e60–e1.
21. Arthur JR, Haglin JM, Makovicka JL, Chhabra A. Anatomy and biomechanics of the posterior cruciate ligament and their surgical implications. Sports Med Arthrosc Rev. 2020;28(1):e1–e10.
22. Logterman SL, Wydra FB, Frank RM. Posterior cruciate ligament: anatomy and biomechanics. Curr Rev Musculoskelet Med. 2018;11(3):510–4.
23. Vaquero-Picado A, Rodriguez-Merchan EC. Isolated posterior cruciate ligament tears: an update of management. EFORT Open Rev. 2017;2(4):89–96.
24. Patel A, Singh R, Johnson B, Smith A. Compression neuropathy of the common peroneal nerve by the fabella. BMJ Case Rep. 2013;2013.
25. Geiger D, Chang EY, Pathria MN, Chung CB. Posterolateral and posteromedial corner injuries of the knee. Magn Reson Imaging Clin N Am. 2014;22(4):581–99.
26. Grawe B, Schroeder AJ, Kakazu R, Messer MS. Lateral collateral ligament injury about the knee: anatomy, evaluation, and management. J Am Acad Orthop Surg. 2018;26(6):e120–e7.
27. Reicher MA, Hartzman S, Duckwiler GR, Bassett LW, Anderson LJ, Gold RH. Meniscal injuries: detection using MR imaging. Radiology. 1986;159(3):753–7.
28. Blanke F, Vavken P, Haenle M, von Wehren L, Pagenstert G, Majewski M. Percutaneous injections of platelet rich plasma for treatment of intrasubstance meniscal lesions. Muscles Ligaments Tendons J. 2015;5(3):162–6.
29. Matthieu, Ollivier Julie, Falguières Martine, Pithioux Philippe, Boisrenoult Phillippe, Beaufils Nicolas, Pujol Sectioning of the Anterior Intermeniscal Ligament Changes Knee Loading Mechanics. Arthroscopy: The Journal of Arthroscopic & Related Surgery 2018;34(10):2837–43. https://doi.org/10.1016/j.arthro.2018.03.007

10 Ultrasound-Guided Orthobiologics of the Foot and Ankle

Lauren Vernese, Adam Pourcho,
and Troy P. Henning

Introduction

Chronic pain affects over one-fifth of adults, with an estimated 50% related to chronic musculoskeletal disorders [1, 2]. Over 54 million Americans alone have arthritis, with one in four reporting persistent pain [3]. According to the Centers for Disease Control and Prevention, the total medical costs and lost earnings related to arthritis in 2013 were 3.5 billion US dollars or 1% of the gross domestic product [4]. Tendinopathy affects a large number of athletes and nonathletes and constitutes approximately 30% of consultations for musculoskeletal pain in the general practice setting [5].

For patients who have persistent foot and ankle joint-related pain that is recalcitrant to conservative treatment, corticosteroid injections are typically offered to help alleviate pain. However, numerous studies of corticosteroids have been shown it to be toxic to tenocytes and chondrocytes, as well as increase the risk of infection, lower the immune system response, temporarily raise blood sugar, and increase the risk of tendon rupture [6, 7]. As more evidence emerges revealing long-term and potentially short-term harmful effects of corticosteroid on cartilage, physicians and patients are turning to other injectable options such as prolotherapy, autologous blood products, or placental-derived tissues with the goal of influencing tissue regeneration or disease modulation. The hope of regenerative medicine is to restore the homeostasis of the affected tissue and if possible replace or regenerate human cells or tissues to restore normal function, through stimulation of the body's natural intrinsic pathways [8]. While still an emerging field, regenerative medicine has touched nearly every field of medicine and has been applied to congenital defects, chronic disease, trauma, and aging [9].

Regenerative treatment options in the current musculoskeletal research and clinical practice for management of foot and ankle injuries include autologous blood products such as platelet-rich plasma (PRP), mesenchymal cells ("stem cells") (MSC) derived from bone marrow aspirate concentrate (BMAC) and/or adipose tissue, placental-derived products, prolotherapy, microfracture, and autologous chondrocyte implantation [10–15] (Table 10.1).

Until recently, most insurers in the United States have not included orthobiologic therapies as a covered benefit. However, the use of ortho-

L. Vernese · A. Pourcho
Rehabilitation and Performance Medicine, Swedish Medical Group, Seattle, WA, USA
e-mail: Lauren.Vernese@swedish.org; Adam.Pourcho@swedish.org

T. P. Henning (✉)
Rehabilitation and Performance Medicine, Swedish Medical Group, Seattle, WA, USA

Swedish Rehabilitation and Performance Medicine, Seattle, WA, USA
e-mail: troy.henning@swedish.org

Y. El Miedany (ed.), *Musculoskeletal Ultrasound-Guided Regenerative Medicine*,
https://doi.org/10.1007/978-3-030-98256-0_10

Table 10.1 Types of orthobiologics

Platelet-rich plasma (PRP)	Concentrated autologous platelets: defined as greater than circulating volume, generally four to eight times that found in serum	
Mesenchymal cells (MSC)	Bone marrow aspirate concentrate (BMAC)	Autologous concentrated MSCs and PRP
	Adipose derived	Autologous MSCs mechanically separated from fat tissue
Placental derived (amnion and amniotic fluid)	Allogenic commercially available product; available as sheets of tissue or injectable solution	

biologics may be more cost effective and less invasive than alternatives when compared head-to-head. In fact, a recent meta-analysis of level 1 randomized controlled trials (RCTs) assessing PRP in the treatment of knee arthritis estimated it would be on average $1192.08 less annually than hyaluronic acid or saline injections [16]. Further comparisons of other regenerative options are needed to substantiate these results.

Before reviewing the current literature available for clinic-based musculoskeletal regenerative medicine about the foot and ankle, this chapter will review pertinent anatomy of the foot and ankle structures that may be amenable to regenerative techniques.

Ankle Anatomy

Osseous and Ligamentous Anatomy

The ankle complex is composed of three joints from the lower leg and the foot: the talocrural, subtalar, and inferior tibiofibular joint.

The ankle joint proper, also known as the talocrural or tibiotalar joint, is a hinged synovial joint formed by the articulation between the talus and the distal tibia and fibula. The malleoli of the tibia and fibula provide constraint for this hinge joint, resulting in primarily dorsiflexion and plantarflexion motion [17] (see Fig. 10.1a).

Three major ligamentous complexes are required for dynamic stability of the ankle mortice: the tibiofibular syndesmosis, the lateral collateral ligament, and the medial collateral (or deltoid) ligaments. The tibiofibular syndesmosis consists of the anterior inferior tibiofibular ligament (AITFL), the posterior tibiofibular ligament, and the interosseous membrane. The lateral collateral ligaments include the anterior talofibular ligament (ATFL), calcaneofibular ligament (CFL), and posterior talofibular ligament (PTFL). The medial collateral ligaments include the anterior and posterior tibiotalar, tibionavicular, and tibiocalcaneal portions of the deltoid ligament complex. Distal to the talocrural joint is the subtalar joint, a tri-planar, uniaxial joint between the talus and the calcaneus (Fig. 10.1b).

The foot is divided by regions: the hindfoot (talus and calcaneus), midfoot (navicular, cuboid, and cuneiforms), and forefoot (metatarsals and phalanges). The hindfoot and midfoot consist of seven irregularly shaped tarsal bones that are further organized into three rows: proximal, intermediate, and distal. The proximal row includes the talus and calcaneus.

The calcaneus is the largest of the tarsal bones. It has two joints including the subtalar (talocalcaneal) joint superiorly and the calcaneocuboid joint anteriorly. Its posterior aspect, the calcaneal tuberosity, is the attachment site of the Achilles tendon. Its medial aspect has a shelf-like facet known as the sustentaculum, to which the talus rests on as well as the calcaneonavicular "spring ligament" (CNL) complex attaches (Fig. 10.2a, b).

The next row (intermediate) contains the navicular bone and its articulation with the talus posteriorly, the three cuneiforms anteriorly, and the cuboid laterally. The navicular bone's medial plantar surface has a tuberosity that serves as an attachment site for the posterior tibialis tendon (PTT). The distal row of the midfoot contains the three cuneiforms (lateral, intermediate, and medial) and the cuboid. The cuneiforms articulate with the first through third metatarsals. The

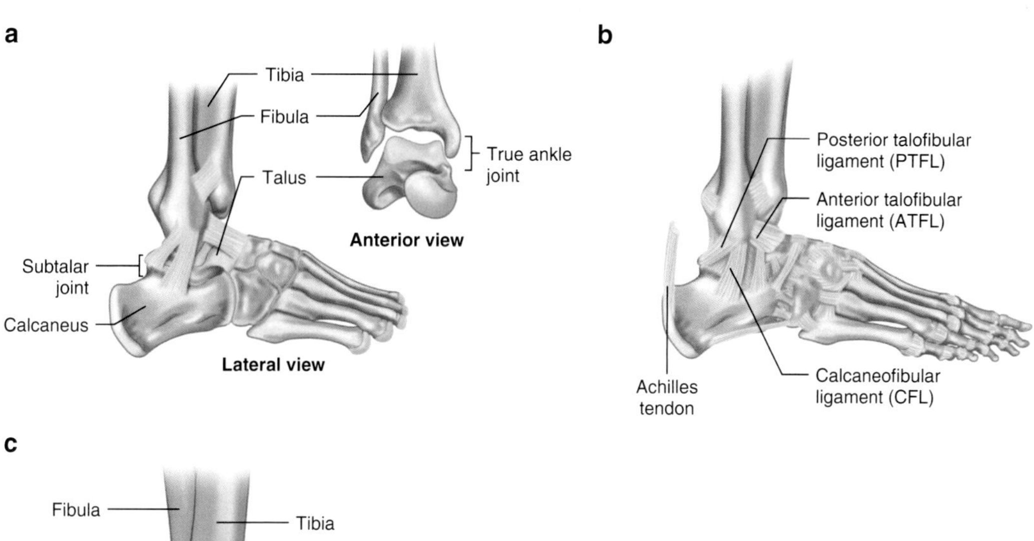

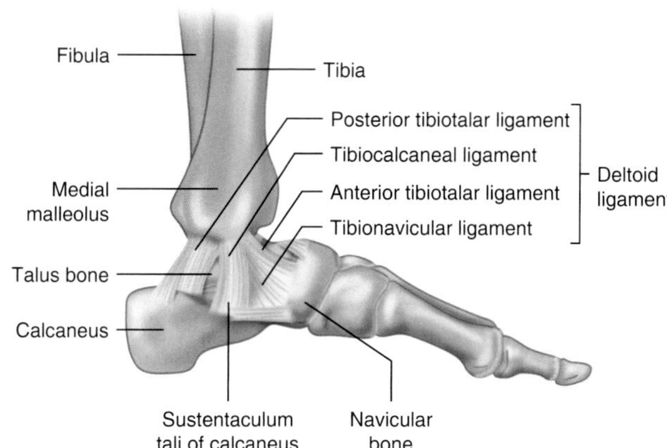

Fig. 10.1 Ankle bony and ligamentous anatomy. (**a**) Anatomy of bones of the ankle from lateral and anterior views, demonstrating the tibiotalar (ankle joint) and talocalcaneal (subtalar joint). (**b**) Lateral ligamentous anatomy of the ankle. (**c**) Medial ligamentous anatomy demonstrating the deltoid ligamentous complex

cuboid, the most lateral bone, sits proximal to the fourth and fifth metatarsals. The tarsometatarsal articulations are known as the Lisfranc joint line. The forefoot consists of the metatarsals and their respective phalanges. Important ligamentous complexes of the foot include the CNL and Lisfranc ligaments (Fig. 10.2a).

Muscle, Tendon, and Neurovascular Anatomy

Across the anterior ankle are three main tendons: the tibialis anterior (located medially), the extensor hallucis longus, and the extensor digitorum longus (most lateral). The peroneus tertius is along the anterolateral region and extends from the distal fibula and interosseous membrane to insert on the dorsal base of the fifth metatarsal, although can have varying origin and insertion. It has been found to be absent in 10.5–18.5% of the population [18, 19]. Overlying the anterior tendons is the extensor retinaculum. Important anterior neurovascular structures that travel deep to the extensor retinaculum include the tibial artery and superficial and deep fibular (peroneal) nerves (Fig. 10.3a).

The lateral ankle tendons include the fibularis (peroneus) longus and brevis, and these are covered by the superior and inferior peroneal retinacula. An estimated 5–21% of patients will have a peroneus quartus, an accessory fibular muscle that typically inserts on the retrotrochlear eminence or blends in with the native fibularis longus

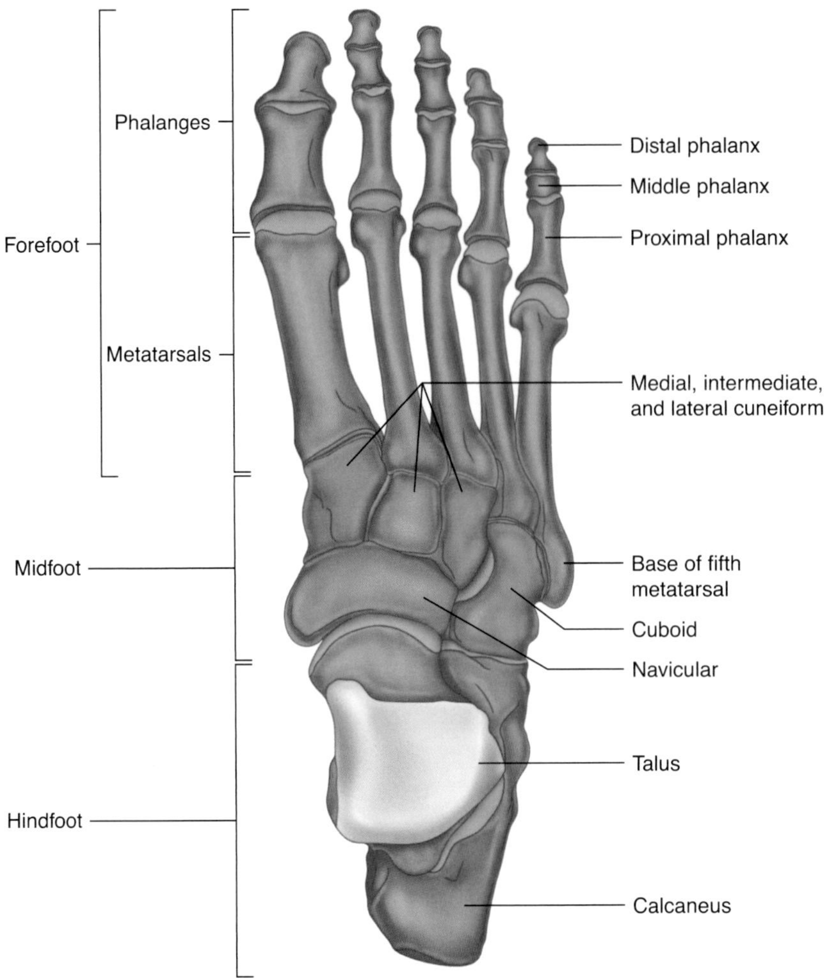

Fig. 10.2 Foot bony anatomy. Anatomy of bones of foot divided into regions, hindfoot, midfoot, and forefoot

[20–22]. The lateral ankle also is the origin for the extensor digitorum brevis muscle, arising from the lateral calcaneus and extensor retinaculum (Fig. 10.3b).

Laterally, the sural nerve moves from midline to the lateral edge of the Achilles tendon in the distal lower leg, then continues to move lateral until it passes posterior to the lateral malleolus. Just distal and posterior to the lateral malleolus it branches into lateral calcaneal, lateral dorsal cutaneous, and medial dorsal cutaneous nerves (Fig. 10.3b).

Tendons at the medial ankle include the PTT (most anterior), flexor digitorum longus (FDL), and flexor hallucis longus (FHL) (most posterior) tendons. Between the flexor digitorum and FHL tendons is the neurovascular bundle – the tibial artery, tibial vein, and tibial nerve. Overlying these structures is the flexor retinaculum, forming the tarsal tunnel.

Just distal to the flexor retinaculum and around the origin of the abductor hallucis, the tibial nerve divides into the medial and lateral plantar nerves. The lateral plantar nerve gives off a branch before traversing the plantar foot, known as the inferior calcaneal (Baxter's) nerve. Rarely, this nerve may come off more proximal from the main tibial nerve [23].

The posterior ankle's main structure is the Achilles tendon, inserting onto the posterior cal-

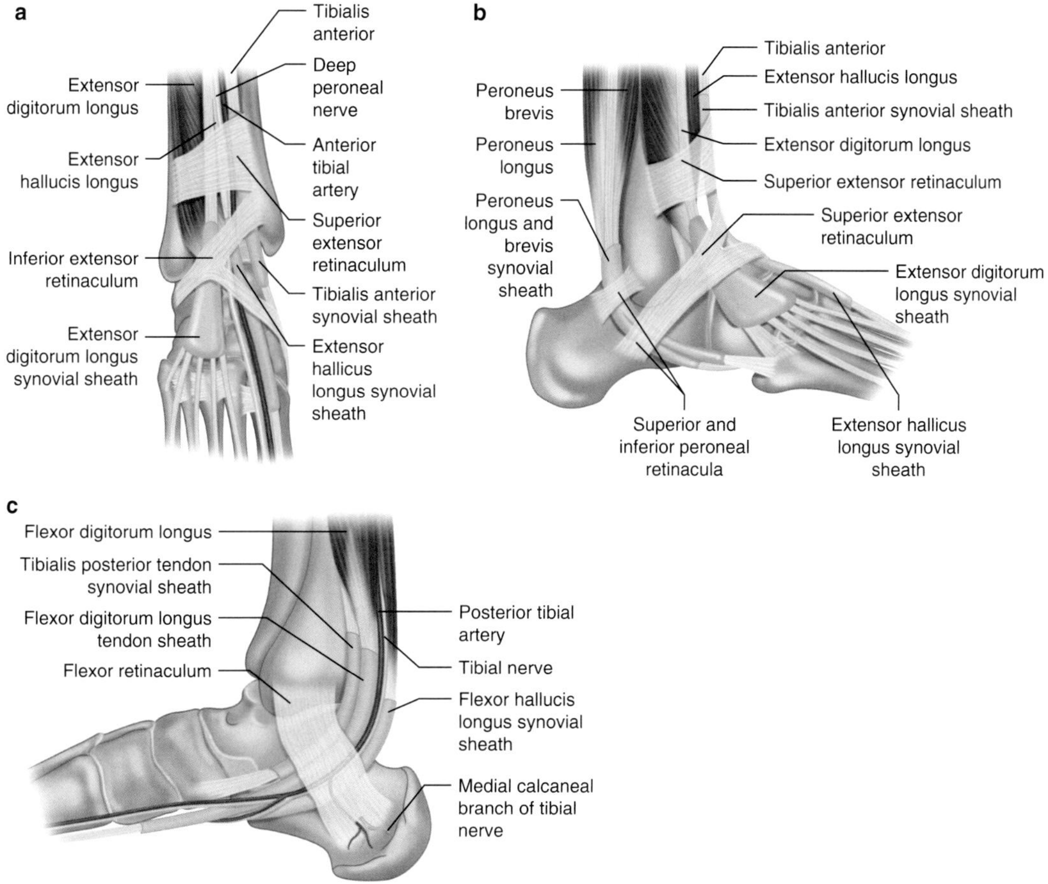

Fig. 10.3 Ankle musculotendinous anatomy. (**a**) Anterior ankle musculotendinous and neurovascular anatomy. (**b**) Lateral ankle musculotendinous anatomy. (**c**) Medial ankle musculotendinous and neurovascular anatomy

caneal tuberosity. Additionally, the plantaris, which can be absent in 7–20% of individuals, can have a variable insertion along the medial Achilles tendon to the calcaneus [24–27] (Fig. 10.3b).

The most common target in the plantar hindfoot for regenerative therapies is the plantar fascia, which originates off the plantar calcaneus as a thick aponeurosis supporting the arch of the plantar foot. The plantar fascia originates from the medial calcaneal tuberosity and has three components: medial, central, and lateral bands [18]. At the posterior heel, the Achilles tendon and plantar fascia remain in continuity by a paratenon ("the windlass mechanism"); however, this is typically lost with age, leaving few if any fibers [28] (Fig. 10.4).

Orthobiologic Use About the Foot and Ankle Interventional Procedures: Joints

The majority of orthobiologic research related to joint disease has focused on the treatment of knee osteoarthritis [13, 29]. Several studies highlight the role of leukocyte concentration in clinical outcomes. Riboh et al.'s meta-analysis comparing leukocyte-poor (LP) to leukocyte-rich (LR) platelet-rich plasma (PRP) to hyaluronic acid (HA) or placebo found the greatest improvements in Western Ontario and McMaster Universities Osteoarthritis Index (WOMAC) scores in the LP group [30]. Conversely, Filardo et al.'s study comparing LR-PRP to HA found no difference

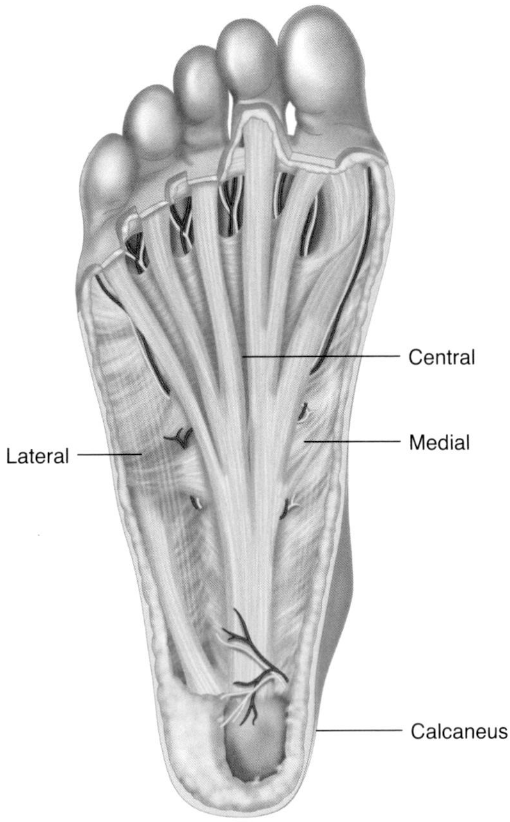

Fig. 10.4 Plantar fascia anatomy. Plantar fascia anatomy. Note the central, medial, and lateral bands of the plantar fascia. The central band is the most commonly affected with plantar fascia pathology

between the treatment groups [31]. Furthermore, Braun et al. found greater synoviocyte death in LR-PRP than LP-PRP suggesting some formulations or PRP may be counterproductive in the treatment of degenerative/arthritic joint diseases [32]. Current evidence for foot and ankle intra-articular injection of these products is limited to a small number of studies, small study population, frequent lack of placebo control, and variability in product preparation and administration [33–35].

A 2012 study by Mei-Dan et al. demonstrated intra-articular tibiotalar therapeutic injections of PRP to be superior to hyaluronate in the management of talar osteochondral defects (OCD) [35]. In this study of 30 patients, there was reduction in pain and stiffness and improved function for both groups. However, there was statistically significant higher reduction from the PRP group in the 28-week follow-up period. A 2015 study by Görmeli et al. demonstrated improved efficacy of PRP versus hyaluronic acid or saline injection for talar OCD lesions following microfracture surgery [34]. Guney et al. also assessed the addition of PRP to microfracture surgery on the talar dome and demonstrated that the combination was superior to microfracture alone for the long-term treatment of symptomatic OCD lesions in terms of pain reduction and functional outcomes [36].

With regard to osteoarthritis about the foot and ankle, Repetto et al. evaluated the effects of four weekly PRP injections on 20 ankles with symptomatic osteoarthritis of the tibiotalar joint and found a significant improvement on pain and function and high patient satisfaction rates, with a mean follow-up of 17.7 months [37]. Fukawa et al. reported similar reduction in pain and improved function following three PRP injections at an interval of 2 weeks on 20 patients with symptomatic ankle osteoarthritis [33]. Neither study reported significant adverse side effects. A 2010 study on prolotherapy for chronic ankle pain demonstrated a significant improvement in pain level, stiffness, and quality of life after an average of 4.4 prolotherapy treatments, with an average follow-up of 21 months [2]. Despite promising results from these studies, interpretation of findings is limited due to small sample sizes, poorly controlled protocols, lack of control for leukocytes or reporting of concentrations, and lack of placebo-controlled interventions.

General considerations when doing treatments about the foot and ankle are as follows:

- Ultrasound guidance (USG) is recommended to ensure accuracy of injectate in treatment target [38].
- No matter the injectate, the injection approach is essentially the same.
- Needle gauge may vary depending on the size/viscosity of the injectate.
  - One study demonstrated that platelets are prematurely lysed and activated when small bore (<21 gauge) needles were used [39].
- Patient and provider positioning are optimized for comfort and proper ergonomics and to facilitate visualization of the needle approaching/entering the target.

- Prior to the injection, the region should be adequately cleansed to reduce the risk of infection.
- Local anesthetic is typically performed using USG along the intended needle pathway.
- Anesthetic infiltration into the target tissue is minimized to ensure optimal functioning of the orthobiologic.
- Linear array high-frequency (optional hockey stick) Tds should allow for optimal visualization of all structures.
- Ability to adjust the focal zones, frequency range, and gain can help optimize image of certain regions such as the plantar fascia.
- In-plane techniques are generally and technically easier to perform.
- Using a gel standoff technique can aid in visualization of the needle and target in regions with less compliant tissue between the skin and target.
- An understanding of at-risk structures and anatomy with pre-scanning prior to any injection is recommended. This will allow the provider to choose the safest path to complete the procedure.
- Consider performing a tibial nerve block prior to plantar fascia procedures to aid in pain reduction during and after procedure.

Ultrasound-Guided Joint Injections of the Foot and Ankle

Positioning

- Patient: supine or lateral recumbent (subtalar joint) with knee straight and foot/ankle in relaxed position

Td Type

- High-frequency linear array

Needle

- Anesthetic: 25–30 gauge, 25–38 mm
- Orthobiologic: 21 gauge or larger, 25–38 mm
- Aspiration: 18 gauge or larger, 38 mm

Injection Volume

- 0.5–5 ml injectate dependent on joint volume size

Approaches

Long Axis to Joint, in-Plane with Td

With the patient in lateral recumbent position with pillow between knees and treatment limb away from the table, the US Td is placed in the sagittal or axial to the long axis of the joint. The needle is then advanced in-plane with the Td into the target joint ensuring the articular cartilage is avoided with the needle. The injectate should then easily flow into the joint under little to no resistance. Care should be taken to monitor pressure while injecting to ensure the joint is not overly distended, which can increase pain following procedure (Fig. 10.5a, b) – example of in-plane ankle injection through anterior talofibular ligament.

Out-of-Plane with Td

The US Td is placed to create an anatomic long-axis view of the desired joint. The needle is then advanced using a walk-down technique from superficial to deep, to a position within the target joint. This can also be done in-plane by turning the transducer 90 degrees (Fig. 10.6a–c).

Ultrasound-Guided Subtalar Joint Injection

Posterior Subtalar (Talocalcaneal) Joint Injection

Given the relative complexity of injecting the subtalar joint over the other joints about the foot and ankle, it will be described here in greater detail. The subtalar joint consists of two facet joints, which do not often communicate when injected [40]. Therefore, positioning to optimally inject the desired facet of the subtalar joint is recommended.

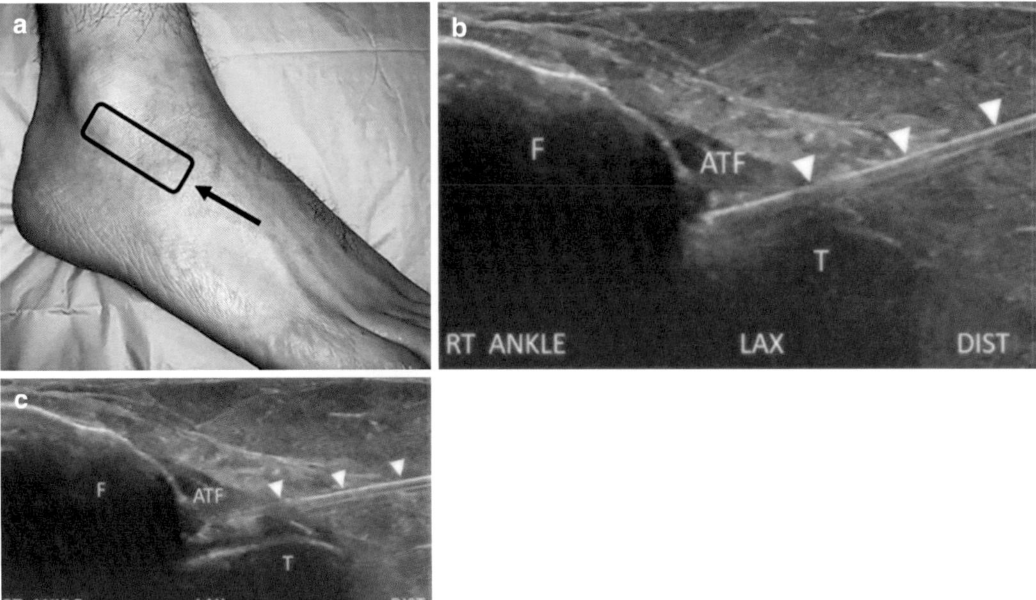

Fig. 10.5 Ultrasound-guided tibiotalar joint injection. (**a**) External view of a right (RT) ankle with Td (*solid rectangle*) placement and needle approach (*solid arrow*) for an in-plane transligamentous injection of the tibiotalar (ankle) joint. (**b**) Ultrasound correlate, with distal (DIST) to the right, showing an in-plane view of hyperechoic needle (*arrowheads*) through the right anterior talofibular (ATF) ligament, within the tibiotalar (ankle) joint. (**c**) US image, with DIST to the right, showing a hyperechoic needle (*arrowheads*) within the RT ATF ligament for orthobiologic injection. *F* fibula, *T* talus, *LAX* long axis, *DIST* distal

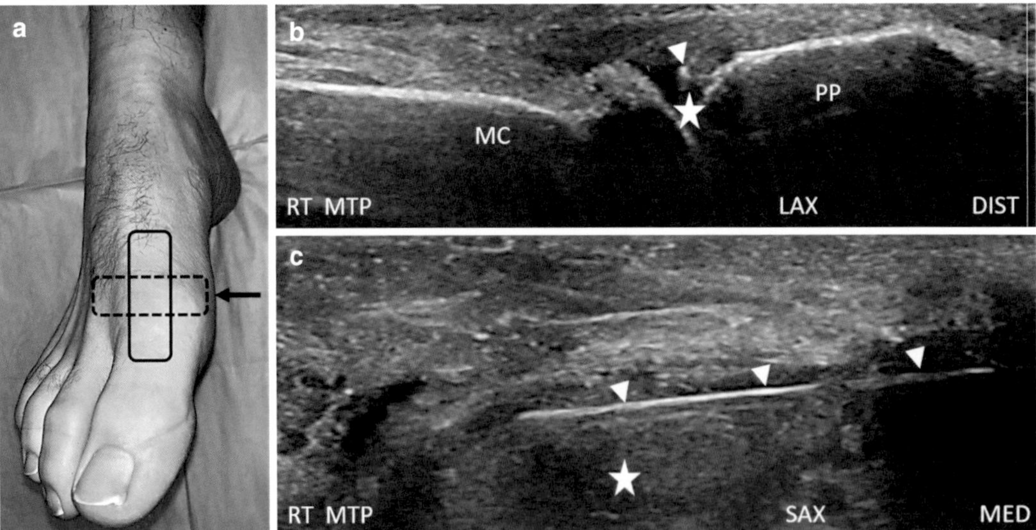

Fig. 10.6 Ultrasound-guided metatarsophalangeal joint injection. (**a**) External view of the right (RT) foot demonstrating Td placement and needle direction (*solid arrow*) for out-of-plane (*solid rectangle*) and in-plane (*dotted rectangle*) medial-to-lateral approach to injecting the first metatarsophalangeal (MTP) joint. (**b**) USG correlate of an out-of-plane medial-to-lateral approach showing a hyperechoic needle tip (*arrowhead*) within the MTP joint (*star*). (**c**) USG correlate of an in-plane approach showing a hyperechoic needle (*arrowheads*) within the MTP joint (*star*). *MC* metacarpal, *PP* proximal phalanx, *MED* medial, *DIST* distal

Approaches

Posteromedial

The patient is in the lateral recumbent position, with involved extremity towards the table and contralateral side bent out of the way. The US Td is placed in the anatomic coronal plane giving a short-axis view of the subtalar joint, overlying the talus and calcaneus. The at-risk tibial artery, nerve, and vein should be noted prior to injection, with needle trajectory adjusted appropriately. The needle is then advanced anterior to posterior in a walk-down technique from superficial to deep, to a position within the subtalar joint (Fig. 10.7a, b).

Anterolateral

The patient is in the lateral recumbent position, with involved side further from the table. The US Td is placed in the anatomic sagittal plane, visualizing the calcaneus, talus, and fibula. The location of the at-risk peroneal tendons should be noted prior to injection. The needle is then advanced anterior to posterior in a walk-down technique from superficial to deep, to a position within the subtalar joint (Fig. 10.8a, b).

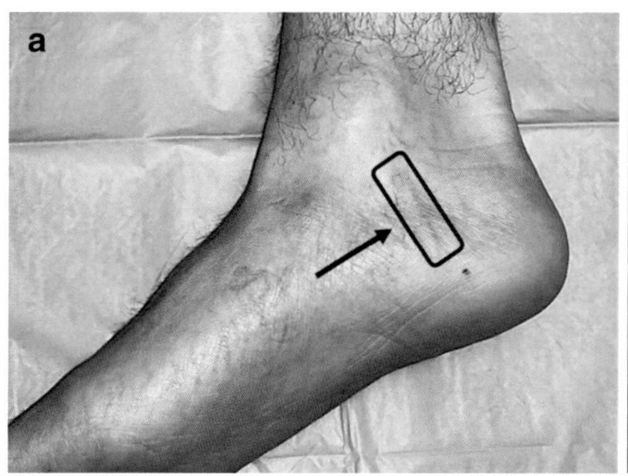

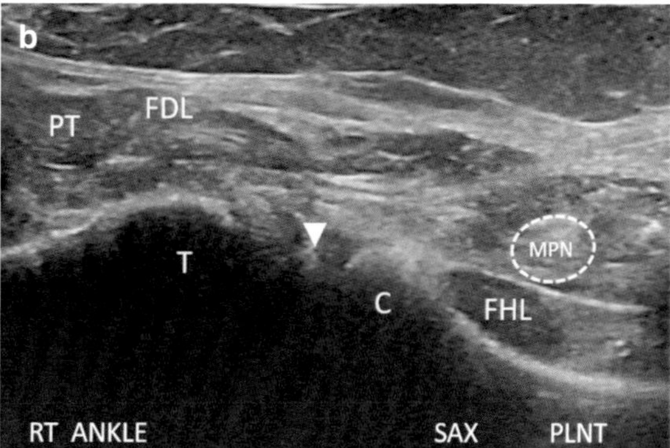

Fig. 10.7 Ultrasound-guided posteromedial subtalar joint injection. (**a**) External photo showing transducer (Td) and needle (*solid arrow*) placement for out-of-plane injection of the right (*RT*) posteromedial subtalar joint from a distal to proximal direction. (**b**) USG correlate showing a hyperechoic needle tip (*arrowhead*) within the subtalar joint via an out-of-plane approach. Note the location of the medial plantar nerve (*MPN*) just plantar (*PLNT*) to the posteromedial subtalar joint as well as the adjacent posterior tibialis (*PT*), flexor digitorum longus (*FDL*), and flexor hallucis longus (*FHL*) tendons. *SAX* short axis, *T* talus, *C* calcaneus

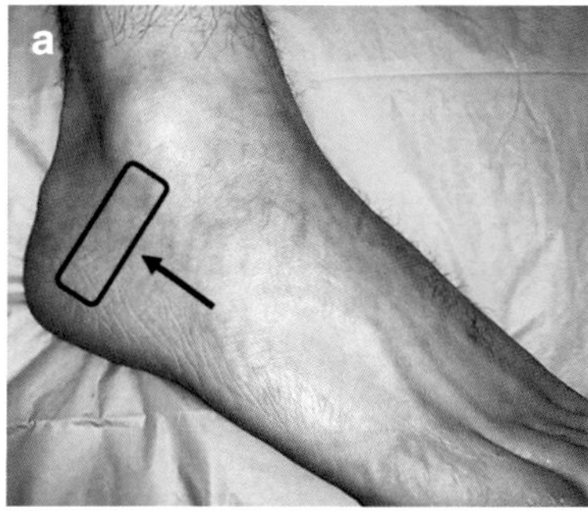

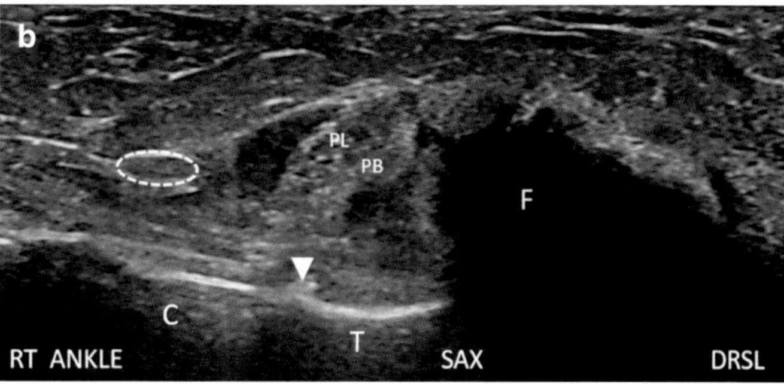

Fig. 10.8 Ultrasound-guided anterolateral subtalar joint injection. (**a**) External photo showing transducer (*solid rectangle*) and needle (*solid arrow*) placement for out-of-plane injection of the right (*RT*) anterolateral subtalar joint from a distal to proximal direction. (**b**) USG correlate showing a hyperechoic needle tip (*arrowhead*) within the subtalar joint via an out-of-plane approach. Note the location of the sural nerve (*dotted arrow*) just plantar to the anterolateral subtalar joint as well as the peroneus brevis (*PB*) and peroneus longs (*PL*) tendons. *SAX* short axis, *F* fibula, *T* talus, *C* calcaneus, *DRSL* dorsal

Interventional Procedures: Soft Tissue Structures – Regenerative Introduction

Tendinopathy has been well established to be less of an inflammatory response and more of a chronic degradation of the tendon, with pathophysiology consisting of degenerative microtearing, collagen fiber disorganization, hypercellularity, and angiofibroblastic hyperplasia of the tendon proper [41]. Chronic tendinopathies affect approximately ten million patients per year, requiring frequent physician visits and a large economic health burden [42, 43]. Often despite months of extensive conservative treatment such as rest, activity modification, physical therapy, oral and topical medications, and orthotics and/or bracing, more advanced treatment options such as injections and surgery are sought for pain relief [42, 43]. Traditionally, corticosteroid injections are offered as the next step in the treatment approach. However, as more evidence emerges revealing potential harms of corticosteroids on soft tissues such as risk of tendon rupture and fat pad atrophy, physicians are turning to other injectable options such as prolotherapy, autologous blood products, or placental-derived products; needle tenotomy with or without orthobiologic injectate; and neovessel ablation [44–50]. The current literature has not revealed the most effective regenerative treatment option but is more consistently demonstrating that a combination approach with an injection plus rehabilitation may be more effective than either alone [51, 52].

Plantar Fascia: Regenerative Evidence

Plantar fasciopathy (PF) is an extremely painful condition classically causing pain with the first few steps out of bed but can persist throughout the day limiting one's function and quality of life [53]. It affects approximately two million people per year with a lifetime prevalence of 10% [53]. Although considered a fascia or aponeurosis, the pathophysiology is thought of as the same as tendinopathies such as Achilles tendinopathy. Rather than an inflammatory issue, microscopic analyses have supported a chronic degenerative process with disruption of collagen matrix, fiber disorganization, microscopic tears, and abnormal blood flow zones [54, 55]. Typical conservative management includes rest, activity modification, stretching, heel cups or orthotics, night splints, immobilization, physical therapy, shock wave therapy, ice, and oral anti-inflammatories. While about 80–90% of patients improve within 9 months of symptom onset, over 10% of patients develop recalcitrant chronic plantar fasciopathy and corticosteroid injections or surgery has been the traditional next step [55, 56]. In refractory cases, surgery with either an open or endoscopic approach has been described with success rates of 67–82% reported in the literature [57, 58]. Surgical release has also demonstrated alteration of the "windlass mechanism" with increased stress risers on the ligaments and bones of the midfoot and forefoot [55]. Emerging treatment options with hopefully fewer adverse effects include regenerative injections such as PRP or prolotherapy and USG tenotomy/fasciotomy [59].

Platelet-Rich Plasma

Many recent studies have compared PRP injection against the more traditional CS injection for chronic PF. At least four trials have demonstrated that a single injection of PRP or CS for chronic PF results in significantly reduced pain and improved function at 3 months [54, 55, 60]. CS typically has similar to slightly superior short-term results as compared to PRP. However, at 12 months, a single injection of PRP results in significantly improved outcomes than CS, while patients receiving CS typically return near baseline [54, 55, 61, 62]. Jimenez-Perez et al. compared two injections of LR-PRP versus CS and found significantly improved pain scores and functional scores at 6 and 12 months, and this effect was sustained in even longer follow-up [56]. Additionally, it was noted that at least 90% of the PRP group at 6 and 12 months had good or excellent outcomes, whereas only 15% of the CS group had good outcomes at 6 months and 0% at 12 months [56]. Tabrizi et al. evaluated 3 weekly injections of PRP versus a single CS injection in obese patients with PF and found that both groups had a better foot function score but CSI had better pain score at 24 weeks [63]. Of note, this study did not restrict oral anti-inflammatory use which is typically considered standard protocol to avoid interference with the PRP's action [64, 65]. The studies used a variety of PRP injectate volumes ranging from 2 ml to 6 ml with variable volumes of anesthetic if used. Most studies implemented a needle tenotomy "peppering" technique with a single skin portal site. Overall, a vast majority of studies support that one to two injections of PRP for chronic PF are as effective as CS at 3 months and have a more durable effect than CS at 1 year [61, 62].

Despite the successes of the abovementioned studies, these studies are not without their limitations. Foremost, most lack a placebo control. There is significant variability among study methods including the PRP composition, injectate volume, injection frequency, and injection approach. Most of the abovementioned studies involve landmark-guided injections rather than USG injections, and it has been suggested that USG injections result in more reliable and successful outcomes [38, 66]. Before drawing conclusions about the effectiveness of PRP to other treatments for reducing pain and improving function in patients with chronic PF, higher-quality RCTs with larger sample sizes are needed. Additionally, it would be beneficial to have RCTs comparing different PRP preparations and applications to determine the most effective PRP composition, volume of injectate, and frequency of injections for chronic PF to improve consistency among comparison trials with other interventions.

Amniotic Membrane Derivatives

Dehydrated human amnion/chorion membrane (dHACM) products have been studied in only a few trials for the treatment of chronic plantar fasciitis. A 2013 feasibility study performed in 45 patients with refractory PF demonstrated that a landmark-guided, single injection of reconstituted dHACM yielded a significant improvement in symptoms at 1 week and at the 8-week study end period as compared to a saline injection [67]. They also assessed different volumes of dHACM injectate and found no difference between 0.5 cc and 1.25 cc [67]. In 2018, Cazzell et al. performed a multicenter study comparing a landmark-guided, single injection of 1 mL micronized dHACM versus 1 ml 0.9% sodium chloride placebo performed in 73 and 72 heels, respectively [68]. The intervention group yielded significantly lower pain scores and improved function scores at a 3-month follow-up [68]. Additionally, they assessed longer-term (12-month) safety, and only three adverse events were considered possibly related to the dHACM product – two cases of postinjection pain at injection site and one case of postinjection itching [68]. Based on so few studies, it is difficult at this time to draw a conclusion on the use of AM derivatives for the treatment of refractory PF.

Prolotherapy

In 2018, Ersen et al. compared three USG prolotherapy (15% dextrose with lidocaine solution) injections with a non-injection, rehabilitation control [69]. A significant improvement in pain and function was achieved in both groups during follow-up, with inter-group comparisons demonstrating superior results in the prolotherapy group at a 42- and 90-day follow-up [69]. At 360 days, there was no significant difference between the two groups [69]. Furthermore, 77% of the treatment group reported good and excellent results, whereas only 17% of the treatment group reported these outcomes [69]. A study by Mansiz-Kaplan et al. demonstrated clinical improvement from prolotherapy as compared to placebo injection in 65 patients with chronic PF [70]. The study included administration of 15% dextrose solution or saline solution two times at 3-week intervals and demonstrated statistically significant superior improvement in the prolotherapy group at a 7- and 15-week follow-up [70]. Kim et al. in 2014 performed a comparison of two USG prolotherapy (15% dextrose/lidocaine solution) versus PRP injections for chronic PF and found that each treatment was effective for improving pain, disability, and activity limitations [71].

In a study comparing USG CS, extracorporeal shockwave therapy (ESWT), PRP, and prolotherapy in 158 patients with chronic PF, CS was most effective in the first 3 months, ESWT is effective in the first 6 months for pain, whereas PRP and prolotherapy effects were seen within 3–12 months [72]. At a 36-month follow-up, no differences were found among the four treatments [72].

Similar to the overall concerns with the PRP research, the prolotherapy investigations have significant variety in terms of volume of injectate and frequency of repeated injections, making comparison between treatments quite challenging. Overall, the studies suggest that prolotherapy is a safe and effective treatment in the short to medium term for chronic PF.

Regenerative Technique: Ultrasound-Guided Plantar Fascia Procedures

Positioning

- Patient: lateral recumbent with treatment side on table and pillow between knees, to facilitate an in-plane medial-to-lateral approach (Fig. 10.9a)
- Provider: seated with US screen directly in front of line of sight

Td Type

- High-frequency linear array

Needle

- Anesthetic: Author's preferred technique is to perform an USG tibial nerve block at the level of the tarsal tunnel with 5–10 ml of local anesthetic ensuring that the medial and lateral plantar and medial calcaneal nerves are adequately encircled with anesthetic solution. Most commonly, USG is used to direct a 27- or 25-gauge, 38 mm needle via a posterior-to-anterior approach adjacent to the tibial nerve complex.
- Additional local anesthetic solution is kept in reserve for local anesthesia of the skin or subcutaneous tissue if the nerve block was not 100% effective.

Approach

- In our experience, the medial-to-lateral approach is easiest to perform as it creates stability of the treatment limb and allows easy manipulation of the needle during performance of the procedure. Furthermore, this prevents the need to puncture the plantar surface of the foot which theoretically increases the risk of infection as well as fat pad atrophy.

Regenerative Medicine/Orthobiologic Injection With or Without Fenestration

Needle: 18–21 gauge, 38–50 mm

Injection Volume: 3–5 mL orthobiologic injectate

Approaches

Medial to Lateral, in-Plane with Td

We recommend the patient is positioned in the previously mentioned lateral recumbent position with the provider seated at the foot of the bed facing the plantar aspect of the foot and US machine. The orthobiologic is typically injected along with fenestration (repeated passing of the needle through the diseased tissue), approximately 15–20 passes. Orthogonal long- and short-axis views can be used to assure proper position of needle and injectate (Fig. 10.9b, c).

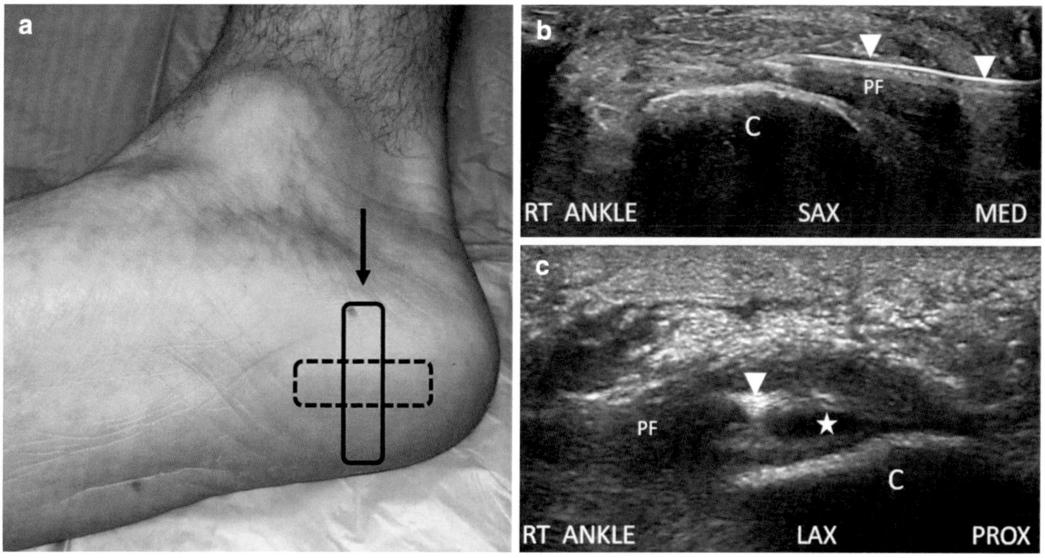

Fig. 10.9 Ultrasound-guided plantar fascia injection. (**a**) External view of the right (RT) foot demonstrating Td placement and needle direction (*solid arrow*) for an in-plane (*solid rectangle*) and out-of-plane (*dotted rectangle*), medial-to-lateral approach to injecting the plantar fascia (*PF*). (**b**) USG correlate of an in-plane, medial-to-lateral approach showing a hyperechoic needle (*arrowheads*) within the central band of the PF. (**c**) USG correlate of an out-of-plane, medial-to-lateral approach showing a hyperechoic needle tip (*arrowhead*) within the central band of the PF with large partial thickness tear (*star*). *C* calcaneus

Achilles Tendon: Introduction

Chronic midportion Achilles tendinopathy (AT) is a common overload injury most commonly seen in running and jumping athletes, affecting 7–9% of active runners [73]. Despite its high incidence, there remains no gold standard in management. This likely reflects a poor understanding of the true pain generator(s) which requires a more comprehensive treatment approach. Based on imaging and histologic analyses, it is believed that chronic overload results in ingrowth of new vessels with associated nerve endings (neurovascularization), intra-tendinous microtears, and chronic degeneration [74, 75, 76]. The most commonly diseased portion of the Achilles tendon is the hypovascular midportion, located about 2–7 cm proximal to the insertion on the calcaneus [75, 76].

Typically, chronic AT has been managed with overload reduction and rehabilitation including progressive tendon loading via eccentric exercises and more recently heavy-slow exercises, along with analgesics, anti-inflammatories, ice, manual therapy, and correction of biomechanics when appropriate [48, 73, 74]. For recalcitrant cases, options may include injection therapy, shock wave therapy, and surgery [76, 77]. Examples of current interventional treatment options include high-volume injection (HVI) or tendon scraping with neovessel ablation, intratendinous platelet-rich plasma (PRP) injection, needle tenotomy, and ultrasonic tenotomy [73, 77–80].

To date, there is no study comparing the efficacy of different treatment options, and therefore no definitive superior method. Therefore, decision on technique remains a personalized decision based on unique patient factors, imaging findings, and provider expertise/comfort level. Despite lack of strong evidence for the modality, a study by Boesen et al. in 2017 demonstrated superiority of the combined effect of injection therapy with progressive eccentric tendon loading compared to either performed independently [73]. This suggests that a comprehensive approach is prudent for patients with chronic AT.

Ultrasound-Guided Achilles Tendon Procedures

Achilles Tendon Injection Technique

Positioning

- Patient: prone position with the feet dangling off the edge of the bed/table (Fig. 10.10a)
- Provider: seated with US screen directly in front of line of sight

Td Type

- High-frequency linear array

Needle

Anesthetic: A 25-gauge 50 mm needle is used to deliver local anesthetic via a preferred medial-to-lateral USG approach

Approaches

Lateral to medial or medial to lateral dependent on the location of the sural nerve.

The needle (18–21 gauge, 38–50 mm) is directed via USG either in-plane or out-of-plane to the Td while fenestrating the diseased portion of the tendon and injecting the orthobiologic or prolotherapy solution (Fig. 10.10b).

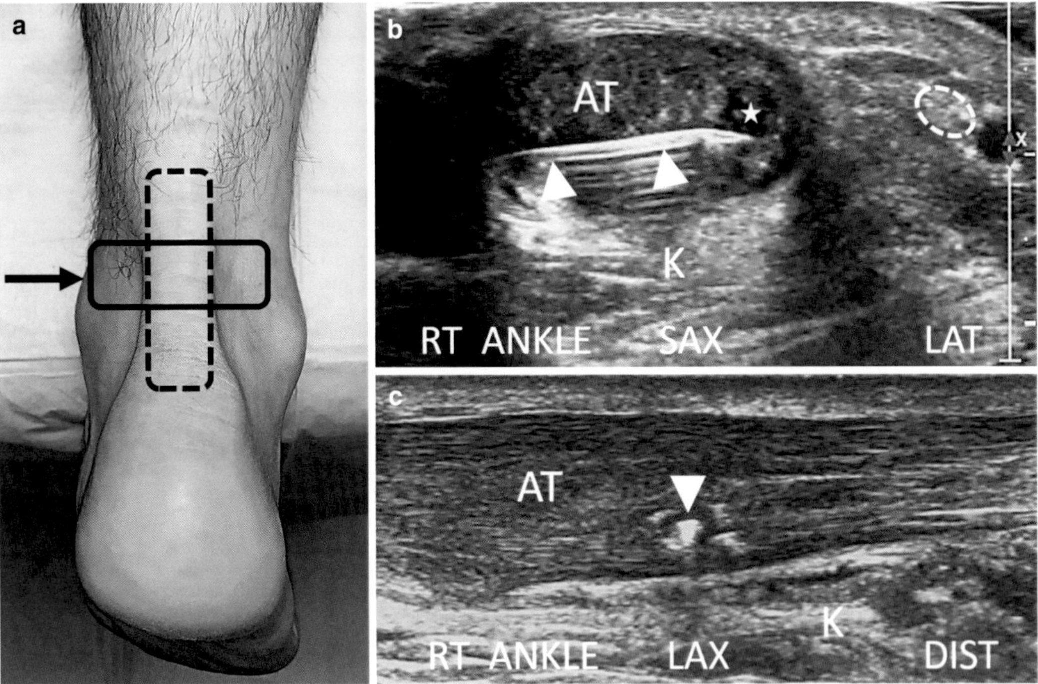

Fig. 10.10 Ultrasound-guided Achilles tendon injection. (**a**) External view of the right (RT) ankle demonstrating Td placement and needle direction (*solid arrow*) for an in-plane (*solid rectangle*) and out-of-plane (*dotted rectangle*), medial-to-lateral approach to injecting the Achilles tendon (*AT*). (**b**) USG correlate of an in-plane, medial-to-lateral approach showing a hyperechoic needle (*arrowheads*) within a partial thickness intra-substance tear (*star*) of the AT. Note the location of the sural nerve (*dotted circle*) just lateral to the Achilles tendon. (**c**) USG correlate of an out-of-plane, medial-to-lateral approach showing a hyperechoic needle tip (*arrowhead*) within the AT. *Lax* long axis, *DIST* distal, *LAT* lateral, *K* Kager's fat pad

Achilles Tendon Neovessel Ablation: High-Volume Injection and Tendon Scraping

Background: With the idea of reduction/ablation of neovessel formation for pain relief from chronic AT, tendon scraping and high-volume paratenon stripping has been suggested as possible treatment avenue for mid-substance AT. Maffulli et al. performed HVI using 10 ml of 0.5% bupivacaine hydrochloride, 25 mg aprotinin, and up to 40 ml of injectable normal saline in a series of 94 athletes with recalcitrant midportion Achilles tendinopathy and showed improved VISA-A scores from baseline 41.7 ± 23.2 to 74.6 ± 21.4 by 12 months [78]. A randomized, placebo-controlled trial by Boesen et al. compared the effectiveness of HVI plus eccentrics, PRP plus eccentrics, and eccentrics alone in 58 middle-aged men with chronic midportion AT [73]. After 12 weeks of the intervention, the injection groups proved more effective in reducing pain symptoms, improving activity level and function, and reducing tendon thickness and intra-tendinous vascularity than eccentric rehabilitation alone [73]. In the short term (6 and 12 weeks), HVI appeared more effective at improving pain, function, and patient satisfaction than PRP, but both had similar outcomes in the long term (24 weeks) [73]. Additionally, HVI only required one injection, whereas the PRP group underwent multiple injections [73].

Hakan Alfredson was the first to demonstrate that neovessel ablation "tendon scraping" technique resulted in decreased pain and improved function in patients with AT [48]. Good results with interval reduction in pain with both open and USG percutaneous neovessel ablation techniques for midportion AT were reported [48]. The same group demonstrated good long-term (2–13 years) clinical outcomes with high satisfaction rates in 241 tendons following the same technique, suggesting that neovessel ablation is a safe and effective treatment for chronic AT [74].

Ultrasound-Guided Achilles Tendon Neovessel Ablation (Scraping) with HVI

Positioning

- Patient: prone position with the feet dangling off the edge of the bed/table (Fig. 10.11a)
- Provider: seated with US screen directly in front of line of sight

Td Type

- High-frequency linear array

Needle

- Anesthetic: A 25-gauge 50 mm needle is used to deliver local anesthetic via a preferred medial-to-lateral USG approach.

Approach

- In general, a medial-to-lateral approach is preferred to avoid the superficial and more posterior (relative to tibial nerve) located sural nerve.
- During procedure – Regardless of approach, the use of orthogonal long- and short-axis views (relative to tendon and device) should be utilized to ensure device location, thus avoiding injury to the respective sural and tibial nerves.

Procedure

Once a decision is made on the approach, a 25-gauge, 50 mm needle is used to anesthetize the skin, Kager's fat pad, and paratenon of the Achilles tendon in the region of abnormality. Using a fanning technique under USG 5–10 ml of local anesthetic, with or without epinephrine, is used to ensure the region is adequately anesthetized. A small stab incision is made with a #11 blade and a dual-bladed meniscotome is introduced through the incision with USG via the same medial-to-lateral approach deep to the ten-

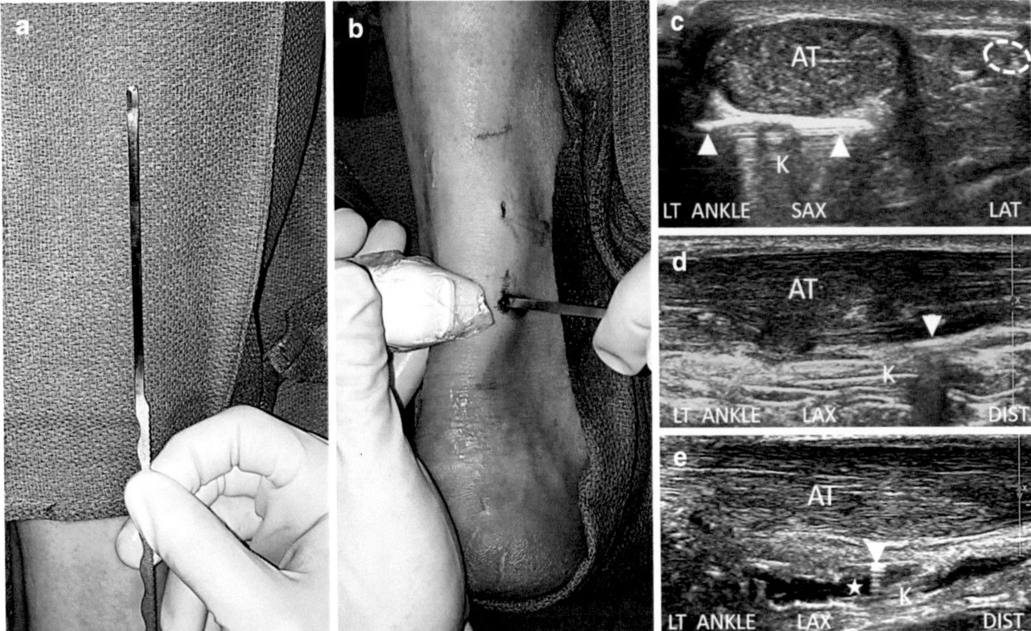

Fig. 10.11 Ultrasound-guided Achilles tendon neovessel ablation (scraping) and high-volume injection. (**a**) Single-use dual-bladed meniscotome. (**b**) External view of the left (LT) ankle demonstrating Td placement and meniscotome insertion via a medial-to-lateral approach for neovessel ablation (tendon scraping) procedure. Note a #11 blade was used to create a stab incision for introduction of the meniscotome. In this patient, the area of pathology required two incision points. (**c**) USG correlate of an in-plane, medial-to-lateral approach showing a hyperechoic meniscotome (*arrowheads*) between the Achilles tendon (AT) and Kager's (*K*) fat pad. Note the location of the sural nerve (*dotted circle*) just lateral to the Achilles tendon. (**d**) USG correlate of an out-of-plane, medial-to-lateral approach showing a hyperechoic meniscotome (*arrowhead*) between the AT and K for tendon scraping procedure. The meniscotome is then toggled distal to proximal to scrape the bottom of the tendon, separating it from Kager's fat pad. (**e**) USG image of a hyperechoic needle tip (*arrowhead*) between the AT and K performing a high-volume injection. Notice the separation of the K from the AT as the injectate (*star*) is injected. *LAX* long axis, *SAX* short axis, *DIST* distal, *LAT* lateral

don between Kager's fat pad and the Achilles tendon. Alternatively, an 18-gauge, 50–89 mm hypodermic needle or a 16-gauge, 38 mm Nokor needle (Becton, Dickinson and Company, Franklin Lakes, New Jersey) may be used for this technique if preferred. Following US confirmation of correct placement, a proximal-to-distal sweeping motion is used to separate the fat pad from the tendon. Once a separation plane is created with the needle, the meniscotome is withdrawn and an 18-gauge 50 mm needle is introduced with USG through the incision. Subsequently, 20–40 mL of 0.9% NS sterile 0.9% normal saline is injected to hydrodissect the fat pad away from the tendon (Fig. 10.11a–e). Orthogonal short- and long-axis views are used to continually confirm correct placement and complete hydrodissection. Care must be taken throughout the procedure to ensure the tip of the needle does not pass too far (lateral or medial) as to avoid injury to the respective sural or tibial nerves.

Achilles Tendon Intra-tendinous Platelet-Rich Plasma (PRP) Injection with or Without Needle Tenotomy

Background: The application of PRP injections for chronic AT has been used clinically to treat chronic AT despite inconsistent evidence for its efficacy in clinical studies. The heterogeneity in preparation of PRP, volume of injectate, number of injections, and postinjection protocol makes comparing studies a challenge. A 2018 meta-analysis of four level 1 randomized controlled trials involving a total of 170 participants (85 treated with PRP injection and eccentric training and 85 treated with saline injection and eccentric training) found no significant difference in outcomes between the two groups at a 1-year follow-up [81]. A 2019 meta-analysis of five RCTs including a total of 189 patients with chronic AT concluded the same [82]. Boesen et al. was the first randomized placebo-controlled trial to demonstrate PRP in combination with eccentric training program had a positive effect when compared with the sham treatment [73]. In this study, 19 tendons were treated with four injections of PRP at 2-week intervals, whereas the other studies performed only one injection, possibly indicating more injections may be superior. Additionally, the recovery and rehabilitation differed from prior studies with early return to eccentric exercises after 10 days rather than 4–6 weeks in other investigations [82]. Further studies with consistent protocols are needed to further support or refute the use of PRP injection for chronic mid-portion AT.

Key Recommendations

- Anesthetizing the periphery of the tendon can help to reduce pain with the procedure.
- Consider performing the neovessel ablation/hydrodissection along with Achilles tendon procedures to address the neovessel formation.
- Location of the at-risk sural nerve and tibial nerves (particularly the medial calcaneal branch) should be noted prior to any procedure about the Achilles tendon.
- In general, a medial-to-lateral approach is preferred to avoid the neurovascular structures.
- During procedure – Regardless of approach, the use of orthogonal long- and short-axis views (relative to tendon and device) should be utilized to ensure device location, thus avoiding injury to the respective sural and tibial nerves.

Tendon Sheath Injections: Regenerative Evidence

Non-Achilles ankle tendinopathies may involve the PTT, anterior tibialis (AT), peroneus longus (PL) and/or brevis (PB), and FHL [83]. The pathology is generally accepted to be that of intra-tendinous microtears and chronic degeneration of the tendon proper, similar to other described tendinopathies [84]. Management of such tendinopathies is similar to the aforementioned Achilles and plantar fasciopathy with a trial of conservative management such as activity modification, immobilization, stretching, oral and topical medications, bracing and orthotics, and physical therapy [84, 85]. Refractory cases such as PTT tendon dysfunction with a rigid adult-acquired flatfoot deformity may progress to surgical fixation [86].

There is a paucity of literature for regenerative treatment options for non-Achilles ankle tendinopathies. Currently, only case reports and small case studies exist for these specific tendon disorders. Angthong et al. assessed the outcomes of PRP injections for four cases of PTT tendinopathy and noted improvement in pain scores but not for SF-36 scores [87]. Finnoff et al. reported USG needle tenotomy and platelet-rich plasma injection resulted in improvements in functional scores and tendon appearance on 31 subjects with lower extremity tendinopathies, including one patient with PTT tendinopathy [88]. Mautner et al. reported on 180 patients with chronic tendinopathy, 1 involving the posterior tibialis, 2 peroneus brevis, and 3 peroneus longus tendons, with 95% of patients reporting no pain at rest and 68% reporting no pain with activities [89]. Oloff and Lam documented successful treatment of PTT in a soccer player with PRP, with improved post-procedure imaging and full return to soccer at 31 weeks [90].

Given the scarcity of data on orthobiologics for less common tendinopathies about the foot and ankle, outcomes regarding these treatments remain unclear.

Posterior Tibial, Achilles, and Peroneal Tendon Injection Technique

Positioning

- Patient (varies depending on the tendon being treated)
  - Anterior tibialis – supine with the ankle in relaxed position
  - Posterior tibialis – lateral recumbent with treatment side on the table
  - Peroneal tendons – lateral recumbent with treatment side up
- Provider: seated with US screen directly in front of line of sight

Td Type

- High-frequency linear array

Needle

- Anesthetic: 25 to 22 gauge, 38 mm
- Procedure: 21 to 18 gauge, 38 mm

Injection Volume

- Anesthetic: 1–2 mL 1% lidocaine
- Orthobiologic injectate: 1–3 mL

Approaches: Posterior Tibialis Tendon

Posterior to Anterior, in-Plane with Td

With the patient in lateral recumbent position with the affected limb on the table and a pillow between the knees, the Td is placed short axis to the tendon in the anatomic axial plane. If needle tenotomy is planned, a tibial nerve block may be performed as documented in the "Plantar Fascia" section above and can be performed prior to a local anesthetic along the target tendon. Following decision adequate anesthesia, the needle is advanced from an anterior to posterior direction, in-plane with the Td, until confirmed in the tendon sheath (Fig. 10.12a, b). Although a posterior approach can be undertaken, the anterior approach is preferred to avoid the tibial neurovascular bundle. Furthermore, the medial malleolus may be used as a bony backstop for the needle.

Tibialis Anterior Tendon

Medial to Lateral, in-Plane with Td

The patient is lateral recumbent with the affected limb on top and pillow between the knees. If needle tenotomy is planned, a fibular nerve block or local anesthetic injection can be performed prior. After anesthetic, the Td is placed short axis to the tendon over the region of primary pathology. The needle is advanced from a posterior to anterior direction, in-plane with the Td, until confirmed within the tendon sheath. This allows the lateral malleolus to be used as a bony backstop.

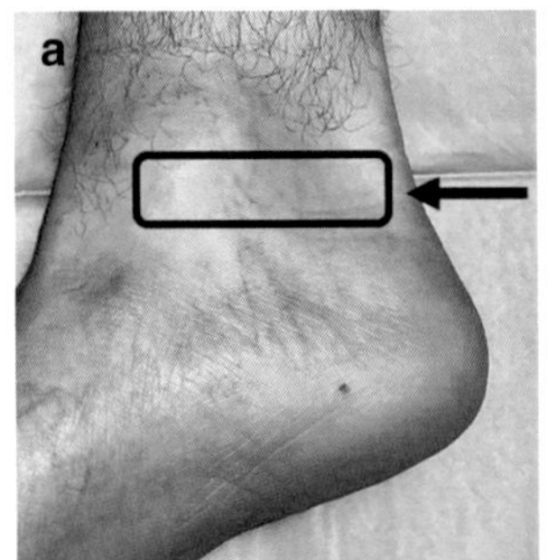

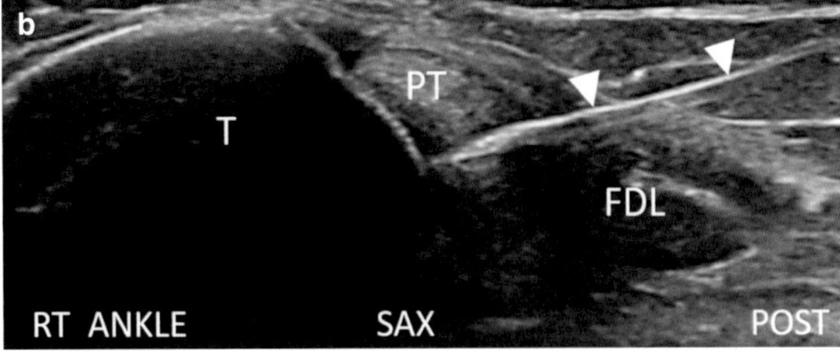

Fig. 10.12 Ultrasound-guided posterior tibialis tendon injection. (**a**) External view of the right (RT) ankle demonstrating Td placement (*solid rectangle*) and needle direction (*solid arrow*) for an in-plane posterior-to-anterior approach to injecting the posterior tibialis (*PT*) tendon. (**b**) USG correlate of an in-plane, posterior-to-anterior approach showing a hyperechoic needle (*arrowheads*) within the PT tendon sheath. *SAX* short axis, *POST* posterior

Peroneus Longus and Brevis Tendon

Posterior to Anterior, in-Plane with Td

The patient is in the lateral decubitus with the lateral ankle of interest superior. The ankle is slightly inverted and plantarflexed, using a towel roll as needed for optimal patient comfort and procedure visualization. The physician sits distal, facing the foot/patient. The Td is placed short axis to the tendon at the retro-malleolar groove as the tendons share a common synovial sheath at this level. The needle is advanced from a posterior to anterior direction, in-plane with the Td, until confirmed within the tendon sheath, taking care to avoid the sural nerve which should be just posterior to the tendons at this level.

Ligament Injections: Regenerative Evidence

Acute ankle sprains account for around 15% of sports-related injuries among collegiate athletes, with rates as high as 3.85 per 1000 basketball players [91, 92]. The majority (up to 60.5–90%) of ankle sprains involve the lateral ligament complex, 73% of which involve the anterior talofibular ligament (ATFL) [93–95]. Syndesmotic "high ankle" sprains involving the anterior inferior tibiofibular ligament (AITFL) and/or medial ankle sprains involving the deltoid ligament complex occur less frequently but often requiring a prolonged treatment course compared to lateral ankle sprains [93–96]. Lateral ankle sprains have a high rate of recurrence and chronic ankle instability. A study of athletes from 25 NCAA sports over 6 academic years found that 1 in 8 lateral ligamentous complex sprains was recurrent [95]. A 7-year follow-up study of patients after an acute inversion ankle sprain found that 212 (32%) of patients reported ongoing ankle disability [97].

Studies to evaluate the effectiveness of orthobiologic interventions on pain reduction and functional improvement after acute ankle sprains are limited and with mixed results. To the best of the authors' knowledge, there are no available studies for the treatment of chronic ankle instability. A 2014 study by Laver et al. was one of the first to report on PRP use for ankle sprains, and they compared two ultrasound-guided PRP injections (separated by 7 days) followed by a rehabilitation program versus rehabilitation alone for grade 3 AITFL injuries [98]. This resulted in a statistically significant earlier return to play (40.8 versus 59.6 days) and improved pain scores in the PRP group. Another study of PRP injections for syndesmotic injuries found that a single ultrasound-guided PRP injection into the AITFL tear resulted in earlier return to play as compared to a historical cohort (48.6 vs. 69.3 days) [99]. A 2015 randomized placebo-controlled trial failed to show a statistical difference in pain or function following a single, ultrasound-guided injection of 3–4 cc of PRP for patients with acute ankle sprains (details of sprain not included in study details) presenting to the emergency department at 3, 8, and 30 days' assessments [100]. A 2019 randomized controlled trial by Blanco-Rivera et al. compared rigid immobilization followed by a rehabilitation protocol with or without a single, landmark-guided 5 ml PRP injection into the ATFL for patients presenting to the emergency department within 48 hours of a grade 2 ankle sprain [101]. Although similar outcomes at 24 weeks, the PRP group demonstrated significant improvements in pain and American Orthopedic Foot and Ankle Scores (AOFAS) at earlier assessment points (3, 5, and 8 weeks) [101]. These studies have numerous limitations, including a small patient population, variable procedure techniques, and relatively short follow-up.

One retrospective observational study reported on the use of prolotherapy for chronic ankle pain and showed favorable outcomes [102]. The authors performed on average 4.4 treatment sessions of 20–30 injections of 0.5–1 cc of a 15% dextrose, 0.2% lidocaine solution around the ankle at areas of tenderness. At least 50% improvement in pain was reported in 90% of patients, and 78% reported full resolution of pain and stiffness.

Anterior Talofibular Ligament and Anterior Inferior Tibiofibular Ligament PRP Injection Techniques

Positioning

- Patient: lateral recumbent with treatment side up
- Provider: seated with US screen directly in front of line of sight

Td Type

- High-frequency linear array

Needle

- Procedure: 21 gauge, 38 mm

Injection Volume

- Orthobiologic injectate: 1–2 mL

Approaches

Anterior Talofibular Ligament

Distal to Proximal, in-Plane with Td

The patient is lateral recumbent with the affected limb on top and pillow between the knees. Anesthetic is often not necessary given superficial position of the ligament and to prevent inhibitory interaction with the orthobiologic. The Td is placed long axis to the ligament, with a gel standoff to improve access to the ligament and visualization of the needle. The needle is advanced from a distal to proximal direction, in-plane with the Td, until confirmed within the edematous ligament or at site of ligament tear.

Anterior Inferior Tibiofibular Ligament

Medial to Lateral, in-Plane with Td

The patient is either supine or in lateral recumbent with the affected limb on top and pillow between the knees (Fig. 10.13a). The ankle should be placed in slight plantarflexion to improve access. Anesthetic is often not necessary given superficial position of the ligament and to

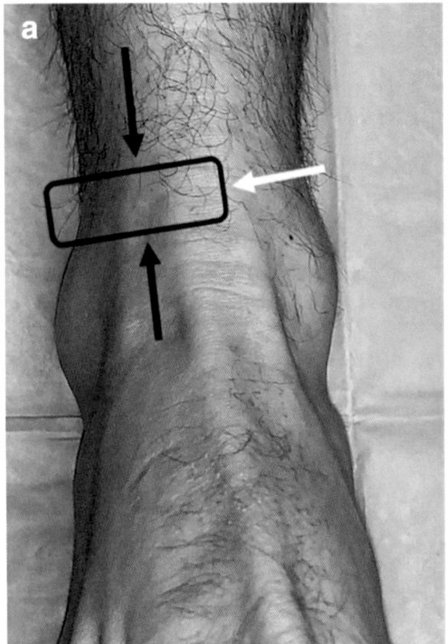

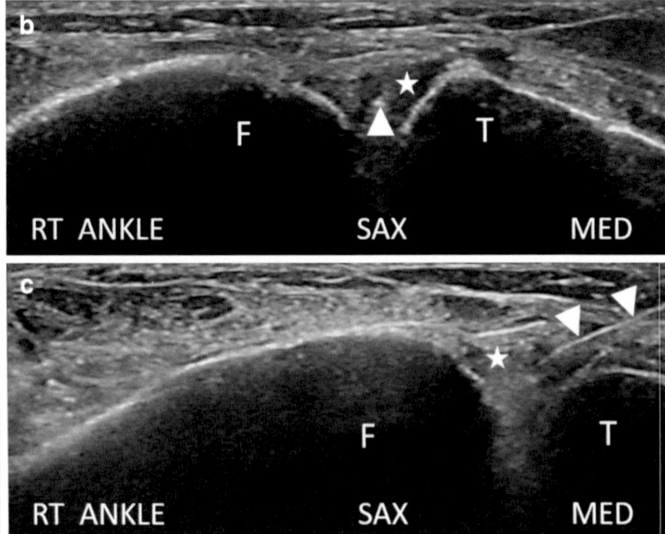

Fig. 10.13 Ultrasound-guided anterior inferior tibiofibular ligament injection. (**a**) External view of the right (RT) ankle demonstrating Td placement (*solid rectangle*) and needle direction for an out-of-plane (*black arrow*) *and* in-plane (*white arrow*) anterior inferior tibiofibular ligament injection. (**b**) USG correlate, with medial (MED) to the right, showing an out-of-plane, distal-to-proximal or proximal-to-distal approach of a hyperechoic needle tip (*arrowhead*) within the ligament (*star*). (**c**) USG correlate of an in-plane, medial-to-lateral approach showing a hyperechoic needle (*arrowheads*) within the ligament (*star*). *SAX* short axis, *F* fibula, *T* tibia

prevent inhibitory interaction with the orthobiologic. The Td is placed long axis to the ligament, with a gel standoff to improve access to the ligament and visualization of the needle. The needle is advanced from a medial to lateral direction, in-plane with the Td, until confirmed within the edematous AITFL or at site of ligament tear (Fig. 10.13b).

Distal to Proximal, Out-of-Plane with Td

Alternatively, with the AITFL imaged in long axis, the needle can be advanced using an out-of-plane, walk-down technique from superficial to deep, to a position within the desired portion of the injured ligament (Fig. 10.13c).

Deltoid Ligament

Anterior to Posterior, Out-of-Plane with Td

The patient is in lateral recumbent with the affected limb on the table (Fig. 10.14a). Anesthetic is often not necessary given superficial position of the ligament and to prevent inhibitory interaction with the orthobiologic. The Td is placed long axis to the ligament. The needle is advanced from an *anterior to posterior* direction, out-of-plane with the Td, until confirmed within the edematous deltoid ligament or at site of ligament tear (Fig. 10.14b).

Anterior to Posterior, in-Plane with Td

Alternatively, with the deltoid ligament imaged in short axis, the needle can be advanced using an in-plane approach from anterior to posterior, to a position within the desired portion of the injured ligament (Fig. 10.14c).

Post-procedure Rehabilitation Protocol

There is no consensus on post-procedure rehabilitation protocols nor activity limitations following any of the aforementioned procedures. Post-procedure activity limitations and weight-bearing status are largely driven by expert opinion and tolerance of the activity by individual patient factors. It is the authors' general practice

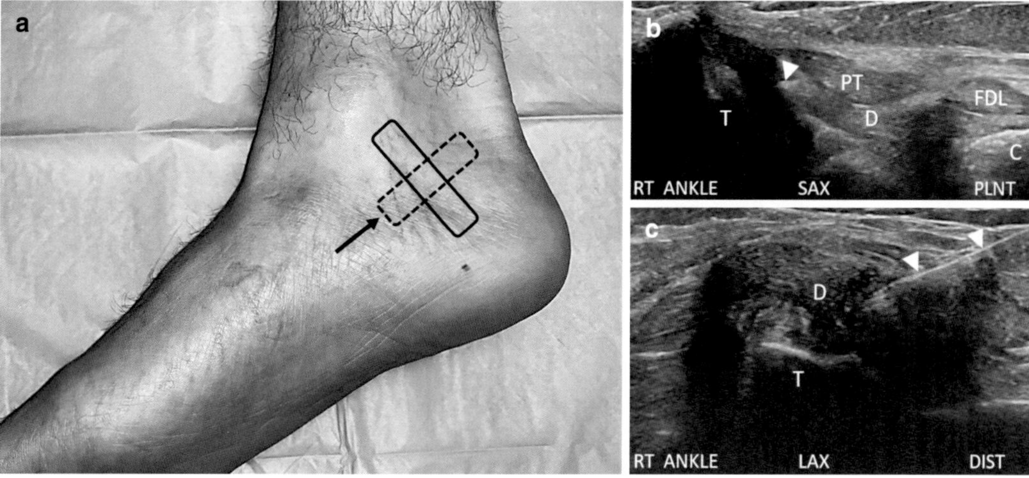

Fig. 10.14 Ultrasound-guided deltoid ligament injection. (**a**) External view of the right (RT) ankle demonstrating Td placement and needle direction (*solid arrow*) for an out-of-plane (*solid rectangle*) and in-plane (*dotted rectangle*) and distal-to-proximal approach to injecting the deltoid ligament. (**b**) USG correlate of an out-of-plane, distal-to-proximal approach showing a hyperechoic needle tip (*arrowhead*) within the tibiocalcaneal portion of the deltoid ligament (*D*). Note the location of the adjacent posterior tibialis (*PT*) and the flexor digitorum longs (*FDL*) tendons. (**c**) USG correlate of an in-plane, distal-to-proximal approach showing a hyperechoic needle (*arrowheads*) within the tibiocalcaneal portion of the deltoid ligament. Note similar approaches can be used to target the posterior and anterior tibiotalar and tibionavicular portions of the deltoid ligament complex. *LAX* long axis, *C* calcaneus, *PLNT* plantar, *DIST* distal

to follow a four-phase protocol after needling of any tendon about the foot or ankle (Achilles tendon, plantar fascia, PTT, etc.). Phase one involves the use of protected weight-bearing device, CAM boot, for 2–4 weeks following tendon needling procedure, regardless of injectate/device used. This is done out of an abundance of caution to reduce the risk of tissue/tendon rupture and help with pain control immediately following the procedure. For isolated Achilles tendon scraping and joint injections, protected weight-bearing is not utilized, and the patient is permitted to engage in activity as tolerated once the needle puncture site has closed. Phase two (weeks 4–5 post-procedure) involves cessation of protected weight-bearing and introduction of isometric exercises to facilitate strength gains and aid in pain modulation [103]. Phase three (weeks 6–12) involves a progress resistance training program (eccentric-concentric, eccentric only, or heavy-slow resistance training) based on individual patient factors such as exercise tolerance and post-rehabilitation goals [104–106]. For example, our 20-year-old soccer player will proceed with heavy-slow resistance training, while our 80-year-old patient will focus on more simplistic eccentric-concentric contractions with an emphasis more on neuromuscular reeducation. Phase four (weeks 10–16) continues with phase three exercise program with addition of sport-/activity-specific exercises.

Conclusion

Although the optimal protocols for orthobiologics about the foot and ankle have yet to be defined, some general conclusions can be drawn from the currently available literatures. First, USG orthobiologics largely appear safe with few reported side effects outside from transiently increased pain following procedure without reported long-term side effects. The autologous nature of some orthobiologics (PRP, fat, and BMAC-derived products) makes them particularly appealing to practitioners and patients alike. Further RCTs accounting for variables such as injection technique, injectate volume, leukocyte concentration, platelet/MSC, dHACM, or dextrose concentration, frequency of injections, and post-procedure protocols are needed to validate the promising early publications on mentioned procedures.

References

1. Dahlhamer J, et al. Prevalence of chronic pain and high-impact chronic pain among adults—United States, 2016. Morb Mortal Wkly Rep. 2018;67(36):1001.
2. Hauser RA, Lackner JB, Steilen-Matias D, Harris DK. A systematic review of dextrose prolotherapy for chronic musculoskeletal pain. Clin Med Insights: Arthritis Musculoskelet Disord. 2016;9:CMAMD. S39160.
3. Centers for Disease Control and Prevention. Arthritis data and statistics. (February 7 2018). Arthritis. cdc.gov/arthritis/data_statistics/national-statistics.htm.
4. Centers for Disease Control and Prevention. The cost of arthritis in US adults. (February 22, 2018). www.cdc.gov/arthritis/data_statistics/cost.htm. Accessed 25 Feb 2020.
5. Kaux J-F, Forthomme B, Goff CL, Crielaard J-M, Croisier J-L. Current opinions on tendinopathy. J Sports Sci Med. 2011;10(2):238–53.
6. Peterson C, Hodler J. Adverse events from diagnostic and therapeutic joint injections: a literature review. Skelet Radiol. 2011;40(1):5–12.
7. Richardson SS, Schairer WW, Sculco TP, Sculco PK. Comparison of infection risk with corticosteroid or hyaluronic acid injection prior to total knee arthroplasty. J Bone Joint Surg Am. 2019;101(2):112–8.
8. Foster TE, Puskas BL, Mandelbaum BR, Gerhardt MB, Rodeo SA. Platelet-rich plasma: from basic science to clinical applications. Am J Sports Med. 2009;37(11):2259–72.
9. Polykandriotis E, Popescu LM, Horch RE. Regenerative medicine: then and now – an update of recent history into future possibilities. J Cell Mol Med. 2010;14(10):2350–8.
10. Anz AW, Bapat A, Murrell WD. Concepts in regenerative medicine: past, present, and future in articular cartilage treatment. J Clin Orthop Trauma. 2016;7(3):137–44.
11. Bruno F, La Marra A, Mariani S, et al. Treatment of supraspinatus tendinopathy: dry needling as a stand-alone procedure vs dry needling and platelet-rich plasma (prp). 2016.
12. Di Matteo B, El Araby MM, D'Angelo A, et al. Adipose-derived stem cell treatments and formulations. Clin Sports Med. 2019;38(1):61–78.
13. Le ADK, Enweze L, DeBaun MR, Dragoo JL. Current clinical recommendations for use of platelet-rich plasma. Curr Rev Musculoskelet Med. 2018;11(4):624–34.

14. Riboh JC, Saltzman BM, Yanke AB, Cole BJ. Human amniotic membrane-derived products in sports medicine: basic science, early results, and potential clinical applications. Am J Sports Med. 2016;44(9):2425–34.
15. Wang S, Qu X, Zhao RC. Clinical applications of mesenchymal stem cells. J Hematol Oncol. 2012;5:19.
16. Bendich I, Rubenstein WJ, Cole BJ, Ma CB, Feeley BT, Lansdown DA. What is the appropriate price for PRP injections for knee osteoarthritis? A cost-effectiveness analysis based on evidence from level 1 randomized controlled trials. Arthroscopy: J Arthroscop Relat Surg. 2020.
17. Brockett CL, Chapman GJ. Biomechanics of the ankle. Orthop Trauma. 2016;30(3):232–8.
18. Joshi S, Joshi S, Athavale S. Morphology of peroneus tertius muscle. Clin Anat. 2006;19(7):611–4.
19. Witvrouw E, Vanden Borre K, Willems TM, Huysmans J, Broos E, De Clercq D. The significance of peroneus tertius muscle in ankle injuries: a prospective study. Am J Sports Med. 2006;34(7):1159–63.
20. Athavale SA, Gupta V, Kotgirwar S, Singh V. The peroneus quartus muscle: clinical correlation with evolutionary importance. Anat Sci Int. 2012;87(2):106–10.
21. Hur M-S, Won H-S, Chung I-H. A new morphological classification for the fibularis quartus muscle. Surg Radiol Anat. 2015;37(1):27–32.
22. Zammit J, Singh D. The peroneus quartus muscle: anatomy and clinical relevance. Bone Joint J. 2003;85(8):1134–7.
23. Govsa F, Bilge O, Ozer MA. Variations in the origin of the medial and inferior calcaneal nerves. Arch Orthop Trauma Surg. 2006;126(1):6–14.
24. van Sterkenburg MN, Kerkhoffs GMMJ, Kleipool RP, Niek van Dijk C. The plantaris tendon and a potential role in mid-portion Achilles tendinopathy: an observational anatomical study. J Anat. 2011;218(3):336–41.
25. Alfredson H. Persistent pain in the Achilles mid-portion? Consider the plantaris tendon as a possible culprit! Br J Sports Med. 2017;51(10):833–4.
26. Alfredson H, Masci L, Spang C. Surgical plantaris tendon removal for patients with plantaris tendon-related pain only and a normal Achilles tendon: a case series. BMJ Open Sport Exerc Med. 2018;4(1):e000462.
27. Spang C, Alfredson H, Docking SI, Masci L, Andersson G. The plantaris tendon: a narrative review focusing on anatomical features and clinical importance. Bone Joint J. 2016;98-B(10):1312–9.
28. Stecco C, Corradin M, Macchi V, et al. Plantar fascia anatomy and its relationship with Achilles tendon and paratenon. J Anat. 2013;223(6):665–76.
29. Pourcho AM, Smith J, Wisniewski SJ, Sellon JL. Intraarticular platelet-rich plasma injection in the treatment of knee osteoarthritis: review and recommendations. Am J Phys Med Rehabil. 2014;93(11 Suppl 3):S108–21.
30. Riboh JC, Saltzman BM, Yanke AB, Fortier L, Cole BJ. Effect of leukocyte concentration on the efficacy of platelet-rich plasma in the treatment of knee osteoarthritis. Am J Sports Med. 2016;44(3):792–800.
31. Filardo G, Di Matteo B, Di Martino A, et al. Platelet-rich plasma intra-articular knee injections show no superiority versus viscosupplementation: a randomized controlled trial. Am J Sports Med. 2015;43(7):1575–82.
32. Braun HJ, Kim HJ, Chu CR, Dragoo JL. The effect of platelet-rich plasma formulations and blood products on human synoviocytes: implications for intra-articular injury and therapy. Am J Sports Med. 2014;42(5):1204–10.
33. Fukawa T, Yamaguchi S, Akatsu Y, Yamamoto Y, Akagi R, Sasho T. Safety and efficacy of intra-articular injection of platelet-rich plasma in patients with ankle osteoarthritis. Foot Ankle Int. 2017;38(6):596–604.
34. Görmeli G, Karakaplan M, Görmeli CA, Sarıkaya B, Elmalı N, Ersoy Y. Clinical effects of platelet-rich plasma and hyaluronic acid as an additional therapy for talar osteochondral lesions treated with microfracture surgery: a prospective randomized clinical trial. Foot Ankle Int. 2015;36(8):891–900.
35. Mei-Dan O, Carmont MR, Laver L, Mann G, Maffulli N, Nyska M. Platelet-rich plasma or hyaluronate in the management of osteochondral lesions of the talus. Am J Sports Med. 2012;40(3):534–41.
36. Guney A, Akar M, Karaman I, Oner M, Guney B. Clinical outcomes of platelet rich plasma (PRP) as an adjunct to microfracture surgery in osteochondral lesions of the talus. Knee Surg Sports Traumatol Arthrosc. 2015;23(8):2384–9.
37. Repetto I, Biti B, Cerruti P, Trentini R, Felli L. Conservative treatment of ankle osteoarthritis: can platelet-rich plasma effectively postpone surgery? J Foot Ankle Surg. 2017;56(2):362–5.
38. Hall MM. The accuracy and efficacy of palpation versus image-guided peripheral injections in sports medicine. Curr Sports Med Rep. 2013;12(5):296–303.
39. Lippi G, Salvagno GL, Montagnana M, Poli G, Guidi GC. Influence of the needle bore size on platelet count and routine coagulation testing. Blood Coagul Fibrinolysis. 2006;17(7):557–61.
40. Henning T, Finnoff JT, Smith J. Sonographically guided posterior subtalar joint injections: anatomic study and validation of 3 approaches. PM&R. 2009;1(10):925–31.
41. Bhabra G, Wang A, Ebert JR, Edwards P, Zheng M, Zheng MH. Lateral elbow tendinopathy: development of a pathophysiology-based treatment algorithm. Orthop J Sports Med. 2016;4(11):2325967116670635.
42. Shiri R, Viikari-Juntura E, Varonen H, Heliövaara M. Prevalence and determinants of lateral and medial

epicondylitis: a population study. Am J Epidemiol. 2006;164(11):1065–74.
43. Fu S-C, Rolf C, Cheuk Y-C, Lui PP, Chan K-M. Deciphering the pathogenesis of tendinopathy: a three-stages process. BMC Sports Sci Med Rehabil. 2010;2(1):30.
44. Basadonna P-T, Rucco V, Gasparini D, Onorato A. Plantar fat pad atrophy after corticosteroid injection for an interdigital neuroma: A case report. Am J Phys Med Rehabil. 1999;78(3):283–5.
45. Reddy PD, Zelicof SB, Ruotolo C, Holder J. Interdigital neuroma. Local cutaneous changes after corticosteroid injection. Clin Orthop Relat Res. 1995;317:185–7.
46. Acevedo JI, Beskin JL. Complications of plantar fascia rupture associated with corticosteroid injection. Foot Ankle Int. 1998;19(2):91–7.
47. Lee HS, Choi YR, Kim SW, Lee JY, Seo JH, Jeong JJ. Risk factors affecting chronic rupture of the plantar fascia. Foot Ankle Int. 2014;35(3):258–63.
48. Alfredson H. Ultrasound and Doppler-guided mini-surgery to treat midportion Achilles tendinosis: results of a large material and a randomised study comparing two scraping techniques. Br J Sports Med. 2011;45(5):407–10.
49. Halpern AA, Horowitz BG, Nagel DA. Tendon ruptures associated with corticosteroid therapy. West J Med. 1977;127(5):378.
50. Ruergard A, Spang C, Alfredson H. Results of minimally invasive Achilles tendon scraping and plantaris tendon removal in patients with chronic midportion Achilles tendinopathy: a longer-term follow-up study. SAGE Open Med. 2019;7:2050312118822642.
51. Kon E, Filardo G, Delcogliano M, et al. Platelet-rich plasma: new clinical application: a pilot study for treatment of jumper's knee. Injury. 2009;40(6):598–603.
52. Virchenko O, Aspenberg P. How can one platelet injection after tendon injury lead to a stronger tendon after 4 weeks?: Interplay between early regeneration and mechanical stimulation. Acta Orthop. 2006;77(5):806–12.
53. Rosenbaum AJ, DiPreta JA, Misener D. Plantar heel pain. Med Clin. 2014;98(2):339–52.
54. Jain K, Murphy PN, Clough TM. Platelet rich plasma versus corticosteroid injection for plantar fasciitis: a comparative study. Foot (Edinb). 2015;25(4):235–7.
55. Monto RR. Platelet-rich plasma efficacy versus corticosteroid injection treatment for chronic severe plantar fasciitis. Foot Ankle Int. 2014;35(4):313–8.
56. Jimenez-Perez AE, Gonzalez-Arabio D, Diaz AS, Maderuelo JA, Ramos-Pascua LR. Clinical and imaging effects of corticosteroids and platelet-rich plasma for the treatment of chronic plantar fasciitis: a comparative non randomized prospective study. Foot Ankle Surg. 2019;25(3):354–60.
57. Lundeen RO, Aziz S, Burks JB, Rose JM. Endoscopic plantar fasciotomy: a retrospective analysis of results in 53 patients. J Foot Ankle Surg. 2000;39(4):208–17.
58. Saxena A, Fournier M, Gerdesmeyer L, Gollwitzer H. Comparison between extracorporeal shockwave therapy, placebo ESWT and endoscopic plantar fasciotomy for the treatment of chronic plantar heel pain in the athlete. Muscles Ligaments Tendons J. 2012;2(4):312.
59. Folman Y, Bartal G, Breitgand A, Shabat S, Ron N. Treatment of recalcitrant plantar fasciitis by sonographically-guided needle fasciotomy. Foot Ankle Surg. 2005;11(4):211–4.
60. Peerbooms JC, Lodder P, den Oudsten BL, Doorgeest K, Schuller HM, Gosens T. Positive effect of platelet-rich plasma on pain in plantar fasciitis: a double-blind multicenter randomized controlled trial. Am J Sports Med. 2019;47(13):3238–46.
61. Ling Y, Wang S. Effects of platelet-rich plasma in the treatment of plantar fasciitis: a meta-analysis of randomized controlled trials. Medicine (Baltimore). 2018;97(37):e12110.
62. Shetty SH, Dhond A, Arora M, Deore S. Platelet-rich plasma has better long-term results than corticosteroids or placebo for chronic plantar fasciitis: randomized control trial. J Foot Ankle Surg. 2019;58(1):42–6.
63. Tabrizi A, Dindarian S, Mohammadi S. The effect of corticosteroid local injection versus platelet-rich plasma for the treatment of plantar fasciitis in obese patients: a single-blind, randomized clinical trial. J Foot Ankle Surg. 2020;59(1):64–8.
64. Scharf RE. Drugs that affect platelet function. Paper presented at: Seminars in thrombosis and hemostasis. 2012;38(08):865–83.
65. Shi S, Klotz U. Clinical use and pharmacological properties of selective COX-2 inhibitors. Eur J Clin Pharmacol. 2008;64(3):233–52.
66. Nair A, Sahoo R. Ultrasound-guided injection for plantar fasciitis: a brief review. Saudi J Anaesth. 2016;10(4):440.
67. Zelen CM, Poka A, Andrews J. Prospective, randomized, blinded, comparative study of injectable micronized dehydrated amniotic/chorionic membrane allograft for plantar fasciitis—a feasibility study. Foot Ankle Int. 2013;34(10):1332–9.
68. Cazzell S, Stewart J, Agnew PS, et al. Randomized controlled trial of micronized dehydrated human amnion/chorion membrane (dHACM) injection compared to placebo for the treatment of plantar fasciitis. Foot Ankle Int. 2018;39(10):1151–61.
69. Ersen Ö, Koca K, Akpancar S, et al. A randomized-controlled trial of prolotherapy injections in the treatment of plantar fasciitis. Turkish J Phys Med Rehabil. 2018;64(1):59.
70. Mansiz-Kaplan B, Nacir B, Pervane-Vural S, Duyur-Cakit B, Genc H. Effect of dextrose prolotherapy on pain intensity, disability and plantar fascia thickness in unilateral plantar fasciitis: a randomized, controlled, double-blind study. Am J Phys Med Rehabil. 2019;99(4):318–24.
71. Kim E, Lee JH. Autologous platelet-rich plasma versus dextrose prolotherapy for the treatment

of chronic recalcitrant plantar fasciitis. PM&R. 2014;6(2):152–8.
72. Uğurlar M, Sönmez MM, Uğurlar ÖY, Adıyeke L, Yıldırım H, Eren OT. Effectiveness of four different treatment modalities in the treatment of chronic plantar fasciitis during a 36-month follow-up period: a randomized controlled trial. J Foot Ankle Surg. 2018;57(5):913–8.
73. Boesen AP, Hansen R, Boesen MI, Malliaras P, Langberg H. Effect of high-volume injection, platelet-rich plasma, and sham treatment in chronic midportion Achilles tendinopathy: a randomized double-blinded prospective study. Am J Sports Med. 2017;45(9):2034–43.
74. Ruergård A, Spang C, Alfredson H. Results of minimally invasive Achilles tendon scraping and plantaris tendon removal in patients with chronic midportion Achilles tendinopathy: a longer-term follow-up study. SAGE Open Med. 2019;7:2050312118822642.
75. Krogh TP, Ellingsen T, Christensen R, Jensen P, Fredberg U. Ultrasound-guided injection therapy of Achilles tendinopathy with platelet-rich plasma or saline: a randomized, blinded, placebo-controlled trial. Am J Sports Med. 2016;44(8):1990–7.
76. Murawski CD, Smyth NA, Newman H, Kennedy JG. A single platelet-rich plasma injection for chronic midsubstance Achilles tendinopathy: a retrospective preliminary analysis. Foot Ankle Spec. 2014;7(5):372–6.
77. Boesen AP, Langberg H, Hansen R, Malliaras P, Boesen MI. High volume injection with and without corticosteroid in chronic midportion Achilles tendinopathy. Scand J Med Sci Sports. 2019;29(8):1223–31.
78. Maffulli N, Spiezia F, Longo UG, Denaro V, Maffulli GD. High volume image guided injections for the management of chronic tendinopathy of the main body of the Achilles tendon. Phys Ther Sport. 2013;14(3):163–7.
79. Wheeler PC, Tattersall C. Novel interventions for recalcitrant Achilles tendinopathy: benefits seen following high-volume image-guided injection or extracorporeal shockwave therapy-a prospective cohort study. Clin J Sport Med. 2020;30(1):14–9.
80. Yeo A, Kendall N, Jayaraman S. Ultrasound-guided dry needling with percutaneous paratenon decompression for chronic Achilles tendinopathy. Knee Surg Sports Traumatol Arthrosc. 2016;24(7):2112–8.
81. Zhang YJ, Xu SZ, Gu PC, et al. Is platelet-rich plasma injection effective for chronic Achilles tendinopathy? A meta-analysis. Clin Orthop Relat Res. 2018;476(8):1633–41.
82. Liu CJ, Yu KL, Bai JB, Tian DH, Liu GL. Platelet-rich plasma injection for the treatment of chronic Achilles tendinopathy: a meta-analysis. Medicine (Baltimore). 2019;98(16):e15278.
83. Simpson MR, Howard TM. Tendinopathies of the foot and ankle. Am Fam Physician. 2009;80(10):1107–14.
84. Maffulli N, Longo UG, Petrillo S, Denaro V. Management of tendinopathies of the foot and ankle. Orthop Trauma. 2012;26(4):259–64.
85. Nakamura T, Sekiya I, Muneta T, Yamamoto H. Active flatfoot phenomenon caused by posterior tibial tendon dysfunction. Int J Foot Ankle. 2017;1(003).
86. Ikpeze TC, Brodell JD Jr, Chen RE, Oh I. Evaluation and treatment of posterior tibialis tendon insufficiency in the elderly patients. Geriatric Orthop Surg Rehabil. 2019;10:2151459318821461.
87. Angthong C, Khadsongkram A, Angthong W. Outcomes and quality of life after platelet-rich plasma therapy in patients with recalcitrant hindfoot and ankle diseases: a preliminary report of 12 patients. J Foot Ankle Surg. 2013;52(4):475–80.
88. Finnoff JT, Fowler SP, Lai JK, et al. Treatment of chronic tendinopathy with ultrasound-guided needle tenotomy and platelet-rich plasma injection. PM R. 2011;3(10):900–11.
89. Mautner K, Colberg RE, Malanga G, et al. Outcomes after ultrasound-guided platelet-rich plasma injections for chronic tendinopathy: a multicenter, retrospective review. PM R. 2013;5(3):169–75.
90. Oloff LD, Lam JD. Does PRP have promise for advanced posterior tibial tendinopathy in athletes? Podiatry Today. 2017;30(12):54–6.
91. Hootman JM, Dick R, Agel J. Epidemiology of collegiate injuries for 15 sports: summary and recommendations for injury prevention initiatives. J Athl Train. 2007;42(2):311–9.
92. McKay GD, Goldie PA, Payne WR, Oakes BW. Ankle injuries in basketball: injury rate and risk factors. Br J Sports Med. 2001;35(2):103–8.
93. Clifton DR, Koldenhoven RM, Hertel J, Onate JA, Dompier TP, Kerr ZY. Epidemiological patterns of ankle sprains in youth, high school, and college football. Am J Sports Med. 2017;45(2):417–25.
94. McCann RS, Kosik KB, Terada M, Gribble PA. Prediction of recurrent injury in the same competitive sport season following return-to-play from an ankle sprain. Int J Athletic Ther Training. 2019;24(2):78–84.
95. Roos KG, Kerr ZY, Mauntel TC, Djoko A, Dompier TP, Wikstrom EA. The epidemiology of lateral ligament complex ankle sprains in National Collegiate Athletic Association sports. Am J Sports Med. 2017;45(1):201–9.
96. Rammelt S, Zwipp H, Grass R. Injuries to the distal tibiofibular syndesmosis: an evidence-based approach to acute and chronic lesions. Foot Ankle Clin. 2008;13(4):611–33.
97. Konradsen L, Bech L, Ehrenbjerg M, Nickelsen T. Seven years follow-up after ankle inversion trauma. Scand J Med Sci Sports. 2002;12(3):129–35.
98. Laver L, Carmont MR, McConkey MO, et al. Plasma rich in growth factors (PRGF) as a treatment for high ankle sprain in elite athletes: a randomized control trial. Knee Surg Sports Traumatol Arthrosc. 2015;23(11):3383–92.

99. Samra DJ, Sman AD, Rae K, Linklater J, Refshauge KM, Hiller CE. Effectiveness of a single platelet-rich plasma injection to promote recovery in rugby players with ankle syndesmosis injury. BMJ Open Sport Exerc Med. 2015;1(1):e000033.
100. Rowden A, Dominici P, D'Orazio J, et al. Double-blind, randomized, placebo-controlled study evaluating the use of platelet-rich plasma therapy (PRP) for acute ankle sprains in the emergency department. J Emerg Med. 2015;49(4):546–51.
101. Blanco-Rivera J, Elizondo-Rodríguez J, Simental-Mendía M, Vilchez-Cavazos F, Peña-Martínez VM, Acosta-Olivo C. Treatment of lateral ankle sprain with platelet-rich plasma: a randomized clinical study. Foot Ankle Surg. 2019.
102. Hauser R, Hauser M, Cukla J. Dextrose Prolotherapy injections for chronic ankle pain. Pract Pain Manag. 2010;10(1):70–6.
103. Rio E, Van Ark M, Docking S, et al. Isometric contractions are more analgesic than isotonic contractions for patellar tendon pain: an in-season randomized clinical trial. Clin J Sport Med. 2017;27(3):253–9.
104. Habets B, van Cingel REH, Backx FJG, Huisstede BMA. Alfredson versus Silbernagel exercise therapy in chronic midportion Achilles tendinopathy: study protocol for a randomized controlled trial. BMC Musculoskelet Disord 2017;18(1):296–296.
105. Kongsgaard M, Qvortrup K, Larsen J, et al. Fibril morphology and tendon mechanical properties in patellar tendinopathy: effects of heavy slow resistance training. Am J Sports Med. 2010;38(4):749–56.
106. Silbernagel KG, Thomeé R, Eriksson BI, Karlsson J. Continued sports activity, using a pain-monitoring model, during rehabilitation in patients with Achilles tendinopathy: a randomized controlled study. Am J Sports Med. 2007;35(6):897–906.

Part III

Back and Spine

Ultrasound-Guided Regenerative Injections for the Spine

11

Donald Tsung-Yung Tang and Chih-Peng Lin

Introduction

Chronic spinal pain is one of the most common complaints encountered in pain clinic. The prevalence and burden of disability has increased markedly in recent decades [1]. In the aging population, the prevalence, severity, and complexity are even more escalated. Diagnosis of spinal pain is usually challenging because of the nonspecific, overlapping clinical presentation. Laboratory and imaging studies could help in ruling out red flags; however, the diagnostic value is less than satisfactory. Therefore, for a definite diagnosis, diagnostic or prognostic injection is usually needed before proceeding to invasive pain management. Regenerative injection, which is based on the concept of regeneration and enhancement of tissue integrity in the biotensegrity model, is one of the modalities in the interventional category. The targets of regenerative injection also include some structures which are not proven pain generators like ligaments and muscle entheses [2]. Therefore, for practitioners of regenerative injection, clinical reasoning with knowledge of anatomy and biomechanics is needed in choosing adequate targets of injection. Ultrasound is one of the imaging modalities used in interventional treatments, with advantages in the cost, portability, and no radiation exposure [3]. For precision and safety injection therapies in ultrasound-guided regenerative injection, comprehensive understanding of the anatomy and sonoanatomy is mandatory. In this chapter, the anatomy, sonoanatomy, and injection techniques for axial structures of cervical, thoracic, and lumbosacral levels will be reviewed.

Neck Pain and Regenerative Medicine

Neck pain is one of the most common complaints and the leading cause of disability worldwide. The estimated mean point, annual, and lifetime prevalence is 7.6%, 37.2%, and 48.5%, respectively [4]. The probable pain generators of the cervical spine are facet joints, intervertebral discs, muscles, ligaments, and nerve root compression or spinal stenosis leading to radicular symptoms [5]. The clinical presentations of different etiologies share certain similarities; therefore, it is usually challenging to make a definite diagnosis without a comprehensive assessment protocol for all possible differential diagnoses. Moreover, these pain-generating structures may have negative impact on biomechanics of the cer-

D. T.-Y. Tang
Department of Pain Managemet, Taichung Tzu Chi Hospital, Taichung, Taiwan

C.-P. Lin (✉)
Department of Anesthesiology, National Taiwan University Hospital and National Taiwan University College of Medicine, Taipei, Taiwan

Y. El Miedany (ed.), *Musculoskeletal Ultrasound-Guided Regenerative Medicine*,
https://doi.org/10.1007/978-3-030-98256-0_11

vical spine, deteriorate the overall stability, and induce another pain generator. Since the history, physical findings, and imaging studies are often not specific, diagnostic block or provocative test is commonly regarded as the standard of making a diagnosis.

The clinical presentation of cervical radicular pain secondary to nerve root compression or spinal stenosis is relatively specific when compared to other cervical spine pain generators. It typically leads to neck pain and/or arm pain in a dermatomal pattern. Herniated disc or spinal stenosis may be revealed by imaging studies like CT or MRI; however, these findings are not specific. To confirm the causative relationship between the image findings and clinical symptoms, electrodiagnostic tests could help. Selective nerve root injection by ultrasound guidance could provide pain relief to the patients, albeit the spread of injectate is not consistent with a transforaminal epidural injection (Fig. 11.1). Although selective cervical nerve root injection is not commonly

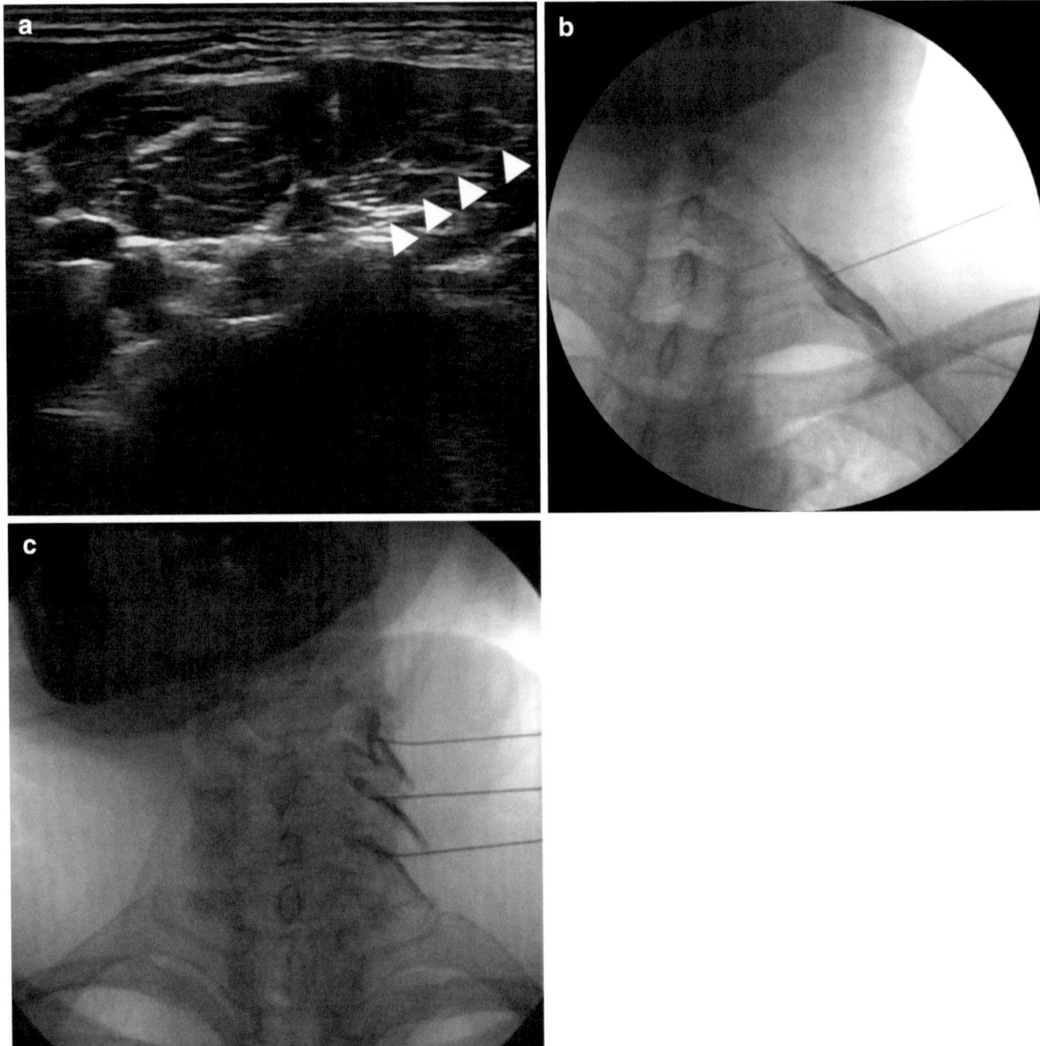

Fig. 11.1 Ultrasound-guided cervical selective nerve root block (SNRB), vs. fluoroscopy-guided transforaminal epidural injection. The injectate is actually out of the neuroforamen when compared to the fluoroscopy-guided transforaminal technique. (**a**) C7 ultrasound-guided SNRB on the posterior tubercle of C7. (**b**) Fluoroscopic demonstration with contrast after (**a**). (**c**) Typical fluoroscopy-guided transforaminal epidural injection

performed in the practice of regenerative medicine, cervical radicular pain is commonly encountered in clinical pain practice, and the technique will be briefly summarized in this chapter.

As a crucial component of the cervical spine biomechanics, cervical facet joint is the most important structure in axial neck pain. In chronic neck pain population, the prevalence of facetogenic pain could be up to 55% [6]. There are several neck muscles inserting onto the cervical facet joint and capsular ligament, responsible for the biomechanical integrity of the posterior cervical spine. The facetogenic pain could be related to the instability, laxity, or weakness of capsular ligaments and neck muscles. Contussional injury to the facet joints or strain of the capsular ligaments caused by whiplash-like injury and may further predispose to the overall biomechanical failure and degeneration [7], which ultimately cause chronic neck and upper back pain and limited range of motion.

For the diagnosis of facetogenic neck pain, clinical diagnosis by physical tests is attempted [8]; however, currently, the gold standard for diagnosis remains diagnostic facet joint injection or medial branch block with local anesthetics [9]. Up to now, in the literature, there is no report regarding the necessity of diagnostic block in regenerative injection. Clinically, diagnostic injection is usually not a routine for clinicians practicing regenerative injection. Future works are needed to clarify the role of diagnostic injection in regenerative injection.

When treating the chronic spinal pain with regenerative injection, choosing the crucial targets is of paramount importance. The choice of targets usually depends on tenderness to palpation, dynamic tests according to the biomechanics, and dynamic ultrasound scanning [10]. In the following section, the sonographic scanning of the cervical spine will be briefly reviewed.

Anatomy and Sonoanatomy of the Cervical Spine

For ultrasound scanning or guidance of intervention of the cervical spine, a high-frequency linear array transducer is usually recommended. For sonographic scanning and injection of the cervical nerve roots, the patient is usually placed in a semi-decubitus or lateral decubitus position. The transducer is placed in the transverse plane of the neck to obtain the short-axis view of the cervical spine. Moving the transducer in cephalad or caudal direction, the transverse process (TP) of the C5, C6, and C7 levels could be visualized (Fig. 11.2). In typical cases, the anterior tubercle of the C6 TP, which is also called Chassaignac's tubercle, is the most prominent anterior tubercle in the lower cervical spine levels. The size of anterior and posterior tubercle of the C5 TP is similar, while at the C7 level, the anterior tubercle is absent or remnant. Ultrasound-guided cervical root injection is performed with an in-plane, posterior-to-anterior approach. Before advancement of the needle, always check blood vessels in the vicinity of the nerve roots with Doppler ultrasound (Fig. 11.1d).

Injection of the cervical facet joint could be performed with either lateral or posterior approach. In the lateral approach, the patient is placed in the lateral decubitus position, with the symptomatic side uppermost. The level is identified by visualizing the TP of C1 and the inferior articular process (AP) of the C2, with the latter presenting as an oblique bony drop-off just cranial to the C2–3 facet joint (Fig. 11.3). The C2–3 facet joint could be used as a starting point to count the following levels. The articular pillar appears as hyperechoic wavy lines, and the facet joint is the anechoic gap between the APs. Facet joint injection on the lateral side could be performed in this long-axis view of the cervical spine with an out-of-plane technique or rotate the transducer 90 degrees to the short-axis view then perform injection with the in-plane technique (Fig. 11.4). In the

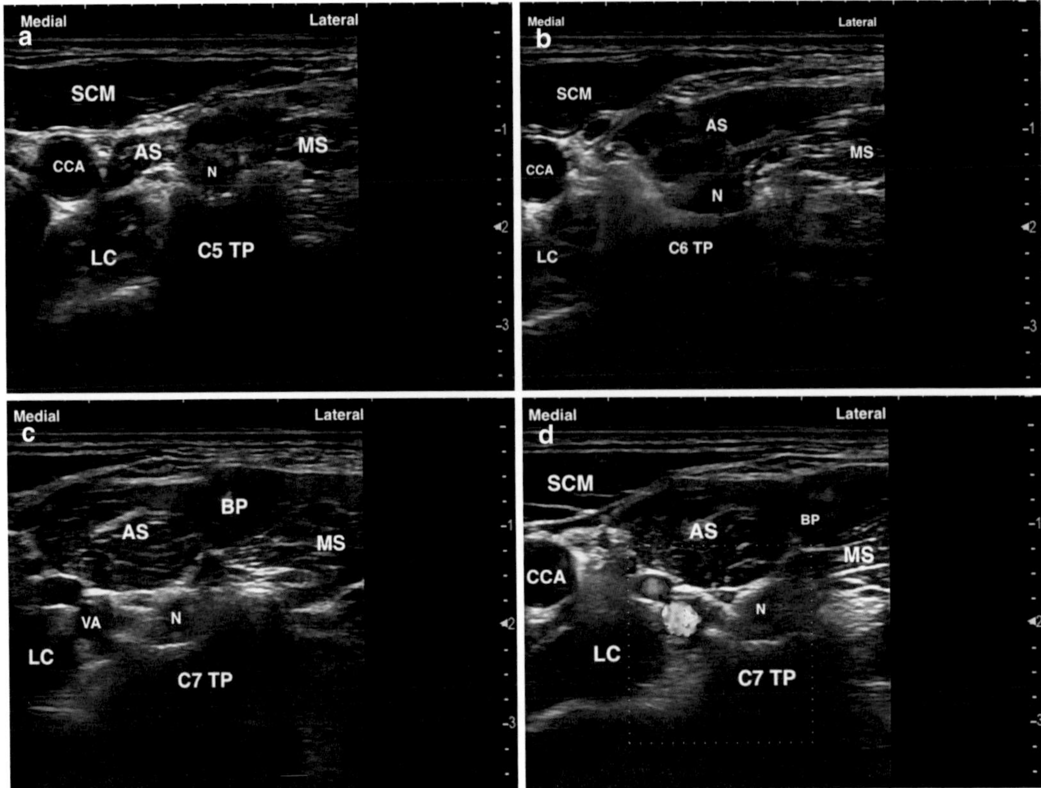

Fig. 11.2 Ultrasound-guided cervical selective nerve root injection. (**a**) Typical C5 appearance: comparable sizes of the anterior and posterior tubercle of the transverse process (TP). (**b**) Typical C6 appearance: prominent anterior tubercle of the TP, which is also named "Chassaignac's tubercle." (**c**) Typical C7 appearance: absent or rudimentary anterior tubercle of the TP. (**d**) Abundant vascularity including the vertebral artery traverse around the C7 nerve root. To avoid intravascular injection or injury to the vessels, Doppler ultrasound scan is highly recommended prior to any cervical spine procedures

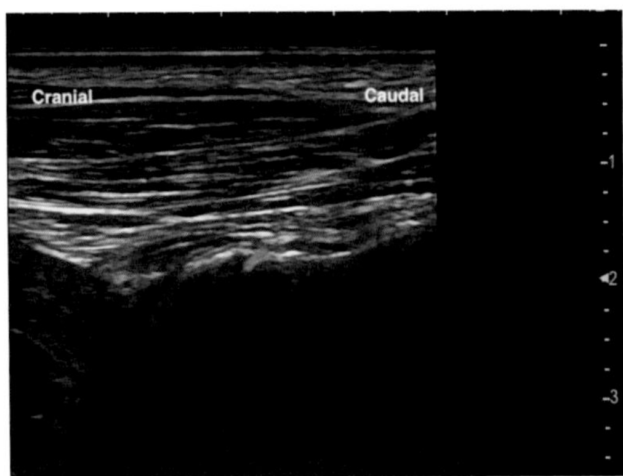

Fig. 11.3 C2–3 facet joint. *Red dashed line* the steep slope of the C2 interior articular process, *yellow line* C2–3 facet joint cleft

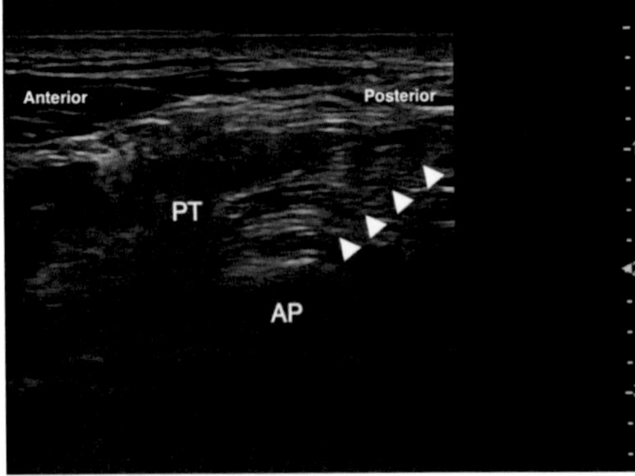

Fig. 11.4 The in-plane, posterior-to-anterior cervical facet injection. *Red overlaying shadow* the articular pillar and the transverse process of the cervical spine

perspectives of regenerative medicine and biotensegrity, the degeneration or symptoms of a joint could be secondary to the injury or laxity of its supporting structures. Winkelstein et al. [11] conducted an anatomical investigation of the human cervical facet capsule and found that 22.4 ± 9.6% of the capsular area was inserted and supported by the paraspinal muscles. Therefore, the in-plane approach, which is performed from posterior to anterior in the short-axis view of the cervical spine, may be more favorable than the out-of-plane approach. This lateral in-plane approach allows more comprehensive treatment on the facet capsule and muscle entheses.

The posterior approach of cervical facet joint injection is performed with the patient placed in the prone position. Bilateral injection could be performed at the same time without changing position. Place the transducer sagittal first on the midline to identify the C1 spinous process, which has no or rudimentary spinous process. The C2 spinous process could be ascertained in the short-axis view by identifying the most rostral bifid of spinous processes. Scanning in the sagittal plane and moving caudally, the level of treatment could be identified. When the level was identified, move the transducer laterally to see the interlaminar space and then the articular pillar of the facet joints (Fig. 11.5). The articular pillar of the facet joints will present as "saw sign" in the sonographic view. The needle is introduced immediately caudal to the transducer, with an in-plane, caudal-to-cranial approach. This approach has three advantages. First, the caudal-to-cranial needle trajectory is parallel to the angulation of the cervical facet joints, which makes it easier to obtain an intra-articular needle placement. Second, it is possible to inject more than one joint in one needle puncture. Last but not least, as we know, there are several muscle insertions on the joint capsule, and these muscles are biomechanically important to the cervical facet joint pain. It is possible to scatter the injectate extensively along the joint capsules and muscular attachments with this posterior approach.

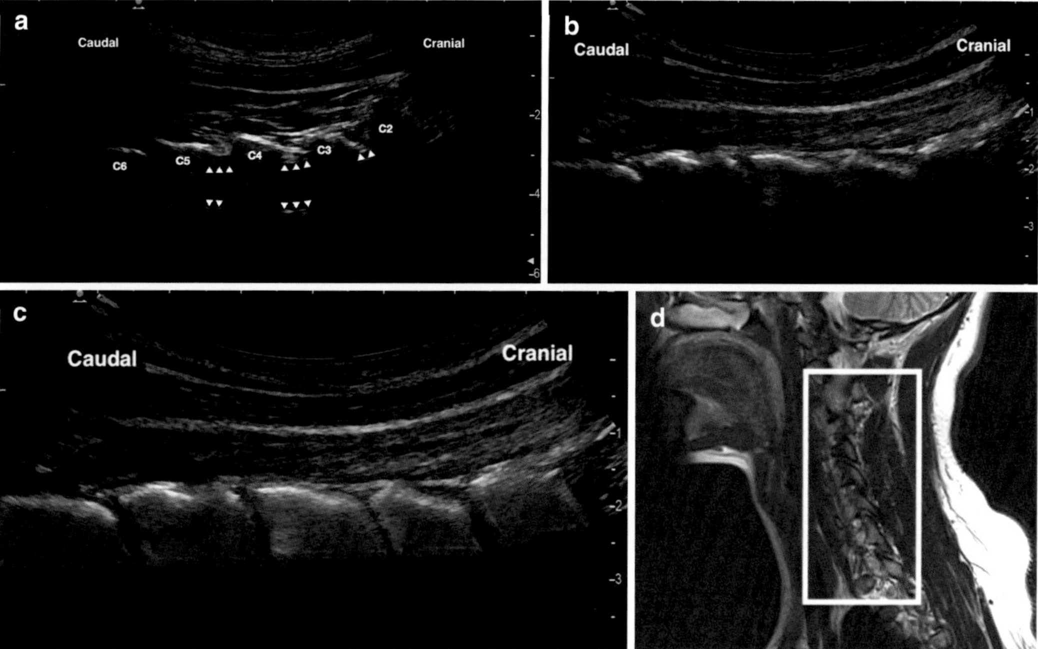

Fig. 11.5 Cervical spine sonoanatomy: posterior approach, sagittal scan of the cervical facet joints. (**a**) Interlaminar plane. *C2, C3, C4, C5, C6* the lamina of the corresponding level, *arrowhead* anterior and posterior dura. (**b**) Cervical facet joints, posterior approach. (**c**) Cervical facet joints, posterior approach, with overlaying shadow indicating the cervical articular pillar. (**d**) Morphology of the cervical articular pillar in MRI

Clinical Pearls of Specific Structures

Cervical Facet Joint

The cervical facet joints are diarthrodial joints, which are formed by the articulation of inferior AP of the above vertebra and the superior AP of the below vertebra. These joints contain synovial cells and joint fluid and are surrounded by a joint capsule, functioning similar to the knee joint [12]. The orientation of the joint is angulated at about 45 degrees at C2–3 cervical facets [13] and getting more vertical, close to the coronal plane at lower cervical facet joints (Fig. 11.6), which lie nearly in the orientation of thoracic facet joints [14]. The orientation of the cervical facet joints provides the freedom of movement of the cervical spine in all three planes. This freedom of movement makes the cervical spine susceptible to acceleration-deceleration, rotation, or compressive injury.

The facet joints are innervated by the articular branches from the medial branches of dorsal rami from the spinal nerves above and below the level. The medial branches lie on the waists of the articular pillars of corresponding vertebrae (Fig. 11.7). Clinically, the pain referral patterns are not dermatomal [15–18] (Fig. 11.8) and usually give rise to the difficulties in the diagnostic process. In clinical assessment, the first step is always ruling out the red flags including neoplastic, infectious, traumatic, or systemic inflammatory disorders. Radicular distribution is usually not presented in facet joint pain patients. Currently, the gold standard for diagnosis is still image-guided diagnostic block. To reduce the false-positive rates, dual or controlled diagnostic blocks with at least 75% pain relief are recommended [19]. The treatment modalities for cervical facetogenic pain are intra-articular injections with steroid, medial branch block, and radiofrequency neurotomy [20]. Regenerative injection for the cervical facet joints with dextrose or orthobiologics, albeit the evidence is less than well established, it could be a novel and promising intervention [12].

Thoracic Back Pain and Regenerative Medicine

Upper or middle back pain without neck or low back pain is relatively less common than neck pain and low back pain in clinical practice. The incidence of thoracic pain ranges from 3% to 26% and the prevalence is from 5% to 34% [21]. The prevalence of thoracic facetogenic pain in

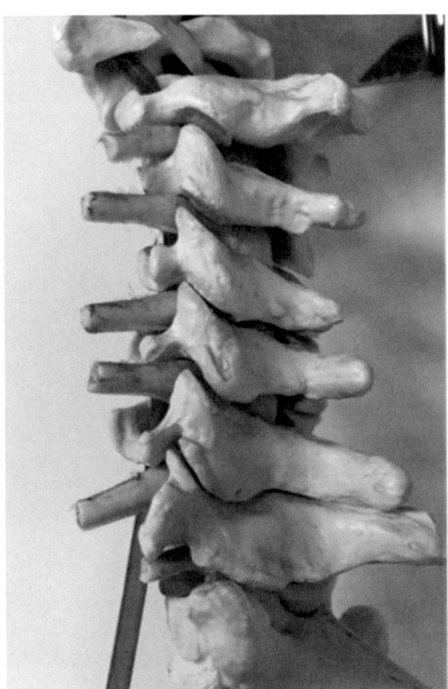

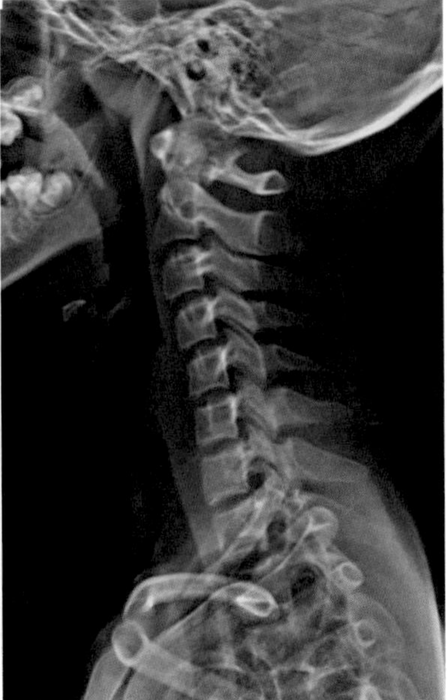

Fig. 11.6 The orientation of the cervical facet joints. The C2–3 facet faces anteroinferior, in 45 degrees from the horizontal plane. In lower cervical facets, the joint lines get more vertical and are close to the coronal plane at lower cervical facet joints, which lie nearly in the orientation of thoracic facet joints

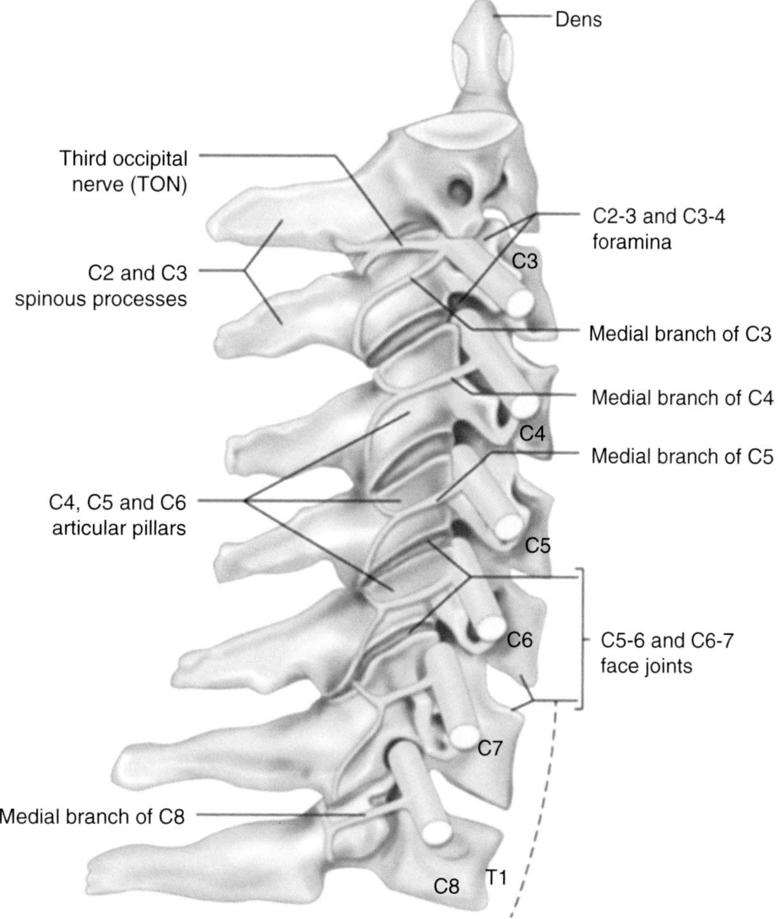

Fig. 11.7 The innervation of the cervical facet joints. Below the C2–3 facet joint, each facet joint was innervated by the medial branch of the dorsal rami from the spinal nerves of the above and below level. (From Manchikanti et al. [75], with permission from Springer)

thoracic spine pain ranges from 34% to 48% [22]. Pain generators other than the facet joints are the thoracic discs, costotransverse joints (CTJ), and costovertebral joints [23–25]. Due to their close proximity, the pain referral patterns from these structures are overlapping and indistinguishable, and usually a definite diagnosis could not be established before a diagnostic or provocative injection. For ultrasound-guided injection, thoracic intervertebral discs and costovertebral joints are hardly accessible due to their deep location and so are beyond the scope of our discussion. Some red flags, like thoracoabdominal visceral pathology, great vessel pathology, neoplasms, or infectious spinal disorders, should always be ruled out first before starting injection therapy.

Anatomy and Sonoanatomy of the Thoracic Spine

For ultrasound-guided thoracic spine regenerative injections, the two most important and viable structures are the thoracic facet joints and the CTJs. Procedures on these two structures are performed in a relatively shallow depth and are relatively simple and easy. However, to avoid complications which could be fetal or permanent, a more comprehensive understanding of the spatial relationship with several vital structures is mandatory and will be described in this section.

In any spine interventions, counting level is of paramount importance. In the thoracic level, the clinician could count the level from the cephalad at the T1 level, at which is the first rib located, or

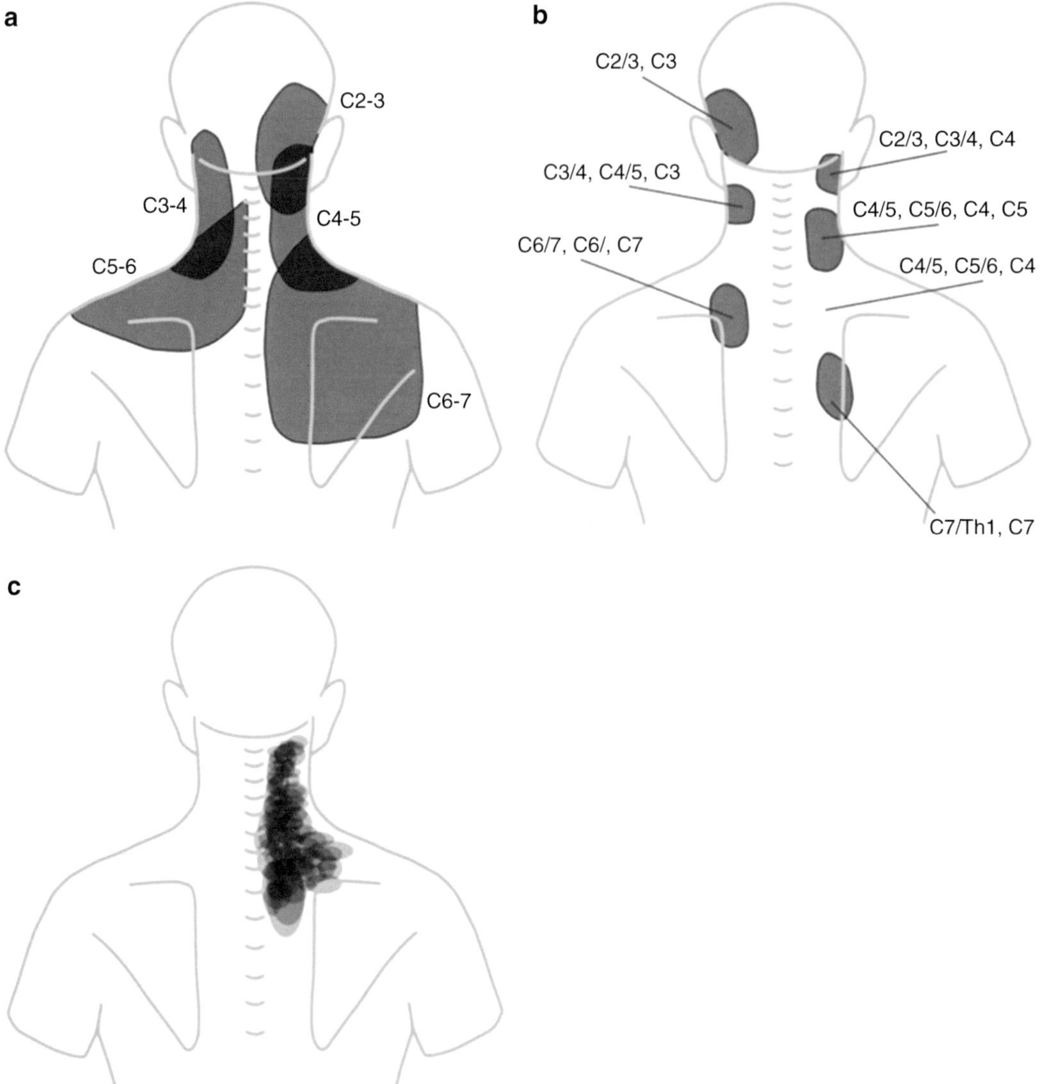

Fig. 11.8 The pain referral patterns from different investigators [16–18]. (**a**) Cervical facet pain distribution in healthy volunteers. (**b**) Pain distributions for the facet joints from C0/C1 to C7/T1 and the dorsal rami C3 to C7. (**c**) The referral patterns of all subjects obtained by minimal threshold stimulation of their right third occipital nerve and C3 to C8 medial branches. (From Manchikanti et al. [75], with permission from Springer)

from the caudad, begin with the most caudal rib at the T12 level or the lumbosacral junction. The scanning usually begins in the sagittal plane at the ribs and the intercostal spaces (Fig. 11.9). The ribs are separated, hyperechoic, round bony structures. The intercostal space, which is located between the ribs, contains the intercostal muscles, vessels, and nerves. The pleura is a hyperechoic line beneath the intercostal space. The intercostal nerve block, which is utilized in both acute and chronic pain management, is usually performed using this view at the area 7–8 cm lateral to the midline. Moving the transducer medially from the intercostal view, when approximating to the midline, a "jump" from the rib to the TP representing the costotransverse junction could be visualized (Fig. 11.10). If the target of injection is the CTJ, rotating the transducer 90 degrees to the transverse plane at this level, the CTJ could be visualized as a small cleft between the rib and the TP (Fig. 11.11). The needle could be advanced with a lateral-to-medial, in-plane approach.

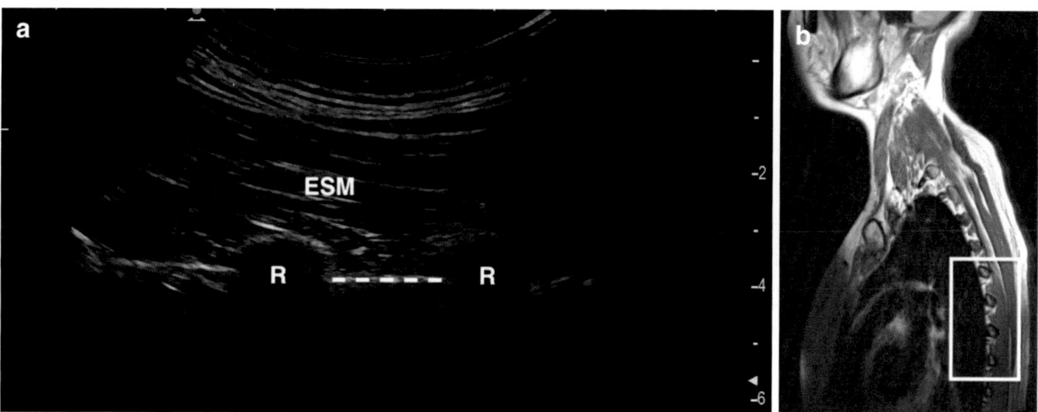

Fig. 11.9 The intercostal spaces in the sagittal plane (**a**) with MR correlation (**b**). *ESM* the erector spinae muscles, *R* rib, *dashed line* the pleura

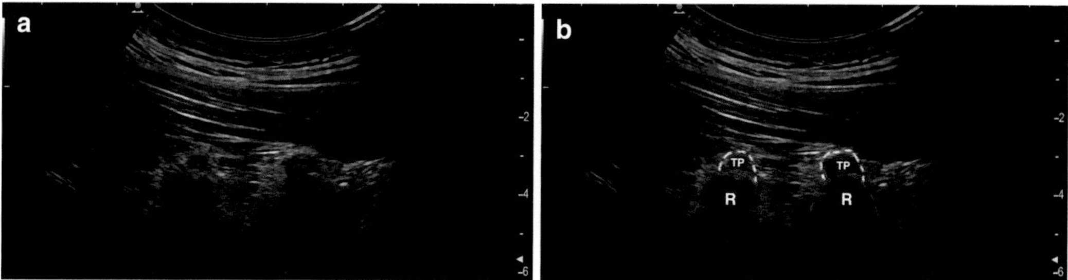

Fig. 11.10 The costotransverse joint in the sagittal scan (**a**) with elucidation by sketch in (**b**). *R* rib, *TP* transverse process

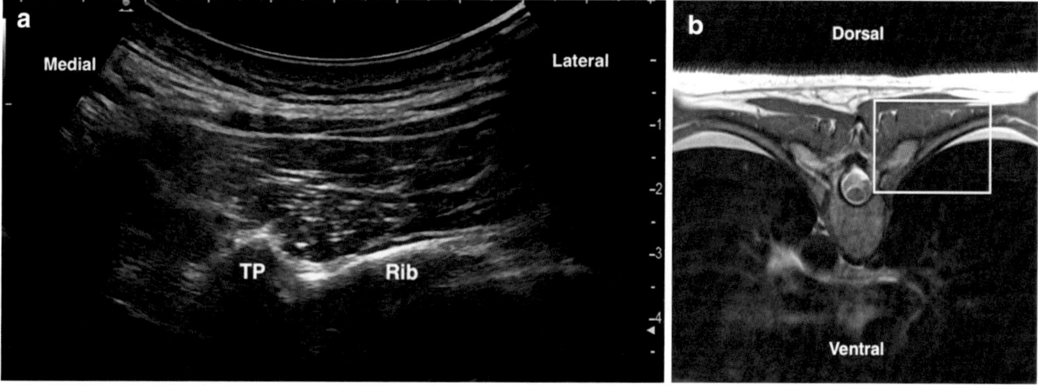

Fig. 11.11 The costotransverse joint in the transverse scan (**a**) with MR correlation (**b**). *R* rib, *TP* transverse process, *red line* the costotransverse joint line

Moving the transducer more medially in the sagittal plane, the transverse process view could be obtained (Fig. 11.12). It is crucial to distinguish ribs from the TP in the preprocedural scan. Besides the anatomical relationship, the morphological appearance could be used as a clue to differentiate the two structures. The sonographic appearance of the ribs appears as hyperechoic semicircular lines, and the TP is in a rectangular shape in the sonographic view (Fig. 11.13). The

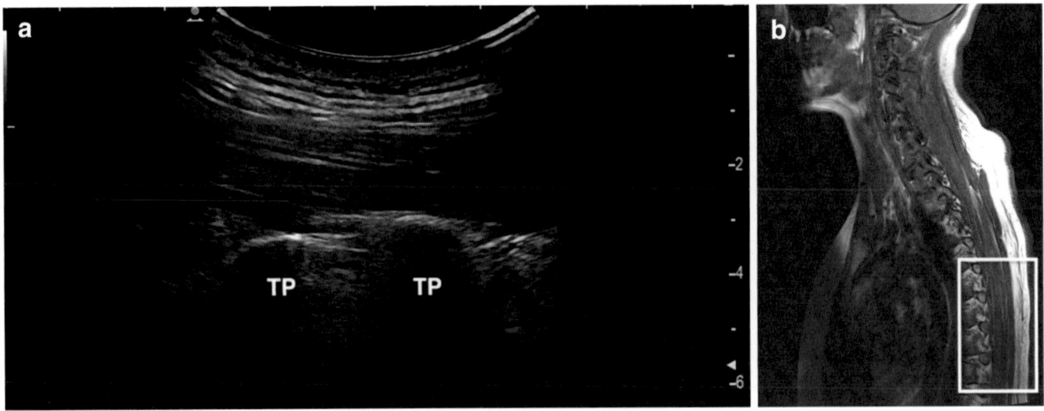

Fig. 11.12 The thoracic transverse processes in the sagittal scan (**a**) with MR correlation (**b**). *TP* transverse process

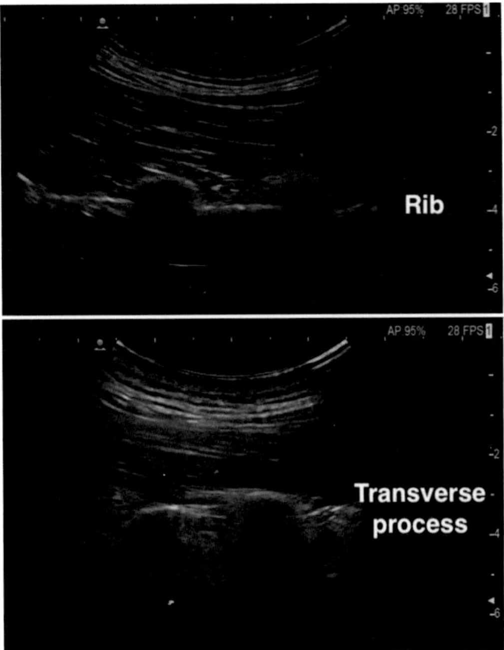

Fig. 11.13 Morphological comparison of the ribs and the transverse processes. Notice the cross section of the ribs is relatively round, while the cross section of the transverse processes is relatively in square

erector spinae plane block (ESPB), which could provide a certain degree of pain relief of myofascial upper back pain [26], is performed in the sagittal transverse process view with an in-plane approach. The choice of target level depends on the indication and level of pain generator. The needle tip is placed on the tip of the TP, obtaining an interfascial spread of injectate between the erector spinae muscles and the TP (Fig. 11.14). Besides the interfascial plane as a target of nerve block, there are several attachments of ligaments and muscle entheses to the TP. The anterior surface was attached by the costotransverse ligament, while the posterior surface was attached by deep back muscles which are crucial to the stability of the thoracic spine. The superior costotransverse ligament connects the ribs to the inferior surface of the TP of the above vertebrae. The intertransverse ligament connecting the adjacent TP also stabilizes the thoracic spine by limiting the lateral flexion [27]. Although there is few evidence in the literature regarding regenerative injection on the thoracic TP, the thoracic TP theoretically could be a good candidate to be "regenerated" based on the concept of biotensegrity.

More medially to the TP, the sagittal thoracic facet joint view could be obtained. The thoracic facet joint space lies almost in the coronal plane, with a certain degree of anterior tilting depending on the level. The sonographic appearance of the thoracic facet joint appears as small cleft between horizontal lines, which are the APs of the thoracic vertebrae (Fig. 11.15). The thoracic facet joint injection is executed in this view. When the targeted facet joint is optimally scanned, the needle is introduced immediately caudal to the transducer and advanced in-plane in a caudal-to-cranial direction. Sometimes an intra-articular needle placement is hindered by the degenerative

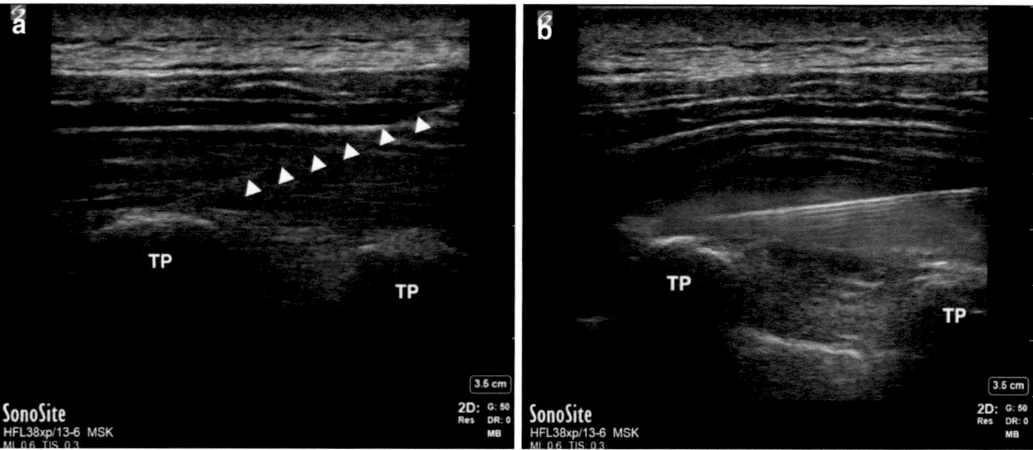

Fig. 11.14 Erector spinae plane block (**a**) and the interfascial spreading of the injectate (**b**). *TP* transverse process, *arrowheads* the needle

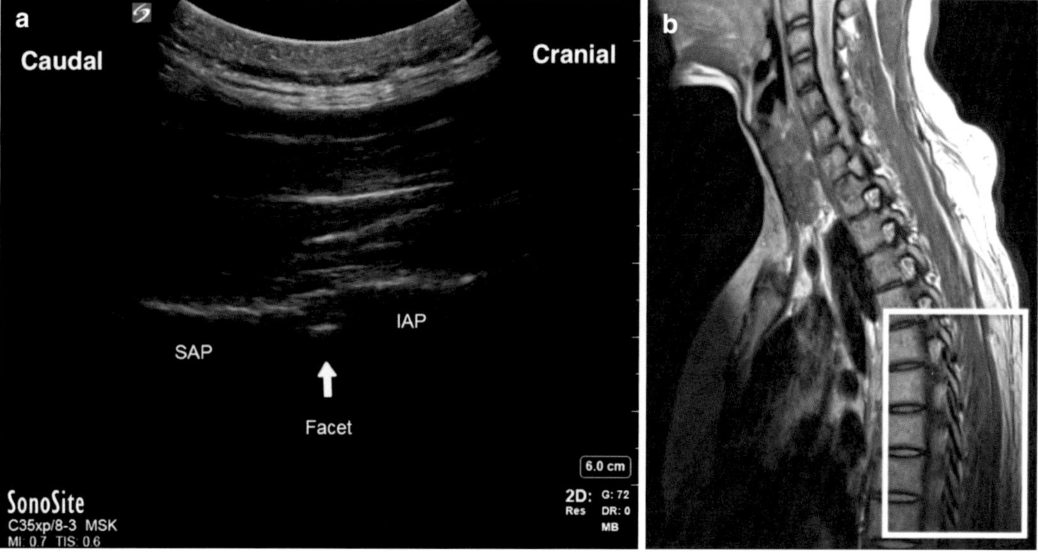

Fig. 11.15 The thoracic facet joint in the sagittal scan (**a**) with MR correlation (**b**). *SAP* superior articular process (of the above level), *IAP* inferior articular process (of the below level)

changes or morphological factors, fine needle adjustment is needed, and fluoroscopy verification should be considered. In our experience, a periarticular injection without penetration of the capsule also gains some therapeutic benefit.

Medial to the facet joint column, the lamina and interlaminar spaces (Fig. 11.16) lie in close proximity to the facet joints. Before injecting a thoracic facet joint, the clinician should always scan more medially to the facets and identify the thoracic interlaminar space, avoiding an inadvertent epidural injection, intrathecal injection, or spinal cord injury. The interspinous ligaments and supraspinous ligaments at the anatomical midline sometimes are targets for regenerative injection. Although landmark-guided injection for these two superficial structures could be performed easily, ultrasound guidance could further optimize the safety and precision of the therapy. The thoracic spinous

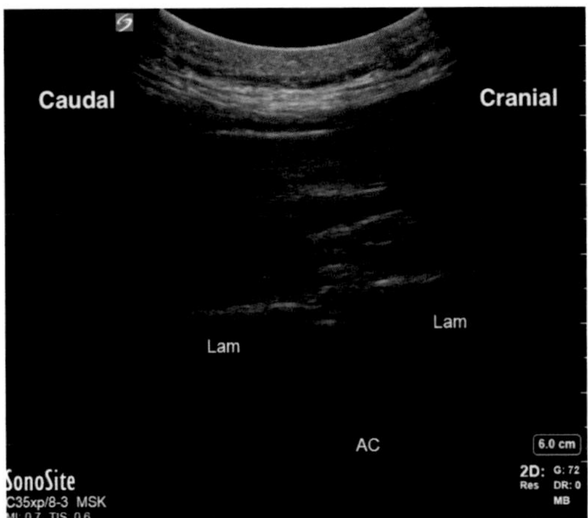

Fig. 11.16 Thoracic interlaminar space: this image could be obtained by medially tilting the ultrasound transducer from the thoracic facet joint view (Fig. 11.15). Scanning this view is crucial to prevent dural puncture in thoracic facet joint injection

process also receives several attachments from muscles and ligaments including the superior and lateral costotransverse ligaments, intertransverse muscles and ligaments, and deep back muscles, which are important for the biomechanical stability of the upper torso. Including the spinous process, interspinous ligaments, and supraspinous ligaments in the regenerative injection protocol would further optimize the therapeutic benefit.

Clinical Pearls of Specific Structures

Thoracic Facet Joint

The thoracic facet joints, like the cervical ones, are formed by the articulation of the inferior AP of the vertebra above and the superior AP of the vertebra below. The superior AP faces posteriorly, superiorly, and laterally [28], with the joints inclined anteriorly about 25–30 degrees from the frontal plane [29]. Each joint receives dual innervation from the medial branches from the dorsal rami of the spinal nerves above and below the joint. The orientation of the facet joint provides the freedom of rotational movement, while the flexion, extension, and lateral flexion movements are limited. The thoracic facet joint could be a pain generator when sustaining degenerative changes, inflammation, infection, or trauma.

Clinically, the patient may present with bilateral or unilateral paravertebral pain without neurologic deficit. The pain worsens with prolonged standing, hyperextension, or rotation of the thoracic spinal column [30]. Paraspinal tenderness to palpation is common yet not specific. Imaging modalities such as CT or MRI could help to exclude red flags such as malignancy or infectious disorder and, however, are not necessary in clinical assessment. Due to the overlapping clinical presentations of different pain generators in the thoracic spine pain, a definite diagnosis of thoracic facet joint pain could not be obtained without a diagnostic block on the medial branches or directly to the joint.

Costotransverse Joint (CTJ)

The CTJ is the joint between the TP and the ipsilateral rib and plays an important role in providing stability to the thoracic spine [31]. While the thoracic facet joints are innervated by the medial branches from the dorsal rami, the CTJs are innervated by the lateral branches of the dorsal rami [32]. It could be one of the pain generators in thoracic back pain, along with the thoracic facet joint and intervertebral disc. In contrast to the thoracic facet joint, the area of tenderness is usually more localized to the joint [33] and is mainly presented with unilateral middle back pain. In some cases, the pain may refer to the anterior chest, leading to atypical chest pain [34].

There are few clinical reports regarding regenerative injection on the CTJ. Besides the joint itself, the main supporting structures to the joint are superior, lateral, posterior, and inferior costotransverse ligaments [32, 35]. These ligaments attach to the lamina, the neck of the rib, the TP, and across the posterior joint capsule, and these structures could theoretically be targets of regenerative injection. The costovertebral joint and CTJ provide biomechanical stability to each other, and it is reasonable to consider a costovertebral joint injection when the tentative diagnosis is CTJ pain. However, costovertebral joint injection under ultrasound guidance could be technically difficult and dangerous due to the acoustic shadow of the TP and rib, the depth of the joint, and its close proximity to the pleura. For safety, regenerative injection for the CTJ should be limited to the joint itself and the supporting ligaments, instead of going deeper to the costovertebral joint.

Low Back Pain and Regenerative Medicine

Low back pain is one of the most common problems in clinical pain practice. The exact prevalence of low back pain is variable among different studies; however, it is a recurrent problem throughout most people's lives and causes significant health care-related burden [36]. Traditionally, on an interventional and anatomical basis, the common pathologies are nerve roots, facet joints, intervertebral discs, and sacroiliac joints (SIJs). As possible pain generators, muscles, ligaments, and tendons are usually overlooked in low back pain. When a definite pain generator could not be identified, the patient is often categorized into myofascial pain syndrome or idiopathic low back pain. The more common scenarios are when a single patient has more than one pain generator, different pathologies may share overlapping clinical features. In this kind of patients, an interplay between different structural deficits may further exaggerate the severity of pain and dysfunction, making a higher failure rate of conservative therapies and lower probability of precise plan of interventional pain management. To conquer this tough situation, the low back pain patient could also be managed in a more comprehensive way by regenerative injection with the concept of biotensegrity.

The key concepts of successful regenerative injection are knowledge of biotensegrity and fascial anatomy. In the model of biotensegrity, the bones float in a tension network, which consists of muscle, tendon, ligament, and fascial system. The bones are moved passively in the network when the dynamics of the tension system change. When there is instability or deficit in the tension network, pain or dysfunction may present. Regenerative injection focuses on "rebuilding" the overall stability of the network, which means the focuses of injection include not only the classic pain generators like facet joints or SIJs but also ligaments, entheses, and fascial systems. In a proof-of-concept review and case description [10], common targets of regenerative injection are described. These structures are thoracolumbar fascia (TLF), aponeurosis of the erector spinae muscles, interspinous ligaments, supraspinous ligaments, insertions of the multifidi, lateral raphe of abdominal wall muscles and lumbar interfascial triangle (LIFT) [37], the origins or insertions of the gluteus muscles. The quadratus lumborum (QL) muscles, lumbar facet joints, iliolumbar ligaments (ILLs), SIJs, and posterior sacroiliac ligaments are also possible pain generators or targets for regenerative injection.

Choosing the correct targets of injection usually depends on tenderness to palpation, dynamic tests according to the biomechanics, and dynamic ultrasound scanning [10]. In this section, the anatomy and sonoanatomy of the lumbosacral spine will be discussed as a fundamental background for ultrasound-guided interventional procedures. The paraspinal muscles, ligaments, and the TLF will also be included. Scanning and injection techniques will be described for different structures. Biomechanics of respective structures are beyond the scope of this chapter.

Anatomy and Sonoanatomy of the Lumbosacral Spine

For ultrasound scanning or guidance of intervention of the lumbosacral spine, a low-frequency curved array transducer is usually recommended due to the depth of the adult lumbosacral neuraxial structures. In scanning the lumbosacral spine, there are seven commonest sonographic views for interventional procedures or neuraxial anesthesia [38]. In the seven views, four are obtained in the sagittal plane and three are in the transverse plane (Table 11.1). While performing regenerative injection, which commonly targets the fascial systems and entheses, we can move the ultrasound transducer more laterally to the junction of the QL muscle and the lateral raphe of the abdominal wall muscles. The lateral extension of scanning could be achieved easily in the transverse plane.

In the series of sagittal scanning, one can begin at the spinous process on the midline, then move the transducer laterally to see the lamina and interlaminar spaces, facet joints and articular pillar, and TPs. A lateral-to-medial scanning protocol, which begins at the TPs and ends on the midline, was used by some clinicians. Our preferred protocol is the medial-to-lateral one. When targeted structures are localized, scanning back and forth to verify the correct position could further optimize the precision of injection.

In the medial-to-lateral approach, the first step is identifying the midline by palpating the spinous process. Placing the transducer on the midline, the hyperechoic line formed by the spinous process could be visualized (Fig. 11.17). The tip of the spinous process is the shallowest part of the lumbosacral bony structures. Sometimes the ultrasound transducer may "slip off" from the spinous process and falls onto the laminar view, especially when the patient is in a thin habitus. When the supraspinous ligaments or the interspinous ligaments are the target of treatment, one can move the transducer back and forth to make sure the location of the spinous process, avoiding mistaking the spinous process for the lamina or vice versa. Moving the transducer laterally with a certain degree of medial tilting, the lamina and interlaminar space could be visualized. In this view, the bony cortex of the lamina looks like horseheads (Fig. 11.18), facing to the caudad of the spine. Ultrasound-guided neuraxial anesthetic procedures are usually performed in this view. When performing an interventional procedure, level counting is of paramount importance for precise treatment. Counting level could be reliably done by using the interlaminar view.

More laterally in the sagittal plane, the lumbar facet joints and articular pillar could be visualized. The bony cortex of the articular pillar is in a wavy appearance, or so-called "camel hump"

Table 11.1 Common sonographic views of the lumbar spine

Sagittal plane
Spinous process view
Interlaminar view
Facet joint view
Transverse process view
Transverse plane
Transverse process view
Interlaminar view
Transverse oblique foraminal view

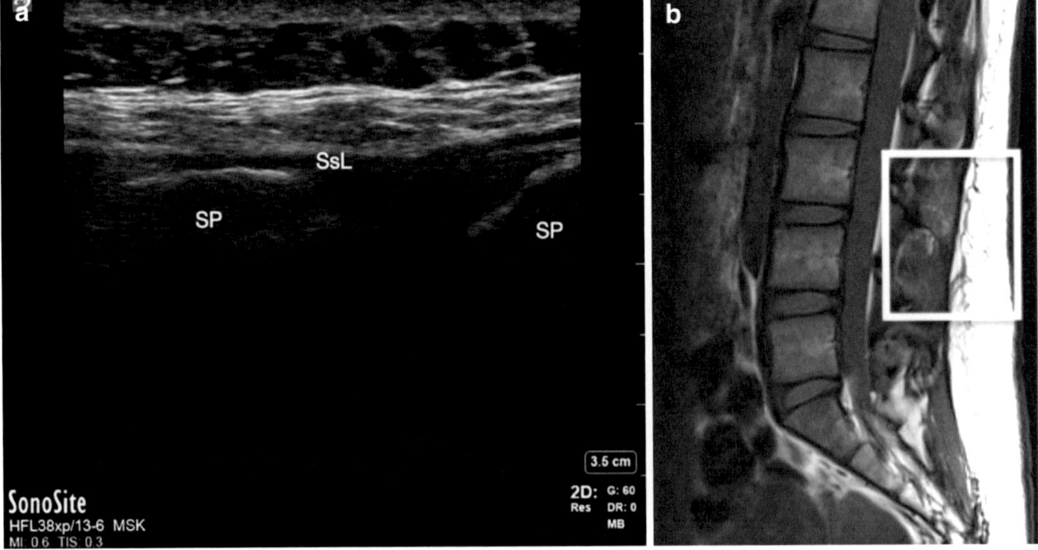

Fig. 11.17 The spinous process view in the sagittal plane of the lumbar spine (**a**) with MR correlation (**b**). *SP* spinous process, *SsL* supraspinous ligament

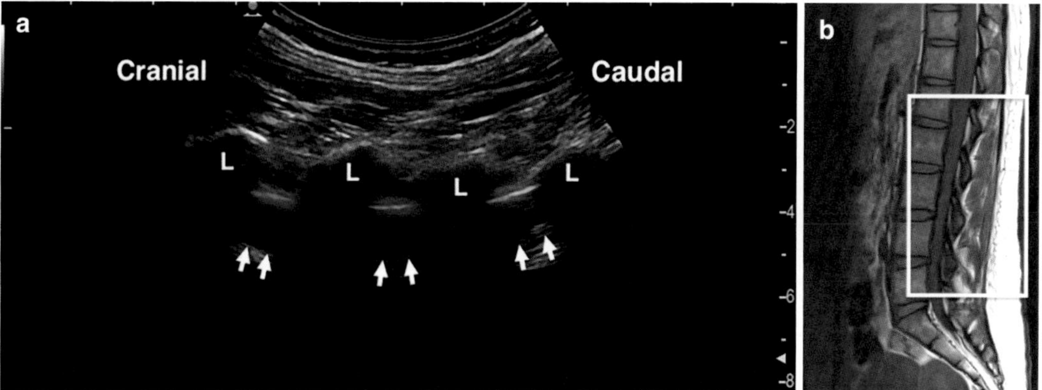

Fig. 11.18 The interlaminar view in the sagittal plane of the lumbar spine (**a**) with MR correlation (**b**). Note the "horsehead" appearance of the lamina. *L* lamina, *yellow shadow* posterior dura, *arrows* anterior complex

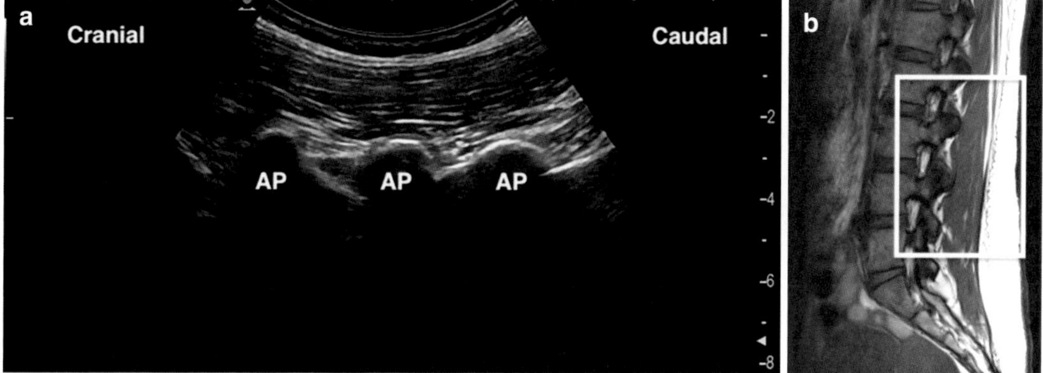

Fig. 11.19 The facet joint view in the sagittal plane of the lumbar spine (**a**) with MR correlation (**b**). Note the "camel hump" appearance of the articular pillar. *AP* articular pillar, *yellow shadow* joint cleft of the lumbar facets

sign (Fig. 11.19). When the lumbar facet joint is the target of treatment and the level is ascertained, one can rotate the transducer 90 degrees to the transverse view; the lumbar facet joint could be visualized as a small cleft between the inferior AP of the level above and the superior AP of the level below. The injection could be done in a lateral-to-medial, in-plane approach. Lateral to the articular pillar, we can visualize the TP in the sagittal plane. The bony cortex of the TP appears as separated round structures, or so-called "trident" sign (Fig. 11.20). Again, counting level is of paramount importance in spinal interventional procedures; the view of the TP could also be used to identify the correct level of treatment. In this view, the muscles above the TP are the erector spinae muscles, and the below is the psoas muscle. ESPB could be performed in this view. It could provide some pain relief in some idiopathic back pain, or when a diagnosis is not clear and the red flags have been ruled out.

The series of transverse views could be scanned when the TP of a certain level is identified. Rotating the transducer 90 degrees into the transverse orientation, the transverse process view (Fig. 11.21) could be obtained. In this view, part of the superior AP and the TP could be visualized. The medial branch of the lumbar dorsal rami is located at the junction of the superior AP and TP. Ultrasound-guided lumbar medial branch block is usually performed in this view, with an in-plane, lateral-to-medial approach. Moving the transducer a little bit cranially, the transverse view of the lumbar facet joint could be visualized (Fig. 11.22). An in-plane, lateral-to-medial facet joint injection could be executed in this view.

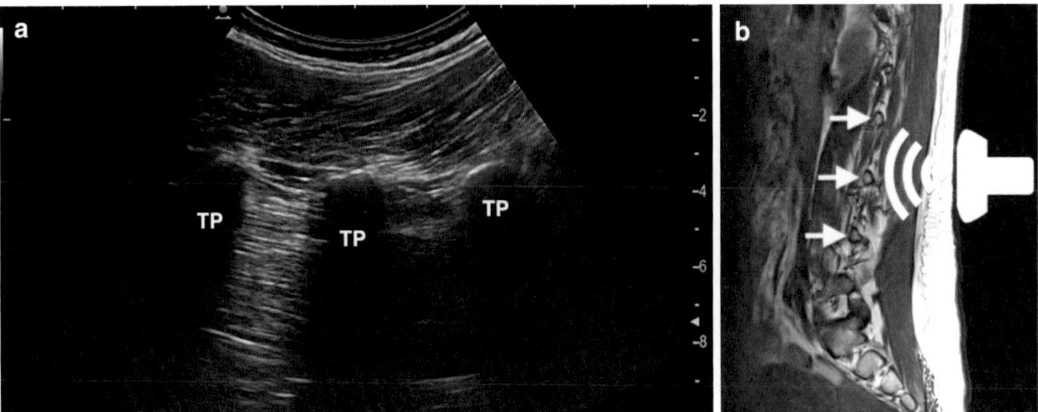

Fig. 11.20 The transverse process view in the sagittal plane of the lumbar spine (**a**) with MR correlation (**b**). Note the "trident" appearance of the transverse processes. *TP and arrows* transverse process

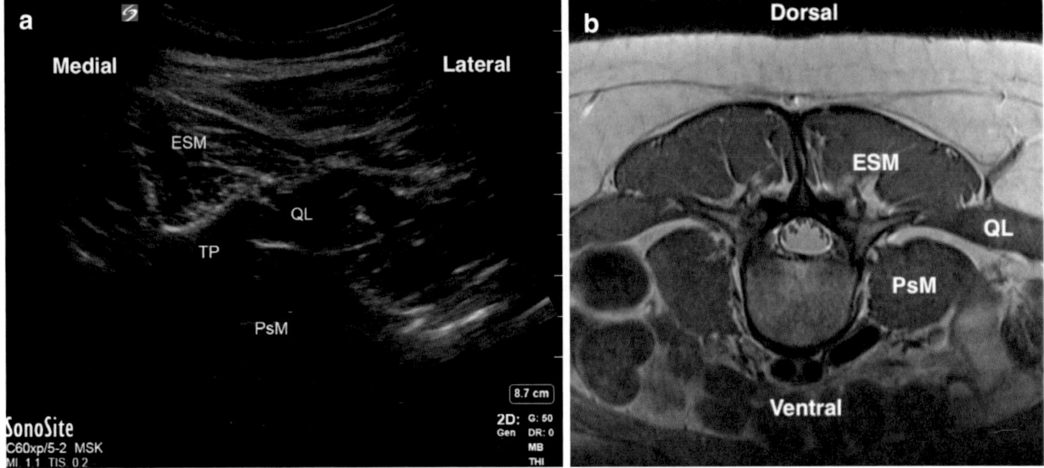

Fig. 11.21 The transverse process view in the transverse plane of the lumbar spine (**a**) with MR correlation (**b**). *ESM* erector spinae muscle, *QL* quadratus lumborum muscle, *PsM* psoas major muscle, *TP* transverse process

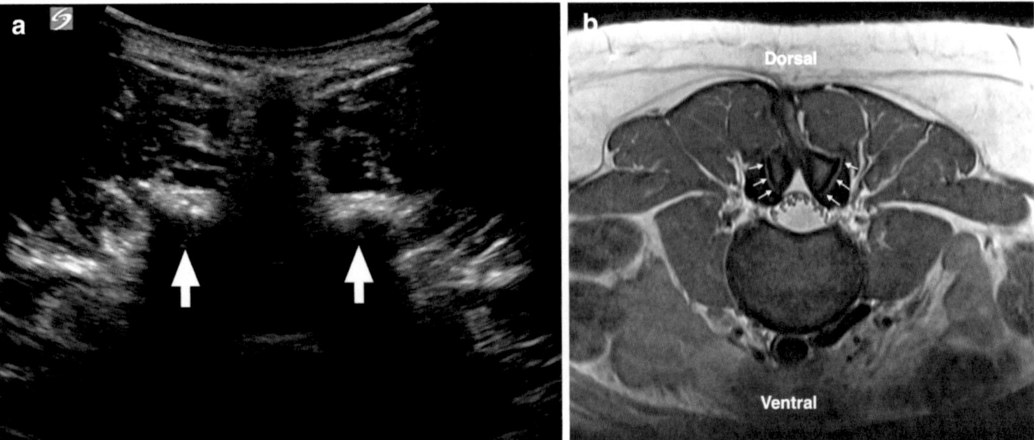

Fig. 11.22 The facet joint view in the transverse plane of the lumbar spine (**a**) with MR correlation (**b**). *Arrows* lumbar facet joint cleft

Moving the transducer in cephalad or caudal direction from the transverse process view, the transverse interlaminar view could be obtained (Fig. 11.23). In this view, the contents in the spinal canal including epidural space, dura, spinal cord, and even vertebral body could be visualized. In the transverse plane, when moving the transducer in a caudal-to-cephalad direction or vice versa, the hyperechoic bony structures could be visualized like a swimmer in the butterfly style, with the period of hands and shoulders up corresponding to the TP and facet joint, and the period diving into the water corresponding to the transverse interlaminar view. Moving the transducer laterally in the transverse plane with medial tilting, one can obtain the transverse oblique foraminal view (Fig. 11.24), which is usually utilized in the peri-radicular or transforaminal injection for lumbar radicular pain. More laterally from the transverse oblique foraminal view at the L3–4 level, the transverse quadratus lumborum view (Fig. 11.25) could be obtained. In this view, the QL muscle is in spindle shape and relatively hypoechoic when compared to the erector spinae muscles and the psoas muscle. Several important pivots in the TLF system, such as the lateral raphe and LIFT, could be visualized in this view and intervened with ultrasound guidance. Placing the QL muscle in the center of the ultrasound scan, rotating the transducer to the long axis of the QL muscle, we can see the enthesis of the QL onto the iliac crest (Fig. 11.26), which is also an important target for regenerative injection. For correctly counting the level in the interventional procedure in the lumbar spine, always remember utilizing both sagittal and transverse views, and validate the precise location by each other.

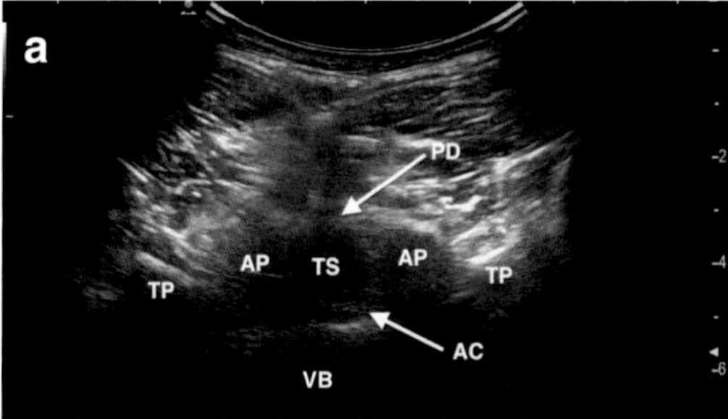

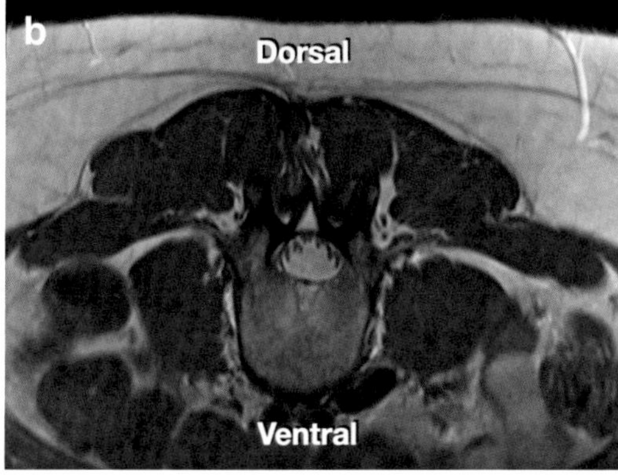

Fig. 11.23 The interlaminar view in the transverse plane of the lumbar spine (**a**) with MR correlation (**b**). *PD* posterior dura, *AP* articular pillar, *TP* transverse process, *TS* thecal sac, *AC* anterior complex, *VB* vertebral body

In addition to the lumbar spine, the SIJ also plays a crucial role in chronic low back pain. The SIJ is a synovial joint between the sacrum and the

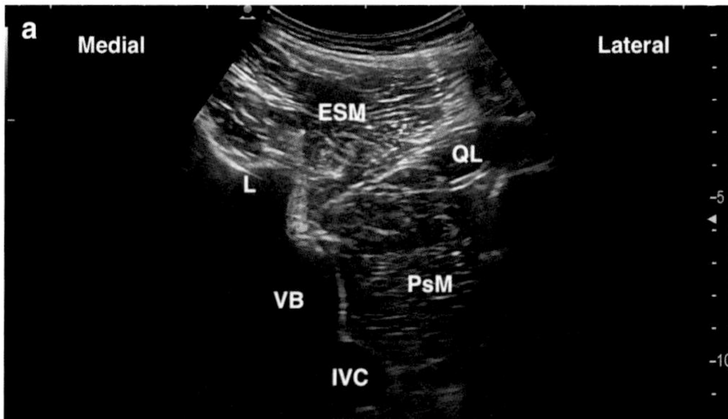

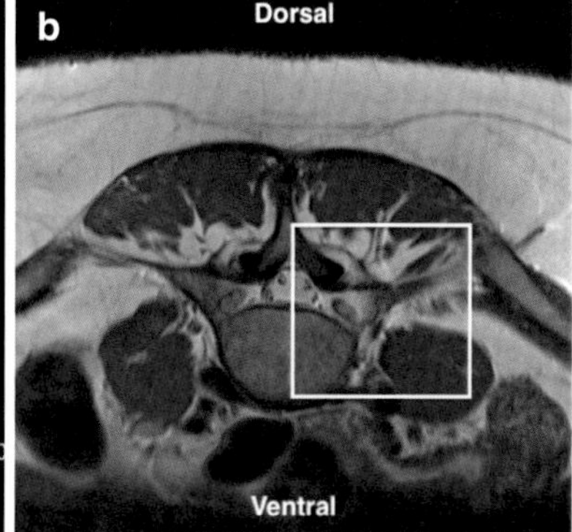

Fig. 11.24 The transverse oblique foraminal view of the lumbar spine (**a**) with MR correlation (**b**). *ESM* erector spinae muscle, *QL* quadratus lumborum muscle, *PsM* psoas major muscle, *L* lamina, *VB* vertebral body, *IVC* inferior vena cava, *yellow shadow* assumed location of the neuroforamen

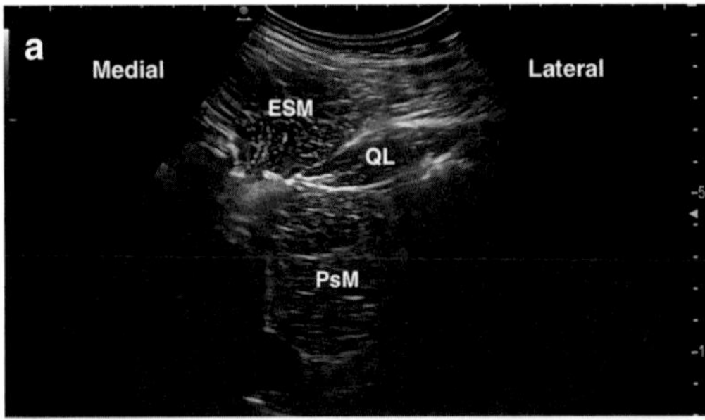

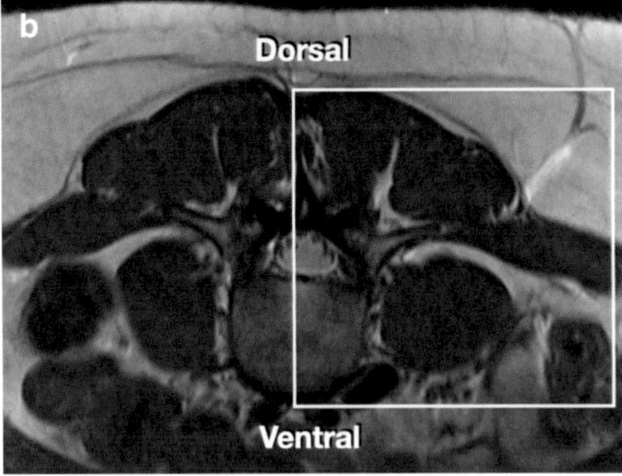

Fig. 11.25 The transverse quadratus lumborum view of the lumbar spine (**a**) with MR correlation (**b**). *ESM* erector spinae muscle, *QL* quadratus lumborum muscle, *PsM* psoas major muscle

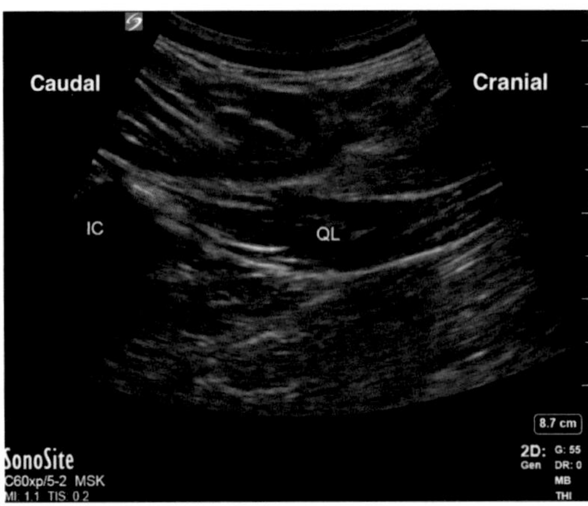

Fig. 11.26 The long-axis view of the quadratus lumborum muscle with its insertion on the iliac crest. *QL* quadratus lumborum muscle

ilium and lies in a posteromedial to anterolateral direction bilaterally. When scanning the SIJ, there are two recommended methods, one is the cranial-to-caudal technique from the posterior superior iliac spine and another is the caudal-to-cranial technique from the caudal hiatus. The final target of an intra-articular injection is the cleft between the hyperechoic bony structures, which are the ilium laterally and the sacrum medially (Fig. 11.27). In some patients, the posterior joint line lies almost in the sagittal plane; as such, an out-of-plane approach of injection should be considered. In the practice of regenerative injection, the dorsal interosseous ligament [39] in the upper pole of the posterior surface of the SIJ is more commonly targeted (Fig. 11.28). Some pitfalls should always be kept in mind when injecting the SIJ: one is the inferior pole of the joint often lies on the same level with the S2 posterior foramen; always move the transducer cranially or caudally to verify the continuation of joint line instead of S2 posterior foramen. Another issue is the volume of the SIJ is quite small. Extravasation of local anesthetics from the joint cavity would probably cause sciatic nerve blockade and motor weakness of the lower limbs; extravasation of high concentration dextrose would induce nerve irritation on the sacral plexus.

Clinical Pearls of Specific Structures

Lumbar Facet Joint

The lumbar spine and lower extremities support the weight of the human torso; therefore, the lumbosacral spine is susceptible to degenerative changes or traumatic injuries. The weight-bearing mechanism consists of the anterior column (vertebral bodies and intervertebral discs) and the posterior pillars (facet joints). The facet joints are diarthrodial and synovial joints and are the principal supporting structure of the lumbar spine. The capsular ligament encloses the facet joints and supports mechanical stability of the joints; therefore, the instability of the capsular ligaments is likely to cause low back pain [40]. Generally, the anterior one-third of the joints are oriented coronally, and the posterior two-thirds of the joints are oriented in sagittal direction [40]. The lower lumbar facet joints tend to orient in the coronal plane when compared to the upper ones; consequently, the lower ones are more susceptible to degenerative changes.

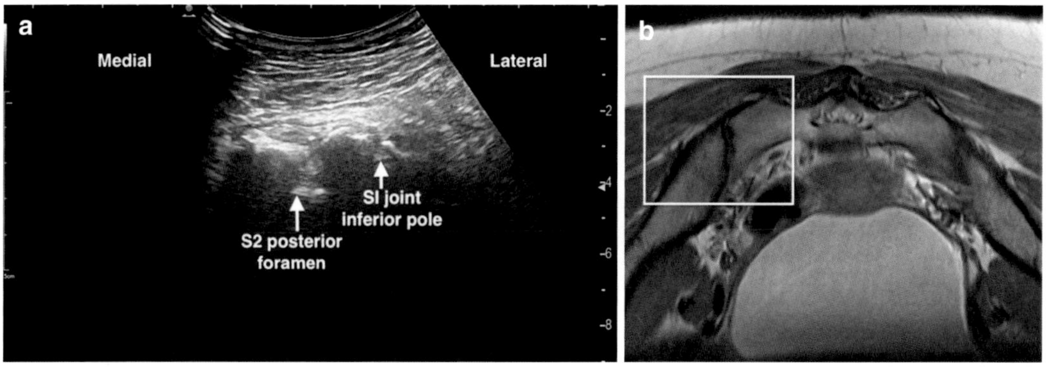

Fig. 11.27 The sonographic appearance of inferior pole of the sacroiliac (SI) joint (**a**) with MR correlation (**b**). Note the SI joint cleft could be in the same transverse plane of the posterior sacral foramen, either S2 or S3. Avoid mistaking the posterior sacral foramen for the SI joint

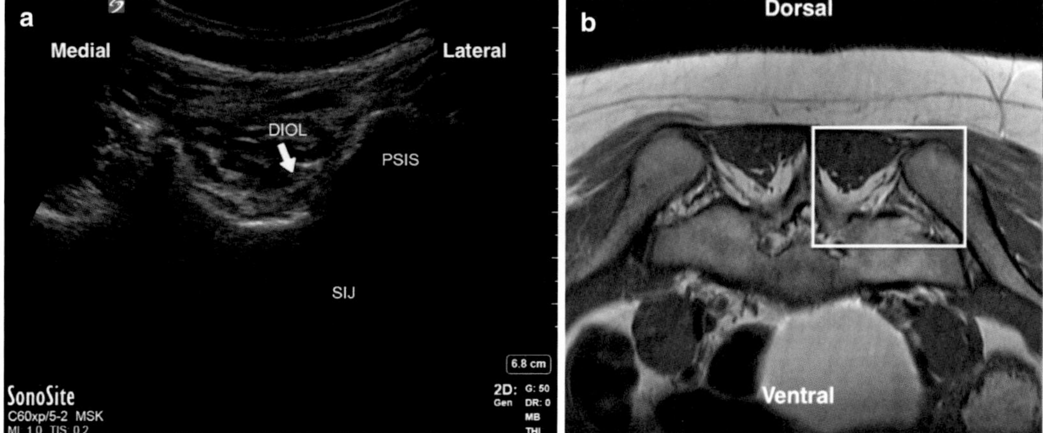

Fig. 11.28 The sonographic appearance of inferior pole of the sacroiliac joint (**a**) with MR correlation (**b**). *DIOL* dorsal interosseous ligament, *PSIS* posterior superior iliac spine, *SIJ* assumed location of the upper pole of the SI joint

The lumbar facet joints are innervated by the medial branches of the dorsal rami from the spinal nerves at the corresponding level and the above level (Fig. 11.29). After departed from the spinal nerves, the dorsal rami divide into lateral, intermediate, and medial branches. For L1 to L4 medial branches, they run between the osseous grooves between the TP and the superior AP and then under the mamilloaccessory ligament. The medial branches innervate the multifidi, interspinous ligaments, and the bony structures along their routes. The trajectory of the L5 dorsal rami is different from other lumbar dorsal rami [41]. It goes along the osseous groove between the S1 superior AP and the sacral ala. The anatomy of the nociceptive innervation of the lumbar facet joints is crucial in performing diagnostic block. Incorrect needle tip placement or excessive volume of local anesthetics would lead to high false-positive rates.

Clinically, lumbar facet joint pain is one of the differential diagnoses in axial low back pain, with the prevalence ranging from 15% to 45% in the low back pain population [42] and higher rates in the aged groups. It is usually unreliable to make a clinical diagnosis of lumbar facetogenic pain with only history and physical exam. Paraspinal tenderness is a common physical sign but is not specific. Imaging studies are usually not specific but could be helpful in excluding red

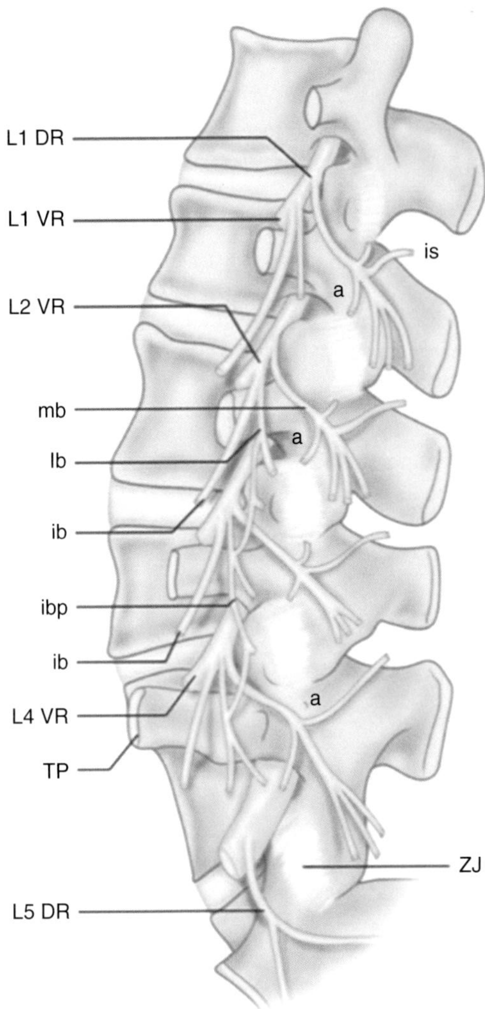

Fig. 11.29 Innervation of the lumbar facet joints. The lumbar facet joints receive dual innervation by the medial branch of the dorsal rami from the above and below spinal nerves. (From Manchikanti et al. [75], with permission from Springer)

flags or other occult pathology. For diagnosis of facetogenic low back pain, either facet joint injection or medial branch block has diagnostic value. Intra-articular injection of corticosteroid with local anesthetics provides limited therapeutic benefit [43], and currently, the mainstay of interventional management of lumbar facet joint pain remains radiofrequency denervation [44] or pulsed radiofrequency neuromodulation of lumbar medial branches [45, 46]. The clinical evidence of prolotherapy for lumbar facetogenic pain is relatively in minority [47, 48] and controversial [49]; however, positive result was obtained from a randomized controlled trial [50]. Platelet-rich plasma, which is a concentrate of whole blood, containing high concentration of platelet and growth factor, demonstrates positive result for facetogenic low back pain, superior to intra-articular corticosteroid injection [51]. The question is, is it correct to treat only the facet joint in a patient with lumbar facetogenic low back pain? Or a more comprehensive and individualized approach is needed? Needless to say, a comprehensive approach meets the principal concept "biotensegrity" much more than a traditional, single-structural approach. When a comprehensive approach is utilized, important structures associated with the TLF system should be considered in the regenerative injection protocol. Not all the related structures should be injected in each patient; the choice of targets depends on clinical assessment. As the treatment algorithm could be optimized and standardized in the future, the benefits of regenerative injection in facetogenic low back pain would probably be more significant.

Thoracolumbar Fascia (TLF) and Paraspinal Muscles [52]

The TLF is a girdling system that is crucial in lumbosacral stability and movement of the lower torso. It is a multilayer, multi-compartment system that separates paraspinal muscles from the muscles of posterior abdominal wall, QL, and psoas major and serves as a bridging system between the trunk and extremities. For this fascial system, both two-layer and three-layer models have been described. Although they are in different nomenclatures, the concepts of both models share much similarities. The middle layer in the three-layer model corresponds to the anterior layer in the two-layer model, while the anterior layer in the three-layer model is the fascia transversalis in the two-layer model. The three-layer model is the most commonly used. In this section, we will discuss the anatomy and its clinical relevance with the three-layer model.

In the three-layer system, the posterior layer is further divided into the superficial lamina and deep lamina. The superficial lamina is the aponeuroses of the latissimus dorsi and serratus posterior inferior, while the deep lamina encapsulates the paraspinal muscles and enhances the stability. The middle layer lies between the paraspinal muscles and the QL and is responsible for the tensional connection between the abdominal wall muscles and paraspinal muscles; the anterior layer runs anterior to the QL and posterior to the psoas major. In the center of the whole fascial system, the paraspinal muscles, which are the iliocostalis, longissimus, and multifidus, are contained in the paraspinal retinacular sheath and reinforced by attachments to the spinous processes and the TPs and stabilize the lumbosacral spine. In the lumbosacral junction, the anterior fascial sheath of the paraspinal muscle fuses with the ILLs and the posterior sacral joint capsule, while the posterior one attaches to the posterior superior iliac spine and extends to and fuses with the gluteus maximus and sacrotuberous ligament. The lower border of the middle layer fuses with the ILL and inserts onto the iliac crest. The lateral extreme of the TLF system is joined by the aponeurosis of the transverse abdominis, forming the anatomical linchpin called the "lateral raphe," and the triangular structure called the lumbar interfacial triangle. The fascia encapsulating the paraspinal muscles also joins the aponeurosis of the transverse abdominis around this area, which means the biomechanics of different parts of the TLF is interconnected and should be considered as a whole when doing regenerative injection.

Based on the above anatomical descriptions and the concept of biotensegrity, the stability of several attachments or connecting structures between muscles, ligaments, bones, and fascia should be considered as targets of regenerative injection. That is why in regenerative injection, structures like the supraspinous ligament, interspinous ligament, lateral raphe, LIFT, ILL, TP (insertion of the QL), and spinous process (insertion of the multifidus muscle) are common targets of treatment.

The Iliolumbar Ligament (ILL)

The ILL is one of the three most important vertebropelvic ligaments; the others are the sacrotuberous and sacrospinous ligaments. It originates from the TP of the L5 vertebrae and inserts on the superomedial part of the iliac crest (Fig. 11.30). The most common description of the subdivision of this ligament is a two-band model, in which there are anterior and posterior bands [53]. The anterior band is broad and flat, with 30–40 mm in length, 5–10 mm in width, and 2–3 mm in thickness [54]. It runs in the coronal plane and blends with the periosteum of the iliac crest. The posterior band is almost in round shape with 10–12 mm in length and 5–7 mm in diameter [54]. It runs

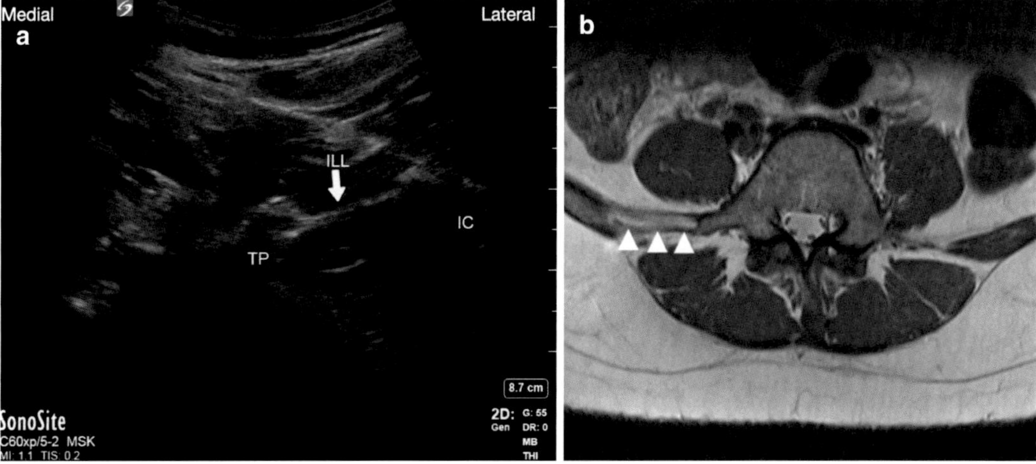

Fig. 11.30 The iliolumbar ligament in sonographic scan (**a**) with MR correlation (**b**). *TP* transverse process, *ILL* iliolumbar ligament, *IC* iliac crest, *arrowheads in the MRI* iliolumbar ligament

obliquely and inserts onto the posterior margin of the crest. The QL muscle is sandwiched between the two bands. The anterior border is the psoas muscle and the posterior border is the erector spinae muscle. Pool-Goudzwaard et al. [55] reported more detailed anatomy of the ILL, in which there are at least seven parts that could be found consistently in the human cadavers.

The presence of the ILL may be related to the upright position of the human beings [56, 57]. Biomechanically, the ILL is responsible for the stability of the lumbosacral junction, in coordination with lumbar discs, ligaments, and facet joints [58]. The anterior band restrains lateral bending [56, 58] and may prevent tilting of the vertebra in the coronal plane; the posterior band controls forward flexion of L5 on S1 and may prevent anterior slipping of the L5 vertebra [53, 56]. Flexion and extension are restricted by bilateral ligaments instead of unilateral control [58]; therefore, when treating the ILL, bilateral injection should be considered. The ILL is also important in maintaining torsional stability of the lumbosacral junction, protecting the L5-S1 disc especially in the presence of unstable lumbar facet column [59]. The presence of the strong ILL may explain why the L4–5 spondylolisthesis is more frequent than the L5-S1 spondylolisthesis. When the disc becomes more degenerative, the biomechanical stability provided by these ligaments becomes more important [57]. Attachment of the ligament to the anterior layer of the TLF was described [52]. When treating musculoskeletal pain or spine pain on a regenerative basis, it is crucial to apply the concept of biotensegrity meticulously and never neglect the continuity and connection of the fascial system in different parts of the human body.

The ILL is one of the primary causes of chronic low back pain because: [60] (1) it is the weakest part of the multifidus triangle; (2) increased susceptibility due to its angulated insertion; (3) it is the primary inhibitor of excessive sacral flexion; (4) it has rich nociceptive and proprioceptive innervation; and (5) the loading to this ligament is increasingLow back painIliolumbar ligament when the lumbosacral disc becomes degenerative. The numbers on the webpage are presented as hyperlinks to the references while it is not. I would like to make sure it is just numbers. The dorsal rami of the lumbar spinal nerves could be entrapped in the edematous or scarred ILL and further exaggerate the symptoms [54]. In a typical case, the patient complains of unilateral, well-localized pain on the posterior iliac crest. The pain could be provoked by prolonged standing or sitting and lateral bending to the unaffected side. Referred pain could be noticed in various areas including the hip, groin, and perineum, with a non-dermatomal nature. No neurologic deficit should be noticed in a typical iliolumbar pain patient. The iliolumbar pain syndrome could be explained by the enthesopathy of the ILL, especially of the insertion on the iliac crest [61]. When treating patients with symptoms from the ILL by regenerative injection, treating the entheses, especially the side of the iliac crest, should not be missed out.

The Sacroiliac Joints (SIJs)

The SIJ is a diarthrodial joint with interosseous portion [62], connecting the sacrum and the pelvis. It is the pivot that transmits the forces from the spine to the lower extremities or vice versa. The superior third of the SIJ is lined by hyaline cartilage and strongly attached to the surrounding ligaments, and the inferior third of the joint has some synovial characteristics [63]. In the low back pain population, the prevalence of SIJ pain is around 15–30% [64]. It is more common in patients after lumbar spinal fusion [65], pregnancy, or trauma [66]. The clinical presentation, like other types of low back pain, is not specific and not diagnostic. Imaging studies are usually not diagnostic and, however, could assist in revealing red flags like malignancy, inflammatory disorders, or occult trauma. The cluster of Laslett [67], in which more than three positive tests in the six clustered tests indicating high probability of SIJ pain.

To obtain a definite diagnosis of SIJ pain, comparative blocks using either different local anesthetics or local anesthetics and saline are mandatory. However, on the basis of regenerative medicine, any musculoskeletal pain or spinal pain should be considered in a whole picture instead of a single structure origin. Therefore, in the framework of "regeneration," performing comparative diagnostic blocks seems not to change the treatment plan a lot and is not a routine practice in regenerative-based pain practice.

Another important issue is the target structure of injection. Traditionally, when treating a painful SIJ, an intra-articular injection is usually the target of treatment, and positive clinical result of intra-articular prolotherapy or PRP has been obtained in a randomized controlled trial [68, 69]. In regenerative pain practice, however, the supporting ligaments [70] including the anterior sacroiliac ligament, the posterior sacroiliac ligament, the long posterior sacroiliac ligament, the ILL, the sacrospinous ligament, and the sacrotuberous ligament should be taken into consideration. Histologic pathology in the ligaments of the SIJs has been correlated to SIJ pain [71]. The anterior side is hard to inject due to the vicinity of pelvic viscera; however, the posterior structures could be treated thoroughly with ultrasound guidance. The posterior layer of the TLF system [72–74], which has rich connections with the sacrum, posterior superior iliac crest, LPSL, and the aponeurosis of the erector spinae muscle group, may be injected on the attaching point to the sacroiliac area. For intra-articular injection, the joint is about 1–2 mm in width [66]; therefore, an intra-articular injection sometimes could be difficult and hindered by the osteophytes, either by ultrasound or fluoroscopic guidance.

Conclusion

Chronic spine pain is a common complaint in pain clinic, and the prevalence is even higher in the aging population. In clinical assessment, the clinician could hardly make a definite diagnosis by history and physical exams. Imaging studies usually reveal nonspecific degenerative changes and are not diagnostic. For some validated pain generators like facet joints, the diagnosis usually depends on diagnostic block with local anesthetics. Traditionally, the interventional therapy consists of injection of corticosteroid and/or local anesthetics, neuromodulation, or radiofrequency denervation, and these interventions usually target single specific painful structure. Structures like muscle entheses, ligaments, or fascial systems are not recognized as valid pain generators; however, they play a certain role in the anatomy and biomechanics of spine pain and could be targets of treatment in regenerative injection. In recent decades, thanks to the rapidly evolving ultrasound-guided interventional technique, accurate injection on delicate yet pivotal structures like attachment of fascia or muscle enthesis is possible. Although the evidence is not yet fully established in the literature, with the knowledge of anatomy and biomechanics and precision of injection technique with ultrasound guidance, regenerative injection could potentially be a powerful treatment modality for chronic spinal pain in the future.

References

1. Hurwitz EL, Randhawa K, Yu H, Cote P, Haldeman S. The global spine care initiative: a summary of the global burden of low back and neck pain studies. Eur Spine J. 2018;27(Suppl 6):796–801.
2. Felix S, Linetsky LM. Regenerative injection therapy for axial pain. Techn Reg Anesth Pain Manag. 2005;9:40–9.
3. Wang D. Image guidance technologies for interventional pain procedures: ultrasound, fluoroscopy, and CT. Curr Pain Headache Rep. 2018;22(1):6.
4. Fejer R, Kyvik KO, Hartvigsen J. The prevalence of neck pain in the world population: a systematic critical review of the literature. Eur Spine J. 2006;15(6):834–48.
5. Cohen SP, Hooten WM. Advances in the diagnosis and management of neck pain. BMJ. 2017;358:j3221.
6. Manchikanti L, Boswell MV, Singh V, Pampati V, Damron KS, Beyer CD. Prevalence of facet joint pain in chronic spinal pain of cervical, thoracic, and lumbar regions. BMC Musculoskelet Disord. 2004;5:15.
7. Pearson AM, Ivancic PC, Ito S, Panjabi MM. Facet joint kinematics and injury mechanisms during simulated whiplash. Spine (Phila Pa 1976). 2004;29(4):390–7.
8. Usunier K, Hynes M, Schuster JM, Cornelio-Jin Suen A, Sadi J, Walton D. Clinical diagnostic tests versus medial branch blocks for adults with persisting cervical zygapophyseal joint pain: a systematic review and meta-analysis. Physiother Can. 2018;70(2):179–87.
9. Falco FJ, Erhart S, Wargo BW, Bryce DA, Atluri S, Datta S, et al. Systematic review of diagnostic util-

ity and therapeutic effectiveness of cervical facet joint interventions. Pain Physician. 2009;12(2):323–44.
10. Fullerton BD. Prolotherapy for the thoracolumbar myofascial system. Phys Med Rehabil Clin N Am. 2018;29(1):125–38.
11. Winkelstein BA, McLendon RE, Barbir A, Myers BS. An anatomical investigation of the human cervical facet capsule, quantifying muscle insertion area. J Anat. 2001;198(Pt 4):455–61.
12. Steilen D, Hauser R, Woldin B, Sawyer S. Chronic neck pain: making the connection between capsular ligament laxity and cervical instability. Open Orthop J. 2014;8:326–45.
13. Gellhorn AC, Katz JN, Suri P. Osteoarthritis of the spine: the facet joints. Nat Rev Rheumatol. 2013;9(4):216–24.
14. Rong X, Liu Z, Wang B, Chen H, Liu H. The facet orientation of the subaxial cervical spine and the implications for cervical movements and clinical conditions. Spine (Phila Pa 1976). 2017;42(6):E320–E5.
15. van Eerd M, Patijn J, Lataster A, Rosenquist RW, van Kleef M, Mekhail N, et al. 5. Cervical facet pain. Pain Pract. 2010;10(2):113–23.
16. Dwyer A, Aprill C, Bogduk N. Cervical zygapophyseal joint pain patterns. I: A study in normal volunteers. Spine (Phila Pa 1976). 1990;15(6):453–7.
17. Fukui S, Ohseto K, Shiotani M, Ohno K, Karasawa H, Naganuma Y, et al. Referred pain distribution of the cervical zygapophyseal joints and cervical dorsal rami. Pain. 1996;68(1):79–83.
18. Windsor RE, Nagula D, Storm S, Overton A, Jahnke S. Electrical stimulation induced cervical medial branch referral patterns. Pain Physician. 2003;6(4):411–8.
19. Falco FJ, Datta S, Manchikanti L, Sehgal N, Geffert S, Singh V, et al. An updated review of the diagnostic utility of cervical facet joint injections. Pain Physician. 2012;15(6):E807–38.
20. Falco FJ, Manchikanti L, Datta S, Wargo BW, Geffert S, Bryce DA, et al. Systematic review of the therapeutic effectiveness of cervical facet joint interventions: an update. Pain Physician. 2012;15(6):E839–68.
21. Manchikanti L, Boswell MV, Singh V, Benyamin RM, Fellows B, Abdi S, et al. Comprehensive evidence-based guidelines for interventional techniques in the management of chronic spinal pain. Pain Physician. 2009;12(4):699–802.
22. Manchikanti L, Helm S, Singh V, Benyamin RM, Datta S, Hayek SM, et al. An algorithmic approach for clinical management of chronic spinal pain. Pain Physician. 2009;12(4):E225–64.
23. Manchikanti L, Singh V, Pampati V, Beyer CD, Damron KS. Evaluation of the prevalence of facet joint pain in chronic thoracic pain. Pain Physician. 2002;5(4):354–9.
24. Fruth SJ. Differential diagnosis and treatment in a patient with posterior upper thoracic pain. Phys Ther. 2006;86(2):254–68.
25. Singh V, Manchikanti L, Shah RV, Dunbar EE, Glaser SE. Systematic review of thoracic discography as a diagnostic test for chronic spinal pain. Pain Physician. 2008;11(5):631–42.
26. Tulgar S, Thomas DT, Suslu H. Ultrasound guided erector spinae plane block relieves lower cervical and interscapular myofascial pain, a new indication. J Clin Anesth. 2019;53:74.
27. Standring S. Gray's anatomy : the anatomical basis of clinical practice. 41st ed. New York: Elsevier Limited; 2016. xviii, 1562 pages
28. Cramer GD, Darby SA, Cramer GD. Clinical anatomy of the spine, spinal cord, and ANS. 3rd ed. St. Louis: Elsevier; 2014. xv, 672 p
29. Masharawi Y, Rothschild B, Dar G, Peleg S, Robinson D, Been E, et al. Facet orientation in the thoracolumbar spine: three-dimensional anatomic and biomechanical analysis. Spine (Phila Pa 1976). 2004;29(16):1755–63.
30. van Kleef M, Stolker RJ, Lataster A, Geurts J, Benzon HT, Mekhail N. 10. Thoracic pain. Pain Pract. 2010;10(4):327–38.
31. Oda I, Abumi K, Lu D, Shono Y, Kaneda K. Biomechanical role of the posterior elements, costovertebral joints, and rib cage in the stability of the thoracic spine. Spine (Phila Pa 1976). 1996;21(12):1423–9.
32. Dedrick GS, Sizer PS, Sawyer BG, Brismee JM, Smith MP. Immunohistochemical study of human costotransverse joints: a preliminary investigation. Clin Anat. 2011;24(6):741–7.
33. Young BA, Gill HE, Wainner RS, Flynn TW. Thoracic costotransverse joint pain patterns: a study in normal volunteers. BMC Musculoskelet Disord. 2008;9:140.
34. Arroyo JF, Jolliet P, Junod AF. Costovertebral joint dysfunction: another misdiagnosed cause of atypical chest pain. Postgrad Med J. 1992;68(802):655–9.
35. Ibrahim AF, Darwish HH. The costotransverse ligaments in human: a detailed anatomical study. Clin Anat. 2005;18(5):340–5.
36. Hoy D, March L, Brooks P, Blyth F, Woolf A, Bain C, et al. The global burden of low back pain: estimates from the global burden of disease 2010 study. Ann Rheum Dis. 2014;73(6):968–74.
37. Schuenke MD, Vleeming A, Van Hoof T, Willard FH. A description of the lumbar interfascial triangle and its relation with the lateral raphe: anatomical constituents of load transfer through the lateral margin of the thoracolumbar fascia. J Anat. 2012;221(6):568–76.
38. Provenzano DA, Narouze S. Sonographically guided lumbar spine procedures. J Ultrasound Med. 2013;32(7):1109–16.
39. Cusi M, Saunders J, Hungerford B, Wisbey-Roth T, Lucas P, Wilson S. The use of prolotherapy in the sacroiliac joint. Br J Sports Med. 2010;44(2):100–4.
40. Bermel EA, Barocas VH, Ellingson AM. The role of the facet capsular ligament in providing spinal stability. Comput Methods Biomech Biomed Engin. 2018;21(13):712–21.

41. Greher M, Moriggl B, Peng PW, Minella CE, Zacchino M, Eichenberger U. Ultrasound-guided approach for L5 dorsal ramus block and fluoroscopic evaluation in unpreselected cadavers. Reg Anesth Pain Med. 2015;40(6):713–7.
42. Manchikanti L, Manchikanti KN, Cash KA, Singh V, Giordano J. Age-related prevalence of facet-joint involvement in chronic neck and low back pain. Pain Physician. 2008;11(1):67–75.
43. Cohen SP, Doshi TL, Constantinescu OC, Zhao Z, Kurihara C, Larkin TM, et al. Effectiveness of lumbar facet joint blocks and predictive value before radiofrequency denervation: the facet treatment study (FACTS), a randomized, controlled clinical trial. Anesthesiology. 2018;129(3):517–35.
44. Lee CH, Chung CK, Kim CH. The efficacy of conventional radiofrequency denervation in patients with chronic low back pain originating from the facet joints: a meta-analysis of randomized controlled trials. Spine J. 2017;17(11):1770–80.
45. Lindner R, Sluijter ME, Schleinzer W. Pulsed radiofrequency treatment of the lumbar medial branch for facet pain: a retrospective analysis. Pain Med. 2006;7(5):435–9.
46. Cetin A, Yektas A. Evaluation of the short- and long-term effectiveness of pulsed radiofrequency and conventional radiofrequency performed for medial branch block in patients with lumbar facet joint pain. Pain Res Manag. 2018;2018:7492753.
47. Hooper RA, Ding M. Retrospective case series on patients with chronic spinal pain treated with dextrose prolotherapy. J Altern Complement Med. 2004;10(4):670–4.
48. Solmaz I, Akpancar S, Orscelik A, Yener-Karasimav O, Gul D. Dextrose injections for failed back surgery syndrome: a consecutive case series. Eur Spine J. 2019;28(7):1610–7.
49. Yelland MJ, Glasziou PP, Bogduk N, Schluter PJ, McKernon M. Prolotherapy injections, saline injections, and exercises for chronic low-back pain: a randomized trial. Spine (Phila Pa 1976). 2004;29(1):9–16; discussion
50. Klein RG, Eek BC, DeLong WB, Mooney V. A randomized double-blind trial of dextrose-glycerine-phenol injections for chronic, low back pain. J Spinal Disord. 1993;6(1):23–33.
51. Wu J, Zhou J, Liu C, Zhang J, Xiong W, Lv Y, et al. A prospective study comparing platelet-rich plasma and local anesthetic (LA)/corticosteroid in intra-articular injection for the treatment of lumbar facet joint syndrome. Pain Pract. 2017;17(7):914–24.
52. Willard FH, Vleeming A, Schuenke MD, Danneels L, Schleip R. The thoracolumbar fascia: anatomy, function and clinical considerations. J Anat. 2012;221(6):507–36.
53. Luk KD, Ho HC, Leong JC. The iliolumbar ligament. A study of its anatomy, development and clinical significance. J Bone Joint Surg Br. 1986;68(2):197–200.
54. Sims JA, Moorman SJ. The role of the iliolumbar ligament in low back pain. Med Hypotheses. 1996;46(6):511–5.
55. Pool-Goudzwaard AL, Kleinrensink GJ, Snijders CJ, Entius C, Stoeckart R. The sacroiliac part of the iliolumbar ligament. J Anat. 2001;199(Pt 4):457–63.
56. Pun WK, Luk KD, Leong JC. Influence of the erect posture on the development of the lumbosacral region. A comparative study on the lumbosacral junction of the monkey, dog, rabbit and rat. Surg Radiol Anat. 1987;9(1):69–73.
57. Leong JC, Luk KD, Chow DH, Woo CW. The biomechanical functions of the iliolumbar ligament in maintaining stability of the lumbosacral junction. Spine (Phila Pa 1976). 1987;12(7):669–74.
58. Yamamoto I, Panjabi MM, Oxland TR, Crisco JJ. The role of the iliolumbar ligament in the lumbosacral junction. Spine (Phila Pa 1976). 1990;15(11):1138–41.
59. Chow DH, Luk KD, Leong JC, Woo CW. Torsional stability of the lumbosacral junction. Significance of the iliolumbar ligament. Spine (Phila Pa 1976). 1989;14(6):611–5.
60. Kiter E, Karaboyun T, Tufan AC, Acar K. Immunohistochemical demonstration of nerve endings in iliolumbar ligament. Spine (Phila Pa 1976). 2010;35(4):E101–4.
61. Basadonna PT, Gasparini D, Rucco V. Iliolumbar ligament insertions. In vivo anatomic study. Spine (Phila Pa 1976). 1996;21(20):2313–6.
62. Walker JM. The sacroiliac joint: a critical review. Phys Ther. 1992;72(12):903–16.
63. Puhakka KB, Melsen F, Jurik AG, Boel LW, Vesterby A, Egund N. MR imaging of the normal sacroiliac joint with correlation to histology. Skelet Radiol. 2004;33(1):15–28.
64. Cohen SP, Chen Y, Neufeld NJ. Sacroiliac joint pain: a comprehensive review of epidemiology, diagnosis and treatment. Expert Rev Neurother. 2013;13(1):99–116.
65. Lee YC, Lee R, Harman C. The incidence of new onset sacroiliac joint pain following lumbar fusion. J Spine Surg. 2019;5(3):310–4.
66. Foley BS, Buschbacher RM. Sacroiliac joint pain: anatomy, biomechanics, diagnosis, and treatment. Am J Phys Med Rehabil. 2006;85(12):997–1006.
67. Laslett M, Aprill CN, McDonald B, Young SB. Diagnosis of sacroiliac joint pain: validity of individual provocation tests and composites of tests. Man Ther. 2005;10(3):207–18.
68. Kim WM, Lee HG, Jeong CW, Kim CM, Yoon MH. A randomized controlled trial of intra-articular prolotherapy versus steroid injection for sacroiliac joint pain. J Altern Complement Med. 2010;16(12):1285–90.
69. Singla V, Batra YK, Bharti N, Goni VG, Marwaha N. Steroid vs. platelet-rich plasma in ultrasound-guided sacroiliac joint injection for chronic low Back pain. Pain Pract. 2017;17(6):782–91.
70. Poilliot AJ, Zwirner J, Doyle T, Hammer N. A systematic review of the normal sacroiliac joint anatomy and

adjacent tissues for pain physicians. Pain Physician. 2019;22(4):E247–E74.

71. Hammer N, Ondruschka B, Fuchs V. Sacroiliac joint ligaments and sacroiliac pain: a case-control study on micro- and ultrastructural findings on morphologic alterations. Pain Physician. 2019;22(6):E615–E25.
72. Barker PJ, Briggs CA. Attachments of the posterior layer of lumbar fascia. Spine (Phila Pa 1976). 1999;24(17):1757–64.
73. Vleeming A, Pool-Goudzwaard AL, Stoeckart R, van Wingerden JP, Snijders CJ. The posterior layer of the thoracolumbar fascia. Its function in load transfer from spine to legs. Spine (Phila Pa 1976). 1995;20(7):753–8.
74. Vleeming A, Pool-Goudzwaard AL, Hammudoghlu D, Stoeckart R, Snijders CJ, Mens JM. The function of the long dorsal sacroiliac ligament: its implication for understanding low back pain. Spine (Phila Pa 1976). 1996;21(5):556–62.
75. Manchikanti L, et al. Essentials of interventional techniques in managing chronic pain. Cham: Springer; 2018.

12 Spinal Regenerative Medicine

Jeffrey D. Gross

Introduction

Following just a close step behind the rapidly advancing successes in applying regenerative medical treatments to the extremity joints and related structures, a blossoming field with encouraging results in applying similar therapies to spinal structures serves as the impetus for the present manuscript. Slow to be adopted by mainstream medical policy, regenerative approaches to the spine represent a disruptive and paradigm shifting biotechnology with the potential to meaningfully reduce pain and dysfunction of spinal origin, with less dependence on surgical reconstruction. This chapter outlines the current cutting edge in biological spinal regenerative medicine (exclusive of prolotherapy), surely but excitingly to be at least partially outdated by the time of publication. The presentation here is a general overview of the practical and clinical considerations involving the spine and is not intended to review the scientific foundation of regenerative biology and medicine. This chapter serves more specifically to review regenerative targets of painful pathologies of the spine, short of neuro-regeneration, and therefore does not include review of a large body of study on addressing spinal cord pathologies. Additionally, this chapter does not take up the topic of spinal fusion, which is a surgical augmentative process enhanced by regenerative products for the better part of two decades.

The organization of this chapter is designed to break down the differing anato-physiological regenerative medicine targets of the spine, sub-organized by a review of the specific biologics which have been applied to these spinal targets. When mixed biologics are described having been delivered to a spinal element, they are discussed as grouped with their more potently perceived element (PRP and growth factors first, extracellular matrix and other amniotic supportive contents, next followed by cellular therapies, and then exosomal biologics). There is not yet uniformity whereby each regenerative method has been comparatively applied to all structures of the spine, let alone adequate blinded, randomized trials. This comment is not meant to be critical, but instead is an observation as to the analytic cautions and limitations to the present availability of scientifically grounded studies [1].

As always, clinicians are recommended to use best judgment in acting in a patient's best interest with a clear and thorough description of all options and the pros and cons of each as part of a fully informed consent process.

J. D. Gross (✉)
Stem Cell Whisperer, SPINE & ReCELLebrate, Henderson, NV, USA
e-mail: jdgross@theultimateinhealth.com

Y. El Miedany (ed.), *Musculoskeletal Ultrasound-Guided Regenerative Medicine*, https://doi.org/10.1007/978-3-030-98256-0_12

Regenerative Medicine by Spinal Target

The following section serves to review regenerative approaches to the spine by location(s). These targets include paraspinal myofascial structures, facetogenic structures, epidural spaces, intradiscal targets, and intervertebral/subchondral targets. Each area is discussed with both a rationale for the approach and a review of related study results. Most studies are noted to be anecdotal collections and serve as a starting place, as did most great advances in any field of medicine or other discipline. Given that this chapter is focused on clinical aspects applying regenerative therapies to the spine, the topic of the biological advantage of such approaches (including anti-inflammatory, analgesic, rehabilitative, and anato-physiological restorative augmentation) is deferred.

Regenerative Facet and/or Paraspinal Injections

It is well understood that a common source of spinal pain and dysfunction, involving all segments of the spine, can be facetogenic: arising of the facet joint(s) and their surrounding structures [2, 3]. Traditional treatment beyond physical rehabilitation and anti-inflammatory (or stronger) medications include injections into the facet joint, into the facet joint capsule, and/or targeting by injection and/or denervation the local innervation by way of the medial branch nerves [3]. Although said treatments are reasonably effective, often measured for up to months in the case of repeat rhizotomies [4–10], regenerative approaches seek to enhance and restore anatomical and/or physiological defects causing facetogenic pain and dysfunction without the need for degenerative or neuro-ablative treatments, which themselves may beget cumulative and accelerated degeneration. Not considered in this chapter are the many studies referencing use of biologics more generically for any joint(s); however, it is reasonable to extrapolate those findings to facet joints [11].

Perhaps the most frequent and robust foundation in support of regenerative approaches to the spine involves treatment with platelet-rich plasma (PRP). Beginning with facet intra-articular injections, Wu et al. [12] reported on 15 of 19 patients having received intra-articular facet PRP injections. It was concluded that such a procedure is safe and effective in a 3-month time frame. The study was limited for lack of a control group, limited outcome measures (5-point benefit scale), and relatively short follow-up. The same group in 2017 compared intra-articular facet joint PRP to traditional corticosteroid/local anesthetic injection, finding statistically significant improvement in the PRP group as far as 6 months after injection, whereas the non-regenerative group results waned over time [13]. Although not suitable for referencing, there is a large additional body of anecdotal support for using PRP for facetogenic pain. However, a meta-analysis concluded that facet joint PRP may be effective in managing discogenic, radicular, and facet joint pain [14]. It is not trivial that delivering PRP to facet joints has been shown to assist with other pain generators of the spine. The American Society of Interventional Pain Physicians Guidelines indicate PRP treatment for facet joints is based upon class IV evidence [15]. Each year, the scientific evidence improves to support PRP and other regenerative approaches to the spine [16].

Growth factors (a component of PRP) have been studied as injected into facet joints, but only when combined with other spinal areas (see below). Aufiero et al. reported on the benefits in a series of three PRP injections to the facet joints and surrounding ligaments via ultrasound guidance, finding meaningful pain reduction measured at 6 months and up to 12 months in some of the cases [17]. Cameron et al. also injected PRP into the lateral masses, facet joints, lateral gutters, spinal ligaments, and related posterior spinal structures for herniated disc-related pain, finding significant pain reduction for a mean of 5 years [18]. This study however suffers from lack of confirmation of a pain generator prior to treatment.

Few have reported on the use of stem cell preparations in any form delivered to facet joint structures. One report contained a treatment arm of bone marrow concentrate (BMC) to the facet joints, ligaments, and sacroiliac joints [19]. Although the results were not positive, this study's main limitations in the present context include a problematic assumption that all discogram-negative patients had facetogenic pain and that more than just the facet joints were injected. There are no identifiable scientific studies looking at adipose, or adipose-derived stem cells for use in the posterior spinal elements, inclusive of facet joints, although such procedures are clinically available.

Bennett reported on the use of cryopreserved amniotic membrane and umbilical cord (AMUC) particulate for facet joint syndrome [20]. He found statistically significant pain reduction as far as 6 months posttreatment. Other more generic studies dealing with amniotic products for joint pain may be practically extrapolated to facet joints [20].

Extracellular vesicles/exosomes have also been used to address facetogenic spinal pain. In 2019, Li et al. demonstrated the utility of bone marrow-derived stem cell exosomes to address lumbar pain behavior in an animal facetogenic injury model, whereby the subchondral facet joint bone was injected [20]. The facet bone marrow is known to house stem cells and has relation to the health of local ligaments [21]. As exosomes act to vitalize the metabolism of cells within reach, facet joint bone marrow health can be most directly influenced by subchondral injection, although also reachable by capsular, intra-articular, and paraspinal approaches, perhaps due to shared blood flow. Further discussion and reference to the therapeutic potential of exosomes deal with joints in general [22].

Regenerative paraspinal injections have also been utilized to address spinal pain. These are discussed in the facetogenic pain section, being so closely anatomically related to the facet joints, and due to a shared vascularity with same. Additionally, paraspinal injections often also involve the facet joint capsules and local peri-facetal ligamentous structures. Regenerative paraspinal injections for spinal pain with spinal muscular atrophy (as part of a "self-sustained vicious cycle which start with an injury to either the disc, muscle," or the facet joint...can lead to further injury to the other two components") as reported by Hussein and Hussein [23] demonstrated continued pain reduction at 24 months in 74/104 patients, although began soon after injection, in theoretical relation to serotonin release. Additionally, MSCs (mesenchymal stem cells) have been used to address spinal (and limb) muscular atrophy in Duchenne's muscular dystrophy successfully [24]. At the time of this writing, there is an open study looking in part at the use of paraspinally delivered BMC for spinal cord injury [25, 26]. Regenerative approaches to paraspinal muscles are also being looked at to address adolescent idiopathic scoliosis [27] and amyotrophic lateral sclerosis [28].

Direct injection of growth factors (particularly PRGF-Endoret) to facet articulations has also been described [29]. Statistically significant pain reduction was found, lasting to 6 months. Drawbacks of this study include the 6-month (short) end point.

Clinical considerations for applying regenerative strategies to facet joint structures include first confirming the presence of facetogenic pain clinically and/or by local block. Such can be more efficiently accomplished with imaging guidance for more specific localization of the spinal levels. Fluoroscopy and ultrasound are the more efficient methods, with ultrasound making in-office procedures more accessible. Biological theory supports subchondral injections as being the most direct and effective, but it is not fully known if such is practically superior to intra-articular, peri-facetal, or even paraspinal injections. The choice of biologics is left to the good judgment of an individual clinician, with considerable nonclinical factors of cost, accessibility, and governmental regulation(s). Another factor for consideration is the number of injections to offer. It appears most reasonable to start with one series and observe the result before offering any accumulative booster treatments.

As I hope other clinicians have experienced anecdotally, I continue to be amazed by the results of the rather simple application of regenerative biologics to facet/paraspinal structures. It is my opinion, and I look forward to a more robust, large trial of study, in which concentrated perinatal sourced exosome-containing preparations delivered to the facet capsule and its surrounding myoligamentous structures provide the multimodal anti-inflammatory and regenerative cellular activity transformations to support anatomical and physiological improvements to facet joints and local muscles for which pain and related dysfunction are mitigated.

It is almost too perfectly simplistic that the biological rehabilitation of spinal muscles (paraspinal, multifidus) has a benefit in addressing spinal pain of various sources. Although traditionally addressed through physical rehabilitation, biological augmentation can be delivered with ultrasound or without guidance in a clinician's office without much ado. This has been my personal experience as well.

Regenerative Epidural Injections

The following section considers epidural placement of regenerative biological preparations, including by various delivered routes (interlaminar, transforaminal). Such endeavors embody the helpful alternative strategies versus corticosteroid injections and/or surgical approaches to related spinal pain and dysfunction.

Epidural PRP has been utilized in multiple studies for different types of pain of spinal origin (including discal pathologies) and/or neurological/radicular involvement. Brian Lemper, DO reported on the use of epidural PRP in a pregnant woman to avoid the use of corticosteroids [30]. He noted lumbar pain was resolved by 3 months. Bhatia et al. described the use of PRP via interlaminar injection for pain associated with prolapsed intervertebral disc [31]. Improvements in pain measures were seen at 3 months, although this study was also limited by its short follow-up period. Radicular pain was addressed by transforaminal or interlaminar lumbar epidural injection of platelet lysate in another study resulting in significantly less radicular pain (and improved function) through 24 months, although progressing with additional and progressive improvement beginning at the 6-month mark [32].

A double-blind, randomized trial in comparing fluoroscopically delivered caudal leukocyte-rich PRP to corticosteroids was reported by Ruiz-Lopez and Tsai [33]. In this study, PRP had a longer pain-relieving effect and longer improvement in quality of life. Bise et al. [34] reported on CT-guided interlaminar PRP vs. steroid injections for radicular pain, but the end point measure was oddly limited to 6 weeks, which is not logical for a regenerative medicine study. Nonetheless, PRP was found to produce similar results when compared to steroidal injections in this referenced study.

PRP and epidural platelet lysate were delivered to two patients by an interlaminar approach, one with an acute large lumbar extruded disc. The procedure was repeated 3 months later. These anecdotal results described significant resorption of disc herniation and resolution of radicular symptoms [35] (Fig. 12.1) is reproduced from this reference to demonstrate significant but not complete resorption of the extruded L4–5 disc (although the particular imaging slices are not identical when comparing the before treatment vs. after treatment views). The reactive immune activity in the epidural space and the impact of regenerative strategies appear to imbue more efficacy on sequestered disc herniations than on protrusions. An enhanced understanding in this particular arena will be clinically useful [36, 37]. Additionally, the pain reduction benefits of interlaminar epidural injections have been confirmed by Correa et al. [38] in supporting regenerative over "palliative" medicine for the treatment of lower back pain. More recently, Xu et al. [39] published on a comparison of lumbar transforaminal epidural PRP vs. steroid injection for lumbar disc herniation by ultrasound guidance, demonstrating equivalent benefit to pain and function at a 1-year follow-up (Fig. 12.2). PRP has also been delivered via the caudal epidural approach to address complex chronic degenerative spinal pain [40].

Therefore, although further study is needed, various epidural deliveries appear useful in addressing lower back pain and radicular pain,

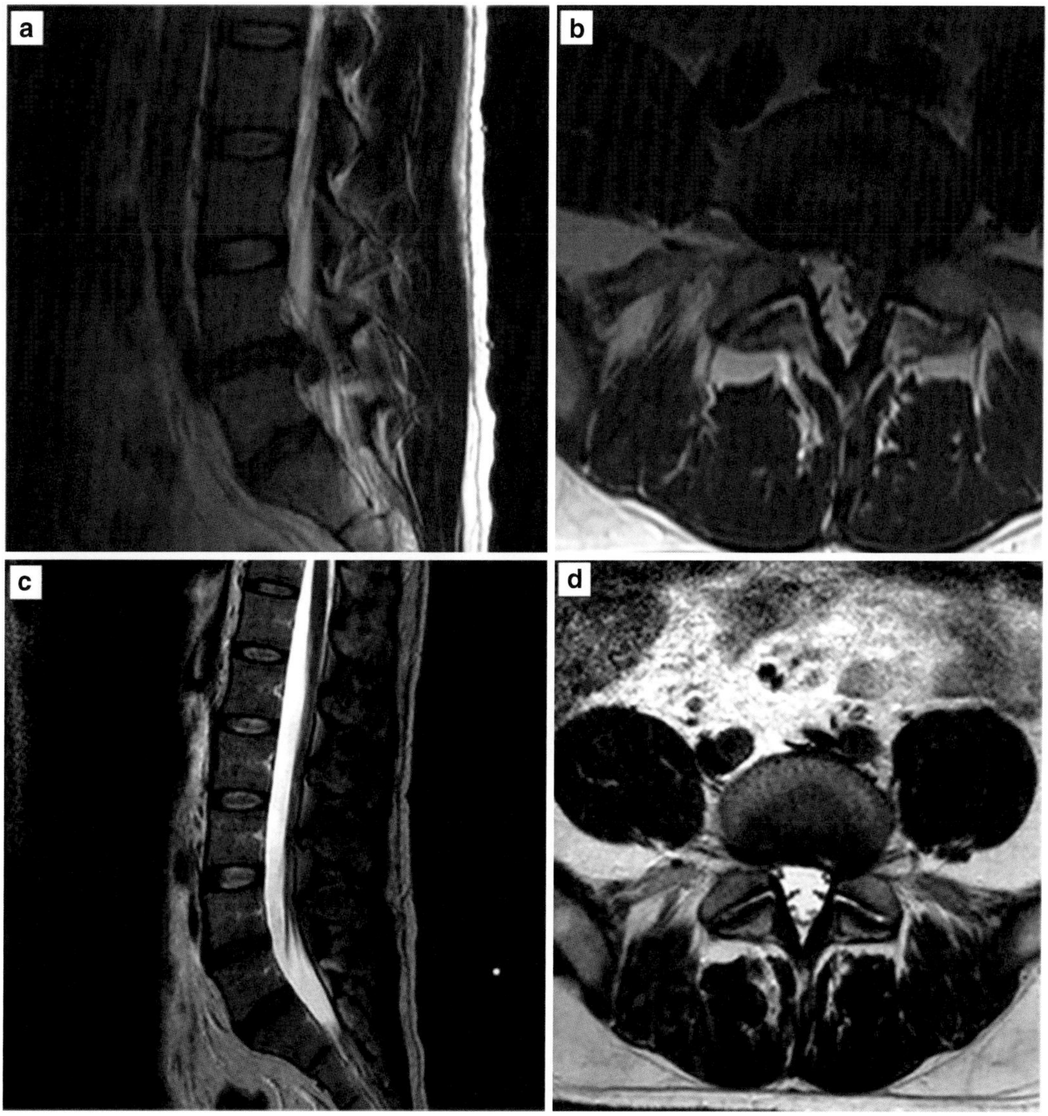

Fig. 12.1 (**a–d**) Top row is prior to PRP. Bottom row was taken 3 months after the second of two interlaminar epidural PRP injections

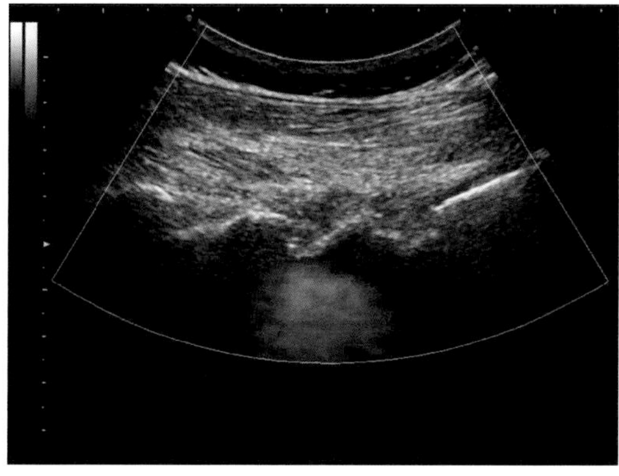

Fig. 12.2 Spinal ultrasound from Xu et al. [39]

both with radicular pain taking longer to respond. Although longer studies are desired, clinical benefits appear to be less acute, but more sustained when compared to corticosteroids, but not less than equivalent to steroidal injections in some studies. Epidural delivery of PRP is also helpful to address lower back and radicular pain associated with discal herniation (and possibly accelerate and encourage resorption of herniated fragments). PRP has also been used to address symptoms related to CSF leak-related symptoms [41, 42] and to prevent postsurgical scar formation in the epidural space [43].

There are no identifiable studies of amniotic components, extracellular matrix, or noncellular elements applied to the epidural space. Despite anecdotal unpublished experiences, there are no present studies of epidural exosomal stem or cell applications published for review. However, it is not unreasonable to consider these regenerative biologics for use in the epidural space, as it appears that steroid injections are not superior, at least in the case of PRP-type preparations. Clinical factors may allow the inclusion of those with discal herniations and/or radiculopathy, independent from pain of spinal origin. In an effort to be complete, it is worthy of mention that exosomes have been used in a cellulose membrane to successfully prevent epidural fibrosus in a rabbit model [44] and are a quickly blossoming area for clinical research and trial.

Regenerative Intradiscal Injections

Perhaps the most robust area in reported application of regenerative treatments to the spine is for discogenic pain and pathology. Not unlike large lower extremity joints, the spinal disc is exposed to daily, cumulative, and injurious stresses and is uniquely susceptible. This section remains agnostic to intradiscal regenerative procedures being an adjunct of surgery, or separate, de novo percutaneous treatment, with the clinical goals uniformly being pain reduction and improved function [45] and with additional benefits such as improved disc hydration and height (at the treated and even adjacent discs).

Platelet-rich plasma has been reported for the purpose of addressing intervertebral disc degeneration-related pain on the heels of a large number of in vitro and animal studies. Masuda, Akeda, and their colleagues have reported clinical improvement in pain sustained through 6 months of observation after intradiscal injection (by fluoroscopic guidance) in patients with discographically confirmed discogenic lower back pain. MRIs taken after treatment did not demonstrate significant change [45–48]. Navani et al. reported 50% pain reduction and increased function by 3 months, and for 6 months and beyond, and a small number of patients had improvement in MRI findings after intradiscal PRP injection [49]. The results of pain reduction from intradiscal PRP were reproduced by Levi et al. [50]. A randomized controlled study of intradiscal PRP also confirmed significant pain reduction at 8 weeks through 1 year [51]. Uncontrolled follow-up for 2 years demonstrated sustained clinical benefit [51]. Furthermore, Lutz [52] reported improved MRI findings (consistent with better discal hydration) 1 year after intradiscal PRP (Fig. 12.3). The same group published a 5–9-year follow-up, extending the promising results for this approach [53].

Buck injected amniotic membrane and umbilical particulate into discs of patients with positive discograms. He found progressive pain reduction through the 6 months of the study in most of the patients [1].

Studies demonstrating the clinical outcomes from intradiscal delivery of stem cells are limited [54]. After a failed trial by Haufe and Mork [55] in 2006, the earliest related beneficial studies are European: Meisel et al. [56, 57] and Hohaus et al. [58] reported intradiscal autologous culture-expanded disc cell transplantation as an adjunct to (although 12 weeks after) lumbar discectomy surgery. The treatment group fared better with pain reduction, increased discal hydration on MRI, and with adjacent segment disc hydration on MRI at 2 years. These results were confirmed by Mochida et al. through a 3-year follow-up [59]. Other stem cell types, including juvenile chondrocytes [60] and nasal chondrocytes, have also shown promise [61]. Additionally, MSC-encapsulated hydrogels have been shown to be chondrogenic [62]. Noriega et al. [63] trialed allogenic intradiscal MSCs, followed for 1 year, finding quick and significant reduction in pain and improvement in function in 40% of the treatment group when compared to controls. Discal appearance on MRI improved in the treatment group while worsening in the control group. This clinical result echoed animal models, demonstrating the same [64]. Others have confirmed similar results: intradiscal culture-expanded MSCs were found to be safe when delivered by fluoroscopy [65] and showed continued benefits

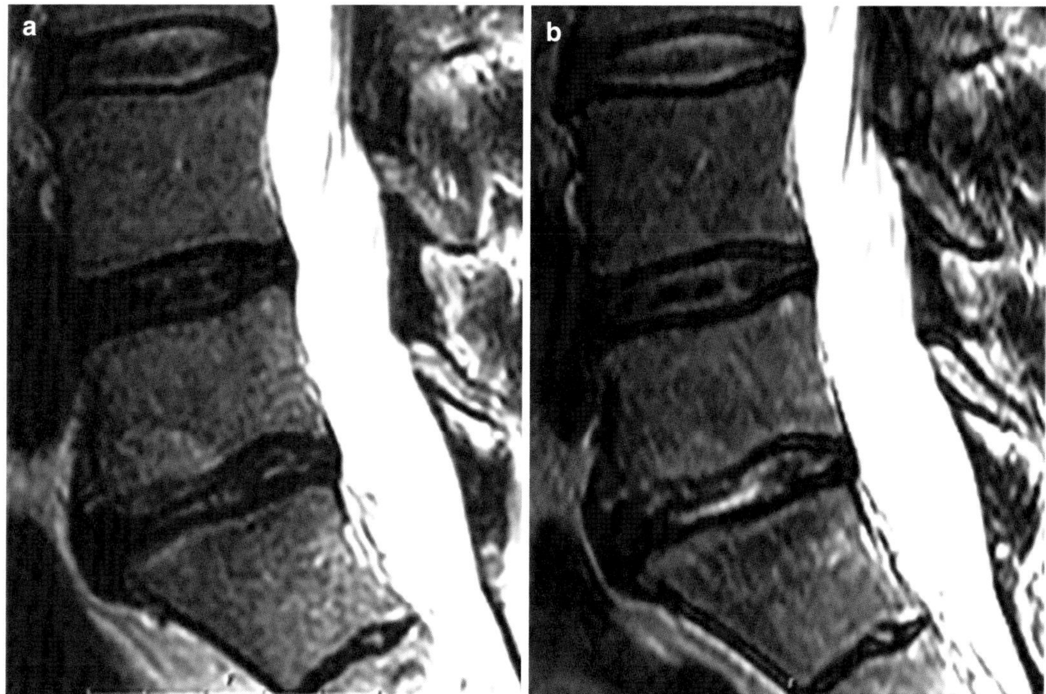

Fig. 12.3 (**a**, **b**) From Lutz et al. [52] showing improved hydration after intradiscal injection of PRP. (The left panel is prior to treatment. The right panel is posttreatment showing increased T2 signal, consistent with improved hydration)

as far out as 72 months [66, 67]. Disc "bulge" size reduction was observed in the majority of patients who underwent post-procedural MRI. Wolff et al. published on the use of fluoroscopically guided intradiscal autologous BMC, finding improvement of at least 50% in pain in up to 38.9% of 33 patients (limited to those with positive discography but without full thickness annular tears) followed to 1 year, most notably for those with higher initial pain [68].

Autologous implanted intradiscal MSCs demonstrated clinical improvement by 3 months, and when measured at 1 year, as reported by Orozco et al. [45]. At the last metric, this group found improved discal hydration on MRI, but not improved discal height. Another group performed a similar study with culture-expanded MSCs for radicular pain, finding beneficial results as far as 6 years after treatment [66]. Notable for this study was reduction in the size of disc "bulge" in a portion of the patients who underwent post-treatment MRI. The same group also had good results with hypoxic cultured MSCs [67].

Perhaps the most notable clinical series of intradiscal MSCs is reported by Pettine et al., who have published their results at the 1-, 2-, 3-, and 5-year marks. The 5-year outcomes were superior to a 2-year post-fusion comparative with the stem cell treatment group having persistent pain reduction, improvement in function, and improvement in MRI appearance [69]. Yoshikawa et al. [70] reported on two patients receiving intradiscal autologous MSCs with clinical improvement in lower back and lower extremity symptoms at 2 years and improvement in vacuum phenomenon on x-ray and CT imaging.

As referenced above, El-Kadiry et al. recently published their findings in utilizing BMAC targeted delivery to either intradiscal (with positive discography) or to the facet joints and their surrounding structures (if discography was negative) [19]. The intradiscally treated population exhibited improved disc height and canal space size, and clinically reduced pain (and reduced opioid use), from 1 to 12 months posttreatment and at all metrics in between.

All of these relevant studies utilized bone marrow-derived stem cells. There are not yet any clinical studies identifiable reporting on adipose-derived stem cells, or pluripotent cells for intradiscal therapy, except as a combined therapy (see below). However, Pang et al. described the intradiscal use of amniotic MSCs in two patients with discographically confirmed discal pain. The results included pain reduction and improved signal on T2-weighted MRI, although the study was limited to two patients [71]. There is not yet enough information to conclude as to the best source of naturally occurring stem cells for intradiscal efficacy. There is some evidence that a cell population might best include notochordal lineage, being the source of the nucleus of an intervertebral disc; however, the studies identified and described herein are all MSC based.

Combined intradiscal therapies have also been described. Kumar et al. injected adipose-derived stem cells plus hyaluronic acid to the intervertebral discs [72] with results of clinical improvement in six of ten patients sustained to 1 year (the end point of the study) and disc rehydration suggested in half of six patients. Combined use of stromal vascular fraction (SVF) and PRP for fluoroscopically guided intradiscal application was reported by Comella et al. [73]. Improvement in pain was seen in over 6 months; however, the pre-procedural pain generator was not confirmed by discography, and there was no imaging metric in this study.

Although not yet clinically described, there is much discussion of growth factors and scaffolding to support intradiscal stem cell-based treatments [74–76]. The disc is generally thought to be inhospitable to cells, which is also a foundation for intravertebral injections (see next section) [72, 75–77]. However, some authors theorize that combined intradiscal biological therapies to the spine will be best form of delivery [74, 75]. Although not yet clinically confirmed, in an animal disc injury model, intradiscal delivery of MSCs prevented multifidus muscle degeneration [78].

Broadly, clinical results appear promising as described herein. Intradiscal delivery being deeper and requiring navigation around neurological structures is advised to be guided by fluoroscopy or tomographic scanning, although there are experienced ultrasonographers who can localize the intervertebral discs [79]. Until a practical alternative replacement is identified, provocative discography remains the best method to confirm discogenic spinal pain and can be performed simultaneously with an intradiscal injection procedure. However, one can theorize that even if in the presence of negative discography, preventative (and sealant) reasoning exists to support further investigation and applications of intradiscal regenerative treatment.

Regenerative Subchondral Intravertebral Injections

Not yet published, but worthy of discussion here, is the vertebral endplate as treatment target. Based upon the work of Hernigou, and stemming from his study in following patients with knee osteoarthritis for 15 years, one can find references to anecdotal analogous treatments of vertebrae [80, 81]. The logic behind this approach is that the disc receives its nutrients and health from the vertebral endplate, mostly by diffusion. Healthier vertebral endplates and nearby subchondral bone marrow subserve a healthy condition for the intervertebral disc, and theoretically with that, less pain, and improved viscoelastic function of the disc/endplate complex. This appears to be a strong candidate for the future direction in treating the symptomatic degeneration of discs.

Conclusions

The explosion of scientific advancements in biomedicine is coming back full circle to a more logically bioactive and less pharmaceutical approach, addressing cellular metabolism directly, instead of the indirect downstream extracellular and organismal effects of inflammatory changes. The clinical observations catalogued herein demonstrate a broad demonstration of relative safety and success without prejudice for a biological or anatomical treatment approach. Although further studies are needed [82, 83] to more specifically address confirmed anatophysiological problems of spinal origin and to compare the differing available biologics, there is adequate support for further refining and mainstreaming the described treatment as a beneficial step prior to considering more invasive, including surgical endeavors for many patients.

References

1. Buck D. Amniotic umbilical cord particulate for discogenic pain. J Am Osteopath Assoc. 2019;119(12):814–9.
2. Falco FJ, Manchikanti L, Datta S, Sehgal N, Geffert S, Onyewu O, Zhu J, Coubarous S, Hameed M, Ward SP, Sharma M, Hameed H, Singh V, Boswell MV. An update of the effectiveness of therapeutic lumbar facet joint interventions. Pain Physician. 2012;15(6):E909–53.
3. Perolat R, Kastler A, Nicot B, Pellat JM, Tahon F, Attye A, Heck O, Boubagra K, Grand S, Krainik A. Facet joint syndrome: from diagnosis to interventional management. Insights Imaging. 2018;9(5):773–89.
4. Smuck M, et al. Success of initial and repeated medical branch neurotomy for zygapophysial joint pain: a systematic review. Physical Med Rehabil. 2012;49(9):686–92.
5. Husted D. Effectiveness of repeated radiofrequency neurotomy for cervical facet joint pain. Proceedings of NASS, 22nd Annual Meeting. Spine J. 2007;7:87S.
6. Sharma A: Radiofrequency denervation. Spineline. 2011:30–5.
7. Schofferman J, Kine G. Effectiveness of repeated radiofrequency neurotomy for lumbar facet pain. Spine. 2004;29(21):2471–3.
8. Van Kleef M, et al. Randomized trial of radiofrequency lumbar facet denervation for chronic low back pain. Spine. 1999;24(18):1937–42.
9. Bogduk N. ISIS (now SIS) practice guidelines for spinal diagnostic and treatment procedures. 2nd ed. Medial Branch Thermal Radiofrequency Neurotomy; 2013.
10. Abd-Elsayed A, et al. The long-term efficacy of radiofrequency ablation with and without steroid injection. Psychoparmacol Bull. 2020;40(4 Suppl 1):11–6.
11. Kristjansson B, Honsawek S. Mesenchymal stem cells for cartilage regeneration in osteoarthritis. World J Orthop. 2017;8(9):674–80.
12. Wu J, Du Z, Lv Y, Zhang J, Xiong W, Wang R, Liu R, Xhang G, Liu Q. A new technique for the treatment of lumbar facet joint syndrome using intra-articular injection with autologous platelet rich plasma. Pain Physician. 2016;19(8):617–25.
13. Wu J, Zhou J, Liu C, Zhang J, Xiong W, Lv Y, Liu R, Wang R, Du Z, Zhang G, Liu Q. A prospective study comparing platelet-rich plasma and local anesthetic (LA)/ corticosteroid in intra-articular injection for the treatment of lumbar facet syndrome. Pain Pract. 2017;17(7):914–24.
14. Sanapati J, Manchikanti L, Atluri S, Jordan S, Albers AL, Pappolla MA, Kaye AD, Candido KD, Pampati V, Hirsch JA. Do regenerative medicine therapies provide long-term relief in chronic low back pain: a systematic review and metaanalysis. Pain Physician. 2018;21:515–40.
15. Navani A, Manchikanti L, Albers SL, Latchaw RE, Sanapati J, Kaye AD, Atluri S, Jordan S, Gupta A, Cedeno D, Vallejo A, Fellows B, Knezevic NN, Pappolla M, Diwan S, Trescot AM, Soin A, Kaye AM, Aydin SM, Calodney AK, Candido KD, Bakshi S, Benyamin RM, Vallejo R, Watanabe A, Beall D, Stitik TP, Foye PM, Helander EM, Hirsch JA. Responsible, safe, and effective use of biologics in the management of low back pain: American Society of Interventional Pain Physicians (ASIPP) guidelines. Pain Physician. 2019;22(1S):S1–S74.
16. Desai MJ, Mansfield JT, Robinson DM, Miller BC, Borg-Stein J. Regenerative medicine for axial and radicular spine-related pain: a narrative review. Pain Pract. 2020;20(4):437–53.
17. Aufiero D, Vincent H, Sampson S, Bodor M. Regenerative injection treatment in the spine: review and case series with platelet rich plasma. J Stem Cells Res Review Rep. 2015;2(1):1019.
18. Cameron JA, Thielen KM. Autologous platelet rich plasma for neck and lower back pain secondary to spinal disc herniation: midterm results. Spine Res. 2017;3(2):10.
19. El Hakim El Kadiry A, Lumbao C, Rafei M, Shammaa R. Autologous BMAC therapy improves spinal degenerative joint disease in lower back pain patients. Front Med. 2021;8:309.
20. Bennett DS. Cryopreserved amniotic membrane and umbilical cord particulate for managing pain caused by facet joint syndrome: a case series. Medicine (Baltimore). 2019;98(10):e14745.
21. Krisjansson B, Limthongful W, Yingsakmongkol W, Thantiworasit P, Jirathanathornnukul N, Honsawek S. Isolation and characterization of human mesenchymal stem cells from facet joints and interspinous ligaments. Spine. 2016;41(1):E1–7.
22. Ni Z, Zhou S, Li S, Kuang L, Chen H, Luo X, Ouyang J, He M, Du X, Chen L. Exosomes: roles and therapeutic potential in osteoarthritis. Bone Res. 2020;8:25.
23. Hussein M, Hussein T. Effect of autologous platelet leukocyte rich plasma injections on atrophied lumbar multifidus muscle in low back pain patients with monosegmental degenerative disc disease. SICOT-J. 2016;2:12.
24. Rajpu BS, Chakrabarti SK, Dongare VS, Ramirez CM, Deb KD. Human umbilical cord mesenchymal stem cells in the treatment of Duchenne muscular dys-

trophy: safety and feasibility study in India. J Stem Cells. 2015;10(2):141–56.
25. ClinicalTrials.gov [Internet]. Bethesda (MD): National Library of Medicine (US). 2000 Feb 29. Identifier NCT03225625, Stem Cell Spinal Cord Injury Exoskeleton and Virtual Reality Treatment Study (SciExVR); 2017 July 17 [cited 2021 July 10]; [about 5 screens]. Available from: https://clinicaltrials.gov/ct2/show/NCT03225625.
26. Platt A, David BT, Fessler RG. Stem cell clinical trials in spinal cord injury: a brief review of studies in the United States. Medicines (Basel). 2020;7(5):27.
27. Brzoska E, Kalkowski L, Kowalski K, Michalski P, Kowalczyk P, Mierzejewski B, Walczak P, Ciemerych MA, Janowski M. Muscular contribution to adolescent idiopathic scoliosis from the perspective of stem cell-based regenerative medicine. Stem Cells Dev. 2019;28:1059–77.
28. Chen KS, McGinley LM, Kashlan ON, Hayes JM, Bruno ES, Chang JS, Mendelson FE, Tabbey MA, Johe K, Sakowski SA, Feldman EL. Targeted intraspinal injections to assess therapies in rodent models of neurological disorders. Nat Protoc. 2019;14:331–49.
29. Kirchner F, Anitua E. Intradiscal and intra-articular facet infiltrations with plasma rich in growth factors reduce pain in patients with chronic low back pain. J Craniovertebr Junction Spine. 2016;7(4):250–6.
30. Lemper BA, Rhodes S, Njoroge BK, Yurgelon JT, Klassen LJ. Chronic pain management and pregnancy a platelet rich plasma epidural case study. http://www.aaomed.org/AAOM/files/ccLibraryFiles/Filename/000000000115/PRP%20Case%20Study%20-%20Pregnancy.pdf.
31. Bhatia R, Chopra G. Efficacy of platelet rich plasma via lumbar epidural route in chronic prolapsed intervertebral disc patients-a pilot study. J Clin Diagn Res. 2016;10(9):UC05–7.
32. Centeno C, Markle J, Dodson E, Stemper I, Hyzy M, Williams C, Freeman M. The use of lumbar epidural injection of platelet lysate for treatment of radicular pain. J Exp Ortho. 2017;4:38.
33. Ruiz-Lopez R, Tsai YC. A randomized double-blind controlled pilot study comparing leucocyte-rich platelet-rich plasma and corticosteroid in caudal epidural injection for complex chronic degenerative spinal pain. Pain Pract. 2020;20:639–46.
34. Bise S, Dallaudiere B, Pesquer L, Pedram M, Meyer P, Antoun MB, Hocquelet A, Silvestre A. Comparison of interlaminar CT-guided epidural platelet-rich plasma versus steroid injection in patients with lumbar radicular pain. Eur Radiol. 2020;30:3152–60.
35. Rawson B. Platelet-rich plasma and epidural platelet lysate: novel treatment for lumbar disk herniation. J Am Osteopath Assoc. 2020;120(3):201–2017.
36. Cunha C, Almeida CR, Almeida MI, Silva AM, Molinos M, Lamas S, Pereira CL, Teixeira GQ, Monteiro AT, Santos SG, Goncalves RM, Barbosa MA. Systemic delivery of bone marrow mesenchymal stem cells for in situ intervertebral disc regeneration. Stem Cell Transl Med. 2016;5:1–11.
37. Virri J, Gronblad M, Seitsalo S, Habtemariam A, Kappa E, Karaharju E. Comparison of the prevalence of inflammatory cells in subtypes of disc herniations and associations with straight leg raising. Spine (Phila Pa 1967). 2001;26(21):2311–5.
38. Correa J, Cortes H, Abella P, Garcia E. Epidural plasma rich in growth factors for degenerative disc disease: a valuable alternative to conventional "palliative medicine". Int J Anesthesia Clin Med. 2019;7(1):1–6.
39. Xu Z, Wu S, Li X, Liu C, Fan S, Ma C, Ultrasound-guided transforaminal injections of platelet-rich plasma compared with steroid in lumbar disc herniation: a prospective, randomized, controlled study. Neural Plast. 2021;2021. Article ID 5558138, 11 pages.
40. Xu Z, Wu S, Li X, Liu C, Fan S, Ma C, Ultrasound-guided transforaminal injections of platelet-rich plasma compared with steroid in lumbar disc herniation: a prospective, randomized, controlled study. Neural Plasticity. 2021;2021. Article ID 5558138, 11 pages.
41. Gunaydin B, Acar M, Emmez G, Akcali D, Tokgoz N. Epidural patch with autologous platelet rich plasma: a novel approach. J Anesth. 2017;31(6):907–10.
42. Quereshi A, Ahrar A, Jadhav V, Wallery SS. Epidural injection of platelet rich plasma for postlumbar puncture headaches. J Neurosurg Anesthesiol. 2018;30(3):276–8.
43. Guler S, Akcali O, Sen B, Micili SC, Sanli NK, Cankaya D. Effect of platelet-rich plasma, fat pad and dural matrix in preventing epidural fibrosis. Acta Ortop Bras. 2020;28(1):31–5.
44. Wang B, Li P, Shangguan L, Ma J, Mao KZ, Zhang Q, Wang YG, Liu ZY, Mao KY. A novel bacterial cellulose membrane immobilized with human umbilical cord mesenchymal stem cells-derived exosome prevents epidural fibrosis. Int J Nanomedicine. 2018;13:5257–73.
45. Orozco L, Soler R, Morera C, Alberca M, Sanchez A, Garcia-Sancho J. Intervertebral disc repair by autologous mesenchymal bone marrow cells: a pilot study. Transplantation. 2011;92(7):822–8.
46. Akeda K, OHishi K, Masuda K, Bae WC, Takegami N, Yamada J, Nakamura T, Sakakibara T, Kasai Y, Sudo A. Intradiscal injection of autologous platelet-rich plasma releasate to treat discogenic low back pain : a preliminary clinical trial. Asian Spine J. 2017;11(3):380–9.
47. Akeda K, Imanishi T, Ohishi K, Masuda K, Uchida A, Sakakibara T, Kasai Y, Sudo A. Intradiscal injection of autologous serum isolated from platelet-rich-plasma for the treatment of discogenic low back pain: preliminary prospective clinical trial: GP141. Spine J Meeting Abstracts. October 2011.
48. Akeda K, Yamada J, Linn ET, Sudo A, Masuda K. Platelet-rich plasma in the management of chronic low back pain: a critical review. J Pain Res. 2019;12:753–67.
49. Navani A, Hames A. Platelet-rich plasma injections for lumbar discogenic pain: a preliminary assessment

of structural and functional changes. Tech Regional Anesth Pain Manage. 2015;19(1–2):38–44.

50. Levi D, Horn S, Tyszko S, Levin J, Hecht-Leavitt C, Walko E. Intradiscal platelet-rich plasma injection for chronic discogenic low back pain: preliminary results from a prospective trial. Pain Med. 2016;17(6):1010–22.
51. Tuakli-Wosornu YA, Terry A, Boachie-Adjei K, Harrison JR, Gribbin CK, LaSalle EE, Nguyen JT, Solomon JL, Lutz GE. Lumbar intradiskal platelet-rich plasma (PRP) injections: a prospective, double-blind, randomized controlled study. PM&R J Injury Function Rehabil. 2016;8(1):1–10.
52. Lutz GE. Increased nuclear T2 signal intensity and improved function and pain in a patient one year after an intradiscal platelet-rich plasma injection. Pain Med. 2017;18(6):1197–9.
53. Cheng J, Santiago K, Nguyen J, Solomon J, Lutz G. Treatment of symptomatic degenerative intervertebral discs with autologous platelet-rich plasma: follow-up at 5–9 years. Regen Med. 2019;14(9):831–40.
54. Oehme D, Goldschlager T, Ghosh P, Rosenfeld JV, Jenkin G. Cell-based therapies used to treat lumbar degenerative disc disease: a systematic review of animal studies and human clinical trials. Stem Cells Int. 2015;2015:946031.
55. Haufe SMW, Mork AR. Intradiscal injection of hematopoietic stem cells in an attempt to rejuvenate the intervertebral discs. Stem Cells Dev. 2006;15(1):136–7.
56. Meisel HJ, Agarwal N, Hsieh PC, Skelly A, Park JB, Brodke D, Wang JC, Yoon ST, Buser Z. Cell therapy for treatment of intervertebral disc degeneration: a systematic review. Global Spine J. 2019;9(1suppl):39S–52S.
57. Meisel HJ, Siodla V, Ganey T, Minkus Y, Hutton WC, Alasevic OJ. Clinical experience in cell-based therapeutics: disc chondrocyte transplantation: a treatment for degenerated or damaged intervertebral disc. Biomol Eng. 2007;25(1):5–21.
58. Hohaus C, Ganey TM, Minkus Y, Meisel HJ. Cell transportation in lumbar spine disc degeneration disease. Eur Spine J. 2008;17(4):492–503.
59. Mochida J, Sakai D, Nakamura Y, Watanabe T, Yamamoto Y, Kato S. Intervertebral disc repair with activated nucleus pulposus cell transplantation: a three-year, prospective clinical study of its safety. Eur Cell Mater. 2015;29:202–12; discussion 212.
60. Acosta F Jr, Metz L, Liu J, Carruthers-Liebenberg E, Adkisson HD, Maloney M, Lotz J. Juvenile chondrocytes are superior to undifferentiated mesenchymal stem cells for porcine intervertebral disc repair. Spine J. 2008;8(5)50S:8.
61. Vedicherla S, Buckley CT. In vitro extracellular matrix accumulation of nasal and articular chondrocytes for intervertebral disc repair. Tissue Cell. 2017;49(4):503–13.
62. Tsaryk R, Silva-Correia J, Oliveira JM, Unger RE, Landes C, Brochhausen C, Ghanaati S, Reis RL, Kirkpatrick CJ. Biological performance of cell-encapsulated methacrylated gellan gum-based hydrogels for nucleus pulposus regeneration. J Tissue Eng Regen Med. 2017;11:637–48.
63. Noriega DC, Ardura F, Hernandez-Ramajo R, Martin-Ferrero MA, Sanchez-Lite I, Toribio B, Alberca M, Garcia V, Moraleda JM, Sanchez A, Garcia-Sancho J. Intervertebral disc repair by allogeneic mesenchymal bone marrow cells: a randomized controlled trial. Transplantation. 2017;101:1945–51.
64. Daly C, Ghosh P, Jenkin G, Oehme D, Goldschlager T. A review of animal models of intervertebral disc degeneration: pathophysiology, regeneration, and translation to the clinic. Biomed Res Int. 2016;2016:5952165.
65. Centeno CJ, Schultz JR, Cheever M, Freeman M, Faulkner S, Robinson B, Hanson R. Safety and complications reporting update on the re-implantation of culture-expanded mesenchymal stem cells using autologous platelet lysate technique. Curr Stem Cell Res Ther. 2011;6(4):368–78.
66. Centeno C, Markle J, Dodson E, Stemper I, Williams CJ, Hyzy M, Ichim T, Freeman M. Treatment of lumbar degenerative disc disease-associated radicular pain with culture-expanded autologous mesenchymal stem cells: a pilot study on safety and efficacy. J Transl Med. 2017;15(197).
67. Elabd C, Centeno CJ, Schultz JR, et al. Intradiscal injection of autologous, hypoxic cultured bone marrow-derived mesenchymal stem cells in five patients with chronic lower back pain: a long-term safety and feasibility study. J Transl Med. 2016;14:253.
68. Wolff M, Shillington J, Rathbone C, Piasecki S, Barnes B. Injections of concentrated bone marrow aspirate as treatment for discogenic pain: a retrospective analysis. BMC Musculoskelet Disord. 2020;21:135.
69. Pettine K, Dordevic M, Hasz M. Reducing lumbar discogenic back pain and disability with intradiscal injection of bone marrow concentrate: 5-year follow-up. Am J Stem Cell Res. 2018;2(1):1–4.
70. Yoshikawa T, Ueda Y, Miyazaki K, Koizumi M, Takakura Y. Disc regeneration therapy using marrow mesenchymal cell transplantation: a report of two case studies. Spine. 2010;35(11):E475–80.
71. Pang X, Yang H, Peng B. Human umbilical cord mesenchymal stem cell transplantation for the treatment of chronic discogenic low back pain. Pain Physician. 2014;17:E525–30.
72. Kumar H, Ha DH, Lee EJ, Park JH, Shim JH, Ahn TK, Kim KT, Ropper AE, Sohn S, Kim CH, Thakor DK, Lee SH, Han IB. Safety and tolerability of intradiscal implantation of combined autologous adipose-derived mesenchymal stem cells and hyaluronic acid in patients with chronic discogenic low back pain: 1-year follow-up of a phase I study. Stem Cell Res Ther. 2017;8:262.
73. Comella K, Silbert R, Parlo M. Effects of the intradiscal implantation of stromal vascular fraction plus platelet rich plasma in patient with degenerative disc disease. J Transl Med. 2017;15:12.

74. Barakat AH, Elwell VA, Lam KS. Stem cell therapy in discogenic back pain. J Spine Surg. 2019;5(4):561–83.
75. Richardson SM, Kalamegam G, Pushparaj PN, Matta C, Memic A, Khademhosseini A, Mobasheri R, Poletti FL, Hoyland JA, Mobasheri A. Mesenchymal stem cells in regenerative medicine: focus on articular cartilage and intervertebral disc regeneration. Methods. 2016;99:69–80.
76. Mohammed S, Yu J. Platelet-rich plasma injections: an emerging therapy for chronic discogenic low back pain. J Spine Surg. 2018;4(1):115–22.
77. Gou S, Oxentenko SC, Eldrige JS, Xiao L, Pingree MJ, Wang Z, Perez-Terzic C, Qu W. Stem cell therapy for intervertebral disk regeneration. Am J Phys Med Rehabil. 2014;93(11 Suppl 3):S122–31.
78. James G, Blomster L, Hall L, Schmid AB, Shu CC, Little CB, Melrose J, Hodges PW. Mesenchymal stem cell treatment of intervertebral disc lesion prevents fatty infiltration and fibrosis of the multifidus muscle, but not cytokine and muscle fiber changes. Spine (Phila Pa 1976). 2016;41(15):1208–17.
79. Wu TJ, Hung CY, Lee CW, Lam S, Clark TB, Chang KV. Ultrasound-guided lumbar intradiscal injection for discogenic pain: technical innovation and presentation of two cases. J Pain Res. 2020;13:1103–7.
80. Hernigou P, Bouthors C, Bastard C, Flouzat Lachaniette CH, Rouard H, Dubory A. Subchondral bone or intra-articular injection of bone marrow concentrate mesenchymal stem cells in bilateral knee osteoarthritis: what better postpone knee arthroplasty at fifteen years? A randomized study. Int Orthop. 2021;45(2):391–9.
81. Delgado D, Garate A, Vincent H, Bilbao AM, Patel R, Fiz N, Sampson S, Sanchez M. Current concepts in intraosseous platelet-rich plasma injections for knee osteoarthritis [published correction appears in J Clin Orthop Trauma. 2020;11(6):1169–1171. J Clin Orthop Trauma. 2019;10(1):36–41.
82. Baig MZ, Abdullah UEH, Muhammad A, Aziz A, Syed MJ, Darbar A. Use of platelet-rich plasma in treating low back pain: a review of the current literature. Asian Spine J. 2021;15(1):117–26.
83. Valimahomed A, Haffey P, Urman R, Kaye A, Yong R. Regenerative techniques for neuraxial back pain: a systematic review. Curr Pain Headache Rep. 2019;23(3):20.

Part IV

Dentistry

Regenerative Medicine in Dentistry

13

Samia Elazab

Introduction

Stem cell assortment from bone marrow, blood, fetal material, and umbilical cords presents exceptional practical and conflicting ethical challenges [1, 2]. However, the discovery of postnatal stem cell populations in the tooth pulp by Gronthos et al. [3] about two decades ago opened up new horizons to dental stem cell research and pushed the dental profession further into the exciting field of regenerative medicine.

Regenerative medicine research has exploded in the last few decades; in turn dentistry, as a major segment of medicine, would have its fair share of research attempting to make new scientific breakthroughs in this field. In dentistry, adult mesenchymal stem cells (MSCs) have been detected in several oral and maxillofacial tissues. These cells have participation in regenerative therapies and consequently have attracted significantly increasing clinical interest [4].

Many research groups have therefore used dental stem cells (DSCs) to elucidate various biological phenomena and to establish their potential clinical applications [5, 6]. However, these cells are heterogeneous with various differentiation states as they may include true "stem" cells, progenitor cells, and possibly fibroblasts [7]. Thus, it is necessary to effectively classify and purify these cells to prevent unexpected clinical results.

Stem cells that fit for regenerative medicine/dentistry must be exposed to complete control of cell fate in the body to ensure the safety of the patient. In this regard, only adult MSCs, as that obtained from oral tissues, currently have faithful clinical potential. Certainly, the regeneration of bone and periodontal tissues by MSCs has been extensively evaluated, with some studies already applied in the dental clinic [8].

With regard to accessibility, bone marrow aspiration from the iliac crest and liposuction from extra-oral tissue is not an easy operation for dentists because of the limitations of the dental license and the dental specialization. In contrast, orofacial bone marrow, periosteum, salivary glands, and dental tissues are accessible stem cell sources for dentists. Thus, appropriate stem cells for dental tissue engineering should not only be able to differentiate into the target tissue/organ but also should be easily collected and prepared, and probable immunomodulatory properties have to be used to provide a further benefit. In this scenario, human oral tissue-derived MSCs have low inherent immunogenicity [9].

A great number of patients all over the world experience tooth loss due to irreparable damage of the periodontium caused by deep severe periodontal diseases or trauma. Inappropriately, con-

S. Elazab (✉)
Galala University, Suez, Egypt

Faculty of Dentistry, Cairo University, Giza, Egypt
e-mail: samia.elazab@gu.edu.eg

Y. El Miedany (ed.), *Musculoskeletal Ultrasound-Guided Regenerative Medicine*,
https://doi.org/10.1007/978-3-030-98256-0_13

ventional therapies such as scaling and root planning are frequently only palliative. Consequently, the decisive goal of the treatment for periodontitis is to restore disrupted periodontium to its original shape and function [10]. The periodontium is a complex tissue composed mainly of two soft tissues and two hard tissues; the former comprises the periodontal ligament (PDL) tissue and gingival tissue, and the latter includes alveolar bone and cementum covering the tooth root. PDL is a unique dynamic connective tissue that is exposed to frequent adaptation to maintain tissue size and width, as well as structural integrity of ligament fiber attachment in the alveolar bone. The primary function of PDL is to retain the tooth within its bony socket and protecting it from injury by mechanical loading. Actually, reconstruction of PDL using stem cells is valuable in regenerative dentistry [11].

The new era in regenerative dentistry not only constitute stem cells but also use ultrasound and law density laser for enhancing proliferation and bio-stimulation [12–14]. Herein this chapter, there will be emphasis on the characteristics, preservation, and multiple roles of DSCs and its potential impact on clinical settings. These novel insights of the regenerative capacity of DSCs appear hopeful to explore their abilities in a wide diversity of pathologies. Besides, DSCs are becoming very related to tissue engineering and regenerative medicine. Moreover, the advantages of using DSCs over stem cells derived from other parts of the body will be declared.

Sources of Dental Stem Cells (DSCs)

Recent stem cell studies in the dental field have recognized many adult stem cell sources in the oral and maxillofacial region. These cells are thought to present in a precise zone of mesenchymal tissue, referred as "stem cell niche," and these cells are collectively referred to as multipotent MSCs [15]. DSCs are MSC-like populations with self-renewal capacity and multi-differentiation potential. At present, there are five main DSCs, the first type was isolated from the human pulp tissue and termed "postnatal dental pulp stem cells" (DPSCs) [16]. Afterward, three more types of DSCs populations were isolated and characterized: stem cells from exfoliated deciduous teeth (SHED) [17], periodontal ligament stem cells (PDLSCs) [7], and stem cells from apical papilla (SCAP) [18, 19]. Recent studies have identified a fifth dental-tissue-derived progenitor cell population, referred to as "dental follicle precursor cells" (DFPCs) [(20)]. These cells had phenotypic characteristics similar to those of BMSCs [21].

Alternatively, it was reported that two types of adult stem cells have been characterized in dental tissues: epithelial stem cells and MSC-like cells. An adult epithelial stem cell niche in teeth was first established in 1999 [22] through organ culture of the apical end of the mouse incisor. The niche is located in the cervical loop of the tooth apex and possibly contains dental epithelial stem cells, which can notably differentiate into enamel-producing ameloblasts [23].

Although the epithelial stem cell niche is valuable for the fate of stem cells in tooth development, no data is available for dental epithelial stem cells in humans. This niche may be specific to rodents because their incisors differ from all human teeth in that they erupt continuously throughout the life of the animal. On the other hand, mesenchymal progenitor or stem cells have also long been assumed to exist in dental tissues [24, 25] and can regenerate or form reparative dentin to protect the pulp against invading irritants [26, 27]. Ikeda et al. [28] identified distinctive stem cells in the dental mesenchyme of the third molar tooth germ at the late bell stage (tooth germ progenitor cells: TGPCs) with high proliferation activity and the capability to differentiate in vitro into lineages of the three germ layers including osteoblasts, neural cells, and hepatocytes [15].

DSCs are enormously nearby, prevail during all life, and own a remarkable multipotency. In the past decade, DPSCs and SHED have been meticulously studied in regenerative medicine and tissue engineering as autologous stem cell therapies and have shown amazing therapeutic abilities in orofacial, neurologic, corneal, cardiovascular, hepatic, diabetic, renal, muscular dystrophy, and auto-immune conditions, in both animal and human models, and lately some of them proceeded to human clinical trials [29]. Interestingly, DSCs not only have potent capacities to differentiate into odontogenic cells but also have the ability to give rise to other distinct cell lineages: osteo-/odontogenic, adipogenic, and neurogenic as well as endothelial cell lineages [30, 31].

Recent reports verified that DSCs also secrete nanoscale extracellular vesicles that may add to their therapeutic functions [32, 33]. These vesicles transfer specifically packaged proteins, lipids, and small RNA species and are taken up by, and capable of reprogramming, target cells [34]. Yet, although stem cells from early tooth buds can generate entirely new teeth, and while DSCs may remediate specific lesions, growing any other replacement organs from these accessible DSCs may yet be just out of reach [35, 36]. On the other hand, there are the oral mucosa-derived stem cells (OMSCs), besides stem cells that could be harvested from alveolar periosteum, salivary glands, as well as oral adipose tissue [37].

Dental Pulp Stem Cells (DPSCs)

Postnatal stem cells present in pulp could be obtained from adult premolar teeth extracted for orthodontic purposes as well as surgically removed impacted third molars (wisdom teeth). One significant character of pulp cells is their odontoblastic differentiation potential. Human pulp cells could be induced in vitro to differentiate into cells of odontoblastic phenotype with polarized cell bodies and accumulation of mineralized nodules [38].

From the pulp tissues, DPSCs are extracted with enzyme treatment [39]. There are diverse cell densities of the resultant colonies, supposing that each cell clone may have a dissimilar growth rate [40]. Inside the same colony, different cell sizes and morphologies might be observed. Besides, ectopic pulp-dentin-like tissue complexes were formed in immunocompromised mice when ex vivo expanded DPSCs mixed with hydroxyapatite/tricalcium phosphate were transplanted [3]. These pools of heterogeneous DPSCs form vascularized pulp-like tissue and are surrounded by a layer of odontoblast-like cells that produces dentin with dentinal tubules mimicking natural dentin that, over time, thickened [41]. Moreover, if DPSCs are seeded onto human dentin surfaces and implanted into immunocompromised mice, reparative dentin-like structure is deposited on the dentin surface [42]. In addition to their dentinogenic potential, subpopulations of DPSCs have adipogenic and neurogenic differentiation capacities as well, by exhibiting adipocyte- and neuronal-like cell morphologies and expressing their corresponding gene markers [40]. More recently, DPSCs were similarly found to undergo osteogenic, chondrogenic, and myogenic differentiation in vitro [43–45]. It was reported that DSC therapy primarily involves DPSCs found in the core of baby teeth and wisdom teeth. DPSCs are considered as naturally produced "raw materials" that can multiply, differentiate, and even grow to new tissue. They are primarily intended to promote healing injuries in the teeth or gums. However, current research efforts are proposed to use DPSCs in healing injuries throughout the human body [46].

Nowadays, so-called stem cell banking is a flourishing business with several companies everywhere in the world offering to extract and cryogenically preserve children's DPSCs. These companies claim that stem cells could be effectively used after being stored for 22 years for a diversity of applications. They additionally suppose that the donor could use the stocked cells for medical problems including metabolic disorders, cardiovascular disease, multiple sclerosis, as well as cancer [47, 48]. Furthermore, DPSCs might be used autologously (extracted from and applied to the same person); this means that immune response is extremely nil. A few studies over the last decade have indicated that DPSCs could serve in treating or aiding recovery from traumatic spinal cord and brain injury, retinal damage, as well as glaucoma, stroke, and more [49]. Similarly, it's reasonable to assume – and the trials appear to confirm – that because of their influential capabilities, DPSCs possibly will be used in tissue engineering to regenerate the liver, esophagus, bladder, bone, and other body parts. Moreover, DPSCs have already shown promise in preliminary trials to regrow teeth and may shortly find their way into clinical practice for this application. Collectively, DPSCs are considered to be unique among other types of stem cells in that they are present in body parts that are habitually removed for medical reasons or that simply fall out in aged person [50].

Stem Cells from Human Exfoliated Deciduous Teeth (SHED)

Significantly, it was reported that SHED could precisely induce formation of a bone-like matrix with a lamellar structure by recruiting host cells [51]. This distinct character of SHED may be explained by the nature of deciduous teeth, whose root resorption is associated with new bone formation around the root. Although SHED could not differentiate directly into osteoblasts, they seemed to induce new bone formation by establishing an osteoinductive template to recruit murine host osteogenic cells [17]. With the osteoinductive potential, SHED can repair critical-sized calvarial defects in mice with considerable bone formation [51]. These observations suggest that deciduous teeth may not only afford guidance for the eruption of permanent teeth, as mostly supposed, but may also be involved in inducing bone formation during the eruption of permanent teeth. Likewise, it was found that SHED have the capacity to undergo not only osteogenic but also adipogenic differentiation [17]. Furthermore, iPS cells have been generated from SHED where iPS cells may be of particular importance for developing innovative technologies to regenerate missing jaw bones, periodontal tissues, salivary glands, and lost teeth [52].

SHED appear to represent a population of multipotent stem cells that are perhaps more immature than other postnatal stromal stem-cell populations. Kerkis et al. (2006) isolated SHED and termed the cells "immature DPSCs" (IDPSCs), and they found that IDPSCs express the embryonic stem (ES) cell markers as well as tumor recognition antigens. Regarding in vivo engraftment into different tissues, 3 months following the injection of IDPSCs into the intraperitoneal space of nude mice, IDPSCs can be traced in various tissues and organs, including the liver, spleen, and kidney, suggesting their potent differentiation plasticity [53].

Under neurogenic conditions, cultured SHED readily express a variety of neural cell and glial cell markers, which may be related to the neural crest cell origin of the dental pulp. Neural developmental potential was studied by the injection of SHED into the dentate gyrus of the hippocampus of immunocompromised mice [54]. It was reported that SHED could survive for more than 10 days within the mouse brain microenvironment and express neural markers such as neurofilament M. This finding is comparable to what was verified for BMSCs, which are capable of differentiating into neural-like cells subsequent to in vivo transplantation into the rat brain [55].

SHED also exhibit multicytoplasmic processes instead of the typical fibroblastic morphology. Additionally, myogenic and chondrogenic potentials of SHED have been proved as well. Allogeneic SHED, which is easily accessible, appears to be an attractive candidate for periodontium tissue regeneration and may be applied to treat periodontitis in clinics in the near future. Moreover, ex vivo expanded SHED transplanted into immunocompromised mice yield human-specific odontoblast-like cells directly associated with a dentin-like structure. When single-colony-derived SHED clones were transplanted into immunocompromised mice, only one-fourth of the clones had the potential to generate ectopic dentin-like tissue equivalent to that generated by multicolony-derived SHED. However, all single-colony-derived SHED clones tested are capable of inducing bone formation in immunocompromised mice [17].

Periodontal Ligament Stem Cells (PDLSCs)

The perception that stem cells may reside in the periodontal tissues was first anticipated nearly

20 years ago. Since periodontal regeneration is principally a form of reconstrucion of periodontium growth including cytodifferentiation, morphogenesis, extracellular matrix production as well as mineralization, this is supporting the thoucht that PDLSCs are responsible for tissue homeostasis. PDLSCs can even be isolated from extracted teeth. The periodontal ligament is an adult MSC source in dental tissues, and PDLSCs act as a source of renewable progenitor cells generating fibroblasts, osteoblasts, and cementoblasts during adult life [56].

A recent report proposed that the characteristics of the PDLSCs may depend on the harvest location because PDLSCs from the alveolar bone surface exhibited superior alveolar bone regeneration compared with PDLSCs from the root surface. PDLSCs were identified as a specific MSC with expression of array of osteogenic markers like alkaline phosphatase, matrix extracellular phosphoglycoprotein, bone sialoprotein, and osteocalcin as well as tendon marker scleraxis [57].

Electron microscope radio-autography was utilized in an attempt to recognize any association between the location and degree of differentiation of progenitor cells in the periodontal ligament (PDL). Accordingly, PDL fibroblasts were classified on the basis of their nuclear/cytoplasmic ratio and their distance to the closest blood vessel measured. It was determined that an undifferentiated paravascular progenitor cell population exists and that the PDL also contains progenitor cells displaying a range of cytodifferentiation. This demonstrated that postnatal stem cells can be retrieved from solid-frozen human PDL with promising clinical utility of PDLSCs [58].

Stem Cells from Apical Papilla (SCAP)

Apical papilla refers to the soft tissue at the apical part of the roots of developing permanent teeth where there is an apical cell-rich zone lying between the apical papilla and the pulp. Stem cells from the apical papilla (SCAP) are found in this apical papillary tissue [59].

SCAP also demonstrate the capacity to undergo adipogenic differentiation following induction in vitro. Interestingly, without neurogenic stimulation, cultured SCAP show positive staining for several neural markers. After stimulation, additional neural markers are also expressed by SCAP, including glutamic acid decarboxylase, neuronal nuclear antigen, neurofilament M, neuron-specific enolase, and glial markers [60].

Dental Follicle Precursor Cells (DFPCs)

Dental follicle is an ectomesenchymal tissue surrounding the enamel organ and the dental papilla of the developing tooth germ prior to eruption. This tissue contains progenitor cells that form the periodontium, i.e., cementum, PDL, and alveolar bone. Precursor cells have been isolated from human dental follicles of impacted third molars. Similar to other DSCs, these cells form low numbers of adherent clonogenic colonies when released from the tissue following enzymatic digestion [61].

Cells in dental follicles express markers, suggesting the presence of undifferentiated cells. After cells are released from the tissue, only a small number of single dental follicle cells are attached onto the plastic surface. DFPCs show a typical fibroblast-like morphology and express collagen type I, bone sialoprotein, osteocalcin, and fibroblast growth factor receptor. DFPCs demonstrate osteogenic differentiation capacity in vitro after induction. A membrane-like structure forms in DFPC cultures after 5 weeks of stimulation with dexamethasone [62].

Incubation with enamel matrix derivatives (EMD) for 24 hrs. increases the expression of bone morphogenetic protein-2 and protein-7 (BMP-2 and BMP-7, respectively) by DFPCs. Expression of cementum attachment protein and cementum protein-23, two putative cementoblast markers, has been detected in EMD-stimulated whole dental follicle and in cultured DFPCs stimulated with EMD or BMP-2 and BMP-7 [62].

Transplantation of DFPCs generates a structure comprised of fibrous or rigid tissue. These transplants expressed human-specific transcripts and collagen type I. However, there was no dentin, cementum, or bone formation observed in the transplant in vivo. The authors explained that it could be due to the low number of cells in the original cultures [15].

DPSCs vs SHED vs DPSCs vs SCAP

Similar to DPSCs and SHED, ex vivo expanded SCAP can undergo odontogenic differentiation in vitro. However, SCAP express lower levels of matrix extracellular phosphoglycoprotein, transforming growth factor β receptor II, and melanoma-associated glycoprotein in comparison with DPSCs. Significantly, CD24 is expressed by SCAP which is not detected on DPSCs or BMSCs. The expression of CD24 by SCAP is downregulated in response to osteogenic stimulation. However, the biological consequence of this outcome needs additional study. On the other hand, both DPSCs and SHED possess definitive stem cell properties, such as multi-differentiation and self-renewal [40]. Besides, DPSCs have the specific ability to regenerate the dentin-pulp complex when transplanted into immunocompromised mice. Meanwhile, unlike DPSCs, SHED is unable to regenerate a complete dentin pulp-like complex in vivo. Furthermore, one prominent character of SHED is that they have the capacity of inducing recipient murine cells to differentiate into bone-forming cells, which is not a property attributed to DPSCs following transplantation in vivo [17].

Although it seems that there is little functional difference between DPSC and SHED, both of them have the capability to recapitulate dental pulp tissue, regarding endothelial cells and dentin secreting odontoblasts, the critical constituents to regenerate the integrity of a damaged tooth [63]. Therefore, under investigational conditions, SHED and DPSC are able to reconstitute human tissue in general and more complex dental tissues – such as pulp – specifically. DSCs in vivo seem to repair damaged tissue in a variety of ways that comprise direct cell replacement and also release of cytokines and chemokines mediating immunomodulation, vascular remodeling by angiogenesis, synaptogenesis, and apoptosis in target tissue [63]. In addition to tissue repair, these secreted mediators may allow local stem cells to exert an immunomodulatory influence on tissue response to oral pathogens in the progression of oral diseases such as periodontitis [15].

Unlike other mesenchymal stem cells, it looks clear now that DPSCs are derived from neural-crest tissue and that neural cells such as Schwann cells and their precursors have the capacity to migrate into the pulp chamber and be able to produce dentin matrix material [64]. In turn, isolated dental pulp cells – and other neural crest-derived dental stem cells such as PDLSCs, DFSCs, and gingiva-derived stem cells – can become functional neurons with SHED again having a greater capacity to do so than DPSC. In vivo studies have demonstrated that implanted SHED can regenerate functional neurons, which is an exciting clinical prospect if successfully translated [65, 66].

Importantly, it was observed that SHED proliferate faster than DPSCs and BMSCs (SHED > DPSCs > BMSCs) and produce sphere-like clusters when cultured in neurogenic medium. The clusters either adhere to the culture dish or float freely in the culture medium and could be dissociated and subsequently grown on 0.1% gelatin-coated dishes as individual fibroblastic cells. This phenomenon advocates a high proliferative capability, analogous to that of neural stem cells [17]. Concerning DPSCs and SCAP, the distinction between dental pulp and apical papilla is that apical papilla is the precursor tissue of the radicular pulp. From this perspective, it may be speculated that SCAP are similar to stem cells residing in the dental papilla that gives rise to the coronal dentin-producing odontoblasts. Once the apical papilla turns into pulp, whether the SCAP convert into DPSCs or the latter are derived from a different stem cell pool is currently unclear [67].

Nonetheless, previous studies showed that when SCAP and DPSCs are compared in vitro, there are some differences. Overall, SCAP are derived from a developing tissue that may represent a population of early stem/progenitor cells which may be a superior cell source for tissue regeneration. Additionally, these cells also highlight an important fact that developing tissues may contain stem cells distinctive from those of mature tissues [68].

The capacity of SCAP to differentiate into functional dentinogenic cells has been verified by the same approaches as for DPSCs. Likewise, a typical dentin-pulp-like complex is generated when SCAP are transplanted into immunocompromised mice in an appropriate carrier matrix. As mentioned above, SCAP show characteristics similar to, but different from, those of DPSCs. SCAP appear to be the source of primary odontoblasts that are responsible for root dentin formation, whereas DPSCs are likely the source of replacement odontoblasts that form reparative dentin. Again, the apical papilla is different from the pulp in terms of containing less cellular and vascular components than the pulp. Also, the cells in the apical papilla proliferate two- to threefold faster than those in the pulp in organ cultures [15].

Compared with DPSCs, SCAP demonstrate better proliferation in vitro and better regeneration of the dentin matrix when transplanted in immunocompromised mice. These findings support that "developing" dental tissues may provide a better source for immature stem cells than "developed" dental tissues. In a pilot study with minipigs as a model, the surgical removal of the root apical papilla at an early developing stage halted root development, despite the pulp tissue being intact, whereas other roots of the tooth, containing apical papilla, maintained normal growth and development [17].

Oral Mucosa Stem Cells (OMSCs)

The oral mucosa is composed of stratified squamous epithelium and underlying connective tissue consisting of the lamina propria, which is a zone of well-vascularized tissue, and the submucosa, which might involve minor salivary glands, adipose tissue, neurovascular bundles, and lymphatic tissues dependent on the site [69]. One of the oral mucosa-derived stem cells is the oral epithelial progenitor/stem cells, which are a subpopulation of small oral keratinocytes (smaller than 40 μm) [70]. Although these cells seem to be unipotential stem cells, i.e., they can only develop into epithelial cells, they possess clonogenicity and the ability to regenerate a highly stratified and well-organized oral mucosal graft ex vivo [71], which advocates that they may be valuable for intra-oral grafting [72].

In 2009, Zhang et al. [10] first characterized human gingiva-derived MSCs (GMSCs) as other stem cells in the oral mucosa that have been identified in the lamina propria of the gingiva that attaches directly to the periosteum of the underlying bone with no intervening submucosa. This gingival tissue overlying the alveolar ridges and retromolar region is frequently resected during routine dental surgical procedures and can often be obtained as a discarded biological sample [69].

Lately, Marynka-Kalmani et al. [73] reported that a multipotent neural crest stem cell-like population, termed oral mucosa stem cells (OMSCs), can also be reproducibly generated from the lamina propria of the adult human gingiva and can differentiate in vitro into lineages of the three germ layers. The inherent stemness of gingival cells may therefore partly explain the high reprogramming effectiveness of gingiva-derived fibroblastic cell populations during iPS cell generation [74].

The multipotency of GMSCs/OMSCs and their ease of isolation, clinical abundance, and rapid ex vivo expansion provide a great advantage as a stem cell source for potential clinical applications. It was reported that iPS cell generation could be obtained from human gingiva as well. These iPS cells, as in SHED, may be of precise benefit to regenerate missing jaw bones, periodontal tissues, salivary glands, and lost teeth [52]. In a mouse model, iPS cells combined with enamel matrix derivatives provided greatly improved periodontal regeneration by promoting the formation of cementum, alveolar bone, and periodontal ligament. However, the scientific understanding of iPS cells and how to control their differentiation fate is still limited [75].

Alveolar Periosteum Stem/Progenitor Cells

A comparative analysis of canine MSCs/progenitor cells showed that the in vivo potential of periosteum cells to form bone was higher than that of ilium-derived BMSCs [76]. The phenotypic profiles of human maxillary/mandibular periosteum cells were analogous to those of maxillary tuberosity-derived BMSCs, and both cell populations formed ectopic bone after subcutaneous implantation in mice [77]. Agata et al. reported that human periosteal cells proliferated faster than marrow stromal cells, and subcutaneous transplants of periosteal cells treated with a combination of recombinant growth factors formed more new bone than BMSCs in mice [78].

Periosteal grafts have been shown to induce cortical bone formation, whereas bone marrow grafting induced cancellous bone formation with a bone marrow-like structure in a rat calvarial defect model [79], which indicates that the source of the transplanted cells can impact the structural properties of the regenerated bone. The robust osteogenic potential of periosteum-derived cells has inspired dentists to use the periosteum for orofacial bone regeneration. Indeed, the inverted periosteal flap technique [80] has been suggested for alveolar bone augmentation in conjunction with implant placement or in combination with bone graft surgery.

Additionally, cultured periosteum-derived cells have been used for alveolar ridge or maxillary sinus floor augmentation that effectively proved enhanced bone remodeling and lamellar bone formation with subsequent reliable implant insertion [81] and reduced postoperative waiting time after implant placement [82]. Therefore, the alveolar periosteum is a source of stem/progenitor cells for bone regeneration, principally for large defects.

Salivary Gland Stem Cells

Patients aggrieved with head and neck cancer who receive radiotherapy suffer from an irreversible impairment of salivary gland function that results in xerostomia and a compromised quality of life. Therefore, stem cells in the adult salivary gland are expected to be useful for autologous transplantation therapy in the context of tissue engineered salivary glands or direct cell therapy [15]. Even though existence of salivary gland stem cells was proved [83], a single stem cell that gives rise to all epithelial cell types within the gland has not yet been identified. Thus far, the isolation of stem cells in the salivary glands has been attempted through the cell culture of dissociated tissue. Kishi et al. [84] isolated salivary gland stem/progenitor cells from rat submandibular glands and found that the cells are highly proliferative and express acinar, ductal, and myoepithelial cell lineage markers.

Lombaert et al. [85] reported that an in vitro floating sphere culture method could be used to isolate a specific population of cells expressing stem cell markers from dissociated mouse submandibular glands. These cell populations could differentiate into salivary gland duct cells as well as mucin- and amylase-producing acinar cells in vitro. Progenitor/stem cells were also isolated from swine [86] and human [87] salivary glands. Moreover, the intra-glandular transplantation of cells isolated from mouse submandibular glands successfully rescued the salivary function of irradiated salivary glands [88]. These reports recommend that the salivary gland is a promising stem cell source for future therapies targeting irradiated head and neck cancer patients. However, primary cultures of dispersed cells will always contain a number of cells with different origins, such as parenchymal cells, stromal cells, and blood vessel cells, which makes it difficult to select salivary gland stem cells [15].

Indeed, Gorjup et al. [89] isolated primitive MSC-like cells from the human salivary gland, but possibly from stromal tissue, which expressed embryonic and adult stem cell markers and could be guided to differentiate into adipogenic, osteogenic, and chondrogenic cells. To obtain a genuine stem cell population that can be considered to be a true stem cell for the salivary gland, it is necessary to select cells carrying a specific marker or labeled with induced reporter proteins [90].

Adipose Stem Cells (ASCs) from Orofacial Tissues

Adipose-derived MSCs can be readily harvested via lipectomy or from lipoaspirate from areas such as the chin; ASCs exhibit robust osteogenesis and are thus expected to be an alternative source of MSCs for bone regeneration in dentistry. Indeed, the feasibility of using autologous ASCs for orofacial bone regeneration and implant placement has been demonstrated [91]. Pieri et al. demonstrated that the transplantation of autologous ASCs with an inorganic bovine bone scaffold enhanced new bone formation and implant osseointegration following vertical bone augmentation of the calvarial bone of rabbits, which proposes that ASCs may be useful for vertical alveolar bone augmentation for implant insertion [92].

Most recently, periodontal tissue regeneration using ASCs has been successfully verified in a rat experimental animal model [93]. Another in vitro study demonstrated that rat ASCs acquired cementoblast features when cultured in dental follicle cell conditioned medium containing dentin non-collagenous proteins [94]. Furthermore, Ishizaka et al. [95] demonstrated that ASC transplantation induced pulp regeneration in the root canal after pulpectomy in dogs. Additionally, Hung et al. [96] demonstrated that ASC implants were able to grow self-assembled new teeth containing dentin, periodontal ligament, and alveolar bone in adult rabbit extraction sockets with a high success rate. Further studies on the isolation, characterization, and application of ASCs to enhance their efficacy for bone and periodontal regeneration will provide a significant protocol for the use of waste fat tissues in future clinical applications [97].

Scaffolds and Tissue Bioengineering in Dentistry

In recent years, DSCs have gained in popularity for tissue engineering. The highly proliferative and self-renewing population of DSCs with the neural crest origin expands their applicability for regeneration of tissues from both ectochyme and mesenchymal origin. Ease of tissue harvest, high initial yield of cells, low population-doubling time, plasticity, multipotential capabilities, and immunomodulatory characteristics make them an appropriate candidate for tissue engineering applications. Furthermore, immunoregulatory properties of DSCs provide potential for both autologous and allogenic tissue engineering approaches [98].

To engineer and regenerate a complete tooth, the cell source may have to come from tooth buds in which all the needed cell types are retained. To repair partly lost tooth tissues such as PDL, dentin, and pulp, one or two particular types of DSCs could be satisfactory to fulfill the need [11].

Tissue engineering is an emerging field of regenerative medicine, where during the past decade, it has progressed from the use of naked biomaterials just replacing small area of damaged tissue to the use of controlled three-dimensional scaffolds in which cells can be seeded before implantation. These cellularized constructs intend to functionally regenerate large tissue defects [99].

Scaffolds or matrices are specific materials that provide mechanical support to the forming tissue and deliver the cells or signaling molecules to the appropriate anatomic site. The physical and chemical characteristics of a scaffold play a significant role in cell proliferation and tissue ingrowth. Cell-seeding scaffolds are either natural, synthetic, resorbable, or non-resorbable [100].

Among the settled scaffolds is the polymeric hydrogels that proved to be reasonable for jaws' cartilage and bone repair [101]. In contrary, fibrin-based scaffolds have been used for soft tissue engineering and the revascularization of dental pulp as a result of odontoblastic differentiation. For instance, platelet-rich fibrin was applied into the root canal of a necrotic infected immature tooth after total canal disinfection [102].

The use of biomaterial scaffolds and stem cells can be safe and potent for the regeneration of pulp tissue and re-establishment of tooth vitality. Natural and synthetic polymers have distinct advantages and limitations, and in vitro and in vivo testing have produced positive results for cell attachment, proliferation, and angiogenesis [103]. The type of biomaterial used for scaffold fabrication also facilitates stem cell differentiation into odontoblasts. Multiple methods of scaffold design exist for pulp tissue engineering, which demonstrates the variability in tissue engineering applications in endodontics [104]. Delivery of marrow mesenchymal stem cells (MSCs), with or without growth factor, from biodegradable hydrogel composites could be used for the repair of osteochondral defects [105]. Alternatively, in a tooth slice model (horizontal section, 1 mm thick), it was shown that SHED seeded onto synthetic scaffolds seated into the pulp chamber space formed odontoblast-like cells that localized against the existing dentin surface (Cordeiro et al., 2008) [(106)]. However, no orthotopic regeneration of pulp-like tissues in the pulp space has been reported with this approach.

One concern is that implanting stem cells/scaffolds into root canals that have a blood supply only from the apical end may compromise vascularization to support the vitality of the implanted cells in the scaffolds. It has been proposed that, because of the concern of over vascularization, a stepwise insertion of engineered pulp may have to be implemented clinically to achieve the desired pulp tissue regeneration [(107)]. Recent in vitro studies demonstrated the differentiation of mouse iPS cells into ameloblasts [(108)] and odontogenic mesenchymal cells, which may be useful approach for tooth bioengineering strategies [109]. Most recently a new approach was introduced in dentistry using pulsed low-intensity ultrasound displays with an optimistic consequence on cell proliferation and collagen deposition even without growth factor supplements [13].

Regenerative Medicine Versus Regenerative Dentistry

Growing evidence has revealed that regenerative medicine in dentistry is superior in many aspects. For instance, many intra-oral tissues such as deciduous teeth, wisdom teeth, and the gingiva, despite being rich sources of stem cells, they are discarded as biological samples. Consequently, dental specialists must identify the promise of the emergent field of regenerative dentistry and the possibility of obtaining stem cells during conventional dental treatments. These cells could be banked for autologous therapeutic use in the future [20].

Furthermore, it was found that bone marrow stem cells (BMSCs) that obtained from the craniofacial area (membranous bone) for autologous bone grafting provide better bone volume than bone harvested from the iliac crest or rib (endochondral bone) [110]. This finding suggests that different skeletal donor tissues have site-specific regenerative properties that may depend on stem cell type and its niche present in the graft. Embryologically, the maxilla and mandible bones exclusively originate from cranial neural crest cells [111], whereas the iliac crest bone is formed by mesoderm. This variance in embryological origin might consequence in functional phenotypically differences between orofacial and iliac crest human BMSCs. Additionally, Akintoye et al. observed that orofacial BMSCs from the same individuals are of higher proliferation and osteogenic differentiation capacity forming more mineralized bone compared with the iliac crest BMSCs. Also, the adipogenic potential of orofacial BMSCs is less than that of iliac BMSCs, which could decrease unfavorable fat formation during bone regeneration [112].

Interestingly, orofacial bone-derived BMSCs can be obtained not only from young patients but also from relatively aged individuals, indicating that the age of the donor appears to have minute consequence on the BMSC gene expression pattern and the clinical efficacy of bone formation [113]. In contrary, several reports have demonstrated an age-related decline in the osteogenic potential of BMSCs isolated from the human iliac crest and femur [114, 115]. In addition, cultured mesenchymal stem cells obtained from the periodontium, PDLSCs, display almost 30% higher rates of propagation compared to the growth of cultured BMSCs. It appears that these cells preserve this ability of higher growth potential beyond 100 population doublings before in vitro senescence is noticed. It was demonstrated that putative stem cell marker, STRO-1, used to isolate and purify BMSCs, is also expressed by human PDLSCs as well as dental pulp stem cells (DPSCs) [116].

Besides, iPS cells have been generated from several oral mesenchymal cells and found to have a higher reprogramming efficiency than the conventionally skin fibroblasts. This perhaps is due to their high expression of endogenous reprogramming factors and/or ES cell-associated genes [117] along with their high proliferation rate [52]. Accordingly, cells of oral origin are expected to deliver an ideal iPS cell source for dental researchers [15]. The chondrogenic potential of DPSCs appears weak, and both DPSCs and SCAP are weaker in adipogenesis in comparison with BMSCs [18, 19]. Conversely, the neurogenicity of DSCs may be more potent than that of BMSCs, most probably due to their neural crest origin [54]. Furthermore, a similar level of gene expression between DPSCs and BMSCs was found for more than 4000 known human genes, except a few differentially expressed genes, including, for instance, insulin-like growth factor-2 and cyclin-dependent kinase 6, which are highly expressed in DPSCs, whereas insulin-like growth factor binding protein-7 and collagen type I $\alpha 2$ are more highly expressed in BMSCs. The cementum/PDL-like structures are totally different from typical bone/marrow structures generated by BMSCs and dentin/pulp-like structures generated by DPSCs. Collectively, current evidence suggests that biochemical pathways involved in the differentiation of DPSCs into functional odontoblasts are similar to differentiation pathways of BMMSCs into osteoblasts [4].

DPSCs do share a similar pattern of protein expression with BMMSCs in vitro. Furthermore, human GMSCs exhibited clonogenicity, self-renewal, and a multipotent differentiation capacity similar to that of BMSCs. However, GMSCs are uniformly homogenous, proliferate faster than BMSCs, display a stable phenotype, maintain normal karyotype and telomerase activity with extended passaging, and are not tumorigenic and do not lose their MSC characteristics with extended passaging [118].

Tooth Banking

With the promise of cures for conditions as diverse as diabetes, autism, neural degeneration, organ replacement, aging, addiction, as well as cancer, long-term preservation of dental stem cells is a growing market. Banks specialized in stem cells isolated from teeth are relatively new in comparison to stem cell banks collecting bone marrow and placental cord blood. In North America, India, and the United Kingdom in particular, dental stem cell banks are expanding in number. An English language Internet search of the first 100 hits for "tooth + stem + cell + bank" recovered 15 separate tooth-banking services. Though this is not a comprehensive search, other tooth bank companies that work locally, in particular in the United States, extend their banking facilities continentally and globally. It is worth noting that one of the first tooth banks looking at stem cell recovery was started in Hiroshima University in Japan as early as 2004 [119].

Tooth banking concentrates on the collection of a child's baby teeth, as they are shed naturally and it is noninvasive source of autologous stem cells used for therapeutic purposes later on when the child need. In turn, companies and dental offices offer to collect extracted teeth and preserve the DPSCs within teeth. Moreover, associated oral tissue such as epithelium, gingiva (gums), and salivary gland also house unique populations of stem cells [120].

On the other hand, tooth germ progenitor cells (TGPCs) and DFSC present in the tooth bud are stem cells that contribute to the developing tooth and so are not readily accessible for therapeutic use [121]. Indeed, frequent studies have noted that SHED have even greater proliferative properties than DPSC and may have a greater propensity for survival than their adult counterparts [122]. This property is significant when considering the small numbers of stem cells available within the confines of a tooth pulp. One of the primary services provided by dental stem cell banking companies is the expansion of the few cells isolated from the pulp to a number that could be therapeutically useful [123]. Regarding carious teeth as a source for banked stem cells where a percentage of extracted deciduous teeth are carious and so are bacterially infected, tooth-banking companies are alienated over receiving of diseased teeth. Similarly, the scientific literature is split [51].

Werle et al. proved that stem cells extracted from mutually carious and healthy deciduous teeth established equivalent capacity for tissue differentiation [124]. In similar manner, Tsai et al. compared the efficiency of stem cell recovery from deciduous teeth in the presence or absence of caries regarding increasing levels of disease severity [125]. They also concluded that stem cells could be isolated from carious teeth nevertheless with numbers in inverse relation to the clinical severity of the caries. Really, a greater than fourfold variance in fruitful stem cell isolation from healthy versus carious teeth was established. Contrarily, Werle et al. noticed only a 10% difference in successful stem cell isolation from carious versus healthy teeth [124]. Studies of adult stem cells from healthy teeth and post-caries teeth with inflamed pulps confirmed that cell recovery was inferior in the diseased teeth but that both sources of stem cells retained comparable differentiation abilities [125, 126].

Notably, Tsai et al. described an increase in both inflammatory mediator expression and of innate immune system molecules in stem cells from the diseased teeth compared to healthy ones. It is blurred how those alterations may influence the long-term use of SHED or DPSC banked for regenerative purposes; however it is reasonable to be cautious at the very least. The questions around carious teeth obviously highlight the paucity of information regarding teeth as a source of banked stem cells [125].

Collection and Processing for Tooth Banking

Many collection protocols for DSC banks are comparable; so far there are some notable and important differences in both sample requirements and sample processing. The majority of services recommend that a dentist extracts the deciduous tooth as soon as it is loose (174). In contrary, BioEden claim to use a process for collection and transport augmented for naturally exfoliated teeth. Indeed, their transport medium for the tooth is pasteurized cow milk. For the other services they are accepting teeth from home extractions, just requiring the tooth to have an existing blood supply – evidenced by post removal bleeding. However, for all the Indian tooth banks and five of the US tooth banks, extraction by a dental professional is required [127].

Indeed, professional extraction shortens the time the tooth is out of physiological circumstances possibly to preserve the pulp tissue. Long-term success rates for re-implantation of avulsed teeth lost due to physical trauma range from about 20% to above 90% depending on how the tooth was handled and how the patient was treated post implant [128].

Yet, the enthusiasm of an otherwise healthy extracted tooth and the manner in which it is extracted are not the primary factors concerning tooth-banking services. Once a tooth has been extracted or exfoliated, storage for transport has the major impact on living pulp and consequently stem cell survival [129].

Transporting of Dental Stem Cells

A number of studies have assessed different media for efficacious preservation of live teeth though many are ex vivo models and have looked at the specific survival of periodontal ligament cells after tooth storage in the media. One of the described transport media is the balanced salt solutions such as phosphate buffered saline. Alternatively, there is Hank's buffered saline solution (HBSS) that is predominates with some undefined nutrients. As previously declared, BioEden calls for the use of bovine milk as the transport medium [130].

Avulsed teeth are often recommended to be transported to the dentist in milk or even held in the mouth with saliva acting as the carrier [131]. Significantly, tissue drying is the greatest enemy to successful tooth recovery, and similarly, the same is true for stem cell retrieval from banked teeth. Times allocated for transportation vary from overnight up to 48 hours as maximum conveyance times from tooth extraction to receipt by the banking facility. So far, just keeping the tooth hydrated, in water, for instance, is insufficient to that purpose instead an isotonic fluid mimicking physiological conditions is compulsory [132].

Bovine milk offers a number of appropriate standards that are absent from many other media [133]. It is biocompatible, has neutral pH, and is naturally buffered, as well as it is commonly available. Accordingly, if milk is used as a carrier, dental tissue obviously survives in it, and teeth can be successfully re-implanted [134]. This is more imperative for the unplanned loss of teeth by avulsion due to trauma, but still also, conceivably to a lesser extent, for exfoliated teeth where the tooth is shed at home, school, or anywhere other than the dental clinic. Notably, bovine milk is still the most widely recommended preservation media for avulsed tooth storage during transport to the dentist [135].

Other biological media explored for tooth preservation include propolis (a honeybee natural product), soymilk, almond milk, pomegranate and other fruit juices, chicken egg white, coconut water, green tea extract, Gatorade sports drink, and the Brazilian plant extract dragon's blood *Croton lechleri* sap [136–139]. Nevertheless, with the possible exception of Gatorade, these non-defined media have recognized to be viable as tooth tissue preservation vehicles, yet none standing out as consistently better than milk [140].

Closely following bovine milk in frequency of recommendation is HBSS, which is frequently used for tissue and cell preservation and maintenance under in vitro experimental circumstances [129]. Remarkably, HBSS is the medium contained in the tooth preservation kit, Save-a-Tooth™ the kit officially used by the tooth bank Store-A-Tooth [141]. The main apparent benefit of HBSS, and similar saline solutions, is that they are of a distinct and consistent formulation, rather than milk [134]. Ideally, for tooth banking, it is required to use their proprietary collection media kits and preferred extraction by a dentist; it is this matter of consistency that drives the tooth preservation process.

Isolation and Preparation of Dental Stem Cells

Magnificently gaining viable cells is the critical step in banking process. Stem cells are extracted from the pulp by mechanical and enzymatic preparation of single cell populations or alternatively by tissue outgrowth – where cells are permitted to naturally migrate from the extracted pulp onto plastic culture surfaces. In early studies for isolation and characterization of DPSCs, Songtao Shi and Stan Gronthos enzymatically digested the pulp tissue with collagenase type I and dispase – to free cells from the extracellular matrix – then they passed them through a 70 μm sieve. Single cells were able to grow in culture thereafter. This recovery protocol, with rapidity of process, 24–48 h from start to finish, is likely employed basically with no modification two decades later [142, 143].

The primary substitute method described frequently in the literature, tissue outgrowth, is a simpler yet lengthier protocol where the pulp tissue is macerated and then placed in a culture vessel in balanced salt solution with suitable nutrients to maintain stemness. The cells migrate out from the tissue and establish colonies on the plastic culture surface. In both cases, the cell population surviving in culture is greatly enriched in stem cells following two or three rounds of subculture [144].

The existence of stem cells needs both viability testing and flow cytometry. Regarding flow cytometry, it requires only a few thousand cells out of the entire sample [145], yet this is critical as pulp tissue volumes vary between incisors and molars and are consistently small in deciduous teeth. Cells can be concurrently labeled by fluorescent molecular probes or antibodies, which could include markers for viability and stem cell-specific markers as well. All tooth-banking services test cell viability, though stem cell marker testing may not be conducted unless explicitly noted. The reason for this is possibly that excessive handling of the pulp-derived cells in the early stages of isolation could result in loss of stemness or viability [146].

At least one company, the National Dental Pulp Laboratory tooth bank, states that they adhere to the US Food and Drug Administration (FDA) non-binding regulatory guidance on minimal handling of cell and tissue-based products for homologous use. For extracted cells this means, in the words of the FDA, "… processing that does not alter the relevant biological characteristics of cells or tissues" [147].

Cryopreservation of Dental Stem Cells

Once viable cells or pulp tissue have been isolated, they have to be effectively frozen and stored. Cells are suspended in a preservation medium, possibly containing growth factors and a cryoprotectant, commonly dimethyl sulfoxide which inhibits the growth of ice crystals that may disrupt the cell membrane and so reduce overall viability [148]. They are transferred to specialized cryo-vials generally constructed from high-density polypropylene, and then the samples are frozen and placed in low-temperature storage containers filled with liquid nitrogen [149].

The majority of tooth banks store isolated, viable stem cells, but at least one, Store-A-Tooth, mentions the preservation of at least some of the original pulp material along with the isolated cells. Although whole tooth storage for future recovery of stem cells has proven technically possible, the efficiency of stem cell recovery is highly variable, and it is not in general use by commercial banking services [150]. Indeed, both in vitro and in vivo functions are maintained if stem cells are recovered from frozen pulp tissue [151].

Interestingly, Lizier et al. settled a protocol for greatly scaling up the numbers of extracted stem cells from pulp tissue prior to freezing in which the same piece of pulp tissue is transferred from culture plate to culture plate seeding each of them in turn with stem cells over a number of days [152]. Under these circumstances, cells preserved stemness throughout the process indicating that dental stem cells and pulp tissue are relatively resistant to handling and manipulation if done carefully.

Low-Level Laser Therapy (LLLT) and Bone Bio-stimulation

Apart from using stem cells in regenerative dentistry, a recent study was designed to evaluate the effect of low-level laser therapy (LLLT) by means of diode laser bio-stimulation compared to traditional teriparatide therapy in induced osteoporosis (OP) in rats [14]. In 2002, FDA has approved teriparatide (TPTD), the first anabolic agent that stimulates osteoblastic bone formation to improve bone quality and bone mass. To date, it is the only currently available therapeutic agent that increases the formation of new bone and could provide some remediation of the architectural defects in the osteoporotic skeleton. However, it is restricted to second-line usage for OP treatment due to its higher cost than first-line less effective agents such as alendronate [153].

On the other hand, LLLT has gained acceptance in both medical and dental practices in the past few decades. The application of low intensity impacts the cellular behavior through photophysical, photochemical, and photobiological effects on the irradiated cell tissues. Various studies showed that LLLT could be an alternative, co-adjuvant, and noninvasive therapy with a significant effect on the healing process with minimum side effects. Due to the several benefits of LLLT, researchers have attempted to determine its effect on the bone. However, scarce investigations were accomplished to explore the osteogenic potential of LLLT on OP [154].

Accordingly, it was interesting to study the effect of LLLT on OP in rat lower jaws and compare it to the widely approved TPTD, as well as to study their combined effects, using a state-of-art techniques like computed tomography (CT), ordinary light microscope, and scanning electron microscope (SEM) to detect bone pores (Fig. 13.1) and energy dispersive x-ray analyzer (EDAX) and enzyme-linked immunosorbent assay (ELISA) to detect procollagen type I N propeptide (PINP) concentrations. This study was looking forward to widening the variety of the less invasive therapeutic options to improve the OP prognosis and enhance the quality of life for humans, especially elderly patients [14].

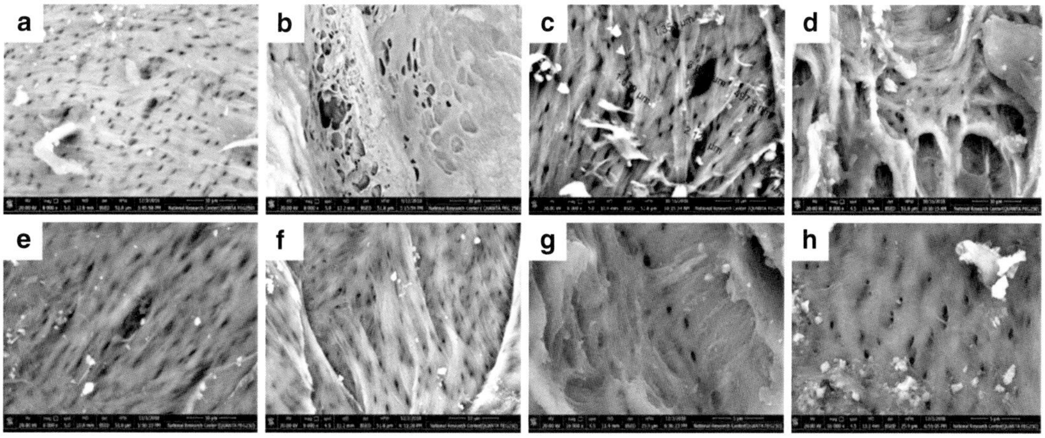

Fig. 13.1 SEM images. (**a**) Normal control group showing normal jawbone architecture with equal and uniform porosity. (**b**) Osteoporotic group displaying increased large and irregular bone pores, (**c**) TPTD group revealing at week 16 bone pores with variation in size. (**d**) LLLT group illustrating at week 16 bone pores that get narrower. (**e**) Combination group presenting at week 16 numerous small regular pores with few large ones (**f**) TPTD group demonstrating at week 24 numerous uniform bone pores, (**g**) LLLT group showing uniform regular bone pores at week 24. (**h**) Combination group presenting at week 24 uniform regular bone pores with some pores are getting completely obscured

The beneficial effect of LLLT on the bone is attributed to its bio-stimulatory action, where it is capable of increasing mitochondrial activity, bone formation, osteocalcin and osteopontin gene expression, as well as alkaline phosphate activity [155]. This is supported by Torstrick et al. [156], who pointed out that LLLT could be utilized to prevent fracture, improve healing, and accelerate implant fixation. The osteogenic potential of LLLT is in harmony with the results of Scalize et al. [154] and Fallahnezhad et al. [157], as they observed new bone formation and improved cell viability of the ovariectomized rat bone marrow mesenchymal stem cells, respectively. Furthermore, through histopathological examination, numerous reversal lines were observed of lased group that reflects the capability of LLLT to induce rapid bone formation and high bone turnover. In this regard, Matsumoto et al. [158] highlighted that experimental group irradiated by LLLT was able to induce woven bone formation faster than the control group. Moreover, the recent study of Suzuki et al. [159] demonstrated that LLLT could independently accelerate the bone remodeling process and in turn accelerate tooth movement during orthodontic treatment.

It was concluded that TPTD has osteogenic potential and is capable to enhance bone architecture by inducing the formation of new well-organized bone with narrower bone pore diameter. LLLT can be used as a good alternative local treatment strategy with minimal side effects and superior outcomes as it can improve bone strength by faster bone deposition and higher calcium content. Additionally, combination of both TPTD and LLLT has a synergistic beneficial effect on bones of experimental rats with induced OP. This can possibly overcome systemic side effects of a high dose of TPTD and the limitations of LLLT application, as well as giving maximum benefit of uniform and speedy new bone formation [14].

Low-Intensity Pulsed Ultrasound Applications in Dentistry

In tissue engineering, mechanical stimulates are required for creating the circumstances appropriate for cell proliferation. In turn, low-intensity pulsed ultrasound (LIPUS) improves cells by effective mechanical interaction. It was found that the mechanical index parameter 0.20 has promoted collagen I expression and cell proliferation [160]. In dentistry, several applications of LIPUS were tried. For instance, LIPUS was evaluated to detect its possible effect on tooth movement and root resorption in orthodontic patients. The study outcome revealed accelerated tooth movement and minimized orthodontically induced tooth root resorption at the same time [161]. Furthermore, there was a clinically significant reduction in the overall orthodontic treatment duration indicating acceleration of new bone formation around the moving teeth [162].

Moreover, LIPUS therapy was investigated to detect whether it stimulates osteogenesis in mandibular distraction in a double-blind trial. It was concluded that LIPUS matures the regenerated tissue by altering the microarchitecture of the newly formed bone [163]. Besides, it was observed that LIPUS accelerates impaired fracture healing suggesting that the mechanism is by increasing osteoid thickness, mineral apposition rate, and bone volume, indicating increased osteoblast activity, at the front of new bony callus formation. Improved stability and/or increased blood flow, but probably not increased angiogenesis, might explain the differences in ossification modes between LIPUS-treated delayed unions and untreated controls [164].

Most recently, LIPUS was demonstrated to promote the formation of periodontal ligament stem cell sheets and enhance ectopic periodontal tissue regeneration. In this regard, LIPUS has been reported as an effective stimulus to regulate cell biological behavior. Collectively, the results of the study indicate that LIPUS not only promotes the formation and osteogenic differentiation of human PDLSCs but also is a potential treatment strategy for periodontal tissue engineering ([165]).

Conclusions

Teeth and oral tissues, that are often discarded in the dental clinic as medical waste, are proved to be a particularly attractive source for stem cells because of their availability and potentiality not only in regenerative dentistry but also for regenerating any tissue in the body.

Stem cells derived from oral and maxillofacial region is superior on other body stem cells in several aspects.

Tissue engineering is among the latest technologies that impacted the field of dentistry and is now being successfully applied in regenerative surgery.

Parents should think twice before throwing away their child's avulsed or extracted tooth which may be a nidus for tooth banking which will serve in autologous regenerative therapies.

New modalities other than stem cells could be utilized for regenerative medicine/dentistry including low-level laser therapy and low-intensity pulsed ultrasound for bio-stimulation and new bone formation as well as dental supporting tissues.

References

1. Rosemann A, Luo HY. Attitudes towards the donation of human embryos for stem cell research among Chinese IVF patients and students. J Bioethic Inq. 2018;15:441–57.
2. Sivaraman MAF. Using surplus embryos and research embryos in stem cell research: ethical viewpoints of buddhist, hindu and catholic leaders in Malaysia on the permissibility of research. Sci Eng Ethics. 2018;24:129–49.
3. Gronthos S, Mankani M, Brahim J, Robey PG, Shi S. Postnatal human dental pulp stem cells (DPSCs) in vitro and in vivo. Proc Natl Acad Sci U S A. 2000;97:13625–30.
4. Shi S, Robey PG, Gronthos S. Comparison of human dental pulp and bone marrow stromal stem cells by cDNA microarray analysis. Bone. 2001;29:532–9.
5. Huang GT, Yamaza T, Shea LD, Djouad F, Kuhn NZ, Tuan RS, et al. Stem/progenitor cell-mediated de novo regeneration of dental pulp with newly deposited continuous layer of dentin in an in vivo model. Tissue Eng. 2010;16:605–15.
6. Liu HC, Wang DS, Su F, Wu X, Shi ZP, et al. Reconstruction of alveolar bone defects using bone morphogenetic protein 2 mediated rabbit dental pulp stem cells seeded on nano-hydroxyapatite/collagen/poly (L-lactide). Tissue Eng. 2011;17:2417–33.
7. Seo M, Miura M, Gronthos S, Bartold PM, Batouli S, Brahim J, et al. Investigation of multipotent postnatal stem cells from human periodontal ligament. Lancet. 2004;364:149–55.

8. Park BW, Kang EJ, Byun JH, Son MG, Kim HJ, Hah YS, et al. In vitro and in vivo osteogenesis of human mesenchymal stem cells derived from skin, bone marrow and dental follicle tissues. Differentiation. 2012;83:249–59.
9. Huang GT, Gronthos S, Shi S. Mesenchymal stem cells derived from dental tissues vs. those from other sources: their biology and role in regenerative medicine. J Dent Res. 2009;88:792–806.
10. Zhang Q, Shi S, Liu Y, Uyanne J, Shi Y, Shi S, et al. Mesenchymal stem cells derived from human gingiva are capable of immunomodulatory functions and ameliorate inflammation-related tissue destruction in experimental colitis. J Immunol. 2009;183:7787–98.
11. Tomokiyo A, Wada N, Maeda H. Periodontal ligament stem cells: regenerative potency in periodontium. Stem Cells Dev. 2019;28:974–85.
12. Bohari SPM, Grover LM, Hukins DWL. Pulsed low-intensity ultrasound increases proliferation and extracelluar matrix production by human dermal fibroblasts in three-dimensional culture. J Tissue Eng. 2015;6:204.
13. Bernardi S, Zeka K, Continenza MA. Application of low-level laser therapy in dentistry: laser biostimulation. JSM Oro Facial Surg. 2016;1:1002.
14. Hamza S, Fathy S, EL-Azab S. Effect of diode laser biostimulation compared to Teriparatide on induced osteoporosis in rats: an animal study from Egypt. Int J Clin Exp Pathol. 2020;13:1970–85.
15. Egusa H, Sonoyama W, MasahiroNishimura IA, Akiyama K. Stem cells in dentistry – Part I: stem cell sources. J Prosthodont Res. 2012;56:151–65.
16. Gronthos S, Mankani M, Brahim J, Robey PG, Shi S. Postnatal human dental pulp stem cells (DPSCs) in vitro and in vivo. Proc Natl Acad Sci. 2000;97:13625–30.
17. Miura M, Gronthos S, Zhao M, Lu B, Fisher LW, Robey PG, et al. SHED: stem cells from human exfoliated deciduous teeth. Proc Natl Acad Sci. 2003;100:5807–12.
18. Sonoyama W, Liu Y, Fang D, Yamaza T, Seo BM, Zhang C, et al. Mesenchymal stem cell mediated functional tooth regeneration in swine. PLoS. 2006;1:79.
19. Sonoyama W, Liu Y, Yamaza T, Tuan RS, Wang S, Shi S, et al. Characterization of the apical papilla and its residing stem cells from human immature permanent teeth: a pilot study. J Endod. 2008;34:166–71.
20. Morsczeck C, Schmalz G, Reichert T, Völlner F, Galler K, Driemel O. Somatic stem cells for regenerative dentistry. Clin Oral Investig. 2008;12:113–8.
21. Papaccio G, Graziano A, d'Aquino R, Graziano MF, Pirozzi G, Menditti D. Long-term cryopreservation of dental pulp stem cells (SBP-DPSCs) and their differentiated osteoblasts: a cell source for tissue repair. J Cell Physiol. 2006;208:319–25.
22. Harada H, Kettunen P, Jung HS, Mustonen T, Wang YA, Thesleff I. Localization of putative stem cells in dental epithelium and their association with Notch and FGF signaling. J Cell Biol. 1999;147:105–20.
23. Ning F, Guo Y, Tang J, Zhou J, Zhang H, Lu W, et al. Differentiation of mouse embryonic stem cells into dental epithelial-like cells induced by ameloblasts serum-free conditioned medium. Biochem Biophys Res Commun. 2010;394:342–7.
24. Butler WT, Ritchie HH, Bronckers AL. Extracellular matrix proteins of dentine. Ciba Found Symp. 1997;205:107–17.
25. Ruch JV. Odontoblast commitment and differentiation. Biochem Cell Biol. 1998;76:923–38.
26. Kitamura C, Kimura K, Nakayama T, Terashita M. Temporal and spatial expression of c-jun and jun-B proto-oncogenes in pulp cells involved with reparative dentinogenesis after cavity preparation of rat molars. J Dent Res. 1999;78:673–80.
27. Kao DW, Fiorellini JP. Regenerative periodontal therapy. Front Oral Biol. 2012;15:149–59.
28. Ikeda E, Yagi K, Kojima M, Yagyuu T, Ohshima A, Sobajima S, et al. Multipotent cells from the human third molar: feasibility of cell-based therapy for liver disease. Differentiation. 2008;76:495–505.
29. Botelho J, Cavacas MA, Machado V, Mendes JJ. Dental stem cells: recent progresses in tissue engineering and regenerative medicine. Ann Meds. 2017;49:644–51.
30. Peng L, Jia Z, Yin X, Zhang X, Liu Y, Chen P, et al. Comparative analysis of mesenchymal stem cells from bone marrow, cartilage, and adipose tissue. Stem Cells Dev. 2008;17:761–73.
31. Christine Sedgley M, Tatiana BM. Dental stem cells and their sources. Dent Clin N Am. 2012;56:549–61.
32. Kang H, Lee MJ, Park SJ, Lee MS. Lipopolysaccharide-preconditioned periodontal ligament stem cells induce M1 polarization of macrophages through extracellular vesicles. Int J Mol Sci. 2018;19:3843.
33. Wu JY, Chen LL, Wang RF, Song Z, Shen ZS, Zhao YM. Exosomes secreted by stem cells from human exfoliated deciduous teeth promote alveolar bone defect repair through the regulation of angiogenesis and osteogenesis. ACS Biomater Sci Eng. 2019;5:3561–71.
34. Warren L, Manos PD, Ahfeldt T, Loh YH, Li H, Lau F, et al. Highly efficient reprogramming to pluripotency and directed differentiation of human cells with synthetic modified mRNA. Cell Stem Cell. 2010;7:618–30.
35. Oshima M, Mizuno M, Imamura A, Ogawa M, Yasukawa M, Yamazaki H. Functional tooth regeneration using a bioengineered tooth unit as a mature organ replacement regenerative therapy. PLoS One. 2011;6.1–11.
36. Ono M, Oshima M, Ogawa M, Sonoyama W, Hara ES, Oida Y. Practical whole-tooth restoration utilizing autologous bioengineered tooth germ transplantation in a postnatal canine model. Sci Rep. 2017;7:44522.

37. Alipour R, Sadeghi F, Hashemi-Beni B, Zarkesh-Esfahani SH, Heydari F, Mousavi SB, et al. Phenotypic characterizations and comparison of adult dental stem cells with adipose-derived stem cells. Int J Prev Med. 2010;1:164–71.
38. Couble ML, Farges JC, Bleicher F, Perrat-Mabillon B, Boudeulle M, Magloire H. Odontoblast differentiation of human dental pulp cells in explant cultures. Calcif Tissue Int. 2000;66:129–38.
39. Huang G, Sonoyama W, Chen J, Park S. In vitro characterization of human dental pulp cells: various isolation methods and culturing environments. Cell Tissue Res. 2006;324:225–36.
40. Gronthos S, Brahim J, Li W, Fisher LW, Cherman N, Boyde A. Stem cell properties of human dental pulp stem cells. J Dent Res. 2002;81:531–5.
41. Batouli S, Miura M, Brahim J, Tsutsui TW, Fisher LW, Gronthos S, et al. Comparison of stem-cell-mediated osteogenesis and dentinogenesis. J Dent Res. 2003;9:976–81.
42. Huang GT, Shagramanova K, Chan SW. Formation of odontoblast-like cells from cultured human dental pulp cells on dentin in vitro. J Endod. 2006;32:1066–73.
43. Laino G, d'Aquino R, Graziano A, Lanza V, Carinci F, Naro F, et al. A new population of human adult dental pulp stem cells: a useful source of living autologous fibrous bone tissue (LAB). J Bone Miner Res. 2005;20:1394–402.
44. Zhang W, Walboomers XF, Shi S, Fan M, Jansen JA. Multilineage differentiation potential of stem cells derived from human dental pulp after cryopreservation. Tissue Eng. 2006;12:2813–23.
45. d'Aquino R, Graziano A, Sampaolesi M, Laino G, Pirozzi G, De Rosa A, et al. Human postnatal dental pulp cells co-differentiate into osteoblasts and endotheliocytes: a pivotal synergy leading to adult bone tissue formation. Cell Death Differ. 2007;14:1162–71.
46. Isaac J, Nassif A, Asselin A, Taihi I, Fohrer-Ting H, Klein C. Involvement of neural crest and paraxial mesoderm in oral mucosal development and healing. Biomaterials. 2018;172:41–53.
47. Yang XR, Li L, Xiao L, Zhang DH. Recycle the dental fairy's package: overview of dental pulp stem cells. Stem Cell Res Ther. 2018;9:347.
48. Anitua E, Troya M, Zalduendo M. Progress in the use of dental pulp stem cells in regenerative medicine. Cytotherapy. 2018;20:479–98.
49. Kobayashi Y, Okada Y, Itakura G, Iwai H, Nishimura S, Yasuda A. Pre-evaluated safe human iPSC-derived neural stem cells promote functional recovery after spinal cord injury in common marmoset without tumorigenicity. PLoS One. 2012;7:1–12.
50. Zeitlin BD. Banking on teeth – Stem cells and the dental office. Biomed J. 2020;43:124–33.
51. Seo BM, Sonoyama W, Yamaza T, Coppe C, Kikuiri T, Akiyama K, et al. SHED repair critical-size calvarial defects in mice. Oral Dis. 2008;14:428–34.
52. Egusa H. iPS cells in dentistry. Clin Calcium. 2012;22:67–73.
53. Kerkis I, Kerkis A, Dozortsev D, Stukart-Parsons SM, Gomes Massironi GC, Pereira LV, et al. Isolation and characterization of a population of immature dental pulp stem cells expressing OCT-4 and other embryonic stem cell markers. Cells Tissues Organs. 2006;184:105–16.
54. Chai Y, Jiang X, Ito Y, Bringas P Jr, Han J, Rowitch DH, et al. Fate of the mammalian cranial neural crest during tooth and mandibular morphogenesis. Development. 2000;127:1671–9.
55. Azizi SA, Stokes D, Augelli BJ, DiGirolamo C, Prockop DJ. Engraftment and migration of human bone marrow stromal cells implanted in the brains of albino rats-similarities to astrocyte grafts. Proc Natl Acad Sci. 1998;95:3908–13.
56. Narang S, Sehgal N. Stem cells: a potential regenerative future in dentistry. Indian J Hum Genet. 2012;18:150–4.
57. Wang L, Shen H, Zheng W, Tang L, Yang Z, Gao Y, et al. Characterization of stem cells from alveolar periodontal ligament. Tissue Eng Part A. 2011;17:1015–26.
58. Hynes K, Menicanin D, Gronthos S, Bartold PM. Clinical utility of stem cells for periodontal regeneration. Periodontol 2000. 2012;59:203–27.
59. Rubio D, Garcia-Castro J, Martin MC, de la Fuente R, Cigudosa JC, Lloyd AC, et al. Spontaneous human adult stem cell transformation. Cancer Res. 2005;65:3035–9; erratum in Cancer Res 2005; 65:4969.
60. Abe S, Yamaguchi S, Amagasa T. Multilineage cells from apical pulp of human tooth with immature apex. Oral Sci Int. 2007;4:13.
61. Morsczeck C, Gotz W, Schierholz J, Zeilhofer F, Kuhn U, Mohl C, et al. Isolation of precursor cells (PCs) from human dental follicle of wisdom teeth. Matrix Biol. 2005;24:155–65.
62. Kémoun P, Laurencin-Dalicieux S, Rue J, Farges J-C, Gennero I, Conte-Auriol F, et al. Human dental follicle cells acquire cementoblast features under stimulation by BMP-2/−7 and enamel matrix derivatives (EMD) in vitro. Cell Tissue Res. 2007;329:283–94.
63. Raza SS, Wagner AP, Hussain YS, Khan MA. Mechanisms underlying dental-derived stem cell-mediated neurorestoration in neurodegenerative disorders. Stem Cell Res Ther. 2018;9:245.
64. Kaukua N, Shahidi MK, Konstantinidou C, Dyachuk V, Kaucka M, Furlan A. Glial origin of mesenchymal stem cells in a tooth model system. Nature. 2014;513:551–4.
65. Pereira LV, Bento RF, Cruz DB, Marchi C, Salomone R, Oiticicca J. Stem cells from human exfoliated deciduous teeth (SHED) differentiate in vivo and promote facial nerve regeneration. Cell Transplant. 2019;28:55–64.
66. Zhang N, Lu X, Wu S, Li X, Duan J, Chen C. Intrastriatal transplantation of stem cells

from human exfoliated deciduous teeth reduces motor defects in Parkinsonian rats. Cytotherapy. 2018;20:670–86.
67. Yamada Y, Fujimoto A, Ito A, Yoshimi R, Ueda M. Cluster analysis and gene expression profiles: a cDNA microarray system-based comparison between human dental pulp stem cells (hDPSCs) and human mesenchymal stem cells (hMSCs) for tissue engineering cell therapy. Biomaterials. 2006;27:3766–81.
68. Yamada Y, Ueda M, Hibi H, Baba S. A novel approach to periodontal tissue regeneration with mesenchymal stem cells and platelet-rich plasma using tissue engineering technology: a clinical case report. Int J Periodontics Restorative Dent. 2006;26:363–9.
69. Garant PR. Oral mucosa. In: Dickson, editor. Oral cells and tissues. Illinois: Quintessence; 2003. p. 81–122, 123–151.
70. Izumi K, Tobita T, Feinberg SE. Isolation of human oral keratinocyte progenitor/stem cells. J Dent Res. 2007;86:341–6.
71. Izumi K, Feinberg SE, Terashi H, Marcelo CL. Evaluation of transplanted tissue-engineered oral mucosa equivalents in severe combined immunodeficient mice. Tissue Eng. 2003;9:163–74.
72. Izumi K, Feinberg SE, Iida A, Yoshizawa M. Intraoral grafting of an ex vivo produced oral mucosa equivalent: a preliminary report. J Oral Maxillofac Surg. 2003;32:188–97.
73. Marynka-Kalmani K, Treves S, Yafee M, Rachima H, Gafni Y, Cohen MA, Pitaru S. The lamina propria of adult human oral mucosa harbors a novel stem cell population. Stem Cells. 2010;28:984–95.
74. Egusa H, Okita K, Kayashima H, Yu G, Fukuyasu S, Saeki M, et al. Gingival fibroblasts as a promising source of induced pluripotent stem cells. PLoS One. 2010;5:12743.
75. Duan X, Tu Q, Zhang J, Ye J, Sommer C, Mostoslavsky G, et al. Application of induced pluripotent stem (iPS) cells in periodontal tissue regeneration. J Cell Physiol. 2011;226:150–7.
76. Zhu SJ, Choi BH, Huh JY, Jung JH, Kim BY, Lee SH. A comparative qualitative histological analysis of tissue-engineered bone using bone marrow mesenchymal stem cells, alveolar bone cells, and periosteal cells. Oral Surg Oral Med Oral Pathol Oral Radiol Endod. 2006;101:164–9.
77. Cicconetti A, Sacchetti B, Bartoli A, Michienzi S, Corsi A, Funari A, et al. Human maxillary tuberosity and jaw periosteum as sources of osteoprogenitor cells for tissue engineering. Oral Surg Oral Med Oral Pathol Oral Radiol Endod. 2007;104:618–8..
78. Agata H, Asahina I, Yamazaki Y, Uchida M, Shinohara Y, Honda MJ, et al. Effective bone engineering with periosteum-derived cells. J Dent Res. 2007;86:79–83.
79. Ueno T, Honda K, Hirata A, Kagawa T, Kanou M, Shirasu N, et al. Histological comparison of bone induced from autogenously grafted periosteum with bone induced from autogenously grafted bone marrow in the rat calvarial defect model. Acta Histochem. 2008;110:217–23.
80. Soltan M, Smiler D, Soltan C. The inverted periosteal flap: a source of stem cells enhancing bone regeneration. Implant Dent. 2009;18:373–9.
81. Schmelzeisen R, Schimming R, Sittinger M. Making bone: implant insertion into tissue-engineered bone for maxillary sinus floor augmentation-a preliminary report. J Craniomaxillofac Surg. 2003;31:34–9.
82. Nagata M, Hoshina H, Li M, Arasawa M, Uematsu K, Ogawa S, et al. A clinical study of alveolar bone tissue engineering with cultured autogenous periosteal cells: coordinated activation of bone formation and resorption. Bone. 2012;50:1123–9.
83. Man YG, Ball WD, Marchetti L, Hand AR. Contributions of intercalated duct cells to the normal parenchyma of submandibular glands of adult rats. Anat Rec. 2001;263:202–14.
84. Kishi T, Takao T, Fujita K, Taniguchi H. Clonal proliferation of multipotent stem/progenitor cells in the neonatal and adult salivary glands. Biochem Biophys Res Commun. 2006;340:544–52.
85. Lombaert IM, Brunsting JF, Wierenga PK, Faber H, Stokman MA, Kok T, et al. Rescue of salivary gland function after stem cell transplantation in irradiated glands. PLoS One. 2008;3:2063.
86. Matsumoto S, Okumura K, Ogata A, Hisatomi Y, Sato A, Hattori K, et al. Isolation of tissue progenitor cells from duct-ligated salivary glands of swine. Cloning Stem Cells. 2007;9:176–90.
87. Sato A, Okumura K, Matsumoto S, Hattori K, Hattori S, Shinohara M, et al. Isolation, tissue localization, and cellular characterization of progenitors derived from adult human salivary glands. Cloning Stem Cells. 2007;9:191–205.
88. Nanduri LS, Maimets SAP, van der Zwaag M, van Os RP, Coppes RP. Regeneration of irradiated salivary glands with stem cell marker expressing cells. Radiother Oncol. 2011;99:367–72.
89. Gorjup E, Danner S, Rotter N, Habermann J, Brassat U, Brummendorf TH, et al. Glandular tissue from human pancreas and salivary gland yields similar stem cell populations. Eur J Cell Biol. 2009;88:409–21.
90. Coppes RP, Stokman MA. Stem cells and the repair of radiation-induced salivary gland damage. Oral Dis. 2011;17:143–53.
91. Kulakov AA, D.V. Clinical study of the efficiency of combined cell transplant on the basis of multipotent mesenchymal stromal adipose tissue cells in patients with pronounced deficit of the maxillary and mandibulary bone tissue. Bull Exp Biol Med. 2008;146:522–5.
92. Pieri F, Lucarelli E, Corinaldesi G, Aldini NN, Fini Parrilli A, et al. Dose-dependent effect of adipose-derived adult stem cells on vertical bone regeneration in rabbit calvarium. Biomaterials. 2010;31:3527–35.
93. Tobita M, Uysal AC, Ogawa R, Hyakusoku H, Mizuno H. Periodontal tissue regeneration with

adipose-derived stem cells. Tissue Eng Part A. 2008;14:945–53.
94. Wen X, Nie X, Zhang L, Liu L, Deng M. Adipose tissue-deprived stem cells acquire cementoblast features treated with dental follicle cell conditioned medium containing dentin non-collagenous proteins in vitro. Biochem Biophys Res Commun. 2011;409:583–9.
95. Ishizaka R, Iohara K, Murakami O, Fukuta M. Nakashima. Regeneration of dental pulp following pulpectomy by fractionated stem/progenitor cells from bone marrow and adipose tissue. Biomaterials. 2012;33:2109–18.
96. Hung CN, Mar K, Chang HC, Chiang YL, Hu HY, Lai CC, et al. A comparison between adipose tissue and dental pulp as sources of MSCs for tooth regeneration. Biomaterials. 2011;32:6995–7005.
97. Dziedzic DSM, Mogharbel BF, Irioda AC, Stricker PEF, Perussolo MC, Franco CRC, Chang H-W, Abdelwahid E, de Carvalho KAT. Adipose-derived stromal cells and mineralized extracellular matrix delivery by a human decellularized amniotic membrane in periodontal tissue engineering. Membranes (Basel). 2021;11:606.
98. Dave JR. Dental tissue-derived mesenchymal stem cells: applications in tissue engineering. Crit Rev Biomed Eng. 2018;46:429–68.
99. Vinatier C, Guicheux J, Daculsi G, Layrolle P, Weiss P. Cartilage and bone tissue engineering using hydrogels. Biomed Mater Eng. 2006;16:107–13.
100. Yu H, Yang X, Cheng J, Wang X, Shen SG. Distraction osteogenesis combined with tissue-engineered cartilage in the reconstruction of condylar osteochondral defect. J Oral Maxillofac Surg. 2011;69:558–64.
101. Holland TA, Bodde EWH, Baggett LS, Tabata Y, Mikos AG, Jansen JA. Osteochondral repair in the rabbit model utilizing bilayered, degradable oligo (poly (ethylene glycol) fumarate) hydrogel scaffolds. J Biomed Mater Res A. 2005;75:156–67.
102. Jazayeri HE, Lee S-M, Kuhn L, Fahimipour F, Tahriri M, Tayebi L. Polymeric scaffolds for dental pulp tissue engineering: a review. Dent Mater. 2020;36:47–58.
103. Cordeiro MM, Dong Z, Kaneko T, Zhang Z, Miyazawa M, Shi S. Dental pulp tissue engineering with stem cells from exfoliated deciduous teeth. J Endod Dent Pulp Tissue Eng Stem Cells Exfoliated Deciduous Teeth. 2008;34:962–9.
104. Huang GT. A paradigm shift in endodontic management of immature teeth: conservation of stem cells for regeneration. J Dent. 2008;36:379–86.
105. Arakaki M, Ishikawa M, Nakamura T, Iwamoto T, Yamada A, Fukumoto E, et al. Role of epithelial-stem cell interactions during dental cell differentiation. J Biol Chem. 2012;287:10590–601.
106. Otsu K, Kishigami R, Oikawa-Sasaki A, Fukumoto S, Yamada A, Fujiwara N, et al. Differentiation of induced pluripotent stem cells into dental mesenchymal cells. Stem Cells Dev. 2011;21:1156–64.
107. Crespi R, Vinci R, Cappare P, Gherlone E, Romanos GE. Calvarial versus iliac crest for autologous bone graft material for a sinus lift procedure: a histomorphometric study. Int J Oral Maxillofac Implants. 2007;22:527–32.
108. Huang GT, Sonoyama W, Liu Y, Liu H, Wang S, Shi S. The hidden treasure in apical papilla: the potential role in pulp/dentin regeneration and bioroot engineering. J Endod. 2008;34:645–5.
109. Koki Yoshida, Jun Sato, Rie Takai, Osamu Uehara, Yoshihito Kurashige, Michiko Nishimura et al. Differentiation of mouse iPS cells into ameloblast-like cells in cultures using medium conditioned by epithelial cell rests of Malassez and gelatincoated dishes. Med Mol Morphol. 2015;48:138–45.
110. Dixin Cui, Hongyu Li, Mian Wan, Yiran Peng, Xin Xu, Xuedong Zhou, Liwei Zheng. The origin and identification of mesenchymal stem cells in teeth: from odontogenic to non-odontogenic. Curr Stem Cell Res Ther. 2018;13:39–45.
111. Chung IH, Yamaza T, Zhao H, Choung PH, Shi S, Chai Y. Stem cell property of postmigratory cranial neural crest cells and their utility in alveolar bone regeneration and tooth development. Stem Cells. 2009;27:866–77.
112. Akintoye SO, Lam T, Shi S, Brahim J, Collins MT, Robey PG. Skeletal site-specific characterization of orofacial and iliac crest human bone marrow stromal cells in same individuals. Bone. 2006;38:758–68.
113. Han J, Okada H, Takai H, Nakayama Y, Maeda T, Ogata Y. Collection and culture of alveolar bone marrow multipotent mesenchymal stromal cells from older individuals. J Cell Biochem. 2009;107:1198–204.
114. Mueller SM, Glowacki J. Age-related decline in the osteogenic potential of human bone marrow cells cultured in three-dimensional collagen sponges. J Cell Biochem. 2001;82:583–90.
115. Mendes SC, Tibbe JM, Veenhof M, Bakker K, Both S, Platenburg PP, et al. Bone tissue-engineered implants using human bone marrow stromal cells: effect of culture conditions and donor age. Tissue Eng. 2002;8:911–20.
116. Ikeda E, Morita R, Nakao K, Ishida K, Nakamura T, Takano-Yamamoto T, et al. Fully functional bioengineered tooth replacement as an organ replacement therapy. Proc Natl Acad Sci. 2009;106:13475–80.
117. Tamaoki N, Takahashi K, Tanaka T, Ichisaka T, Aoki H, Takeda-Kawaguchi T, et al. Dental pulp cells for induced pluripotent stem cell banking. J Dent Res. 2010;89:773–8.
118. Tomar GB, Srivastava RK, Gupta N, Barhanpurkar AP, Pote ST, Jhaveri HM, et al. Human gingiva-derived mesenchymal stem cells are superior to bone marrow-derived mesenchymal stem cells for cell therapy in regenerative medicine. Biochem Biophys Res Commun. 2010;393:377–83.
119. Kaku M, Kamada H, Kawata T, Koseki H, Abedini S, Kojima S. Cryopreservation of periodontal ligament cells with magnetic field for tooth banking. Cryobiology. 2010;61:73–8.

120. Nakamura S, Yamada Y, Katagiri W, Sugito T, Ito K, Ueda M. Stem cell proliferation pathways comparison between human exfoliated deciduous teeth and dental pulp stem cells by gene expression profile from promising dental pulp. J Endod. 2009;35:1536–42.
121. Karaoz E, Demircan PC, Saglam O, Aksoy A, Kaymaz F, Duruksu G. Human dental pulp stem cells demonstrate better neural and epithelial stem cell properties than bone marrow-derived mesenchymal stem cells. Histochem Cell Biol. 2011;136:455–73.
122. Kaukua N, Chen M, Guarnieri P, Dahl M, Lim ML, Yucel-Lindberg T. Molecular differences between stromal cell populations from deciduous and permanent human teeth. Stem Cell Res Ther. 2015;6:59.
123. Majumdar D, Kanafi M, Bhonde R, Gupta P, Datta I. Differential neuronal plasticity of dental pulp stem cells from exfoliated deciduous and permanent teeth towards dopaminergic neurons. J Cell Physiol. 2016;231:2048–63.
124. Werle SB, Lindemann D, Steffens D, Demarco FF, de Araujo FB, Pranke P. Carious deciduous teeth are a potential source for dental pulp stem cells. Clin Oral Invest. 2016;20:75–81.
125. Tsai AI, Hong HH, Lin WR, Fu JF, Chang CC, Wang IK. Isolation of mesenchymal stem cells from human deciduous teeth pulp. Biomed Res Int. 2017;3:1–9.
126. Pereira LO, Rubini MR, Silva JR, Oliveira DM, Silva IC, Pocas-Fonseca MJ. Comparison of stem cell properties of cells isolated from normal and inflamed dental pulps. Int Endod J. 2012;45:1080–90.
127. Wang G, Wang C, Qin M. A retrospective study of survival of 196 replanted permanent teeth in children. Dent Traumatol. 2019;35:251–8.
128. Krasner P. Treatment of avulsed teeth by oral and maxillofacial surgeons. J Oral Maxillofac Surg. 2010;68:2888–92.
129. Adnan S, Lone MM, Khan FR, Hussain SM, Nagi SE. Which is the most recommended medium for the storage and transport of avulsed teeth? A systematic review. Dent Traumatol. 2018;34:59–70.
130. Moazami F, Mirhadi H, Geramizadeh B, Sahebi S. Comparison of soymilk, powdered milk, Hank's balanced salt solution and tap water on periodontal ligament cell survival. Dent Traumatol. 2012;28:132–5.
131. Andersson L, Andreasen JO, Day P, Heithersay G, Trope M, Diangelis AJ. International Association of Dental Traumatology guidelines for the management of traumatic dental injuries: 2. Avulsion of permanent teeth. Dent Traumatol. 2012;28:88–96.
132. Chen FB, Qi SC, Yang QX, Zhang X, Xu YZ, Wang RR. Effect of temperature and six storage media on human dental pulp cells. Acta Med Mediterr. 2019;35:461–6.
133. Courts FJ, Mueller WA, Tabeling HJ. Milk as an interim storage medium for avulsed teeth. Pediatr Dent. 1983;5:183–6.
134. Hasan MR, Takebe H, Shalehin N, Obara N, Saito T, Irie K. Effects of tooth storage media on periodontal ligament preservation. Dent Traumatol. 2017;33:383–92.
135. Sottovia AD, Sottovia D, Poi WR, Panzarini SR, Luize DS, Sonoda CK. Tooth replantation after use of euro-coffins solution or bovine milk as storage medium: a histomorphometric analysis in dogs. J Oral Maxillofac Surg. 2010;68:111–9.
136. Hwang JY, Choi SC, Park JH, Kang SW. The use of green tea extract as a storage medium for the avulsed tooth. J Endod. 2011;37:962–7.
137. Martins CM, Hamanaka EF, Hoshida TY, Sell AM, Hidalgo MM, Silveira CS. Dragon's blood sap (Croton Lechleri) as storage medium for avulsed teeth: in vitro study of cell viability. Braz Dent J. 2016;27:751–6.
138. Ozan F, Polat ZA, Er K, Ozan U, Deger O. Effect of propolis on survival of periodontal ligament cells: new storage media for avulsed teeth. J Endod. 2007;33:570–3.
139. Babaji P, Melkundi M, Devanna R, Suresh SB, Chaurasia VR, Gopinath PV. In vitro comparative evaluation of different storage media (hank's balanced salt solution, propolis, Aloe vera, and pomegranate juice) for preservation of avulsed tooth. Eur J Dermatol. 2017;11:71–5.
140. Sinpreechanon P, Boonzong U, Sricholpech M. Comparative evaluation of periodontal ligament fibroblasts stored in different types of milk: effects on viability and biosynthesis of collagen. Eur J Oral Sci. 2019;127:323–32.
141. Souza BD, Luckemeyer DD, Felippe WT, Simoes CM, Felippe MC. Effect of temperature and storage media on human periodontal ligament fibroblast viability. Dent Traumatol. 2010;26:271–5.
142. Piva E, Susan AT, Jacques EN, Zou D, Hatfield E, Guinn T. Dental pulp tissue regeneration using dental pulp stem cells isolated and expanded in human serum. J Endod Dent Pulp Tiss Regen Using Dental Pulp Stem Cells Isolated Expand Hum Serum. 2017;43:568–74.
143. Suchanek J, Kleplova TS, Rehacek V, Browne KZ, Soukup T. Proliferative capacity and phenotypical alteration of multipotent ecto-mesenchymal stem cells from human exfoliated deciduous teeth cultured in xenogeneic and allogeneic media. Folia Biol-Prague. 2016;62:1–14.
144. Nowwarote N, Pavasant P, Osathanon T. Role of endogenous basic fibroblast growth factor in stem cells isolated from human exfoliated deciduous teeth. Archives Oral Biol Role Endogenous Basic Fibroblast Growth Factor Stem Cells Isolated Hum Exfoliated Deciduous Teeth. 2015;60:408–15.
145. Adan A, Alizada G, Kiraz Y, Baran Y, Nalbant A. Flow cytometry: basic principles and applications. Crit Rev Biotechnol. 2017;37:163–76.
146. Woods EJ, Perry BC, Hockema JJ, Larson L, Zhou D, Goebel WS. Optimized cryopreservation method for human dental pulp-derived stem cells and their tissues of origin for banking and clinical use. Cryobiology. 2009;59:150–7.

147. Sunil PM, Manikandan R, Muthumurugan TRY, Sivakumar M. Harvesting dental stem cells – overview. J Pharm Bioallied Sci. 2015;7:S384–6.
148. Lee HS, Jeon M, Kim SO, Kim SH, Lee JH, Ahn SJ. Characteristics of stem cells from human exfoliated deciduous teeth (SHED) from intact cryopreserved deciduous teeth. Cryobiology. 2015;71:374–83.
149. Gioventu S, Andriolo G, Bonino F, Frasca S, Lazzari L, Montelatici E. A novel method for banking dental pulp stem cells. Transfus Apher Sci. 2012;47:199–206.
150. Huynh NCN, Le SH, Doan VN, Ngo LTQ, Tran HLB. Simplified conditions for storing and cryopreservation of dental pulp stem cells. Arch Oral Biol. 2017;84:74–81.
151. Ma L, Makino Y, Yamaza H, Akiyama K, Hoshino Y, Song G. Cryopreserved dental pulp tissues of exfoliated deciduous teeth are a feasible stem cell resource for regenerative medicine. PLoS One. 2012;7–13.
152. Lizier NF, Kerkis A, Gomes CM, Hebling J, Oliveira CF, Caplan AI. Scaling-up of dental pulp stem cells isolated from multiple niches. PLoS One. 2012;7:1–12
153. Eastell R, Walsh JS. Anabolic treatment for osteoporosis: teriparatide. Clin Cases Miner Bone Metab. 2017;14:173.
154. Scalize PH, de Sousa LG, Regalo SC, Semprini M, Pitol DL, da Silva GA, de Almeida CJ, Coppi AA, Laad AA, Prado KF, Siessere S. Low-level laser therapy improves bone formation: stereology findings for osteoporosis in rat model. Lasers Med Sci. 2015;30:1599–607.
155. Bossini PS, Rennó AC, Ribeiro DA, Fangel R, Ribeiro AC, Lahoz Mde A, Parizotto NA. Low level laser therapy (830 nm) improves bone repair in osteoporotic rats: similar outcomes at two different dosages. Exp Gerontol. 2012;47:136–42.
156. Torstrick FB, Guldberg RE. Local strategies to prevent and treat osteoporosis. Curr Osteoporos Rep. 2014;12:33–40.
157. Fallahnezhad S, Piryaei A, Darbandi H, Amini A, Ghoreishi SK, Jalalifirouzkouhi R, Bayat M. Effect of low-level laser therapy and oxytocin on osteoporotic bone marrow-derived mesenchymal stem cells. J Cell Biochem. 2018;119:983–97.
158. Matsumoto MA, Ferino RV, Monteleone GF, Ribeiro DA. Low-level laser therapy modulates cyclo-oxygenase-2 expression during bone repair in rats. Lasers Med Sci. 2009;24:195–201.
159. Suzuki SS, Garcez AS, Reese PO, Suzuki H, Ribeiro MS, Moon W. Effects of corticopuncture (CP) and low-level laser therapy (LLLT) on the rate of tooth movement and root resorption in rats using micro-CT evaluation. Lasers Med Sci. 2018;33:811–21.
160. Xia B, Yang Z, Xu Z, Yonggang LV. Gene expression profiling analysis of the effects of low-intensity pulsed ultrasound on induced pluripotent stem cell-derived neural crest stem cells. Biotechnol Appl Biochem. 2017;64:927–37.
161. El-Bialy T, Farouk K, Carlyle TD, Wiltshire W, Drummond R, Dumore T, Knowlton K, Tompson B. Effect of low intensity pulsed ultrasound (LIPUS) on tooth movement and root resorption: a prospective multi-center randomized controlled trial. J Clin Med. 2020;9:804.
162. Kaur H, El-Bialy T. Shortening of overall orthodontic treatment duration with low-intensity pulsed ultrasound (LIPUS). J Clin Med. 2020;9:1303.
163. Lou S, Lv H, Li Z, Tang P, Wang Y. Effect of low-intensity pulsed ultrasound on distraction osteogenesis: a systematic review and meta-analysis of randomized controlled trials. J Orthop Surg Res. 2018;13:205.
164. Inubushi T, Tanaka E, Rego EB. Effects of ultrasound on the proliferation and differentiation of cementoblast lineage cells. J Periodontol. 2008;79:1984–90.
165. Li H, Zhou J, Zhu M, Ying S, Li L, Chen D, Li J, Song J. Low-intensity pulsed ultrasound promotes the formation of periodontal ligament stem cell sheets and ectopic periodontal tissue regeneration. J Biomed Mater Res A. 2021;109:1101–12.

Part V

Musculoskeletal Ultrasound in Regenerative Medicine

14 Regenerative Medicine Procedures Under Ultrasound Guidance

Jeimylo C. de Castro

Introduction

Regenerative injection therapy is an evolving interventional treatment that provides alternative solutions for different musculoskeletal conditions. Recent advances in research and scientific knowledge regarding regenerative therapies for neuromusculoskeletal conditions have evolved from a mere alternative therapy to a more specific treatment of musculoskeletal conditions. In fact, the surge in research on regenerative medicine have shown the varied interest of different specialties on the potential of this treatment. The gap between conservative and surgical options has been bridged with the advent of this technology, allowing physicians to postpone an operative procedure in favor of this intervention with some operative procedures incorporating the use of regenerative therapies either to shorten the time of recovery or return to play especially for some elite athletes. Although this treatment modality has been challenged by some physicians and accepted by others, the amount of progress in the development of new approaches in the preparation, isolation, administration of regenerative products, and the understanding of its biologic mechanisms and molecular components shift the momentum in favor of its use as a modern tool for treating different musculoskeletal injuries. The lack of long-term efficacy of existing therapies also contributes to why there is an increasing interest in its use. In addition, patients and healthcare providers alike raise a common concern about the safety of oral medications for prolonged use in the presence of comorbidities. Thus, regenerative therapies, being an autologous source have the potential of providing the needed answer to these concerns with an added advantage of minimal safety issues, ease of administration and less immune reactions. Additionally, the advent of musculoskeletal ultrasound complements the procedure by its portability and dynamic feature. A better view of the target site makes it a point of care modality assuring both patients and physicians that the intended injection site with the regenerative solutions are precisely delivered. it also ensures that no vital structures were affected during the injection procedure. While it is true that regenerative injection therapy is a modern intervention used in addressing musculoskeletal conditions, the use of ultrasound is a much needed tool to ensure that the solution is delivered appropriately.

J. C. de Castro (✉)
Chair, Physical Medicine and Rehabilitation Department, The Medical City-South Luzon, Sta. Rosa, Laguna, Philippines

Medical Director/CEO, SMARTMD Center for Non-Surgical Pain Interventions, Makati City, Philippines

Y. El Miedany (ed.), *Musculoskeletal Ultrasound-Guided Regenerative Medicine*,
https://doi.org/10.1007/978-3-030-98256-0_14

General Guidelines for Regenerative Intervention

Just like any procedure, it is always important to provide safety procedures in the process of preparing patients for the treatment procedure. Be it platelet-rich plasma (PRP), bone marrow concentrate (BMC), or lipoaspirate (LA), the value of skill and safety cannot be overemphasized. Although each of these procedures has its unique harvesting technique, it is important to be familiar with these techniques and ensure that patients are oriented as to the process of harvesting, the amount of time needed for the procedure, and where exactly it will be injected and how it will be injected. This information, therefore, sets the expectation of patients before the actual procedure is done. Several studies confirmed the accuracy and superiority of ultrasound-guided procedures over palpation-guided procedures in any part of the musculoskeletal system [1–4], although some would also use and prefer fluoroscopy [5] in doing procedures. Thus, to enhance safety and accuracy, I would like to suggest that imaging must be done in any of these procedures [6].

Platelet-Rich Plasma (PRP)

The use of platelet-rich plasma (PRP) in the musculoskeletal system could be traced back to the 1990s when Marx et al. initially demonstrated an improved density of mandibular defects with PRP-enhanced autografts versus autografts alone and has since stimulated other practitioners to investigate its potential effects in driving an effective and faster healing process [7]. Anitua demonstrated the application of PRP in dental procedures to enhance bone regeneration in future sites of tooth extraction site implants [8]. In sports medicine, Mishra and Pavelko recognized the value of PRP in chronic lateral elbow tendinosis [9]. Since then, the use of PRP was expanded to include other musculoskeletal injuries [10, 11].

PRP is an autologous plasma enriched with platelet and growth factors with varying concentrations of 2.5 to 3× to about 5× to 7× (about 1.5 million/μL) baseline from what is normally found in the whole blood [12, 13, 16]. It is basically prepared by centrifuging autologous, anticoagulated whole blood to separate its plasma components based on their densities and to concentrate platelets above their baseline levels [10, 11, 13]. Depending on the systems used, the protocols may include one or two-steps centrifugation to separate the different layers of the whole blood, based on their sedimentation rates [14]. The effectivity of PRP depends on the number of growth factors and cytokines released from the alpha granules of platelets and the accuracy of the injection sites, whether it be tendons, joints, muscles, nerves, or any part of the musculoskeletal system, thus providing a regenerative stimulus to augment healing and repair in the target tissues [9, 10, 15–17]. Thus, the "ideal" PRP concentration depends on various factors like the type of tissues being treated and the stage of the disease (Fig. 14.1).

The potential of PRP to enhance healing is due to the presence of growth factors and cytokines. The basic cytokines include insulin-like growth factor-1 (IGF-1), transforming growth factor β (TGFβ), platelet-derived growth factor (PDGF), fibroblast growth factor (FGF), epidermal growth factor (EGF), and vascular endothelial growth factor (VEGF) [18, 19]. In vitro studies have shown that 1.5×10^6 platelets/μL (5× to 7× baseline) was optimal in promoting human umbilical vein endothelial cell proliferation, motility, and morphology with greater or lower concentration causing lower angiogenic potential [17]. Depending on which tissues to treat, the concentration of platelets has been observed to vary in its effectivity. For instance, in vitro platelet preparation containing 0.494×10^6 platelet/μL can induce hyaluronic acid secretion in the joints among osteoarthritic patients [20]. No benefit however was observed in rotator cuff tears when the platelet concentration is greater than 2.0×10^6 platelets/μL [21].

Leukocytes play a major role in the inflammatory process where growth factors from the platelets during the initial stage of healing attract and activate neutrophils and macrophages to the site of injury. Thus, it may contribute to the pro-inflammatory effects in the tissues once it is

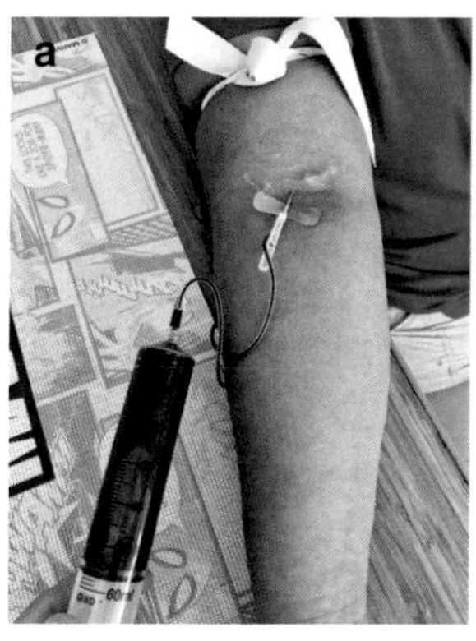
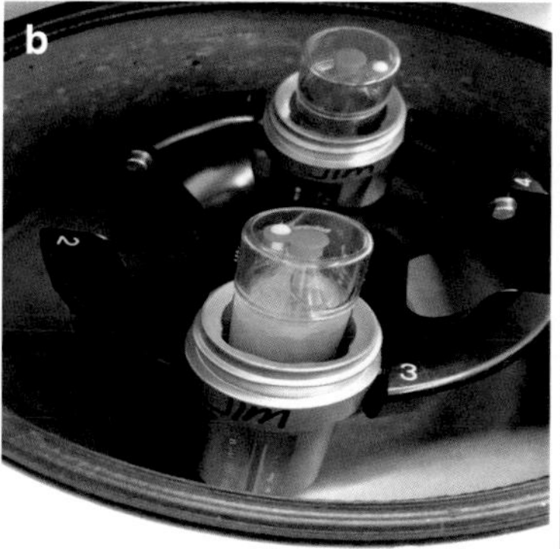
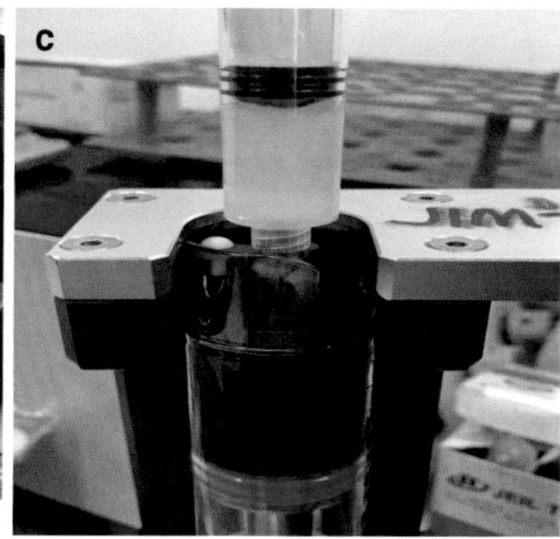

Fig. 14.1 Preparing a PRP solution. (**a**) Extracting 60 cc of anticoagulated peripheral venous blood. (**b**) Using a swing-out centrifuge to separate the cellular components from plasma, 3800 rpm. (**c**) Platelet-poor plasma is extracted initially from the topmost layer, and then the lower layer of plasma is the platelet-rich plasma

injected. Braun et al. have shown that a leukocyte-rich PRP (LR-PRP) with red blood cells (RBC) formulations administered intra-articularly resulted in cell death in the synovium and pro-inflammatory mediator production [22]. Consequently, there is a significant increase in other pro-inflammatory mediators such as interleukin-1β (IL-1β), interleukin-6 (IL-6), interferon-λ (IFN-λ), tumor necrosis factor-α (TNF-α), and greater matrix metalloproteinases (MMP-9), which lead to cartilage degeneration in the joints [19, 22]. By releasing anti-inflammatory mediators, namely IL-4 and IL-10, leukocyte-poor PRP and RBC-free formulations may be considered when injecting intra-articularly and thus may be ideal for joint pathologies [22]. LR-PRP, however, may be beneficial to tendinopathies [23]. Furthermore, Mirosnychenko et al. showed in their studies that non-neutrophil-containing PRP or platelet-poor plasma (PPP), after an additional spin to remove platelets, stimulates myoblast differentiation, which is important in skeletal muscle regeneration [24]. Intentionally slowing and shortening the spin regimens when processing PRP can result in lowering and excluding of the leukocytes. Subsequently, the reverse is true when producing a higher concentration of leukocytes and red blood cells [15, 22].

On a similar note, red blood cells in PRP have a negative effect on chondrocytes with hemarthrosis from either traumatic knee injuries or hemophilia and consequently may result in a higher incidence of arthritis [25, 26].

With varied methods used in the preparation of PRP come different classification systems. This comes because of diligent research and while this technology is still evolving there will always be change that will take place over the years. Part of standardizing the practices for PRP is the proposed classification system to enable practitioners to identify what type of method to follow. The classification systems have been proposed to improve practices and clinical results. In 2012, DeLong et al. proposed the PAW (Platelet-Activation-White Blood Cell) Classification System [27]. This classification is based on three variables namely the absolute number of platelets, the manner of platelet activation, and the presence or absence of leukocytes or white blood cells [27].

The PLRA System proposed by Mautner et al. (Fig. 14.2) includes four variables which include platelet count, leukocyte content, red blood cell content, and whether it is exogenously activated or not [28]. In 2017, Lana et al. proposed another classification called MARSPILL which include additional variables including the harvest method, activation, red blood cells, number of spins, image guidance, leukocyte number, and the use of light activation [29] (Fig. 14.3). Interestingly, the function of monocytes and all their plasticity which is a potential property for regeneration of tissue are discussed in this classification system [29]. Other PRP classification includes the

PLRA Classification			
		Criteria	Final Score
P	Platelet count	______ P	______ M
		Volume injected	Cells/μL
L	Leucocyte count*	>1%	+
		<1%	–
R	Red blood cell content	>1%	+
		<1%	–
A	Activation[+]	Yes	+
		No	–

Table created by Drs. Patrick Nguyen and Walter Sussman
* If white blood cells are present (+), the percentage of neutrophils should also be reported.
[+]The method of exogenous activation should be reported.

Fig. 14.2 PLRA classification. (Used with permission from Dr. Kenneth Mautner; Source: Mautner et al [28])

MARSPILL Classification		
Letter	**Relates to**	**Type**
M	Method	Handmade (H) Machine (M)
A	Activation	Activated (A+) Not activated (A-)
R	Red blood cells	Rich (RBC-R) Poor (RBC -P)
S	Spin	One spin (Sp1) Two spins (Sp2)
P	Platelet number (folds basal)	PL 2-3 PL 6-8 PL 4-6 PL 8-10
I	Image guided	Guided (G+) Not guided (G-)
L	Leukocyte concentration.	Rich (Lc-R) Poor (Lc-P)
L	Light activation.	Activated(A+) Not activated (A-)

Lc: leucocyte concentration; PL: platelet concentration; RBC: red blood cell

Fig. 14.3 MARSPILL classification. (Used with permission from Dr. Joseph Purita; Source: Lana et al. [29])

Mishra Classification [11] and Dohan Ehrenfest Classification [30].

Preparation Methods for PRP

It is very important that patients are properly instructed about the pre-procedure preparation, the procedure itself, and to orient them as to the level of expectation during the early stage of healing after the procedure.

During the pre-procedure instruction, patients must avoid any intake of non-steroidal anti-inflammatory medications (NSAIDs) for at least 2 weeks prior to the procedure. NSAIDs are known to inhibit the prostaglandin pathway and thus reduce the release of growth factors [31]. The use of blood thinners must be noted, and it is prudent to obtain an International Normalized Ratio (INR) to ensure that values are within normal therapeutic levels. Patients with bleeding tendencies and those with neoplastic findings need to get medical clearance from their physicians before undergoing this procedure.

In the beginning, a venipuncture is performed from the patients usually at the brachial area of the arm. To ensure easy blood extraction, especially for obese patients, an ultrasound-guided extraction is suggested. Depending on what system is used or the number of sites to be injected, blood extraction volume can vary from 20 cc to about 120 cc. Different systems come with their unique packaging kits. Some kits have pre-filled anticoagulants in their tubes. Others have separate anticoagulants and must be filled into their respective tubes. The anticoagulant solution in many prefabricated PRP kits that are commonly used is acid citrate dextrose (ACD), sodium citrate (SC), or ethylenediaminetetraacetic acid (EDTA). These different anticoagulants may affect the normal physiologic tissue pH, platelet count, and growth factor content [32]. The use of EDTA resulted in higher platelet yield in whole blood. However, it induced an increase in the mean platelet volume (MPV) when centrifuging for PRP purposes. EDTA had the lowest overall growth factor release and can damage the platelet membrane [32]. When using SC, PRP obtained a higher platelet recovery at 81% during the first centrifugation step as compared to EDTA (76%). SC also showed the highest TGF release and is suggested by the authors to be the preferred anticoagulant for PRP purposes. ACD however showed the highest VEGF concentration [32].

PRP is processed by means of differential centrifugation using a swing-out centrifuge rotor instead of the fixed angle rotor [33]. The acceleration force is adjusted to sediment certain cellular constituents based on their respective specific gravity [32]. There are two methods of preparing PRP: the PRP method and the buffy-coat method. The PRP method is a dual-spin centrifugation (soft spin) procedure, where the first spin separates the plasma from the red blood cells followed by a second spin where the platelet is concentrated. During the first spin, three layers will be seen: the topmost layer which contains mostly platelets and leukocytes, an intermediate layer known as the buffy coat which is rich in leukocytes, and the bottom layer which is mostly made up of red blood cells. A leukocyte-rich PRP is obtained by extracting the topmost and intermediate layers and a second spin is performed. Once the second spin is done, about two-thirds of the upper layer are removed, which in this case is mostly made up of platelet-poor plasma (PPP), and the lower third is extracted without getting the red blood cell that sticks at the bottom of the tube and is homogenized to obtain a PRP [33]. In the second method, otherwise called the buffy coat, whole blood collected is centrifuged (high spin) at a high speed. Similarly, the three layers of platelet-poor plasma (uppermost) and the middle (buffet coat layer) and the bottom (red blood cell) layers can be seen. The uppermost portion is removed up to the level just above the buffy coat. And then the buffy coat is collected and transferred to another sterile tube. Leukocytes can be separated from the buffy coat using a leukocyte filtration filter or centrifuge at a low speed. This method obtains a high concentration of leukocytes [33]. Platelet activation can be done by using either calcium chloride or thrombin. This is referred to as exogenous activation. Thus, there is prompt release of 70–95% growth factors for about 10 minutes [10, 11]. In endogenous activation, the collagen in the tissue where it is injected activates the release of growth factors through exposure [11, 33]. Whatever system is preferred, despite their variations, the generic sequence of blood collection, centrifugation (single- or dual spin), and activation is followed prior to the injection proper [33].

Injection Procedure of PRP

Once the PRP solution is ready, it is important to identify the specific location of the approach on the patient so that patient can be positioned in such a way that will be convenient for both the patient and the physician doing the procedure. Ideally, but not obligatory, the line of needle approach together with the position of the ultrasound monitor should be in one place where the physician is at one end and the ultrasound machine on the direct opposite end with the target on the patient at the middle, for as long as it is ergonomically advantageous for both patient and physician.

Ultrasound scanning and ultrasound-guided injection (Fig. 14.4) allow the physician to see and identify specific structures for injection with improved accuracy [4]. Pre-scanning of the area or regions to be injected prior to injection must be performed. This allows the physician to plan their approach as to whether to perform an in-plane or out-of-plane approach and for uneven surfaces a stand-off approach. It is also important to determine what type of transducer to use, the length and size of the needle, and its trajectory during the procedure. The use of Doppler will also help avoid neurovascular structures along the needle path but at the same time provide you with information about the existence of an inflammatory process [34] (Fig. 14.5).

A sterile movable table can be used to secure the PRP solution, alcohol-based chlorhexidine solution [35], needles, syringes, sterile gloves, masks, sterile anesthetic ultrasound gel, and local anesthetics and must be in proximity with the physician during the procedure. Ensure that consent forms are properly read and signed by the patient.

Draw up all the necessary medications needed for the procedure including the PRP solution and local anesthetics. Determine appropriate ultrasound probes to be used and ensure to maintain sterile technique during the procedure. A sterile

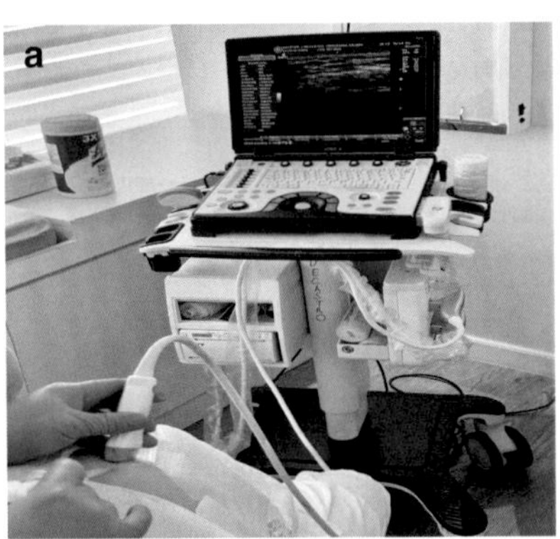

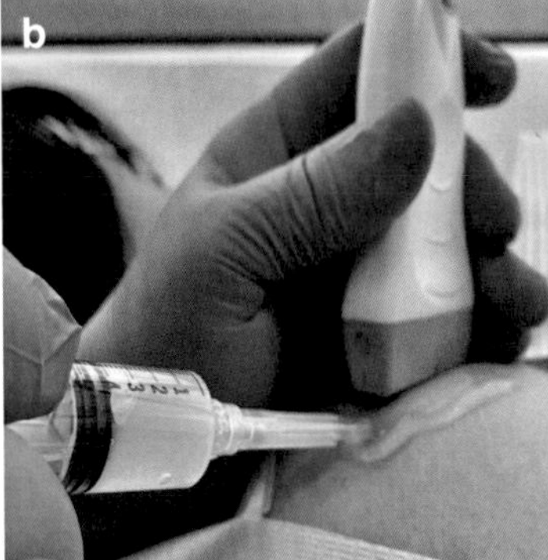

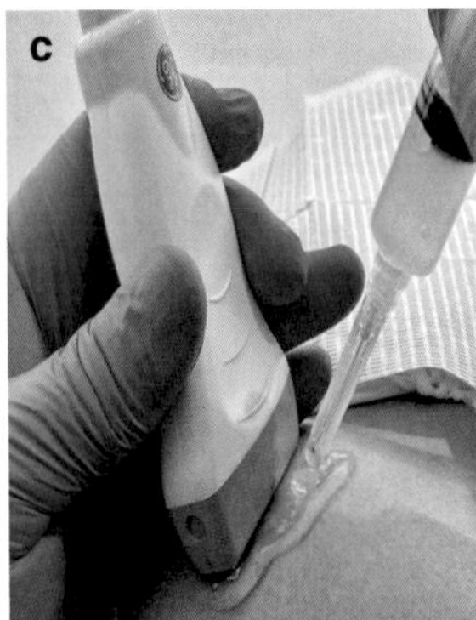

Fig. 14.4 Ultrasound-guided PRP injection. (**a**) Ultrasound-guided PRP injection allows every physician to plan his approach during an injection. (**b**) An in-plane approach will ensure easy visualization of the target, the needle, and the track of the needle. (**c**) The out-of-plane approach uses the walk-down method toward the target

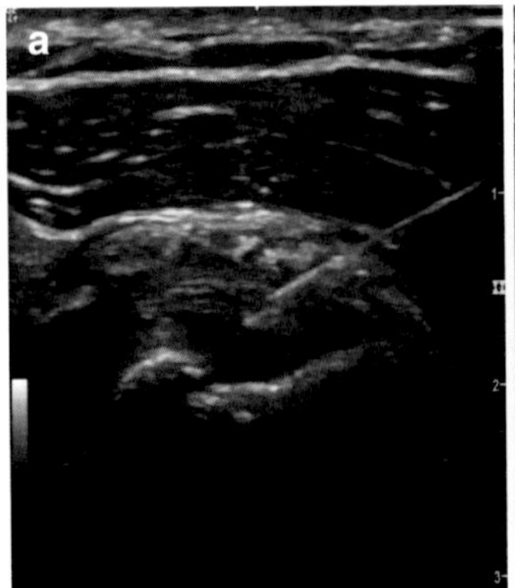

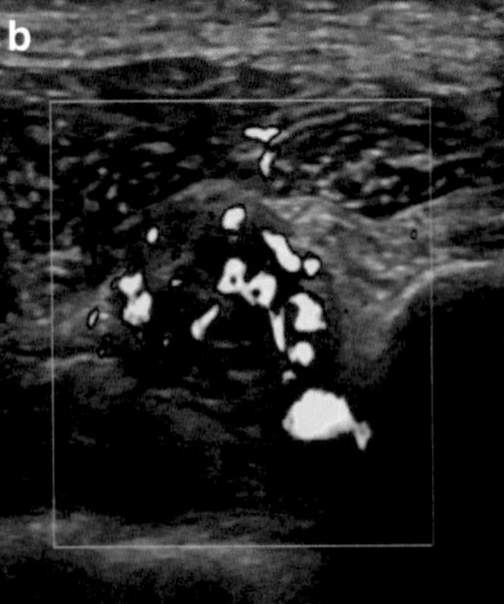

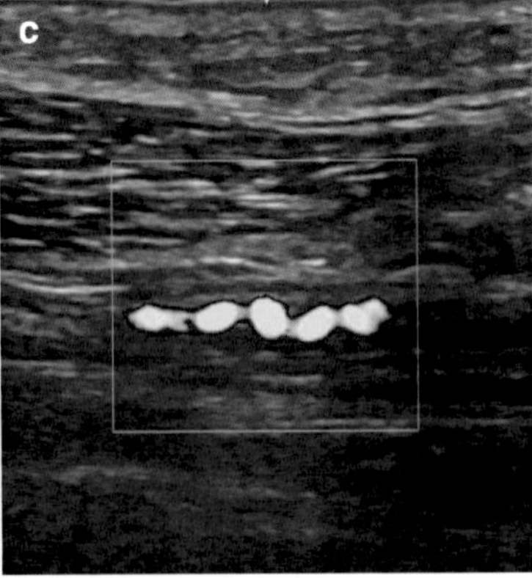

Fig. 14.5 Ultrasound images of the (**a**) in-plane approach during an injection procedure. An out-of-plane image simply shows a dot in the ultrasound image. (**b**) Power Doppler is a very useful feature in ultrasound to visualize the degree of inflammation in short-axis view (SAX). (**c**) Long-axis view of the image with power Doppler

condom cover for the ultrasound probe is an excellent way for making sure that a sterile interface during the procedure is assured [36, 37]. Skin preparations using alcohol-based chlorhexidine must be used and a sterile drape on top of the area to be injected [35] be placed.

Bone Marrow Aspirate Concentrate (BMAC)

Bone marrow aspirate concentrate (BMAC) is another method of regenerative injection therapy procedure (Fig. 14.6). Bone marrow has long been used as a primitive cell source for fracture healing and bone grafting dating back to the 1800s [38]. It is a major source of two major progenitor and adult stem cells namely mesenchymal stem cells (MSCs) and hematopoietic stem cells (HSCs) [39]. IN 1960, MSCs were discovered in the marrow through fibroblastic colony-forming unit (CFU-F) assays [40] and can differentiate into multiple different musculoskeletal lineages (multipotent) in vitro and regenerate bone in vivo (not multipotent) [39]. Over time as we age, however, the MSCs' proliferative capacity and telomere length are diminished [41]. Conversely, hematopoietic stem cells (HSC) are characterized by their positive expression of surface marker CD34+ (cluster of differentiation) which can differentiate into their respective blood cell types. HSCs were first identified in the 1980s although bone marrow transplantation began around the 1950s primarily for patients suffering from the effects of radiation and chemotherapy [42–44]. In contrast to MSCs, HSCs have been considered exempt from the aging process, although extensive studies in cycling kinetics [45], ontogeny-related studies [46], and ex vivo expansion trials [47] strongly suggest a certain

ACH Classification:		
Letter	**Relates to**	**Classification**
A	BMA	1 – Collection and injection
		2 – Description of harvesting
		3 – Cell count
		4 – Dosage of cytokines (GF and/or IL)
		5 – CFU
		6 – MSC and HSC phenotyping
		7 – Differentiation evaluation
		8 – Functional assays
C	BMAC	1 – Collection and injection
		2 – Description and harvesting
		3 – Cell count
		4 – Dosage of cytokines (GF and/or IL)
		6 – HSC and/or MSC phenotyping
		7 – Differentiation evaluation
		8 – Functional assays
H	BMA + BMAC used together	1 – collection and injection
		2 – Description of harvesting
		3 – Cell count
		4 – Dosage of cytokines (GF and/or IL)
		5 – CFU
		6 – HSC and/or MSC phenotyping
		7 – Differentiation evaluation
		8 – Functional assays

Fig. 14.6 The ACH classification. BMA Bone marrow aspirate, BMAC bone marrow aspirate concentrate, CFU colony-forming unit, MSC mesenchymal stem cell, HSC hematopoietic stem cell, A aspirate, C concentrated, H hybrid. (Source: Purita et al. [398])

degree of aging in the most primitive stem cell population. The HSC pool dynamics could be affected by programmed cell death within the HSC population and HSC pool size might be feedback regulated [48]. In the bone marrow aspirate, around 0.001–0.01% of all nucleated cells are MSCs and 0.01–1% are HSCs characterized by CFU-F and CD34+ expression, respectively [39, 49]. While HSCs may be available in the bloodstream by means of activation during a bone injury, transplantation, and stimulation with drugs like GCSF (granulocyte colony-stimulating factor), MSCs are not inherently available in the bloodstream. Thus, when a BMAC is delivered on the site of injury, direct cellular therapy is performed [39].

It was Arnold Caplan in 1991 who popularized and coined "mesenchymal stem cells" to refer to the spindle-shaped plastic-adherent cells isolated from bone marrow, adipose, and other tissue sources such as pericytes on the outside of blood vessels with multipotent capacity in vitro [49–51]. It is characterized in the literature in the 1950s and isolated later by Friedenstein et al. [52]. in 1970. Despite Caplan's proposal that these cells can differentiate into bone, cartilage, tendon, ligament, marrow stroma, adipocytes, dermis, muscle, and connective tissue [50], convincing data to support "stemness" of these cells were not forthcoming and isolated MSCs are not the homogeneous population of stem cells, although a bona fide stem cell may reside within the adherent cell compartment of marrow. Thus, the International Society for Cellular Therapy (ISCT) has recommended that MSCs be termed "mesenchymal stromal cells" and that "mesenchymal stem cells" should be reserved for the subset of mesenchymal cells that demonstrate stem cell activity [53]. To use this term appropriately, the single most characteristic feature of MSCs is their capacity to differentiate between osteoblasts, adipocytes, and chondroblasts in vitro [51]. Another characteristic feature of MSCs is that they escaped immune recognition (immune-privileged) and may secrete immunosuppressive molecules while being recognized by an allogeneic immune system (immunosuppressive) [51]. As to its ability to home to diseased tissues while administered intravenously, there is little data to support such a hypothesis, although MSCs may arrive and incorporate in the desired tissue to generate clinical benefits [51]. MSCs secrete a variety of cytokines inducing other MSCs to the area, promoting cellular differentiation to target tissue sites, promoting new tissue formation and angiogenesis, reducing fibrosis and inflammation, preventing apoptosis, and suppressing catabolic activity [54]. Bone marrow and its concentrate contain several growth factors like vascular endothelial growth factor (VEGF), platelet-derived growth factor (PDGF), transforming growth factor β (TGF-β), bone morphogenic proteins (BMP), interleukin-8 (IL-8), and interleukin-1 receptor antagonist [55]. Thus, bone marrow aspirate concentrate (BMAC) with its MSCs has enormous potential as cell therapy for tissue regeneration, immune modulation, and anti-tumor agents [51].

Several bones in the body can be a source of these mesenchymal progenitor cells such as the vertebral body, iliac crest, tibia, and calcaneus. The iliac crest yielded a higher mean concentration of osteoblastic progenitor cells compared with tibia and calcaneus [56]. Advanced age has been shown to reduce the colony-forming units (CFU-F), and hence, stem cells may have reduced efficacy in the elderly population [56, 57].

The quality of iliac crest harvesting is technique-dependent, and failures happen due to inconsistent aspiration techniques. It is suggested that targeting the posterior superior iliac spine yields more MSCs [58] than in any other site. Further, the quality of MSCs decreases as you increase the volume being aspirated. In fact, the first 4–5 ml contains MSCs of high quality, and withdrawal of bigger volumes leads to dilution with peripheral blood [55]. Thus, it is suggested that drawing blood from multiple sites increases MSC yield rather than more volumes from a single bone site [59–61]. This is since MSCs reside in the subcortical areas and pericytes reside around blood vessels, and so drawing from more sites and not necessarily from manipulating the trocar with one entry in different sites maximizes MSC yield and allows access to pericytes [62, 63]. Pericytes around blood vessels can differentiate into MSCs when injuries occur and are recruited from the bone marrow for neovasculogenesis [64, 65].

Crisan and colleagues in their landmark study showed that MSCs are derived from perivascular cells (pericytes) from several human tissues such as fat, skin, heart, liver, and muscle [66–69] and not from the connective tissue (stroma) of marrow or the stroma of other tissues [70, 71]. Furthermore, mesenchymal cells (pericytes) that exhibit the properties of MSC can be isolated between the tunica media and tunica intima of large blood vessels [71–73], small vessels, and capillaries. Each pericytes coming from different tissue origin are morphologically tissue- and vessel-specific and have shown to have different chemistries and reactivities, although embryologically the vascular endothelial cells have not been proven to be the progenitors of pericytes [71]. Pericyte is expressed by its markers (CD146, PDGFRβ, NG2, αSMA) [74]. In addition, MSCs secrete "trophic factors" that inhibit scar formation, inhibit ischemia-caused apoptosis, stimulate angiogenesis, stimulate the mitosis of tissue-specific, tissue-inherent stem cells, and guard against viruses and bacteria. Thus, Caplan would like to call MSC a "medicinal signaling cell" [71]. Pericytes are sourced from the abluminal surface of the blood vessel, anchored at the basement membrane through the PDGF-BB, and its sympathetic innervation is not associated with the vascular endothelial cell but with the pericytes-MSCs. In an injury, the pericytes differentiate into MSCs and can be squeezed in due to its sympathetic innervation and contractile apparatus and can respond accordingly [71]. It, therefore, plays a fundamental role in angiogenesis, blood vessel homeostasis, regulation of blood vessel integrity, permeability, blood flow, immune response, and their regenerative application in the musculoskeletal system especially in wound healing and inflammation becoming collagen type 1-producing fibroblasts and can differentiate into skeletal muscle [70, 71, 74, 75].

In 2006, the Mesenchymal and Tissue Stem Cell Committee of the International Society of Cellular Therapy (ISCT) cited the following minimum criteria for defining MSCs: cells must (1) adhere to plastic, (2) express cell surface antigens (CD105, CD73, and CD90) and (3) not express the cell surface antigens CD45, CD34, CD14, CD11B, CD79α, CD19, or HLA-DR, and (4) differentiate into osteoblasts, adipocytes, and chondroblasts in vitro [76].

Preparation Methods of BMAC

To ensure safety, informed consent must be required from all patients. It should detail the name of the patient, date, time, home address, phone number, name of the procedure, name of physician and assists, and the involved risks and benefits of the procedure. A detailed statement regarding the procedure must be included in the consent form, to allow time for the patient to read and understand the procedure. Once the consent form is read and understood, the patient needs to sign at the bottom page to accede to the given procedure. Since this is not a standard care procedure, the risks of the procedures must be included in the statement, like hematoma, fracture, or infection [77]. Caution as to the use of steroids and non-steroidal anti-inflammatory drugs (NSAIDS) must be emphasized prior to the start of the procedure. Studies have shown that these medications interfere with the results of the treatment and thus are best to be discontinued during the treatment period [78]. Patients with asthma using injectable steroids need to delay the procedure for about 8 weeks prior to the procedure while inhaled steroids should be temporarily discontinued [79, 80]. Interestingly, short-term fasting (minimum of 12 hours) or calorie restriction (20–40% reduction of calorie intake) was shown to enhance stem cell function in multiple tissues and slow the ravages of aging with a high-fat diet reducing hematopoietic stem cells activity. The ketogenic diet however did not show any effect on stem cell function [81–83].

Basic laboratory examination like complete blood count could provide the adequacy of hematocrit and hemoglobin levels. Prothrombin time/partial thromboplastin time (PT/PTT) together with HBA1C may serve as useful references to ensure the patient would not have bleeding tendencies. Patients under anticoagulants should be properly weighed in terms of benefits versus risks as withdrawing such drugs might cause more harm than good [77].

When doing the posterior superior iliac spine approach, it is important that one is familiar with the anatomy of the pelvis. The location of the following structures must be scanned carefully namely sacroiliac joint, sacral foramina, sciatic nerve, superior cluneal nerves, lumbar nerve roots, superior gluteal nerve, and blood vessels and must be thoroughly marked out using a pen [84]. To ensure a safe and reliable procedure, Hernigou and colleagues constructed a sector system where the neural and vascular structures are located. Six equal sectors or lines were drawn between the anterior and superior iliac spines and converge at the center of the hip where sector 1 is anterior and sector 6 is the most posterior (Fig. 14.7). The space between the lines of the sector drawn is used as a reference for the placement of the trocar. When the trocar is placed in the most posterior superior portion (sector 6), there is a possibility that it may puncture the sciatic nerve and the superior gluteal nerve and vessels. If the trocar is pushed more than 6 cm, perforation of the bone might occur. Thus, the safest sector to put the trocar is around sector 6. Factors that may give rise to complications include the thickness of the iliac crest with subsequent breaching of the lateral and medial table of the ilium and injury to the sciatic nerve and superior gluteal nerves and blood vessels [85].

In another study, Hernigou and colleagues evaluated the size of the trocar in relation to the thickness of the ilium specifically the spongy bone in an iliac wing (transverse thickness between two tables) on vertical sections relevant for bone aspiration to ensure safe placement of the trocar between the two tables and to evaluate the risk of reaching vascular and neurologic structures. For instance, when the spongious bone transverse thickness of the iliac wing is <3 mm, it would be difficult to use an 8- gauge trocar (3.26 mm). Six equal sectors were drawn as explained in the previous study above with number 1 as the most anterior and 6 as the most posterior. In between these sectors are lines with

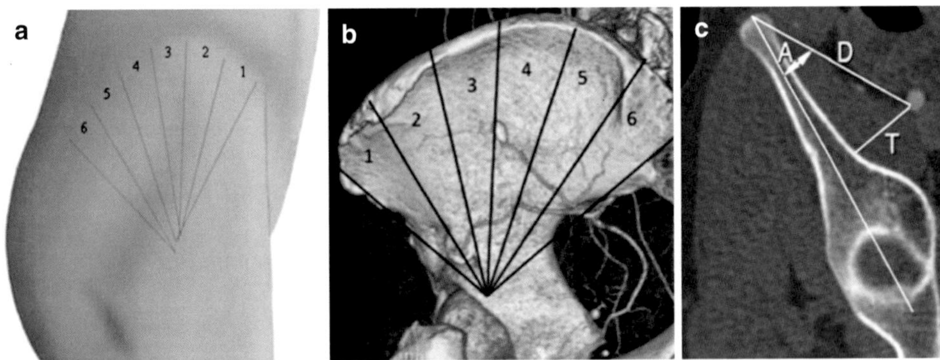

Fig. 14.7 (**a**) The corresponding sectors can be found and marked on the patient by using the same technique and corresponding in clinical practice to different zones of bone marrow aspiration according to the position of the patient. Three different approaches can be used to harvest bone marrow from the iliac crest: patient supine and anterior crest approach (sectors 1, 2, and 3), patient prone and posterior iliac crest approach (sectors 4, 5, and 6), and patient in the left or right lateral position allowing easier middle iliac crest approach (sectors 3 and 4). (**b**) The iliac wing (three-dimensional construction) was divided by drawing lines from equidistant portions spaced along the rim of the iliac crest to the center of the hip. These lines were approximately perpendicular to the curve of the iliac crest. Six sectors were defined by these lines. Sectors 1 and 2 are anterior parts of the iliac bone, sectors 3 and 4 centers are part of the iliac bone, and sectors 5 and 6 are posterior parts of the iliac bone. (**c**) Radial CT scan cuts of the hemipelvis. The transverse distance (*T*) of the external iliac artery from the inner pelvic table, the distance (*D*) between the iliac crest and external iliac artery, and the angle (*A*) between the iliac wing direction and the line joining the external iliac artery to the iliac crest (Used with permission from Springer); Source: Hernigou et al. [85])

letter A between 1 and 2 sectors and letter E between 5 and 6 sectors. Pelvic CT scans were done to measure the transverse thickness of the iliac wing. Results of the study showed that sector 6 had the greatest spongious bone thickness close to the entry point followed by sectors 2 and 3. The trocar of 3 mm can be safely penetrated up to 9 cm as the thickness of the spongious is >3 mm. There was no correlation between the thickness of the iliac crest in each sector and sex, age, side (left or right), height, and BMI [86] (Fig. 14.8).

In Denmark, Gronkjaer and colleagues assessed two techniques of bone aspiration using either an R-technique or an S-technique. The R-technique is a quick pull, creating a high differential pressure for 1 second in a 10 ml syringe, while the S-technique is a slow, low differential pressure. The uniform pull of a 10-ml syringe for approximately 5–15 seconds in the posterior superior iliac spine provides for the extraction of 1.5–3.0 ml of bone marrow under local anesthesia. The results of the study showed a better specimen quality of the R-technique as compared to the S-technique, except for the pain intensity which is higher in the R-technique. Thus, pain could be generated from inadequate anesthesia or from the results of negative pressure from the pull of the trocar during bone marrow aspiration [87].

The use of local anesthetics in bone marrow aspiration procedures is an acceptable method for rendering the approach to bone marrow aspiration less painful if not totally anesthetized. In 2003, Vanhelleputte and colleagues reported 84% of procedural pain which was less than anticipated but disappeared within 10 minutes after the procedure. Younger patients and longer procedures, however, emerged as independent predictors of pain [88]. Levels of local anesthetic toxicity are also one concern and physicians should properly administer an acceptable therapeutic dose. There is no concern for anesthetics to affect the cells of the bone marrow as it is outside the bone marrow. For lidocaine, 4.5 mg/kg is the maximum dose, up to 300 mg lidocaine without epinephrine, or 7 mg/kg or 500 mg lidocaine with epinephrine. The maximum recommended volume for a 70 kg male is between 32 ml and 45 ml of 1% lidocaine depending on the reference chosen [89].

Contraindications to bone marrow procedure include infection at the graft site with its symptoms, bleeding tendencies, hemophilia, dissemi-

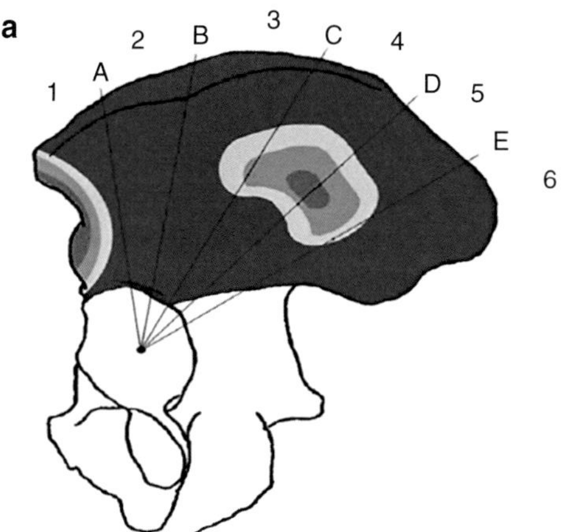

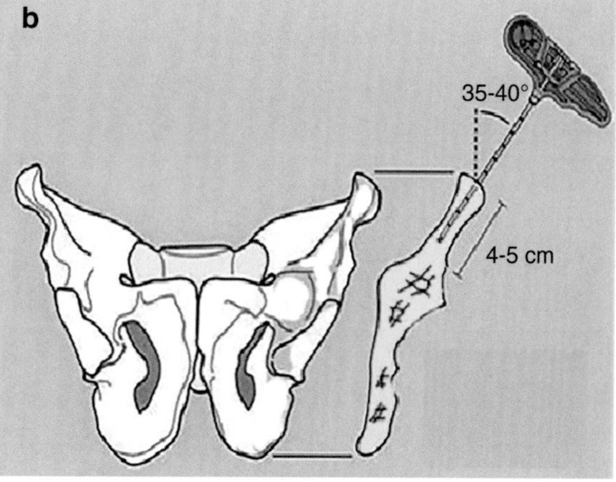

Fig. 14.8 (**a**) Map of the ilium. The blue zone is the part of the ilium where the thickness of the spongios is always >3 mm. The yellow area corresponds to the zone wherein 50% cases of the thickness is <3 mm but >2 mm. The orange area corresponds to the zone wherein 25% cases of the thickness is <2 mm but >1 mm. The red corresponds to the zone wherein 20% of cases of the thickness is <1 mm. The yellow, orange, and red zones are in sectors 1, 4, and 5. Line A is the border between sectors 1 and 2 and line B is the border between sectors 2 and 3, and so forth. (**b**) Trocars are introduced between the two tables of the ilium. (Used with permission from Springer; Source: Hernigou et al. [86])

nated intravascular coagulation, and neoplastic conditions [90]. Other relative contraindications may include the use of anticoagulant medications, those with atrial fibrillations, and other blood dyscrasias [91].

Injection Procedure of BMAC

Aseptic technique for any procedure applies for bone marrow aspiration. Sterile gloves, masks, hair caps, drapes, and towels and other equipment should be used to ensure that pathogens do not get in the way. It is preferable to use chlorhexidine-alcohol solution to clean the area of approach [35, 92] in this procedure. Other supplies should include a scalpel blade if a drill is to be used to incise the skin prior to drilling at the posterior superior iliac spine (PSIS). The choice between 11-gauge Jamshidi trocars and a similar power drill with a bit must be made depending on the familiarity of the physician. Friedlis and Centeno suggested the use of 20 ml 0.5% ropivacaine, 27-gauge 0.5-in skin needle, 22-gauge 3.5–4.0 11-/16-in needle, 5 ml syringe with 5000 units of heparin in normal saline, Steri-Strips (3 M, St Paul MN), gauze and tape [93]. Alternative medication includes 1% lidocaine without epinephrine that would be used through the skin before the skin incision. Marcaine and lidocaine however are toxic and should not be used when injecting the periosteum of the ileum before the trocar is drilled through the bone. In this case, ropivacaine is safer in lower concentrations [94]. The trocar to be used must be rinsed thoroughly with 1000 IU/ml solution of heparin together with the syringes to ensure that no clot is formed, [89] as clots can trap stem cells and render them ineffective for their intended use [93]. The syringes (10-ml) to be used for bone marrow extraction must also be thoroughly heparinized. Leave at least 1 ml of heparin inside the syringe to serve as an anticoagulant during bone marrow extraction.

The patient preparing for this procedure should be lying in a prone position, with a head cut out. The area for bone marrow aspiration must be cleaned using the chlorhexidine-alcohol solution. The target area at the PSIS must be prepped and draped appropriately. A pillow under the abdomen is useful to minimize lordosis of the spine. The table preferably must be stable and movable to allow it to move in different positions [89, 93] (Fig. 14.9).

Image guidance either by means of ultrasound or fluoroscopy allows the precision of the targeted areas during trocar placement. While ultrasound offers a convenient way of imaging with no exposure to radiation, fluoroscopy facilitates placement of the trocar within the anesthetized area and provides less soft tissue penetration due to its steeper approach with easier trocar manipu-

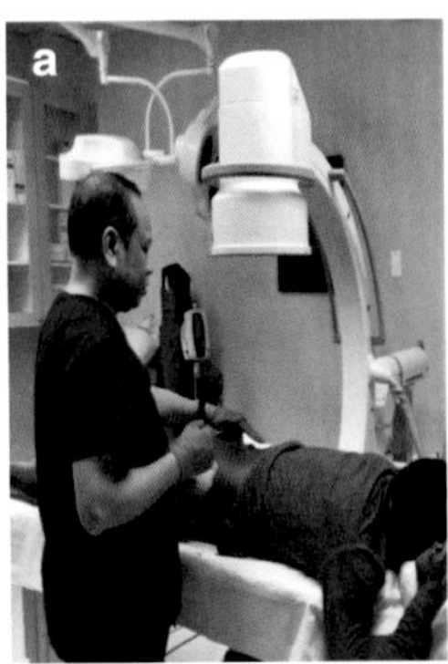
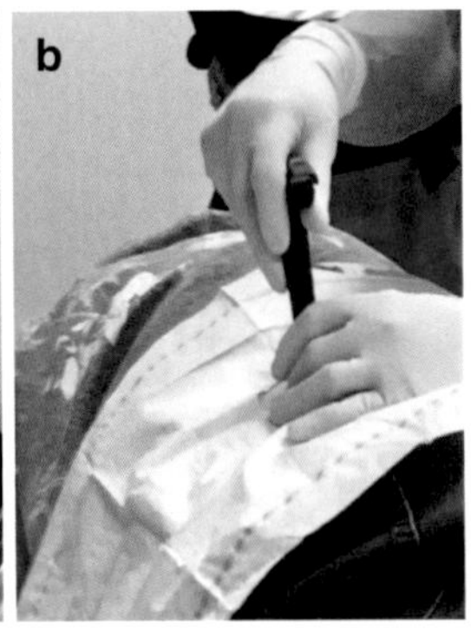
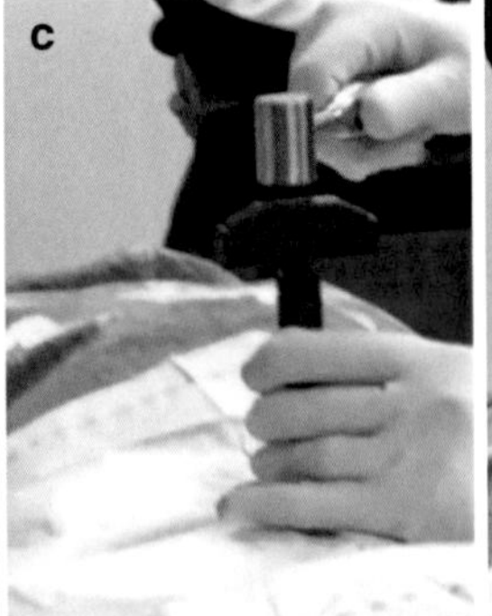
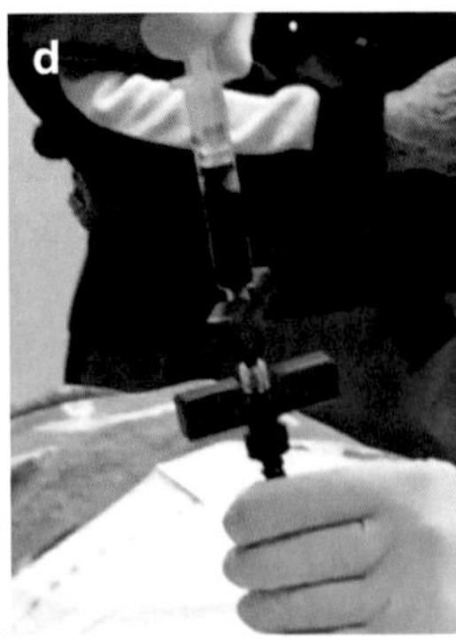

Fig. 14.9 Fluoroscopic-guided aspiration of bone marrow aspirate. (**a**) The patient is positioned in a prone position with the beam oriented to about 15° to 30° ipsilateral oblique and caudal tilt with PSIS as the target. (**b**) The trocar is inserted toward the PSIS between the two tables of the ilium. (**c**) Once PSIS is reached, gently tap the trocar with a mallet until a give is felt and the trocar is inserted to a depth of about 4–5 cm. (**d**) Once the marrow cavity is reached, unscrew the top portion of the trocar, insert a sterile 10 cc syringe and begin the aspiration of the bone marrow aspirate. (Courtesy of Dr. Joseph Purita)

lation [93]. Ultrasound however requires a larger area of local anesthetics as the trocar will have to travel a longer distance through the soft tissue but with no procedural suit needed [93]. When using an ultrasound, the location of the PSIS is scanned and marked first and then the iliac crest is marked all the way to about 4 cm toward the anterolateral portion from the PSIS. A linear probe may be sufficient for a thinner individual but a curvilinear probe for obese patients is better for greater depth in any bony identification [89] (Fig. 14.10). Three approaches are possible: the parallel, perpendicular, and ultrasound-assisted approaches. In a parallel approach, PSIS is drawn and marked out as indicated above. The trocar is inserted from inferior to superior at a steep angle, in the plane to the probe. In the perpendicular approach, the medial part of the probe is placed on the PSIS and the lateral portion points to the greater trochanter. The trocar is inserted from lateral to medial about 1–2 cm from the iliac crest for bone marrow aspiration. For the ultrasound-assisted parallel approach, the PSIS, medial and lateral, are thoroughly marked out on the skin but with no direct visualization with the trocar entry at the PSIS mark [89]. In all these approaches, a skin incision by a scalpel must be made on the target entry point prior to the trocar insertion to enable a smooth entry of the trocar into the PSIS.

If fluoroscopy is preferred, orient the beam to about 15°–30° ipsilateral oblique and caudal tilt to help visualize the target site at the PSIS. A radiopaque marker can help identify the area 1 cm lateral to the PSIS, and a hub view is done once the needle is inserted for perpendicular approach [89, 93]. Care should be taken to avoid going beyond the superolateral area to avoid hitting the superior cluneal nerve. Conversely, avoid going too inferior towards the sacroiliac joint to avoid hitting the the superior gluteal neurovascular structures [89]. Anesthetize the area in a circular manner about 2 cm in diameter with about 7 ml of anesthetics for the injection point and the track leading to the periosteum. The second target must be about 2 cm from the first one and 1 cm from the edge of the ilium and anesthetized like the first one [93] (Fig. 14.11).

The area of the target is spherical. Drilling on a curve surface is a bit challenging. Care should be taken to prevent the trocar from sliding down to areas that are not anesthetized as it may cause pain and complications. To prevent unnecessary errors, approach the ilium at right angles to the surface of the curvature. If you are harvesting from different sectors, be conscious of the different neurovascular structures around it as each area will have a different curvature. Another aspect of drilling is deciding on what type of aspiration tool to use, whether a manual tool or a power-driven rotary device. When using a manual drill, firm pressure must be applied and 180° rotation must be applied at the target site in the PSIS, alternating in both clockwise and counterclockwise directions. A mallet could also be used

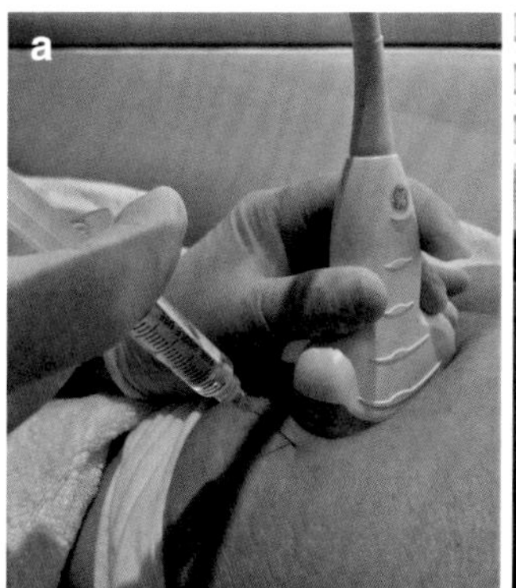

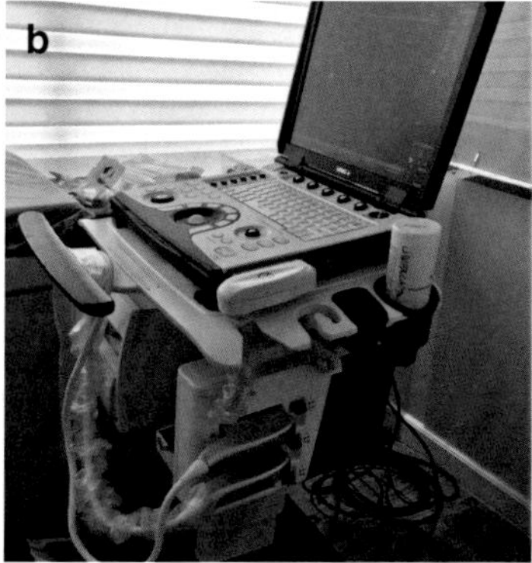

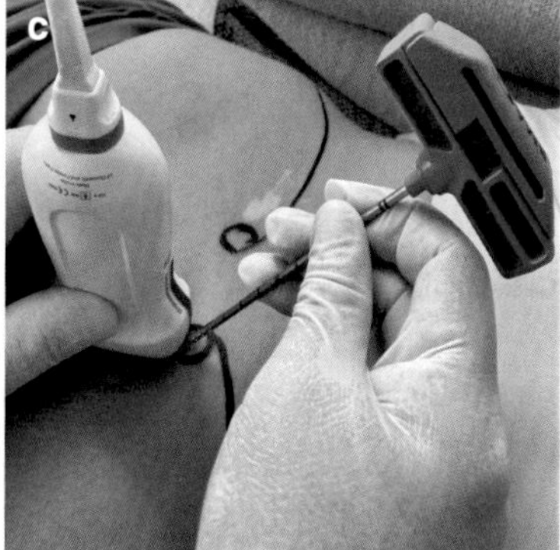

Fig. 14.10 Ultrasound-guided approach to the PSIS. (**a**) Anesthetic is administered over the area of approach at the PSIS. (**b**) Ultrasound is used to pre-scan the area to ensure a correct approach. (**c**) Ultrasound-guided entry into the PSIS 30° lateral and about 15° cephalad. (Courtesy of Zarah Francine de Castro)

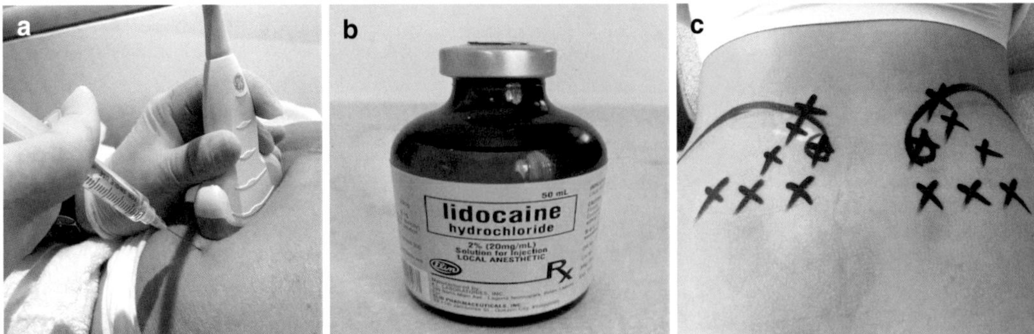

Fig. 14.11 Target sites for anesthesia. (**a**) Anesthesia is applied over the PSIS until the periosteum is reached using 2% lidocaine (**b**) Then you may do other injection points in marked areas, as shown here (**c**) Sites for anesthesia injection

while the trocar is touching the target site to enable it to enter the marrow cavity [89, 93]. A moderate tap may be used in the beginning as it allows entry into the PSIS and a sense of "give" is felt indicating the entrance into the marrow (Fig. 14.9). Hernigou and colleagues [85] cautioned the practitioner about the risk when the tip of the trocar (10 cm) is accessible to the sector and a deviation of 20° from the plane of the iliac wing. Also, as the trocar enters the marrow, the patient usually feels the pressure, but not the pain, unless the trocar goes out of the anesthetized area. In that case, redirect the trocar for appropriate direction and target [93]. When using the powered rotary device, a specialized needle fits into the battery-powered handle. This type of aspiration tool is more ideal for younger patients. By using a smaller 15-gauge needle, less axial force is required with associated less procedure time, and the chance of sliding is also reduced. Less pain was also observed using the power rotary device. It is suggested that it must be operated continuously rather than by pulse to sense the sound of the drill as it transitions from the cortex to the marrow cavity. Once it reaches the marrow cavity, the trocar is usually stuck firmly in the bone. If it is loose, continuous drilling is done until the trocar is solidly in the bone. You can test it by tapping gently showing a solid feel which means that it has reached the bone. Take note of the 1-cm marking on the trocar to ensure that the depth is acceptable [93].

The purpose of bone aspiration is to get as many nucleated cells as possible. Most of the MSCs are found mostly in the trabeculae [60, 95]. Various studies note the advantage of smaller volumes of 2–4 ml of bone marrow aspirate over bigger volumes which will cause peripheral blood dilution [60, 96]. A study by Hernigou and colleagues examined the higher concentration of MSCs using 10 ml syringes compared to that of 50 ml syringes [97]. Thus, for the purpose of maximizing the quality of MSCs harvested, a smaller volume from multiple sites is ideal for bone marrow aspiration than the bigger volumes. Furthermore, in the process of extracting the bone marrow using a syringe, it is important to pull gently in a pulse-wise fashion but not oblivious to the pressure that might be felt by the patient. After completing the extraction of bone marrow from at least 3 sites, remove the syringe and cap it, and allow the syringe to be moved continuously to prevent clotting. Then withdraw the trocar quickly and apply pressure into the wound to prevent bleeding [93]. Tegaderm (3 M, St. Paul, MN) is an ideal dressing for the wound to be kept until the following day, after which the patient can clean the area and replace it with a simple dressing or Band-Aid (Johnson & Johnson Consumer Inc, New Brunswick, NJ). For post-procedural pain, 500 mg/tablet of paracetamol or acetaminophen is taken once a day up to a maximum of thrice a day be taken until pain subsides. The patient can stay on the table for a sufficient period while the sample is being processed and to make it ready for injection. Repeat the same process if there is a need to get more samples at the opposite side of the ilium.

Adipose-Derived Stem/Stromal Cells (ADSC)

Liposuction is a popular procedure among aesthetic and plastic surgeons for a variety of clinical conditions (Fig. 14.12). Most of these procedures are intended for aesthetic purposes but only recently have they found it to be equally effective for degenerative musculoskeletal conditions. The isolation of adipose-derived stem cells is a novel therapy in regenerative medicine that caught the attention of a lot of practitioners due to its potential regenerating capacity in an aging musculoskeletal region. Adipose-derived stem cells (ADSC) are a ubiquitous solution for aesthetic and reconstructive problems because of tissue volume loss secondary to aging or radiation-induced loss of tissue pliability and vascularity [98].

Adipose tissue, otherwise known as "white adipose tissue," to distinguish it from infantile, thermoregulatory "brown adipose tissue," is an energy store and an endocrine organ secreting several adipokine hormones [99]. ADSC (white adipose tissue) is said to be multipotent as it can differentiate into a range of different adult cell types such as adipocytes, osteoblasts, myocytes, and neurons but within the same lineage [98, 100]. Mature adipocytes are sensitive to ischemic changes while their precursors (ADSC) are resistant to ischemia, a feature that makes it very ideal for tissue grafting. Their popularity stemmed from its potential to address a host of therapeutic benefits with a higher cell yield per unit of tissue substrate than bone marrow MSCs. It is estimated that a given adipose has a frequency yield of about 1:100 to 1:1500, while bone marrow yields about 1:100,000 nucleated cells and their quantity decline over time as one ages [98, 101]. They are also genetically stable and relatively resistant to senescence in culture as compared to bone marrow MSCs [98]. Because of its stability, it can be cryopreserved and stored for long periods but with a finite lifespan and clinically is ideal for tissue repair and regrowth in several pathologies. Thus, they can be called progenitor cells, which reflects their ability to renew over a longer period while committed to a certain lineage. However, to date, stem cell research and clinical trials are yet to be ascertained [98, 102].

Adipose stem cells (ASC) then are mesenchymal, adult stem cells that reside in the stromal vascular component of adipose tissue, with a primary function of tissue repair and expansion [103]. Like bone marrow-derived stem cells, it is immunosuppressive and upon systemic injection, it can home to specific injured areas, in response to hypoxia, apoptosis, or inflammation [100, 103]. The International Society for Cellular Therapy (ISCT) introduced a minimum criterion for MSCs expressing the following cell surface markers CD70, CD90, CD105, and HLA-ABC but negative for the other markers such as the pan hematopoietic marker CD45; the monocyte/macrophage markers CD 11B or CD14; the B cell markers CD79α and CD19; and primitive

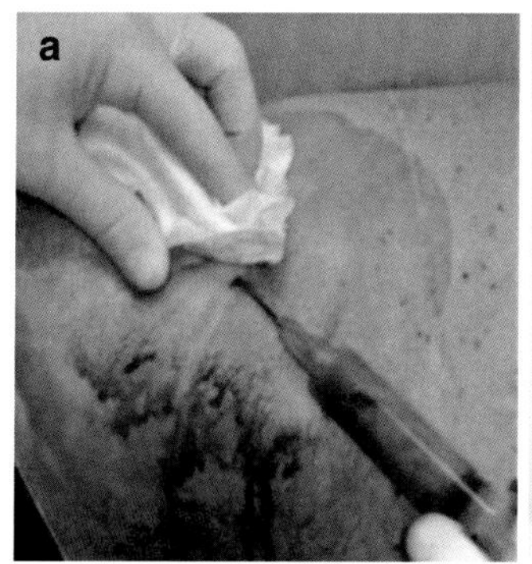

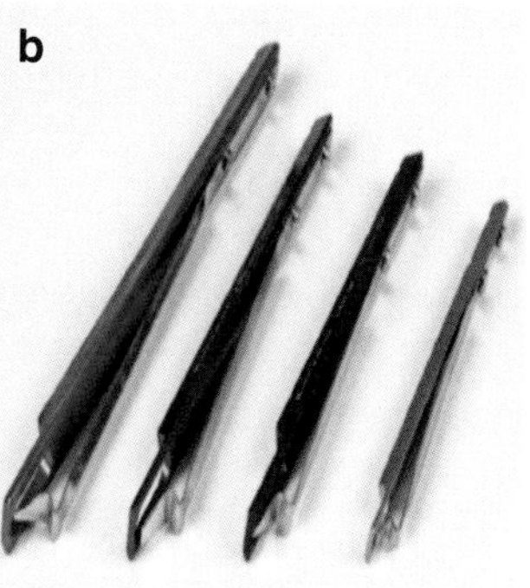

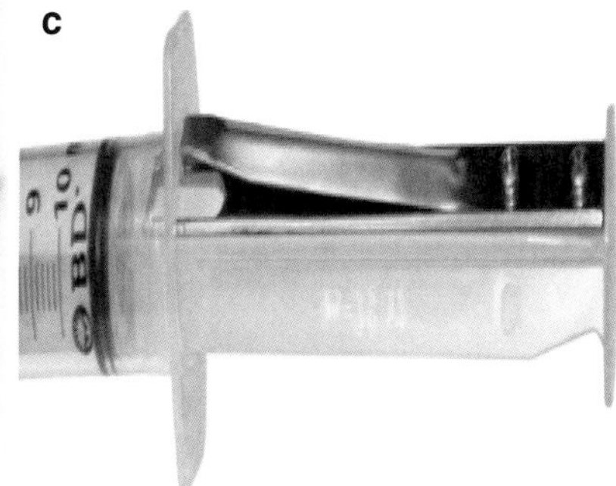

Fig. 14.12 Simple liposuction procedure. (**a**) Simple manual liposuction procedure using a 23-gauge needle to harvest fat at the posterior pelvis. (**b**) Snap Lok device (Tulip®) in different sizes to accommodate various syringes. (**c**) Snap Lok device (Tulip®) inserted into the plunger to create a vacuum during the harvesting of fats

hematopoietic progenitors and endothelial cell markers CD34 and HLA-DR [98, 102, 103]. Other positive markers for ADSC-MSCs are CD10 [104], CD13 [104–106], CD29 [104–108], CD44 [105–107], and CD166 [105, 106, 108]. They also secrete growth factors such as basic fibroblast growth factor (bFGF), keratinocyte growth factor (KGF), transforming growth factor-beta (TGF-β), hepatocyte growth factor (HGF), and vascular endothelial growth factor (VEGF) [101].

Before we go any further to discuss some details regarding the harvesting procedures and isolation of the ADSC, let me share the regulation that governs this type of procedure. In the United States, adipose stem cells are regulated under the broader category Human Cells, Tissues, and Cellular and Tissue-Based Products (HCT/Ps). Other countries prescribed their own regulation after the United States. This is further subdivided into 361 or 351 products which determine how stringent the Food and Drug Administration (FDA) allows their access into the markets. The 351 products are considered drugs and as such they are regulated like pharmaceutical products subject to stringent clinical trials before gaining market accessibility. In contrast, 361 products are not regulated like pharmaceutical products but need to comply with the Public Health Services Act and Current Good Tissue Practice Legislations, under the Code of Federal Regulations, Title 21, Part 1271 [100, 109]. A 361 product must be only minimally manipulated, intended for homologous use, and not used in conjunction with another article. FDA defines minimal manipulation as cutting; grinding; shaping; centrifugation; soaking in antibiotic solution; sterilization by ethylene oxide treatment or irradiation; cell separation; density gradient separation; lyophilization; freezing; cryopreservation; and selective removal of B cells, T cells, malignant cells, red blood cells, or platelets. Except for autologous cells, the product must have no systemic effects or rely on the metabolic effect of the patient's living cells [100]. With this in view, ADSC is a 351 product, and a stromal vascular fraction (SVF) should be treated and regulated as a drug [100]. Adistem™ extracts stromal cells by dissolving lipids and connective tissue from a lipoaspirate and may not be compliant with the US FDA, whereas Lipogems® and Puregraft® are closed systems, provide autologous fat for lipofilling and are delivered percutaneously, do not extract from stromal vascular fraction, and are compliant with the US FDA [89]. As a word of caution, please do not rely on a commercial company or its medical representative without verifying such information as to the US FDA guidelines.

In the European Union, cell-based therapies are regulated as advanced therapy medical products (ATMPs) and are subject to European Medicines Agency (EMA) regulation and require market approval. ATMPs are further subdivided into gene therapy medicinal product (GTMP), somatic cell therapy medicinal product (SCTMP), tissue-engineered product (TEP), or a combination. Cell-based products like ADSC may only be subject to public health legislation if they are homologous, not manipulated substantially, and not combined with any article. Interestingly, there are products in the United States that fall under non-ATMPs in the EU, thus causing some safety concerns if these products have unproven effects for different indications. The approval system therefore could be circumvented [100].

In Japan and much in Asia, they have their own regulatory bodies which may be patterned after the US or EU regulations. In Japan, they fall under a separate regulatory body called "cell/tissue-engineered product." To encourage the use of new regenerative products, they provide incentives during the clinical trials with conditional market approval. Data are collected for the next 7 years for monitoring and reevaluation and for final market approval [100].

Rodbell and colleagues in the 1960s were the first to isolate cells from adipose tissue using minced rat fat pads [110]. Subsequently, with the potential of this procedure, it was modified for the isolation of cells from human adipose tissue specimens. This procedure was minced using hands, but with the development of liposuction, this procedure has been simplified [111, 112]. In humans, fat is usually harvested from the lower abdomen, lateral gluteal region, medial and lateral thigh, posterior hip, or flank with the greatest number of viable cells taken from the lower abdomen followed by the thigh [113]. Lim and colleagues together with the study by Choudhery and colleagues did not show any difference in the quality of MSCs from different sites taken from the same donor showing unaffected differentiation capacity [114, 115]. Although previous studies indicate that abdominal sources are resistant to apoptosis, the arm has the highest yield of cells and the inguinal area has the greatest plasticity [116]. Ultrasound imaging can be used to assess the thickness of adipose tissue prior to harvesting of the adipose tissue.

Preparation Methods for Adipose Aspirate

Usually, the patient is prepped by choosing the appropriate area for liposuction [113–115]. My personal preference is at the posterior hip and lower abdomen. When the area is chosen, the patient is draped in an aseptic manner. An anesthetic solution of about 3 cc is delivered over the skin to form a wheal at the entry site. A dermatologist in California named Dr. Jeffrey Klein described a tumescent solution for liposuction which is composed of lignocaine, epinephrine, and large amounts of saline. The saline balloons the fat tissue; epinephrine causes vasoconstriction and decreased bleeding, and lignocaine induces anesthesia [117, 118]. This tumescent solution is infiltrated at the collection sites in the skin by creating a skin nick by a scalpel. A blunt cannula is used to deliver about 180–300 ml of the tumescent fluid into the subcutaneous fat layer. After delivering the solution, 15–20 minutes is allowed for the diffusion of the tumescent solution. Then, the cannula is inserted where the skin nick was made into the subcutaneous fat layer, and by using a 10-cc syringe with a locking device to create a vacuum, begin the aspiration process. Lipoaspiration using a 20 ml or 60 ml syringe is more difficult. A total volume of about 20 ml of lipoaspirate is obtained. Repeat the aspiration when necessary. Trivisonno and colleagues found higher stromal and vascular cells with blunt microcannula (2 mm diameter, with 5 rounded ports on each side, 1 mm in size each) as compared with 3 mm blunt cannula with a single port on the side (3 × 9 mm) [119]. The lipoaspirate is then transferred to a sterile test tube from the syringes (Fig. 14.13). Other methods use automated aspirating devices, but there are findings that it could damage the cells. No significant difference of cells aspirated was found though when comparing manual versus automated processing systems [120].

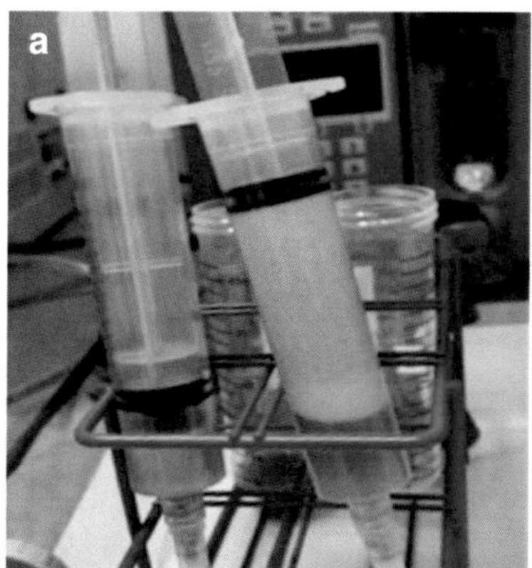

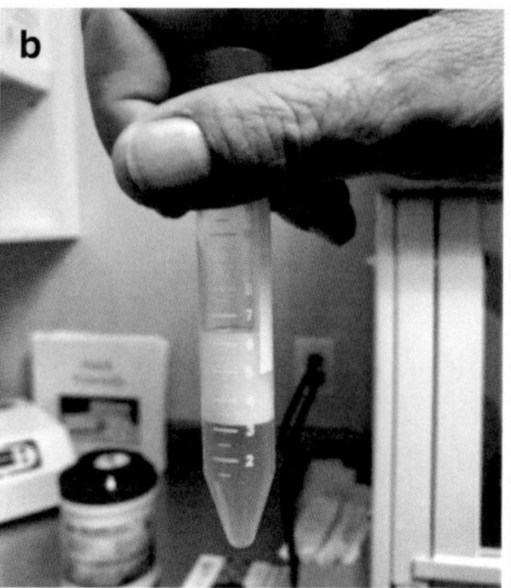

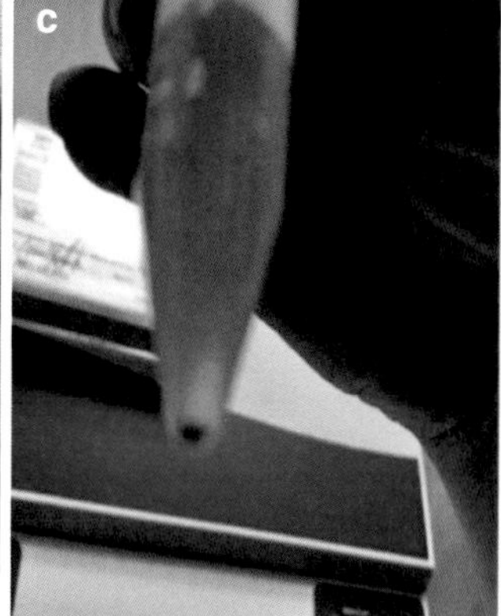

Fig. 14.13 Lipoaspirate. (**a**) Simple separation of the lipoaspirate to gravity separate without centrifugation to remove excess fluid at the bottom admixed with blood. The middle portion is a concentrated adipose tissue. The uppermost layer is made up of oil and lipid fractions. Additional washing with sterile normal saline is done until the adipose tissue becomes homogeneous. (**b**) After centrifugation, there is a clear delineation of the infranatant fluid at the lower layer of the tube. The adipose tissue remains at the top layer. (**c**) Sediments settle at the bottom of the tube

After the aspiration of fat, the cannula is withdrawn, and pressure is applied in the area with a 2 × 2 gauze and a Tegaderm patch. The area must be kept dry while the area is still healing. It might take not less than 2 days before the area of injection will fully recover. The patient must watch out for any sign of infection or any untoward signs and symptoms [89].

As discussed earlier, there are regulations that govern whatever the final product of the lipoaspirate would be. The use of enzymes such as collagenase in the processing of lipoaspirate with the resultant stromal vascular fraction (SVF) is considered a 351 product [89, 100, 109], while minimal manipulation for homologous use falls under a 361 product. Thus, the removal of red blood cells and oil that can interfere with healing is minimal manipulation and is done with the goal of preserving the optimum amounts of multipotent cells and growth factors. Adipose tissue cannot be kept at room temperature for more than 24 hours [111].

A stromal vascular fraction (SVF) is done by collecting the lipoaspirate and mixing it with a physiological solution. Adipose tissue is washed repeatedly using phosphate-buffered solution (PBS) until a clear lipoaspirate without red cells and fat is removed. This then will be mixed with a digestion solution containing 2 mg/ml of collagenase A, with or without trypsin dissolved in (PBS) solution (1:1 ratio). Digestion is done by agitation at 37 °C for 30 minutes. After this process, 1 volume of PBS is added, and the solution is filtered through a 40-μm cell strainer. Then centrifugation is done at low speed (500 g) or at 2000 rpm for 5 minutes and then washed twice with PBS [111, 119]. Other methods include agitating the cells after centrifugation, disrupting the pellet, and mixing the cells. This completes the separation of stromal cells from the primary adipocytes. Then repeat the centrifugation process again, and after the spin, remove all the solution above without disturbing the cells at the bottom of the tube. The resultant cell pellet is called stromal vascular fraction (SVF). The pellet is resuspended in a cell culture medium and seeded into a culture plate. In vitro differential adhesion cell culture technique is used to isolate ADSC from SVF. ADSC is identified as the spindle-shaped cells adherent to the plate after it is placed in a humidifier atmosphere of 5% $C0_2$ at 37 °C [98, 111]. At present, this is not allowed by law and, therefore, is treated as a drug, subject to strict clinical trials before being allowed access to the market.

Four SVF isolation systems are identified: MultiStation (PNC International, Gyeonggido, Republic of Korea), Cytori StemSource 900/MB System (Cytori Therapeutics, Inc., San Diego, California), LipoKit Platform (Medi-Khan Inc., Irwindale, California), and GID SVF-2 Platform (The GID Group, Inc, Louisville, CO). The choice of which system is to be used depends upon the type of clinical practices of the physicians [121]. To overcome the issue of enzymatic digestion which is not allowed by law, van Dongen and colleagues developed a technique called the fractionation of adipose tissue (FAT) procedure. This procedure can be done within 10–12 minutes with isolation of 1 ml of SVF from a 10 ml centrifuged adipose tissue. However, based on histological stainings, interdonor variation exists which might result in different therapeutic effects. Thus, it is too early to say that this could be effectively used for the treatment and at the same time be allowed by the FDA [122].

Commercial kits for adipose tissue processing are also available. These include AdiPrep® from Harvest®, Adistem™, Lipogems®, Puregraft®, and Tulip®. The Lipogems® is a system that is designed to harvest, process, and transfer refined adipose tissue without the use of enzymes. Adipose tissue is micro fragmented gently and washed from pro-inflammatory oil and blood residues, whose end-product contains pericytes which are retained within an intact stromal vascular niche and thereby activated as MSCs as it interacts with the target tissues [123]. Like Lipogems®, Puregraft® is a closed system and provides autologous fat for lipofilling and is delivered to the patient percutaneously. Adistem™ uses enzymes in processing the lipoaspirate and thus its clinical use at this point may not be compliant with the US FDA [89].

Liposuction is not without any complications. Although rare, the list is extensive. It may include bleeding, hematoma, chronic edema, depression, fat embolism, fibrosis, hyperpigmentation, scars, seroma, thromboembolism, infection, lidocaine anaphylaxis and toxicity, loose skin, necrosis, neurologic problems, injury of vessels, perforation of a hollow viscus, pulmonary edema, and skin burns [124]. The most common of this complication is sepsis due to necrotizing fasciitis. The mortality rate is about 19–20 per 100,000 [125, 126]. Tumescent liposuction, however, is the safest method of fat removal with the fewest complications [127]. In a review of literature done by Boni, there were no reported fatalities in tumescent liposuction, while very rarely, fatalities were reported in intravenous sedation or under general anesthesia [128]. The current FDA limit of 7 mg/kg lidocaine is a non-significant risk of harm to patients. Also, a dose of 55 mg/kg of tumescent lidocaine is remarkably safe for liposuction, although the standard recommended dose of about 35 mg/kg as presented by Klein is recommended. With liposuction, the dose range of epinephrine ranged from 1.2 mg to 4.3 mg, and with this dose, there was no clinical evidence of epinephrine toxicity [129, 130]. Furthermore, the tumescent solution did not also alter the quality of fat grafts and did not influence the viability of the adipocytes [131]. Bupivacaine was reported to show the highest cell viability but has to be properly dosed to be safe and effective [129, 132].

Lipoaspiration and tumescent liposuction are safe procedures when done under a controlled environment where all precautions are put in place assuming also that this procedure is done mainly for healthy individuals. Although much of the research done is derived from aesthetic and cosmetic procedures, we can use their data to our own advantage. Those patients taking anticoagulants are advised to discontinue the medications 2 weeks prior to the procedure. Ask for any allergies to medications so unnecessary reactions could be avoided [89].

Alpha-2-Macroglobulin (A2M)

The human ultrastructure of alpha-2-macroglobulin was first identified by Hoglund and Levin in 1965, by Bloth et al. in 1968, by Gauthier et al. in 1974, and then by Lebreton de Vonne and Mouray in 1974 [133]. It is a high molecular weight homotetrameric glycoprotein that can inhibit matrix metalloproteases (MMPs) or any protease without the direct blockage of protease active sites [134, 135]. It is one of the members of protease inhibitors family (alpha$_1$ antitrypsin or α_1_AT, C_1-inhibitor, alpha$_1$-antichymotrypsin, etc.). It is synthesized by the liver, astroglia, and blood cells in humans. It forms an irreversible complex and transports of cytokine interleukin-6 (IL-6) and growth factors [134, 136]. Alpha-2-macroglobulin (A2M) has been identified in the luminal surfaces of the endothelial cells of arteries, veins, and lymphatics. It was found to inhibit a broad spectrum of plasma proteases, thus having a protective role against injurious plasma and cellular enzymes [137]. It is a 718-kDa protein and is found in the plasma and extracellular spaces at a concentration of about 2–4 mg/ml [138].

Peptidases trigger a massive conformational rearrangement of alpha-2-macroglobulin after cutting in a highly flexible bait region such that A2M being a broad-spectrum endopeptidase inhibitor causes their entrapment described as "Venus flytrap" or "snap-trap" mechanisms. A second action may take place among other homologs that involve a highly reactive β-cysteinyl-γ-glutamyl thioester bond, which covalently binds cleaving peptidases which further stabilizes the enzyme–inhibitor complex. Although active, trapped peptidases have limited access to their substrates. This way, A2M (the active form is S; inactive form is F) homolog regulates proteolysis in complex biological processes such as nutrition, signaling, and tissue remodeling and at the same time protects the host organisms against attacks by external toxins and other virulence factors during infection and envenomation. Further, it can inhibit pro-inflammatory cytokines, inhibits a broad spectrum of serine, threonine, and metalloproteases, and modifies hormones and growth factors [139, 140]. Therefore, it has the potential to treat cartilage-based pathology, inflammatory painful arthritides [140], alter the course of peripheral nerve injury [141], and has the potential to treat neuropathic pains [134]. A recent study in 2019 by Orhurhu and colleagues also showed that A2M is an active inhibitor of joint degeneration and cartilage preservation, and improves the quality of life for patients with knee osteoarthritis [142]. In fact, early intra-articular A2M exerts an anti-inflammatory effect and attenuates cartilage and bone damage [143]. Huang and colleagues in 2019 have also demonstrated that supplemental A2M has beneficial effects on cartilaginous endplates (CEP) that slow the progression of intervertebral disk (IV) degeneration by inhibiting effects of proinflammatory cytokines [144]. Vincenzetti and colleagues have observed that A2M in neuropathic pains is decreased and that treatment with gabapentin reverses the condition [145]. Similarly, alpha-2 macroglobulin inhibits proinflammatory cytokines such as interleukin-1, tumor necrosis factor-α (TNF-α), and interleukin-6 [134] which are predominant in peripheral nerve injury [141] and inhibits matrix metalloproteases and other proteases in addition to other enzymes involved in joint pathologies [140]. It has also been found that A2M exhibited a protective effect against radiation injury in human bone marrow mesenchymal stem cells and is a potential therapeutic agent for the prevention and treatment of osteoradionecrosis of the jaws during radiation therapy [146].

Peripheral nerve injury, whether partial or complete, may result in a series of complicated responses. While it is true that regeneration follows an inflammatory process, fulminant inflammation may cause unnecessary axonal damage and neuropathic pain [141, 147]. This peripheral nerve injury will in turn cause the release of tumor necrosis factor-α (TNF-α) and interleukin-1β (IL-1β) with associated infiltration of neutrophils and pro-inflammatory M_1 monocytes/macrophages in the distal stump [134, 148]. In a study by Wagner and Myers, direct injection of TNF-α in an uninjured nerve causes demyelination, macrophage infiltration, and pain mimicking changes seen in an injury [149]. The activation of p38 mitogen-activated protein kinase (MAPK) by TNF-α in Schwann cells, consequently, leads to increased expression of IL-1β [147]. The peripheral nerve injury also leads to release of pro-inflammatory cytokines like interleukin-6 (IL-6), interferon-γ (IFN-γ), interleukin-10 (IL-10), and interleukin-18 (IL-18) [134, 150–153]. In fact, TNF-α is used as a biomarker of Wallerian degeneration in an injured peripheral nerve [154]. Wallerian degeneration upregulates other factors such as chemokines and transcription factors in a peripheral nerve injury with both beneficial and detrimental effects in a regenerating nerve or neuropathic pain induction [155].

Alpha-2-macroglobulin (A2M) can regulate the distribution and activity of pro-inflammatory cytokines such as transforming growth factor-β (TGF-β), TNF-α, platelet-derived growth factor (PDGF), IL-6, nerve growth factor (NGF), fibroblast growth factor (βFGF), and IL-1β [156]. In a study, Arandjelovic [141] prepared three preparations for A2M namely human A2M, activated A2M (methylamine-activated α2-macroglobulin – α2M-A), and MAC, where a native α2M was treated with 0.6 mmol/L cis-Pt for 6 hours at 37 °C and then with MA (methylamine HCl), by dialysis. Like TNF-α, IL-1β binds with increased affinity with MAC [157] and has been reported to play an important role in peripheral nerve injury [151]. Other proinflammatory cytokines such as IL-6 and IL-18 have a close affinity with MAC as compared with α2M-A and human α2M, with IL-6 binding exclusively with MAC [152, 153]. Such α2M derivative (MAC) is very active in suppressing inflammation and in altering the course of peripheral nerve injury by acting against the proinflammatory cytokines, thereby directly addressing neuropathic pains [141]. Electron microscopy studies, however, suggest that naturally occurring A2M conformational intermediates may be like MAC [158] with similar effects when done in vivo, causing a direct anti-inflammatory activity in peripheral nerve injuries [134, 141], thus relieving neuropathic pains.

Known to be a non-inflammatory joint process, osteoarthritis presents however with significant joint inflammation as shown by the presence of proinflammatory cytokines. Cells originating from the synovium (synoviocytes), cartilage (chondrocytes), and leucocytes participate in the pathogenesis of the disease. During the early stages of osteoarthritis, the synovial cells release proinflammatory cytokines especially TNF-α, IL-1β [159, 160], IL-6, and several other cytokines and chemokines [161]. These proinflammatory cytokines, in turn, cause the release of lysosomal enzymes and matrix metalloproteinases (MMPs) from the synoviocytes, chondrocytes, and infiltrating leukocytes, which collectively degrade the cartilage proteoglycan, collagen, and matrix [162, 163]. These proinflammatory cytokines namely, TNF-alpha and IL-1β stimulate the mRNA expression of catabolic cytokines, such as MMP-1, MMP-3, MMP-9, and MMP-13 thus degrading structural components of extracellular matrix (ECM) such as the aggrecan and collagen and causing changes in chondrocyte viability and GAG (glycosaminoglycans) release [164–167, 174]. Further, catabolic factors such as disintegrin and metalloproteinase with thrombospondin motifs (ADAMTS), cathepsins, and receptor activator of nuclear factor κB ligand (RANKL) affect bone and cartilage metabolism and ultimately erode the bone [168, 169] which are activated by TNF-α and IL-1β. Fragments of fibronectin and collagen are reported to further stimulate the release of proinflammatory cytokines and their production, chemokines, and MMPs, thus resulting in a vicious cycle of increased protease production [140]. Aggrecan, which is a large multidomain proteoglycan component of articular cartilage, provides cartilage compressibility and elasticity under normal circumstances, but it then deteriorates over time as one ages. In an osteoarthritic condition, proteases that cleave to aggrecan can trigger the release of its G3 domain (MMP-2, MMP-7, MMP-9, and MMP-13) and which ultimately form the fibronectin-aggrecan complex (FAC). Loss of aggrecan is a critical event in an early degenerative process, beginning at the surface and eventually affecting the deeper layers of the articular cartilage. FAC can then stimulate cytokines and the release of MMPs. The by-product which is fibronectin-aggrecan complex (FAC) is a good indicator of a joint pathology, as well as those patients undergoing microdiscectomy who are FAC+ prior to the operation. A therapeutic agent that can prevent the release of the G3 domain from aggrecan reduces the chance of FAC formation, thus affording relief from pain in the degenerative process [140]. With this information, the potential of α2-macroglobulin as a multipurpose protease inhibitor and anti-inflammatory mediator is seen [140].

TNF-α is involved in acute phase reaction and systemic inflammation and disrupts the normal turnover of the extracellular matrix which degrades the cartilage and thereby causes pain [170, 171]. In fact, TNFα is also involved in osteophyte formation and in muscle and tendon damage in osteoarthritis [172, 173]. In addition, these proinflammatory cytokines will also induce the release of other biologically active substances such as prostaglandin E_2 (PGE_2) and nitric oxide (NO) by inducing nuclear factor-κB (NF-κB) and mitogen-activated protein kinase (MAPK), which then contribute to the pathogenesis of osteoarthritis [174]. Recently, there are findings seen in the subchondral bone area which may be due to an imbalance in remodelling between bone resorption and bone formation which may result in diminished tissue mineralization, loss of stiffness, and bone thickening [175, 176]. Certain neuropeptides from the synoviocytes such as Substance P contribute to inflammation and pain inside the joint. Growth factors such as TGF-1β and IGF-1 are also involved in the disease process [163].

Another interesting finding in osteoarthritis is the release of exosomes from neutrophils and synovial fibroblasts which have been detected in OA and RA synovial fluid. Exosomes occur naturally from many tissues and cells arising via the endocytic pathway from the endosomal cell compartment where they are stored in multivesicular bodies of late endosomes and are released in short bursts by exocytosis upon fusion with the cell membrane. They are responsible for cell-cell communication and epigenetic modifications. Exosomes could modulate joint pathology especially because their release is influenced by senescence and hypoxia which are present in osteoarthritis [175]. MSC-derived exosomes stimulated repair of osteochondral defects in animal models and cartilage damage in chondrocyte cultures which involved increased cellular proliferation and infiltration [175, 177].

Preparation and Clinical Application of α2-Macroglobulin

Several methods are available in the preparation of autologous α2-macroglobulin. This is usually an office-based procedure approved by the Food and Drug Administration for different types of musculoskeletal conditions. It is referred to as Autologous Platelet Integrated Concentrate (APIC) protein-rich plasma (Cytonics) (Fig. 14.14). The system concentrates α2-macroglobulin via centrifugation and ultrafiltration with a tangential flow filter after drawing 45 ml of peripheral blood [140]. Treatment of α2-macroglobulin is based on its multipurpose protease inhibiting ability. Wang and colleagues have shown that α2M is a powerful inhibitor of many cartilages catabolic factors and it can attenuate posttraumatic OA cartilage degeneration. It inhibits MMP-13 in a dose-dependent manner and further decreases cartilage catabolic cytokines and enzymes including IL-1β, IL-8, TNF-α, GM-CSF, MMP-3, and MMP-9 [178]. Studies have also shown that α2M inhibits ADAMTS-4, ADAMTS-5, ADAMTS-7, and ADAMTS-12 which is upregulated by IL-1β [178–180]. ADAMTS-5 and MMP-13 specifically degrade collagen type II where ADAMTS-5 is released during the early phase of an injury and MMP-13 shows a delayed response. In the spine, Kang and colleagues found that herniated nucleus pulposus (HNP) has elevated levels of MMPs, nitric oxide (NO), prostaglandin-E, and IL-6 [181]. In a related study, the cartilage degration products FAC is found to be associated with pain due to inflammation. The presence of FAC indicates that lumbar epidural steroid injection will respond positively to patients with radiculopathy secondary to a disc herniation. Similarly, significant clinical improvements are also observed following surgical microdiscectomy [182]. In hip OA and femoroacetabular impingement (FAI), FAC together with cartilage oligomeric matrix protein (COMP) was also used as biomarkers with potential utility in the clinical diagnosis and clinical management [183]. With this inflammatory component in the joints and around it, autologous α2-macroglobulin-rich concentrate injection has shown successful results, especially for those positive with FAC, against proinflammatory cytokines especially TNF-α and IL-1β, IL-6, against metalloproteinases, and against neurotrophic factors in the neuromusculoskeletal system [134, 140–145, 178–180].

Cytonics (Cytonics, West Palm Beach, Florida) Autologous Platelet Integrated Concentration (APIC™) System is an autologous α2M treatment system with the intent of halting cartilage degeneration. The CYT-108 is an α2M recombinant drug that can help slow the progression of osteoarthritis in preclinical models [184]. A company named PuRxCell™

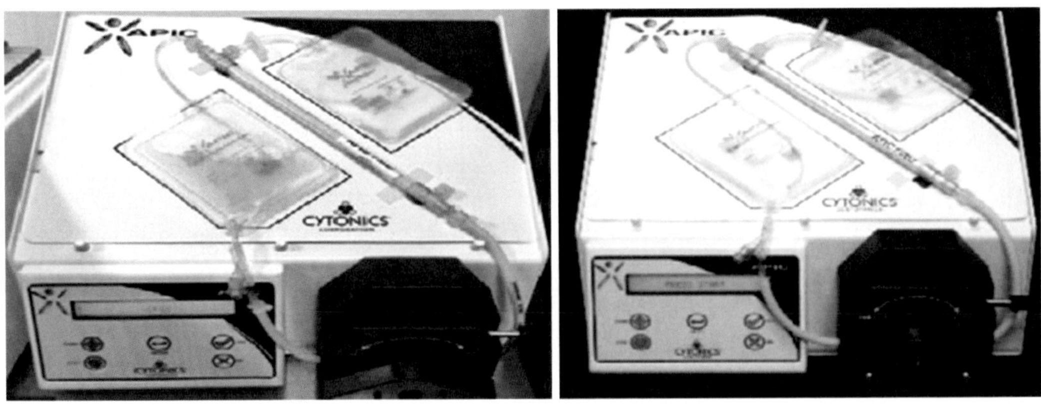

Fig. 14.14 Cytonics Corporation (Jupiter, FL, USA) processes alpha-2-macroglobulin (6× concentration) from autologous blood using an Autologous Platelet Integrated Concentration (APIC™) System

located at 200 Glades Road, Boca Raton, Florida prepares PuRx-A2M kits. This company uses rapid platelet-poor plasma (PPP) ultrafiltration processing kit to be able to extract α2-macroglobulin (Fig. 14.15). This preparation is primarily used for peripheral nerve injuries with associated neuropathic pains acting against the proinflammatory cytokines such as TNF-α, IL-1β, and IL-6. This is also used for degenerative joint diseases [134]. Research is underway to be able to understand better its specific mechanisms on peripheral nerve injuries and the dramatic success especially when it is injected in affected nerves in an entrapment, age-related, and metabolic neuropathies using ultrasound-guided hydrodissection procedures.

Interleukin-1 Receptor Antagonist Protein (IRAP)

Due to the proinflammatory cytokines that predominate an inflammatory process, such as TNF-α and IL-1β in the joints and peripheral nerves, there was a growing interest in addressing how these cytokines can be inhibited to counteract a degenerative process. Interleukin-1 receptor antagonist (IL-1ra) protein is a naturally occurring modulator of inflammatory and immune response and is an important therapeutic cytokine that acts as a receptor-binding antagonist against IL-1a and IL-1b [185]. The amino acid sequence of IL-1ra is said to be 26% identical to IL-1β [186]. By binding to the IL-1 receptor, IL-1 acti-

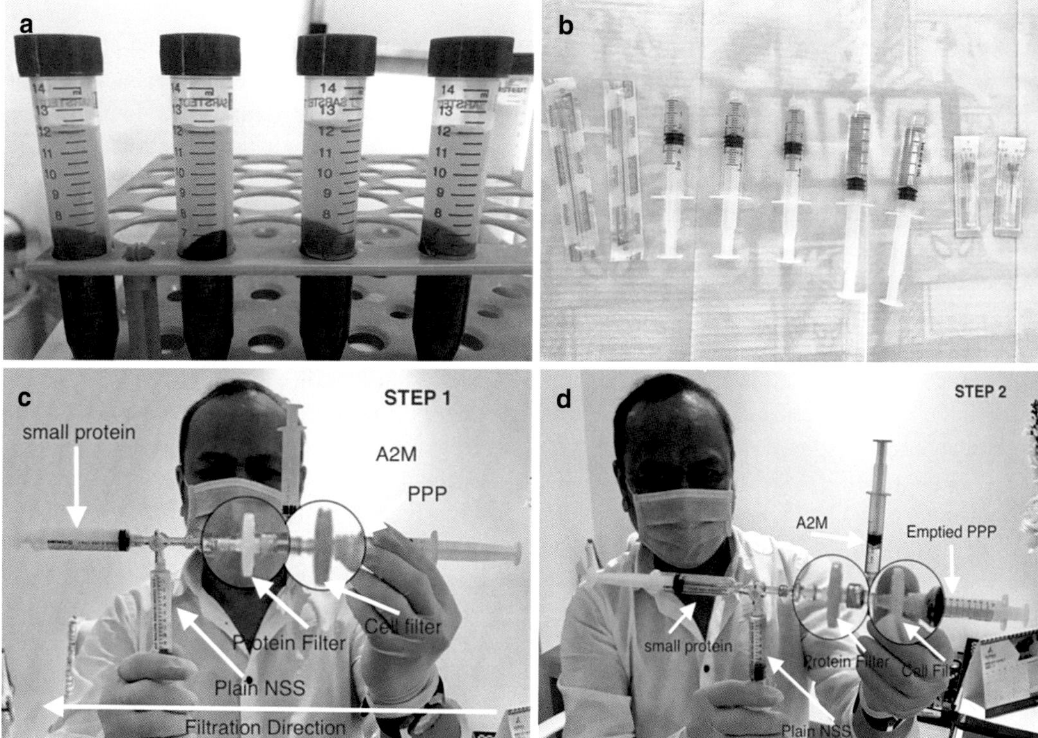

Fig. 14.15 Preparing an A2M solution (PuRxCell): (**a**) Platelet-poor plasma (PPP) is extracted from about 40 cc of venous peripheral blood. (**b**) A total of about 8 cc of A2M is extracted from PPP. (**c**) Using the PuRxCell technology, PPP is filtered passing through two separate filters: the first one is a cellular filter that filters out cellular elements as it is gently pushed to the opposite side, and the next one is a protein filter that filters in the alpha-2-macroglobulin (A2M) protein and filters out the smaller proteins. (**d**) After the filtration process, the stopcock in between filters is directed in such a way that the Plain NSS will push back the A2M trapped in the protein filter back to the designated syringe and the process is completed

vates the nuclear factor kappa B (NFκB) pathway, triggering the transcription of genes for proteins involved in the inflammatory process such as cytokines and prostaglandins [187]. It is also associated with activation of macrophages, monocytes, and stimulation of osteoclasts which subsequently breaks down the bone and cartilage matrix [188]. IL-1Ra is normally produced by monocytes or mononuclear cells which could be found at the synovial tissue and from keratinocytes [189, 190]. In fact, the IL-1Ra of the peripheral blood mononuclear cells (PBMCs) may be a useful marker for untreated early RA [187, 191]. There is an equilibrium that exists between IL-1 and IL-1Ra which maintains a healthy balance in the tissues of the joints under normal circumstances. During an inflammatory process, TNF-α is thought to have a role in early RA, while IL-1, being a more potent cytokine, will shift the equilibrium, and thus, a catabolic process ensues with subsequent destruction of the cartilage inside the joint associated with bone erosion [192, 193].

The IL-1 family consists of two inflammatory agonists namely IL-1α and IL-1β and one naturally occurring interleukin-1 receptor antagonist (IL-1Ra). The two inflammatory agonists bind to the same signaling receptor and exert comparable biological effects on target cells. In vivo, however, IL-1β is actively secreted and functions as an extracellular cytokine while most of the IL-1α is not processed to its mature form and remains intracellular. Two different cell-surface receptors are available for IL-1 – type I (IL-1RI) and type II (IL-1RII) [193]. IL-1RI is responsible for transducing the IL-1 signal to the cell [194]. With its long cytoplasmic tail, it binds with IL-1 by forming a complex with IL-1 accessory protein (IL-1AcP). This bond activates a series of intracellular phosphorylation events amplifying the IL-1 signal and dictating the specific response of the cell [195]. On the other hand, the type II (IL-1RII) receptor with its short cytoplasmic tail only serves as a decoy molecule that binds with IL-1 and locally titrates its activity [196]. As discussed earlier, IL-1Ra is a competitive inhibitor of IL-1. IL-1Ra preferentially binds with type I (IL-1RI) without the stimulatory activity we see in IL-1. Once bound, it simply prevents the IL-1 from interacting with IL-1AcP, thus impeding the signaling capacity of the receptor [193, 197]. Nature however has endowed IL-1 the advantage of transducing a signal to the cell even in an extremely low concentration. It has been calculated that even with a 5% IL-1 availability, full biological response can already be triggered. This means that an excessively high amount of IL-1Ra must be available to inhibit the actions of IL-1, which is at least 10–100 times the concentration of IL-1 [193, 198].

The therapeutic efficacy of a recombinant molecule of IL-1Ra named anakinra, derived from *Escherichia coli*, has been evaluated to treat RA. It is available in combination with methotrexate and is approved by the US Food and Drug Administration for the treatment of rheumatoid arthritis and is marketed as Kineret. It is self-administered subcutaneously at a daily dose of 100 mg [199]. In the European Monotherapy Study, which is a 24-week, placebo-controlled, randomized, double-blind, multicenter study, the safety and efficacy of anakinra at 150 mg per day was examined. The study revealed that 43% of patients who took 150 mg/day achieved a clinical response (ACR20) compared with 27% of the placebo group. It showed a superior response in RA for several indices of disease including the number of swollen joints, number of tender joints, Health Assessment Questionnaire, erythrocyte sedimentation rate (ESR), and C-reactive protein (CRP). Clinical responses (via ACR20) were noted to occur after 2 weeks of therapy [200]. Radiologic images also confirmed a statistically significant improvement in joint space narrowing and several joint erosions as compared to placebo at 24- and 48-week follow-up. Further, the improvement was stable both clinically and radiologically even up to 76 weeks [193, 200] of anakinra therapy. Consequently, the rate of bone erosions is reduced as treatment is continued. This treatment can be singly or in combination with methotrexate is well tolerated and is safe for patients with RA [201], although the frequency of serious infection was slightly higher with its use which is about 2.1% [202]. A newer drug such as canakinumab shares a similar effect with anakinra, and the safety and efficacy of both the drugs on prolonged usage against RA remain elusive [203].

The possible beneficial effects of anakinra in osteoarthritis do not extend for more than a month due to its limited persistence in the joint space when injected intraarticularly. It could however dampen pain and swelling in an erosive OA of the hand [204–207].

Autologous Conditioned Serum (ACS)

Autologous conditioned serum (ACS) has been developed in 1998 and used clinically to treat OA, RA, and spine disorders. ACS is prepared from peripheral white blood cells by initially drawing 60 ml of peripheral venous blood and then placed into a syringe containing glass beads with $CrSO_4$ to initiate monocyte activation. The specimen is incubated for 24 h at 37 °C and blood is recovered, clarified by centrifugation, filtered, and returned to the patient. The resulting autologous is now selectively enriched for anti-inflammatory cytokines IL-1Ra, IL-4, and IL-10 and returned to the patient. ACS is injected six times over a 21-day period, with each 2 ml solution injected into the knee joints [199, 208–210]. For epidural use, 1 ml each for 3 injections was injected over a 21-day period [199]. This product is marketed as Orthokine (Orthokine, Dusseldorf, Germany) in a Good Manufacturing Process (GMP) facility [199]. Since IL-1β is active at low concentrations, it is important that a minimum ratio of 1:10 (IL-1β to IL-1Ra) is required to inhibit IL-1β activity [193, 211]. This process also produces other beneficial growth factors and cytokines embedded in ACS such as vascular endothelial growth factors (VEGF), platelet-derived growth factors (PDGF) AB, hepatocyte growth factor (HGF), insulin-like growth factor-1 (IGF-1), fibroblast growth factor-2 (FGF-2), and transforming growth factor (TGF) [199, 212]. ACS is based on studies that revealed that macrophages and monocytes are endogenous sources of IL-1Ra [199, 213, 214]. Other data showed however the presence of TNF-α in ACS [215].

Three studies on ACS showed conflicting results on OA. Auw Yang and colleagues formed the current cohort and found statistically significant improvement of Knee Injury and Osteoarthritis Outcome Score (KOOS) symptom and sport parameters. However, at 12-month follow-up, the expected clinical improvement was not achieved and thus the use of Orthokine could not be recommended [216]. In 2009, Baltzer and colleagues did a controlled clinical trial with an observer-blinded follow-up of 104 weeks after treatment with Orthokine. In this study, Orthokine showed a statistically significant improvement based on Patient Reported Outcome Measures (PROM) compared to saline and hyaluronic acid [217]. In 2010, an in vitro study was conducted by Rutgers and colleagues to investigate the effect of Orthokine on cartilage proteoglycan metabolism and cytokine production. The aim was to evaluate possible disease-modifying and chondroprotective effects. The study showed no difference between Orthokine and saline administration [215]. Although considered to be an option prior to arthroplasty, Orthokine still seemed to provide a potential treatment for patients suffering from degenerative joint diseases. With the predominance of inflammatory cytokines in advance cases, there is a need to then modify the approach of therapy toward the early stage of OA [218]. Other options such as α2-macroglobulin and mesenchymal stem cells as discussed earlier may offer better results. Strumper conducted an unblinded, uncontrolled retrospective cohort study to evaluate the effect of Orthokine in 47 patients with pain diagnosed with meniscal lesions. Results showed a significant reduction in knee pain but with no evidence of meniscal repair [219]. Another study was carried out in 2015 with 118 patients suffering from OA, whose chronic pain made them eligible for surgery, but who chose treatment with ACS and physiotherapy. By 24 months, all patients reported more than 60–80% improvement in pain with only one opting for a knee replacement [220]. In a subgroup analysis, ACS was found out to be effective regardless of age, weight, sex and disease grade highlighting its potential to address different sets of patient population [221].

Patients undergoing ACL reconstruction of the knee usually present with elevated pro-inflammatory cytokines, of which majority is IL-1β. In fact, there is evidence that IL-1β plays an important role in the pathogenesis of bone tunnel enlargement following ACL reconstruction. Studies have shown that IL-1β are elevated following that procedure and continue to be elevated several weeks thereafter [222–224]. In a study by Darabos and colleagues, it has been observed that IL-1β is increased up to 10 days postoperatively causing an osteoclastic activity following ACL injuries at the graft-bone tunnel interface. Application of ACS intraarticularly showed a healing effect on the ACL reconstruction of the knee with a decreasing level of IL-1β concentration. After 10 days, the values of IL-1β become equal or even below the concentration compared to the normal knee [222]. In a related study, Darabos and colleagues published a level 1 therapeutic randomized controlled trial study demonstrating that ACS reduced bone enlargement with four injections after ACL reconstruction [225].

The incidence of Achilles tendon rupture is about 18/10,000 and is commonly seen among middle-aged men who exercise. Surgical intervention is very common to treat the tendon. Novel intervention however is available to treat such a condition. A study done by Genc and colleagues showed that injection of ACS showed positive histopathological healing on day 15 and 30 and biomechanical healing on day 15 in rat Achilles tendon. ACS treatment is said to lower the collagen type 3 density by day 30 [226]. In a related study, Muller and colleagues showed the importance of paratenon in the Achilles tendon for the effective healing of an injured tendon. Growth factors cannot replace the absence of paratenon in the healing process as it is limited in restoring blood supply nor providing local progenitor cells [227]. Earlier studies by Majewski and colleagues among rat Achilles tendons showed that ACS-treated tendons showed a thicker tendon with more type 1 collagen and it presents with the accelerated recovery of tendon stiffness and maturity of repair tissue. However, it did not show any advantage as to its ability to withstand a load as compared to the untreated group [228].

Goni described the effect of ACS among 40 randomized patients with cervical disk herniation radiculopathy versus epidural application with methylprednisolone over a 6-month study period. Results showed gradual and sustained improvement among those treated with ACS, while those receiving steroids showed improvement initially but then showed deterioration over the 6-month study period [229]. A separate trial for patients with lumbar disk herniation radiculopathy comparing ACS against triamcinolone showed favorable responses in the ACS group for both pain and disability over a 6-month study period [230]. In a related study, Kumar and colleagues showed improvement among patients diagnosed with lumbar radiculopathy treated with ACS presenting with a 6-week duration of painful radiculopathy but with absent motor deficits, no epidural injections done 3 months prior, and no opioids given 6 months prior to intervention [231].

One of the most common sport injuries is muscle contusion followed by muscle strain. The presence of a muscle strain, however, takes a toll on an athlete, limiting his/her ability to return to sports or if severe enough also affecting his/her full recovery. In a study by Wright-Carpenter and colleagues, the use of ACS was evaluated in second-degree muscle strains based on MRI findings. Due to its inherent capacity to contribute specific growth factors which are essential for muscle regeneration, ACS was used in this experimental study using a control against Actovegin/Traumeel. Results showed a faster recovery time in the ACS group which was also confirmed by MRI with an observed acceleration of the lesion [232]. In another study, this time on muscle contusion done with mice, Wright-Carpenter and colleagues assessed ACS in stimulating growth factors to improve the proliferative activity of myogenic precursor cells. Mice were subjected to experimental contusion injury at the gastrocnemius muscle. One group received ACS at 2 hours, 24 hours, and 48 hours post-injury against a control group that received saline injections. The histology results showed that satellite cell activation at 30/48 hours post-injury was accelerated and the diameter of the regenerating myofibers was increased during the first week as compared with the saline control group. ELISA results confirmed an elevation of fibroblast growth factor (FGF-2) (460%) and transforming growth factor-β1 (TGF-β1) (82%) as compared to controls. The study concluded the advantage of ACS in reducing the time of recovery from muscle injury [233].

Specific Regenerative Interventions uUnder Ultrasound Guidance

In this section, I will discuss which regenerative interventions will be appropriate and for what indications. I will also include some techniques on how to approach it under ultrasound guidance. I will not include all musculoskeletal areas as they will be discussed separately and elaborately in some parts of this book. Hopefully, this approach will help readers and practitioners choose the right regenerative interventions based on scientific clinical evidence. As this field is still evolving, I expect that some indications will continue to change over the years as we continue to understand the specific roles of each regenerative intervention with newer techniques and newer regenerative procedures discovered and studied.

Joints

Among the most common indications for doing regenerative injection therapy is osteoarthritis. About 10% of men and 13% of women over 60 years of age show a certain degree of symptomatic knee [1, 234]. The total cost of total knee arthroplasty is about US$57,000 with a mortality rate of approximately 0.25% and post-op complications ranging from deep vein thrombosis, infection, and chronic pain [235]. With the projected increase of about 601% by 2030 annually for a total knee replacement, it is imperative that we have a clearer understanding of the different factors contributing to its development together with an earlier and better detection to lower its progression [236]. On the other hand, non-surgical treatments such as physical therapy, anti-inflammatory, and analgesics medications have all modest and short-term efficacy at best [237]. Such is the need to find new, effective, and sustainable ways of treating osteoarthritis.

Different regenerative treatments are available for treating osteoarthritis, the most common of which is platelet-rich plasma (PRP) therapy (Fig. 14.16). Depending on the platelet concentration, it could be an autologous conditioned plasma (ACP) where the platelet concentration is about two- to threefold greater than baseline or a platelet-rich plasma where the platelet concentration is about four- to sixfold greater than baseline [238]. Leucocyte concentrations of the PRP are further subdivided into leucocyte rich (LR) or leucocyte poor (LP) depending on the concentration of granulocyte or neutrophil but with high mononu-

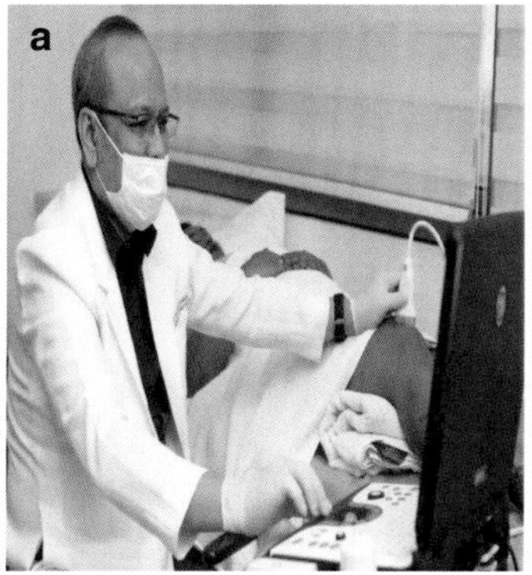

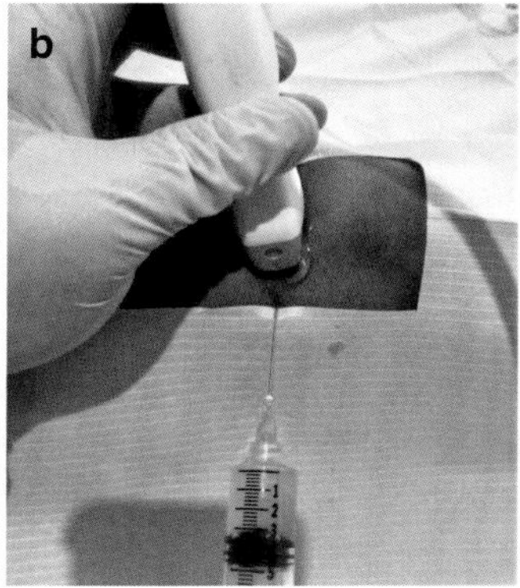

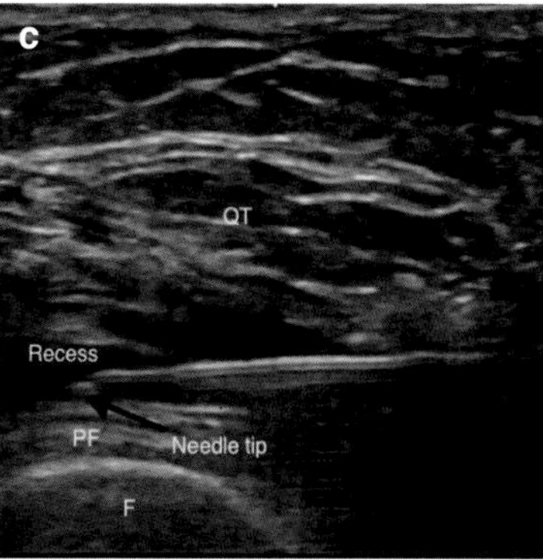

Fig. 14.16 Ultrasound-guided joint injection of the knee. (**a**) Planning the approach for ultrasound-guided injection of the knee. (**b**) Ultrasound-guided injection of the knee, in-plane to the probe but short axis to the knee at the level of the suprapatellar recess, lateral to medial approach. (**c**) Needle is slowly inserted into the suprapatellar recess with the bevel of the needle facing upward. Ensure that the ultrasound probe is parallel to the needle during the needle injection. QT quadriceps tendon, PF prefemoral fat pad, F femur

clear cell concentration [238, 239]. Bone marrow concentrate (BMC) and its MSCs with or without PRP is another option. Moreover, adipose-derived stem cells (ADSC) with or without cellular expansion or ADSC which requires collagenase for enzymatic digestion are an equally important option [238]. Autologous chondrocyte transplantation which is another option for a focal defect OA has showed limitations in its effectivity and necessitates the development of a new treatment paradigm for it to be useful [240].

Chang and colleagues published a level 1 systematic review and meta-analysis showing the effectiveness of PRP over hyaluronic acid (HA) and the results showed that patients with less severe OA achieved a superior outcome than those with advanced OA [241]. Riboh and colleagues in 2015 performed a level 1 meta-analysis comparing LR-PRP and LP-PRP. This study did not show any statistical difference between LR-PRP and LP-PRP, although LP-PRP treatment is ranked the highest based on the WOMAC (Western Ontario and McMaster Universities Osteoarthritis Index) and IKDC (International Knee Documentation Committee) scores [242]. The decrease in pain and improved functional status for knee OA because of PRP injection, however, showed a consistent decline in improvement 12 months after injection based on the systematic review done by Souzdalnitski and colleagues adding that the decline is still better than the pre-injection scores [243]. A combination treatment of PRP and injectable HA hydrogel in a study done by Yan and colleagues showed hyaline-like cartilage (type II collagen) without formation of hypertrophic cartilage in a porcine model evaluated at 6-month period [244]. Dallari and colleagues have shown favorable outcomes of PRP in hip joint OA as compared to HA, based on the visual analog scale, WOMAC, and Harris Hip Score with 1-, 3-, and 6-month follow-ups but not at 12 months [245]. Singh and colleagues in a retrospective analysis of 36 patients showed that those with Kellgren-Lawrence grade 1 and grade 2 hip OA responded to PRP at 6 months with 86% and 82% pain relief, respectively [246].

Adipose stem cells (ASC) exhibit a superior ability than bone marrow stem cells (BMSC) in differentiating into cartilage tissue [247]. Therefore, ASCs differentiate into cartilage cells and fill the defects in the cartilage as well as treat OA. Exosomes in the ASC acting as paracrine mediators help treat OA by downregulating TNF-α, IL-6, PGE_2, and nitrogen monoxide which cause inflammatory response and thus prevent cartilage degradation. Cho and colleagues in their recent study on knee OA showed a decrease in pain, improved joint range, and decreased defect size in the short term after directly injecting the joint using a combination of ASC and PRP. No enhanced recovery however was seen in a 1-year and 2-year follow-ups [248]. Infrapatellar fat pad (IPFP)-derived stem cell is also an excellent source for cartilage regeneration with an easy harvesting access [249].

Bone marrow stem cell (BMSC) is another great source of treatment for OA. Shapiro and colleagues in a randomized controlled trial compared the effects of BMAC with saline in OA using VAS and ICOAP constant pain and ICOAP Intermittent pain scores during pre-injection, 1-week, 3-month, and 6-month period on the knee. The study showed significant pain reduction from pre-injection pain scores [250]. Bone marrow stem cells were used in the knee by Centeno and colleagues with signficant improvement in pain as shown in the outcomes scores. No added benefit therefore was noticed when lipoaspirate was added. Females tend to benefit from pain and functionality and those with higher body mass index reported improvement in function [251]. Thus, the most common source of MSCs right now is BMAC for OA. Adipose with its enzymatic process producing SVF is not allowed by the FDA [252]. Also, another advantage of BMAC is its low oxygen tension which is advantageous for bone marrow stem cell induction activity for chondrocytes which is kept at 2–3% oxygen tension [253]. In a study by Kokubo and colleagues, greater proliferation by chondrocytes in the joint was noted when the oxygen tension is at 2% which is the same environment deep within the cartilage as compared with the ambient environment (21% oxygen tension). Normally, the joint has an oxygen tension of 10% at the surface and 2% at the deep layer close to the bone [254].

Pro-inflammatory cytokines originating from synviocytes of the synovial layer inside the joint, chondrocytes in the cartilage, and leucocytes that infiltrate during the inflammatory process may be found in OA. In the early stages of inflammation, TNF-α and IL-1β cause a cascade of reactions which in turn release the chemokines and neurotrophic factors that cause additional pain and inflammation [161]. It is for this purpose that α2-macroglobulin is used to counteract the effects of pro-inflammatory cytokines [134, 141] and inhibit matrix metalloproteinases from the damaged cartilage [140].

Among the exercise for the knee joint, joint distraction seemed to be the most plausible technique for enhancing chondrocyte regeneration using a pull traction device. It was found out that it promoted cartilage repair of osteochondral defects in weight-bearing joints [255].

Joint Injection Technique

The use of either ultrasound or fluoroscopy is a vital tool in ensuring that the area being targeted is correctly injected and that the solution reaches the area appropriately (Fig. 14.17).

For regenerative treatment to have its optimal and beneficial effect, mild to moderate joint degeneration with fibrocartilage tears and degeneration is warranted. Severe osteoarthritis associated with osteophyte formation causing bony impingement and osteocartilagenous loose bodies with loss of range of motion is contraindicated [256]. Ideally, physical therapy should precede any regenerative procedures to improve the range of motion and muscle is reeducated. A separate chapter in this book will discuss the details of injection in every joint.

Tendons and Ligaments

Tendons are tissues that are interposed between muscles and tendons containing highly specialized cells and a unique structure composed of long type 1 collagen fibrils (70–80%) and a few elastic fibers. Most of the cells are made up of highly metabolically active fibroblasts called tenoblast which over time mature into less metabolically active tenocytes [257]. Collectively, these cells comprise 90–95% of the cells in the tendons. An abundant extracellular matrix made up of glycosaminoglycans and proteoglycans surrounds the collagen and tenocytes. Tendons are maintained by a dynamic interaction between matrix metalloproteinases (MMPs) and their inhibitors. Cytokines, mechanical load, and sys-

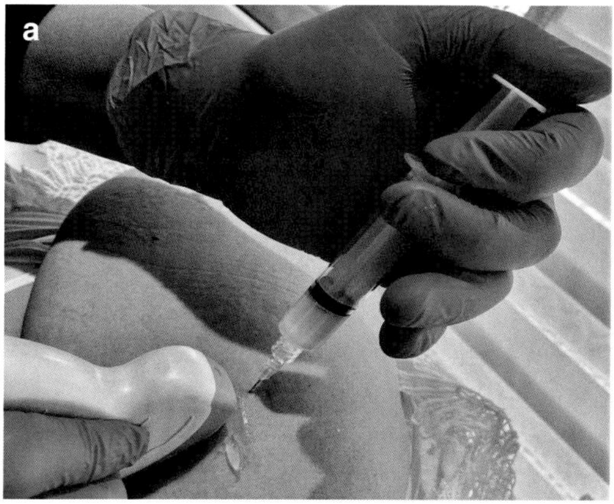

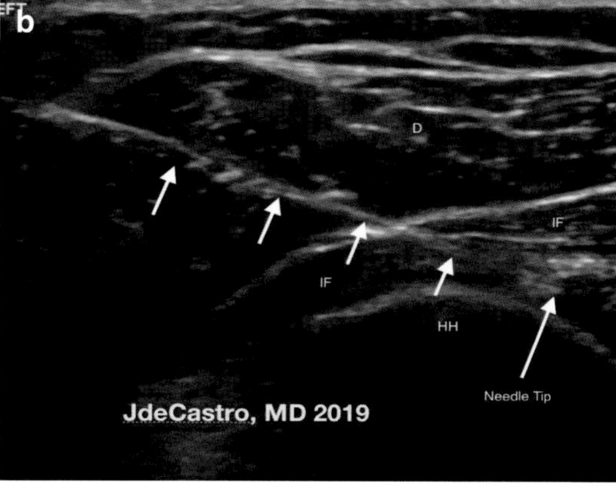

Fig. 14.17 Ultrasound-guided injection of the posterior glenohumeral joint of the shoulder. (**a**) Patient is positioned in lateral decubitus position with the shoulder to be injected in adducted and retracted position. A linear ultrasound is used and positioned just below the spine of the scapula with the probe tilted to visualize the entry of the needle. Needle is injected from lateral to medial approach, in-plane with the probe. (**b**) Needle is injected from lateral to medial, in about 45° angle targeting the posterior glenohumeral joint. D deltoid, IF infraspinatus muscle and tendon, HH humeral head

temic conditions affect the tendon environment [258]. When this balance is disrupted due to injuries or trauma, there is tendon inflammation, tendinopathy, or tendon injury, all of which can cause pain. Remodeling of tendon after an injury usually takes 2 years to complete healing, but full tendon regeneration is never completed [259]. Sedentary individuals surprisingly have a higher level of proinflammatory factors such as TNFα, IL-1β, VEGF, and low levels of collagen-1. This in turn stimulates an increase of MMPs (MMP-2, MMP-9, and MMP-13) activity with the onset of low state of inflammation resulting in a higher risk of tendon rupture [260]. Inflammation appears to be strongly influenced by exercise in animal models [261, 262]. This highlights the role of early mobilization (about 3–7 days) in injured tendons. Without inflammation, the healing process and the subsequent changes that characterize chronic inflammation (>12 weeks) cannot take place. Therefore, exercise still represents one of the best ways to influence tendon healing [263, 264]. Early physical therapy with eccentric and concentric exercise after tendon injury or surgery is strongly recommended [259]. Caution, however, should be observed when stretching the tendons as their elasticity is lost and becomes more rigid because of inflammation, which is why exercise at this point becomes more challenging [265]. The ruptured force of healed tendons is only 56.7% of normal tendons [266]. Further, healed tendon also has 80% of normal tendon strength, 80% of normal tendon stiffness, 40% of normal tendon stress [267].

Like tendons, ligaments are made up of type I collagen, which is usually densely packed and cross-linked and therefore provides stability and strength to this structure [268]. It is also relatively avascular with little innate ability for healing [269]. The ligament has a lower percentage of collagen as compared to tendon but has a higher percentage of elastin, proteoglycans, and water [270]. In a ligamentous injury, fibroblasts during the proliferative phase synthesize collagen III rather than type I but with a lesser volume during this phase of healing [271]. Like tendons, the fibroblast in ligaments is also responsible for the synthesis of collagen, proteoglycan, and other components of the extracellular matrix. This collagen synthesis continues up to the remodeling phase. Type I collagen increased its production during the modeling phase which usually occurs 6 weeks following the injury. It is aligned in the direction of stress until it is fully matured and usually would last for a year [272]. Ligamentous laxity is part of the consequence of ligamentous injury during the healing phase. There is greater stress relaxation as was shown in an experimental study of the medial collateral ligament and which will ultimately lead to posttraumatic osteoarthritis of the joint [268], especially among athletes. The joint instability resulting from the ligament injury together with the shear motion in the joint surfaces is the primary factor that causes osteoarthritis [273].

Platelet-rich plasma (PRP) therapy is one of the most common regenerative interventions used for tendon and ligament injuries. PRP-treated structures showed better collagen organization and increased metabolic activity, histologically [274]. Sanchez and colleagues showed excellent results for midportion tendinopathy injection as compared to only good results in insertional tendinopathy [275]. A recent meta-analysis by Hurley and colleagues examined 18 randomized controlled trials comparing PRP to arthroscopic repair alone of a rotator cuff injury with 1147 patients. The study showed that patients treated with PRP had significantly decreased rates of incomplete tendon healing for small-medium and medium-complete tears. They also found out that the visual analog scale for PRP-treated patients was low at 30 days and final follow-up as compared to the control group [276]. Liddle and colleagues in a systematic review done on the patellar tendon showed an overall improvement in pain and function with 81% of patients able to return to their pre-symptom level of activity [277]. Lateral epicondylitis is one of the most common areas being studied for PRP treatments. In a recent systematic review by Ben-Nafa and colleagues, PRP showed a slower onset of efficacy as compared with steroids. PRP, however, showed a longer-lasting clinical effect as compared with steroids that lasted up to 2 years [278]. The kind of PRP preparation also matters in this treatment. Mishra and colleagues found that leucocyte-rich PRP yielded better long-term results than the local anesthetic injection and dry needling for tendinopathy [279]. In fact, Fitzpatrick and colleagues in a systematic review and meta-analysis study showed the advantage of using leucocyte-rich PRP for tendinopathies under ultrasound guidance with a single injection [280].

No randomized controlled trial is available for injuries affecting the ulnar collateral ligament of the elbow using PRP. Surgery provides 83–90% success rate for a complete ulnar collateral ligament injury and a return to play for 9–12 months post-surgery [281]. Other than the conservative treatments for partial ulnar collateral ligament injury, PRP holds promise as a possible treatment for the elbow. In a study by Dines and colleagues, PRP showed 73% success rate among baseball players treated due to partial UCL injury and a return to play in 12 weeks [282].

Sports injury on the knee with anterior cruciate ligament tear (ACL) is usually treated with surgery to restore functionality. PRP can be incorporated during an ACL surgery, but studies show that they found no significant effect with no difference in healing at the intraarticular portion of the ACL on MRI at 12 months [283]. However, in a partial ACL injury, Di Matteo and colleagues in a systematic review that between 70% and 85% of PRP-treated partial ACL injury patients return to their previous level of activity without surgery [284]. In another recent study by Walters and colleagues, there was no difference noted in kneeling pain after a bone-patellar-bone-tendon (BPTB) autograft ACL reconstruction with intra-operative administration of PRP [285]. There are varied results in PRP efficacy in tendons and ligaments, and one way to address this difference is to standardized preparation of PRP, in terms of composition, quantity, and frequency to optimize results to induce maximal amount of healing [286]. Despite its promise effect, we are yet to see a definitive proof of efficacy in ligaments and tendons healing when using PRP. Multiple factors contribute to this issue such as varied formulations from different physicians and peculiar ways of isolating PRP from different vendors. With its low risk during the treatment, it remains a viable conservative treatment [287].

Mesenchymal stem cells (MSCs) from bone marrow or adipose tissue are another option for tendon and ligament regenerative recovery. They have been shown to indirectly stimulate tissue repair by secreting trophic factors which activate residual recipient cells or modulate local immune response. MSCs rarely if ever contribute to tissue regeneration [287, 288].

The more recent approach for tendon and ligament regenerative treatment is the use of tissue-engineered approach where MSCs are seeded into a scaffold prior to implantation or the use of culture method where MSCs are cultured on a scaffold in vitro to produce a neotendon before they are implanted into an injured tissue. This approach provides a mechanical support to the injured structure. The scaffold provides mechanical stability and 3D template for regenerative tissue growth. To augment ligament and tendon healing, PRP or growth factors are incorporated into the scaffold. The following are parameters to ensure an effective administration of regenerative products through tissue engineering and this includes the choice of cells, quantity of cell delivered, type of growth factor, drug delivery system, and type of biologically active molecules and scaffold. The goal of tissue-engineered substitute is to provide a temporary functional tissue while awaiting the natural regenerative process to set in [272, 287]. Another good source of stem cells comes from tendon-derived stem cells (TDSCs) or endogenous ligament-derived stem cells (LDSCs) [287]. Some studies refer to this as a resident tendon stem/progenitor cell (TSPCs). But even if they have potential for tissue regeneration in vitro, it is unclear why TSPCs do not regenerate tendon under normal conditions [289]. They have been found out, however, to have superior tenogenic capacity in vitro with superior tendon healing as compared with MSCs. These types of stem cells however have limited supply. Leong and colleagues in their review note that despite this progress, the only accepted treatments to date are still surgery and physical therapy [287]. Previous studies by Mautner and

Blazuk also confirmed conflicting results with regard to the use of stem cell in muscle, ligaments, and tendons [290].

Ultrasound-Guided Injection of the Tendon and Ligaments

Ultrasound-guided injection of the tendon and ligaments provides a precision-guided intervention to ensure that the needle is correctly placed, the injured tissues are accurately targeted, vital structures are avoided and adverse side effects are prevented (Fig. 14.18). Ultrasound plays a major role in demonstrating the pathophysiologic state of a tendon or ligament. A high-resolution ultrasound can display the different phases of healing with its detectable echo density and echogenic changes and can further check the integrity of the tendons and ligaments by performing dynamic imaging [268, 291, 292]. Often the use of power Doppler imaging can help identify the inflammatory status of the tendons with signs of hyperemia and color Doppler during injection to avoid injecting vital neurovascular structures [293].

When injecting a tendon under ultrasound guidance diagnosed with tendinosis, patients are treated by injecting into the tendon sheath (Fig. 14.19). In the case of an A1 pulley where it is diagnosed with acute stenosing tenosynovitis (trigger finger), the purpose of the injection is to minimize inflammation and to reduce pain. For other solutions like steroids, it is important that direct tendon injection must be avoided to prevent secondary damage to the tendon [294]. However, PRP solution can be injected directly through the intratendinous substance [295].

Muscle Injuries

Muscle injuries are quite common among athletes, the most common of which is muscle strain representing 12–16% [296]. One-third of these athletes will usually suffer any one of the muscle injuries in their lifetime with the lower extremity representing 92% of all these injuries [1, 297]. In a 12-year study of the European professional soccer leagues, injuries occurred in these four muscle groups: the hamstrings, hip adductors, quadriceps, and calf muscles in decreasing order [298]. Hamstring injuries being the most injured muscle of the lower extremity have a reinjury rate of about 12–21% [299] with some studies reporting as high as 39% within the same season [1].

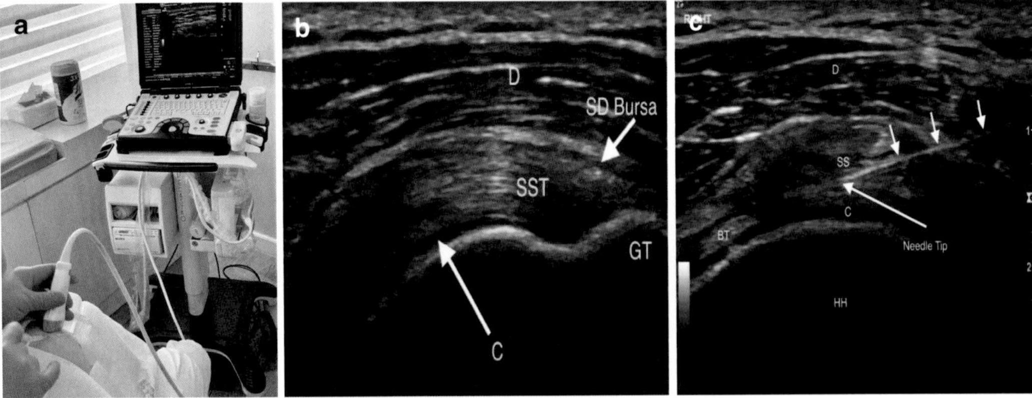

Fig. 14.18 Ultrasound-guided injection of the supraspinatus tendon. (**a**) The patient is in a sitting position with her right shoulder in a modified Crass position. An ultrasound probe is positioned in a coronal oblique plane, a short axis to the supraspinatus tendon. (**b**) Normal long-axis ultrasound image of the supraspinatus tendon (SST) inserted into the greater tuberosity (GT) of the humerus. (**c**) The shoulder of the patient is in modified Crass position. An ultrasound probe is in a coronal oblique plane with the needle approaching from superolateral to inferomedial direction targeting the supraspinatus tendon. D deltoid, SS supraspinatus tendon, C cartilage, GT greater tuberosity, SD bursa subdeltoid bursa, BT biceps tendon

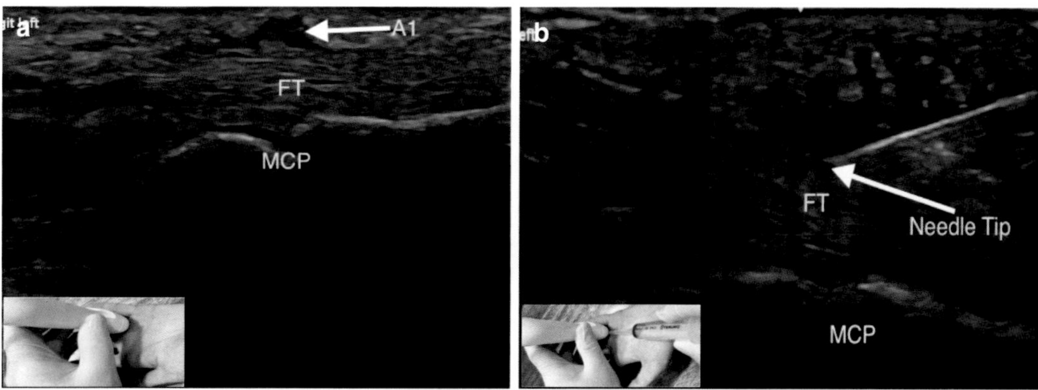

Fig. 14.19 Ultrasound-guided injection of the A1-pulley of the 4th digit. (**a**) Hypoechoic swelling of the A1 pulley of the flexor tendon at the level of the metacarpophalangeal joint. (**b**) Ultrasound-guided injection of the A1-pulley and flexor tendon sheath, in-plane approach, long axis to the flexor tendon using PRP

In a muscle injury, two subsequent stages of responses are observed at the muscle level. In the first phase, which is referred to as degeneration, a given muscle injury leads to death at the cellular level. There is increased permeability of the sarcolemma of affected myofibers with subsequent release of cytokines. These cytokines can stimulate immune and inflammatory cells into the area which is primarily made up of neutrophils during the acute stage and subsequently followed by macrophages (M1) after 48 hours. These early macrophages (M1) stimulate inflammatory cytokines such as TNF-α, IL-1β, and interferon gamma (IFN-γ). These cytokines increase cell proliferation and satellite cell activation. This initial inflammatory response is followed by the proliferation of M2 macrophages. It is in this second phase that these macrophages (M2) are associated with tissue repair and satellite cell differentiation. It ultimately suppresses inflammation and phagocytizes unwanted debris from the necrotic muscles [300]. In the second phase, macrophages (M2) play an active role by secreting cytokines that activate muscle cell precursors to repair the damaged tissues. Examples of these cytokines include fibroblast growth factor (FGFβ), transforming growth factor-β (TGF-β), IL-4, IL-10, and IL-6. These help in the growth and differentiation of muscle stem cells or activated myogenic cells. These precursor cells may include satellite cells and non-muscle stem cells. As it is activated, these cells proliferate and differentiate into myoblasts which are also stimulated by IL-4 and Il-10 in vitro. These myoblasts will eventually fuse with one another, replacing the injured muscle tissue [301]. Satellite cells are usually found between the plasma membrane and the basal lamina surrounding the muscle fibers and this plays a crucial role in the regeneration process. With each regeneration, these satellite cells return to a stage of quiescence until such time that it is needed again [302]. Other non-muscle stem cells are also capable of regeneration. Finally, when regeneration is fully completed, which is usually within a month, the new muscle cells are indistinguishable from existing mature muscle cells [303]. Interestingly, physical exercise promotes regeneration of muscle tissue through rebalance of M1 and M2, but at the same time increases their numbers by exercise [304, 305]. An exception to this type of regeneration is during a volumetric muscle loss (VML), which is usually secondary to combat injury, trauma such as in car accidents, tumor ablation, bone fracture fixation, and degenerative diseases [306]. This type of muscle injury is caused by a persistent functional deficit, and unlike other injuries which fully recover, untreated VML does not regain its full functional capacity [307]. To date, vascularized skeletal muscle tissue engineering and neural regeneration are used for VML treatment together with rehabilitative exercises [306]. A major deterrent in muscle regeneration is the predominance of fibrosis and dense scar formation which eventually leads to muscle contracture and chronic pain. Fibrotic lesion formations are stimulated by TGF-β of which its member, myostatin or otherwise called growth/differentiation factor-8, inhibits skeletal muscle maturation and persistent activation of inflammatory cells and cytokines [308]. A natural inhibitor of TGF-β including myostatin referred to as follistatin was found in animal models which promotes an increased muscle mass [309]. Another interesting case is a denervated muscle tissue where the satellite cells begin to be depleted over 7 months post-injury. During the first few months after denervation, satellite cells usually increased in number suggesting activation from the quiescent stage to a proliferative stage. However, by the seventh month post-denervation, the satellite cells decreased significantly. This satellite cell depletion then exacerbates muscle atrophy and worsens reinnervation. Wong and colleagues then proposed a reinnervation process and satellite cell transplantation process following 3-month denervation in mice models [310].

PRP for muscle injuries to regenerate muscle tissue and speed return to play provides minimal support based on the clinical evidence (Fig. 14.20). In a systematic review, Grassi and colleagues showed that the use of PRP did not promote muscle healing, and although the return to sport is shorter in the PRP group than the control group, there was no significant statistical difference noted considering that the clinical trials were regarded as very low in quality. Thus, there is a need for a larger number of high-quality trials [311]. Although these studies support the potential of PRP as a regenerative solution to treat muscle injuries, no clear benefit was seen in this retrospective study done by Sateyeshi and colleagues [312]. Rossi and colleagues in a randomized controlled trial however showed that a single PRP injection shortened the time to return to play after an acute grade 2 muscle injury when combined with physical rehabilitation [296].

A comparative study of bone marrow aspirate concentrate (BMAC) and PRP and its components by Ziegler and colleagues has shown the high concentration of IL-1Ra which is ideal for muscle strain treatment [232] followed by LR-PRP. They have suggested that in cases where vascularity and healing are desired for pathological or injured tissues, LR-PRP is a good choice due to the high concentration of PDGF, TGF-β, EGF, VEGF, and soluble CD40 ligand [313].

The mesenchymal stem cell is a good source of regenerative intervention. Intramuscular trans-

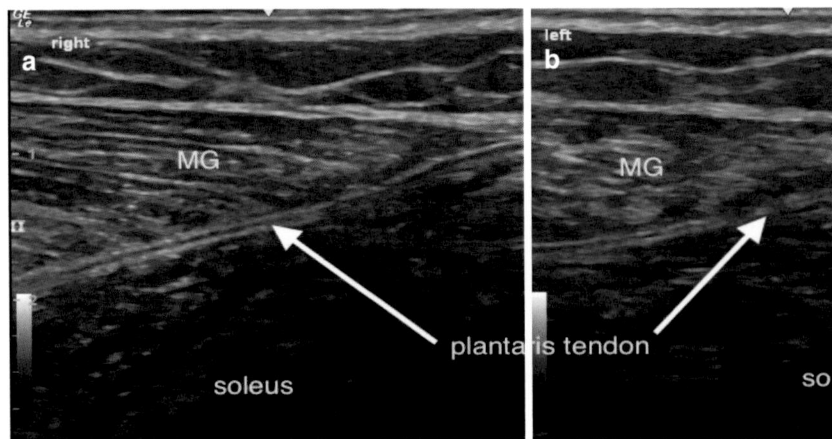

Fig. 14.20 Ultrasound of the medial gastrocnemius muscle. (**a**) Normal ultrasound image of the medial gastrocnemius muscle. Note the uniform "starry-night" appearance of the muscle fibers. (**b**) Ultrasound appearance of the affected side of a 44-year-old male with a history of calf pain after landing on one leg while playing basketball. He complained of persistent discomfort over the medial side of the calf muscle. The patient was given two sessions of PRP 2 weeks apart with complete relief after 1 month

plantation of human bone marrow-derived stem cells in dystrophic mice restored dystrophin expression, although it did not improve contractile function [314]. Another source is the muscle-derived MSCs that are administered intramuscularly. This technique shows an increase in Pax7 (marker of muscle satellite cells) satellite cell quantity, myofiber hypertrophy, and arteriogenesis in mouse hindlimb muscle [301]. Adipose-derived stem cells in contrast to human bone marrow stem cells showed myogenic potential in vitro and have greater myogenic differentiation, and thus aid in muscle regeneration by modulating the inflammatory and fibrotic process. With all that has been recommended, a successful strategy for muscle regeneration at present has yet to be found [315].

Ultrasound-Guided Injection of the Muscles

One of the most common muscle injuries that require ultrasound-guided regenerative injection therapy is the hamstring muscle. In one study by Hamid and colleagues, a single-blinded RCT has shown that PRP reduces pain over 10 weeks and reduces time to return to sports by 16 days for an acute hamstring partial tear [316]. A retrospective study by Park comparing PRP and steroid for grade 2 proximal hamstring injuries favors the efficacy of PRP in a short-term pain relief [317]. A single injection of PRP for grade 2 hamstring injuries among National Football League Players revealed a shorter time of retrun to play [318]. A recent, single-blinded, randomized controlled trial among 20 injured athletes with grade 2 hamstring injuries showed that PRP combined with physical rehabilitation has reduced time to return to play and increased the concentration of growth factors compared to physical rehabilitation alone [319]. In another study, however, by Manduca and colleague, a literature review showed no significant effect on return to play when using PRP compared to rehabilitation alone [320]. Similarly, a larger, double-blind RCT using single PRP injection with physical rehabilitation did not show any benefit as compared to physical rehabilitation alone to accelerate return to sport, improve muscle strength, or influence reinjury rates after 2 and 6 months among athletes after an acute hamstring injury [321]. In a retrospective study in 2020, among National Football League Players with grade 2 acute hamstring injuries, Bradley and colleagues showed that athletes who received leukocyte-poor PRP showed a faster return to play, although there is no significant difference in days missed or time to return to practice [322].

Ultrasound-guided injection of the hamstring muscle is very challenging because most of the major structures are deeply situated. To visualize the appropriate target muscle, a curvilinear probe is needed for better penetrance. It is also possible to initially use a curvilinear probe, and depending on the depth of the pathology, a shift to a linear high frequency probe could be used for superficial lesions. Both short- and long-axis scanning must be done first to ensure the dimension of the muscle injury. In the case of a hamstring injury, the most common area of pathology is usually found at the biceps femoris long head (BFlh) which usually happens during an eccentric contraction [323]. Initially, an examination of the affected part may not be possible due to the intensity of pain, although a palpable defect distal to the ischial tuberosity may be a clue. A large ecchymosis may appear only about 2–4 days after the injury [324]. When this occurs, it is important to evaluate the patient sonographically. More than half of the injuries are intramuscular, whose size and presence by ultrasound have not been shown to correlate with the prognosis of return to sports activity. An increase of echogenicity combined with fiber rupture, hemorrhage, and/or edema is the main sonographic finding. Ideally, 1–10 days are required to examine by ultrasound the injury since no abnormalities may be seen if the timing is too soon or too long [325]. Hall suggested a rational timing for doing an ultrasound of between 2 and 48 hours post-injury [326]. Theoretically, the size of the edema and bleeding will be increased during the first few hours/days after an injury and gradually normalized in subsequent days and weeks [325]. The most common location for hamstring injuries is at the midsubstance [327] typically at the proximal muscle-tendon junction of the long head of the biceps femoris (BFlh) as seen in the setting of excessive lengthening of the hamstrings [328].

Regenerative Treatments for Spinal Conditions

Spine conditions represent a significant burden upon aging populations. And even though they exist in the general population, a whole spectrum of spine conditions can have an impact on the mobility and quality of life of everyone. An injury of the intervertebral discs (IVD) may be the beginning of the end of the spine described as an IVD degeneration cascade. This structural wear alters the stability of the motion segment of the spine and consequently results in diseases affecting the disks, facets, and nerves in between the spine. As had been observed, this spine degeneration (IVD) can lead to degenerative disk disease (DDD), spinal stenosis, radiculopathy, disc herniation, facet joint arthropathy, instability, degenerative spondylolisthesis, and sacroiliac joint pain. Symptoms arising from these conditions may include axial back pain, neuropathic pains, or neurologic symptoms with loss of sensory and/or motor function [329, 330] (Fig. 14.21).

At least 90% of patients over 60 years old have degenerative disk change on imaging with a small minority requiring spine surgery highlighting the ubiquitous nature of this condition [331]. In 2005, the self-reported functional limitations due to neck and back pain are about 24.7% of the US population which is like other developed nations in Europe. In a recent report among Americans who have reported work disability, 30.3% stated that their disability was a function of neck and back problems [332]. Although imaging studies have found an association between IVD degeneration and severity of low back pain, not all individuals with IVD degeneration are symptomatic, and gradual progression of IVD degeneration is part of the aging process [330]. However, Jensen and colleagues observed that 3% of disc bulges and 38% of focal protrusions may resolve spontaneously. Broad-based disc protrusions, extrusions, and sequestrations showed a better prognosis with approximately 75–100% resolving spontaneously [333].

The intervertebral disk is composed of three structures namely the cartilaginous endplates, the nucleus pulposus, and the annulus fibrosus. It is the largest avascular tissue in the body and has a very extensive extracellular matrix with a paucity of cells with which to regenerate that matrix. It relies on passive diffusion from adjacent endplate vessels for nutrition, with resultant poor healing potential. The center of the disk has very low

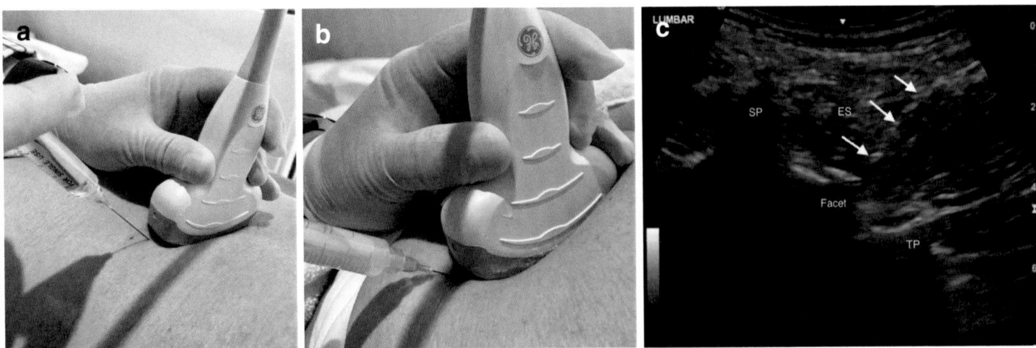

Fig. 14.21 Ultrasound-guided lumbar spine injection. (**a**) Anesthetic applied over the entry site prior to the injection of the regenerative injection therapy. (**b**) Ultrasound-guided injection over the facet joint at the L4L5 level. (**c**) Ultrasound image of the injection site (using A2M) at the L4L5 level facet joint using a curvilinear probe in a lateral to medial approach, in-plane to the probe but short axis to the lumbar spine. SP spinous process, TP transverse process, ES erector spinae

oxygen and glucose concentration and high lactate level resulting in a low pH [334–336]. The IVD is made up of an outer annulus fibrosus and a central nucleus pulposus. The outer annulus fibrosus is composed of tough lamellae of fibrous ring made from type I collagen fibers while the central nucleus pulposus consists of hydrophilic proteoglycan, elastin fibers, aggrecan, and type II collagen. The former provides tensile force resistance while the latter distributes the force radially during a compression [334, 337]. The functional cells within the nucleus pulposus produce the extracellular matrix (ECM) that binds to water. It is bounded superiorly and inferiorly by cartilaginous endplates which are securely attached to the vertebral bodies [334]. Bioactive proteins and growth factors participate in the maintenance of IVD. Transforming growth factor (TGF-β) is associated with the synthesis of collagen and proteoglycans, playing an important role in ECM accumulation. In fact, TGF-β is needed for endplate (EP) growth at the postnatal stage [338]. Bone morphogenetic protein (BMP), which belongs to TGF-β superfamily, promotes the proliferation and differentiation of multiple cell lines. Together with IVD cells, BMP increases the synthesis of proteoglycan, upregulates the mRNA expression of type II collagen, and serves as the mitotic agent of IVD [338, 339].

Intervertebral disk degeneration (IDD) with its non-healing annular fissures has been implicated as one of the major causes of chronic low back pain. With advanced aging, cartilaginous endplates have decreased permeability and blood supply leading to alterations in the microenvironment of IVD that favors catabolism. Changes characteristics of IDD include progressive loss of proteoglycans and water content leading to a less hydrated IVD and replacement of chondrocyte-like cells in the nucleus pulposus [336, 337, 340]. Collagen type I fibers in the inner annulus fibrosus and nucleus pulposus replaced the normal collagen type II. There is also an upregulation of proinflammatory cytokines from the IVD cells, such as IL-1 and TNF-α, which leads to an increased sensitization of the rich network of nerve fibers around the annulus fibrosus causing pain during normal activities of daily living [336, 337, 340]. The IL-1 and TNF-α expression increase matrix-degrading enzyme production while TNF-α stimulates nerve ingrowth [337]. The nerve endings' ingrowth extends into the annulus. They are unmyelinated nerve fibers and are susceptible to stromal changes, inflammatory mediators, and pain information along with the sensory nerve signals. Consequently, the abnormal spinal nerve can cause abnormal spastic pain signals inducing low back pains [341]. As IVD degenerates, the disc space height diminishes, with loading more pronounced posteriorly and consequently leads to asymmetric deformity, and then spinal stenosis sets in [337].

Factors that affect the degeneration process of the IVD include genetic factors, environmental factors, cigarette smoking, and biochemical factors. Surprisingly, 70% of this is caused by genetic factors [342, 343]. Studies indicate that a BMI > 25 mg/m^2 was an independent risk factor for degenerative disk disease (DDD), and obesity at a young age was a strong risk factor for future increases in the number of degenerated disks [342, 344]. It was also shown in another study that there is an increased IL-6 and proinflammatory cytokines among obese patients that could further contribute to disk degeneration [336, 344, 345]. From the biochemical standpoint, the early breakdown of aggrecan leads to loss of hydration of the disk which eventually leads to structural damage of the IVD over time. As degeneration progresses, the catabolic agents (MMPs, ADAMTS, HRTA1, etc.) and the inhibitors of anabolism (TGF-β) favor the extracellular matrix breakdown. This catabolic environment contributes to a degenerative cascade which in turn triggers the production of inflammatory mediators leading to further matrix degradation products. As the severity worsens over time, production of MMPs 1, 3, and 13 and ADAMTS-4 also increased [336]. A by-product of cartilage degeneration is referred to as fibronectin-aggrecan complex (FAC) and this can be used as biomarkers for degenerative disk disease and radicular symptoms from herniated nucleus pulposus [345]. FAC can further stimulate proinflammatory cytokines and release MMPs [140]. There is a positive predictive value for response to lumbar steroid injection when FAC is isolated in the epidural space [346].

Discogenic low back pain because of intervertebral disc (IVD) degeneration is usually chronic and persistent. IVD degeneration usually represents ≥40% of chronic low back pain [347]. Peng and colleagues in their prospective clinical study of 4 years showed that 68.8% of patients with chronic back pain did not show any change in pain and disability from their original pain. The study also showed a longer period of low back pain [348]. For herniated and bulging discs with signs of compressed nerves, a microdiscectomy is a favorable option. For patients requiring a complete IVD replacement either by fusion surgery or by total disc arthroplasty, challenges are on the horizon [349]. In a retrospective cohort study undergoing fusion surgery, the return-to-work rate was reported as 67% for non-treated patients compared to 26% of fusion-treated patients. Moreover, 27% of the fusion-treated patients required reoperation with 11% progressing to permanent disability compared to 2% in the non-surgical group [350]. With this background, a more comprehensive option must be considered with the goal of restoring and reestablishing a healthy IVD under a safe and effective intervention with long-term pain alleviation results (>6 months). With regenerative treatments, there is a need to focus on either stimulating the production of extracellular matrix or inhibiting the inflammatory cytokines that upregulate the matrix-degrading enzymes [337]. An agent that inhibits the formation of FAC will also be efficacious in the treatment of low back pain [346].

There is mounting evidence that PRP injected intradiscally for intervertebral disc degeneration, with its rich content of growth factors, may help injured and degenerative discs during the early stages of degeneration (Fig. 14.22). The remaining functional cells in the IVD once exposed to these growth factors will respond with proliferation and ECM accumulation, thus restoring the function and preserving the structure of the degenerated IVD. Several studies showed coherent evidence supporting the use of PRP intradiscally by fluoroscopic guidance, while at the same time preventing surgery [351–353]. Further studies also showed PRP to be effective in facet joint arthropathy, degenerative disc disease, and sacroiliac joint-related pain [354]. In a prospective, randomized, open-blinded endpoint study, they compare PRP with steroids among 40 patients with sacroiliac joint pain. The study showed that the PRP was more effective in 60% and 90% of patients, while steroids were effective in 75% and 25% of patients at 2 weeks and 3 months respectively [355]. A systematic review comparing PRP with posterior lumbar interbody fusion versus posterior lumbar interbody fusion in patients with low back pain showed lower low

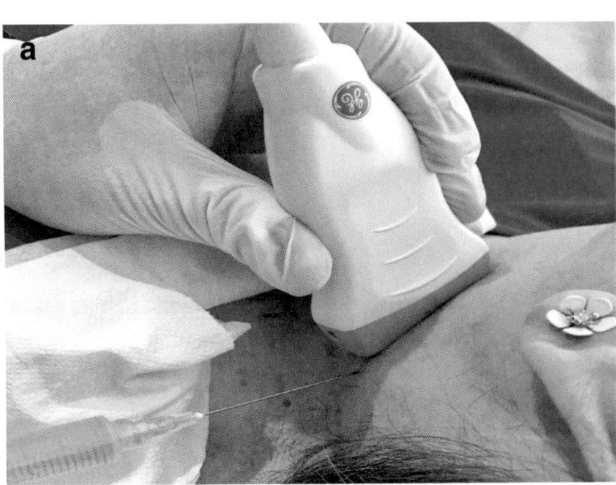

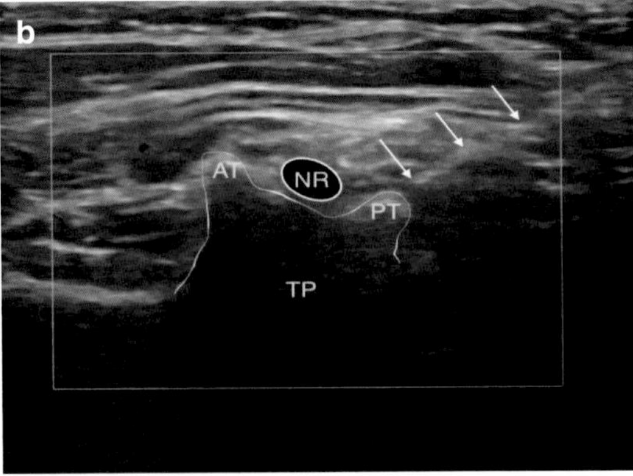

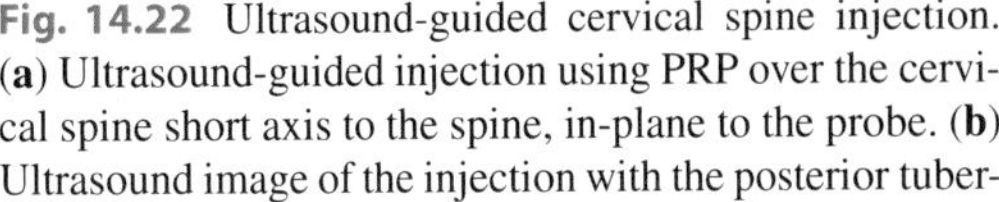
Fig. 14.22 Ultrasound-guided cervical spine injection. (**a**) Ultrasound-guided injection using PRP over the cervical spine short axis to the spine, in-plane to the probe. (**b**) Ultrasound image of the injection with the posterior tubercle as the reference toward the C6 nerve root using PRP. Note the needle tracking (white arrows) close to the posterior tubercle. AT anterior tubercle, PT posterior tubercle, TP transverse process, NR nerve root

back pain and faster bone union time among patients with PRP with autologous bone graft than autologous bone graft alone [356]. An in vitro study found that PRP can suppress the proinflammatory degrading cytokines (TNF-α AND IL-1) and its mediators in the nucleus pulposus cells, thereby stabilizing nucleus pulposus cell differentiation [357]. Further, the growth factors in PRP have confirmed their promising efficacy in the treatment of intervertebral disc degeneration by preserving water content, upregulating the expression of ECM, and maintaining disc height [338].

Alpha-2-macroglobulin (A2M) is a protease inhibitor native to plasma that may help prevent the formation of the fibronectin-aggrecan complex (FAC), which is a product of cartilage degradation, thus relieving low back pain in patients with degenerative disc disease (DDD) [346]. In the study by Montesano and colleagues, patients who are FAC+ within the disk, are more likely to demonstrate clinical improvement following intradiscal injection of autologous platelet-poor plasma rich in A2M [358]. This group of patients also responds with microdiscectomy from disc herniation and epidural steroid injection [182].

Since pain generators in low back pain can also arise from proinflammatory cytokines such as TNF-α, IL-1, and nerve growth factor (NGF), recent preclinical and clinical observations may lead to the development of biologic agents targeting these specific cytokines [359]. Disc degeneration with hypermobility or sometimes referred to as disc dynamic compression accelerates sensory innervation of lumbar IVD and increases the levels of proinflammatory cytokines (TNF-α, IL-6, IL-8, IL-1, NGF), thereby initiating a cascade of inflammatory reactions that causes low back pain [360, 361]. In addition, NGF promotes nerve ingrowth into the disc, sensitizes dorsal root ganglion (DRG) neurons, and causes neuronal sprouting into the dorsal horn. In fact, NGF is higher in painful discs [362]. The presence of nerve ingrowth into the pathological and degenerated IVD is shown also by the presence of growth-associated protein (GAP-43), which is under the influence of its key factor, the NGF. GAP-43 is recognized as the pathological marker of axonal growth in a degenerated IVD [363]. Interestingly, these proinflammatory cytokines are blocked by A2M and thus reversing the inflammatory process [134, 145, 148]. A2M also slows the progression of intervertebral disk (IV) degeneration by inhibiting the effects of proinflammatory cytokines [144]. Furthermore, A2M prevents sensitization of nerve fibers in the IVD and suppresses proinflammatory cytokines. Limiting mobility in the spine in a discogenic low back pain will further help in pain control [361] (Fig. 14.21).

Percutaneous injection of stem cells is one of the promising treatments to slow or reverse disc degeneration or an alternative to disc arthroplasty or spinal fusion procedures. Studies have shown that current surgical procedures fail to address the proinflammatory milieu of the discs, loss of functional cells and tissues, and the loss of matrix anabolism. The elimination of tissues or fixating it by surgery will alter spine biomechanics and would not allow the opportunity for regeneration [364]. Studies have consistently shown that intradiscal stem cell procedures can restore the extracellular matrix of the disc, including the proteoglycan content of the nucleus pulposus [365–368]. One of the criteria for injecting stem cells intradiscally is to choose a cell carrier to effectively carry the progenitor cells into the nucleus pulposus to protect the cells from the harsh environment of the disc, promote engraftment, prevent cell leakage, and restore mechanical properties while regeneration is taking place [365]. An example of a cell carrier to support MSCs delivery into the disc is PRP/hyaluronic acid/Batroxobin gel (PRP/HA/BTX) for cellular disc regeneration [369]. An undesirable migration of MSCs can occur if the cell leakage is not prevented. It could lead to an osteophyte formation. Thus, it is important to ensure a secured sealing technology in the annulus fibrosus and a stable cell carrier system [370]. Prior to the procedure, the integrity of the IVD structure must be assessed to ensure that it is preserved as this kind of interventional treatment will work only in mild to moderate grades of disc degeneration [365].

In some cases, it is also possible to home the MSCs to the IVD cells instead of injecting directly into the IVD to enhance the regenerative capacity of the IVD cells as an alternative procedure to MSC injection. Using a Tie-2-positive progenitor cell population, MSC homing enhances the survival and regenerative capacity of IVD cells. This Tie-2-positive progenitor cells however decrease with aging and thus this strategy could be used instead to prevent the onset of the degenerative cascade in IVDs [371].

Intradiscal fibrin sealant is used as a functioning physical barrier between inflammatory constituents of the annulus fibrosus and the disc's nociceptors [337]. It is also used as a treatment for IVD-related symptoms in an injured annulus fibrosus. Since the nucleus pulposus can leak inflammatory cells into spinal nerves through a defective annulus fibrosus during a pathologic condition, fibrin sealant can serve as a barrier limiting the outflow of these inflammatory constituents into the dura, meninges, and spinal nerves. Further, while intradiscal biologic therapy such as mesenchymal stem cells or PRP is intended to treat and repair degenerated IVD, iatrogenic leakage may be incurred such that the use of a fibrin is important to prevent such a scenario from happening [337, 370]. Fibrin therefore can act as a scaffold to prevent the leak from happening while the stem cells are injected to repair the degenerated IVD. Fibrin is a biocompatible composite hydrogel of fibrin and thrombin acting as a hemostatic agent, sealant, and cell carrier [337, 372]. Intradiscal fibrin injection is safe and effective for patients with low back pain due to degenerative disc disease [373].

Low back pain secondary to IVD degeneration is one of the most disabling conditions contributing to the number of days lost in work and to the rising health conditions. The need to be prudent in diagnosing the problems and identifying the most effective interventional treatment with the goal of relieving the pain and addressing the cause of the pain seems to be the most logical approach to do. Spine intervention targeting the painful annular fissures early will help a long way in preventing the secondary effects of spinal deformities. A well-informed patient regarding possible treatments will help us identify which ones will have to be done first in the process of managing back pains. The surgical option is not an immediate answer to an intractable pain condition. There is a risk of adjacent level of degeneration as observed in spinal fusion [374]. Regenerative medicine offers a great alternative not only for those unwilling to undergo surgery but also for those patients who are refractory to pain management. There is still a lot of work and research to do in regenerative medicine for degenerative disc disease, but to a large degree, a greater tendency is noted toward more conservative but effective regenerative interventions [337].

Regenerative Treatment for Peripheral Nerve Injury

Peripheral nerve injuries represent a major clinical and public health problem that leads to functional impairment and permanent disability. Roughly 3% of all trauma patients have peripheral nerve injuries [375]. Unlike in the central nervous system where damaged neurons are incapable of regenerating, axons in the peripheral nerves can regenerate after an injury though the process is incomplete. This condition, however, can lead eventually to neuropathic pains which are characteristics of a fulminant inflammatory process [376]. The terminal stump of the transected peripheral nerve usually undergoes Wallerian degeneration which begins within 2–3 days post-injury moving in both antegrade and retrograde manner [377, 378]. Schwann cells in the peripheral nervous system provide for a conducive microenvironment for the regeneration of an injured nerve [379]. The process involves dedifferentiation of the Schwann cells with proliferation and migration to build the bands of Bungner, which is a column of Schwann cells within the endoneurial sheath, and then to redifferentiate again to form new Schwann cells around a regenerated unmyelinated peripheral nerve [380, 381]. In fact, proliferating Schwann cells take the lead, and the regenerating axons follow from the proximal terminal stump across the injury into the distal nerve stump [382, 383]. Myelin debris is also cleared by the Schwann cells and together with macrophages are recruited to the injury site and the terminal stump within 3 days to begin the complex process of axonal regeneration and to release the growth factors, chemokines, cytokines, and extracellular matrix (ECM) proteins [384, 385]. Other important growth factors also include the nerve growth factor (NGF), glial cell line-derived neurotrophic factor (GDNF), and brain-derived neurotrophic factor (BDNF) [386]. Peripheral nerve injury regrowth continues at a rate of 1–3 mm/day provided there are no deterrents during the process [378]. The inflammatory process in an injured peripheral nerve will also release proinflammatory cytokines including TNF-α, IL-1β, IL-6, IFN-γ, and IL-18 [134, 141, 152, 377]. TNF-α serves as a biomarker of Wallerian degeneration in an injured peripheral nerve [134, 141].

Although peripheral nerve injury has different types, depending on whether one uses the Seddon Classification or Sunderland Classification, it is very important to know that types 1 and 2 of the Sunderland Classification will show full recovery, while the rest may need surgical intervention for healing of the injured nerve to take place. Surgeons may need 8–10 weeks post-injury to do a surgical intervention to ensure that healing does not improve spontaneously [387, 388]. By that time, if no regeneration occurred, a surgical repair can be done to coaptate the nerve stump that was severed.

The time lapse for a nerve to fully regenerate in the absence of surgical intervention will take a toll on the regeneration process. Most likely, the regenerating axons will fail to reinnervate the denervated skeletal muscle with subsequent fat infiltration. The consequence in the nerve could be any of the following: chronic axotomy of the neurons, which is a denervated axon isolated from their neurons; chronic Schwann cell denervation, which is denervation of Schwann cells in the distal nerve stumps; and chronic skeletal muscle denervation, which is denervation of the muscle due to a prolong severance of the peripheral nerve into the skeletal muscle [389]. As a result of this observation, the delay in any treatment for the injured peripheral nerve could be detrimental to the regeneration of the terminal stump and thus the chances of the distal stump recovery will decline over time, even affecting the denervated skeletal muscle in its recovery [389].

Neuropathic pain represents 7–10% of the population. It is secondary to metabolic diseases such as diabetes mellitus and degenerative peripheral neuropathy. Among diabetic patients, neuropathic pain represents about 10–26% [390]. Among patients undergoing a surgical procedure, 73% of those complaining of persistent pain were identified to be suffering from neuropathic pain [391]. Although this will not be fully discussed in this chapter, the existence of this condition is of primary consideration in pain discussions. Consequently, neuropathic pain, sensory loss, and skeletal muscle denervation become a functional impairment in patients with peripheral nerve injury. Thus, a novel interventional regenerative procedure is a vital treatment option for patients with these conditions.

In a study by Yu and colleagues on platelet-rich plasma, the use of PRP could promote nerve regeneration and repair in patients with peripheral nerve injury [392]. Also, in another study, PRP showed positive effects on healing in the nerve function as well as histological improvements in an injured peripheral nerve. However, more studies are needed to come up with more consistent evidence-based conclusions [393]. The use of PRP on peripheral nerve injury together with appropriate rehabilitation exercises seems to have a promising future [394].

In a preliminary study by Lopez and colleagues using PRP among 45 patients with a 3-month history of neuropathic pain, it showed a pain reduction of 50% one-month post-PRP injection and 70% at the end of the 3-month period. Half of the patients reported complete resolution of pain [395].

Alpha-2-macroglobulin (A2M) is a promising intervention for patients with peripheral nerve injuries with associated neuropathic pains. A2M interacts with and neutralizes the pro-inflammatory cytokines which are one of the causes of pain in peripheral nerve injuires as shown in preclinical studies and reviews [134, 141]. A2M can be safely delivered into an

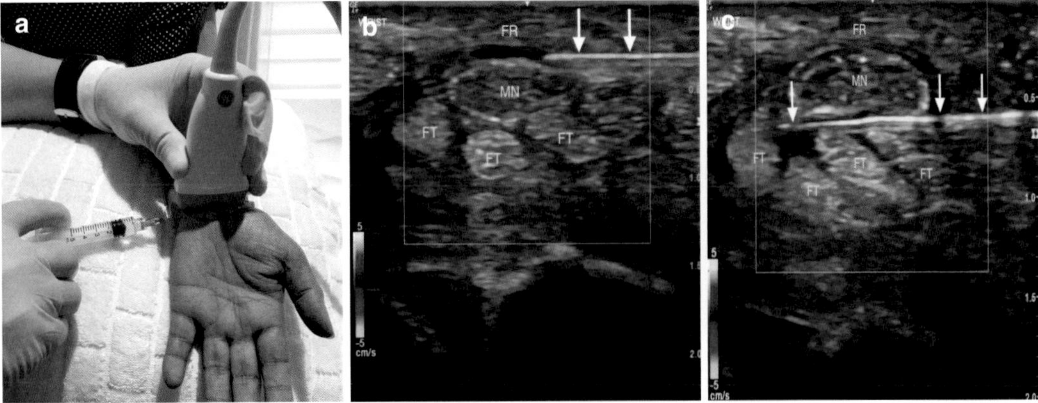

Fig. 14.23 Ultrasound-guided injection of the peripheral nerve. (**a**) Ultrasound-guided injection of the median nerve, medial approach, in-plane to the probe but short axis to the nerve, using alpha-2-macroglobulin (A2M). (**b**) The needle initially hydrodissects the uppermost layer of the perineurium to peel it off from the surrounding connective tissue and retinaculum of the median nerve. (**c**) The needle is redirected to hydrodissect the lower portion of the median nerve at the epineurium. MN median nerve, FT flexor tendons, FR flexor retinaculum, the white arrow represents the needle track

affected peripheral nerve via an ultrasound-guided peripheral nerve hydrodissection procedure [396] (Fig. 14.23). This technique is safe and can deliver the solution for therapeutic purposes [397].

Regenerative medicine is an evolving field that has attracted the attention of a lot of practitioners due to its potential to treat patients in a non-surgical way. But much to its promise of effective results, shorter recovery periods, and other breakthroughs, it is necessary for practitioners to provide patients with informed consent, a well-educated explanation of the procedures, and an end-point expectation of what the procedure can offer. There is still a great need for hard evidence-based research such as determining the length of the treatment, knowing the frequency of the treatment, and identifying the composition of an ideal regenerative solution for a given condition. Since these procedures are at their nascent stage, careful consideration must be given to acceptable standard treatments during the initial treatment. It is also important that regenerative practitioners must achieve a certain level of competence to perform the procedure. It is recommended that such procedures must be performed under image guidance such as ultrasound or fluoroscopy. Further research is needed, however, in ensuring the effectiveness of regenerative procedures in addressing musculoskeletal conditions.

Acknowledgment First and foremost, to the Faithful God who allowed me to finish this manuscript during these challenging times of COVID19 pandemic, who kept me busy writing but at the same time keeping us safe from infection.

My family: my wife Kyna de Castro and two kids, Rafael Bennett and Zarah Francine de Castro, for their constant and unwavering support.

To my colleagues who inspired me to move on.

Psalm 84:11 – "For the Lord God is a sun and shield; the Lord bestows favor and honor. No good thing does He withhold from those who walk uprightly."

References

1. Finnoff ND, Henning P, Hollman J, Smith J. Accuracy of ultrasound-guided versus unguided pes anserine bursa injections. PM & R. 2010;8:732–9.
2. Hashiuchi T, Sakurai G, Morimoto M, Komei T, Yoshinori T, Tanaka Y. Accuracy of the biceps tendon sheath injection: ultrasound-guided or unguided injection? A randomized controlled trial. J Shoulder Elb Surg. 2011;20(7):1069–73.
3. Peck E, Lai JK, Pawlina W, Smith J. Accuracy of ultrasound-guided versus palpation guided acromioclavicular joint injections: a cadaveric study. PM & R. 2010;2(9):817–21.

4. Daley E, Bajaj S, Bisson L, Cole B. Improving injection accuracy of the elbow, knee, and shoulder; does injection site and imaging make a difference? A systematic review. Am J Sports Med. 2011;39:656–62.
5. Furtado RN, Pereira DF, Rodriguez da Luz K, dos Santos MF, Konal MS, SDV M, Rosenfeld A, ARC F, Natour J. Effectiveness of imaging-guided intraarcticular injection: a comparison study between fluoroscopy and ultrasound. Rev Bras Reumatol. 2013;53(6):476–82.
6. Koski JM, Hammer HB. Ultrasound-guided procedures: techniques and usefulness in controlling inflammation and disease progression. Rheumatology. 2012;51:731–5.
7. Marx RE, Carlson ER, Eichstaedt RM, Schimmele SR, Strauss JE, Georgeff KR. Platelet-rich plasma: growth factor enhancement for bone grafts. Oral Surg Oral Med Oral Pathol Oral Radiol Endod. 1998;85(6):638–46.
8. Anitua E. Plasma rich in growth factors: preliminary results of use in the preparation of future sites for implants. Int J Oral Maxillofac Implants. 1999;14(4):529–35.
9. Mishra A, Pavelko T. Treatment of chronic elbow tendinosis with buffered platelet-rich plasma. Am J Sports Med. 2006;34(11):1774–8.
10. Nguyen RT, Borg-stein J, McInnis K. Applications of platelet-rich plasma in musculoskeletal and sports medicine: an evidence-based approach. PM & R. 2011;3(3):226–50.
11. Mishra A, Harmon K, Woodall J, Vieira A. Sports medicine applications of platelet-rich plasma. Curr Pharma Biotechnol. 2012;13(7):1185–95.
12. Malanga GA, Goldin M. PRP: review of the current evidence for musculoskeletal conditions. Curr Phys Med Rehabil Rep. 2014;2:1–5.
13. Marx RE. Platelet-rich plasma (PRP): what is PRP and what is not PRP? Implant Dent. 2001;10(4):225–8.
14. Cerciello S, Beitzel K, Howlett N, Russell RP, Apostolakos J, McCarthy MB, Cote MP, Mazzocca AD. The use of platelet-rich plasma preparations in the treatment of musculoskeletal injuries in orthopaedic sports medicine. Op Tech Orthop. 2013:23(2):69–74.
15. Oh JH, Kim W, Park KU, et al. Comparison of the cellular composition and cytokine-release kinetics of various platelet-rich plasma preparations. Am J Sports Med. 2015;43(12):3062–70.
16. Kevy S, Jacobson M, Mandle R. Defining the composition and healing effect of platelet-rich plasma. Presented at the Platelet-rich Plasma Symposium, New York, 5 Aug 2010.
17. Giusti RA, D'Ascenzo S, Millimaggi D, Pavan A, Dell'Orso L, Dolo V. Identification of an optimal concentration of platelet gel for promoting angiogenesis in human endothelial cells. Transfusion. 2009;49(4):771–8.
18. Foster TE, Puskas BL, Mendelbaum BR, et al. Platelet-rich plasma: from basic science to clinical applications. Am J Sports Med. 2009;37:2259–72.
19. Wasterlain AS, Braun HJ, Dragoo JL. Contents and formulations of platelet-rich plasma. Op Tech Orthop. 2012;22(1):33–42.
20. Anitua E, Sanchez M, Nurden AT, Zalduendo MM, de la Fuente M, Azofra J, Andia I. Platelet-released growth factors enhance the secretion of hyaluronic acid and induce hepatocyte growth factor production by synovial fibroblasts from arthritic patients. Rheumatology. 2007;46(12):1769–72.
21. Jo CH, Kim JE, Yoon KS, Shin S. Platelet-rich plasma stimulates cell proliferation and enhances matrix gene expression and synthesis in tenocytes from human rotator cuff tendons with degenerative tears. Am J Sports Med. 2012;40(5):1035–45.
22. Braun HJ, Kim HJ, Chu CR, Dragoo JL. The effect of platelet-rich plasma formulations and blood products on human synoviocytes implications for intra-articular injury and therapy. Am J Sports Med. 2014;42(5):1204–10.
23. Fitzpatrick J, Bulsara MK, O'Donnell J, Zheng MH. Leucocyte-rich platelet-rich plasma treatment of gluteus medius and minimus tendinopathy: a double-blind randomized controlled trial with 2-year follow-up. Am J Sports Med. 2019;47(5):1130–7.
24. Miroshnychenko O, Chang WT, Dragoo JL. The use of platelet-rich plasma and platelet-poor plasma to enhance differentiation of skeletal myoblasts: implications for the use of autologous blood products for muscle regeneration. Am J Sports Med. 2017;45(4):945–53.
25. Hooiveld M, Roosendaal G, Wenting MJG, van den Berg HM. Short-term exposure of cartilage to blood results in chondrocyte apoptosis. Am J Pathol. 2003;162(3):943–51.
26. Roosendaal G, Vianen ME, Marx JJ, et al. Blood-induced joint damage: a human in vitro study. Arthritis Rheuma. 1999;42(5):1025–32.
27. DeLong JM, Russell RP, Mazzocca AD. Platelet-rich plasma: the PAW classification system. Arthroscopy. 2012;28(7):998–1009.
28. Mautner K, Malanga GA, Smith J, Shiple B. A call for a standard classification system for future biologic research: the rationale for new PRP nomenclature. PM & R. 2015;7(4 Suppl):S53–9.
29. Lana JF, Purita J, Paulus C, Huber SC, Rodrigues B, Rodrigues AA, Santana MH, Madureira JL, Luzo ACM, Belangero WD, Annichino-Bizzacchi JM. Contributions for classification of platelet-rich plasma--proposal of a new classification: MARSPILL. Regen Med. 2017;12(5):565–74.
30. Dohan Ehrenfest DM, Rasmussen L, et al. Classification of platelet concentrates; from pure platelet-rich plasma (P-PRP) to leucocyte- and platelet-rich fibrin (L-PRF). Trends Biotechnol. 2009;27(3):158–67.
31. Schippinger G, Pruller F, Divjak M, et al. Autologous platelet-rich plasma preparation influence of nonsteroidal anti-inflammatory drugs on platelet function. Orthop J Sports Med. 2015;3:6.

32. Amaral R, Silva N, Haddad N, Lopes L, Ferreira F, Filho R, Cappelletti P, de Mello W, Cordeiro-Spinetti E, Balduino A. Platelet-rich plasma obtained with different anticoagulants and their effect on platelet numbers and mesenchymal stromal behavior in vitro. Stem Cells Int. 2016;2016:7414036.
33. Dhurat R, Sukesh M. Principles and methods of preparation of platelet-rich plasma: a review of author's perspective. J Cutan Asthetic Surg. 2014;7(4):189–97.
34. Smith J, Finnoff JT. Diagnostic and interventional musculoskeletal ultrasound: part 1. Fundamentals PM & R. 2009;1(1):64–75.
35. Krobbuaban B, Diregpoke S, Prasan S, et al. Alcohol-based chlorhexidine vs. povidine iodine in reducing skin colonization prior to regional anesthesia procedure. J Med Assoc Thail. 2011;41(11):807–12.
36. Nazarian L, et al. AIUM practice guidelines for the performance of the musculoskeletal ultrasound examination. AIUM Practice Guidelines. 2007; 1–13.
37. Baima J, Isaac Z. Clean versus sterile technique for common joint injection: a review from the physiatry perspective. Curr Rev Musculoskelet Med. 2008;1:88–91.
38. Cohnheim J. Ueber entzu ndung und eiterung. Arch fu'r Pathol Anat und Physiol und fu'r Klin Med. 1867;40:1–79.
39. Murphy MB, Terrazas JA, Buford DA. Bone marrow concentrate and platelet-rich plasma acquisition and preparation. Tech Reg Anesth Pain Manag. 2015;19(1,2):19–25.
40. Friedenstein AJ, Chailakhyan RK, Latsinik NV, et al. Stromal cells responsible for transferring the microenvironment of the hemopoietic tissues. Cloning in vitro and retransplantation in vivo. Transplatation. 1974;17(4):331–40.
41. Golpanian S, El-Khorazaty Y, Mendizabal A, DiFede DL, Suncion VY, Karantalis V, Fishman JE, Ghersin E, Balkan W, Hare JM. Effect of aging on human mesenchymal stem cell therapy in ischemic cardiomyopathy patients. J Am Coll Cardiol. 2015;65(2):125–32.
42. Civin CI, Strauss LC, Brovali C, Fackler MJ, Schwartz JF, Shaper JH. Antigenic analysis of hematopoietic progenitor cell surface antigen defined by a monoclonal antibody raised against KG-1a cells. J Immunol. 1984;133(1):156–65.
43. Tindle RW, Nichols RA, Chan I, et al. A novel monoclonal antibody BI-3C5 recognises myeloblasts and non-B non-T lymphoblasts in acute leukemias and CGL blasts crises, and reacts with immature cells in normal bone marrow. Leuk Res. 1985;9(1):1–9.
44. Thomas ED, Storb R, Cliff RA, et al. Bone-marrow transplantation. N Engl J Med. 1975;292(17):895–902.
45. Phillips RL, Reinhart AJ, Van Zant G. Genetic control of murine hematopoietic stem cell pool sizes and cycling kinetics. Proc Natl Acad Sci U S A. 1992;89:11607–11.
46. Landsdorp PM, Dragowska W, Mayani H. Ontogeny-related changes in proliferative potential of human hematopoietic cells. J Exp Med. 1993;178:787–91.
47. Nygren JM, Bryder D, Jacobsen SE. Prolonged cell cycle transit is a defining and developmentally conserved hemopoietic stem cell property. J Immunol. 2006;177:201–8.
48. Kim MJ, Kim MH, Kim SA, Chang JS. Age-related deterioration of hematopoietic stem cells. Int J Stem Cells. 2008;1(1):55–63.
49. Murphy MB, Moncivas K, Kaplan AI. Mesenchymal stem cells environmentally responsive therapeutics for regenerative medicine. Exp Mol Med. 2013;45(11):e54.
50. Caplan AI. Mesenchymal stem cells. J Orthop Res. 1991;9(5):641–50.
51. Horwitz EM, Andreef M, Frassoni F. Mesenchymal stromal cells. Curr Opin Hematol. 2006;13(6):419–25.
52. Friedenstein AK, Chailakhjan RK, Lalykina KS. The development of fibroblast colonies in monolayer cultures of guinea-pig bone marrow and spleen cells. Cell Tissue Kinet. 1970;3(4):393–403.
53. Horwitz E, Le Blanc K, Dominici M, et al. Clarification of the nomenclature for MSC: the International Society for Cellular Therapy position statement. Cytotherapy. 2005;7:393–5.
54. Finnoff JT. Regenerative rehabilitative medicine for joints and muscles. Curr PM & R Rep. 2020;8:8–16.
55. Salamanna F, Contartese D, Aldini NN, Brodano GB, Griffoni C, Gasbarrini A, Fini M. Bone marrow aspirate clot: a technical complication or a smart approach for musculoskeletal regeneration? J Cell Physiol. 2018;233:2723–32.
56. Hyer CF, Berlet GC, Bussewitz BW, Hankins T, Ziegler HL, Philbin TM. Quantitative assessment of the yield of osteoblastic connective tissue progenitors in bone marrow aspirate from iliac crest, tibia and calcaneus. J Bone Joint Surg Am. 2013;95:1312–6.
57. Iman MA, Mahmoud SSS, Holton J, Abouelmaati D, Elsherbini Y, Snow M. A systematic review of the concept and clinical applications of bone marrow aspirate concentrate in orthopedics. SICOT J. 2017;17(3):1–8.
58. Marx RE, Tursun R. A qualitative and quantitative analysis of autologous human multipotent adult stem cells derived from three anatomic areas by marrow aspiration: tibia, anterior ilium and posterior ilium. Int J Oral Maxillofac Implants. 2013;28(5):e290–4.
59. Fennema EM, Renard AJS, Leusink A, et al. The effect of bone marrow aspiration strategy on the yield and quality of human mesenchymal stem cells. Acta Orthop. 2009;80(5):618–21.
60. Muschler GF, Boehm C, Easley K. Aspiration to obtain osteoblast progenitor cells from human bone marrow: the influence of aspiration volume. J Bone Joint Surg Am. 1997;79(11):1699–709.
61. Batinic D, Marusic M, Pavletic Z, et al. Relationship between differing volumes of bone marrow aspi-

rates and their cellular composition. Bone Marrow Transplant. 1990;6(2):103–7.
62. Ehringer A, Trumpp A. The bone marrow stem cell niche grows up: mesenchymal stem cells and macrophages move in. J Exp Med. 2011;208(3):421–8.
63. Scarpone M, Kuebler D, Harrell DB. Marrow cellution bone marrow aspiration system and related concentrations of stem and progenitor cells. Allegheny Health Network Annual Orthopedic Update. 2016;8-10.
64. Lamagna C, Bergers G. The bone marrow constitutes a reservoir of pericytes progenitors. J LeoKoc Biol. 2006;80(4):677–81.
65. Caplan AI. All MSCs are pericytes? Cell Stem Cell. 2008;3(3):229–30.
66. Hong SJ, Traktuev DO. Therapeutic potential of adipose-derived stem cells in vascular growth and tissue repair. Curr Opin Organ Transplant. 2010;15:86–91.
67. Kuhl T, Mezger M, Hausser I, et al. High local concentrations of intradermal MSCs restore skin integrity and facilitate wound healing in dystrophic epidermolysis bullosa. Mol Ther. 2015;23:1368–79.
68. Peng H, Huard J. Muscle-derived stem cells for musculoskeletal tissue regeneration and repair. Transpl Immunol. 2004;12:311–9.
69. Wang Y, Yu X, Chen E, et al. Liver-derived human mesenchymal stem cells: a novel therapeutic source for liver diseases. Stem Cell Res Ther. 2016;7:71.
70. Crisan M, Yap S, Casteilla L, et al. A perivascular origin for mesenchymal stem cells in multiple human organs. Cell Stem Cell. 2008;3:301–13.
71. Caplan AI. New MSCs: MSCs as pericytes are sentinels and gatekeepers. J Orthop Res. 2017;35:1151–9.
72. Murray IR, Peault B. Q & A: mesenchymal stem cells—where do they come from and is it important? BMC Biol. 2015;13:99.
73. Baily JE, Chen WC, Khan N, et al. Isolation of perivascular multipotent precursor cell populations from human cardiac tissue. J Vis Exp. 2016;116:e54252.
74. Esteves CL, Donadeu FX. Pericytes and their potential in regenerative medicine across species. Cytometry. 2018;93(1):50–9.
75. Gokcinar-Yagci B, Uckan-Cetinkaya D, Celebi-Saltik B. Pericytes: properties, functions and applications in tissue engineering. Stem Cell Rev Rep. 2015;11(4):549–59.
76. Dominici M, et al. Minimal criteria for defining multipotent mesenchymal stromal cells. The international society for cellular therapy position statement. Cytotherapy. 2006;8(4):315–7.
77. Bowen JE. Technical issues in harvesting and concentrating stem cells (bone marrow and adipose). PM & R. 2015;7(4 suppl):S8–S18.
78. Van Esch RW, Kool MM, van As S. NSAIDs can have adverse effects on bone healing. Med Hypothesis. 2003;81(2):343–6.
79. Kitajama M, Shigematsu M, Ogawa K, Sugihara H, Hotokebuchi T. Effect of glucocorticoid on adipocyte size in human bone marrow. Med Mol Morphol. 2007;40:150–6.
80. Lipworth BJ. Systemic adverse effects of inhaled corticosteroid therapy: a systematic review and meta-analysis. Arch Intern Med. 1999;159(9):941–55.
81. Ramos FJ, Kaeberlein M. A healthy diet for stem cells. Nature. Jun 2012;486:477–8.
82. Wilkinson AC, Yamazaki S. Hematopoietic stem cell diet. Int J of Hematol. 2018;107:634–41.
83. Mana MD, Kuo EY, Yilmaz OH. Dietary regulation of adult stem cells. Curr Stem Cell Rep. 2017;3:1–8.
84. Sittitavornwong S, Falconer DS, Shah R, et al. Anatomic considerations for posterior superior iliac crest bone procurement. J Oral Maxillofac Surg. 2013;71:1777–88.
85. Hernigou J, Picard L, Alves A, Silvera J, Homma Y. Understanding bone safety zones during bone marrow aspiration from the iliac crest: the sector rule. Int Orthop. 2014;38(11):2377–84.
86. Hernigou J, Alves A, Homma Y, Guissou I, Hernigou P. Anatomy of the ilium for bone marrow aspiration: map of sectors and implication for safe trocar placement. Int Orthop. 2014;38(12):2585–90.
87. Gronkjaer M, Hasselgren CF, Ostergaerd AS, Johansen P, Korup J, Bogsted M, Bilgrau AE, Jensen P. Bone marrow aspiration: a randomized controlled trial assessing the quality of bone marrow specimens using slow and rapid aspiration techniques and evaluating pain intensity. Acta Haematol. 2016;135(2):81–7.
88. Vanhelleputte P, Nijs K, Delforge M, Evers G, Vanderschueren S. Pain during bone marrow aspiration: prevalence and prevention. J Pain Symptom Manag. 2003;26(3):860–6.
89. Malanga GA, Ibrahim V (eds). Regenerative treatments in sports and orthopedic medicine. Springer Publishing Company; 2017.
90. Zehnder JL, Schrier S, Rosmarin AG. Bone marrow aspiration and biopsy: indications and technique. Website: http://www.uptodate.com/contents/bone--marrowaspiration-and-biopsy-indication-and-tec... 2011.
91. Melampati S, Joshi S, Lai S, Braner DAV, Tegtmeyer K. Bone marrow aspiration and biopsy. N Engl J Med. 2009;361:e28.
92. Miller HJ, Awad SS, Crosby CT, et al. Chlorhexidine-alcohol versus povidone-iodine for surgical site antisepsis. N Engl J Med. 2010;362:18–26.
93. Friedlis MF, Centeno CJ. Performing a better bone marrow aspiration. Phys Med Rehabil Clin N Am. 2016;27:919–39.
94. Rahnama R, Wang M, Dang AC, et al. Cytotoxicity of local anesthetics on human mesenchymal stem cells. J Bone Jt Surg. 2013;95(2):132–7.
95. Caplan AI. Why are MSCs therapeutic? New data: new insight. J Pathol. 2009;217(2):318–24.
96. Hernigou P, Matthieu G, Poignard A, et al. Percutaneous autologous bone marrow grafting for

nonunions: surgical technique. J Bone Joint Surg Am. 2006;88(suppl 1):322–7.
97. Hernigou P, Homma Y, Flouzat Lachaniette CH, et al. Benefits of small volume and small syringe for bone marrow aspirations of mesenchymal stem cells. Int Orthop. 2013;37(11):2279–87.
98. Glass GE, Ferretti P. Adipose-derived stem cells in aesthetic surgery. Aesth Surg J. 2019;39(4):423–38.
99. Salgado AJBOG, Reis RLG, Sousa NJC, Gimble JM. Adipose tissue derived stem cells secretome: soluble factors and their roles in regenerative medicine. Curr Stem Cell Res Ther. 2010;5(2):103–10.
100. Arshad Z, Halioua-Haubold C, Roberts M, Fulvio U, Branford OA, Brindley DA, Davies BM, Pettitt D. Adipose-derived stem cells in asthetic surgery: a mixed methods evaluation of the current clinical trial, intellectual property, and regulatory landscape. Aesth Surg J. 2018;38(2):199–210.
101. Zollino I, Zuolo M, Gianesini S, Pedriali M, Sibilla MG, Tessari M, Carinci F, Occhionorelli S, Zamboni P. Autologous adipose-derived stem cells: basic science, technique, and rationale for application in ulcer and wound healing. Phlebol. 2017;32(3):160–71.
102. Nicoletti GF, De Francesco F, D'Andrea F, Ferraro GA. Methods and procedures in adipose stem cells: state of the art perspective for translational medicine. J Cell Physiol. 2015;230(4):489–95.
103. Kokai L, Traktuev D, Zhang L, Merfeld-Clauss S, DiBernardo G, Lu H, Marra K, Donnenberg A, Donnenberg V, Meyer E, Fodor P, March K, Rubin J. Adipose stem cell function maintained with age: an intra-subject study of long-term cryopreserved cells. Aesthet Surg J. 2017;37(4):454–63.
104. Bourin P, Bunnell BA, Casteilla L, et al. Stromal cells from the adipose tissue-derived stromal vascular fraction and culture expanded adipose tissue-derived stromal /stem cells: a joint statement of the International Federation fir Adipose Therapeutics and Science (IFATS) and the International Society for Cellular Therapy (ISCT). Cytotherapy. 2013;15(6):641–8.
105. De Ugarte DA, Alfonso Z, Zuk PA, et al. Differential expression of stem cell mobilization associated molecules on multi-lineage cells from adipose tissue and bone marrow. Immunol Lett. 2003;89(2–3):267–70.
106. Mitchell JB, McIntosh K, Zvonic S, et al. Immunophenotype of human adipose-derived cells: temporal changes in stromal-associated and stem-cell associated markers. Stem Cells. 2006;24(2):376–85.
107. Kern S, Eicher H, Stoeve J, Kluter H, Bieback K. Comparative analysis of mesenchymal stem cells from bone marrow, umbilical cord blood or adipose tissue. Stem Cells. 2006;24(5):1294–301.
108. Gimble JM, Katz AJ, Bunnell BA. Adipose-derived stem cells for regenerative medicine. Circ Res. 2007;100(9):1249–60.
109. Contributors V. (Brousseau Z.) Fundamentals of US Regulatory Affairs, 10th Ed. Rockville: Regulatory Affairs Professionals Society. 2017.
110. Rodbell M, Jones AB. J Biol Chem. 1966;241:40–142.
111. Bunnell BA, Flaat M, Gagliardi C, Patel B, Ripoll C. Adipose-derived stem cells: isolation, expansion and differentiation. Methods. 2008;45(2):115–20.
112. Bjorntorp P, Karlsson H, Pertoft H, Pettersson P, Sjostrom U, Smith U. J Lipid Res. 1978;19(1978):316–24.
113. Padoin AV, Braga-Silva J, Martins P, et al. Sources of processed lipoaspirate cells: influence of donot site on cell concentration. Plast Reconstr Surg. 2008;122(2):614–8.
114. Lim AA, Fan K, Allam KA, et al. Autologous fat transplantation in the craniofacial patient: the UCLA experience. J Craniofac Surg. 2012;23(4):1061–6.
115. Choudhery MS, Badowski M, Muise A, et al. Subcutaneous adipose-derived stem cell utility is independent of anatomical harvest site. Biores Open Access. 2015;4(1):131–45.
116. Jurgens WJFM, et al. Effect of tissue harvesting site on yield of stem cells derived from adipose tissue: implications for cell-based therapies. Cell Tiss Res. 2008;323(3):415–26.
117. Klein JA. The tumescent technique: anesthesia and modified liposuction technique. Dermatol Clin. 1990;8:425–37.
118. Venkataram J. Tumescent liposuction: a review. J Cutan Aesth Surg. 2008;1(2):49–57.
119. Trivisonno A, Di Rocco G, Cannistra C, Finocchi V, Farr ST, Monti M, Toietta G. Harvest of superficial layers of fat with a microcannula and isolation of adipose tissue-derived stromal and vascular cells. Aesthe Surg J. 2014;34(4):601–13.
120. Doi K, Tanaka S, Lida H, et al. Stromal vascular fraction isolated from lipo-aspirates using an automated processing system: bench and bed analysis. J Tissue Eng Regen Med. 2012;7(11):864–70.
121. Aronowitz J, Lockhart R, Hakakian C, Birnbaum Z. Adipose-derived vascular fraction isolation. Ann Plastic Surg. 2016;77(3):354–62.
122. Van Dongen J, Harmsen M, Stevens H. Isolation of stromal vascular fraction by fractionation of adipose tissue. Methods Mol Biol. 1993;2020:91–103.
123. Tremolada C, Colombo V, Ventura C. Adipose tissue and mesenchymal stem cells: state of the art and Lipogems® technology development. Curr Stem Cell Rep. 2016;2(3):304–12.
124. Teimourian B, Rogers WB. A national survey of complications associated with suction lipectomy: a comparative study. Plast Reconstr Surg. 1989;84:628.
125. Ezzeddine H, Husari A, Nassar H, Kanso M, El Nounou G, Khalife M, Faraj W. Life threatening complications post-liposuction. Aesth Plast Surg. 2018;42:384–7.
126. Grazer FM, de Jong RH. Fatal outcomes from liposuction: census survey of cosmetic surgeons. Plast Reconstr Surg. 2000;105(1):436–46.
127. Coldiron B, Coleman W, Cox SE, Jacob C, Lawrence N, Kaminer M, Narins RS. ASDS guidelines of care for tumescent liposuction. Liposuction Council Bull Dermatol Surg. 2006;32:709–16.

128. Boni R. Safety of tumescent liposuction compared with liposuction in systemic sedation or general anesthesia—a review of the literature. Am J Cosm Surg. 2007;24(3):139–42.
129. Klein JA, Jeske DR. Estimated maximal safe dosages of tumescent lidocaine. Anesth Analg. 2016;122(5):1350–9.
130. Klein JA. Tumescent technique for regional anesthesia permits lidocaine doses of 35 mg/kg for liposuction. J Dermatol Surg Oncol. 1990;16:248–63.
131. Shoshani O, Berger J, Fodor L, et al. The effect of lidocaine and adrenaline on the viability of injected adipose tissue: an experimental study in nude mice. J Drugs Dermatol. 2005;4(3):311–6.
132. Keck M, Zeyda M, Gollinger K, et al. Local anesthetics have a major impact on viability of preadipocytes and their differentiation into adipocytes. Plast Reconstr Surg. 2010;126(5):1500–5.
133. Tapon-Bretaudiere J, Bros A, Couture-Tose E, Delain E. Electron microscopy of the conformational changes of alpha-2-macroglobulin from human plasma. EMBO J. 1985;4(1):85–9.
134. De Castro JC. Alpha-2-macroglobulin: the new weapon for neuropathic pains. J Anesth Pain Relief Manag. 2019; https://doi.org/10.31579/JAPM.2019/002.
135. Rehman AA, Khan FH, Ahsan H. Alpha-2 macroglobulin: a physiological guardian. J Cell Physiol. 2013;228:16651675.
136. Ritchie R, Palomaki G, Neveux L, Navolotskaia O, Ledue T, Craig W. Reference distributions for alpha 2-macroglobulin: a practical, simple and clinically relevant approach in a large cohort. J Clin Lab Analy. 2004;18(2):139–47.
137. Becker C, Harpel P. Alpha-2-macroglobulin on human vascular endothelium. J Exp Med. 1976;144(1):1–9.
138. Sottrup-Jensen L. In the plasma proteins. Academic Press. 1987;5:192–291.
139. Garcia-Ferrer I, Marrero A, Gomis-Ruth FX, Goulas T. Alpha-2-macroglobulins: structure and function. Subcell Biochem. 2017;83:149–83.
140. Cuellar JM, Cuellar VG, Gabrovsky V, Scuderi GJ. Alpha-2-macroglobulin: autologous protease inhibition technology. PM & R Clin N Am. 2016;27(4):9098–918.
141. Arandjelovic S, Dragojlovic N, Li X, Myers RR, Campana WM, Gonias SL. A derivative of the plasma protease inhibitor Alpha-2-macroglobulin regulates the response to peripheral nerve injury. J Neurochem. 2007;103(2):694–705.
142. Orhurhu V, Schwartz R, Potts J, Peck J, Urits I, Orhurhu MS, Odonkor C, Viswanath O, Kaye AD, Gill J. Role of alpha-2-macroglobulin in the treatment of osteoarthritic knee pain: a brief review of the literature. Curr Pain Headache Rep. 2020;24(3):9.
143. Li S, Xiang C, Wei X, Sun X, Li R, Li P, Sun J, Wei D, Chen Y, Zhang Y, Wei L. Early supplemental α2-macroglobulin attenuates cartilage and bone damage by inhibiting inflammation in collagen-II induced arthritis model. Int J Rheuma Dis. 2019;22(4):654–65.
144. Huang B, Chen J, Zhang X, Wang J, Zheng Z, Shan Z, Liu J, Zhu Z, Zhao F. Alpha-2-macroglobulin as dual regulator for both anabolism and catabolism in the cartilaginous endplate of intervertebral disc. Spine (Phila Pa 1976). 2019;44(6):E338–47.
145. Vincenzetti S, Pucciarelli S, Huang Y, Ricciutelli M, Lambertucci C, Volpini R, Scuppa G, Soverchia L, Ubaldi M, Polzonetti V. Biomarkers mapping of neuropathic pain in a nerve chronic constriction injury mice model. Biochimie. 2019;158:172–9.
146. Liu Y, Cao W, Kong X, Li J, Chen X, Ge Y, Zhong W, Fang S. Protective effects of α-2-macroglobulin on human bone marrow mesenchymal stem cells in radiation injury. Mol Med Rep. 2018;18(5):4219–28.
147. Myers RR, Sekiguchi Y, Kikuchi S, Scott B, Medicherla S, Protter A, Campana WM. Inhibition of p38 MAP kinase activity enhances axonal regeneration. Exp Neurol. 2003;184:606–14.
148. Nadeau S, Fillali M, Zhang J, Kerr BJ, Rivest S, Vaccari JPR, Keane RW, Lacroix S. Functional recovery after peripheral nerve injury is dependent on the proinflammatory cytokines IL-1β and TNF: implications for neuropathic pain. J Neurosc. 2011;31-35:12533–42.
149. Wagner R, Myers RR. Endoneurial injection of TNF-α produces neuropathic pain behaviours. Neuroreport. 1996;7:2867–901.
150. Taskinen HS, Olsson T, Bucht A, Khademi M, Svelander L, et al. Peripheral nerve injury induces endoneurial expression of IFN-γ, IL-10, TNF-α, mRNA. J Neuroimmunol. 2000;102:17–25.
151. Shamash S, Reichert F, Rotschenker S. The cytokine network of Wallerian degeneration: tumor necrosis factor-α, interleukin-1α, and interleukin-1β. J Neurosci. 2002;22:3052–60.
152. Menge T, Jander S, Stoll G. Induction of the proinflammatory cytokine interleukin-18 by axonal injury. J Neurosci. 2001;65:332–9.
153. Reichert F, Levitzky R, Rotshenker S. Interleukin-6 in intact and injured mouse peripheral nerves. Eur J Neurosci. 1996;8:530–5.
154. Myers RR, Campana WM, Shubayev VL. The role of neuroinflammation in neuropathic pain; mechanisms and therapeutic targets. Drugs Disc Today. 2006;11:8–20.
155. Dubovy P. Wallerian degeneration and peripheral nerve conditions for both axonal regeneration and neuropathic pain induction. Ann Anat. 2011;193(4):267–75.
156. LaMarre J, Wollenberg GK, Gonias SL, Hayes MA. Cytokine binding and clearance properties of proteinase-activated α2-macroglobulins. Lab Investig. 1991;65(1):3–14.
157. Webb DJ, Gonias SL. A modified human alpha-2-macroglobulin derivative that binds tumor necrosis factor-alpha and interleukin-1 beta with high affinity in vitro and reverses lipopolysaccharide toxicity in vivo in mice. Lab Investig. 1998;78:939–48.

158. Gonias SL, Pizzo SV. Altered clearance of human alpha-2-macroglobulin complexes following reaction with cis-dichlorodiamineplatinum(II). Biochem Biophys Acta. 1981;678:268–74.
159. Benito MJ, Veale DJ, Fitzgerald O, van den Berg WB, Bresnihan B. Synovial tissue inflammation in early and late osteoarthritis. Ann Rheuma Dis. 2005;64:1263–7.
160. Todhunter PG, Kincaid SA, Todhunter RJ, Kammerman JR, Johnstone B, Baird AN, Hanson RR, Wright JM, Lin HC, Purohit RC. Immunohistochemical analysis of an equine model of synovitis-induced arthritis. Am J Vet Res. 1996;57:1080–93.
161. Lefebvre V, Pefers-Joris C, Vaes G. Modulation by interleukin 1 and tumor necrosis factor alpha of production of collagenase, tissue inhibitor of metalloproteinases and collagen types in differentiated and dedifferentiated articular chondrocytes. Biochim Biophys Acta. 1990;1052(3):366–78.
162. Clegg PD, Burke RM, Coughlan AR, Riggs CM, Carter SD. Characteristics of equine matrix metalloproteinase 2 and 9 and identification of the cellular sources of these enzymes in joints. Equine Vet J. 1997a;29:335–42.
163. Sutton S, Clutterbuck A, Harris P, Gent T, Freeman S, Foster N, Barrett-Jolly R, Mobasheri A. The contribution of the synovium, synovial derived inflammatory cytokines and neuropeptides to the pathogenesis of osteoarthritis. Vet J. 2009;179(1):10–24.
164. Ohtori S, Inoue G, Miyagi M, et al. Pathomechanisms of discogenic low back pain in humans and animal models. Spine J. 2015;15(6):1347–55.
165. Saal J, Saal JS. Nonoperative treatment of herniated lumbar intervertebral disc with radiculopathy: an outcome study. Spine (Phila Pa 1976). 1989;14:431–7.
166. Tetlow LC, Adlam DJ, Wooley DE. Matrix metalloproteinases and proinflammatory cytokine production by chondrocytes of human osteoarthritic cartilage: associations with degenerative changes. Arthritis Rheum. 2001;44(3):585–94.
167. Baker JF, Walsh PM, Byrne DP, Mulhall KJ. Pravastatin suppresses matrix metalloproteinase expression and activity in human articular chondrocytes stimulated by interkeukin-1β. J Orthop Traumatol. 2012;13(3):119–23.
168. Garnero P, Landewe R, Chapurlat RD. The role of biochemical markers of joint tissue remodeling to predict progression and treatment efficacy in inflammatory rheumatic diseases. Rheuma. 2020;0:1–11.
169. Kapoor M, Martel-Pelletier J, Lajeunesse D, Pelletier JP, Fahmi H. Role of proinflammatory cytokines in the pathophysiology of osteoarthritis. Nat Rev. 2011;7(1):33–42.
170. Wajant H, Pfizenmaier K, Scheurich P. Tumor necrosis factor signaling. Cell Death Differ. 2003;10(1):45–65.
171. Huang T, Wu C, Yu J, Sumi S, Yang K. l-lysine regulates tumor necrosis factor-alpha and matrix metalloproteinases-3 expression in human osteoarthritic chondrocytes. Process Biochem. 2016;51(7):904–11.
172. Larsson S, Englund M, Struglics A, Lohmander LS. Interleukin-6 and tumor necrosis factor alpha in synovial fluid are associated with progression of radiographic knee osteoarthritis in subjects with previous meniscectomy. Osteoarth Cart. 2015;23:1906–14.
173. Schulze-Tanzil G, Al-Sadi O, Wiegand E, et al. The role of proinflammatory and immunoregulatory cytokines in tendon healing and rupture: new insights. Scand J Med Sci Sports. 2011;21:337–51.
174. Chen W, Jin G, Xiong Y, Hu P, Bao J, Wu L. Rosmarinic acid down-regulated=s NO and PGE_2 expression via MAPK pathway in rat chondrocytes. J Cell Mol Med. 2018;22(1):346–53.
175. Asghar S, Litherland GJ, Lockhart JC, Goodyear CS, Crilly A. Exosomes in intercellular communication and implications for osteoarthritis. Rheuma. 2020;59(1):57–68.
176. Goldring SR, Goldring MB. Clinical aspects, pathology and pathophysiology of osteoarthritis. J Musculoskelet Neuronal Interact. 2006;6:376–8.
177. Zhang S, Chuah SJ, Lai RC, et al. MSC exosomes mediate cartilage repair by enhancing proliferation, attenuating apoptosis and modulating immune reactivity. Biomaterials. 2018;156:16–27.
178. Wang S, Wei X, Zhou J, Zhang J, Li K, Chen Q, Terek R, Fleming BC, Goldring MB, Ehrlich MG, Zhang G, Wei L. Identification of α2-macroglobulin as a master inhibitor of cartilage-degrading factors that attenuates the progression of posttraumatic osteoarthritis. Arthritis Rheumatol. 2014;66(7):1843–53.
179. Tortorella MD, Arner EC, Hills R, Easton A, Korte-Sarfaty J, Fok K, et al. α2-macroglobulin is a novel substrate for ADAMTS-5 and represents and endogenous inhibitor of these enzymes. J Biol Chem. 2004;279:7554–61.
180. Luan Y, Kong L, Howell DR, Ilalov K, Fajardo M, Bai XH, et al. Inhibition of ADAMTS-7 and ADAMTS-12 degradation of cartilage oligomeric matrix protein by α2-macroglobulin. Osteoarthr Cartil. 2008;16:1413–20.
181. Kang JD, Georgescu HI, McIntyre-Larkin L, et al. Herniated lumbar intervertebral discs spontaneously produced matrix metalloproteinases, nitric oxide, interleukin-6 and prostaglandin-E_2. Spine. 1996;21:271–7.
182. Smith MW, Ith A, Carragee EJ, Cheng I, Alamin TF, Golish SR, Mitsunaga K, Scuderi GJ, Smuck M. Does the presence of the fibronectin-aggrecan complex predict outcomes from lumbar discectomy for disc herniation? Spine J. 2019;19(2):e28–33.
183. Lynch TS, O'Connor M, Minkara AA. Biomarkers for femoroacetabular impingement and hip osteoarthritis. Am J Sports Med. 2019;47(9):2242–50.
184. Zhang Y, Wei X, Browning S, Scuderi G, Hanna LS, Wei L. Targeted designed variants of alpha-2-macroglobulin attenuate cartilage degeneration in a rat model of osteoarthritis induced by anterior

cruciate ligament transection. Arthritis Res Ther. 2017;19:75.

185. Latypov RF, Harvey TS, Liu D, Bondarenko PV, Kohno T, Fachini RA II, Rosenfield RD, Ketchem RR, Brems DN, Raibekas AA. Biophysical characterization of structural proteins and folding of interleukin-1 receptor antagonist. J Mol Biol. 2007;368:1187–201.
186. Eisenberg SP, Evans RJ, Arend WP, Verderber E, Brewer MT, Hannum CH, Thompson RC. Primary structure and functional expression from complementary DNA of a human interleukin-1 receptor antagonist. Nature. 1990;343:341–6.
187. Thierry L, Vittecoq O, le Loet X. What is role of interleukin-1 receptor antagonist in rheumatic disease? Joint Bone Spine. 2007;74(3):223–6.
188. Dinarello CA, Thompson RC. Blocking IL-1: interleukin-1 receptor antagonist in vivo and in vitro. Immunol Today. 1991;12(11):4040–410.
189. Corradi A, Bajetto A, Cozzolino F, Rubartelli A. Production and secretion of interleukin-1 receptor antagonist in monocytes and keratinocytes. Cytotechnology. 1993;11:S50–2.
190. Bresnihan B. The safety and efficacy of interleukin-receptor antagonist in the treatment of rheumatoid arthritis. Sem Arthritis Rheuma. 2001;30(5):17–20.
191. Vittecoq O, Jacquot S, Jouen-Beades F, Pouplin S, Thomas M, Dutot I, et al. Potential diagnostic value of IL-1RA production by whole blood cells from community-recruited patients with very early arthritis. Results of the VErA study. Arthritis Rheuma. 2003;48(Suppl):542.
192. O'Shaughnessey K, Matuska A, Hoeppner J, et al. Autologous protein solution prepared from the blood of osteoarthritic patients contains an enhanced profile of anti-ibflammatory cytokines and anabolic growth factors. J Orthop Res. 2014;32(10):1349–55.
193. Ghivizzani S, Gouze E, Watson R, Saran J, Kay K, Bush M, Levings P, Gouze J. Interleukin-1 in rheumatoid arthritis: its inhibition by interleukin-1Ra and Anakinra. J Pharm Tech. 2007;23(2):86–94.
194. Sims JE, Gayle MA, Slack JL, et al. Interleukin-1 signaling occurs exclusively via the type I receptor. Proc Natl Acad Sci U S A. 1993;90:6155–9.
195. Wesche H, Korherr C, Kracht M, Falk W, Resch K, Martin MU. The interleukin-1 receptor accessory protein (IL-1RAcP) is essential for IL-1-induced activation of interleukin-1 receptor-associated kinase (IRAK) and stress-activated protein kinases (SAP kinases). J Biol Chem. 1997;272:7727–31.
196. Colotta F, Dower SK, Sims JE, Montovani A. The type II 'decoy' receptor: a novel regulatory pathway for interleukin-1. Immunol Today. 1994;15:562–6.
197. Dinarello CA. Biologic basis for interleukin-1 in disease. Blood. 1996;87:2095–147.
198. Gouze JN, Gouze E, Palmer GD, et al. A comparative study of the inhibitory effects of interleukin-1 receptor antagonist following administration as a recombinant protein or by gene transfer. Arthritis Res Ther. 2003;5:301–9.
199. Evans CH, Chevalier X, Wehling P. Autologous conditioned serum. Phys Med Rehabil Clin N Am. 2016;27:893–908.
200. Bresnihan B, Alvaro-Gracia JM, Cobby M, et al. Treatment of rheumatoid arthritis with recombinant human interleukin-1 receptor antagonist. Arthritis Rheuma. 1998;41:2196–204.
201. Schiff M. Durability and rapidity of response to anakinra in patients with rheumatoid arthritis. Drugs. 2012;64(22):2493–501.
202. Fleischman R, Schechtman J, Bennett R, Handel M, Burmester G, Tesser J, Modafferi D, Poulakos J, Sun G. Anakinra, a recombinant human interleukin-1 receptor antagonist (r-metHulL-1ra), in patients with rheumatoid arthritis: a large, international, multicenter, placebo-controlled trial. Arthritis Rheuma. 2003;48(4):927–34.
203. Dinesh P, Rasool M. Multifaceted role of interleukin-21 in rheumatoid arthritis: current understanding and future perspective. J Cell Physiol. 2018;233(5):3918–28.
204. Chevalier X, Giraudeau B, Conrozier T, et al. Safety study of intraarticular injection of interleukin-1 receptor antagonist in patients with painful knee osteoarthritis: a multicenter study. J Rheumatol. 2005;32:1317–23.
205. Chevalier X, Goupille P, Beaulieu AD, et al. Intraarticular injection of anakinra in osteoarthritis of the knee: a multicenter, randomized, double-blind, placebo-controlled study. Arthritis Rheum. 2009;61:344–52.
206. Bacconnier L, Jorgensen C, Fabre S. Erosive osteoarthritis of the hand: clinical experience with anakinra. Ann Rheum Dis. 2009;68:1078–9.
207. Cavalli G, Dinarello C. Treating rheumatological diseases and comorbidities with interleukin-1 blocking therapies. Rheumatology. 2015;54(12):2134–44.
208. Magalon J, Bausset O, Veran J, Giraudo L, Serratrice N, Magalon G, Dignat-George F, Sabatier F. Physico-chemical factors influencing autologous conditioned serum purification. Biores Open Access. 2014;3(1):35–8.
209. Arend WP, Leung DY. IgG induction of IL-1 receptor antagonist production by human monocytes. Immunol Rev. 1994;139:71–8.
210. Meijer H, Reinecke J, Becker C, Tholen G, Wehling P. The production of anti-inflammatory cytokines in whole blood by physico-chemical induction. Inflamm Res. 2003;52:404–7.
211. Granowitz EV, Clark BD, Mancilla J, Dinarello CA. Interleukin-1 receptor antagonist competitively inhibits the binding of interleukin-1 to the type II interleukin-1 receptor. J Biol Chem. 1991;266:14147–50.
212. Wehling P, Moser C, Frisbie D, et al. Autologous conditioned serum in the treatment of orthopedic diseases: the orthokine therapy. BioDrugs. 2007;21(5):323–32.
213. Hannum CH, Wilcox CJ, Arend WP, et al. Interleukin-1 receptor antagonist activity of a human interleukin-1 inhibitor. Nature. 1990;343:336–40.

214. Carter DB, Deibel MR Jr, Dunn CJ, et al. Purification, cloning, expression, and biological characterization of an interleukin-1 receptor antagonist protein. Nature. 1990;344:633–8.
215. Rutgers M, Saris DB, Dhert WJA, Creemers LB. Cytokine profile of autologous conditioned serum for treatment of osteoarthritis, in vitro effects on cartilage metabolism and intra-articular levels after injection. Arthritis Res Ther. 2010;12:R114.
216. Auw Yang KG, Raijmakers NJH, Van Arkel ERA, Caron JJ, Rijk PC, Willems WJ, et al. Autologous interleukin-1 receptor antagonist improves function and symptoms in osteoarthritis when compared to placebo in a prospective randomized controlled trial. Osteoarthr Cartil. 2008;16:498–505.
217. Baltzer AWA, Moser C, Jansen SA, Krauspe R. Autologous conditioned serum (Orthokine) is an effective treatment for knee osteoarthritis. Osteoarthr Cartil. 2009;17:152–60.
218. Zarringam D, Bekkers J, Saris D. Long term effect of injection treatment for osteoarthritis in the knee by Orthokin autologous conditioned serum. Cartilage. 2018;9(2):140–5.
219. Strumper R. Intraarticular injections of autologous conditioned serum to treat pain from meniscal lesions. Sports Med Int Open. 2017;1(6):E200–5.
220. Baselga GEJ, Miguel HTP. Treatment of osteoarthritis with a combination of autologous conditioned serum and physiotherapy: a two-year observational study. PLoS One. 2015;10(12):e0145551.
221. Wehling P, Evans C, Wehling J, Maixner W. Effectiveness of intraarticular therapies in osteoarthritis: a literature review. Therap Adv Musculoskel Dis. 2017;9(8):183–96.
222. Darabos N, Hundric-Haspl Z, Haspl M, Markotic A, Darabos A, Moser C. Correlation between synovial fluid and serum IL-1β levels after ACL surgery: a preliminary report. Int Orthop. 2008;33(2):413–8.
223. Cameron M, Buchgraber A, Passler H, Vogt M, Thonar E, Fu F, Evans CH. The natural history of anterior ligament deficient knee. Changes in synovial fluid cytokine and keratan sulfate concentrations. Am J Sports Med. 1997;25:751–4.
224. Marks P, Cameron M. Inflammatory cytokine profiles correlate with the degree of chondrosis in the chronic anterior cruciate ligament deficient knee. ACL study meeting. 2000; Rhodes, Greece.
225. Darabos N, Haspl M, Moser C, et al. Intraarticular application of autologous-conditioned serum (ACS) reduces bone tunnel widening after ACL reconstructive surgery in a randomized controlled trial. Knee Surg Sports Traumatol Arthrosc. 2011;19(Suppl):536–46.
226. Genc E, Beytemur O, Yuksel S, Eren Y, Caglar A, Kucukyildirim B, Gulec M. Investigation of the biomechanical and histopathological effects of autologous conditioned serum on healing of achilles tendon. Acta Orthop Traumatol Turc. 2018;52(3):226–31.
227. Muller S, Quirk N, Muller-Lebschi J, Heisterbach P, Durselen L, Majewski M, Evans C. Response of the injured tendon to growth factors in the presence or absence of paratenon. Am J Sports Med. 2019;47(2):462–7.
228. Majewski M, Ochsner PE, Liu F, et al. Accelerated healing of the rat Achilles tendon in response to autologous conditioned serum. Am J Sports Med. 2009;37(11):2117–25.
229. Goni VG, Singh Jhala S, Gopinathan NR, et al. Efficacy of epidural perineural injection of autologous conditioned serum in unilateral cervical radiculopathy: a pilot study. Spine. 2015;40:E915–21.
230. Becker C, Heidersdorf S, Drewlo S, de Rodriguez SZ, Kramer J, Wilburger RE. Efficacy of epidural injections with autologous conditioned serum for lumbar radicular compression: an investigator-initiated, prospective, double-blind, reference-controlled study. Spine. 2007;32:1803–8.
231. Ravi Kumar HS, Goni VG, Batra YK. Autologous conditioned serum as a novel alternative option in the treatment of unilateral lumbar radiculopathy: a prospective study. Asian Spine J. 2015;9:916–22.
232. Wright-Carpenter T, Klein P, Schaferhoff P, Appell H, Mir L, Wehling P. Treatment of muscle injuries by local administration by autologous conditioned serum: a pilot study on sportsmen with muscle strains. Int J Sports Med. 2005;25(8):588–93.
233. Wright-Carpenter T, Opolon P, Appell H, Meijer H, Wehling P, Mir L. Treatment of muscle injuries by local administration by autologous conditioned serum: animal experiments using a muscle contusion model. Int J Sports Med. 2005;25(8):582–7.
234. Zhang Y, Jordan JM. Epidemiology of osteoarthritis. Clin Geriatr Med. 2010;26(3):355–69.
235. Sakellariou V, Poultsides LA, Ma Y, et al. Risk assessment for chronic pain and patient satisfaction after total knee arthroplasty. Orthopedics. 2016;39(1):55–62.
236. Singh J. Epidemiology of knee and hip arthroplasty: a systematic review. Open Orthop J. 2011;5:80–5.
237. De Girolamo L, Kon E, Filardo G, Marmotti AG, Soler F, Peretti GM, Vannini F, Madry H, Chubinskaya S. Regenerative approaches for the treatment of early OA. Knee Surg Sports Traumatol Arthrosc. 2016;24:1826–35.
238. Crane DM, Oliver KS, Bayes MC. Orthobiologics and knee osteoarthritis: a recent literature review, treatment algorithm, and pathophysiology discussion. Phys Med Rehabil Clin N Am. 2016;27:985–1002.
239. Mascarenhas R, Saltzman B, Fortier L, et al. Role of platelet-rich plasma in articular cartilage injury and disease. J Knee Surg. 2014;28(1):3–10.
240. Block TJ, Garza JR. Regenerative cells for the management of osteoarthritis and joint disorders: a concise literature review. Aesth Surg J. 2017;37(53):S9–S15.
241. Chang KV, Hung CY, Aliwarga F, et al. Comparative effectiveness of platelet-rich plasma injections for treating knee joint cartilage degenerative pathology: a systematic review and meta-analysis. Arch Phys Med Rehabil. 2014;95(3):562–75.

242. Riboh JC, Saltzman BM, Yanke AB, et al. Effect of leucocyte concentration on the efficacy of platelet-rich plasma in the treatment of knee osteoarthritis. Am J Sports Med. 2016;44(3):792–800.
243. Souzdalnitski D, Narouze S, Lerman I, Calodney A. Platelet-rich plasma injections for knee osteoarthritis: systematic review of duration of clinical benefits. Tech Reg Anesth Pain Manag. 2015;19(1):67–72.
244. Yan W, Xu X, Xu Q, Sun Z, Jiang Q, Shi D. Platelet-rich plasma in combination with injectable hyaluronic acid hydrogel for porcine cartilage regeneration: a 6-month follow-up. Regen Biomater. 2020;7(1):77–90.
245. Dallari D, Stagni C, Rani N, et al. Ultrasound-guided injection of platelet-rich plasma and hyaluronic acid, separately and in combination, for hip osteoarthritis: a randomized-controlled study. Am J Sports Med. 2016;44(3):664–71.
246. Singh JR, Haffey P, Valimahomed A, Gelhorn AC. The effectiveness of autologous platelet-rich plasma for osteoarthritis of the hip: a retrospective analysis. Pain Med. 2019;20(8):1611–8.
247. Zuk PAM, Zhu H, Mizuno H, Huang J, Futrell JW, Katz AJ, Benhaim P, Lorenz P, Hedrick H. Multilineage cells from human adipose tissue: implications for cell-based therapies. Tissue. 2001;7:211–28.
248. Cho H, Kim H, Kim Y, Kim K. Recent clinical trials in adipose-derived stem cell-mediated osteoarthritis treatment. Biotechnol Bioproc. 2020;24(6):839–53.
249. Sun Y, Chen S, Pei M. Comparative advantages of infrapatellar fat pad: an emerging stem cell source for regenerative medicine. Rheumatology. 2018;57(12):2072–86.
250. Shapiro SA, Kazmerchak SE, Heckman MG, Zubair AC, O'Connor MI. A prospective, single-blind, placebo-controlled trial of bone marrow aspirate for knee osteoarthritis. Am J Sports Med. 2017;45(1):82–90.
251. Centeno C, Pitts J, Al-Sayegh H, Freeman M. Efficacy of autologous bone marrow concentrate for knee osteoarthritis with or without adipose graft. Biomed Res Int. 2014; 370621.
252. Law L, Hunt CL, Nassr A, Larson AN, Eldrige JS, Mauck WD, Pingree MJ, Yang J, Muir CW, Erwin PJ, Bydon M, Qu W. Office-based mesenchymal stem cell therapy for the treatment of musculoskeletal diseases: a systematic review of recent human studies. Pain Med. 2019;20(8):1570–83.
253. Tsaipalis D, Zeugolis D. Hypoxia preconditioning of bone marrow stem cells before implantation in orthopedics. Am J Orthop Surg. 2019;27(23):e1040–2.
254. Kokubo M, Sato M, Yamato M, Mitani G, Uchiyama Y, Mochida J, Okano T. Characterization of layered chondrocyte sheets created in a co-culture system with synviocytes in a hypoxic environment. J Tiss Eng Regen Med. 2017;11(10):2885–94.
255. Tiku ML, Sabaawy HE. Cartilage regeneration for treatment of osteoarthritis: a paradigm for non-surgical intervention. Ther Adv Musculoskel Dis. 2015;7(3):76–87.
256. Siddiqui AJ, Mazzola TJ, Shiple BJ. Techniques for performing regenerative procedures for orthopedic conditions. Regen Treat Sports Orthop Conditions. 2018:221–56.
257. Sharma P, Maffulli N, Maffulli N. Tendon structure biology of tendon injury: healing, modeling and remodeling. J Musculoskelet Neuronal Interact. 2006;6:181–90.
258. Sakabe T, Sakai T. Musculoskeletal diseases—tendon. Br Med Bull. 2011;99:211–25.
259. Chisari E, Rehak L, Khan WS, Maffulli N. Tendon healing in presence of chronic low-level inflammation: a systematic review. Br Med Bull. 2019;132:97–116.
260. Abate M, Gravare-Silbernagel K, Siljeholm C, et al. Pathogenesis of tendinopathies: inflammation or degeneration? Arthritis Res Ther. 2009;11:235.
261. Hammerman M, Blomgram P, Dansac A, et al. Different gene response to mechanical loading during early and late phases of rat Achilles tendon healing. J Appl Physiol. 2017;123:800–15.
262. Hammerman M, Dietrich-Zagonel F, Blomgran P, et al. Different mechanisms activated by mild versus strong loading in rat achilles tendon healing. PLoS One. 2018;13:e0201211.
263. Hammerman M, Aspenberg P, Eliasson P. Microtrauma stimulates rat Achilles tendon healing via an early gene expression pattern similar to mechanical loading. J Appl Phyiol. 2014;116:54–60.
264. Schepull T, Aspenberg P. Early controlled tension improves the material properties of healing human achilles tendon after ruptures: a randomized trial. Am J Sports Med. 2013;41:2550–7.
265. Rack P, Ross H. The tendon of flexor pollicis longus: its effect on the muscular control of force and position at the human thumb. J Physiol. 1984;351:99–110.
266. Bruns J, Kampen J, Kahrs J, Plitz W. Achilles tendon rupture: experimental results in spontaneous repair in a sheep-model. Knee Surg Sports Traumatol Arthrosc. 2000;8:364–9.
267. Geremia GM, Bobbert MF, Casa Nova M, Ott RD, Lemos Fde A, Lupion Rde O, et al. The structural and mechanical properties of the Achilles tendon 2 years after surgical repair. Clin Biomech (Bristol, Avon). 2015;30:485–92.
268. Brown MN, Shiple BJ, Scarpone M. Regenerative approaches to tendon and ligament conditions. Phys Med Rehabil Clin N Am. 2016;27:941–84.
269. Petersen W, Tillman B. Structure and vascularization of the cruciate ligaments of the human knee joint. Anat Embryol (Berl). 1999;200(3):325–44.
270. Robi K, Jakob N, Matevz K, Matjaz B. The physiology of sports injuries and repair processes. In: Hamlin M, Draper N, Kathiravel Y, editors. Current issues in sports and exercise medicine. London: IntechOpen; 2013.
271. Galatz L, Ball C, Teefey S, et al. The outcome and repair of integrity of completely arthroscopically

repaired large and massive rotator cuff tears. J Bone Joint Surg Am. 2004;86:219–24.
272. Lim WL, Liau LL, Ng MH, Chowdhury SR, Law JX. Current progress in tendon and ligament tissue engineering. Tissue Eng Regen Med. 2019;16(6):549–71.
273. Fleming B, Hulstyn M, Oksendahl HL, et al. Ligament injury, reconstruction and osteoarthritis. Curr Opin Orthop. 2005;16(5):354–62.
274. Bosch G, Van Shie H, de Groot M, et al. Effects of platelet-rich plasma on the quality of repair of mechanically induced core lesions in equine superficial digital flexor tendons: a placebo-controlled experimental study. J Orthop Res. 2010;28:211–7.
275. Sanchez M, Albillos J, Angulo F, Santisteban J, Andia I. Platelet-rich plasma in muscle and tendon healing. Oper Tech Orthop. 2012;22(1):16–24.
276. Hurley ET, Lim Fat D, Moran CJ, Mullet H. The efficacy of platelet-rich plasma and platelet-rich fibrin in arthroscopic rotator cuff repair: a meta-analysis of randomized controlled trials. Am J Sports Med. 2019;47(3):753–61.
277. Liddle AD, Rodriguez-Merchan C. Platelet-rich plasma in the treatment of patellar tendinopathy: a systematic review. Am J Sports Med. 2015;43(10):2583–90.
278. Ben-Nafa W, Munro W. The effect of corticosteroid versus platelet-rich plasma injection therapies for the management of lateral epicondylitis: a systematic review. SICOT-J. 2018;4:11.
279. Mishra AK, Skrepnik NV, Edwards SG, Jones JL, Sampsons S, Vermillion DA, et al. Efficacy of platelet-rich plasma for chronic tennis elbow: a double-blind, prospective, multicenter, randomized controlled trial of 230 patients. Am J Sports Med. 2014;42(2):463–71.
280. Fitzpatrick J, Bulsara M, Zheng M. The effectiveness of platelet-rich plasma in the treatment of tendinopathy: a meta-analysis of randomized controlled clinical trial. Am J Sports Med. 2017;45(1):226–33.
281. Clark NJ, Desai VS, Dines JD, Morrey ME, Camp CL. Nonreconstruction options for treating medial ulnar collateral ligament of the elbow in overhead athletes. Curr Rev Musculosket Med. 2018;11(1):48–54.
282. Dines JS, Williams PN, ElAttrache N, Conte S, Ahmad CS, et al. Platelet-rich plasma can be used to successfully treat elbow ulnar collateral ligament insufficiency in high-level throwers. Am J Orthop. 2016;45(5):296–300.
283. Vogrin M, Rupreht M, Crnjac A, Dinevski D, Krajnc C, Recnik G. The effect of platelet-derived growth factors on stability after anterior cruciate ligament reconstruction: a prospective randomized clinical study. Wien Klin Wochenschrift. 2010;122(S2):91–5.
284. Di Matteo B, Loibl M, Andriolo L, et al. Biologic agents for anterior cruciate ligament healing: a systematic review. World J Orthop. 2016;7(9):592–603.
285. Walters B, Porter D, Hobart S, Bedford B, Hogan D, McHugh M, Klein D, Harousseau K, Nicholas S. Effect of intra-operative platelet-rich plasma treatment on post-operative donor site knee pain in patellar tendon autograft anterior cruciate ligament reconstruction: a double-blind randomized controlled trial. Am J Sports Med. 2018;46(8):1827–35.
286. Kia C, Baldino J, Bell R, Ramji A, Uyeki C, Mazzocca A. Platelet-rich plasma: review of current literature on its use for tendon and ligament pathology. Curr Rev Musculosket Med. 2018;11(4):566–72.
287. Leong N, Kator J, Clemens T, James A, Enamoto-Iwamoto M, Jiang J. Tendon and ligament healing and current approaches to tendon and ligament regeneration. J Orthop Res. 2020;38(1):7–12.
288. Fu Y, Karbaat L, Wu L, et al. Trophic effects of mesenchymal stem cells in tissue regeneration. Tissue Eng Part B Rev. 2017;23:515–28.
289. Walia B, Huang A. Tendon stem progenitor cells: understanding the biology to inform therapeutic strategies for tendon repair. J Orthop Res. 2019;37(6):1270–80.
290. Mautner K, Blazuk J. Where do injectable stem cell treatments apply in treatment of muscle, tendon and ligament injuries? PM & R. 2016;7(4 suppl):S33–40.
291. Mei-Dan O, Kots E, Barchilon V, et al. A dynamic ultrasound examination for the diagnosis of ankle syndesmotic injury in professional athletes. Am J Sports Med. 2009;37(5):1009–16.
292. Gutierrez M. Ultrasound-guided procedures in rheumatology: what is the evidence? J Clin Rheumatol. 2015;21(4):201–10.
293. Thain L, Adler R. Sonography of the rotator cuff and biceps tendon: technique, normal anatomy, and pathology. J Clin Ultrasound. 1999;27(8):446–58.
294. Malanga GA, Axtman M, Mautner KR. The rationale and evidence for performing ultrasound-guided injections. Atlas Ultrasound-guided Musculoskel Inject. 2014:18–22.
295. Wilson JJ, Lee KS, Chamberlain C, DeWall R, Baer GS, Greatens M, Kamps N. Intratendinous injections of platelet-rich plasma: feasibility and effect on tendon pathology and mechanics. J Exp Orthop. 2015;2(1):5.
296. Rossi LA, Romoli ARM, Altiere BAB, Flor JAB, Scordo WE, Elizondo CM. Does platelet-rich plasma decrease time to return to sports in acute muscle tear? A randomized controlled trial. Knee Surg Sports Traumatol Arthrosc. 2017;25:3319–25.
297. Ekstrand J, Hagglund M, Walden M. Epidemiology of muscle injuries in professional football (soccer). Am J Sports Med. 2011;39(6):1226–32.
298. Hallen A, Ekstrand J. Return to play following muscle injuries in professional footballers. J Sports Sci. 2014;32(13):1229–36.
299. Ahmad CS, Redler LH, Ciccotti MG, Maffuli N, Longo UG, Bradley J. Evaluation and management of hamstring injuries. Am J Sports Med. 2013;41(12):2933–47.
300. Wong S, Ning A, Lee C, Feeley B. Return to sports after muscle injury. Curr Rev Musculoskelet Med. 2015;8(2):168–75.

301. Boppart MD, De Lisio M, Zou K, Huntsman HD. Defining a role for non-satellite stem cells in the regulation of muscle repair following exercise. Front Physiol. 2013;4:310.
302. Motahashi N, Asakura A. Muscle satellite cell heterogeneity and self-renewal. Front Cell Dev Biol. 2014;2:1.
303. Karalaki M, Fili S, Philippou A, Koutsilieres M. Muscle regeneration: cellular and molecular events. In Vivo. 2009;23(5):779–96.
304. Perandini L, Chimin P, Lutkemeyer D, Camara N. Chronic inflammation in skeletal muscle impairs satellite cells function during regeneration: can physical exercise restore the satellite cell niche? Febs J. 2018;285(11):1973–84.
305. Yumiko O, Ichiro M. Macrophages in inflammation, repair and regeneration. Int Immunol. 2018;30:11.
306. Gilbert-Honick J, Grayson W. Vascularized and innervated skeletal muscle tissue engineering. Adv Healthc Mater. 2020;9(1):1–27.
307. Corona BT, Wenke JC, Ward CL. Cells Tissues Organs. 2016;202:180.
308. Yosef B, Zhou Y, Mouschouris K, Poteracki J, Soker S, Criswell T. N-acetyl-L-cysteine reduces fibrosis and improves muscle function after acute compartment syndrome injury. Military Med. 2020;185(Suppl1):25–34.
309. Amthor H, Nicolas G, McKinnell I, Kemp CF, Sharma M, Kambadur R, Patel K. Follistatin complexes myostatin and antagonizes myostatin-mediated inhibition of myogenesis. Dev Biol. 2004;270:19–30.
310. Wong A, Pomerantz J. The role of muscle stem cells in regeneration and recovery after denervation: a review. Plast Reconstr Surg. 2019;143(3):779–88.
311. Grassi A, Napoli F, Romandini I, Samuelsson K, Zaffagnini S, Candrian C, Filardo G. Is platelet-rich plasma (PRP) effective in the treatment of acute muscle injuries? A systematic review and meta-analysis. Sports Med. 2018;48(4):971–89.
312. Setayesh K, Villarreal A, Gottschalk A, Tokish J, Choate W. Treatment of muscle injuries with platelet-rich plasma: a review of the literature. Curr Rev Musculoskelet Med. 2018;11(4):635–42.
313. Ziegler C, Van Sloun R, Gonzalez S, Whitney K, DePhillipo N, Kennedy M, Dornan G, Evans T, Huard J, LaPrade R. Characterization of growth factors, cytokines and chemokines in bone marrow concentrate and platelet-rich plasma: a prospective analysis. Am J Sports Med. 2019;47(9):2174–87.
314. Gang EJ, Darabi R, Bosnakovski D, et al. Engraftment of mesenchymal stem cells into dystrophin-deficient mice is not accompanied by functional recovery. Exp Cell Res. 2009;315:2624–36.
315. Dunn A, Talovic M, Patel K, Patel A, Marcinczyk M, Garg K. Biomaterial and stem-cell based strategies for skeletal muscle regeneration. J Orthop Res. 2019;37(6):1246–62.
316. Hamid AM, Mohamed Ali MR, Yusof A, et al. Platelet- rich plasma injections for the treatment of hamstring injuries: a randomized controlled trial. Am J Sports Med. 2014;42(10):2410–8.
317. Park P, Cai C, Bawa P, Kumaravel M. Platelet-rich plasma vs. steroid injections for hamstring injury: is there really a choice? Skelet Radiol. 2018;48(4):577–82.
318. Arner J, Lawyer T, Mauro C, Bradley J. Platelet-rich plasma shortens return to play in National Football League (NFL) Players with acute hamstring injuries. Orthop J Sports Med. 2019;7(7 suppl 5):1.
319. Gaballah A, Elgeidi A, Bressel E, Shakrah N, Abd-Alghany A. Rehabilitation of hamstring strains: does a single injection of platelet-rich plasma improve outcomes? (Clinical Study). Sports Sci Health. 2018;14(2):439–47.
320. Manduca M, Straub S. Effectiveness of PRP injection in reducing recovery time of acute hamstring injury: a critically appraised topic. J Sport Rehabil. 2018;27(5):4870–484.
321. Hamilton B, Tol JL, Almusa E, et al. Platelet-rich plasma does not enhance return to play in hamstring injuries: a randomized controlled trial. Br J Sports Med. 2015;49(14):943–50.
322. Bradley JP, Lawyer TJ, Ruef S, Towers JD, Arner JW. Platelet-rich plasma shortens return to play in National Football League Players with acute hamstring injuries. Orthop J Sports Med. 2020;8(4):1–5.
323. Evangelidis P, Massey G, Ferguson R, Wheeler P, Pain M, Folland J. The functional significance of hamstrings composition: is it really a "fast" muscle group? Scand J Med Sci Sports. 2017;27(11):1181–9.
324. Bentzen R, Ma O, Herzka A. Point of care ultrasound diagnosis of proximal hamstring rupture. J Emerg Med. 2018;54(2):225–8.
325. Peterson J, Thorborg K, Nielsen M, Skjodt T, Bolvig L, Bang N, Holmich P. The diagnostic and prognostic value of ultrasonography in soccer players with acute hamstring injuries. Am J Sports Med. 2014;42(2):399–404.
326. Hall M. Return to play after thigh muscle injury: utility of serial ultrasound in guiding clinical progression. Curr Sports Med Rep. 2018;17(9):296–301.
327. Alzahrani M, Aldebeyan S, Abduljabbar F, Martineau P. Hamstring injuries in athletes: diagnosis and treatment. JBJS Rev. 2015;3(6):11.
328. Chu S, Rho M. Hamstring injuries in the athlete: diagnosis, treatment and return to play. Curr Sports Med Rep. 2016;15(3):184–90.
329. Kubrova E, van Wijnen A, Qu W. Spine disorders and regenerative rehabilitation. Curr Physical Med Rehabil Rep. 2020;8(1):30–6.
330. Sakai D, Andersson G. Stem cell therapy for intervertebral disk regeneration: obstacles and solutions. Nat Rev Rheumatol. 2015;11(4):243–56.
331. Hicks GE, Morone N, Weiner DK. Degenerative lumbar disk and facet disease in older adults: prevalence and clinical correlates. Spine (Phila Pa 1976). 2009;34(12):1301–6.
332. Theis KA, Roblin DW, Helmick CG, Luo R. Prevalence and cause of work disability among

work-age US adults, 2011-2013. NHIS Disabil Health J. 2018;11(1):108–15.

333. Jensen TS, Albert HB, Soerensen JS, et al. Natural course of disc morphology in patients with sciatica: an MRI study using a standardized qualitative classification system. Spine (Phila Pa 1976). 2006;31(14):1606–12.
334. Sowa G. Using biology to define optimal treatments for low back pain opportunities for physiatrists. Am J Phys Med Rehabil. 2013;92(10):841–8.
335. Bogduk M. Clinical anatomy of the lumbar spine and sacrum. 4th ed. New York: Elsevier; 2005. p. 147–8.
336. Dowdell J, Erwin M, Choma T, Vaccaro A, Iatridis J, Cho SK. Intervertebral disk degeneration and repair. Neurosurgery. 2017;80(3S):S46–54.
337. Mascarinas A, Harrison J, Boachie-Adjie K, Lutz G. Regenerative treatments for spinal conditions. Phys Med Rehabil Clin N Am. 2016;27:1003–17.
338. Wang S, Chang Q, Lu J, Wang C. Growth factors and platelet-rich plasma: promising biological strategies for early intervertebral disc degeneration. Int Orthop. 2015;39(5):927–34.
339. Le Maitre CL, Richardson SM, Baird P, et al. Expression of receptors for putative anabolic growth factors in human intervertebral disc: implications for repair and regeneration of the disc. J Pathol. 2005;207:445–52.
340. Vadala G, Sowa G, Hubert M, Gilbertson L, Denaro V, Kang J. Mesenchymal stem cells injection in degenerated intervertebral disc: cell leakage may induce osteophyte formation. J Tiss Engg Regen Med. 2012;6(5):348–55.
341. Zhao L, Manchikanti L, Kaye A, Abd-Elsayed A. Treatment of discogenic low back pain: current treatment strategies and future options—a literature review. Curr Pain Headache Rep. 2019;23(11):1–9.
342. Livshits V, Popham M, Malkin I, et al. Lumbar disc degeneration and genetic factors are the main risk factors for low back pain in women: the UK twin spine study. Ann Rheum Dis. 2011;70(10):1740–5.
343. Kalichman L, Hunter DJ. The genetics of intervertebral disc degeneration. Familial disposition and heritability estimation. Joint Bone Spine. 2008;75(4):383–7.
344. Liuke M, Solovieva S, Lamminen A, et al. Disk degeneration of the lumbar spine in relation to overweight. Int J Obes. 2005;29(8):903–8.
345. Greenberg AS, Obin MS. Obesity and the role of adipose tissue in inflammation and metabolism. Am J Clin Nutr. 2006;83(2):461S–5S.
346. Valimahomed A, Haffey P, Urman R, Kaye A, Yong R. Regenerative techniques for neuraxial back pain: a systematic review. Curr Pain Headache Rep. 2019;23(3):1–11.
347. Schwarzer AC, Aprill CN, Derby R, Fortin J, Kine G, Bogduk N. The prevalence and clinical features of internal disc disruption in patients with low back pain. Spine. 1995;20(17):1878–83.
348. Peng B, Fu X, Pang X, Li D, Liu W, Gao C, et al. Prospective clinical study on natural history of discogenic low back pain at 4 years of follow-up. Pain Physician. 2012;15:525–32.
349. Schol J, Sakai D. Cell therapy for intervertebral disc herniation and degenerative disc disease: clinical trials. Int Orthop. 2018;43(4):1011–25.
350. Nguyen TH, Randolph DC, Talmage J, Succop P, Travis R. Long term outcomes of lumbar fusion among workers' compensation subjects: a historical cohort study. Spine. 2011;36(4):320–31.
351. Monfett M, Harrison J, Boachie-Adjei K, Lutz G. Intradiscal platelet-rich plasma (PRP) injections for discogenic low back pain: an update. Int Orthop. 2016;40(6):1321–8.
352. Burnham T, Conger A, Tate Q, Cushman D, Kendall R, Schneider B, McCormick Z. The effectiveness and safety of percutaneous platelet-rich plasma and bone marrow aspirate concentrate for the treatment of suspected of discogenic low back pain: a comprehensive review. Curr Phys Med Rehabil Rep. 2019;7(4):372–84.
353. Levi D, Horn S, Tyszko S, Levin J, Hecht-Leavitt C, Walko E. Intradiscal platelet-rich plasma injection for chronic discogenic low back pain: preliminary results from a prospective trial. Pain Med. 2016;17(6):1010–22.
354. Urits I, Viswanath O, Galasso A, Sottosani E, Mahan K, Aiudi C, Kaye A, Orhurhu V. Platelet-rich plasma for the treatment of low back pain: a comprehensive review. Curr Pain Headache Rep. 2019;23(7):1–11.
355. Singla B, Batra Y, Bharti N, Goni V, Marwaha N. Steroid versus platelet-rich plasma in ultrasound-guided sacroiliac joint injection for chronic low back pain. Pain Pract. 2017;17(6):782–91.
356. Pairuchvej S, Muljadi J, Arirachakaran A, Kongtharvonskul J. Efficacy of platelet-rich plasma in posterior lumbar interbody fusion: systematic review and meta-analysis. Eur J Orthop Surg Traumatol. 2020;30(4):583–93.
357. Kim H, Yeom J, Koh Y, Yeo J, Kang K, Kang Y, Chang B, Lee C. Anti-inflammatory effect of platelet-rich plasma on nucleus pulposus cells with response of TNF-α and IL-1. J Orthop Res. 2014;32(4):551–6.
358. Montesano PX, Cuellar JM, Scuderi GJ. Intradiscal injection of an autologous alpha-2-macroglobulin (A2M) concentrate alleviates back pain in FAC-positive patients. Orthop Rheumatol. 2017;4(2):555634.
359. Dimitroulas T, Lambe T, Raphael JH, Kitas GD, Duarte RV. Biologic drugs as analgesics for the management of low back pain and sciatica. Pain Med. 2019;20(9):1678–86.
360. Takahashi K, Ohtori S. Perspectives of treatment of low back pain. Glob Spine J. 2017;4(1_suppl):s-0034.
361. Ohtori S, Miyagi M, Inoue G. Sensory nerve ingrowth, cytokines, and instability of discogenic low back pain: a review. Spine Surg Relat Res. 2018;2(1):11–7.
362. Takahashi K, Aoki Y, Ohtori S. Resolving discogenic pain. Eur Spine J. 2008;17(4):428–31.

363. Ohtori S, Aoki Y, Orita S. Pain generators and pathways of degenerative disc disease. Lumbar Spine Online Textbook. JBJS. Section 2, Chapter 4. 2018.
364. Urits I, Capuco A, Sharma M, Kaye A, Viswanath O, Cornett E, Orhurhu V. Stem cell therapies for treatment of discogenic low back pain: a comprehensive review. Pain Headache Rep. 2019;23(9):1–12.
365. Oehmi D, Goldschlager T, Rosenfeld J, Ghosh P, Jenken G. The role of stem cell therapies in degenerative lumbar spine disease: a review. Neurosurg Rev. 2015;38(3):429–45.
366. Feng G, Zhao X, Liu H, Zhang H, Chen X, Shi R, et al. Transplantation of mesenchymal stem cells and nucleus pulposus cells in a degenerative disc model in rabbits: a comparison of 2 cell types as potential candidates for disc regeneration. J Neurosurg Spine. 2011;14(3):322–9.
367. Henriksson HB, Svanvik T, Jonsson M, Hagman M, Horn M, Lindahl A, et al. Transplantation of human mesenchymal cells into intervertebral discs in a xenogeneic porcine model. Spine (Phila Pa 1976). 2009;34(2):141–8.
368. Hiyama A, Mochida J, Iwashina T, Omi H, Watanabe T, Serigano K, et al. Transplantation of mesenchymal stem cells in a canine disc degeneration model. J Orthop Res. 2008;26(5):589–600.
369. Vadala G, Russo F, Musumeci M, D'Este M, Cattani C, Catanzaro G, et al. Clinically relevant hydrogel-based on hyaluronic acid and platelet-rich plasma as a carrier for mesenchymal stem cells: rheological and biological characterization. J Orthop Res. 2017;35(10):2109–16.
370. Vadala G, Sowa G, Hubert M, Gilbertson L, Denaro V, Kang G. Mesenchymal stem cells injection in degenerated intervertebral disc: cell leakage may induce osteophyte formation. J Tiss Engg Regen Med. 2012;6(5):348–55.
371. Wangler S, Peroglio M, Menzel U, Benneker L, HaglunD L, Sakai D, Alini M, Grad S. Mesenchymal stem cell homing into intervertebral discs enhances the tie-2 positive progenitor cell population, prevents cell death, and induces a proliferative response. Spine. 2019;44(23):1613–22.
372. Colombini A, Ceriani C, Banfi G, et al. Fibrin in intervertebral disc tissue engineering. Tissue Eng Part B Rev. 2014;20(6):713–21.
373. Yin W, Pauza K, Olan W, Doerzbacher J, Thorne K. Intradiscal injection of fibrin sealant for the treatment of symptomatic lumbar internal disc disruption: results of a prospective multicenter pilot study with 24-month follow up. Pain Med. 2014;15(1):16–31.
374. Zhang C, Berven SH, Fortin M, et al. Adjacent segment degeneration versus disease after lumbar spine fusion for degenerative pathology: a systematic review with meta-analysis of the literature. Clin Spine Surg. 2016;29(1):21–9.
375. Taylor CA, Braza D, Rice JB, Dillingham T. The incidence of peripheral nerve injury in extremity trauma. Am J Phys Med Rehabil. 2008;87(5):381–5.
376. Benowitz LI, Popovich PG. Inflammation and axon regeneration. Curr Opin Neurol. 2011;24:577–83.
377. Stoll G, Jander S, Myers RR. Degeneration and regeneration of the peripheral nervous system: from Augustus Waller's observations to neuroinflammation. J Peripheral Nerve Syst. 2002;7:13–27.
378. Deumens R, Bozkurt A, Meek MF, et al. Repairing injured peripheral nerves: bridging the gap. Prog Neurobiol. 2010;92(3):245–76.
379. Carr MJ, Johnston AP. Schwann cells as drivers of tissue repair and regeneration. Curr Opin Neurobiol. 2017;47:52–7.
380. Ide C. Peripheral nerve regeneration. Neurosci Res. 1996;25:101–21.
381. Gaudet AD, Popovich PG, Ramer MS. Wallerian degeneration: gaining perspective on inflammatory events after peripheral nerve injury. J Neuroinflammation. 2011;8:110.
382. Webber C, Zochodne D. The nerve regenerative microenvironment: early behavior and partnership of axons and Schwann cells. Exp Neurol. 2010;223:51–9.
383. Fu SY, Gordon T. The cellular and molecular basis of peripheral nerve regeneration. Mol Neurobiol. 1997;14:67–116.
384. Schneidt P, Friede RL. Myelin phagocytosis in Wallerian degeneration. Properties of millipore diffusion chambers and immunohistochemical identification of cell populations. Acta Neuropathol. 1987;75:77–84.
385. Chen P, Piao X, Bonaldo P. Role of macrophages in Wallerian degeneration and axonal regeneration after peripheral nerve injury. Acta Neuropathol. 2015;130(5):605–18.
386. Shin Y, Gu X, Zhang R, Qian T, Li S, Yi S. Biological characteristics of dynamic expression of nerve regeneration related to growth factors in dorsal root ganglia after peripheral nerve injury. Neural Regen Res. 2020;15(8):1502–9.
387. Seddon HJ. Peripheral nerve injuries. Medical Research Council. Medical Report Series 282. London: Her Majesty's Stationery Office; 1954.
388. Sunderland S. Rate of regeneration of I: sensory fibers and II: motor fibers. Arch Neurol Psychiatr. 1947;58:1–14.
389. Gordon T. Electrical stimulation to enhance axon regeneration after peripheral nerve injuries in the animal models and humans. Neurotherapeutics. 2016;13(2):295–310.
390. Colloca L, Ludman T, Bouhassira D, Baron R, et al. Neuropathic pain. Nat Rev Dis Primers. 2017;16(3):17002.
391. Miclescu A, Straamann A, Gkatziani P, Butler S, Karlsten R, Gordh T. Chronic neuropathic pain after traumatic peripheral nerve injuries in the upper extremity: prevalence, demographic and surgical determinants, impact on health and on pain medications. Scand J Pain. 2019;20(1):95–108.
392. Yu W, Wang J, Yin J. Platelet-rich plasma: a promising product for treatment of peripheral nerve regeneration after nerve injury. Int J Neurosci. 2012;121(4):176–80.

393. Bastami F, Vares P, Khojasteh A. Healing effects of platelet-rich plasma on peripheral nerve injuries. J Craniofac Surg. 2017;28(1):e49–57.
394. Afsar SI, Yemisci OU, Cetin N. The role of platelet-rich plasma in peripheral nerve injuries. J Clin Anal Med. 2015;6(suppl 6):905–8.
395. Lopez JC, Cortes H, Ceballos EG, Pizarro LQ. Platelet-rich plasma in treating peripheral neuropathic pain. Preliminary report. Rev Soc Esp Dolor. 2018;25(5):263–70.
396. Cass S. Ultrasound-guided nerve hydrodissection: what is it? A review of literature. Curr Sports Med Rep. 2016;15(1):20–2.
397. Nwawka K, Miller TT. Ultrasound-guided peripheral nerve injection techniques. Am J Roentgen. 2016;207(3):507–16.
398. Purita J, Lana JFSD, Kolber M, Rodriguez BL, Mosaner T, Santos GS, Caliari-Oliveira C, Huber SC. Bone marrow-derived products: a classification proposal –bone marrow aspirate, bone marrow aspirate concentrate or hybrid? World J Stem Cells. 2020;12(4):1–9.

15 Ultrasound-Guided Nerve Hydrodissection for Pain Management: From Anatomy to Techniques

King Hei Stanley Lam, Yung-Tsan Wu, and Kenneth Dean Reeves

Introduction

The technique of ultrasound-guided hydrodissection (HD) of peripheral nerves has become one of the commonly used methods to treat neuropathic pain in the pain, sports, and musculoskeletal medicine fields. There were randomized control trials published in high impact journals showing that this technique can safely and effectively treat carpal tunnel syndrome (CTS) [1–6]. Notably, the 20th edition of *Harrison's Principles of Internal Medicine* textbook now lists injection of 5% dextrose as an alternative local treatment that does not have the side effects of corticosteroid for CTS. The most extensively studied clinical condition treated by ultrasound-guided HD of peripheral nerves is CTS [1–10]. Other clinical studies have also used this technique to treat neuropathic pain related to deep nervous structures or neuro-axial spine [11], ulnar neuropathy at elbow [12], radial nerve palsy [13], and meralgia paresthetica [14]. There was also review articles available which summarize the rationale, methods, current literature, and theoretical mechanisms of this technique [reference]. The aim of this chapter is to provide an introduction and overview to this technique in order to assist physicians in better utilizing this ultrasound-guided HD for the treatment neuropathic or nerve-related pain. However, it is by all means not a replacement of hands-on fresh cadaver workshops which the author believe is the best way to learn and practice this technique before using it to treat real patients.

Nerve HD is a technique which uses high-resolution ultrasound-guided fluid injection to separate nerves from a surrounding or adjacent structure, usually the fascia, which is believed to constrict or irritate the nerve either during movement or at rest [15, 16]. The vulnerability of mixed sensory/motor nerves for circumferential

Supplementary Information The online version contains supplementary material available at [https://doi.org/10.1007/978-3-030-98256-0_15].

K. H. S. Lam (✉)
The Hong Kong Institute of Musculoskeletal Medicine, Kowloon, Hong Kong

Department of Family Medicine, The Faculty of Medicine, The Chinese University of Hong Kong, New Territory, Hong Kong

Department of Family Medicine, The Faculty of Medicine, The University of Hong Kong, Hong Kong, Hong Kong

Y.-T. Wu
Department of Physical Medicine and Rehabilitation, Tri-Service General Hospital, School of Medicine, National Defense Medical Center, Taipei, Taiwan

Integrated Pain Management Center, Tri-Service General Hospital, School of Medicine, National Defense Medical Center, Taipei, Taiwan

K. D. Reeves
Private Practice of Physical Medicine and Rehabilitation, Roeland Park, KS, USA

Y. El Miedany (ed.), *Musculoskeletal Ultrasound-Guided Regenerative Medicine*,
https://doi.org/10.1007/978-3-030-98256-0_15

compression was demonstrated by Bennett [17], who developed the most commonly used animal model of neuropathic pain by placing self-dissolving ligatures about the sciatic nerve of rats. A key aspect of his approach was the exclusive use of light constriction to prevent the restriction of epineural blood flow; moreover, the ligatures could be moved up and down the nerve to ensure minimal indentation [18]. This light constriction led to prominent and rapid reactive morphological changes, and development of allodynia and hyperesthesia, therefore, provided a reliable animal model. Additionally, this model provided a rationale to suspect that in humans, the peripheral nerves may be more vulnerable to light compression and entrapment effects at multiple locations than that previously reported.

Nerve HD techniques can be used to treat neuropathic pain, or pain caused by nerve entrapment/ injuries in the following conditions. These are listed alongside their proposed, but as yet, unconfirmed mechanisms.

1. Sports injuries: sudden nerve elongation during sprain or strain injuries, which exceeds the stretch limit of the semi-elastic nerve components of a nerve or forced nerve movement through areas of fascial constrictions or through the bony prominences, e.g., forced movement of the common peroneal nerve about the fibular head during an inversion sprain injury.
2. Osteophytosis/tendinosis/other degenerative changes with osteophytic changes which alters the course of a nerve or causes friction or nerve irritation within the areas of chronic tendinosis, ligamentosis, or osteophytosis which subsequently sensitizes the innervating peripheral nerves or alters the free movement of the related nerves because of reduced flexibility when innervating through areas of degenerated tissues.
3. Post-fracture or post-surgical pain: uncontrolled pain leading to central and/or peripheral sensitization; stretching of nerves to facilitate surgical access or to avoid inadvertent nerve lysis, contusions at the time of injury with secondary nerve swelling resulting in abnormal friction/compression during nerve movement, altered gait patterns because of limited ability to bear weight or antalgia, and formation of scars or fibrosis about a surgical/fracture site.
4. Idiopathic acute or chronic neuropathic pain without an apparent cause.

Neuropathic pain is defined as pain caused by a lesion or disease of the somatosensory system [19, 20]. It usually has the following characteristics:

1. Deep-seated pain with poor localization of the source of pain.
2. The degree of pain is usually not proportional to the degree of tissue/nerve damage.
3. The pain can be sore, numb, or with electric shock; presence of hyperalgesia and/or allodynia.
4. A sensation of cold or heat can be felt on the affected region, and the skin on the affected area may appear bluish, similar in appearance to venous stasis.

A potential benefit of separation of nerves from the surrounding soft tissue with fluid and with the fluid flushing, or enclosing the nerve to treat neuropathic pain, is the release of pressure on the "free nerves supplying the main nerves," which are called "nervi nervorum" [21–25], outside the epineurium. These "nervi nervorum" innervate and regulate the function and discharge of the main nerves.

Additionally, "vasa nervorum," which are small blood vessels on the surface of the nerves are also present; the arteries supply nutrients to the main nerve, and the veins drain away the metabolites from these main nerves [26–28]. Entrapment of the vasa nervorum would likely result in stasis and ischemia and the potential accumulation of toxins at the affected part of the nerve. In addition, it is postulated that lymphatic drainage might be present outside the epineurium (Fig. 15.1). Therefore, the primary objective of HD is to release the entrapment of the peripheral nerves by hydrodissecting the nerves.

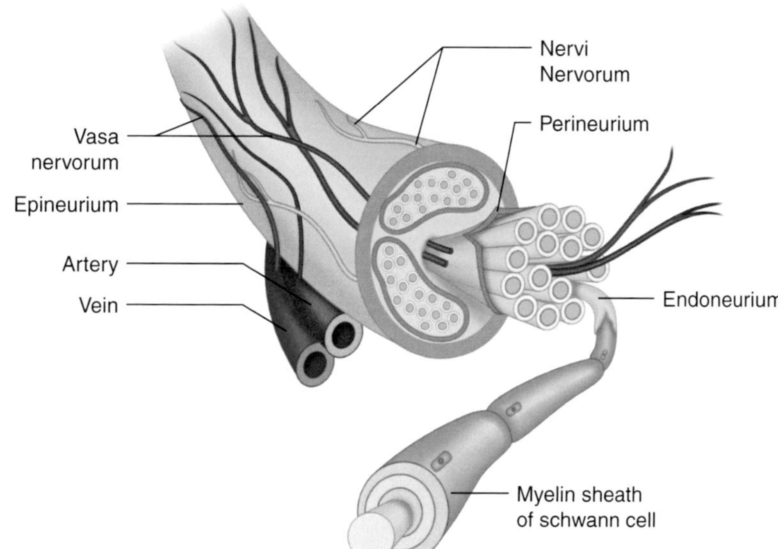

Fig. 15.1 Diagram shows "nervi nervorum," "vasa nervorum," outside the epineurium [21]

Current Methodology

Ultrasonography (US) is usually used in nerve HD to guide needles and fluid (hydro) used to separate (dissect/ release) the nerves from the surrounding entrapped soft tissues.

There are two methods of US-guided HD of the nervous systems [29, 30].

Method 1 (In-Plane Approach, Needle Perpendicular to the Long Axis of the Nerve)

Generally, when using method 1 for HD of nerves, the needle is perpendicular to the long axis of the nerve, and the probe is perpendicular to the short axis of the nerve. The needle is in-plane to the transducer, and the tissues above and below the nerves are hydrodissected. The needle first approaches the inferior surface of the nerve, with the needle bevel positioned up, and the pressure of the injectate is used to open the soft tissues around the nerve layer by layer until the epineurium is surrounded by the injectate. The same process is repeated with the needle approaching from the superior surface of the nerve, with the needle bevel positioned down (Fig. 15.2). The hydrodissected nerve looks oval and surrounded by anechoic fluid on US. A 25-gauge, 2-inch needle or a 22-gauge, 2¾-inch needle is typically used, or a 22-gauge, 4-inch needle is used especially for performing hydrodissections of deeply seated nerves.

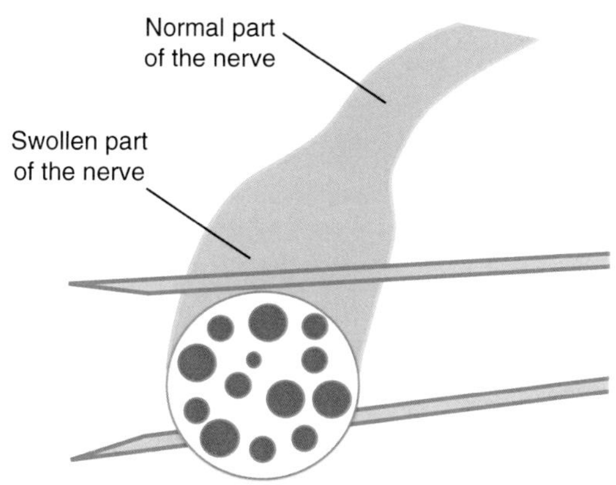

Fig. 15.2 Illustrates the needle position for method 1 of hydrodissection of nerves. With "in-plane" technique, first, the inferior surface of the nerve is hydrodissected with the needle bevel positioned up; and thereafter, the superior surface of the nerve is hydrodissected with the needle bevel positioned down

Real Practice of This Technique

The following links shows the real practice of this technique in clinical situations.

https://www.dropbox.com/s/320rd6ncih6e73w/RN%20HD%20combine%20%2B%20%20name%20.mp4?dl=0

The following link shows the real practice of ultrasound-guided hydrodissection of the radial nerve, using method 1.

https://www.dropbox.com/s/kszoldfrkmjtkx8/CPN%20HD%20new%20with%20name%20.mp4?dl=0

The following link shows the real practice of ultrasound-guided hydrodissection of the common fibular nerve, using method 1.

Clinical Pearls

1. The basic principle of US-guided HD of nervous structure is that the fluid/injectate but not the needle is the actual tool used to separate the soft tissues. Therefore, after administering local anesthetics at the superficial entry point of the needle, it is essential to visualize the needle at all times during the procedure, particularly during needle advancement, during which time the physician will continually inject the fluid. The injectate separates the soft tissues in front of the needle, and the needle just moves through and into the space separated by the fluid.
2. Pay special attention to the beveling of the needle; if the bevel of the hypodermic needle is positioned up, the injectate points and flows upward, whereas the tracking of the needle is downward, especially if a long and thin needle is used (Fig. 15.3).
3. If the bevel of the hypodermic needle is positioned down, the injectate points and flows downward and the tracking of the needle is upward, especially if a long and thin needle is used (Fig. 15.4).
4. Usually, HD of the nerve is initiated from the site where the nerve is most severely damaged or trapped. If the diseased nerve or the damaged/entrapped part of the nerve is long, the same entry point can be used, with the transducer and needle pivoted to the proximal part of the nerve and, thereafter, to the distal part of the nerve to repeat the HD process (Fig. 15.5).

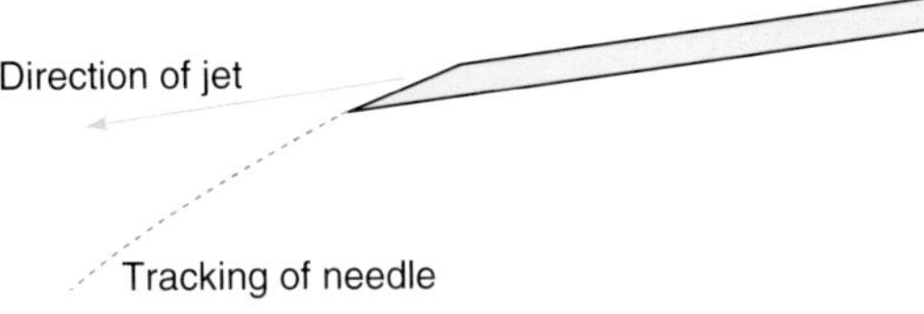

Fig. 15.3 Illustrates the effect of bevel up position on the direction of flow of the injectate and tracking of the needle

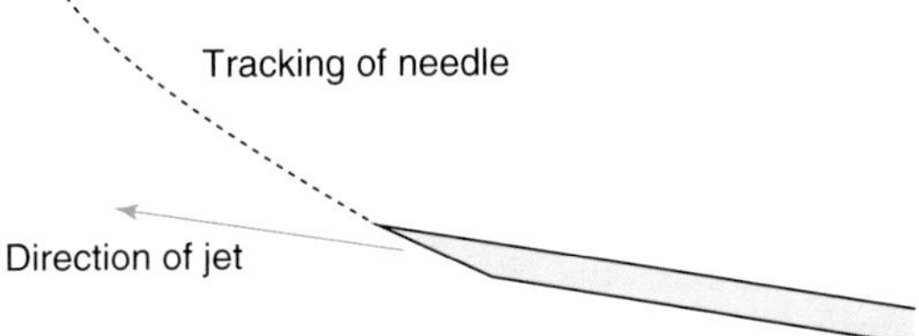

Fig. 15.4 Illustrates the effect of the bevel down position on the direction of flow of the injectate and tracking of the needle

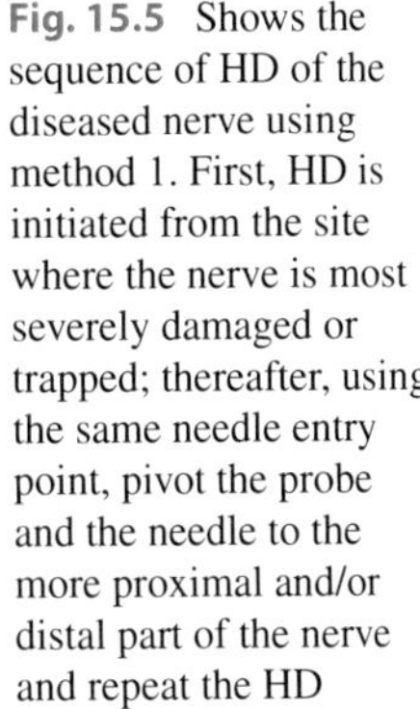

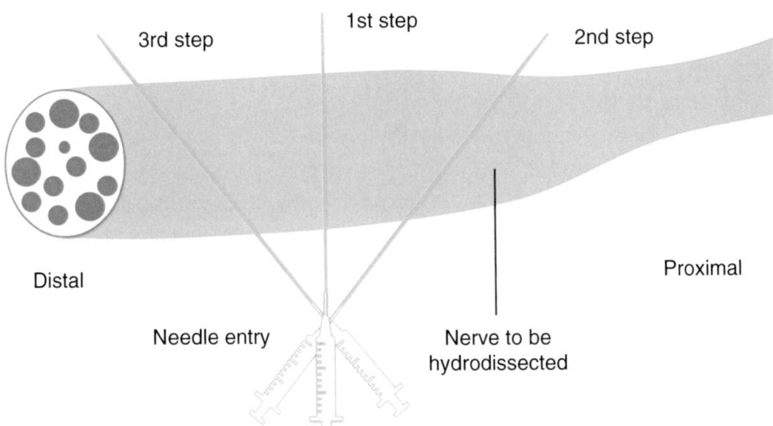

Fig. 15.5 Shows the sequence of HD of the diseased nerve using method 1. First, HD is initiated from the site where the nerve is most severely damaged or trapped; thereafter, using the same needle entry point, pivot the probe and the needle to the more proximal and/or distal part of the nerve and repeat the HD

5. This method can be used for HD of 2–3 nerves running parallel to each other and if all nerves require treatment simultaneously (Fig. 15.6).

https://www.dropbox.com/s/qqmmmk9atl-5ghpv/HD%20TN%20to%20CPN%20com-bine%20%2B%20name%20.mp4?dl=0

The above link shows the use of method 1 to treat 2 or 3 diseased nerves running parallel to each other in real clinical practice.

Method 2 (Out-of-Plane with Subsequent In-Plane Approach)

The needle is parallel to the long axis of the nerve; the probe is first perpendicular and thereafter parallel to the long axis of the nerve. First, an "out-of-plane" technique is used for HD of the nerve from the surrounding tissues. The nerve should be confirmed to be freed from the surrounding soft tissues by visualizing the anechoic fluid surrounding the nerve (both above and below the nerve). Thereafter, the needle is guided back to the top of the nerve, and the probe is turned "in-plane" toward the nerve to inject the fluid above it, with the bevel positioned down when approaching the nerve to avoid making accidental contact with the nerve (Fig. 15.7). The injected fluid should be visualized to be tracking above and below the nerve.

The real clinical practice of method 2 for HD of nerves shown in the following link:

https://www.dropbox.com/s/9uchgjfwfskgsrp/MN%20HD%20SAX%20to%20LAX%20with%20Name.mov?dl=0

Clinical Pearls

1. Method 2 for HD of nerves requires good "out-of-plane" and "in-plane" techniques. Therefore, we suggest extensive practice of this technique on fresh cadavers. A doctor is not proficient in method 2 but with good method 1 skill can still perform in-plane HD perpendicular to the short-axis of the nerve first, followed by HD of the nerve in-plane with the needle and transducer parallel to the long axis of the nerve through another needle entry point.

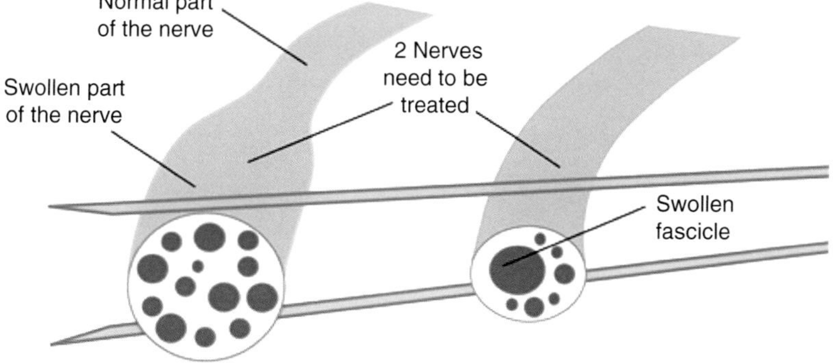

Fig. 15.6 Showing the method for using 1 needle entry for HD of two nerves running parallel to each other, when both need to be treated simultaneously, e.g., the common peroneal nerve lateral to the tibial nerve, at the level of the distal hamstring

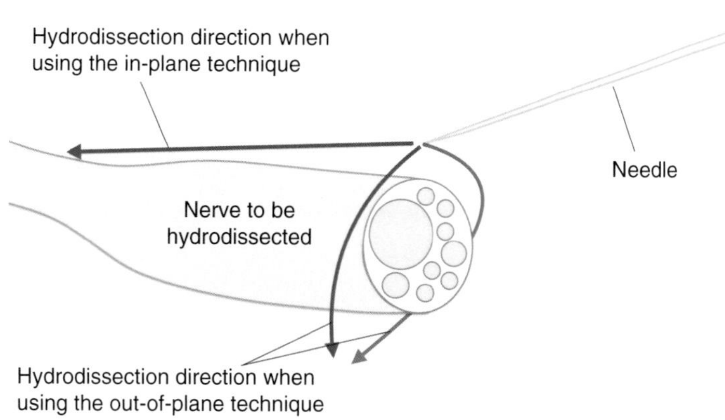

Fig. 15.7 Diagram shows the relative direction and movement of the needle with the nerve with method 2 for HD of nerves

2. Generally, method 2 for HD can separate a comparatively longer length of nerves from the surrounding soft tissues. The end target is the separation of the nerve from the surrounding soft tissues and visualization of the anechoic injectate above, below, proximal, and distal to the hydrodissected nerve.

Identification of Nerve(s) Indicated for Treatment

1. The pathologic nerves/entrapped nerves are usually more swollen compared to the healthy counterpart. The cross-sectional areas of the entrapped nerves are usually found to be double or even triple in size in comparison to the healthy nerves (Figs. 15.8, 15.9, and 15.10).
2. One of the fascicles of the entrapped/diseased nerve is swollen and much bigger than the rest of the fascicles within the same nerve (Figs. 15.11, 15.12, and 15.13).

The following link shows the tracking of common peroneal nerve (CPN) from the distal to proximal end and shows a swollen fascicle.

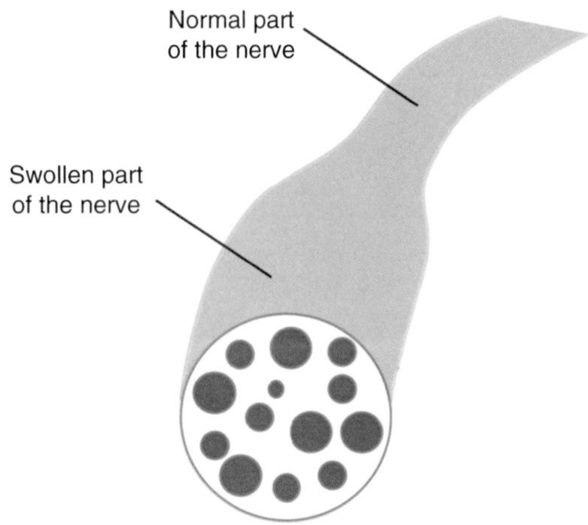

Fig. 15.8 Illustrates a swollen pathologic nerve with twice the cross-sectional area of the healthy nerve

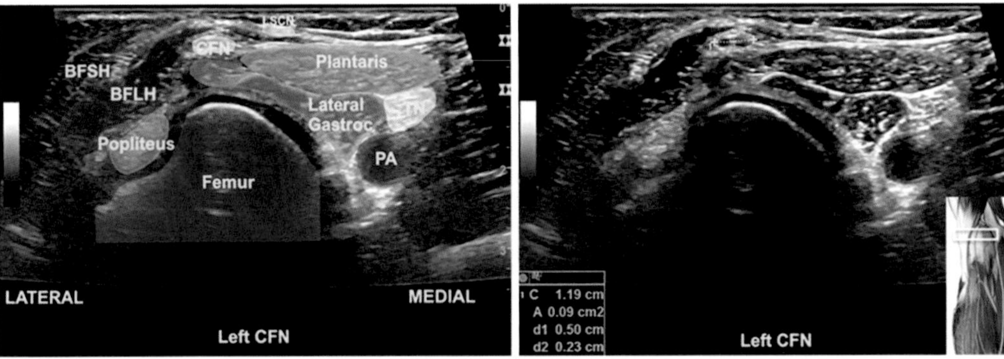

Fig. 15.9 Shows normal common fibular nerve with a normal cross-sectional area of 9 mm²

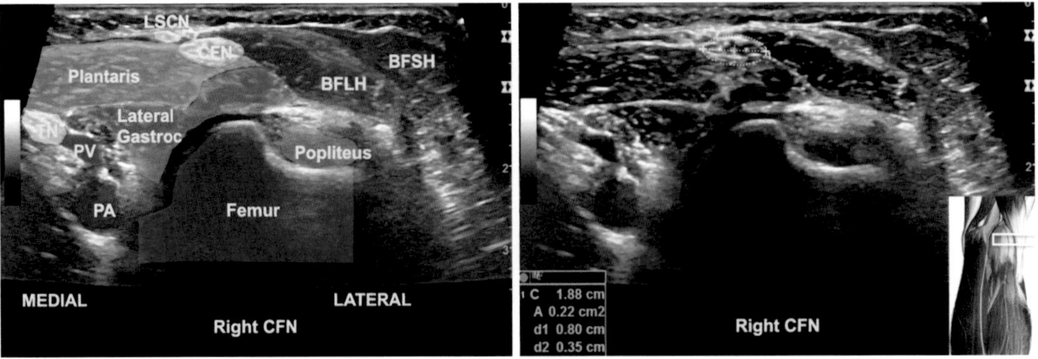

Fig. 15.10 Shows an abnormal/swollen common fibular nerve with a cross-sectional area of 22 mm²

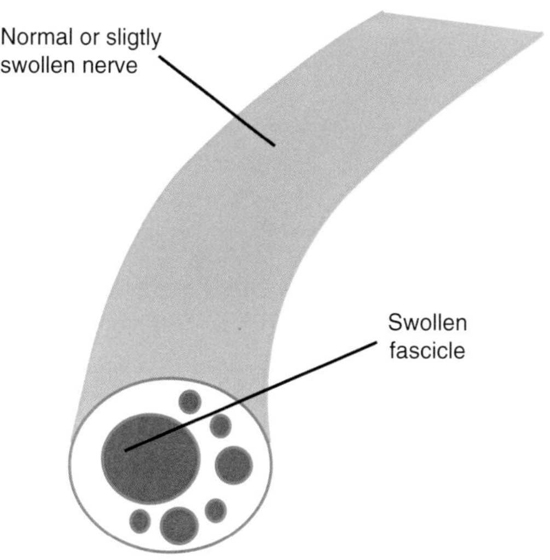

Fig. 15.11 Shows one or more of the fascicles with a cross-sectional (CSA) of more than 2 mm²; the whole nerve may have a normal CSA or may be slightly swollen

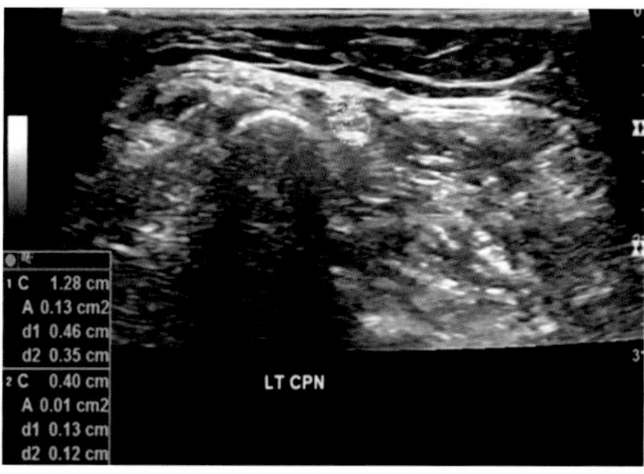

Fig. 15.12 Shows the normal nerve with normal fascicles

https://www.dropbox.com/s/igv46wgl8qch3cc/CPN%20from%20distal%20to%20proximal%201.mp4?dl=0

3. Direct digital/ transducer palpation of the suspected swollen nerve or suspected nerve with swollen fascicles reproduces the neuropathic pain experienced by the patient.
4. Using continuous dynamic US, a snapping/ sudden motion of a nerve against a surrounding bone, ligament, muscle, or tendon is observed, and it reproduces the neuropathic pain experienced by the patient.

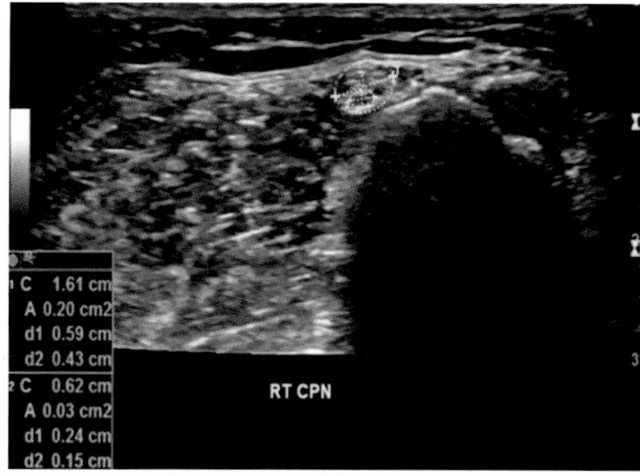

Fig. 15.13 Shows slightly swollen nerve with swollen nerve fasicle with a cross-sectional area of 3 mm²

The following link shows direct transducer palpation and snapping of the superficial radial nerve against the first compartment wrist extensor and reproduce the neuropathic pain the patient is usually experiencing with the proximal intersection syndrome.

https://www.dropbox.com/s/nnfjt0idvb7e32g/Proximal%20intersection%202%20no%20sound%20.mp4?dl=0

Dynamic US of the nerves shows lost relative movement of the some of the nerves to the surrounding structures. The major example is the loss of the "seesaw sign" of the tibial nerve and common peroneal nerve in the sciatic nerve sleeve during the ankle-planter flexion and dorsiflexion [31, 32].

The following link shows the dynamic US visualization of the loss of the "seesaw sign" of the tibial nerve and the CPN in the sciatic nerve sleeve during the ankle-planter flexion and dorsiflexion.

https://www.dropbox.com/s/q586l7wjpa6aynj/Seesaw%20sign%20combine%201.mp4?dl=0

Elastography may show the whole or part of the nerve with fibrosis or the hardened nerve (Fig. 15.14) [10, 33].

If the patient has no phobia of needles, US-guided dry needling can be utilized. The dry needle is placed as close as possible to the diseased part of the nerve and stimulate by vibration or electricity to assess the reproducibility of neuropathic pain experienced by the patient.

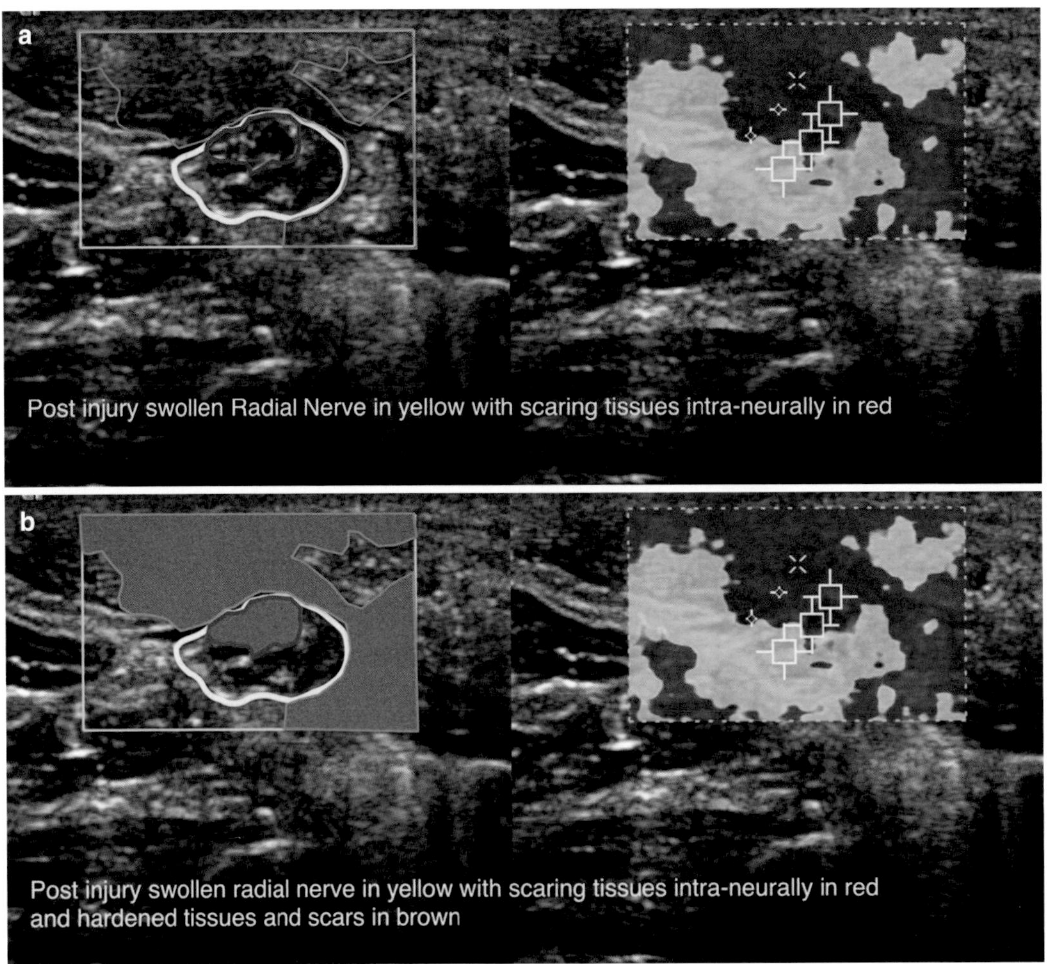

Fig. 15.14 Elastography image of the swollen radial nerve after injury with scar tissues. (**a**) Shows the left-side B-mode image; the yellow circle outlines the swollen radial nerve with the swollen fascicles in red circle; the panel on the right is the elastography image showing the relative hardness of the tissues enclosed in the square under the present scanning conditions, corresponding to the B mode image on the left; the brown regions show that the scanned structure has a high density, and the green regions represent soft tissues. (**b**) The red circular part of the radial nerve shows similar hardness as compared to the scar tissue near the swollen radial nerve

The following link shows the dry needle stimulation of the pathologic lateral sural cutaneous nerve under US guidance; both of the two maneuvers reproduced patient's usual neuropathic pain over the lateral gastrocnemius.

https://www.dropbox.com/s/pney930r-bj15j64/Dry%20needle%20stimmulation%20of%20LSCN1.mp4?dl=0

Injectate for HD

Traditionally, a large volume of normal saline and a small volume of steroids and local anesthetic solution are used for HD of nerves [7, 9]. Recently, other injectate such as 5% dextrose, platelet-rich plasma (PRP), and hyaluronic acid were also used for HD [34].

HD alone appears to be beneficial, as shown in a clinical trial of patients with mild-to-moderate CTS, which compared the effect of HD with saline injected to the intracarpal region (interventional group) and to the subcutaneous area beyond carpal tunnel (sham group). The results show significantly improved the Boston Carpal Tunnel Syndrome Questionnaire score and cross-sectional area (CSA) in the interventional group [4]. Wu et al. compared HD with 5% dextrose and HD with saline in patients with CTS and found 5% dextrose to be more effective in treating median nerve entrapment [2]. In addition, Wu et al. showed that HD with 5% dextrose is more effective than HD with steroid for treating CTS [1]. Hence, the 20th edition of *Harrison's Principles of Internal Medicine* textbook lists HD of 5% dextrose as an alternative local treatment that does not have the side effects of corticosteroids for CTS. Moreover, Shen et al. [5] revealed a single HD with PRP was more effective in reducing the CSA of the median nerve than HD of single 5% dextrose for moderate CTS.

Su et al. [35] also reported HD with hyaluronic acid has more short-term efficacy than HD with saline for CTS.

Other studies have supported the use and efficacy of dextrose solution to treat neuropathic pain [36]. Injection of 5% dextrose into the caudal epidural space has been demonstrated by Smigel et al. to result in prompt and consistent multi-segmental post-injection analgesia and a cumulative analgesic effect in patients with chronic low back pain with radiation to buttock or leg [37]. In a retrospective data collection of consecutive patients with severe neuropathic pain, Lam et al. demonstrated both the safety and efficacy of 5% dextrose solution without the use of lidocaine to treat neuropathic pain caused by nerve roots or plexi in consecutive patients [11]. Chen et al. [12] show HD with 5% dextrose was as effective as HD of steroid for ulnar neuropathy at elbow. Two case reports also revealed HD with 5% dextrose was effective for treating radial nerve palsy [13] and Meralgia paresthetica [14]. This is of particular interest as in the absence of lidocaine, optimal HD volumes can be utilized without the concern for lidocaine toxicity [11]. Given the benefit of injection at the nerve root and plexi level, a mechanism of action of 5% dextrose injection at the somatosensory system at the dorsal root level has been proposed [37].

Several hypotheses have been proposed to explain the effect of dextrose solution on treating neuropathic pain such as the following.

Downregulation of the Transient Receptor Potential Vanilloid Receptor-1 (TRPV1) Ion Channel

The TRPV1 ion channel has been postulated to be associated with chronic neuropathic pain [38]. Its upregulation is directly associated with persistent of chronic neuropathic pain, and dextrose may directly or indirectly antagonize the TRPV1 upregulation effects. The TRPV1 ion channel was previously called the capsaicin receptor (Fig. 15.15) because it is the only capsaicin receptor-containing TRP ion channel [39]. Capsaicin causes characteristic burning sensation by upregulating the TRPV1 channel. Mannitol, a 6-carbon-atom sugar, has been found to reduce the burning sensation after exposure to capsaicin, suggesting an antagonistic (calming) effect on TRPV1 upregulation. Dextrose, similar in structure to mannitol, has empirically been observed to have similar effect, although it has not been formally tested using the capsaicin model developed by Bertrand et al. [40].

Chronic neuropathic pain may signify glycopenia around the corresponding nerve(s). Injecting dextrose may promptly correct this glycopenia and consequently reduce neuropathic pain. Moreover, 40% of our peripheral somatosensory nervous system are small capsaicin-sensitive nerves (nerves with the TRPV1 ion channels on their surface), which are predominantly C fibers, and have an apparent homeostatic role in monitoring the level of systemic dextrose [41]. Both the brain and peripheral nerves have high and constant requirement for glucose [16]. When isolated C fibers are exposed to a hypoglycemic environment by substituting D-glucose with non-metabolizable L-glucose, it demonstrated a dramatic (653 ± 23%) increase in discharge frequency, within 5 minutes and maximized after 15 minutes [42]. Hypoglycemia results in the reduction of high energy substrates, e.g., ATP, leading to reduced activity of the ATP-dependent Na + -K+ pump, resulting in progressive nerve depolarization and hyperexcitability. Replacement of D-glucose can rapidly correct the above-said effects [42].

Dextrose injection may hyperpolarize nerve cells responsible for neuropathic pain and reduce

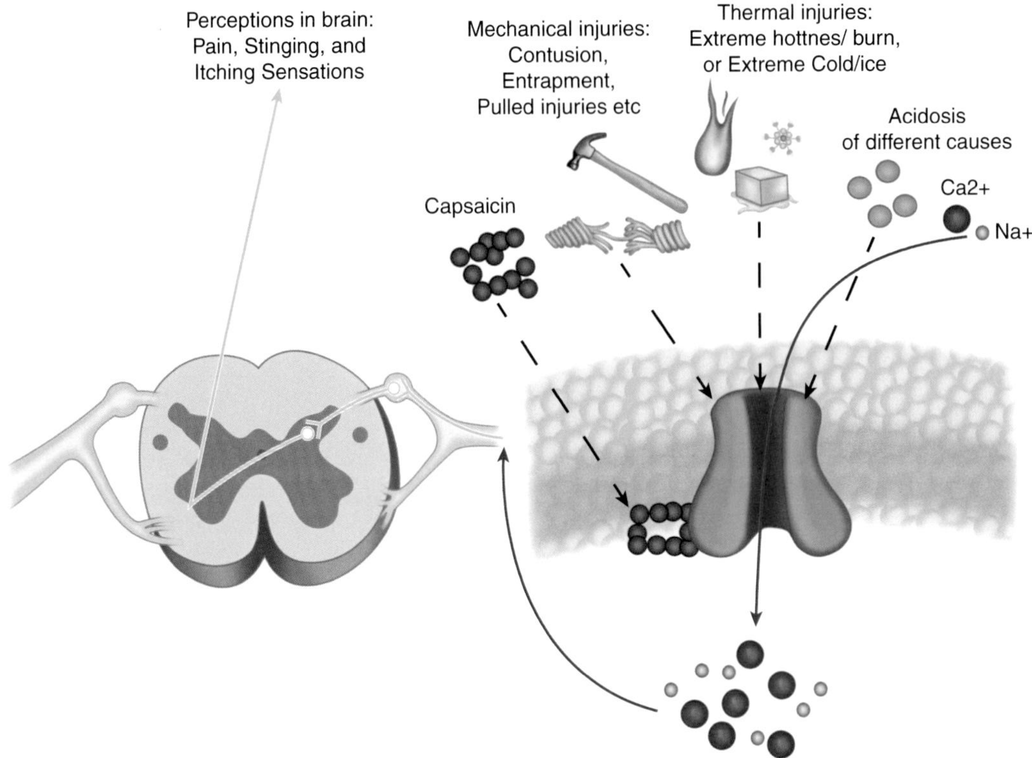

Fig. 15.15 Figure showing different stimuli, including mechanical stimuli (which include entrapment, pulled injuries, direct trauma), heat, ice, acidosis, capsaicin, will cause influx of sodium and calcium and thence depolarization of the nerves, leading to signal perceived in the brain

their depolarization and pain generating ability. There are both potassium channels and TRVP1 channels localized on capsaicin-sensitive nerves [43]. These potassium channels have receptors for dextrose. The attachment of dextrose to the receptor leads to opening of the potassium channel and thence transports potassium out from the cell and hyperpolarizes the nerve cell [43].

In summary, when performing HD of nerves, the needle is guided by US to approach the nerves. The skin is anesthetized by skin bleb by administering local anesthetics. Once the needle is under the skin, the patient usually does not feel the needle movement if continuous HD with 5% dextrose solution is maintained. A key feature of the technique is that the advancement of the injectate/solution dissects the soft tissues in front of the needle, without the involvement of the needle. It is the injectate that opens the fascia or spaces in front of the needle. Needle advancement ceases just outside the epineurium, and the injectate dissects and releases the entrapped soft tissues around the nerves. It is crucial to have the nervi nervorum and vasa nervorum fully released from the entrapment or abnormal external stimuli and to be surrounded by the injectate. Therefore, the soft tissues surrounding the nerve will be hydrodissected layer by layer until the epineurium has no further layers of fascia surrounding it. A key observation here is that the nerve should appear rounded rather than fusiform and is free floating. Along with the release of the nerve, the injection of dextrose is expected to induce a calming effect on the effects of TRPV1 upregulation and improves the vascular supply and venous drainage (may be lymphatic drainage as well) of the main nerves.

Acknowledgments The authors need to acknowledge Dr. Dick Hui for drawing the illustrating pictures.

Conflicts of Interest Declare conflicts of interest or state "The authors declare no conflict of interest."

References

1. Wu YT, et al. Randomized double-blinded clinical trial of 5% dextrose versus triamcinolone injection for carpal tunnel syndrome patients. Ann Neurol. 2018;84(4):601–10.
2. Wu YT, et al. Six-month efficacy of perineural dextrose for carpal tunnel syndrome: a prospective, randomized, double-blind, controlled trial. Mayo Clin Proc. 2017;92(8):1179–89.
3. Wu YT, et al. Six-month efficacy of platelet-rich plasma for carpal tunnel syndrome: a prospective randomized, single-blind controlled trial. Sci Rep. 2017;7(1):94.
4. Wu YT, et al. Nerve hydrodissection for carpal tunnel syndrome: a prospective, randomized, double-blind, controlled trial. Muscle Nerve. 2019;59(2):174–80.
5. Shen YP, et al. Comparison of perineural platelet-rich plasma and dextrose injections for moderate carpal tunnel syndrome: a prospective randomized, single-blind, head-to-head comparative trial. J Tissue Eng Regen Med. 2019;13(11):2009–17.
6. Chen SR, Shen YP, Ho TY, Li TY, Su YC, Chou YC, Chen LC, Wu WT. One-year efficacy of platelet-rich plasma for moderate-to-severe carpal tunnel syndrome: a prospective, randomized, double-blind, controlled trial. Arch Phys Med Rehabil. 2021;102(5):951–8.
7. Wei DGMBC. Ultrasound-guided percutaneous injection, hydrodissection, and fenestration for carpal tunnel syndrome: description of a new technique. J Appl Res. 2010;10(3):107–14.
8. Tran TA, et al. Prospective pilot study comparing pre- and postsurgical CTSAQ and Neuro-QoL Questionnaire with median nerve high-resolution ultrasound cross-sectional areas. J Hand Surg Am. 2018;43(2):184 e1–9.
9. McShane JM, et al. Sonographically guided percutaneous needle release of the carpal tunnel for treatment of carpal tunnel syndrome: preliminary report. J Ultrasound Med. 2012;31(9):1341–9.
10. Lin CP, et al. Utility of ultrasound elastography in evaluation of carpal tunnel syndrome: a systematic review and meta-analysis. Ultrasound Med Biol. 2019;45(11):2855–65.
11. Lam SKH, Reeves KD, Cheng AL. Transition from deep regional blocks toward deep nerve hydrodissection in the upper body and torso: method description and results from a retrospective chart review of the analgesic effect of 5% dextrose water as the primary hydrodissection injectate to enhance safety. Biomed Res Int. 2017;2017:7920438.
12. Chen LC, et al. Perineural dextrose and corticosteroid injections for ulnar neuropathy at the elbow: a randomized double-blind trial. Arch Phys Med Rehabil. 2020;101(8):1296–303.
13. Chen SR, et al. Ultrasound-guided perineural injection with dextrose for treatment of radial nerve palsy: a case report. Medicine (Baltimore). 2018;97(23):e10978.
14. Su YC, et al. Efficacy of nerve hydrodissection with 5% dextrose in chronic meralgia paresthetica. Pain Pract. 2020;20(5):566–7.
15. Cass SP. Ultrasound-guided nerve hydrodissection: what is it? A review of the literature. Curr Sports Med Rep. 2016;15(1):20–2.
16. Andreone BJ, Lacoste B, Gu C. Neuronal and vascular interactions. Annu Rev Neurosci. 2015;38:25–46.
17. Bennett GJ, Xie XY. A peripheral mononeuropathy in rat that produces disorders of pain sensation like those seen in man. Pain. 1988;33:87–107.
18. Bennett GJ, Chung JM, Honore M, Seltzer Z. Models of neuropathic pain in the rat. Curr Protoc Neurosci. 2003, 2003. Chapter 9.
19. Finnerup NB, et al. Neuropathic pain: an updated grading system for research and clinical practice. Pain. 2016;157(8):1599–606.
20. Treede RD, et al. Neuropathic pain: redefinition and a grading system for clinical and research purposes. Neurology. 2008;70(18):1630–5.
21. Marshall J. Nerve_stretching for the relief or cure of pain. Br Med J. 1883;15:1173–9.
22. Sugar O. Victor Horsley, John Marshall, nerve stretching, and the nervi nervorum. Surg Neurol. 1990;34(3):184–7.
23. Victor H. Preliminary communication on the existence of sensory nerves in nerve trunks. True "nervi nervorum". Br Med J. 1884;1:166.
24. Carrero G. Fascicular anatomy, nervi nervorum, and paresthesia. Reg Anesth Pain Med. 2003;1:72–3.
25. Vilensky JA, Gilman S, Casey K. Sir Victor Horsley, Mr John Marshall, the nervi nervorum, and pain: more than a century ahead of their time. Arch Neurol. 2005;62(3):499–501.
26. Mizisin PA, Weerasuriya A. Homeostatic regulation of the endoneurial microenvironment during development, aging and in response to trauma, disease and toxic insult. Acta Neuropathol. 2011;121(3):291–312.
27. Jia Y, Baumann TK, Wang RK. Label-free 3D optical microangiography imaging of functional vasa nervorum and peripheral microvascular tree in the hind limb of diabetic mice. J Innov Opt Health Sci. 2010;13(4):307–13.
28. Felten DL, Maida MS. Peripheral nervous system. In: Netter's atlas of neuroscience. Anesthesiology and pain medicine. The Official Journal of Iranian Society of Regional Anesthesia and Pain Medicine (ISRAPM). 3rd ed; 2016. p. 153–231.
29. Lam KHS, et al. Ultrasound-guided nerve hydrodissection for pain management: rationale, methods, current literature, and theoretical mechanisms. J Pain Res. 2020;13:1957–68.
30. Hei Stanley Lam K, et al. Practical considerations for ultrasound-guided hydrodissection in pronator Teres syndrome. Pain Med. 2022;23(1):221–3.

31. Lam SKH, Hung CY, Clark TB. Loss of the "Seesaw Sign" of the sciatic nerve in a Marathon runner complaining of hamstring cramping. Pain Med. 2020;21(2):e247–8.
32. Hung CY, Lam KHS, Wu YT, Dynamic ultrasound for carpal tunnel syndrome caused by squeezed median nerve between the flexor Pollicis longus and flexor Digitorum tendons. Pain Med, 2021.
33. Su DC, Chang KV, Lam SKH. Shear wave elastography to guide perineural hydrodissection: two case reports. Diagnostics (Basel). 2020;10(6):348.
34. Wu YT, Lam KHS, Lai CY, Chen SR, Shen YP, Su YC, Wu C-H. Novel motor-sparing ultrasound-guided neural injection in severe carpal tunnel syndrome: a comparison of four injectates. Biomed Res Int. 2022;2022:9745322.
35. Su YC, Shen YP, Li TY, Ho TY, Chen LC, Wu YT. The efficacy of hyaluronic acid for carpal tunnel syndrome: a randomized double-blind trial. Pain Med. 2021;22(11):2676–85.
36. Wu YT, et al. Efficacy of 5% dextrose water injection for peripheral entrapment neuropathy: a narrative review. Int J Mol Sci. 2021;22(22):12358.
37. Maniquis-Smigel L, Dean Reeves K, Jeffrey Rosen H, Lyftogt J, Graham-Coleman C, Cheng AL, Rabago D. Short term analgesic effects of 5% dextrose epidural injections for chronic low back pain: A randomized controlled trial. Anesth Pain Med. 2016;7(1):e42550. https://doi.org/10.5812/aapm.42550. PMID: 28920043; PMCID: PMC5554430.
38. Malek N, et al. The importance of TRPV1-sensitisation factors for the development of neuropathic pain. Mol Cell Neurosci. 2015;65(Mar):1–10.
39. Szolcsányi JL, Sándor Z. Multisteric TRPV1 nocisensor: a target for analgesics. Trends Pharmacol Sci. 2012;33:646–55.
40. Bertrand H, et al. Topical mannitol reduces capsaicin-induced pain: results of a pilot-level, double-blind, randomized controlled trial. PM R. 2015;7(11):1111–7.
41. Fujita S, Bohland M, Sanchez-Watts G, Watts A, Donovan C. Hypoglycemic detection at the portal vein is mediated by capsaicin-sensitive primary sensory neurons. Am J Physiol Endocrinol Metab. 2007;293:96–101.
42. MacIver MB, Tanelian DL. Activation of C fibers by metabolic perturbations associated with tourniquet ischemia. Anesthesiology. 1992;76(4):617–23.
43. Burdakov D, et al. Tandem-pore K+ channels mediate inhibition of orexin neurons by glucose. Neuron. 2006;50(5):711–22.

16 High-Frequency Peripheral Nerve Ultrasound

Jeffrey A. Strakowski

Introduction

High-frequency ultrasound has become the modality of choice for visualizing most peripheral nerves. It has a number of advantages over other imaging modalities that include its relative portability, low cost, lack of ionizing radiation, and dynamic capabilities that facilitate seeing moving tissue in real time [42]. In addition, ultrasound has higher resolution for superficial structures than conventional magnetic resonance imaging. The more recent development of ultra-high-frequency transducers has led to unprecedented visualization of superficial nerves [8]. Another advantage is that the ultrasound systems are generally portable and can be used in an office setting. This allows convenient and rapid acquisition of information. Evaluations do not have to be performed in imaging centers, and the point-of-care imaging results in the ability to obtain a diagnosis without delay. There are no problems with patient claustrophobia such as is often experience with magnetic resonance imaging (MRI). There is also no limitation due to metallic prosthesis, fragments, or medical implants [31, 38]. The use of Doppler imaging for assessing vascular structures also provides a significant advantage over other types of imaging modalities. Another advantage of ultrasound over conventionally used imaging modalities is that the peripheral nerve inspection is continuous and does not require the use of the reconstruction of sliced images [65].

One limitation to the assessment of peripheral nerves with ultrasound includes substantial dependence upon the skill of the operator. This is a factor with all types of peripheral nerve imaging; however, ultrasound requires considerable training for both image acquisition and interpretation. This also serves as an advantage with highly skilled practitioners because with ultrasound, the clinical assessment can be performed simultaneously with the imaging. This alleviates the need from adhering to a very strict imaging protocol and allows on-the-spot changes in the regions visualized as needed, including side-to-side comparisons. This is particularly advantageous when the findings are different than the initial expectations.

Other limitations of conventional ultrasound include the inability to penetrate bone and decreased resolution with deeper structures including anatomic structures in patients with a higher body mass index [24]. Ultrasound is not effective for visualization of the spinal cord or the portions of the spinal nerves that are encased in bone. It can be used effectively, however, for the identification of anatomic landmarks as the spinal nerves exit the spinal foramen. Improving

J. A. Strakowski (✉)
Department of PM&R, The Ohio State University, OhioHealth Riverside Methodist Hospital, Columbus, OH, USA

Y. El Miedany (ed.), *Musculoskeletal Ultrasound-Guided Regenerative Medicine*, https://doi.org/10.1007/978-3-030-98256-0_16

technology has also allowing progressively better imaging for deeper peripheral nerves.

Electrodiagnosis has traditionally been the modality of choice for peripheral nerve assessment for both focal and generalized neuropathies [21]. The value of ultrasound in this role and increasingly more apparent and its use has become routine in many centers for this purpose. The modalities are complementary when used to diagnose peripheral nerve disease.

Successful sonographic imaging of peripheral nerves requires an in-depth knowledge of peripheral nerve anatomy as well as the surrounding tissue. Image optimization and proper scanning techniques are needed for appropriate visualization. Ability to accurately measure nerves is needed for distinguishing normal and abnormal anatomy [58]. Other visible internal characteristics can be used to help distinguish normal and diseased peripheral nerve. Ultrasound can be valuable for the assessment of both focal and generalized neuropathies. The dynamic capability of ultrasound also makes it the ideal imaging modality for guided peripheral nerve procedures [27].

Electrodiagnostic techniques and high-frequency ultrasound provide complimentary diagnostic information for assessing focal neuropathies. Electrodiagnosis provides primarily physiologic information about nerve function. Ultrasound is primarily an anatomic assessment. Both together can provide detailed information that in summation has more practical value in many cases than either one alone. Both modalities require extensive training and reasonable experience for an appropriate interpretation of the findings. The testing, in all cases, should be performed as an extension of an appropriately detailed history and physical.

Integrating Electrodiagnosis and Ultrasound for Diagnosis of Peripheral Neuropathies

Electrodiagnosis

The proper use of electrodiagnostic techniques can improve localization, define relative severity, and provide additional objective information in disorders of peripheral nerve over history and physical alone. Techniques are available that can provide relatively good localization of abnormalities of most nerves and examination of even very distal segments of nerves [22]. When used in proper context, electrodiagnosis should be used to refine and narrow a differential diagnosis that has already been established with the history and physical.

Conventional nerve conduction studies (NCS) are of primary importance for the assessment of focal neuropathies [34]. When possible, the nerve being examined should be stimulated on both sides of a suspected lesion to assess for both focal slowing and change in the duration and amplitude of the waveform. This provides the most sensitive measure for the identification of both the presence of a neuropathy and the best indication of relative severity [41]. Distinguishing the extent of neurapraxia versus axonotmesis of a focal neuropathy should be considered one of the most valuable contributions of electrophysiologic testing. This is a distinction that cannot be reliably provided by imaging modalities. A relative weakness of electrodiagnostic testing is that it is not able to reliably distinguish between neurotmesis and a complete functional axonotmesis.

When NCS abnormalities are discovered, sufficient testing should be performed to localize the lesion with the most precision possible. When possible, the nerve should always be tested above and below the level of the lesion to assess severity. The most valuable prognostic information is often the compound muscle action potential and sensory nerve action potential amplitudes distal to the level of the lesion. Enough sampling of both normal and abnormal nerves should also be done to determine if there is a more generalized polyneuropathy present [15, 43].

Needle electromyography (EMG) provides the advantage of allowing investigation with additional techniques of the physiologic function of motor nerves, including those that are less accessible for conventional nerve conduction studies [19]. Features of the EMG findings can often provide a general sense of the chronicity of nerve disease and sometimes help distinguish neurogenic atrophy from other sources of muscle atrophy. The electrodiagnostic information should never be used independently from the clinical presentation, but instead integrated with the clinical scenario to derive the correct diagnosis.

Peripheral Nerve Ultrasonography

Virtually all peripheral nerves that can be evaluated with electrophysiologic techniques can be visualized with high-frequency ultrasound [53]. The exception to this is peripheral nerve structures that are obscured by bone such as spinal nerves. Ultrasound cannot effectively penetrate bony cortex. Ultrasound can serve as an adjunct to electrophysiologic testing as an aid in both performing the test and providing unique diagnostic clues. Ultrasound can be used to facilitate accuracy of needle placement in needle EMG as well as assist in the localization for NCS for less commonly tested nerves [7]. It is also helpful for identifying anatomic variants as well as surgical or traumatic alteration.

Whereas electrodiagnostic techniques provide information on nerve function in focal neuropathies, high-frequency ultrasound provides anatomic information. Identification of changes in peripheral nerves in pathologic conditions as well as surrounding anatomic structures can often provide more precise localization of an injury than other methods. It additionally can provide anatomic detail that explains the source of neuropathy. Ultrasound can be used to assist in the diagnosis of focal neuropathies due to compression, trauma, and tumors. In some situations, it can provide information about the type and severity of the injury.

Comparison of Electrophysiology and Peripheral Nerve Ultrasonography

Ultrasound has some strengths and weaknesses relative to electrodiagnosis in the assessment focal neuropathies. Ultrasound is often better for more precise localization of a focal neuropathy with resolution in the order of microns. This facilitates recognition of structural nerve changes over portions of millimeters (Fig. 16.1). Electrodiagnostic techniques do not provide localization with anywhere near that level of precision for most nerves.

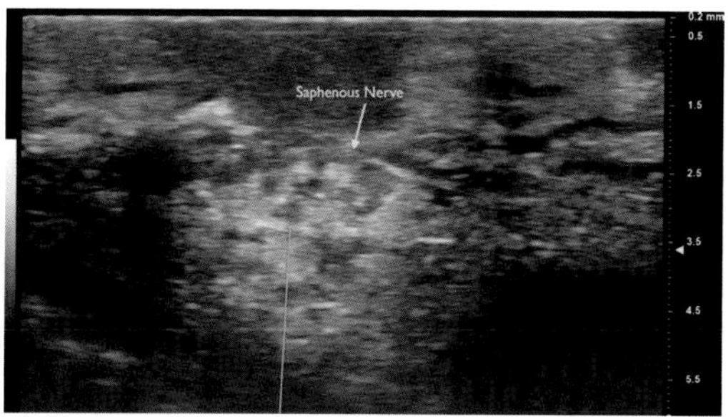

Fig. 16.1 Ultra-high-frequency (70 MHz) sonogram of a short-axis view of an injured saphenous nerve at the level of the proximal foot demonstrating enlargement and disruption of the internal fascicles and scarring of the epineurium. This level of resolution facilitates inspection of changes within portions of a millimeter. Note that the depth of the entire image is 6 mm

By contrast however, electrodiagnostic studies can more easily provide a better overview of the health of the peripheral nervous system and therefore more effectively localize the neuropathy to a certain region of the limb. The meticulous nature of ultrasound scanning for anatomic nerve abnormalities makes this more challenging if the general site of the lesion is not readily apparent from the history and physical. For this reason, it is recommended to perform electrodiagnostic testing prior to ultrasound scanning when it is anticipated that both modalities will be used.

Electrodiagnosis is more effective for assessing the severity of a neuropathy. Despite some tendencies of appearance in axonal injury and neurapraxic lesions previously mentioned, this has not been consistently shown to be a reliable indicator. There is significant variation seen with peripheral nerves displaying conduction block. There can be focal swelling of the entire nerve at the site of the injury, enlargement of a single fascicle, or even a subtle fusiform enlargement (Fig. 16.2). In general, distinction between neurapraxic and axonal injuries are much more reliably made with electrodiagnostic techniques than ultrasound.

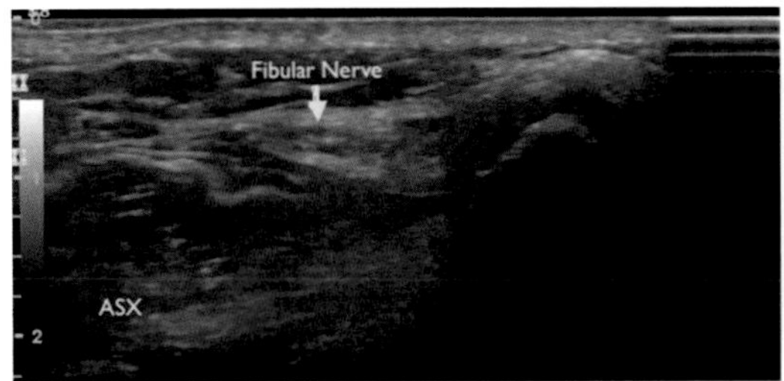

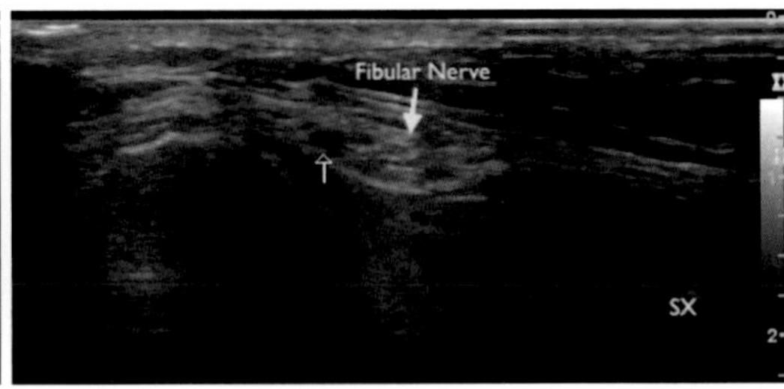

Fig. 16.2 Sonogram of side-to-side comparisons of a short-axis view of the fibular nerve at the fibular head. The normal asymptomatic (ASX) side is shown on the left, and the abnormal symptomatic side (SX) with neuropathy is shown on the right. The symptomatic side has both enlargement of the entire nerve and internal fascicular enlargement (yellow arrow)

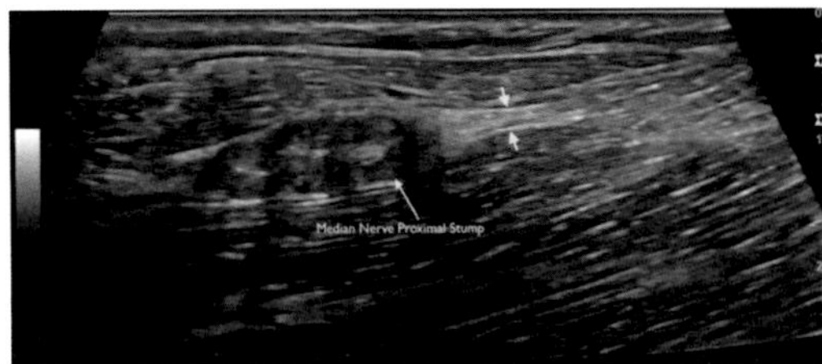

Fig. 16.3 Sonogram of a long-axis view of a complete neurotmesis of the median nerve in the forearm. Note the enlarged appearance of the proximal stump and the "empty bed" appearance of the residual sheath void of nerve tissue (arrowheads)

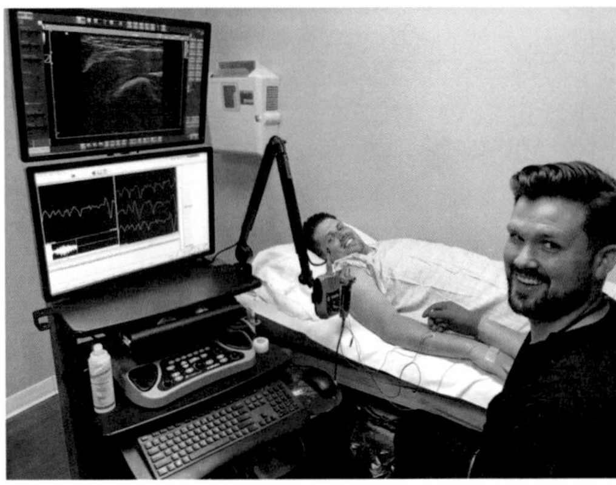

Fig. 16.4 Integration of electrophysiology and ultrasonography

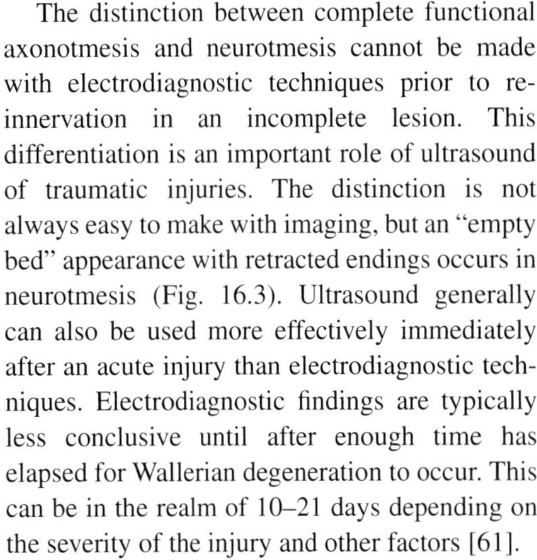

The distinction between complete functional axonotmesis and neurotmesis cannot be made with electrodiagnostic techniques prior to re-innervation in an incomplete lesion. This differentiation is an important role of ultrasound of traumatic injuries. The distinction is not always easy to make with imaging, but an "empty bed" appearance with retracted endings occurs in neurotmesis (Fig. 16.3). Ultrasound generally can also be used more effectively immediately after an acute injury than electrodiagnostic techniques. Electrodiagnostic findings are typically less conclusive until after enough time has elapsed for Wallerian degeneration to occur. This can be in the realm of 10–21 days depending on the severity of the injury and other factors [61].

The clear advantage of ultrasound in focal neuropathies is that it can demonstrate the anatomic source of the neuropathy. It can demonstrate areas of constriction, focal mass lesions, post-traumatic scarring, anatomic variability, and even vascular abnormalities. This knowledge can be invaluable when contemplating treatment options. There is clear value in both modalities, and many authors have concluded that ultrasound should be considered an integral part of routine testing in an electrophysiological assessment [57]. Some of the electrophysiologic instruments are now being created to have integrated ultrasonography (Fig. 16.4).

Peripheral Nerve Anatomy and Sonographic Appearance

Peripheral nerves have an uninterrupted fascicular pattern on ultrasound (Fig. 16.5). This differs from the intercalated fibrillar pattern typical of tendons [10] (Fig. 16.6). The dark (hypoechoic) nerve fascicles are intermixed with brighter (hyperechoic)

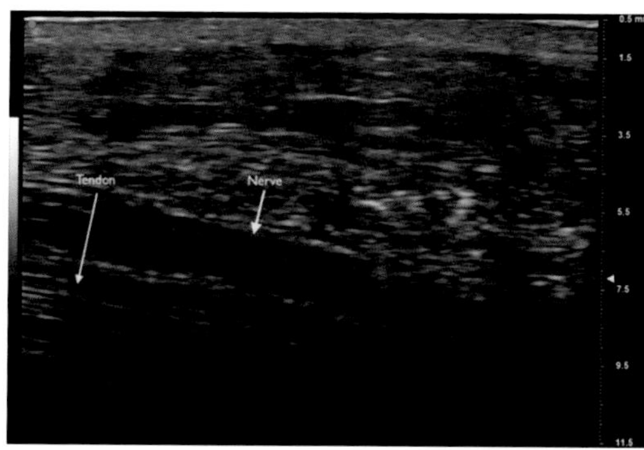

Fig. 16.5 Ultra-high-frequency (48 MHz) sonogram of a long-axis view of the median nerve overlying the flexor tendons. Note the uninterrupted fascicular pattern of the of the nerve in contrast to the intercalated fibular pattern of the tendons

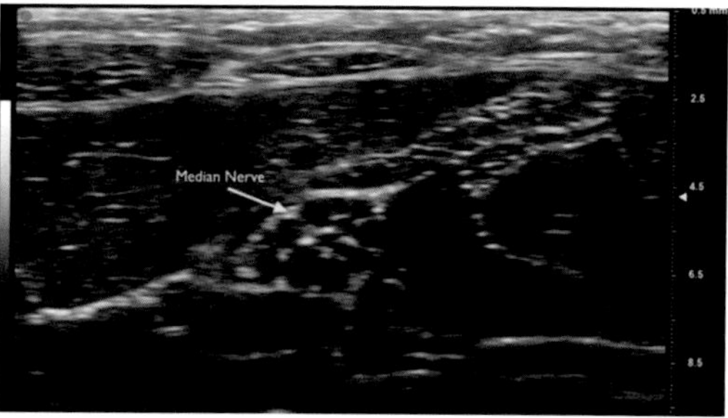

Fig. 16.7 Ultra-high-frequency (48 MHz) sonogram of a short-axis view of the median nerve in the forearm. The fascicular pattern and epineurium are highly conspicuous and in contrast to the hypoechoic surrounding muscle. The hypoechoic fascicles and hyperechoic epineurium give the nerve a "honeycomb" appearance

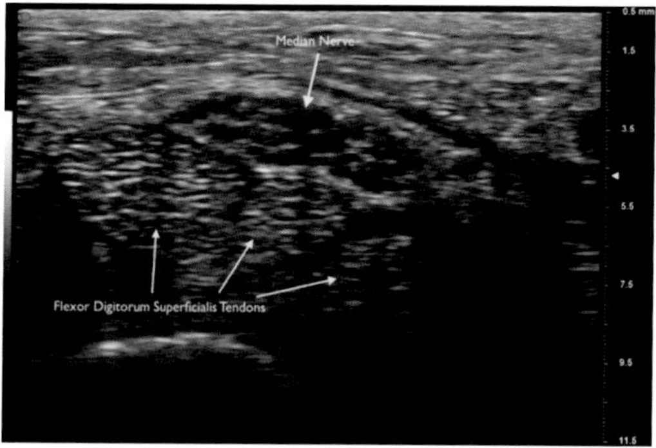

Fig. 16.6 Ultra-high-frequency (48 MHz) sonogram of a short-axis view of the median nerve overlying the flexor digitorum superficialis tendons. Note the fascicular pattern of the of the nerve in contrast to the fine fibular pattern of the tendons

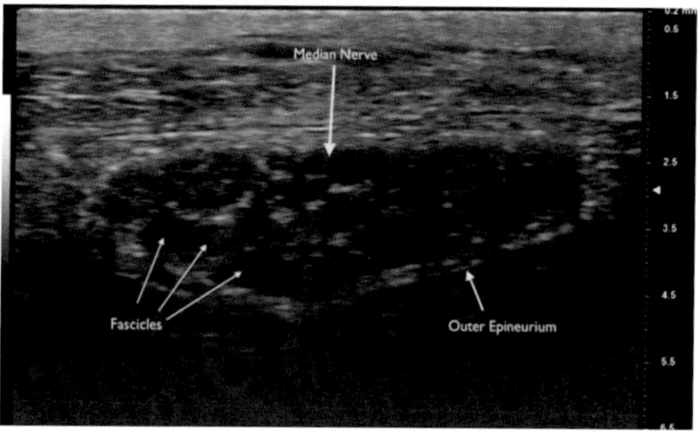

Fig. 16.8 Ultra-high-frequency (48 MHz) sonogram of a short-axis view of the median nerve in the forearm. The fascicular pattern and epineurium are highly conspicuous and in contrast to the hypoechoic surrounding muscle. The hypoechoic fascicles and hyperechoic epineurium give the nerve a "honeycomb" appearance

connective tissue creating what is often referred to as a "honeycomb" appearance when viewed in short axis [47] (Fig. 16.7). The fascicles consist of bundles of individual nerve fibers that are each enveloped by the endoneurium. The perineurium surrounds the bundle of nerve fibers creating the fascicle [49]. The size and number of fascicles seen in nerves are highly variable depending on the nerve size and its location in the body [5, 42], (Peer, 2008) (Fig. 16.8). The external sheath of the nerve is the outer hyperechoic epineurium. The tissue that lies inside the outer epineurium between the fascicles is often called the "inner epineurium" [12]. The short-axis view of the nerve is typically the best orientation to differentiate it from other surrounding tissue [9]. It also assists to understand the relationship to adjacent structures (Fig. 16.9). Longitudinal views also provide valuable information but are more difficult to obtain as they frequently curve out of the field of view (Fig. 16.10). Slight movement of the transducer should be performed with this view, including medially and laterally to visualize the entire width, as well as heel-to-toe rocking to remain reduces anisotropic artifact.

Peripheral nerves are accompanied by an extensive vascular supply. The surrounding arteries and veins are relatively easy to identify, particularly in larger nerves. Power and color Doppler can be used to assess flow (Fig. 16.11). Nerves also have an internal network of vessels

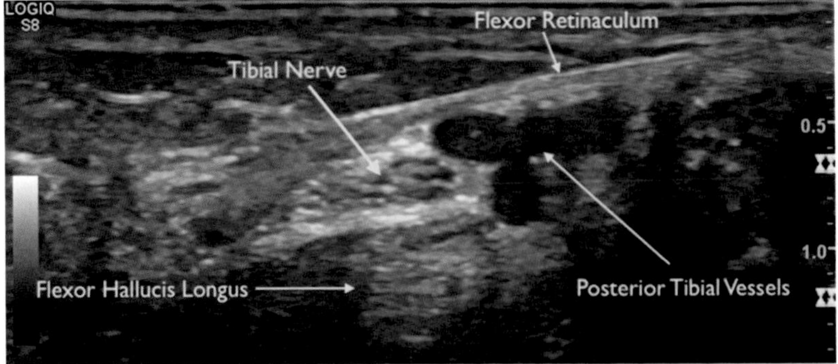

Fig. 16.9 Sonogram of a short-axis view of the tibial nerve at the level of the tarsal tunnel. The short-axis perspective allows detailed inspection of all of the surrounding tissue and structures. In this view, the entire width of the nerve (which has begun to split into medial and lateral plantar nerves) and position of the neighboring posterior tibial artery and veins, flexor hallucis longus tendon (hyperechoic) and surrounding muscle (hypoechoic), and overlying flexor retinaculum can be easily identified. The fascicular pattern and epineurium are highly conspicuous and in contrast to the hypoechoic surrounding muscle. The hypoechoic fascicles and hyperechoic epineurium give the nerve a "honeycomb" appearance

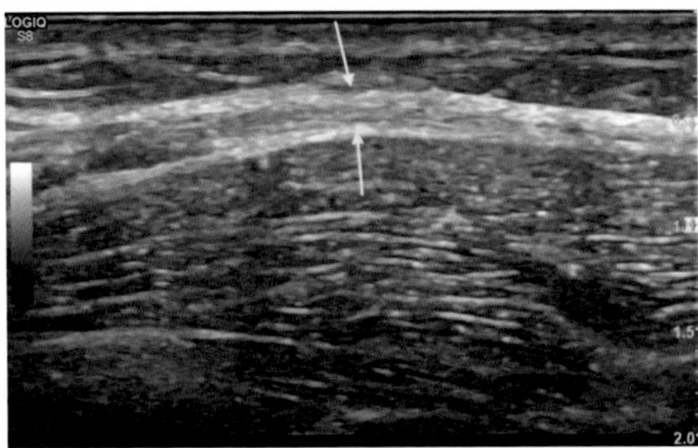

Fig. 16.10 Sonogram of a long-axis view of a nerve with surrounding muscle. Long-axis views are somewhat more challenging for creating still images, and movement of the transducer is required to visualize the width of the nerve, as well as add clarity to the proximal and distal ends if the nerve curves away from a 90-degree relationship to the incident sound waves from the transducer

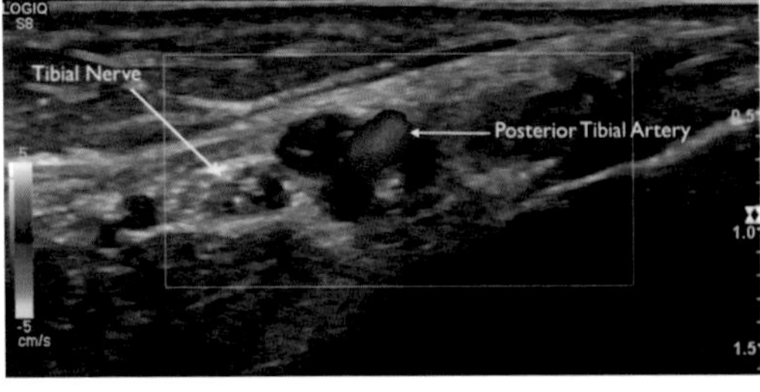

Fig. 16.11 Color Doppler sonogram of a short-axis view of the tibial nerve at the level of the tarsal tunnel. The Doppler flow is seen in the posterior tibial artery. The hypoechoic veins are seen surrounding the artery. Flow can be demonstrated in the veins by alternating transducer pressure

contained within their internal epineurium with endoneurial vessels that traverse into the fascicles [62]. The veins are compressible with alternating transducer pressure, and the arteries can be identified by their pulsations (Fig. 16.12).

Imaging Strategies

Goals of imaging include reliably identifying the nerve and distinguishing it from other tissue. Learning effective scanning techniques to improve nerve conspicuity will enhance the identification of normal and abnormal nerve. The image should also be optimized for reliable assessments and measurements as well as assessment of the fascicular architecture. The nerve, along with the surrounding tissue, should also be compared in both short- and long-axis views. The examiner should be familiar with the often more conspicuous surrounding bony, soft tissue, and vascular landmarks. Doppler imaging can be helpful for distinguishing vessels from small nerves [46]. Nerves are generally more conspicuous when they are surrounded by tissue with different echogenicity. When a nerve is surrounded by other hyperechoic structures, it is often more difficult to identify. In that circumstance, it is helpful to follow the nerve to a location where it is readily visible and trace it back to the region of interest (Fig. 16.13).

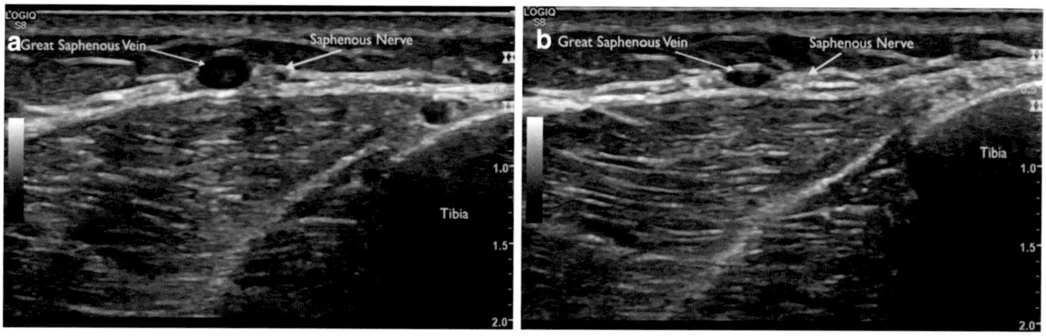

Fig. 16.12 Sonograms demonstrating short-axis views of the great saphenous vein in the medial leg with varying transducer pressure. Veins will collapse with increased transducer pressure. (**a**) Light transducer pressure. (**b**) Slightly increased transducer pressure showing partial collapse of the vein. Veins are often more conspicuous than the smaller nerves. In this case, the great saphenous vein can be used to identify the less conspicuous neighboring saphenous nerve

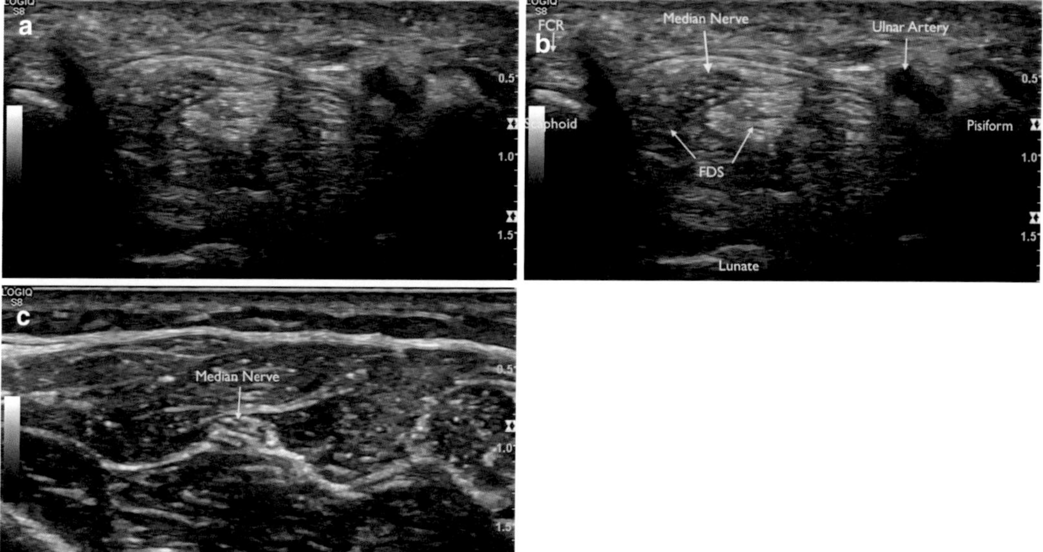

Fig. 16.13 Sonograms demonstrating the relative conspicuity of a nerve in different locations. Short-axis views of the median nerve are shown. (**a**) Unlabeled at the carpal tunnel inlet. Because the nerve is neighboring relatively isoechoic tendons, the median nerve can be more challenging to identify for a less experienced observer. (**b**) Labeled structures at the carpal tunnel inlet including the flexor digitorum superficialis (FDS) and flexor carpi radialis (FCR) tendons, which are relatively isoechoic relative to the median nerve. (**c**) The median nerve at the level of the mid-forearm. At this location, the nerve is much more conspicuous because it is surrounded by hypoechoic muscle. When faced with a scenario in which the nerve is challenging to distinguish from the surrounding tissue, it can be identified in a more conspicuous region and then followed to the area of interest

Developing skill with the ultrasound transducer will also increase success with peripheral nerve scanning. The transducer should be held with a comfortable grip at the base that allows easy movement and good control and prevents fatigue (Fig. 16.14). Scanning quickly but with good control can enhance the contrast between the nerve and surrounding tissue more than moving the transducer slowly [13]. Tracing back and forth rapidly when looking at branch points, smaller nerves, and focal abnormalities within the nerve also improves visualization. A liberal use of conduction gel can facilitate rapid movement of the transducer while maintaining a clear image (Fig. 16.15).

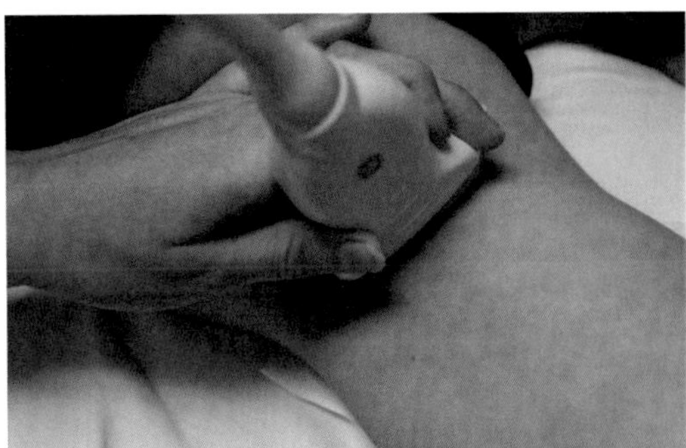

Fig. 16.14 Demonstration of appropriate grip on the base of the transducer for optimum control.

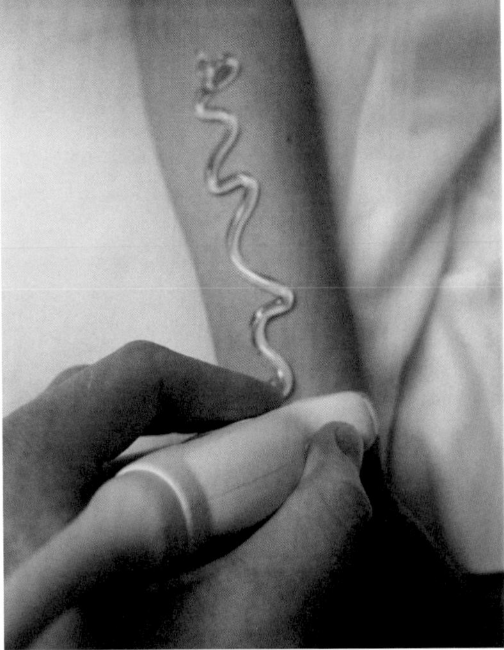

Fig. 16.15 Demonstration of the use of a liberal amount of transducer gel to facilitate rapid scanning for nerves of the forearm.

Changing the direction of the incident sound waves from the transducer has significant impact on the appearance of the tissue. The underlying tissue is seen in the greatest detail when the incident sound waves are orthogonal to the tissue. Any deviation from that leads to increased refraction of the returning sound waves away from the transducer and therefore less detail. The loss of clarity of the image resulting from a deviation from perpendicular incident sound waves is termed anisotropic artifact [11]. It can be challenging at times to minimize anisotropic artifact when moving the transducer because body tissue is rarely completely in a straight line. Movements of the transducer termed "toggling" and "heel-to-toe rocking" can be used to create a perpendicular incident sound beam through the tissue.

Toggling can be used in some circumstances to distinguish nerve from other tissue. A nerve can sometimes be difficult to distinguish from surrounding highly reflective tendons. Tendons generally have a greater amount of anisotropic artifact. Because of this property, toggling can be used to help distinguish similar-appearing tendon from a neighboring nerve. As the incident beam is directed away from a perpendicular position to the tissue, the nerve tends to maintain its appearance better than the tendons [30] (Fig. 16.16).

The examiner should be attentive to the amount of transducer pressure that is being placed on the tissue. It is generally preferable to

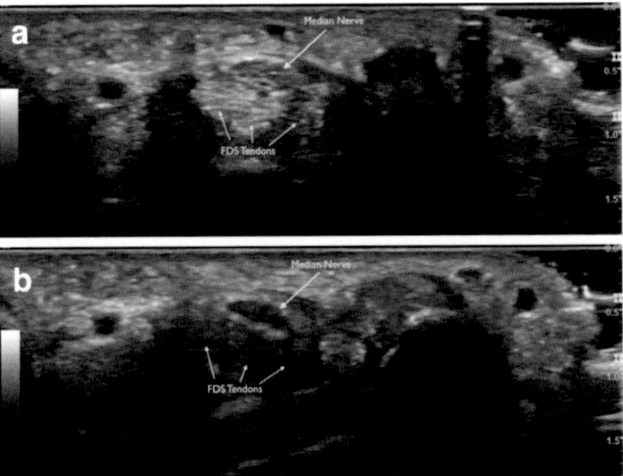

Fig. 16.16 Sonograms demonstrating the effect of toggling the transducer and anisotropic artifact. This is a short-axis view of the median nerve at the carpal tunnel also demonstrating the highly reflective tendons of the flexor digitorum superficialis (FDS). (**a**) The transducer is orthogonal to the carpal tunnel revealing the details of both the nerve and the tendons. Both tissue types are relatively isoechoic, creating some challenge in reliably distinguishing the border of the outer epineurium of the median nerve. (**b**) The transducer is toggled to cause the incident sound waves to approach at a less than orthogonal position resulting in anisotropic artifact. The tendons are prone to more anisotropy than the nerve. This, therefore, results in greater conspicuity of the outer epineurium of the median nerve. This shows the potential value of toggling when assessing the borders of peripheral nerves

use liberal coupling gel and light pressure. Excessive pressure will deform the nerve as well as the surrounding tissue. This is important when assessing the shape of a peripheral nerve, particularly when performing measurements and assessing flattening ratios in tunnel entrapments [17]. The effect of the pressure can be even more pronounced when the nerve is pressed against unyielding bone such as the radial nerve at the spiral groove (Fig. 16.17). In some circumstances, greater transducer pressure can improve the visualization of the nerve by compressing the overlying tissue. This is particularly true of deeper nerves [49]. Actively moving the surrounding muscles and tendons can also be helpful for improving nerve conspicuity.

Detailed knowledge of the ultrasound machine is also critical for optimizing the image. This includes applying the appropriate frequency, image depth, focal zone, grayscale gain, and mapping. These concepts are discussed in more detail in other portions of the book. Some ultrasound machines have a general setting for nerves, and some allow these features to be adjusted with high precision.

The frequency is measurement in millions of hertz (cycles per second) designated megahertz (MHz). High-frequency waves allow better resolution of superficial structures but do not penetrate tissue as deeply as low-frequency waves [24]. Most peripheral nerves should be assessed at the highest transducer frequency available that still provides adequate depth of penetration. A comprehensive assessment might involve visualization at different frequencies to inspect the surrounding tissue in detail (Fig. 16.18).

The depth should be set so the structures of interest encompass the majority of the screen. Having the depth set too high can leave wasted space and decrease the resolution of the nerve.

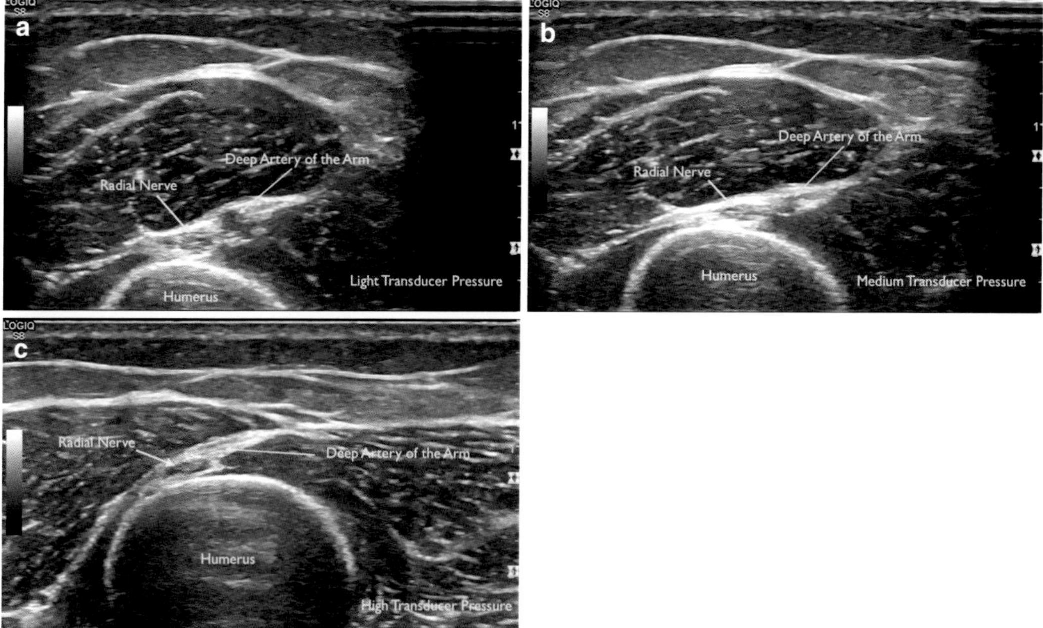

Fig. 16.17 Sonograms demonstrating the effect of transducer pressure on the image. This is a short-axis view of the radial nerve at the level of the arm. (**a**) Light transducer pressure results in the nerve being further from the surface. There is no deformation of the nerve and the surrounding vascularity. (**b**) Medium transducer pressure shows the nerve is closer to the surface and a greater amount of the underlying humerus is seen as the tissue is compressed. The veins surrounding the artery are collapsed and the nerve displays flattening. (**c**) High transducer pressure brings the nerve even closer to the surface as the tissue is flattened. The effect of the transducer pressure also slightly changes the position of the nerve and neighboring muscle. The examiner should be vigilant about the extent of transducer being applied and the effect on the image

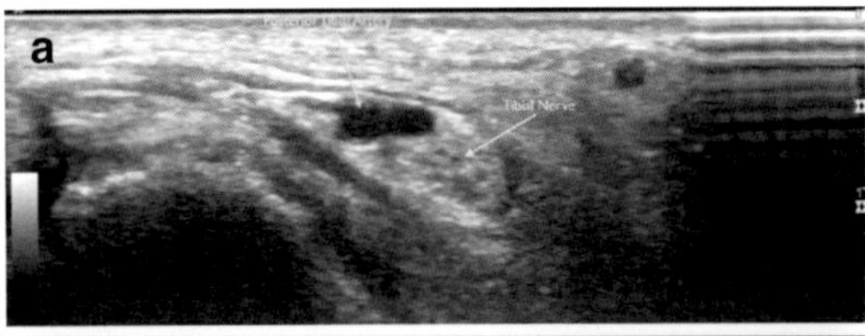

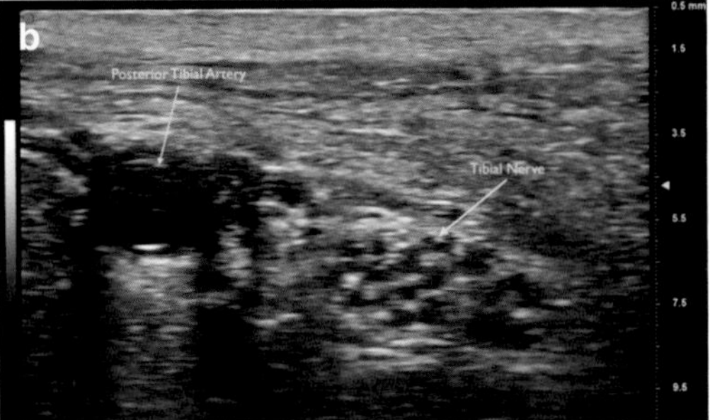

Fig. 16.18 Sonograms demonstrating the effect of frequency differences on the appearance of a short-axis view of the tibial nerve at the tarsal tunnel. (**a**) 12 MHz image demonstrating the nerve and some of the surrounding anatomy. (**b**) Ultra-high-frequency (48MH) image. There is considerably better visualization of the detail of the nerve with the higher frequency. The lower-frequency image demonstrates a broader view of the tissue surrounding the nerve

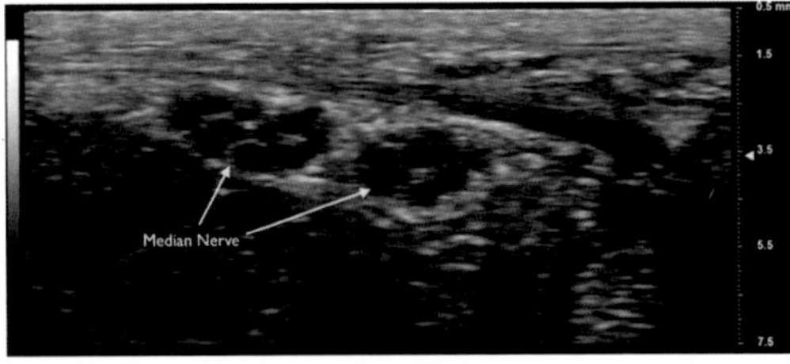

Fig. 16.19 Ultra-high-frequency (70 MHz) sonogram of the median nerve with an early bifurcation. Note that the depth is set so that the nerve of interest encompasses a large portion of the screen

With most peripheral nerves, the depth setting is very superficial (Fig. 16.19). The focal zone refers to the location where the ultrasound beam converges and is typically the site of the clearest image. This feature is not present on every type of ultrasound machine, but when available, it should be placed at the level of the nerve being inspected (Fig. 16.20).

The grayscale gain affects the brightness of the image. This term is not to be confused with the gain on EMG machines, which essentially affects the depth of the screen. The grayscale gain is more analogous to the loudness of a radio. It is used to affect the brightness of the image, and its setting is often personal preference for the degree of contrast between tissues (Fig. 16.21). Grayscale mapping can be altered to affect the contrast between tissues and is also typically a matter of personal preference.

Nerve Measurement

Nerves can be precisely measured with most ultrasound systems. This is an important tool when assessing nerve enlargement or compression in pathologic circumstances. Cross-sectional area measurement of the nerve in short axis with perimeter tracing is generally considered to be the most reliable and reproducible method for the detection of enlargement [2] (Fig. 16.22). This has been shown to also correlate well with measurements in cadaveric studies. This technique is performed by tracing around the margin of the hypoechoic nerve fascicles and inside the hyperechoic border of the outer epineurium with an electronic caliper [36, 37, 45].

The transducer must be placed perpendicular to the nerve to obtain an accurate cross-sectional area measurement. An oblique view will result in an inaccurately large measurement. Generally, the smallest cross-sectional area measurement that can be obtained in short axis reflects the greatest accuracy [37, 51, 60].

Cross-sectional area can be performed by an indirect method with the use of digital calipers. With this method, an ellipse is created to produce the measurement. This method has good inter-rater reliability; however, many nerves have an irregular circumference, particularly at entrapment sites, making them difficult to fit perfectly into an ellipse. The manual tracing method is recommended for greater precision and accuracy [29].

The diameter of the nerve can also be measured in long axis. This view and measurement should always be included and compared to the short-axis view when performing clinical assess-

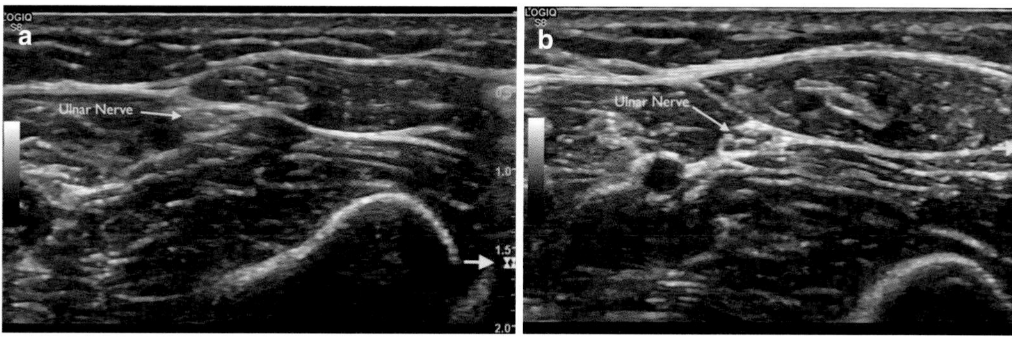

Fig. 16.20 Sonograms demonstrating the effect of the focal zone position on the appearance of a peripheral nerve. A short-axis view of an ulnar nerve in the forearm is shown. (**a**) The focal zone (yellow arrowhead) is significantly deep to the level of the nerve with relatively poor clarity. (**b**) The focal zone is placed at the level of the nerve with significantly improved clarity

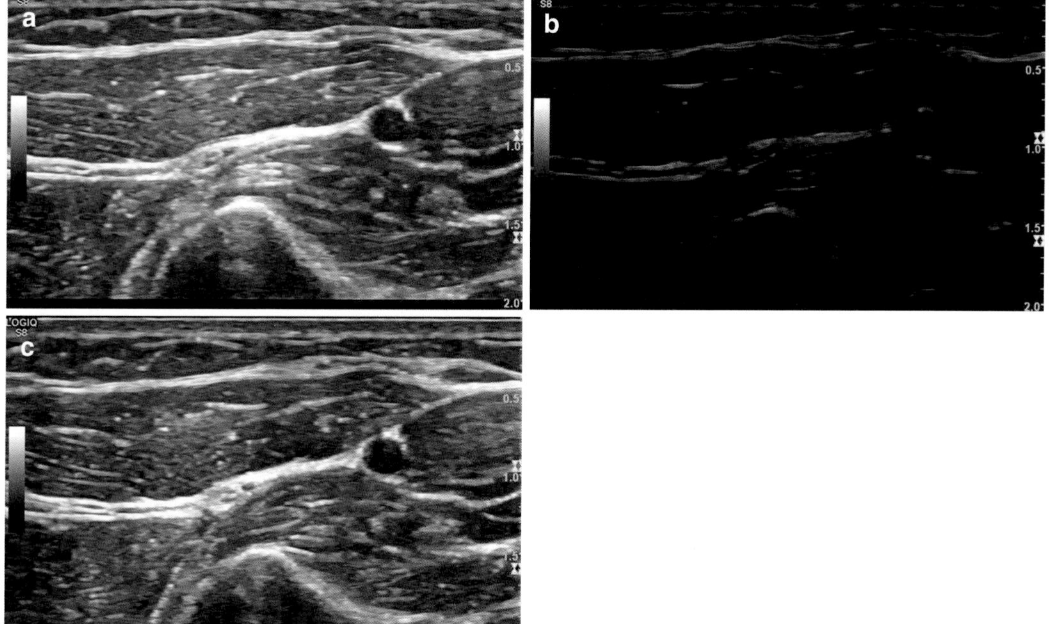

Fig. 16.21 Sonograms demonstrating the effect of changes in the grayscale gain on the appearance of the short-axis view of nerve and muscle. (**a**) The image with the gain slightly high with less contrast between the nerve and surrounding muscle. (**b**) The gain is excessively low, with poor clarity as the image to too dark. (**c**) The gain setting to create the optimum contrast between the nerve and muscle

ments. It is sometimes more challenging to obtain, particularly in smaller nerves. A technique of first localizing the nerve in short axis and then slowly rotating the transducer to a long view can be used to make this easier.

Because the diameter measurement should reflect the center of the nerve, the largest measurement obtained in long-axis view reflects the most accurate (Fig. 16.23).

The surrounding tissue should be inspected in detail, and it should be confirmed that only nerve tissue is being measured. The long-axis diameter measurements should be correlated with the short-axis measurements to confirm accuracy.

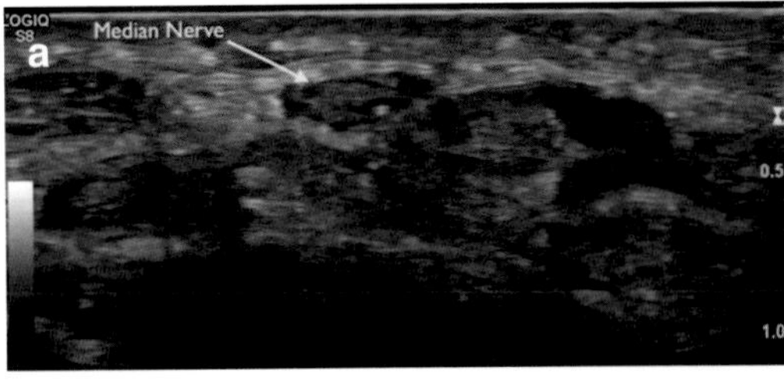

Fig. 16.22 Sonograms demonstrating the direct-tracing method for obtaining cross-sectional area. (**a**) Short-axis view of the median nerve. (**b**) Direct tracing of the nerve at the inner border of the outer epineurium. From this measurement, the cross-sectional area is calculated

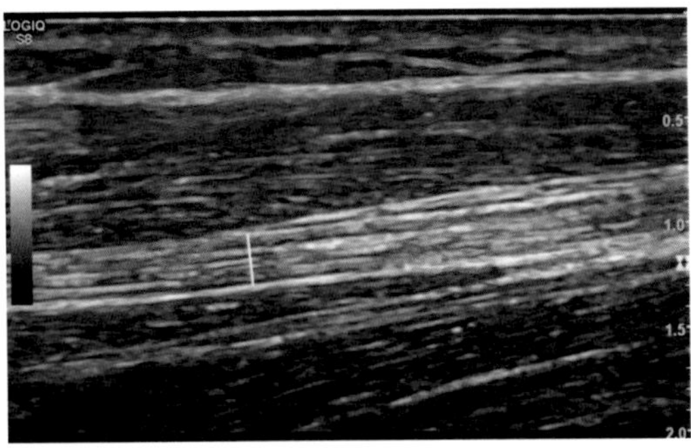

Fig. 16.23 Sonograms demonstrating the diameter measurement (yellow line) of a nerve in long axis. The measurement is made from the inner border of the outer epineurium

Nerve size generally decreases when imaged from proximally to distally as the branches leave the main nerve trunk. The cross-sectional area of nerves tends to be larger in taller individuals and smaller in women. Nerve cross-sectional area also generally increases with age. For this reason, the nerve should be investigated over sufficient length and different levels for adequate comparison when focal enlargement is suspected. Side-to-side comparisons are also helpful in unilateral disease.

Evaluation of Focal Neuropathies

Ultrasound can provide valuable information when assessing focal neuropathies and is an excellent complement to the physiologic information provided by electrodiagnosis. It can be used to localize focal injury with good accuracy and precision, even within millimeters [23]. It also provides anatomic information that can help to identify the source of the neuropathy. This can include nerve distortion in tunnel entrapments, surrounding tissue injury, scarring, and compressive masses [3, 25, 32] (Fig. 16.24). The dynamic capabilities of ultrasound provide an advantage over other imaging modalities. Dynamic compression or subluxation of nerves can be seen in circumstances where no abnormality would be identified in a static image (Fig. 16.25).

Although ultrasound can provide some information about relative severity of a focal neuropathy, electrodiagnosis is generally the most effective modality for this role. Proper use of nerve conduction studies, with stimulation both proximally and distally to a lesion, can be used to distinguish a neurapraxic injury versus one with axonal loss. Ultrasound has an advantage over electrodiagnosis in some traumatic injuries. It can be used to differentiate a functionally complete axonotmesis from neurotmesis (Fig. 16.3). These conditions cannot be distinguished with electrodiagnosis. In addition, some electrodiagnostic clues, such as fibrillations and distal sensory nerve action potential (SNAP) and compound muscle action potential (CMAP) amplitude loss, are not present until the development of Wallerian degeneration, which can often take many days after an acute injury. Ultrasound findings are rarely limited by temporal factors to a significant extent.

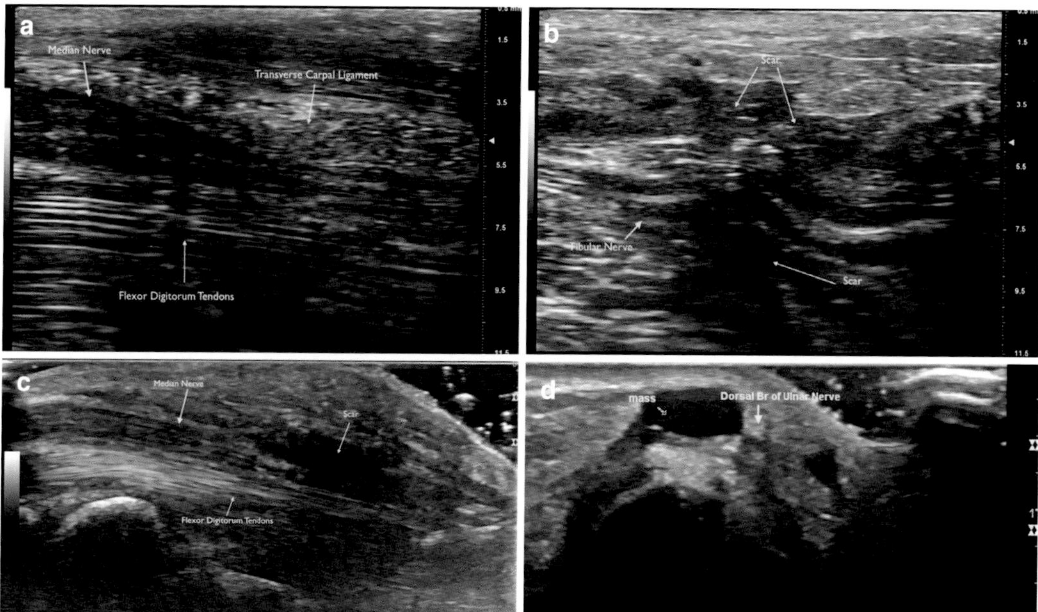

Fig. 16.24 Sonograms demonstrating examples of sources of peripheral nerve compression. (**a**) An ultra-high-frequency (48 MHz) sonogram of a long-axis view of the median nerve at the carpal tunnel being compressed at the level of the carpal tunnel outlet by the overlying transverse carpal ligament. (**b**) An ultra-high-frequency (48 MHz) sonogram of a long-axis view of the common fibular nerve at the knee tunnel being compressed and distorted by post-traumatic laceration tissue injury. (**c**) Sonogram of a long-axis view of the median nerve at the carpal tunnel being compressed at the level of the carpal tunnel outlet by post-surgical scar. (**d**) Short-axis view of the dorsal branch of the ulnar nerve being compressed by a neighboring ganglion cyst (mass)

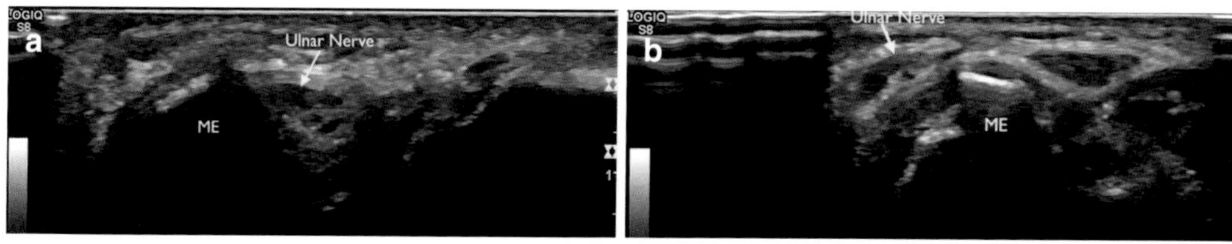

Fig. 16.25 Sonograms demonstrating short-axis views of the ulnar nerve dislocating over the medial epicondyle (ME) with elbow flexion. (**a**) The ulnar nerve is in the ulnar groove with the elbow in relative extension. (**b**) The ulnar nerve has dislocated anterior to the medial epicondyle with elbow flexion

Identifying Focal Nerve Abnormalities

The appearance of focal nerve injury is typically a result of the nature of the injury. Peripheral nerves often display changes in size at levels of focal neuropathy. Entrapment neuropathies usually present with narrowing or deformation at the site of compression and focal swelling just proximal to that area [23] (Fig. 16.26). Median neuropathy at the carpal tunnel is the most common focal entrapment neuropathy and has been studied to the greatest extent. Measuring the nerve for abnormal swelling is the most reliably way to identify abnormality [16]. The precise pathophysiology behind the enlargement is a source of ongoing debate, but theories include the blocking of axoplasmic flow at the entrap-

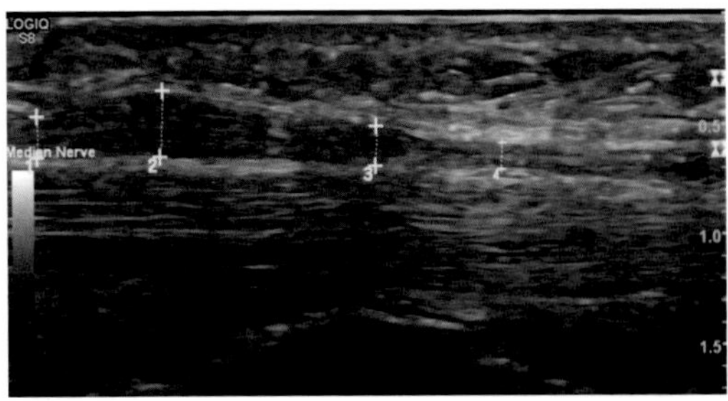

Fig. 16.26 Sonogram of a long-axis view of an abnormal median nerve with compression at the carpal tunnel. Note the narrowing of the nerve at the site of compression (3 and 4) and also the enlargement of the caliper of the nerve proximal to the site of compression (2)

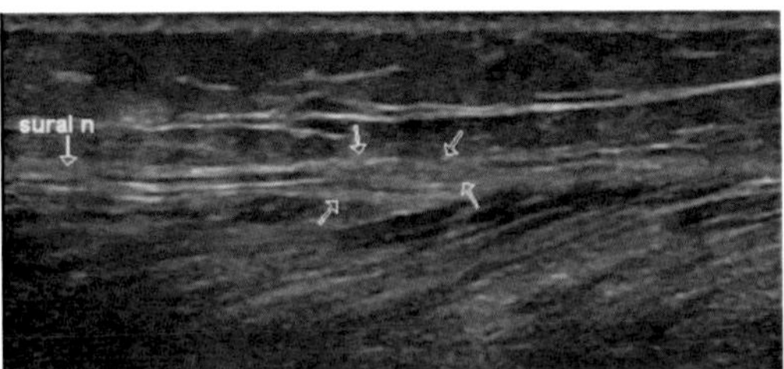

Fig. 16.27 Sonogram of a long-axis view of an abnormal sural nerve with focal injury. The site of neuropathy is identified by the focal enlargement (yellow arrows). This region can be compared to the caliper at other areas of the nerve to help identify the abnormality

ment site and resulting endoneural edema [14]. Cross-sectional areas of nerves can be compared to standardized normal measurements to determine abnormal enlargement. There is considerable variation in the literature, particularly with less commonly studied nerves. The enlargement should always be assessed in both short- and long-axis views. Use of diameter measurement in short axis is preferred in smaller nerves in which a reliable cross-sectional area cannot be obtained.

Comparison of the unaffected course of the nerve can be used to help with this assessment (Fig. 16.27) [63]. This should be performed with caution in more severe injuries as the enlargement can potentially extend over greater lengths of the nerve. In such cases, it can be helpful to compare the neighboring unaffected nerves or use side-to-side comparisons (Fig. 16.28).

Loss or change of normal fascicular architecture is another clue for peripheral neuropathy (Fig. 16.29) [52]. This can be the sole imaging abnormality in some neuropathies. The destruction of the normal fascicular pattern is often associated with more severe injuries and can reflect axonal injury [6, 26]. Demyelinating lesions frequently will appear enlarged without loss of the fascicular architecture. In stretch injuries, the nerve abnormalities can be relatively inconspicuous or notably more diffuse. As with looking for enlargement, techniques of inspecting the nerve proximally and distally with side-to-sides comparisons should also be incorporated for investigating areas for echotexture change.

Color and power Doppler imaging can be used to assess for increased intraneural vascularity. The endoneurial and epineurial vessels accompanying most nerves have slow flow velocities and are ordinarily not seen with conventional ultrasound imaging. Detectable flow signals should be considered to represent increased vascularity, associated with neuropathy [4]. This increased flow has been shown in some entrapment neuropathies including median neuropathy at the carpal tunnel and even polyneuropathies [1, 18]. Care should be used to avoid confusion of normal vessel flow with pathologic increased vascularity (Fig. 16.30).

Relative mobility and excursion of the nerve should also be noted. Anatomic variants should also be identified. In post-operative or post-trauma situations, the region should be assessed for scarring or other potential sources of nerve compression [48]. The course of the nerve should also be inspected for intraneural or extraneural tumors when a neuropathy is suspected (Fig. 16.31).

Evaluation of Generalized Neuropathies

As with focal neuropathies, ultrasound is gaining an increasing role in the assessment of more generalized neuropathies [59]. Ultrasound is a relatively practical and effective imaging modality to distinguish anatomic features to correlate with clinical and electrodiagnostic findings. Additional historical and laboratory data are often needed to

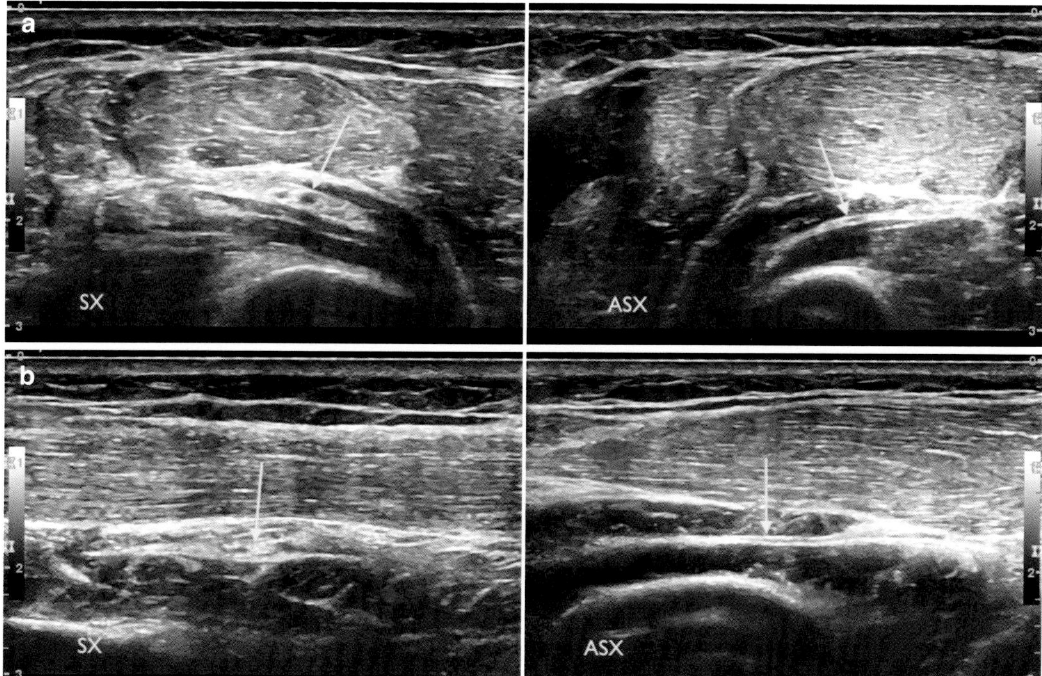

Fig. 16.28 Sonograms of side-to-side comparisons of the deep branch of the radial nerve (yellow arrow) in (**a**) short-axis and (**b**) long-axis in the area of the radial tunnel between the superficial and deep heads of the supinator. The enlarged abnormal nerve is seen on the symptomatic side (SX), and the normal comparison from the asymptomatic side (ASX) is shown for comparison. Side-to-side comparisons are helpful for distinguishing differences, particularly with nerves that are less frequently scanned

reliably determine the source of neuropathy. Despite this, sonographic appearance of peripheral nerves can often provide valuable clues toward the nature of the neuropathy, the areas of involvement, and even the identification of focal neuropathies in the context of more generalized disease.

Ultrasound should be considered an adjunctive tool that can be used to enhance the diagnostic information provided by clinical and electrophysiologic assessments. A goal with clinical and electrodiagnostic testing is to determine if the neuropathy is hereditary or acquired and assess the relative effect on sensory and motor nerves and in some cases autonomic function. Efforts should be made to determine if the neuropathy is acute or chronic, symmetrical or asymmetrical, and axonal or demyelinating.

A role of electrodiagnostic testing in the assessment of generalized peripheral neuropathies includes determining the relative severity, distribution of abnormality, and extent of conduction blocking, conduction slowing, and axonal loss. To reliably do this, sufficient testing of sensory and motor nerve conductions should be performed in multiple limbs to establish the pattern of abnormality [44]. Identification of concomitant nerve entrapments at common sites, including radiculopathies, should be considered in this assessment.

Sonographically, identified morphologic characteristics of peripheral nerves can potentially be used to help characterize the neuropathy, but this has some limitations. The peripheral nerve appearance in many generalized peripheral neuropathies is non-specific and does not reliably identify the underlying condition [28]. Despite this, there are patterns of changes typically seen in some neuropathies that can provide clinical clues [40]. Demyelinating neuropathies, such as

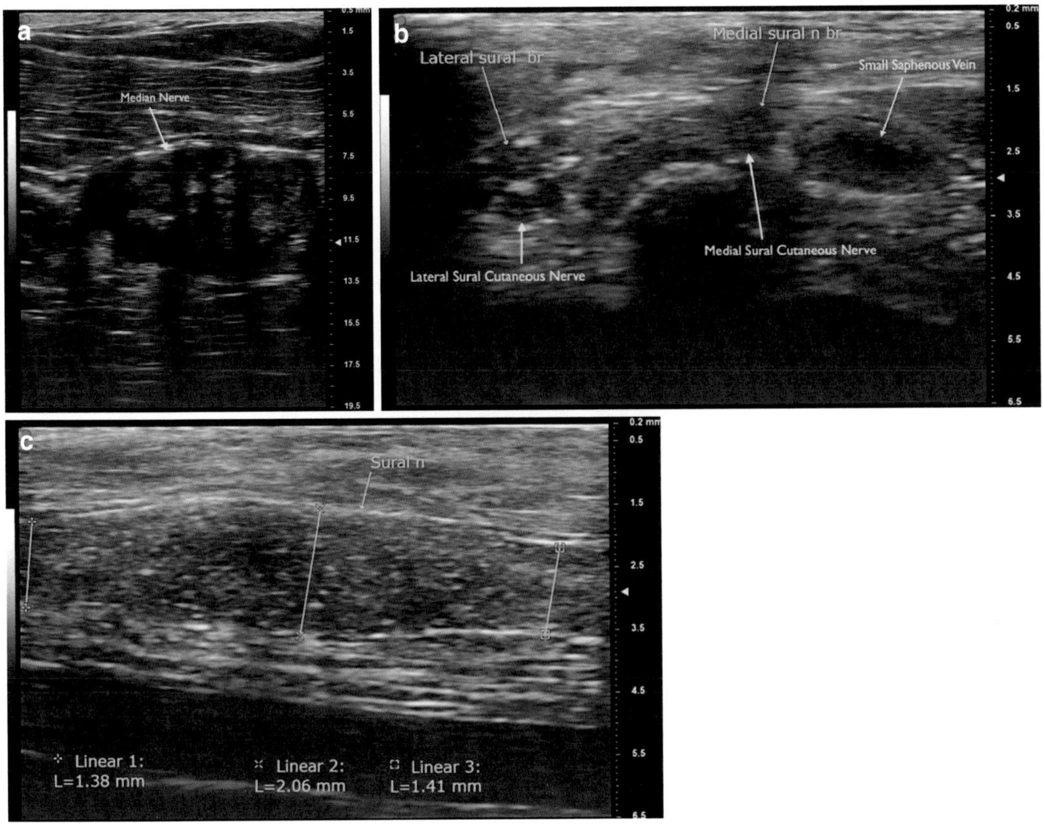

Fig. 16.29 Sonograms demonstrating examples of focal neuropathies with severe axonal loss, identified by the disruption of the normal internal fascicular architecture. (**a**) An ultra-high-frequency (48 MHz) sonogram of a short-axis view of the median nerve in the forearm injured by trauma. Note the enlargement of the fascicles as well as the hyperechoic change in some, reflecting loss of normal axons. (**b**) An ultra-high-frequency (70 MHz) sonogram of short-axis views of the medial and lateral sural cutaneous nerves. In this case, there is a selective injury to the medial sural cutaneous nerve reflected by the loss of the normal internal echotexture. A preserved fascicular pattern is seen in the healthy lateral sural cutaneous nerve. (**c**) An ultra-high-frequency (70 MHz) sonogram of a long-axis view of an injured sural nerve showing complete loss of the normal fascicular architecture

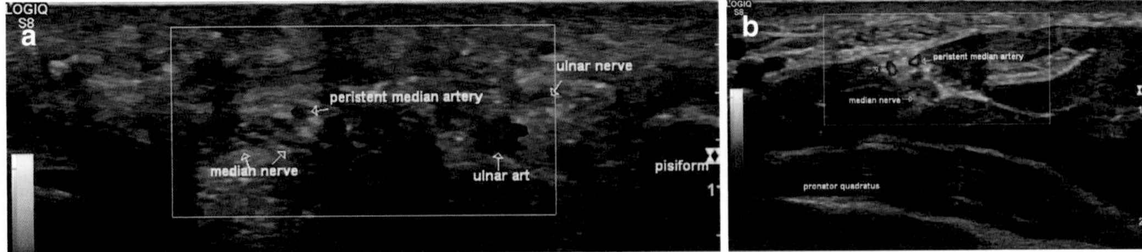

Fig. 16.30 Sonograms demonstrating examples of normal vascularity that could potentially be confused with pathologic neovascularization. (**a**) Short-axis view of a bifid median nerve at the carpal tunnel shows increased vascular flow. This represents flow from a persistent median artery, which is a normal anatomic variation. (**b**) Short-axis view of the same median nerve and persistent median artery more proximally at the level of the pronator quadratus. Following the Doppler flow outside of the region can confirm that the signal is arising from a healthy vessel as opposed to neovascularization at a focal entrapment site. Suspected abnormal vascularization should also ideally be identified within the outer epineurium of the nerve in both short- and long-axis views

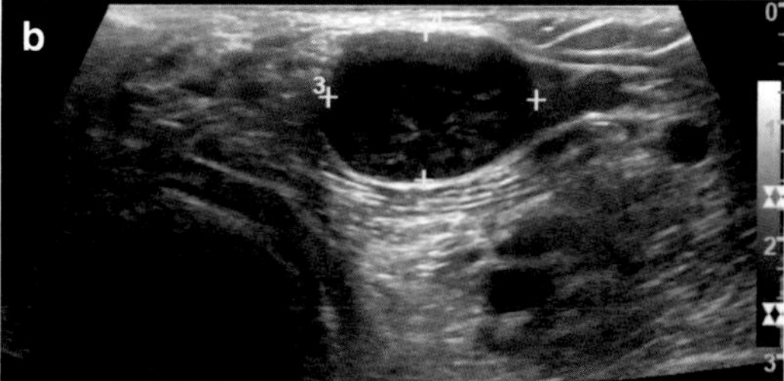

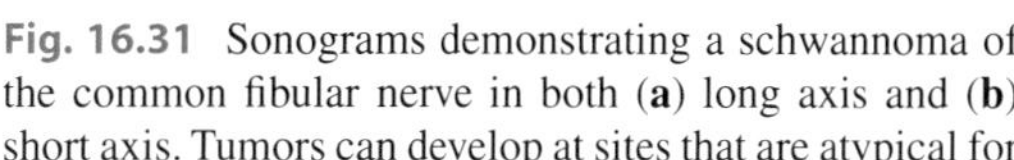

Fig. 16.31 Sonograms demonstrating a schwannoma of the common fibular nerve in both (**a**) long axis and (**b**) short axis. Tumors can develop at sites that are atypical for entrapments. Ultrasound facilitates the rapid inspection of large segments of peripheral nerves to enable screening for unusual sources of neuropathy

acute inflammatory demyelinating polyradiculoneuropathy (AIDP) and chronic inflammatory demyelinating polyradiculoneuropathy (CIDP), have a tendency toward nerve enlargement to a much greater extent than predominantly axonal neuropathies [20, 64].

Patients with chronic inflammatory demyelinating polyradiculoneuropathy have shown dramatic enlargement of multiple peripheral nerves at sites that are not typical for entrapment, including the brachial plexus and cervical roots [33, 55]. This can include nerve enlargement greater than two times normal size. Studies of these conditions have shown good correlation with abnormal nerve sizes measured with ultrasound compared to MRI and autopsy evaluations [35, 56]. Some studies have demonstrated that cross-sectional area enlargement frequently correlates with nerve conduction slowing, but rarely other measures of electrophysiologic assessment. Limited studies have been performed to qualify the extent of peripheral nerve internal derangement which is often more characteristic of axonal neuropathies. Further work is needed in this area to better define morphologic characteristics seen with ultrasound in comparison to electrophysiologic findings.

Ultrasound-Guided Peripheral Nerve Procedures

In addition to use in diagnosis of peripheral nerve disorders, ultrasound is an ideal modality for performing guided nerve procedures. This includes anesthetic and therapeutic blocks, nerve ablation techniques, hydrodissections, and other guided interventional procedures [7]. Ultrasound allows live guidance throughout the procedure while using high-resolution imaging of the peripheral nerve. Details of various ultrasound-guided procedures are discussed throughout the book in other chapters.

The general guidelines for all ultrasound-guided injections should be used for peripheral nerves. Peripheral nerve procedures require special consideration because of the vulnerability of the target. It is recommended that peripheral nerve procedures should be performed with a short-axis view of the nerve and in-plane view of the needle. The needle tip should be visualized at all times throughout the procedures as should the flow of the injectate [50] (Fig. 16.32). In some circumstances, it can be helpful to assess the procedure in both short and long axis to gain full appreciation of the movement of the injectate. This is particularly helpful in higher-volume hydrodissections. The introduction of the injectate should stop while rotating the transducer to view a different plane.

The image of the peripheral nerve should be optimized with guided procedures in the fashion as when performing diagnostic assessments [39]. The goal is to accurately identify the border of the outer epineurium to allow the injectate to be placed close to the nerve but avoid an inadvertent intraneural injection. In general, the highest-frequency transducer that will still allow sufficient penetration should be used for greatest resolution, but consideration should also be given to needle conspicuity. An exception to using higher resolution is deeper peripheral nerves in which bony landmarks are used for identification.

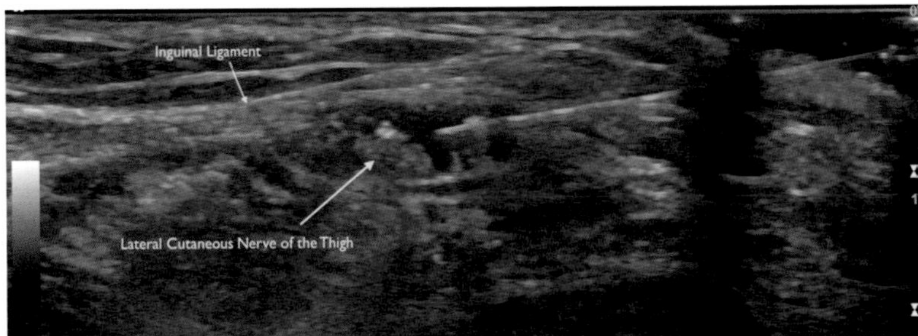

Fig. 16.32 Sonograms demonstrating an in-plane injection with a short-axis view of the lateral cutaneous nerve of the thigh. The needle tip is seen with the in-plane view, and the injectate can be seen creating a hypoechoic halo around the nerve

Pre-scanning of the region around the nerve should also be performed prior to the injection. Doppler imaging can be used to assess for surrounding vascularity.

During the injection, caution should be used to avoid obliquity of the needle relative to the transducer. This can give the false impression that the portion of the needle crossing the transducer is the needle tip. The flow of the injectate should constantly be monitored to establish that the injectate is moving into the desired area [54]. Doppler imaging can also be used to illuminate the flow of the injectate. It is also helpful to initially introduce a small amount of the injectate to increase the conspicuity of the border of the nerve prior to proceeding with the entire injection.

Summary

High-frequency ultrasound has become the imaging modality of choice for most peripheral nerve applications. Its high resolution, portability, lack of ionizing radiation, and magnetic fields as well as dynamic capabilities make it highly practical and effective as a diagnostic and therapeutic tool. It is an excellent adjunct to electrodiagnostic assessments, and both modalities have great value for assessing focal and generalized neuropathies, and the information obtained is additive when they are used together. Ultrasound can provide anatomic information about not only the nerve but also the surrounding tissue, including the surrounding vasculature. Improvements in resolution with development of ultrasound scanning symptoms, including ultra-high-frequency transducers, have led to unprecedented visualization of both normal nerve and pathologic conditions. Advancements in the understanding of the nature of focal and more generalized neuropathies will lead to more effective management decisions.

References

1. Akcar N, Ozkan S, Mehmetoglu O, Calisir C, Adapinar B. Value of power Doppler and gray-scale US in the diagnosis of carpal tunnel syndrome: contribution of cross-sectional area just before the tunnel inlet as compared with the cross-sectional area at the tunnel. Korean J Radiol. 2010;11(6):632–9. Epub 2010 Oct 29
2. Alemán L, Berná JD, Reus M, Martínez F, Doménech-Ratto G, Campos M. Reproducibility of sonographic measurements of the median nerve. J Ultrasound Med. 2008;27(2):193–7.
3. Ali ZS, Pisapia JM, Ma TS, Zager EL, Heuer GG, Khoury V. Ultrasonographic evaluation of peripheral nerves. World Neurosurg. 2016;85:333–9.
4. Bianchi S. Ultrasound of the peripheral nerves. Joint Bone Spine. 2008;75(6):643–9.
5. Bianchi S, Martinoli C. Ultrasound of the musculoskeletal system. Heidelberg: Springer-Verlag; 2007.
6. Boom J, Visser LH. Quantitative assessment of nerve echogenicity: comparison of methods for evaluating nerve echogenicity in ulnar neuropathy at the elbow. Clin Neurophysiol. 2012;123(7):1446–53.
7. Boon AJ, Oney-Marlow TM, Murthy NS, Harper CM, McNamara TR, Smith J. Accuracy of electromyography needle placement in cadavers: non-guided vs. ultrasound guided. Muscle Nerve. 2011;44(1):45–9.

8. Cartwright MS, Baute V, Caress JB, Walker FO. Ultrahigh-frequency ultrasound of fascicles in the median nerve at the wrist. Muscle Nerve. 2017;56(4):819–22.
9. Cartwright MS, Shin HW, Passmore LV, Walker FO. Ultrasonographic findings of the normal ulnar nerve in adults. Arch Phys Med Rehabil. 2007;88(3):394–6.
10. Chiou HJ, Chou YH, Chiou SY, Liu JB, Chang CY. Peripheral nerve lesions: role of high-resolution US. Radiographics. 2003;23(6):e15. Epub 2003 Aug 25
11. Connolly D, Berman L, McNally E. The use of beam angulation to overcome anisotropy when viewing human tendon with high frequency linear array ultrasound. Br J Radiol. 2001;74:183–5.
12. Cre'teur V, Bacq C, Widelec J. Sonography of peripheral nerves. Part I: upper limbs. J Radiol. 2004;85:1887e99.
13. Créteur V, Bacq C, Fumière E, Bissen L, Delcour C. Echographie des nerfs périphériques – Deuxième partie: membre inférieur [Sonography of peripheral nerves. Part II: lower limbs]. J Radiol. 2007;88(3 Pt 1):349–60.
14. Dahlin LB. Aspects on pathophysiology of nerve entrapments and nerve compression injuries. Neurosurg Clin N Am. 1991;2(1):21–9.
15. Dumitru D, Amato AA, Zwarts MJ. Electrodiagnostic medicine. 2nd edn. Hanley & Belfus. Dumitru, Philadelphia. 2002.
16. Duncan I, Sullivan P, Lomas F. Sonography in the diagnosis of carpal tunnel syndrome. AJR Am J Roentgenol. 1999;173:681–4.
17. El-Karabaty H, Hetzel A, Galla TJ, Horch RE, Lücking CH, Glocker FX. The effect of carpal tunnel release on median nerve flattening and nerve conduction. Electromyogr Clin Neurophysiol. 2005;45(4):223–7.
18. Ghasemi-Esfe AR, Khalilzadeh O, Mazloumi M, et al. Combination of high-resolution and color Doppler ultrasound in diagnosis of carpal tunnel syndrome. Acta Radiol. 2011;52:191–7.
19. Johnson EW. The EMG examination. In: Johnson EW, editor. Practical electromyography. Baltimore: Williams & Wilkins; 1988. p. 1–12.
20. Grimm A, Décard BF, Bischof A, Axer H. Ultrasound of the peripheral nerves in systemic vasculitic neuropathies. J Neurol Sci. 2014;347(1–2):44–9.
21. Kimura J. Electromyography and nerve stimulation techniques: clinical applications. Tokyo: Igaku-Shoin; 1990.
22. Kimura J. Electrodiagnosis in diseases of nerve and muscle: principles and practice. 4th ed. Oxford University Press; Kimura - New York. 2013.
23. Koenig RW, Pedro MT, Heinen CP, Schmidt T, Richter HP, Antoniadis G, Kretschmer T. High-resolution ultrasonography in evaluating peripheral nerve entrapment and trauma. Neurosurg Focus. 2009;26(2)
24. Kremkau FW. Diagnostic ultrasound: principles and ultrasound. St. Louis: Sauders; 2002.
25. Lawande AD, Warrier SS, Joshi MS. Role of ultrasound in evaluation of peripheral nerves. Indian J Radiol Imaging. 2014;24(3):254–8.
26. Lee H, Brekelmans GJ, Visser LH. Quantitative assessment of nerve echogenicity as an additional tool for evaluation of common fibular neuropathy. Clin Neurophysiol. 2016;127(1):874–9.
27. Lento PH, Strakowski JA. The use of ultrasound in guiding musculoskeletal interventional procedures. Phys Med Rehabil Clin N Am. 2010;21(3):559–83.
28. Lucchetta M, Pazzaglia C, Granata G, Briani C, Padua L. Ultrasound evaluation of peripheral neuropathy in POEMS syndrome. Muscle Nerve. 2011;44(6):868–72.
29. Mahmood FH, Strakowski JA, Bockbrader MA, Kim D. Accuracy and reliability of peripheral nerve diameter measurement in long axis. J PM&R. 2013;5(9):S217–8.
30. Martinoli C, Bianchi S, Dahmane M, Pugliese F, Bianchi-Zamorani MP, Valle M. Ultrasound of tendons and nerves. Eur Radiol. 2002;12(1):44–55. Epub 2001 Oct 19
31. Martinoli C, Bianchi S, Derchi LE. Tendon and nerve sonography. Radiol Clin N Am. 1999;37(4):691–711, viii.
32. Martinoli C, Bianchi S, Gandolfo N, Valle M, Simonetti S, Derchi LE. US of nerve entrapments in osteofibrous tunnels of the upper and lower limbs. Radiographics. 2000;20 Spec No:S199–213; discussion S213–7.
33. Matsuoka N, Kohriyama T, Ochi K, Nishitani M, Sueda Y, Mimori Y, Nakamura S, Matsumoto M. Detection of cervical nerve root hypertrophy by ultrasonography in chronic inflammatory demyelinating polyradiculoneuropathy. J Neurol Sci. 2004;219(1–2):15–21.
34. Melvin JL, Schuchman JA, Lanese RR. Diagnostic specificity of motor and sensory nerve conduction variables in the carpal tunnel. Arch Phys Med Rehabil. 1973;54:69–74.
35. Mizuno K, Nagamatsu M, Hattori N, Yamamoto M, Goto H, Kuniyoshi K, Sobue G. Chronic inflammatory demyelinating polyradiculoneuropathy with diffuse and massive peripheral nerve hypertrophy: distinctive clinical and magnetic resonance imaging features. Muscle Nerve. 1998;21(6):805–8.
36. Moran L, Perez M, Esteban A, Bellon J, Arranz B, del Cerro M. Sonographic measurement of cross-sectional area of the median nerve in the diagnosis of carpal tunnel syndrome: correlation with nerve conduction studies. J Clin Ultrasound. 2009;37(3):125–31.
37. Nakamichi K, Tachibana S. Ultrasonographic measurement of median nerve cross-sectional area in idiopathic carpal tunnel syndrome: diagnostic accuracy. Muscle Nerve. 2002;26(6):798–803.
38. Nazarian LN. The top 10 reasons musculoskeletal sonography is an important complementary or alternative technique to MRI. AJR Am J Roentgenol. 2008;190(6):1621–6.
39. Nwawka OK, Miller TT. Ultrasound-guided peripheral nerve injection techniques. AJR Am J Roentgenol. 2016;207(3):507–16.

40. Padua L, Paolasso I, Pazzaglia C, Granata G, Lucchetta M, Erra C, Coraci D, De Franco P, Briani C. High ultrasound variability in chronic immune-mediated neuropathies. Review of the literature and personal observations. Rev Neurol (Paris). 2013;169(12):984–90.
41. Pease WS, Lew HL, Johnson EW. Johnson's practical electromyography. Lippincott Williams & Wilkins; Baltimore. 2007.
42. Peer S, Bodner G, editors. High-resolution sonography of the peripheral nervous system. 2nd ed. Berlin: Springer-Verlag; 2008.
43. Raynor EM, Ross MH, Shefner JM, Preston DC. Differentiation between axonal and demyelinating neuropathies: identical segments recorded from proximal and distal muscles. Muscle Nerve. 1995;18:402–8.
44. Robinson LR. Traumatic injury to peripheral nerves. Muscle Nerve. 2000;23:863–73.
45. Roll SC, Case-Smith J, Evans KD. Diagnostic accuracy of ultrasonography vs. electromyography in carpal tunnel syndrome: a systematic review of literature. Ultrasound Med Biol. 2011;37:1539–53.
46. Rubin JM. Musculoskeletal power doppler. Eur Radiol. 1999;9(Suppl 3):S403–6.
47. Silvestri E, Martinoli C, Derchi LE, Bertolotto M, Chiaramondia M, Rosenberg I. Echotexture of peripheral nerves: correlation between US and histologic findings and criteria to differentiate tendons. Radiology. 1995;197(1):291–6.
48. Strakowski JA. Ultrasound evaluation of focal neuropathies: correlation with electrodiagnosis. New York: Demos Medical Publishing; 2013.
49. Strakowski JA. Introduction to musculoskeletal ultrasound: getting started. New York: Demos Medical Publishing; 2015.
50. Strakowski JA. Ultrasound-guided peripheral nerve procedures. Phys Med Rehabil Clin N Am. 2016;27(3):687–715.
51. Suk JI, Walker FO, Cartwright MS. Ultrasound of peripheral nerves. Curr Neurol Neurosci Rep. 2013;13(2):328.
52. Tagliafico AS. Peripheral nerve imaging: not only cross-sectional area. World J Radiol. 2016;8(8):726–8.
53. Walker FO, Cartwright MS. Neuromuscular ultrasound. Philadelphia: Elsevier Saunders; 2011.
54. Tagliafico A, Bodner G, Rosenberg I, et al. Peripheral nerves: ultrasound-guided interventional procedures. Semin Musculoskelet Radiol. 2010;14(5):559–66.
55. Taniguchi N, Itoh K, Wang Y, Omoto K, Shigeta K, Fujii Y, Namekawa M, Muramatsu S, Nakano I. Sonographic detection of diffuse peripheral nerve hypertrophy in chronic inflammatory demyelinating polyradiculoneuropathy. J Clin Ultrasound. 2000;28(9):488–91.
56. Tazawa K, Matsuda M, Yoshida T, Shimojima Y, Gono T, Morita H, Kaneko T, Ueda H, Ikeda S. Spinal nerve root hypertrophy on MRI: clinical significance in the diagnosis of chronic inflammatory demyelinating polyradiculoneuropathy. Intern Med. 2008;47(23):2019–24.
57. Walker FO, Cartwright MS, Alter KE, Visser LH, Hobson-Webb LD, Padua L, Strakowski JA, Preston DC, Boon AJ, Axer H, van Alfen N, Tawfik EA, Wilder-Smith E, Yoon JS, Kim BJ, Breiner A, Bland JDP, Grimm A, Zaidman CM. Indications for neuromuscular ultrasound: expert opinion and review of the literature. Clin Neurophysiol. 2018;129(12):2658–79.
58. Walker FO, Cartwright MS, Wiesler ER, Caress J. Ultrasound of nerve and muscle. Clin Neurophysiol. 2004;115(3):495–507.
59. Watanabe T, Ito H, Sekine A, Katano Y, Nishimura T, Kato Y, Takeda J, Seishima M, Matsuoka T. Sonographic evaluation of the peripheral nerve in diabetic patients: the relationship between nerve conduction studies, echo intensity, and cross-sectional area. J Ultrasound Med. 2010;29(5):697–708.
60. Wiesler ER, Chloros GD, Cartwright MS, Smith BP, Rushing J, Walker FO. The use of diagnostic ultrasound in carpal tunnel syndrome. J Hand Surg [Am]. 2006;31(5):726–32.
61. Wilbourn AJ. Nerve conduction study changes in human nerves undergoing Wallerian degeneration. Neurology. 1981;31:96–7.
62. Wilder-Smith EP, Therimadasamy A, Ghasemi-Esfe AR, Khalilzadeh O. Color and power Doppler US for diagnosing carpal tunnel syndrome and determining its severity. Radiology. 2012;262(3):1043–4. author reply 1044
63. Yoon JS, Walker FO, Cartwright MS. Ultrasonographic swelling ratio in the diagnosis of ulnar neuropathy at the elbow. Muscle Nerve. 2008;38:1231–5.
64. Zaidman CM, Al-Lozi M, Pestronk A. Peripheral nerve size in Normals and patients with polyneuropathy: an ultrasound study. Muscle Nerve. 2009;40:960–6.
65. Zaidman CM, Seelig MJ, Baker JC, Mackinnon SE, Pestronk A. Detection of peripheral nerve pathology: comparison of ultrasound and MRI. Neurology. 2013;80(18):1634–40.

17 Dextrose-Based Perineural Injection Treatment, and Ultrasound Hydrodissection

Liza Maniquis-Smigel, Paschenelle Celis, and Dean Reeves

Introduction

Anyone in pain will say that it needs no definition. It takes over one's whole being and affects activities of daily living, so much so as to make it impossible to be productive in even the simplest of tasks. Throughout the world, one in five adults suffers from severe chronic pain [1]. It affects millions of Americans, hindering many from working, attending school, socializing, and enjoying life [2]. "If all chronic pain conditions were lumped together and considered to be a single disease, as many pain researchers view the problem, it would be the most common, disabling, and expensive health problem in the world" [3].

Traditionally, much of our attention and education in clinical setting is looking at musculoskeletal problems, as it is considered to be the most common cause of chronic pain in the United States, with a 54% proportion of chronic pain related to musculoskeletal conditions [3]. These include osteoarthritis, rheumatoid arthritis, tendinitis, and chronic low back pain. The medical field has classically addressed pain through the use of acetaminophen, nonsteroidal anti-inflammatory drugs, opioids, or in combination, with the expectation of pain resolution once the injury is resolved. Despite addressing and correcting risk factors, many patients report they have "tried everything," but pain persists and becomes a chronic problem.

With the impact of chronic pain, opiate addiction has become a nationwide epidemic in the United States, with drug overdose deaths that continue to increase by twofold in the last decade [4]. National organizations have called for new therapies to address underlying pathologies and to produce improved non-opioid treatment regimens.

Neuropathic pain is a commonly overlooked cause of painful conditions, resulting in pain literally from head to toe. A recent systemic review of epidemiological research on neuropathic pain across the world suggests the prevalence lies between 6.9% and 10% in the general population [5], which in our opinion is a very low percentage given that their criteria only includes specific neurological conditions. Not only is neuropathic pain overlooked, but severity of neuropathic pain can be high. Observational studies in the United States and Europe alone suggest that between 70.0% and 96.0% of patients with neuropathic pain seeking care experience moderate to severe pain [6].

Centralization of pain concepts has dominated the mechanistic explanations for initiation and perpetuation of chronic neuropathic pain, which

L. Maniquis-Smigel (✉)
Hilo, HI, USA

P. Celis
Physical Medicine & Rehabilitation Department, Clinica OS Habitares, Quezon City, Philippines

D. Reeves
Private Practice of Physical Medicine and Rehabilitation, Roeland Park, KS, USA

Y. El Miedany (ed.), *Musculoskeletal Ultrasound-Guided Regenerative Medicine*,
https://doi.org/10.1007/978-3-030-98256-0_17

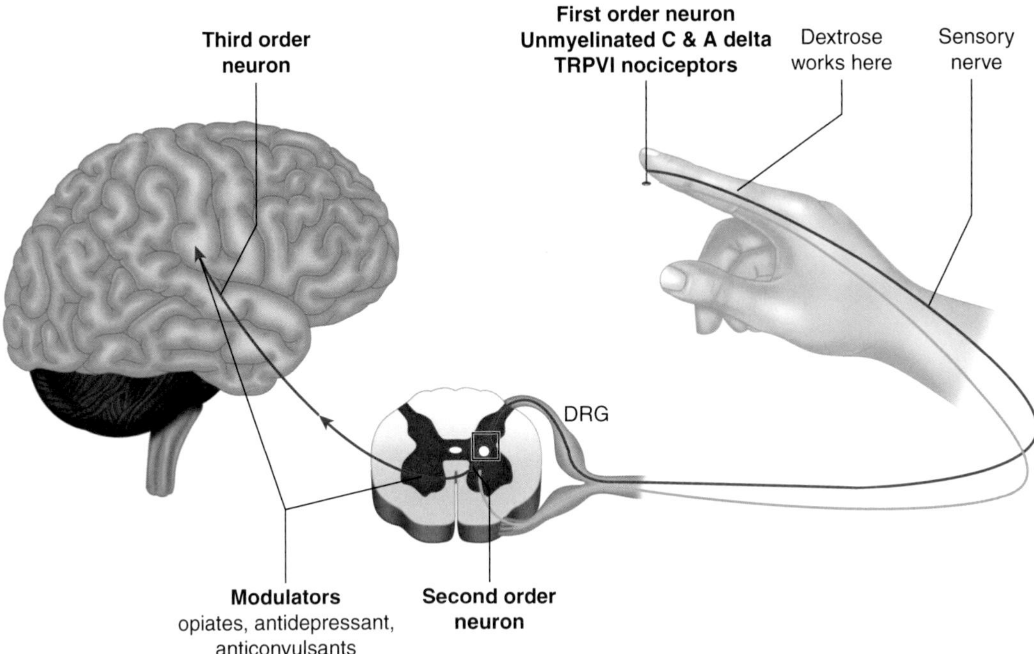

Fig. 17.1 Somatosensory pathway

is thought to result from changes in the properties of neurons in the CNS. The classic explanation of refractory neuropathic pain states that pain signals originating in the periphery migrate centrally, "burn their way" into the CNS, and in time create a permanent trace that is independent of peripheral drive [7]. In other words, it is a state in which neurons in the CNS become hyperexcitable. Treatments have focused on decreasing central sensitization with antidepressants, antiseizure, and opiate medications, which has proven to be unsatisfactory, due to incomplete pain relief and considerable medication side effects.

Change in Neuropathic Pain Definition and Introduction of Perineural Injection Therapy (PIT)

In 2011, the International Association of the Study of Pain proposed a new definition of neuropathic pain, as "pain caused by a lesion or disease of the somatosensory system" [8] (Fig. 17.1). This new definition reflects a general movement to reconsider the importance of peripheral nervous system autonomy as a mechanism for chronic pain [9]. Most clinicians may not be aware that peripheral small fiber nerve abnormalities can lead to debilitating pain, mimicking headaches, adhesive capsulitis, cardiac disease, intra-abdominal pathology, hernia, CRPS, or plantar fasciitis [10]. Localization and effective treatment of these chronic small fiber nerve injuries can prevent unnecessary and expensive diagnostic testing and treatments and help to avoid unnecessary pain and suffering.

PIT is an injection-based treatment for neuropathic pain that has rapidly increased in popularity over the last several years, empirically changing the lives of patients worldwide and directly addressing the peripheral nervous system. Clinically, physicians and patients alike report reduction of pain within seconds after an isotonic dextrose solution (5% dextrose in water; D5W) is injected adjacent to painful peripheral nerves in the subcutaneous tissues or deeper, using a 27G 1/2 inch needle. Repeated treatments have a cumulative effect [11, 12]. Clinical improvement is hypothesized to be due to a sensorineural effect of dextrose on neuropathic pain generators [13].

Somatosensory Pathway starts with the free nerve endings under the skin as unmyelinated C fibers and the A delta fibers, also known as TRPV1 nociceptors, that travel through the whole length of the C fiber nerve with the cell body in the dorsal root ganglion, then enters the spinal cord through the dorsal rami and dorsal horn of the gray matter, then crosses over to contralateral side and ascends up to the thalamus and to the somatic sensory cortex of the brain to perceive pain. Dextrose is postulated to work on the first order neuron/ unmyelinated C fiber nerves.

Many factors have converged to accelerate the growth of PIT worldwide:

1. The lack of long-term efficacy of standard of care for chronic pain, including steroid injections and the rise of the opioid epidemic. There is a push to produce non-opioid treatment that is economical, safe, and effective.
2. Advancements in the scientific understanding of neurogenic inflammation and peripheral sensitization.
3. A clearer understanding of dextrose and its role in chronic pain at its molecular and cellular level.
4. The subsequent escalation of nerve hydrodissection ultrasound techniques that have further enhanced the effects of neural dextrose injections.

The focus of this chapter is:

1. To differentiate dextrose-based treatments
2. To review some of the historical and relevant documentation of neurogenic inflammation and its relationship to pain
3. To explain our current theory of the sensorineural therapeutic effect of D5W at its molecular and cellular level targeting small fiber sensory peripheral nerves in reducing neurogenic pain, hyperalgesia, and allodynia
4. To discuss findings, benefits, and advantages of ultrasound-guided nerve hydrodissection (HD) using dextrose to release peripheral nerves from their encasing fascia in order to provide a decompressive and dextrose sensorineural effect

Differentiating Dextrose-Based Treatments

Although the focus of this chapter is on the perineural injection therapy (PIT), it is important to differentiate this from traditional prolotherapy, two very different dextrose-based treatments.

Dextrose prolotherapy (DPT) uses hypertonic (12.5–25% dose) dextrose solution for regenerative repair of weakened structural tissues. The proposed mechanism is regenerative repair. DPT use began in the 1930s and was originally used in the treatment of ligamentous laxity [14]. In the 1950s, George S. Hackett, a general surgeon in the United States, began performing injections of irritant solutions in an effort to repair joints and hernias [15]. Prolotherapy technique utilizes a combination of palpation and ultrasound scanning to assess anatomical structures that are not routinely emphasized in conventional musculoskeletal medicine (generally ligaments, tendons, and small joints). It is dependent on a highly refined knowledge of neuromusculoskeletal and surface anatomy. Dextrose is predominantly injected in enthesis and intra-articularly in the performance of prolotherapy. One of the pearls of prolotherapy is to always inject on bone as weakness occurs on the enthesis,where the tendon or ligament attaches to the bone[160]. It consists of microinjections into the enthesis whose primary intent is to encourage repair of damaged tissues. The hypertonic dextrose is hypothesized to cause a mild osmotic irritation [9, 13, 16, 17]. This irritation along with needle microtrauma initiates the healing cascade (inflammation, proliferation, and remodeling), with eventual laying down of collagen by fibroblasts and repair of damaged structures, correcting biotensegrity, and relieving pain [9, 13, 16, 17]. However, an immediate benefit after injection of dextrose has been noted frequently, raising questions about whether therapeutic mechanisms of dextrose other than proliferative are at work, such as a neurogenic effect (see below).

Perineural injection treatment (PIT) (formerly known as superficial prolotherapy or neural prolotherapy) is different from DPT. It uses 5% dextrose (D5W), an isotonic concentration, injected subcutaneously, for the treatment of neuropathic pain [18–21]. It first appeared in the medical literature in 2006 [22]. The proposed mechanism is a sensorineural effect of dextrose. Dr. John Lyftogt was the first to observe that injection of subcutaneous dextrose without local anesthetic over painful sensory nerves resulted in relief of pain within seconds of injection of areas of pain. Precise anatomical knowledge of the sensory cutaneous innervation of the body provides the guide to utilize skin gliding palpation technique of the suspected swollen nerves, termed chronic constrictive injuries (CCIs) [23] or Valleix points [24], which reproduces the neuropathic pain experienced by the patient. Every treatment aims to extinguish the pain and has a cumulative effect. Repeated sessions [2, 3, 5–7] may be required, with the aim of complete resolution and to allow return to full function [18] (Figs. 17.2 and 17.3).

Perineural Hydrodissection With Ultrasound Guidance

In recent years, nerve hydrodissection (HD), employing high-resolution ultrasound, has been used for continuous visualization to inject fluid to separate the nerves from fascial layers. The technique is explained in detail in a different chapter of this book (Chap. 13: Peripheral Nerve Hydrodissection by Dr. Stanley Lam). Traditionally, a large volume of normal saline and a small volume of steroids and anesthetic are used for HD of nerves [25]. Since a recent publication evidencing that stand-alone dextrose has an analgesic effect [26], D5W is becoming the solution of choice for USG nerve hydrodissection, as it offers a dual advantage of mechanical hydrodissection and sensorineural effects without the side effects of steroids or the risk of lidocaine toxicity [12]. This is gaining ground as ultrasound technology achieves higher resolution, allowing better visualization of small sensory cutaneous nerves (Fig. 17.4).

There are many advantages of ultrasound guidance (USG). It allows accurate identification of the nerve to facilitate the precise approach required for HD. USG allows visualization of potential areas to avoid, such as vascular structures. One can appreciate pathological nerves which are usually swollen or with thickened epineurium and perineurium compared to healthy nerves. In normal-sized nerves, individual fascicles can be enlarged, signifying pathology as well. Dynamic ultrasound of nerves can show snapping of the nerve against surrounding bone, ligament, or tendon, reproducing pain that is experienced by the patient There is less percentage of error, as compared to palpation-guided needle injection alone, increasing efficiency, and in most cases, this equates to a faster procedure. Ultrasound visualization improves patient comfort and confidence, which increases compliance. Ultrasound documentation, before, during, and after the procedure, can serve as a record of improvement and as a reference for future procedures and plans. Furthermore, use of ultrasound is safe for most patients, including pregnant women or patients with implants [27].

While ultrasound guidance enjoys all these benefits, there are obvious limitations when compared to the palpation-guided PIT. There is a steep learning curve which makes gaining competency a time-intensive training process on the part of the physician. Use of technology will limit the access to patients that can be treated vs PIT, which is palpation-based and can be performed anywhere in the world including third-world countries where ultrasound machines are inaccessible.

With current standard ultrasound machines being used today in the clinical setting, even with extensive training and experience in the part of the physician, the larger nerves are appreciated, but smaller sensory cutaneous fiber nerves cannot be effectively visualized. Therefore, a combination approach combining hydrodissection and injection by palpation guid-

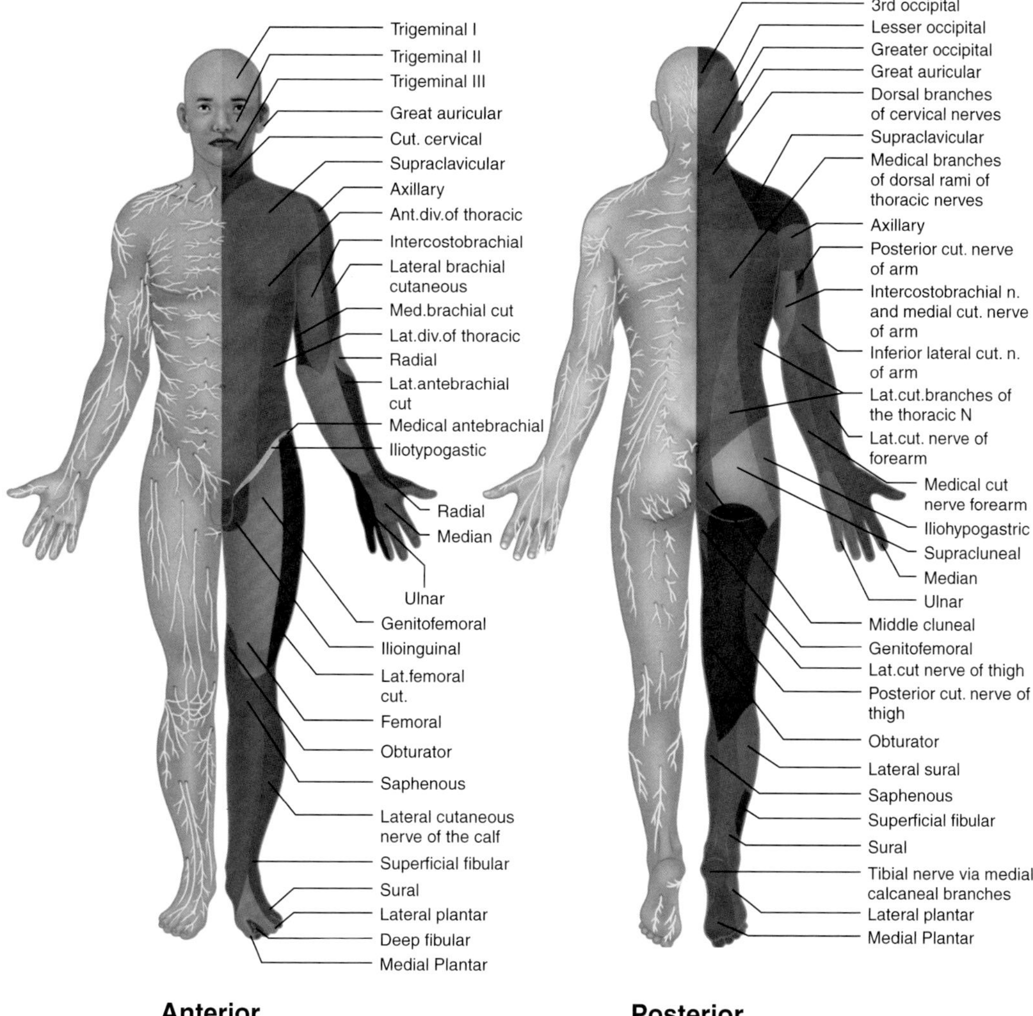

Fig. 17.2 Cutaneous innervation of peripheral nerves provides the guide to identify the area of neuropathic pain region of suspected swollen cutaneous nerves

ance is commonly utilized by clinicians. In the future, as higher-resolution ultrasound technology becomes more available and affordable, improving visualization of small sensory cutaneous nerves, will allow us to be more accurate, effective, and faster in our procedures.

Historical Relationship Between Neurogenic Inflammation and Pain

We are just beginning to understand the scientific rationale for sensorineural effect of dextrose treatments, and the current theory continues to evolve. However, it is important to understand the historical context in which this theory is based. We will review several concepts that are pertinent to our understanding of how glucose works in the peripheral nervous system to reduce pain.

Early Concepts of Pain

Neurogenic inflammation is the inflammation that is produced through the release of substances from the sensory neurons from the periphery, in

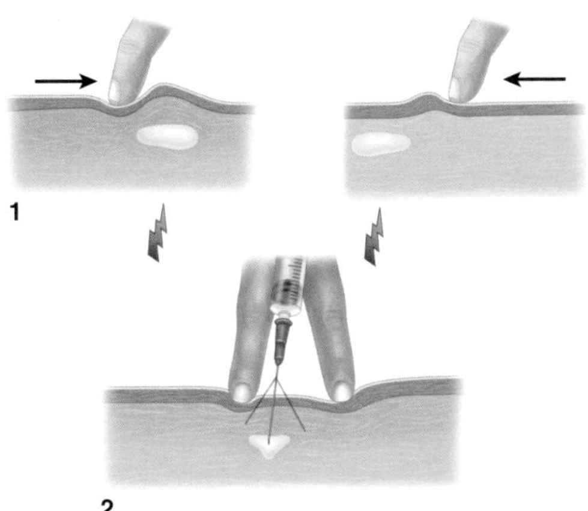

Fig. 17.3 Perineural injection treatment (PIT): 1. Skin gliding palpation over the suspected swollen nerve with tips of fingers; characteristic and localized pain and swelling are present. 2. With the use of the two-finger technique, buffered D5W without local anesthetic is injected perineurally with a 27-gauge, 0.5 inch needle, which results in the relief of pain within seconds of injection

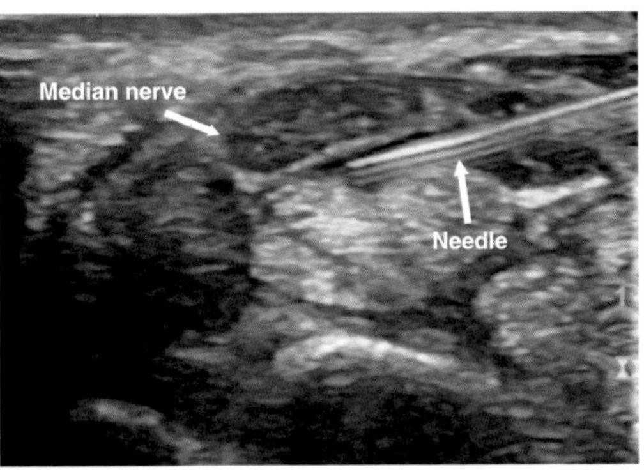

Fig. 17.4 Ultrasound image demonstrating hydrodissection of the median nerve at the carpal tunnel in short-axis, in-plane approach

particular, from A delta and unmyelinated C afferent fibers [28]. In addition to the classic afferent functions of the sensory peripheral nerve, it is now well established that the peripheral nervous system also participates in the regulation of efferent actions on cell proliferation, expression of cytokines and growth factors, inflammation, immune responses, and hormone release. This is called the paradoxical "efferent" role of nociceptive sensory fibers and was suggested already by Baylis in 1901 [29].

Neuralgia and chronic constrictive injury (CCI) were first described by Dr. John Marshall and Sir Victor Horsley In December 15,1883. In their Bradshaw Lecture on Nerve Stretching, they postulated that the nervi nervorum (the small nerve filaments innervating the sheath of a larger nerve) are the cause of neuralgia or neuropathic pain [30, 31].

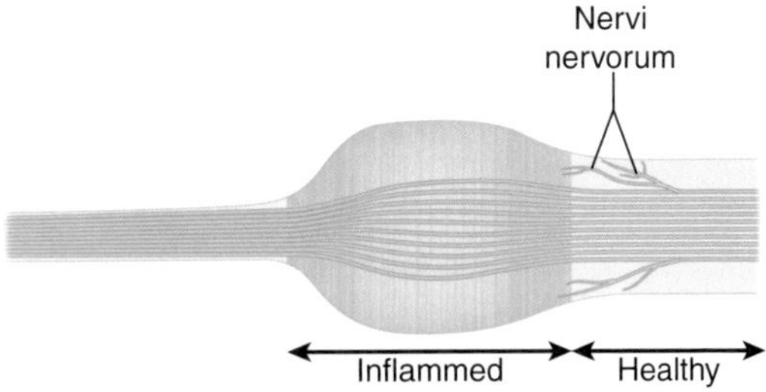

Fig. 17.5 On the right is a normal nerve with nervi nervorum that arises from the nerve trunk itself and branches and extends into the epi-perineurium of nerve trunk. The nervi nervorum, when activated, will result in inflammatory exudates and, ultimately, neural swelling

Their illustration of the healthy nerve shows small nerve endings that arise from the nerve trunk itself (Fig. 17.5). These nerve endings are the nervi nervorum which are intrinsic small fiber nerves that supply the nerve itself and the connective tissue that surrounds the nerve. Nervi nervorum "ramify" in the epi-perineurium of nerve trunks and beyond, and these small fiber nerves can trigger pathological neurogenic inflammation which may result in inflammatory exudates and, ultimately, neural swelling [31].

In the publication "Nerve stretching for the relief or cure of pain," Marshall has inferred that *nervi nervorum* would participate in pain generation mechanisms observed in cases of peripheral nerve compression. Together with Horsley, he has shown that *nervi nervorum* were sensitive to pain, especially to pressure. Dr. Marshall also postulated that "The pain of neuralgia is more severe at certain apertures where the nerve passes out the osseous or fibrous framework of the body, or passes around given points of bone." These neural swellings, which occur at certain small apertures where the nerves pass through, restricting axonal flow and activating the nervi nervorum, he called *chronic constrictive injury* (CCI). When a nerve is subjected to 30 mmHg, there is consistent inhibition, which was even more marked at 60 mmHg and still more at 90 mmHg

[32]. The activated nervi nervorum may, in turn, cause dilation of blood vessels, an increase in blood flow, and swelling which results in neuralgia.

The concept of CCIs is reinforced by Bennett's experimental observation that a peripheral neuropathy is consistently produced when lightly constrictive ligatures are placed around a rat sciatic nerve. This results in functional nerve disruption and an hourglass appearance of nerve, with swelling on either side of the ligature [23]. This sciatic ligature model, commonly used to create neuropathic pain (hyperalgesia and allodynia) in research settings, supports the concept that even minimal compression of nerves in fascial layers can result in clinically important neurogenic inflammation and neuropathic pain [18].

Valleix Points

In the early 1800s, François Louis Isidore Valleix, a French pediatrician, already described the sites of these peripheral nerve swellings, similar to CCIs described by Marshall and Horsley. "Valleix points" are various points in the course of a nerve, at which applied pressure causes pain in cases of neuralgia [24]. These points are enumerated as where the nerve emerges from the bony canal, where it pierces a muscle or aponeurosis to reach the skin, where a superficial nerve rests on a resisting surface where compression is easily made, where the nerve gives off one or more branches, and where the nerve terminates in the skin [24]. PIT practitioners use Valleix points as guide on where to focus palpation to find the swelling of nerves in the subcutaneous tissue.

Concept of Nociceptors

The specificity theory of pain, initially presented by Charles Bell (1774–1842), is one of the first modern theories of pain. It holds that specific pain receptors transmit signals to a "pain center" in the brain that produces the perception of pain [33, 34]. Nociceptors are special cutaneous or subcutaneous nerve cell endings that initiate the perception of pain. They are receptors that respond only to noxious stimuli and generate impulses through nerve pathways along nerve fibers to target centers in the brain, which process the signals to produce the experience of pain [33, 34].

In 1894, Maximilian von Frey made another critical addition to the specificity theory that served to advance the concept. His contribution assigns different types of sensations to different specific pathways. These sensations include cold, pain, heat, and touch [33, 34] (Fig. 17.6). There is a unique receptor for each type of sensation. Frey explained that nociceptors are specialized cells that sense pain or noxious stimuli with no additional influences. He argued that the body has a separate sensory system for perceiving pain, just as it does for hearing and vision. The free nerve endings subserve the pain modality [28, 29]. Thus, it is based on the assumption that the free nerve endings are pain receptors and that the other types of receptors are also specific to a sensory experience. This theory considers pain as an independent sensation, with specialized peripheral sensory receptors (nociceptors), which respond to damage and send signals through nerve fibers to target centers in the brain, which produce the experience of pain [34] (Fig. 17.7).

We now know that peripheral nociceptors (A delta and C fibers) sense three types of noxious impulses: mechanical, mechanothermal, and chemical. The *A delta fibers* are lightly myelinated and respond to intense mechanical or mechanothermal stimuli, while the *C fibers* are the unmyelinated and respond to thermal, mechanical, and chemical stimuli and are therefore polymodal [35].

Sir Charles Scott Sherrington elaborated on the specificity theory of pain. Sherrington's law states "Every nerve can influence the proper and specific activity of a tissue it innervates and has a trophic influence on that tissue" [34, 36]. In other words, sensory nerves have a trophic reparative influence on the tissues that it innervates. In normal physiological conditions, the efferent effect of the sensory system is responsible for tissue maintenance and renewal and has trophic activity [36].

VALLEIX POINT 1841

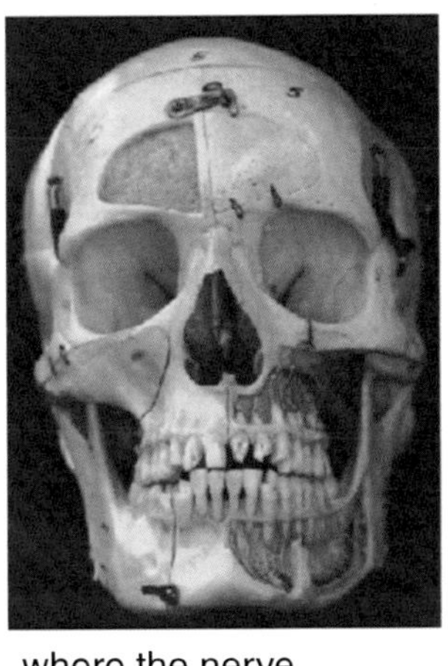

where the nerve emerges from the bony canal

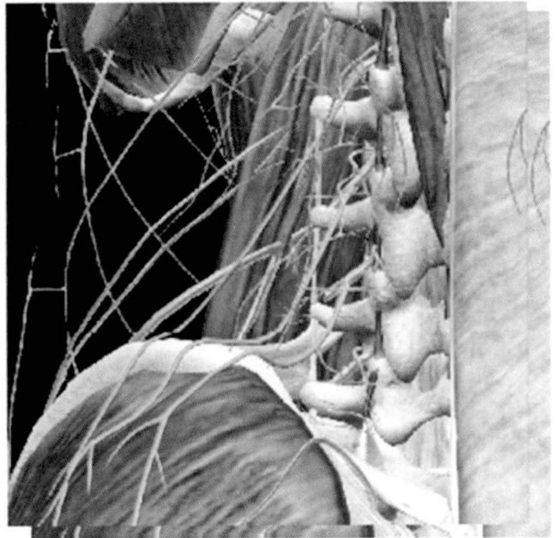

where a superficial nerve rests on a resistingsurface where compression is easily made

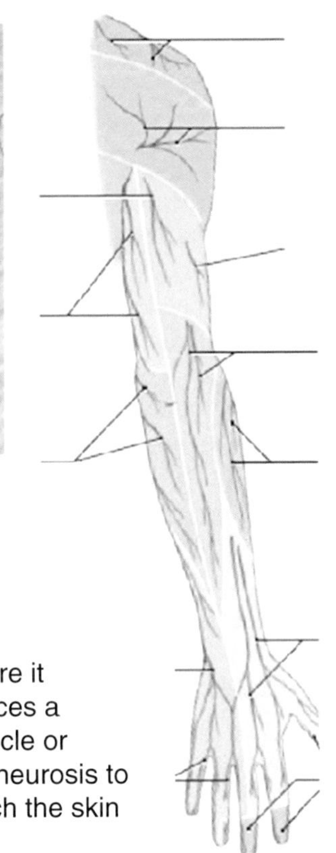

where it pierces a muscle or aponeurosis to reach the skin

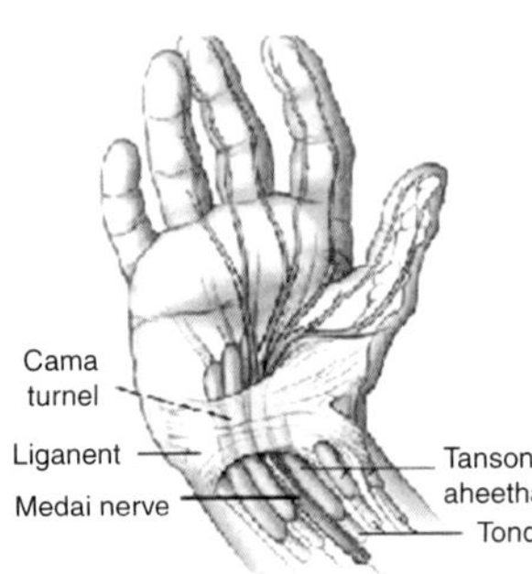

where it is entrapped b/w fibrous tissue

Fig. 17.6 Valleix points are various points in the course of the nerve, about which, when pressure is applied, causes pain in cases of neuralgia

Hilton's Law

HILTON'S LAW 1863

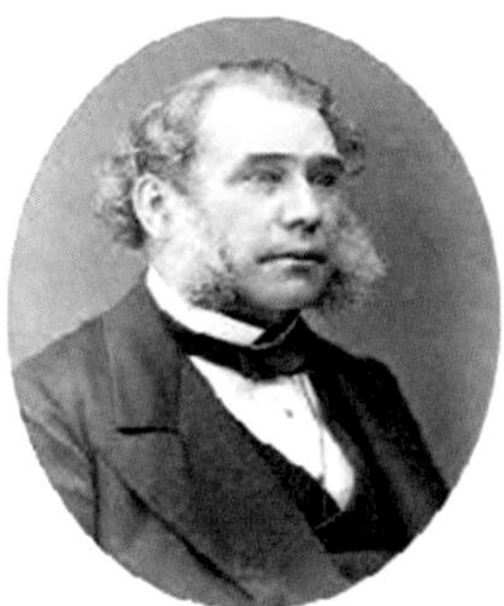

For what we are doing, it is applicable to understand Hilton's law. John Hilton was the foremost anatomist and surgeon of his day. He developed many anatomical principles culminating in a series of lectures on *On Rest and Pain* [32, 33]. He described the organization of peripheral nerves. Hilton's law states "The nerve trunk supplying a joint also supplies the overlying skin and the muscles that move that joint" [37, 38]. This law suggests that in clinical setting, subcutaneous near nerve injections will affect the underlying joint and muscles that they supply (Figs. 17.8 and 17.9).

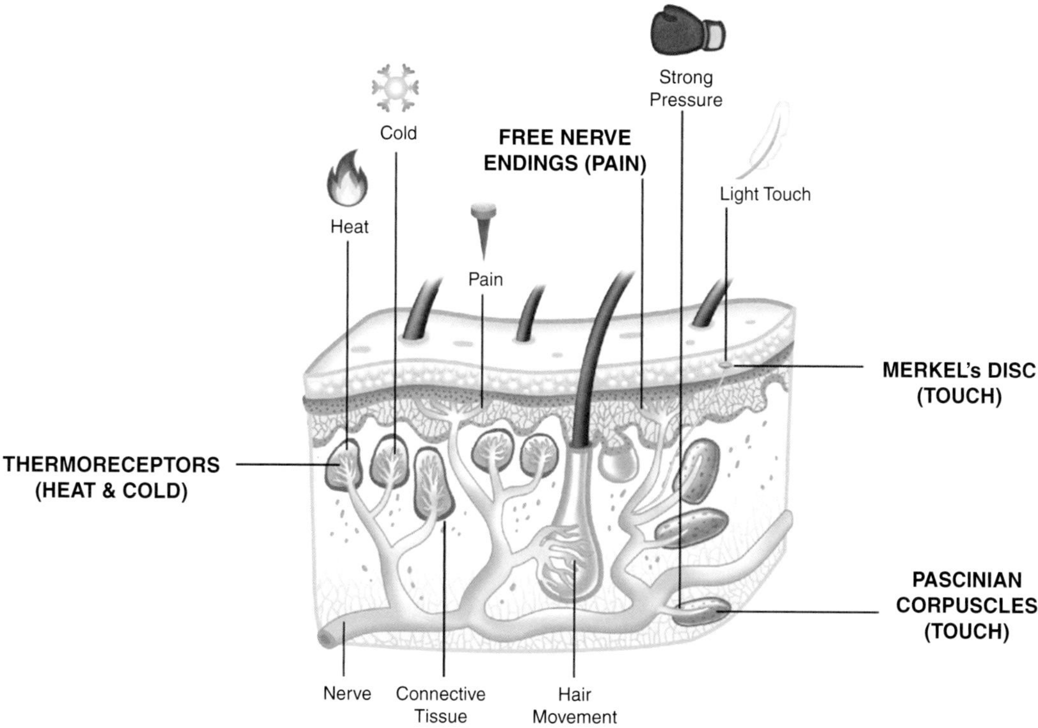

Fig. 17.7 Nociceptors are specialized cells that sense pain or noxious stimuli with no additional influences. The four sensory nociceptor modalities are cold, heat, pain, and touch [29, 34]

PIT subcutaneous injections without intra-articular injections have been empirically reported to relieve pain and improve function of arthritic patients. This may also explain rapid pain reduction after deeper (enthesis or intra-articular) injection in dextrose prolotherapy, since the same pain-producing C fibers are also found in high density on bony cortex [39].

Twenty-First Century: Pain As a Channelopathy

Neuroscientists in the twenty-first century identified complex ion channels on nociceptor membranes. These ion channels found on the sensory axons have an efferent function. This contradicts the classic theory of the unidirectional afferent pathway of sensory nerves, and a bidirectional function for the same side of the sensory nerve is now favored [40]. These recent advances of the role of ion channels in neurons may facilitate our understanding of why dextrose has an instant calming effect on pain sensation. We believe that pain relief has to do with these ion channels through impulse generation (APs), which are heavily influenced by glucopenia and corrected by perineural injection of dextrose (Fig. 17.10).

Ion channels expressed by immune system cells (e.g., P2X7) have been shown to play a pivotal role in changing pain thresholds, while channels involved in sensory transduction (e.g., TRPV1), the regulation of neuronal excitability (potassium channels), action potential propagation (sodium channels), and neurotransmitter release (calcium channels) have all been shown to be potentially selective analgesic drug targets to control pain [34].

Two ion channels and one transport protein system which are of particular importance in neuropathic pain initiation and maintenance, include TRPV1 and potassium ion channels, and the glucose transporters (GLUTs).

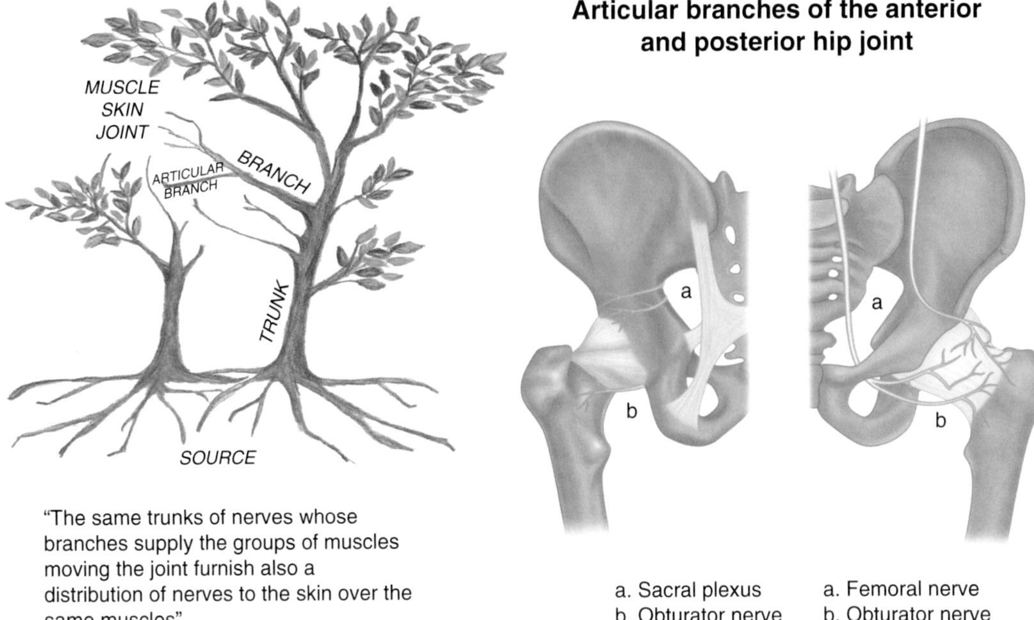

Figs. 17.8 and 17.9 Hilton's law states "The nerve trunk supplying a joint also supplies the overlying skin and the muscles that move that joint" [37, 38]. This law suggests that in clinical setting, subcutaneous near nerve injections will affect the underlying joint and muscles that they supply

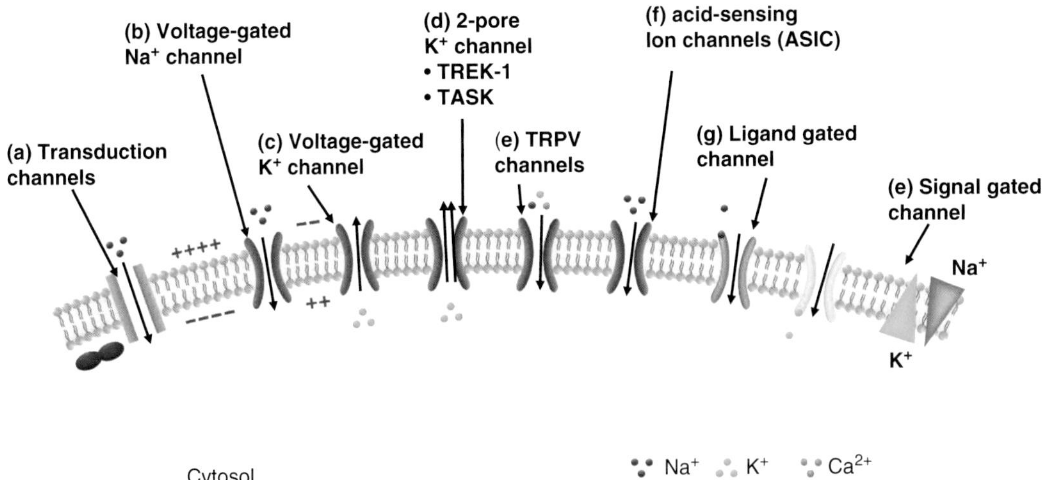

Fig. 17.10 Complex ion channels on nociceptive membrane: Neuroscientists have discovered and identified complex ion channels on nociceptor membranes. The direct activation of most ion channels is triggered by changes in either voltage (voltage-gated channels) or neurotransmitters and hormones (ligand-gated channels). For instance, direct depolarization of neurons by electrical stimuli will open voltage-gated Na+, Ca2+, and K+ channels [34]

TRPV1

The TRPV1 ion channel (formerly known as the "capsaicin receptor") has been postulated to be associated with neuropathic pain [41]. TRPV1 is a member of the vanilloid family of channel receptors that, when stimulated, allow calcium and sodium ions to enter the neuron. There are about 28 TRPV channels that play a role in sensory physiology [42]. TRPV1 is the most studied. It is sensitive to noxious heat; endogenous pro-inflammatory molecules, such as arachidonic acid metabolites; nerve growth factors; bradykinins and protons (tissue acidification). As a result, the neuron becomes depolarized, and if the depolarization passes a certain threshold, it triggers action potentials producing pain. The nociceptor then releases neuropeptides: substance P (SubP) and calcitonin gene-related peptide (CGRP) [43, 44].

Neurogenic inflammation, in this context, refers to the inflammation that is produced through the release of neuropeptides from the small-diameter unmyelinated C fiber nerves that have TRPV ion channels embedded on their membrane [45, 46]. This action is by far the most important source of pathological pain in humans [46] (Fig. 17.11).

What Are the Effects of CGRP and Substance P That Produce Signs and Symptoms of Chronic Pain Syndromes and Degeneration?

Calcitonin gene-related peptide (CGRP), a 37 amino acid peptide, is the most potent microvascular vasodilator currently known. It has a

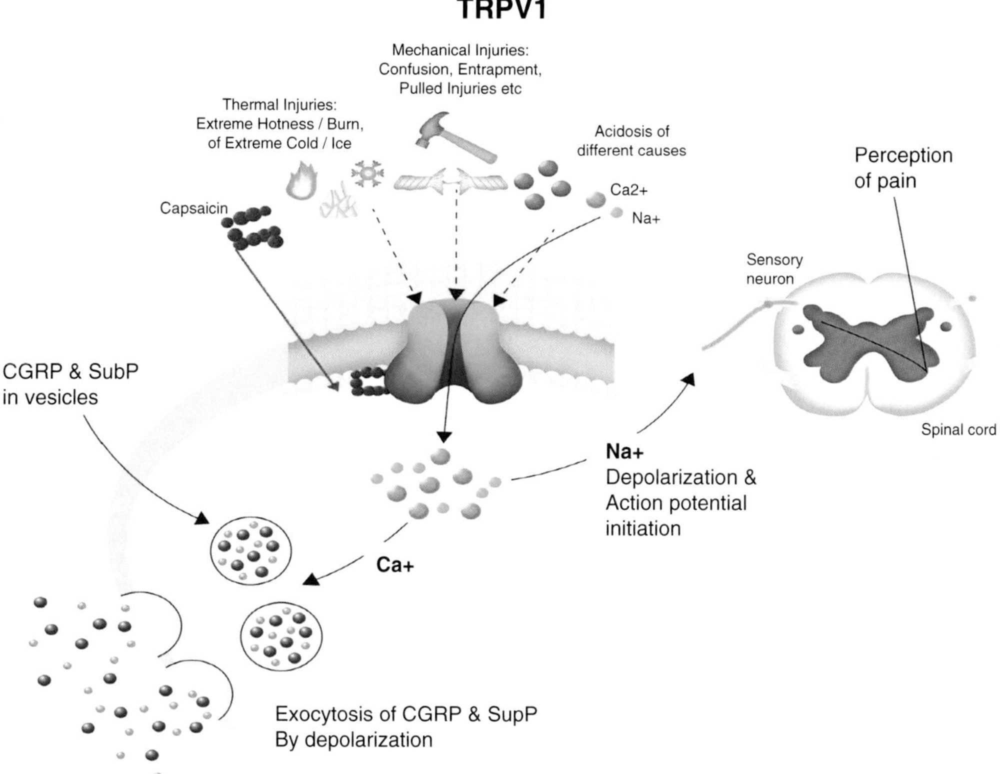

Fig. 17.11 TRPV1 ion channel: TRPV1 is sensitive to mechanical injuries; noxious heat; endogenous pro-inflammatory molecules, such as arachidonic acid metabolites; nerve growth factors; bradykinins; and protons (tissue acidification). When TRPV1 ion channel is activated, there is an influx of Na and Ca into the cells. Na influx causes depolarization of the membrane potential producing pain. Ca influx causes the release of neuropeptides: SubP and CGRP from microvesicles within the cell which are pro-inflammatory mediators of sensory nerves, causing changes in sensory neuron function brought about by these inflammatory transmitters

potency nearly 10-fold higher than the most potent prostaglandins and 10–100 times greater than other vasodilators such as acetylcholine and substance P [47]. It results in increased vascular permeability and plasma extravasation, producing edema formation in skin and joints. It has been known for a long time that arthritic patients have increased levels of CGRP in their plasma and synovial fluid, and CGRP may be a very early mediator in the disease process. CGRP can cause cytokine production from whole blood cells and fibroblasts seen in rheumatoid arthritis (RA) and osteoarthritis (OA) patients. It upregulates vascular endothelial growth factor (VEGF), which leads to neovascularization and neoneurogenesis. VEGF in turn, increases matrix metallopeptidase (MMPI), leading to collagenolysis and tendon and ligament degeneration. It blocks the uptake of calcium by osteoblasts, increasing tissue calcium levels, leading to calcification changes. It stimulates osteoclasts to eventually produce breakdown of bone (dystrophic bone) [47].

Substance P (SubP) is a neuropeptide containing 11 amino acids and belonging to the tachykinin family. Substance P is a key first responder to most noxious stimuli and is regarded as an immediate stress repair-survival system [48]. SubP is also a potent vasodilator in post-capillary venules causing increased vascular permeability and protein extravasation [49, 50]. SubP activates the immune cells to produce cytokines; it binds to mast cells causing degranulation. It is related to the transmission of pain information into the central nervous system. SubP is particularly excitatory to cell growth and multiplication [49]. SubP has been associated with the regulation of mood disorders and anxiety symptoms [51]. It affects the hypothalamus to stimulate the corticotropin-releasing hormone which leads to adrenal fatigue and exhaustion [51]. It also impairs proprioception by delaying antagonist muscle reflex inhibition [39]. Increased SubP can explain the significant negative impact on those afflicted with chronic pain, including decreased activity, fatigue, insomnia, and mood changes such as depression [51].

The TRPV1 ion channel is the only ion channel known to respond to capsaicin [43], which is why it was originally termed the "capsaicin receptor" for years. Dr. Lyftogt observed that that both dextrose (glucose) and a similar 6 carbon atom monosugar, mannitol, reduce burning pain after capsaicin is applied to the human lip (personal communication). This was followed by an RCT by Bertrand et al. which demonstrated that mannitol application (compared to control) reduced the burning pain effect of capsaicin on human lips [52]. Their conclusion was that topical mannitol reduces the effects of TRVP1 channel activation by a downstream mechanism, since mannitol has no receptor on the TRPV1 channel. This study has not been replicated with glucose, which also has no receptor on the TRPV1 channel. The current postulate for further mechanistic research is that there is a class effect of certain monosugars, including dextrose, that antagonizes the effects of TRPV1 activation.

Potassium Channels

Potassium (K^{+}) channels are pertinent to our discussion as they have receptors for dextrose and have a role in energy homeostasis and glucose sensing. This may further clarify the mystery of why dextrose provides instant analgesia.

Ion channels are critical in regulating the membrane potential of neurons [53]. The activation of a specific ion channel will either activate or inhibit a neuron depending on the resting membrane potential (RMP) and the ion's equilibrium. Typically, neurons have RMP of −55 mv. Activation of the ion channel will depolarize the cell as cations will rush into the cell membrane which results in the depolarization of the membrane potential (i.e., Na+ channels, Ca+ channels). By contrast, anions rush in or cations rush out to hyperpolarize the membrane potential when RMP is more positive than the equilibrium potential of an ion (e.g., K+ channels and CL- channels) [53].

Sensory nerves, like all nerves, are high energy users, which is supplied by glucose. A large proportion of energy requirements is used to support neuronal resting membrane potential [53].

To date, glucose sensors in the periphery have been found in the pancreatic β-cell intestine, hepatoportal vein, and carotid body [54]. The portal vein sensory afferents contain CGRP since they are capsaicin sensitive. However, chemosensitivity to CO2 and O2 hampers the interpretation of glucose-sensing afferent signals.

Recent evidence suggests that specialized tandem pore potassium (**K2P**) channels are sensitive to glucose [55]. Glucose-sensing neurons are responsible for regulating energy and glucose homeostasis. The attachment of dextrose to the K2P receptor leads to its activation, which opens the potassium channels, transports potassium outside the cell, and hyperpolarizes the cell membrane. Hyperpolarization of the membrane potential inhibits neuronal activity (associates with pain reduction) [55, 56].

We can therefore hypothesize that the clinical instant relief we observe with perineural dextrose injection has to do with this inhibition of neuronal activity and restoration of perineural glucose levels. This will result in repolarization and hyperpolarization mediated by tandem pore potassium channels, eliminating neuropathic pain and reducing neurogenic inflammation [53].

Glucose Transporter 3 (GLUT3)

The significance of glucose transporters in biology is apparent as they are the gateways for the most important mover of life [51]. The ability to import and metabolize glucose at the cellular level is by a process of facilitative diffusion mediated by members of the GLUT family of membrane transport proteins. The well-established glucose transporter isoforms, GLUTs 1–4, are known to have distinct regulatory and kinetic properties that reflect their specific roles in cellular and whole-body glucose homeostasis. GLUT3, specifically, is the major neuronal glucose transporter, present in both dendrites and axons. GLUT3 has a high affinity for glucose and has the highest number of calculated turnovers of GLUT isoforms, thus ensuring efficient glucose uptake by neurons [57] (Fig. 17.12).

According to GLUTs in the twenty-first-century article by Thorens et al. [58], activation of GLUT3 occurs by glucose-sensing neurons. A decrease in extracellular glucose concentration or hypoglycemia (cellular glucose deprivation) activates ATP-sensitive (K_{ATP}) glucose-sensing K channel neuron, and glucose is transported within the cell by a glucose transporter, which then goes through the glycolysis for ATP production, needed to regulate gene transcription, enzyme activity, hormone secretion, and the activity of glucoregulatory neurons. This has been evidence tested with K_{ATP} channel activation with channel opener diazoxide which amplifies counterregulatory hormone responses to hypoglycemia in normal and recurrently hypoglycemic patients [57] (Fig. 17.13).

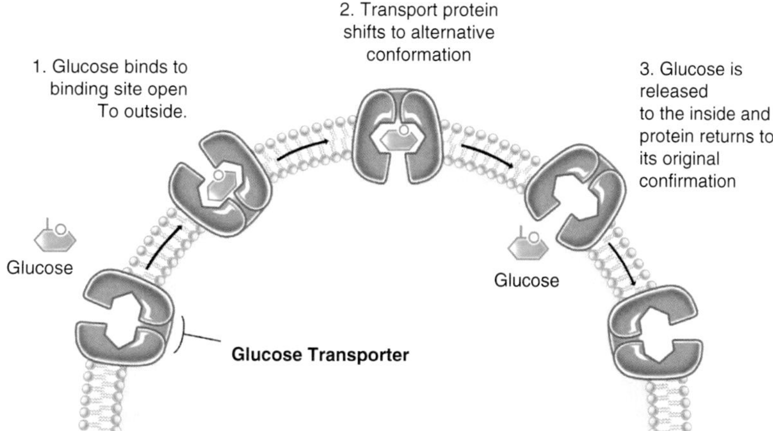

Fig. 17.12 Glucose transporter (GLUT): The ability to import and metabolize glucose at the cellular level is by a process of facilitative diffusion mediated by members of the GLUT family of membrane transport proteins

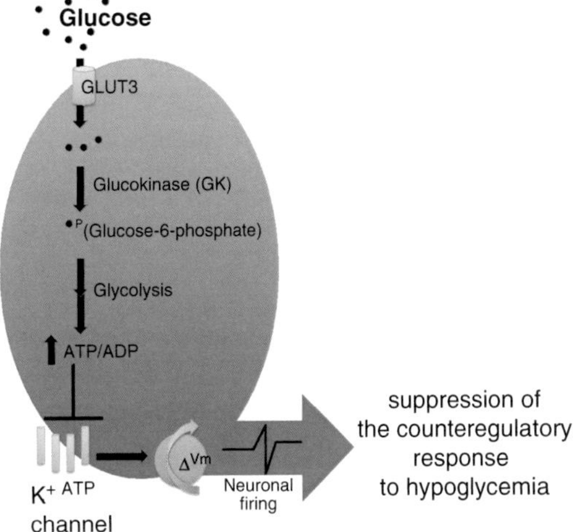

Fig. 17.13 A simplified model of glucose-sensing neuron via ATP-sensitive K+ channels: Glucose sensing in glucose-excited (GE) neuron requires glucose uptake via glucose transporters (GLUTs), glucose phosphorylation by the rate-limiting enzyme glucokinase, and subsequent metabolism of glucose to increase the intracellular ATP-to-ADP ratio. In the setting of glucose sufficiency, ATP-sensitive K+ channels are closed, the membrane is depolarized, and neuronal firing occurs, which suppresses the counterregulatory response while glucose levels are not low. Thus, a rise in plasma glucose increases neuronal activity in GE neurons. However, when glucose levels fall as would occur during hypoglycemia, the decreased metabolism of glucose leads to the opening of K-ATP channels and hyperpolarization of these glucose-excited neurons [59]

The Basic Science on Dextrose Algesia Efficacy

The Maclver study "Activation of C fibers by Metabolic Perturbations" [60] is probably the most important published research study supporting PIT. According to Maclver, the presence or absence of glucose can be detected by small fibers and has been tested by in vitro study in a corneal model of small fibers. Perineural glycopenia results in progressive depolarization and hyperexcitability of nociceptive nerve fibers, presumably through reduced effectiveness of the ATPase pump, which depends on dextrose for ATP production [40]. In this study, nociceptive C fibers exposed to a temporary glycopenia environment demonstrated a 653% ± 23% increase in action potential frequency within 15 min, with prompt reversal to a normal baseline firing rate when dextrose was reintroduced [60, 61].

Dextrose injections may provide analgesia through correction of local glycopenia. However, confirming that the perineural environment is relatively glycopenic will require microdialysis or other analysis methods for confirmation [62] (Figs. 17.14 and 17.15).

Neuronal Energy Deprivation Theory of Pain/Lyftogt Theory of Pain

Dr. John Lyftogt has postulated a "neuronal energy deprivation theory of pain" (personal communication). He hypothesizes that neuropathic pain reflects problems with tissue homeostasis and that pain is due to hypoglycemia, ischemia, or low pH, supported by the Maclver study on the effect of glucose and oxygen level manipulation effects on C fiber firing rate. He postulates that neuropathic pain is an energy failure syndrome due to an oxygen/glucose deprivation state. This triggers C fiber firing through direct or indirect effect through TRPV1 channel activation, triggering release of SubP and CGRP, and subsequent neurogenic inflammation and neuropathic pain. Buffered glucose may resolve neuropathic pain in the absence of hypoxia through correcting local tissue hypoglycemia and acidosis.

Early Clinical Evidence of PIT Efficacy Using Dextrose

Dextrose injected around nerves in reducing neurogenic pain is being supported by a growing number of small but methodologically rigorous clinical studies across many pain conditions [33].

Results of several case studies suggest pain reduction with injection of subcutaneous dextrose over related sensory nerve pathways in shoulder, elbow and knee tendinopathies, also in cases of Achilles tendinopathy and low back pain. [19–21].

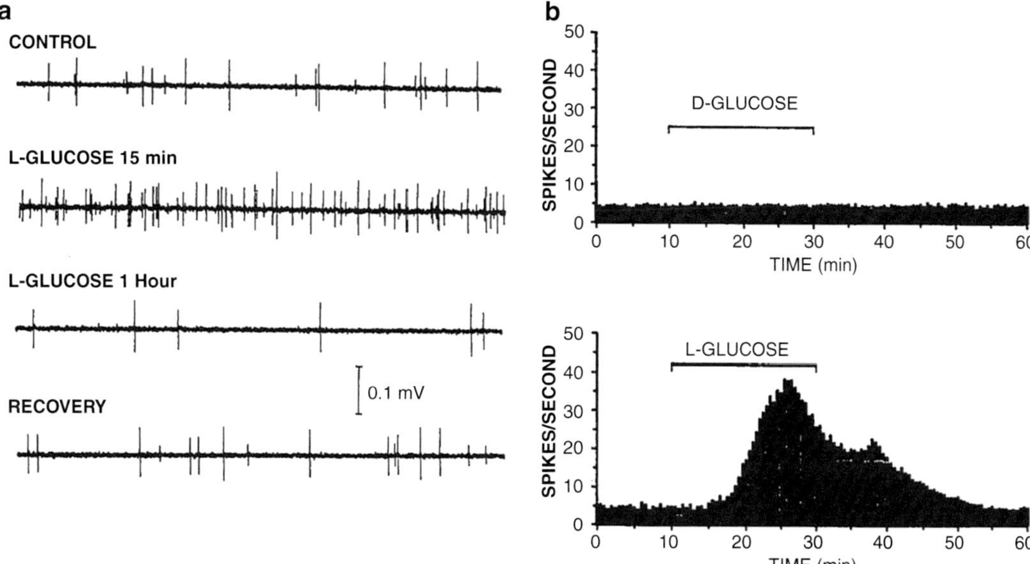

Fig. 17.14 **a** and **b**. Activation of C fibers by metabolic perturbations: Nociceptive C fibers exposed to a temporary hypoglycemia state, by substitution of D-glucose with L-glucose, increases C fiber discharge activity by a 653% ± 23% increase in action potential frequency within 15 minutes, with prompt reversal to a normal baseline firing rate when dextrose was reintroduced. (With permission from Bruce MacIver)

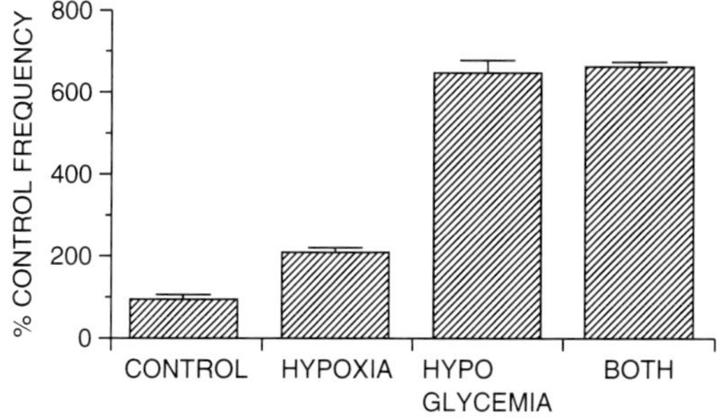

Fig. 17.15 Bar graph comparing cumulative effects of hypoxia and hypoglycemia (L-glucose) on C fiber firing. Hypoglycemia > hypoxia produced statistically significant increase in discharged frequency greater than control. Combined hypoxia and hypoglycemia did not produce a significantly greater increase in discharge frequency compared to hypoglycemia alone. With permission from Bruce MacIver

The primary author of this chapter published a double-blind RCT comparing D5W to saline injection in the caudal epidural space in participants with back and either buttock or leg pain, resulting in significant analgesia of 15 minutes to 48 hours duration [11, 26] (Fig. 17.16). Upon continued open-label treatment, analgesic effects post-injection were consistent, and clinical benefits were cumulative and clinically significant to 1-year follow-up [11, 26] (Fig. 17.17). This is the first study that proves that dextrose is analgesic (Fig. 17.18).

Epidural D5W injection in the absence of anesthetic resulted in consistent post-injection analgesia and clinically significant improvement in pain and disability through 12 months for most participants. The consistent pattern post-injection analgesia suggests potential sensorineural effect of dextrose on neurogenic pain [57]

Another RCT assessing perineural dextrose injection has been performed. Yelland et al. compared subcutaneous dextrose injection to eccentric lengthening exercise (ELE) in Achilles tendinopathy and showed non-inferiority of dextrose injection to the evidence-based ELE approach to Achilles tendinopathies and potential additive benefit from combining both treatments [63].

Recently published RCTs consistently report clinical benefits compared with injection control, including an RCT comparing dextrose to anesthetic in the treatment of temporomandibular dis-

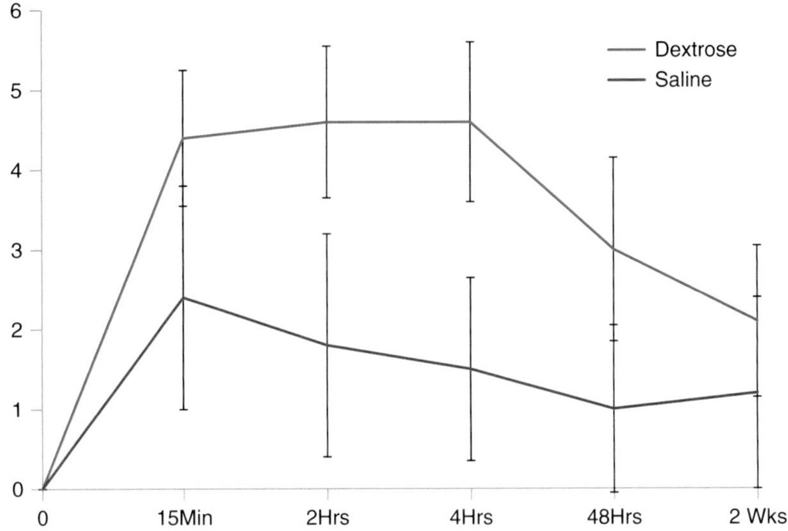

Fig. 17.16 Results of short-term analgesic effects of 5% dextrose epidural injection for chronic low back pain RCT. Change in 0–10 NRS over 2 weeks. Results show significant analgesic effect of dextrose that endured for 48 hours, suggesting a short dextrose-specific biological and clinical effect. Compared with blinded saline, D5W caudal epidural injection resulted in substantial analgesia within 15 minutes that persisted for more than 48 hours among chronic non-surgical LBP patients with buttock and/or leg pain [26]

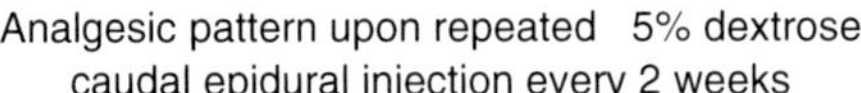

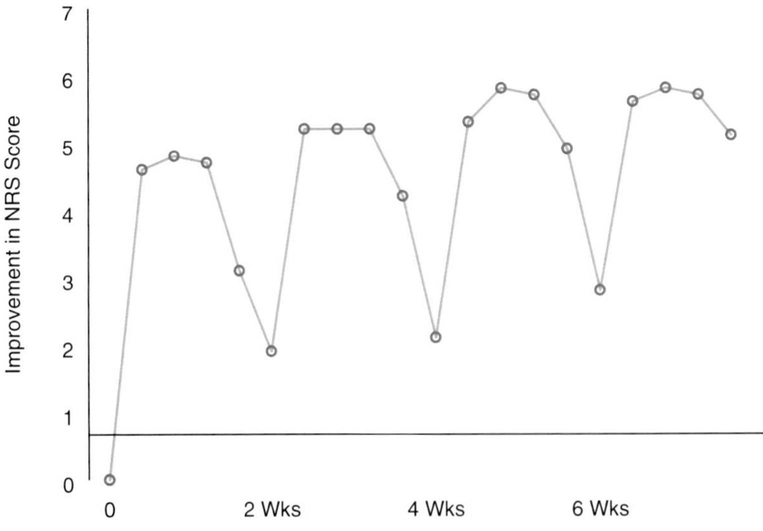

Figs. 17.17 and 17.18 Analgesic response to 5% dextrose caudal epidural injection and long-term pain course. NRS, numerical rating scale. Upon continued open-label treatment, analgesic effects post-injection were consistent, and clinical benefits were cumulative and clinically significant to 1-year follow-up [11]

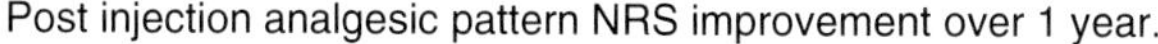

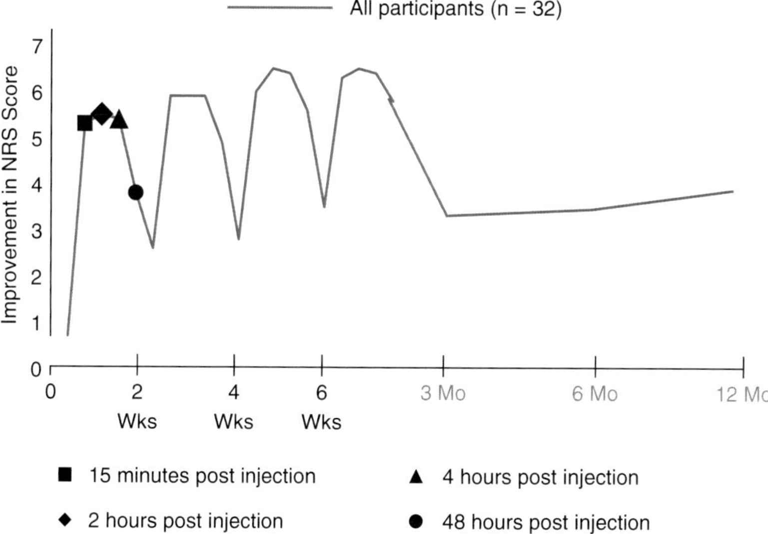

Figs. 17.17 and 17.18 (continued)

order [64], providing increasing evidence of a sensorineural effect of dextrose injection.

Wu et al. demonstrated that hydrodissection of the median nerves in the carpal tunnel with dextrose was clinically effective in reducing symptom of carpal tunnel syndrome compared to saline injection [65]. Wu et al. also demonstrated in other RCTs that hydrodissection with D5W was superior to either hydrodissection with saline [66] or hydrodissection with triamcinolone in saline [67]. Thus, dextrose hydrodissection appears to offer both mechanical hydrodissection and sensorineural effects in carpal tunnel syndrome.

To emphasize the potential generalizability of benefit of hydrodissection for neurogenic pain, Lam et al. hydrodissected a variety of nerves or ganglia in the upper body (stellate ganglion, brachial plexus, cervical nerve roots, and paravertebral spaces) in participants with severe neuropathic pain, and pain reduction exceeded 50% in 26 consecutive participants [12]. This high-volume hydrodissection used only dextrose, and so had no lidocaine toxicity risk. This study supports an effect of D5W on the somatosensory system at the level of the dorsal root/dorsal root ganglion.

Discussion

The rapid analgesic effect of dextrose on pain-producing C fibers following subcutaneous injection is stunning empirically but has not been formally timed except in a study on epidural injection of dextrose versus saline, which has an effect within minutes, slower than that seen with superficial injection of dextrose [26]. The number of clinically based publications related to the effects of D5W on neuropathic pain is growing. We are just beginning to understand the scientific rationale for PIT, and we propose that neuropathic pain is, at least in part, a neuronal energy deprivation disorder. Potential research areas are myriad; e.g., a substantial percentage of those with painful idiopathic neuropathy have empirically benefited clinically from PIT.

In current clinical practice, regenerative/musculoskeletal physicians who are proponents of sensorineural mechanism of dextrose find that adding PIT and US nerve hydrodissection augments the effects of other regenerative injection therapies such as prolotherapy, platelet-rich plasma (PRP), and stem cell therapies. It comprises an intriguing and potentially effective approach to pain and degenerative issues.

Acquisition of procedural skills for PIT requires continuing medical education, through PIT conferences and master workshops by Dr. John Lyftogt or workshops and medical mission and training programs provided by the Hackett Hemwall Patterson Foundation. The use of high-resolution ultrasound is an added and invaluable asset in DPT because it is accurate, efficient, and more comfortable for patients and in PIT because it offers the visualization required for hydrodissection of deeper nerves. Workshops on DPT/PRP injection and hydrodissection are focusing on the development of skill in the use of high-resolution ultrasound.

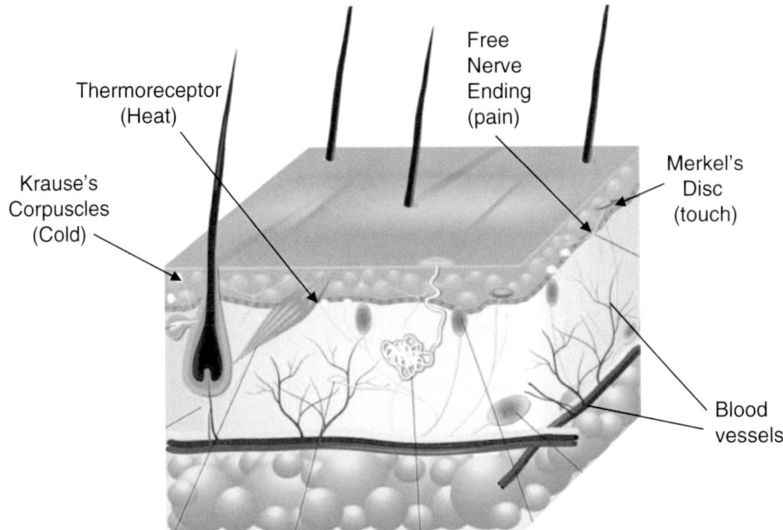

Conclusion

PIT is a simple, extremely effective, and safe treatment for chronic pain and other degenerative conditions. Given the current level B evidence for efficacy of DPT in the treatment of multiple conditions, such as rotator cuff tendinopathy [9, 13, 17, 68–70], temporomandibular dysfunction [71], wrist pain [72], or painful finger/thumb osteoarthritis [9, 13, 17, 68, 73], lateral epicondylosis [9, 13, 17, 68, 74–77], Osgood-Schlatter disease [9, 13, 17, 74, 78], Achilles tendinopathy [9, 13, 17, 74, 78–81], and sacroiliac pain [82], and accumulating evidence of a dextrose analgesic effect [26] and efficacy of hydrodissection for peripheral nerve entrapment [65, 67] and neuropathic pain [12], discussion of treatment options with patients should include mention of dextrose-based therapies.

Further research in these techniques is needed and will help guide their clinical application. In addition, although the peripheral nervous system has the capability for regeneration, much research still needs to be done to optimize the environment for maximum regrowth potential.

References

1. Dahlhamer J, Lucas J, Zelaya C, Nahin R, Mackey S, DeBar L, Kerns R, Von Korff M, Porter L, Helmick C. Prevalence of chronic pain and high-impact chronic pain among adults - United States, 2016. MMWR Morb Mortal Wkly Rep. 2018;67(36):1001–5.
2. Duenas M, Ojeda B, Salazar A, Mico JA, Failde I. A review of chronic pain impact on patients, their social environment and the health care system. J Pain Res. 2016;9:457–67.
3. healthblog.uofmhealth.org/health-management/cost-of-chronic-pain-infographic. University of Michigan; 2017. healthblog.uofmhealth.org/health-management/cost-of-chronic-pain-infographic. Accessed 10 April 2020.
4. Scholl L, Seth P, Kariisa M, Wilson N, Baldwin G. Drug and opioid-involved overdose deaths – United

States, 2013-2017. MMWR Morb Mortal Wkly Rep. 2018;67(5152):1419–27.

5. van Hecke O, Austin SK, Khan RA, Smith BH, Torrance N. Neuropathic pain in the general population: a systematic review of epidemiological studies. Pain. 2014;155(4):654–62.
6. Schaefer C, Sadosky A, Mann R, Daniel S, Parsons B, Tuchman M, Anschel A, Stacey BR, Nalamachu S, Nieshoff E. Pain severity and the economic burden of neuropathic pain in the United States: BEAT neuropathic pain observational study. Clinicoecon Outcomes Res. 2014;6:483–96.
7. Devor M. Centralization, central sensitization and neuropathic pain. Focus on "sciatic chronic constriction injury produces cell-type-specific changes in the electrophysiological properties of rat substantia gelatinosa neurons". J Neurophysiol. 2006;96(2):522–3.
8. Jensen TS, Baron R, Haanpaa M, Kalso E, Loeser JD, Rice AS, Treede RD. A new definition of neuropathic pain. Pain. 2011;152(10):2204–5.
9. Hauser RA, Lackner JB, Steilen-Matias D, Harris DK. A systematic review of dextrose Prolotherapy for chronic musculoskeletal pain. Clin Med Insights Arthritis Musculoskelet Disord. 2016;9:139–59.
10. Trescot AM. Peripheral nerve entrapments: clinical diagnosis and management pg 10. Vol Pg 10. Switzerland: Springer; 2016.
11. Maniquis-Smigel L, Reeves KD, Rosen JH, Coleman C, Lyftogt J, Cheng AL, Rabago D. Analgesic effect and potential cumulative benefit from caudal epidural D5W in consecutive participants with chronic low back and buttock/leg pain. Jnl Alt Compl Med. 2018;12(12):1189–96.
12. Lam SKH, Reeves KD, Cheng AL. Transition from deep regional blocks toward deep nerve hydrodissection in the upper body and torso. Method description and results from a retrospective chart review of the analgesic effect of 5% dextrose water as the primary hydrodissection injectate. Biomed Res Int. 2017:7920438. Available at https://www.hindawi.com/journals/bmri/2017/7920438/.
13. Reeves KD, Sit RWS, Rabago D. Dextrose prolotherapy: a narrative review of basic science and clinical research, and best treatment recommendations. Phys Med Rehabil Clin N Am. 2016;27(4):783–823.
14. Rabago D, Best TM, Zgierska AE, Zeisig E, Ryan M, Crane D. A systematic review of four injection therapies for lateral epicondylosis: prolotherapy, polidocanol, whole blood and platelet-rich plasma. Br J Sports Med. 2009;43(7):471–81.
15. Rabago D, Slattengren A, Zgierska A. Prolotherapy in primary care practice. Prim Care. 2010;37:65–80.
16. Hauser RA, Woldin BA. Joint instability as the cause of chronic musculoskeletal pain and its successful treatment with prolotherapy. In: Korhan O, editor. Anatomy, posture, prevalence, pain, treatment and interventions of musculoskeletal disorders; 2018. https://doi.org/10.5772/intechopen.74384. IntechOpen.
17. Borg-Stein J, Osoaria HL, Hayano T. Regenerative sports medicine: past, present, and future (adapted from the PASSOR legacy award presentation; AAPMR; October 2016). PM R. 2018;10(10):1083–05.
18. Lyftogt J. Pain conundrums: which hypothesis? Central nervous system sensitization versus peripheral nervous system autonomy. Australasian Musculoskeletal Med. 2008;13(11):72–4.
19. Lyftogt J. Subcutaneous prolotherapy for Achilles tendinopathy *Australasian musculoskeletal*. Medicine. 2007;12(11):107–9.
20. Lyftogt J. Subcutaneous prolotherapy treatment of refractory knee, shoulder and lateral elbow pain. Australasian Musculoskeletal Med. 2007;12(2):110–2.
21. Lyftogt J. Prolotherapy for recalcitrant lumbago. Australasian Musculoskeletal Med. 2008; 13(5):18–20.
22. Lyftogt J. Chronic exertional compartment syndrome and prolotherapy. Australasian Musculoskeletal Med. 2006;11:83–5.
23. Bennett GJ, Xie YK. A peripheral mononeuropathy in rat that produces disorders of pain sensation like those seen in man. Pain. 1988;33:87–107.
24. Valleix FLS. Valleix on neuralgia. In: Forbes J, editor. The British and foreign medical review, vol. 13. London: John Churchill Princes Street SOHO; Jan-April, 1942. p. 136–59.
25. Cass SP. Ultrasound-guided nerve Hydrodissection: what is it? A review of the literature. Curr Sports Med Rep. 2016;15(1):20–2.
26. Maniquis-Smigel L, Reeves KD, Rosen JH, Coleman C, Lyftogt J, Cheng AL, Rabago D. Short term analgesic effects of 5% dextrose epidural injection for chronic low back pain. A randomized controlled trial. Anesth Pain Med. 2017;7(1):e42550.
27. Jacobson JA. Fundamentals of musculoskeletal ultrasound, Chapter 9. 2nd ed. Philadelphia: Saunders; 2017. p. 338.
28. Chiu IM, von Hehn CA, Woolf CJ. Neurogenic inflammation and the peripheral nervous system in host defense and immunopathology. Nat Neurosci. 2012;15(8):1063–7.
29. Ackermann PW. Neuronal regulation of tendon homoeostasis. Int J Exp Pathol. 2013;94(4):271–86.
30. Vilensky JA, Gilman S, Casey K. Sir Victor Horsley, Mr John Marshall, the nervi nervorum, and pain: more than a century ahead of their time. Arch Neurol. 2005;62(3):499–501.
31. Marshall J. Bradshaw lecture on nerve-stretching for the relief or cure of pain. Br Med J. 1883;2(1198):1173–9.
32. Hahnenberger RW. Effects of pressure on fast axoplasmic flow. An in vitro study in the vagus nerve of rabbits. Acta Physiol Scand. 1978;104(3):299–308.
33. Trachsel L, Cascella M. Pain theory. Treasure Island, Florida: StatPearls Publishing; 2019 August 12. https://www.ncbi.nlm.nih.gov/books/NBK545194/
34. Moayedi M, Davis KD. Theories of pain: from specificity to gate control. J Neurophysiol. 2013;109(1):5–12.

35. Purves D, Augustine GJ, Fitzpatrick D, Katz LC, LaMantia AS, McNamara JO, Williams SM. Nociceptors. Chapter 3 in neuroscience. Sunderland: Massachusetts; 2001. https://www.ncbi.nlm.nih.gov/books/NBK10965/
36. Sherrington CS. The integrative action of the nervous system. Cambridge: University Press; 1947.
37. Gibson A. John Hilton: "rest and pain". Can Med Assoc J. 1955;73(7):569–72.
38. Hébert-Blouin M, Tubbs RS, Carmichael SW, Spinner RJ. Hiltons' law revisited. Clin Anat. 2014;27(4):548–55.
39. Bachasson D, Singh A, Shah SB, Lane JG, Ward SR. The role of the peripheral and central nervous systems in rotator cuff disease. J Shoulder Elb Surg. 2015;24(8):1322–35.
40. Cregg R, Momin A, Rugiero F, Wood JN, Zhao J. Pain channelopathies. J Physiol. 2010;588(Pt 11):1897–904.
41. Caterina M, Schumacher M, Tominaga M, Rosen T, Levine J, Julius D. The capsaicin receptor: a heat-activated ion channel in the pain pathway. Nature. 1997;389(6653):816–24.
42. Szolcsányi JL, Sándor Z. Multisteric TRPV1 nocisensor: a target for analgesics. Trends Pharmacol Sci. 2012;33(12):646–55.
43. Szallasi A, Cortright DN, Blum CA, Eid SR. The vanilloid receptor TRPV1: 10 years from channel cloning to antagonist proof-of-concept. Nat Rev Drug Discov. 2007;6(5):357–72.
44. Rosenbaum R, Simon SA. TRPV1 receptors and signal transduction. In: Liedtke WB, Heller S, editors. TRP ion channel function in sensory transduction and cellular signaling cascades. Boca Raton, FL: CRC Press; 2007.
45. Ji R, Nackley A, Huh Y, Terrando N, Maixner W. Neuroinflammation and central sensitization in chronic and widespread pain. Anesthesiology. 2018;192(2):343–66.
46. Matsuda M, Huh Y, Ji RR. Roles of inflammation, neurogenic inflammation, and neuroinflammation in pain. J Anesth. 2019;33(1):131–9.
47. Russell FA, King R, Smillie SJ, Kodji X, Brain SD. Calcitonin gene-related peptide: physiology and pathophysiology. Physiol Rev. 2014;94(4):1099–142.
48. O'Connor TM, O'Connell J, O'Brien DI, Goode T, Bredin CP, Shanahan F. The role of substance P in inflammatory disease. J Cell Physiol. 2004;201(2):167–80.
49. Steinhoff MS, von Mentzer B, Geppetti P, Pothoulakis C, Bunnett NW. Tachykinins and their receptors: contributions to physiological control and the mechanisms of disease. Physiol Rev. 2014;94(1):265–301.
50. Koon HW, Zhao D, Na X, Moyer MP, Pothoulakis C. Metalloproteinases and transforming growth factor-alpha mediate substance P-induced mitogen-activated protein kinase activation and proliferation in human colonocytes. J Biol Chem. 2004;279(44):45519–27.
51. Ebner K, Rupniak NM, Saria A, Singewald N. Substance P in the medial amygdala: emotional stress-sensitive release and modulation of anxiety-related behavior in rats. Proc Natl Acad Sci U S A. 2004;101(12):4280–5.
52. Bertrand H, Kyriazis M, Reeves KD, Lyftogt J, Rabago D. Topical mannitol reduces capsaicin-induced pain: results of a pilot level, double-blind randomized controlled trial. PM R. 2015;7(11):1111–7.
53. Sohn JW. Ion channels in the central regulation of energy and glucose homeostasis. Front Neurosci. 2013;7:85.
54. Verbeke G, Molenberghs G. Linear mixed models for longitudinal data. New York: Springer; 2000.
55. Burdakov D, Jensen LT, Alexopoulos H, Williams RH, Fearon IM, O'Kelley I, Gerasimenko O, Fugger L, Verkhratsky A. Tandem-pore K+ channels mediate inhibition of orexin neurons by glucose. Neuron. 2006;50(5):711–22.
56. Scott MM, Marcus JN, Elmquist JK. Orexin neurons and the TASK of glucosensing. Neuron. 2006;50(5):665–7.
57. McTaggart JS, Clark RH, Ashcroft FM. The role of the KATP channel in glucose homeostasis in health and disease: more than meets the islet. J Physiol. 2010;588(Pt 17):3201–9.
58. Thorens B, Mueckler M. Glucose transporters in the 21st century. Am J Physiol Endocrinol Metab. 2010;298(2):E141–5.
59. Diggs-Andrews KA, Silverstein JM, Fisher SJ, Diggs-Andrews KA, Silverstein JM, Fisher SJ. Glucose sensing in the central nervous system. Cyberrounds. 2009; http://www.cyberounds.com/cmecontent/art453.html. Accessed 12 April 2020.
60. MacIver MB, Tanelian DL. Activation of C fibers by metabolic perturbations associated with tourniquet ischemia. Anesthesiology. 1992;76(4):617–23.
61. McCrimmon RJ, Sherwin RS. Hypoglycemia in type 1 diabetes. Diabetes. 2010;59(10):2333–9.
62. Baumeister FA, Hack A, Busch R. Glucose-monitoring with continuous subcutaneous microdialysis in neonatal diabetes mellitus. Klin Padiatr. 2006;218(4):230–2.
63. Yelland MJ, Sweeting KR, Lyftogt JA, Ng SK, Scuffham PA, Evans KA. Prolotherapy injections and eccentric loading exercises for painful Achilles tendinosis: a randomised trial. Br J Sports Med. 2009;45(5):421–8.
64. Louw WF, Burrils F, Reeves KD, Cheng AL, Rabago D. Treatment of temporomandibular dysfunction with dextrose prolotherapy: a randomized controlled trial with long term follow-up. Mayo Clinic Proc. 2019;94(5):820–32.
65. Wu YT, Chen SR, Li TY, Ho TY, Shen YP, Tsai CK, Chen LC. Nerve hydrodissection for carpal tunnel syndrome: a prospective, randomized, double-blind, controlled trial. Muscle Nerve. 2019;59(2):174–80.
66. Wu YT, Ho TY, Chou YC, Ke MJ, Li TY, Tsai CK, Chen LC. Six-month efficacy of perineural dextrose for carpal tunnel syndrome: a prospective, randomized, double-blind, controlled trial. Mayo Clin Proc. 2017;92(8):1179–89.

67. Wu YT, Ke MJ, Ho TY, Li TY, Shen YP, Chen LC. Randomized double-blinded clinical trial of 5% dextrose versus triamcinolone injection for carpal tunnel syndrome patients. Ann Neurol. 2018;84(4):601–10.
68. Dwivedi S, Sobel AD, DaSilva MF, Akelman E. Utility of Prolotherapy for upper extremity pathology. J Hand Surg Am. 2019;44(3):236–9.
69. Catapano M, Zhang K, Mittal N, Sangha H, Onishi K, de Sa D. Effectiveness of dextrose prolotherapy for rotator cuff tendinopathy: a systematic review. PM R. 2019; https://doi.org/10.1002/pmrj.12268.
70. Lin MT, Chiang CF, Wu CH, Huang YT, Tu YK, Wang TG. Comparative effectiveness of injection therapies in rotator cuff tendinopathy: a systematic review, pairwise and network meta-analysis of randomized controlled trials. Arch Phys Med Rehabil. 2019;100(2):336–49.
71. Nagori SA, Jose A, Gopalakrishnan V, Roy ID, Chattopadhyay PK, Roychoudhury A. The efficacy of dextrose prolotherapy over placebo for temporomandibular joint hypermobility: a systematic review and meta-analysis. J Oral Rehabil. 2018; https://doi.org/10.1111/joor.12698. [Epub ahead of print].
72. Hooper RA, Hildebrand K, Faris P, Westaway M, Freiheit E. Randomized controlled trial for the treatment of chronic dorsal wrist pain with dextrose prolotherapy. Int Musculoskeletal Med. 2011;33(3):100–6.
73. Hung CY, Hsiao MY, K.V. C, Han DS, Wang TG. Comparative effectiveness of dextrose prolotherapy versus control injections and exercise in the management of osteoarthritis pain: a systematic review and meta-analysis. J Pain Res. 2016;9:847–57.
74. Covey CJ, Sineath MHJ, Penta JF, Leggit JC. Prolotherapy: can it help your patient? J Fam Pract. 2015;64(12):763–8.
75. Dong W, Goost H, Lin XB, Burger C, Paul C, Wang ZL, Kong FL, Welle K, Jiang ZC, Kabir K. Injection therapies for lateral epicondylalgia: a systematic review and Bayesian network meta-analysis. Br J Sports Med. 2015;50(15):900–8.
76. Bayat M, Raeissadat SA, Mortazavian Babiki M, Rahimi-Dehgolan S. Is dextrose Prolotherapy superior to corticosteroid injection in patients with chronic lateral epicondylitis?: a randomized clinical trial. Orthop Res Rev. 2019;11:167–75.
77. Yelland M, Rabago D, Ryan M, Ng SK, Vithanachchi D, Manickaraj N, Bisset L. Prolotherapy injections and physiotherapy used singly and in combination for lateral epicondylalgia: a single-blinded randomised clinical trial. BMC Musculoskelet Disord. 2019;20(509). https://doi.org/10.1186/s12891-019-2905-5.
78. Sanderson LM, Bryant A. Effectiveness and safety of prolotherapy injections for management of lower limb tendinopathy and fasciopathy: a systematic review. J Foot Ankle Res. 2015;20(8):57.
79. Morath O, Kubocsh EJ, Taeymans J, Zwingmann J, Konstantinidis L, Südkamp NP, Hirschmüller A. The effect of sclerotherapy and prolotherapy on chronic painful Achilles tendinopathy - a systematic review including meta-analysis. Scand J Med Sci Sports. 2018;28(1):4–15.
80. Pavone V, Vescio A, Mobilia G, Dimartino S, Di Stefano G, Culmone A, Testa G. Conservative treatment of chronic Achilles tendinopathy: a systematic review. J Funct Morphol Kinesiol. 2019;4:46.
81. Smith WB, Melton W, Davies J. Midsubstance tendinopathy, percutaneous techniques (platelet-rich plasma, extracorporeal shock wave Therapy, Prolotherapy, radiofrequency ablation). C Podiatr Med Surg. 2017;34(2):161–74.
82. Kim WM, Lee HG, Jeong CW, Kim CM, Yoon MH. A randomized controlled trial of intra-articular prolotherapy versus steroid injection for sacroiliac joint pain. J Altern Complement Med. 2010;16(12):1284–90.

18 Ultrasound-Guided Spinal Procedures

Jonathan Kirschner and Aditya Raghunandan

Regenerative Medicine for Spinal Procedures

Evidence

"Regenerative" and novel orthobiologics in the treatment of spine-related disorders is a relatively new but growing field. The recent guidelines published by the American Society of Interventional Pain Physicians provide the most current data on safe and efficacy of use of the biologics for low back pain [61]. The studies were included based on the PRISMA flow diagram and graded from I to V as described by the Agency for Healthcare Research and Quality (AHRQ). For lumbar disc platelet-rich plasma (PRP), there were one high-quality randomized controlled study (RCT), multiple moderate-quality observational studies, a single-arm meta-analysis, and one systematic review, and the qualitative evidence was assessed as Level III. For lumbar disc medicinal signaling/mesenchymal stem cell (MSCs), there were also only one high-quality RCT, multiple moderate-quality observational studies, a single-arm meta-analysis, and two systematic reviews, with the qualitative evidence also assessed as Level III. For lumbar epidural injections, there were one high-quality RCT, multiple relevant moderate-quality observational studies, and a single-arm meta-analysis, and the qualitative evidence was only assessed as a Level IV. For lumbar facet joint PRP injections, assessment was based on one high-quality RCT and two moderate-quality observational studies with an assessment as Level IV. Finally, for sacroiliac joint injections, there were only one high-quality RCT, one moderate-quality observational study, and one low-quality case report, and the qualitative evidence has been assessed as Level IV. Studies addressing cervical spine-related disorders were not evaluated in this publication, and a search of PubMed reveals a paucity of studies for cervical spine-related orthobiologic interventions.

Contraindications

"Regenerative" or biologic treatments are not without risk; the following contraindications should be kept in mind when selecting appropriate patients for spinal procedures. These include blood dyscrasias, platelet dysfunction, septicemia or fever, cutaneous infections in the area to be injected, anemia (hemoglobin less than 10 g/dl), malignancy (particularly with hematologic or bony involvement), allergy to bovine products if bovine thrombus is to be used, severe psychiatric impairment, or unrealistic expectation [61].

J. Kirschner (✉) · A. Raghunandan
Department of Physiatry, Hospital for Special Surgery, New York, NY, USA

Department of Rehabilitation Medicine, UT Health San Antonio, TX, San Antonio, USA
e-mail: kirschnerj@hss.edu; Raghunandan@uthscsa.edu

Y. El Miedany (ed.), *Musculoskeletal Ultrasound-Guided Regenerative Medicine*,
https://doi.org/10.1007/978-3-030-98256-0_18

Peri-procedural Considerations

Ideally, platelet concentration in the injectate should be at least 2.5 times greater than the baseline plasma concentration [27]. In the USA, the FDA requires "minimal manipulation" and "homologous use." Cells should be used within 24 hours of thawing from a frozen medium [25]; use of 19G needle (or larger bore) is recommended to reduce the incidence of apoptosis of tri-lineage capabilities, differentiation, and viability of MSCs [25]; and a 2 mL syringe is recommended to avoid overinflation [25]. Intra-procedural recommendations are similar to most other procedures in that cell material, patient, joint location, and affected side should be verified prior to injection and performed under direct image-guided visualization. Following the injection, patients should be instructed to rest, and some clinicians partially immobilize the injected body part; to date, there are no specific validated protocols that have been published regarding specific timelines, but about 1 week of activity restriction is a reasonable timeframe to avoid potential sequelae. Patients should also be counseled on avoiding anti-inflammatory medications for at least 1 week pre- and 4 weeks post-injection, since the biological basis of these injections hinges on the utilization of the patient's inflammatory cascade. The risks and benefits for aspirin should also be reviewed with the patient [23, 38, 39].

Cervical Spinal Nerves

Indications

The incidence of cervical radiculopathy is relatively common with an estimated incidence of 107.3 per 100,000 for men and 63.5 per 100,000 for women [68]. Fluoroscopic and CT-guided epidural injections are commonly used to treat cervical radiculitis; however, in a randomized blinded controlled study, there were found to be no difference outcomes in an ultrasound-guided versus fluoroscopy-guided transforaminal injection in the lower cervical spine [40], and similar findings were confirmed by Zhang et al. [78]. The main advantage of utilizing ultrasound for needle placement is that critical blood vessels can be visualized, preventing inadvertent puncture [57]. The important vascular anatomy to be aware of is as follows: in a cadaveric study, it was found that 20% of cervical foramina contained either the deep or ascending cervical artery within 2 mm of the needle target for standard fluoroscopic approach and 33% of the time these arteries entered the posterior foramen [36], radicular artery branches from the ascending or deep cervical arteries traverse the foramen as the course medially [34], and a small study found that there is a small incidence of arteries found in the posterior aspect of the foramen or posterior supply that coursed medially into the foramen [34]. Using the Doppler mode allows optimal visualization of the vasculature and aids in avoiding inadvertent vascular injury [40]. Other complications due to cervical transforaminal injections range from the more common and relatively benign like vasovagal reactions, central steroid response, and transient increase in pain to the rare but serious complications such as spinal cord infarcts, epidural hematomas, quadriparesis, stroke, and even death [70]. These risks are higher with particulate injectates [48], so caution with orthobiologics must be taken.

Scanning Technique and Important Anatomy

The affected side should be exposed by either lying the patient in the lateral decubitus position with the affected side toward the ceiling or lying the patient supine with the head rotated away from the affected side. The prominent posterior tubercle and rudimentary anterior tubercle are identified by placing the transducer in short axis at the C7 level. As the transducer is moved cranially to C6, the anterior and posterior tubercles of the cervical vertebrae as well as the two-humped camel sign become more prominent [50]. Tracing the vertebral artery, which lies anterior to C7 and enters the C6 foramen 90% and further cranial 10% of the time, is another method for identifying the correct cervical level [51]. It is important

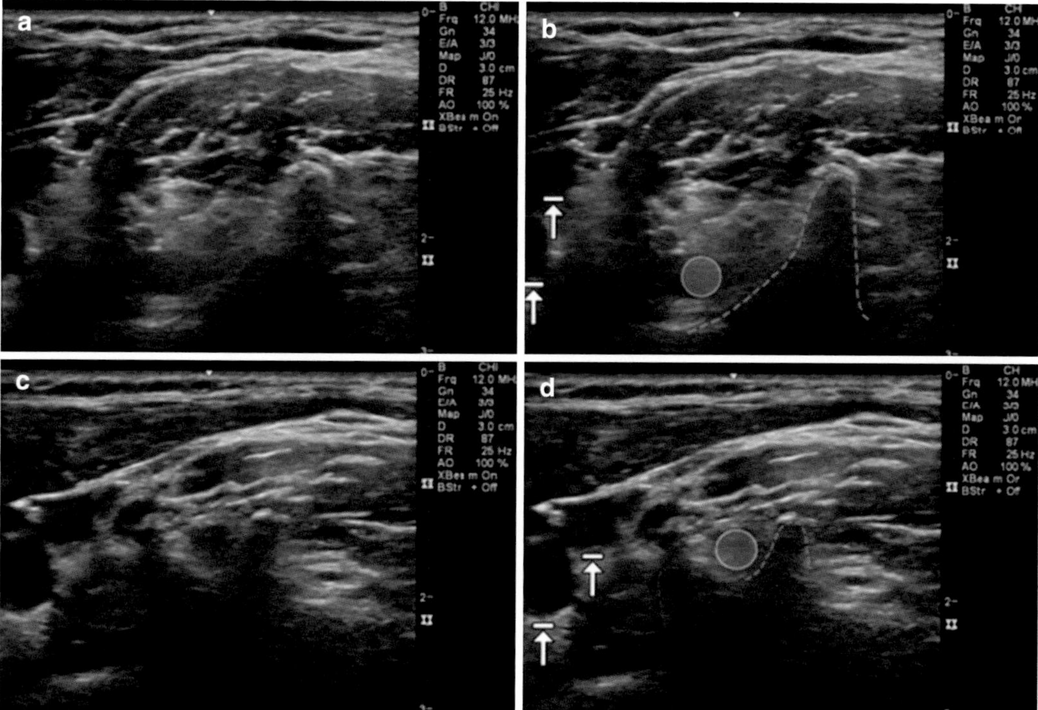

Fig. 18.1 (**a**) Transverse (axial) view over C7; note the prominent posterior tubercle. (**b**) *Dashed orange line* outlines posterior tubercle, *yellow* indicates C7 spinal nerve, and *arrows with stops* indicate carotid artery and internal jugular vein. (**c**) Transverse (axial) view over C6 with prominent anterior and posterior tubercles. (**d**) *Dashed orange line* outlines posterior tubercle, dashed purple line outlines anterior tubercle, yellow indicates C6 spinal nerve, and arrows with stops indicate carotid artery and internal jugular vein

to keep the transducer perpendicular to the cervical level of interest to prevent angling the transducer toward an unintended level. The power Doppler feature should be utilized to identify the significant vascular structures including the carotid artery, vertebral artery, and smaller radicular vessels in and around the foramen (Fig. 18.1).

Injection Technique

- Patient positioning: Lay the patient in the lateral decubitus position with the affected side facing upward with a pillow placed between the patient's legs and one under the arm to facilitate comfort. The patient can also lay supine with the head rotated and side bent away.
- Probe positioning: Place the transducer transverse (short axis) over the C7 vertebrae, visualizing the rudimentary anterior tubercle and prominent posterior tubercle.
- Markings: Identify the transverse process and tubercles of C7 as they differ from the other cervical vertebrae, marking the C7 level. If more than one level injection is planned, use a marker to identify the probe position at the desired vertebral levels and the needle entry site. Mark any vessels that are identified on Doppler to avoid inadvertent injury.
- Needle position: Plan your needle path prior to insertion to avoid any feeding vessels or ones located in the posterior foramen. A blunt needle should be inserted from a posterior to anterior direction. The needle should be kept in-plane directed toward the desired nerve root.
- Safety considerations: Care should be taken to avoid contact with a blood vessel or spinal nerve.

Pearls

- The anterior spinal artery may receive some blood flow from the ascending and deep cervical arteries.
- Keep the transducer perpendicular as you scan to keep your desired vertebral level in site. Angling the transducer may cause you to view up or down a level. Always inject from a posterior to anterior direction to avoid the internal jugular vein, vagus nerve, common carotid artery, and 80% of anterior located radicular arteries in the cervical foramen.
- Doppler mode may help to identify feeding vascular structures in the posterior foramen.

Equipment Needed

- High-frequency linear array transducer
- 22- or 25-gauge spinal needle
- Non-particulate steroid preparation
- 1–2 mL of local anesthetic or normal saline (Fig. 18.2)

Cervical Medial Branch Blocks and Third Occipital Nerve

Indications

Axial neck pain can arise from the cervical zygapophyseal or facet joints. This pain can radiate to the posterior occipital region (commonly the C2–3 joint), the shoulder, or the interscapular region (C5–6, C6–7) [15]. Each cervical facet joint is innervated by two medial branches, and anesthetizing these nerves can provide specificity and a diagnostic benefit [4]. Injection of the joint with corticosteroid may provide therapeutic benefit, but may not be as helpful diagnostically [11]. Cervical medial branch blocks have conventionally been performed via fluoroscopic guidance; however, ultrasound guidance presents some unique advantages [16]. The main advantages of using ultrasound guidance are the direct real-time visualization of vessels and nerves and needle advancement which decreases the number of needle passes and trauma to adjacent structures [16, 17, 73], as well the lack of radiation exposure. Longer-term treatment for cervical facet-mediated pain can be achieved by radiofrequency neurotomy, and ultrasound guidance to perform the procedure has been shown to be a viable option [18, 43].

Scanning Technique and Important Anatomy

The patient should be placed in a lateral decubitus position with the transducer placed in long axis; the superior end should be positioned on the mastoid process. The articular pillars of the cervical vertebrae (C2–7) appear as hills and valleys, the

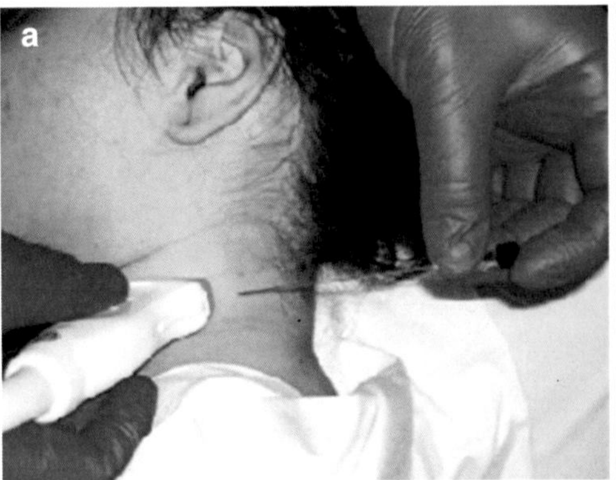

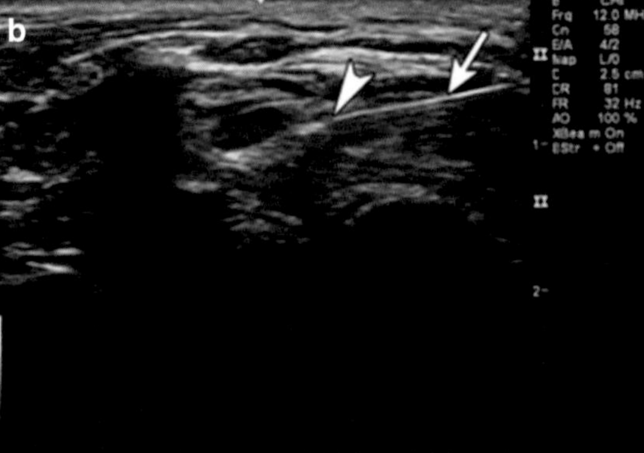

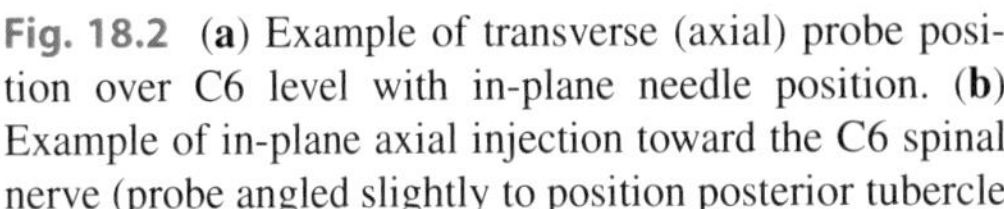

Fig. 18.2 (**a**) Example of transverse (axial) probe position over C6 level with in-plane needle position. (**b**) Example of in-plane axial injection toward the C6 spinal nerve (probe angled slightly to position posterior tubercle out of the field of view to allow for easier needle trajectory); *arrowhead* indicates needle tip, and arrow indicates needle

joint being the hills and the troughs where the medial branches lie, the valleys. The first hill represents the C2–3 zygapophyseal joint. There are two ways to confirm your level, either by visualizing the transverse process of C1 on the cephalad portion of the screen or via use of the Doppler to identify the vertebral artery traversing anteriorly into the C2 foramen [58]. The superficial medial branch of C3 differs from the other cervical medial nerves, because it sits on top of the "hill" at the C2–3 zygapophyseal junction as it travels enroute to becoming a cutaneous nerve; this nerve is also referred to as the third occipital nerve (TON) and also has smaller contributions from the C2 medial branch. The TON can be identified by placing the transducer in long axis, starting at mastoid process and scanning caudally from the transverse process of C1 to the vertebral artery as it traverses into the C2 foramen, and ultimately identified at the top of the "hill" of the C2–3 zygapophyseal junction [73]. The remainder of the cervical medial branches (C4–8) are identified by scanning caudally and visualized as they traverse dorsally in the troughs of the articular pillars to innervate the facet joint at the levels above and below [24] (Fig. 18.3).

Injection Technique

- Patient positioning: Lay the patient in the lateral decubitus position with pillows underneath the head, between the legs, and under the arm.
- Probe positioning: Place the transducer coronally over the mastoid process and view the articular pillar, identifying the levels as you move caudally.
- Markings: Identify and mark the desired cervical levels.
- Needle position: The needle is inserted in-plane toward the medial branch if identified. If the nerve is not visualized, direct straight down between the articular pillars toward the deepest point, touching down on bone. For the TON, the needle is inserted in-plane toward the apex of the C2–3 joint.
- Safety considerations: Keep the transducer and injection posterior and lateral to avoid the anterior vasculature and spinal cord.

Pearls for CMBB

- Aim at the deepest point between the articular pillars.
- The medial branch may be difficult to visualize in an obese patient.
- The cervical medial branch becomes more difficult to identify as you proceed caudally.

Pearls for TON

- Aim at the convexity of the C2–3 joint.
- The C2 level is also identified as having the first bifid spinous process [23]. The transducer can be placed axially over the spinous process of C2, and the lamina of C2 can be traced laterally until the C2–3 joint appears.

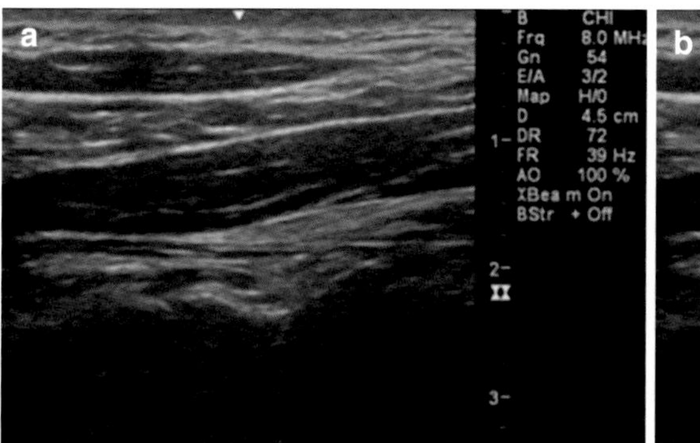

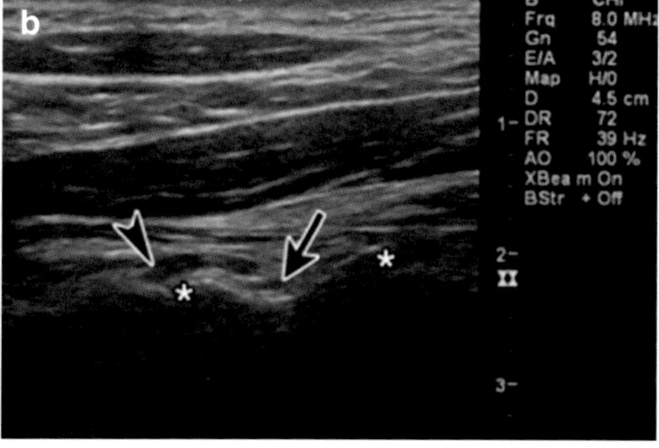

Fig. 18.3 (**a**) Coronal view of the cervical articular pillars. (**b**) *Black arrowhead* indicates TON, black arrow indicates C3 medial branch, and asterisk indicates C2–3 and C3–4 zygapophyseal joint

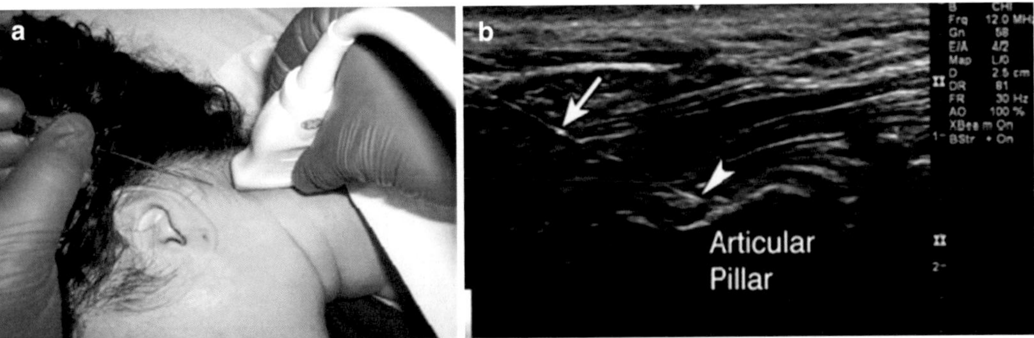

Fig. 18.4 (a) Example of coronal view over the cervical medial branches with in-plane needle position. (b) *Arrowhead* indicates needle tip adjacent to medial branch; *white arrow* indicates needle; articular pillar labeled

Equipment Needed

- High-frequency linear array transducer
- 22 or 25G 2.5–3.5″ spinal needle
- 0–1 mL of steroid preparation per level
- 0.5–1 mL of local anesthetic per level (Fig. 18.4).

Cervical Zygapophyseal Joint

Indications

The cervical zygapophyseal or facet joints are formed by the articulation of the superior and inferior articular pillars of contiguous vertebrae. Intra-articular zygapophyseal joint injections have been shown to have both diagnostic and therapeutic benefits [6, 71], but the evidence is less robust than for MBB and RFA. These procedures are usually performed under either fluoroscopic or CT guidance; however, ultrasound-guided cervical facet joint injections have been found to have the advantages of requiring fewer needle repositions, shorter procedure time, and better pain scores at 1-month follow-up [63]. The main hindrance for using ultrasound guidance compared to fluoroscopy is difficulty in the identification of the correct target and level [22].

Scanning Technique and Important Anatomy

The patient should be placed prone with the transducer placed in long axis in the midline sagittal plane over the cervical spinous processes. The C2 level can be identified as the most cranial cervical vertebra with a bifid spinous process [15]. Each cervical level can be identified by scanning caudally and counting the midline superficial hyperechoic spinous processes. In order to view the desired zygapophyseal joint, identify the corresponding spinous process, and move the transducer laterally to bring the saw-tooth image of the zygapophyseal joint into view. It should be noted that zygapophyseal joints become more vertical as the scan progresses caudally [65, 69] (Fig. 18.5).

Injection Technique

- Patient positioning: Lay the patient in the prone position with a pillow underneath the chest to allow for slight cervical flexion.
- Probe positioning: Place the transducer in the sagittal plane over the cervical spinous processes and move laterally until the facet joints at the desired levels are in view.

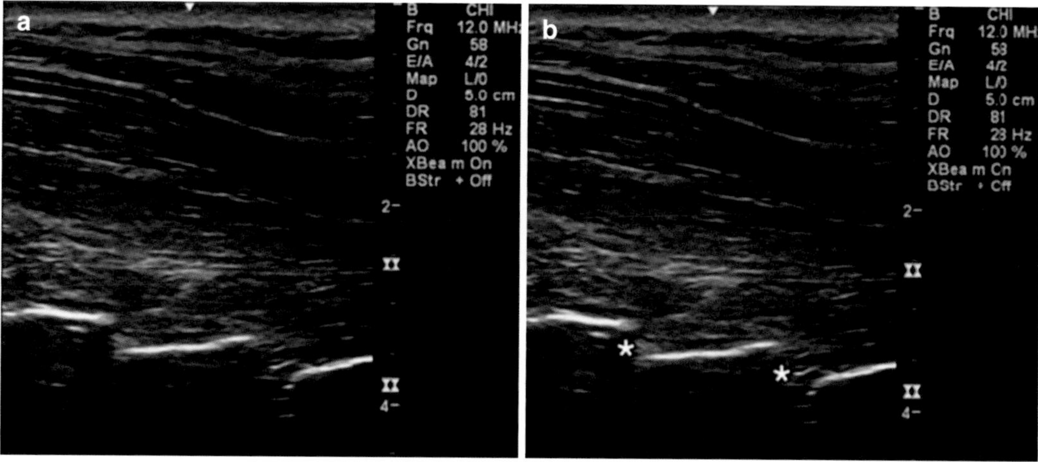

Fig. 18.5 (**a**) Sagittal view of the cervical facet joints. (**b**) *Asterisk* indicates cervical facet joints

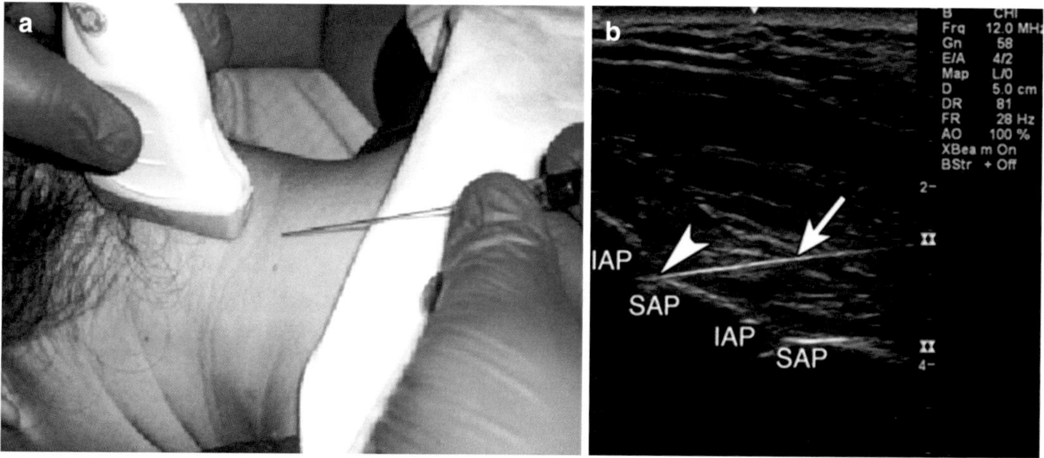

Fig. 18.6 (**a**) Example of sagittal probe position over cervical facet joint with in-plane injection technique. (**b**) *Arrowhead* indicates needle tip entering facet joint; *arrow* indicates needle; *IAP* inferior articular process, *SAP* superior articular process

- Marking: Identify and mark the desired cervical levels.
- Needle position: The needle is inserted in-plane from caudal to cephalad toward the facet joint.
- Safety considerations: Keep the transducer and injection posterior to avoid the anterior vasculature.

Pearls

- The cervical facets appear as shingles on a roof with the probe in the sagittal plane.
- Keeping the needle angle shallow will help to mimic the angle of the facet joint and ease the approach and needle placement for an intra-articular injection.
- The C2 vertebra has the first bifid spinous process.

Equipment Needed

- High-frequency linear transducer
- 22-gauge, 1.5–3.5″ needle
- 0.5–1 mL of steroid preparation per level
- 0.5–1 mL of local anesthetic per level (Fig. 18.6).

Stellate Ganglion

Indications

The stellate ganglion block (SGB) is the oldest and most common sympathetic block. It has many indications including complex regional pain syndrome (types I and II), postherpetic neuralgia, intractable angina, post-traumatic stress disorder, hyperhidrosis, arrhythmias, hot flashes, and Raynaud's disease [1, 2, 31, 33, 45, 47, 64]. The original procedure was described as being performed under palpation guidance in which the needle target was the anterior aspect of the C6 transverse process, named Chassaignac's tubercle [44]. Various imaging-guided techniques for SGB have also been described including fluoroscopy, computerized tomography, magnetic resonance imaging, and radionucleotide tracers. The main issue with these techniques, however, is that they may not be practical in a clinical setting, due to increased time, cost, and radiation exposure. Use of ultrasound guidance provides the benefit of direct visualization of the needle path, vasculature close to the stellate ganglion, as well as important adjacent soft tissue structures [26]. The stellate ganglion, or cervicothoracic ganglion, is the fusion of the inferior cervical ganglion and the first thoracic ganglion. It lies posterior and lateral to the trachea, esophagus, and thyroid; medial to the common carotid artery and internal jugular vein; just lateral to the inferior thyroid artery and recurrent laryngeal nerve; and anterior to the vertebral artery and longus colli muscle [35]. Dimensions of the stellate ganglion are usually 2.5 cm long, 1 cm wide, and 0.5 cm thick [59].

Scanning Technique and Important Anatomy

The patient should be placed in supine position with the head placed in slight extension and rotated away from the affected side. Start by placing the transducer over the cricoid cartilage in the axial plane, and scan laterally until the prominent anterior tubercle of the C6 transverse process is visualized. It is important to identify and avoid the following structures: carotid artery, internal jugular vein, cricoid cartilage, and longus colli muscle. The Doppler should be utilized to identify and avoid the inferior thyroid artery and a vertebral artery. To confirm the level, identify the C7 level, which has a prominent posterior and rudimentary anterior tubercle; this differs from the more cranial C6 level which has prominent posterior and anterior tubercles [67] (Fig. 18.7).

Injection Technique

- Patient positioning: Lay the patient supine with the neck in slight extension and slight rotation away.

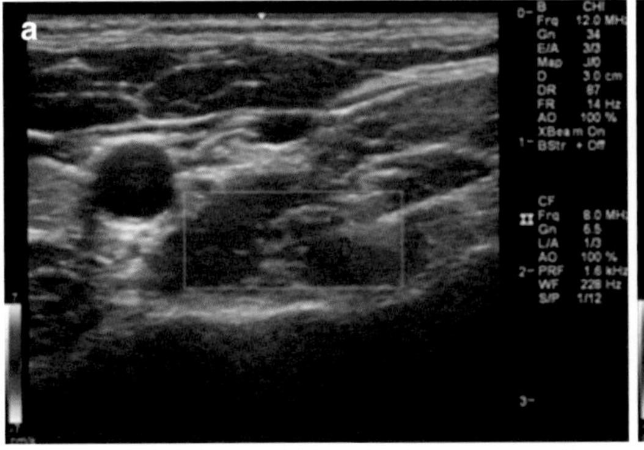

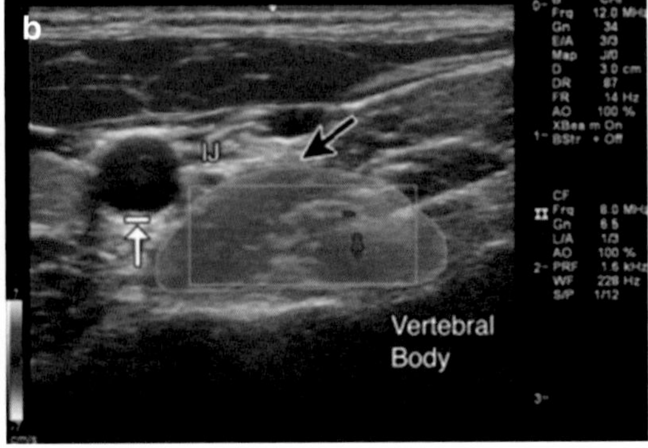

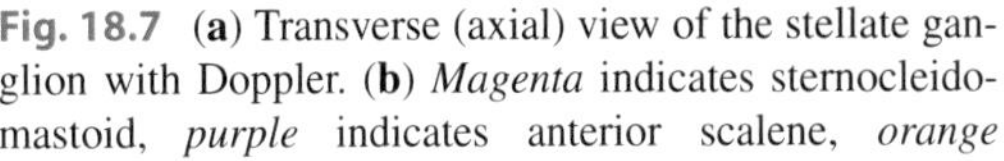

Fig. 18.7 (**a**) Transverse (axial) view of the stellate ganglion with Doppler. (**b**) *Magenta* indicates sternocleidomastoid, *purple* indicates anterior scalene, *orange* indicates longus colli, *black arrow* indicates location of stellate ganglion, and *arrow with stop* indicates carotid artery; *IJ* internal jugular vein

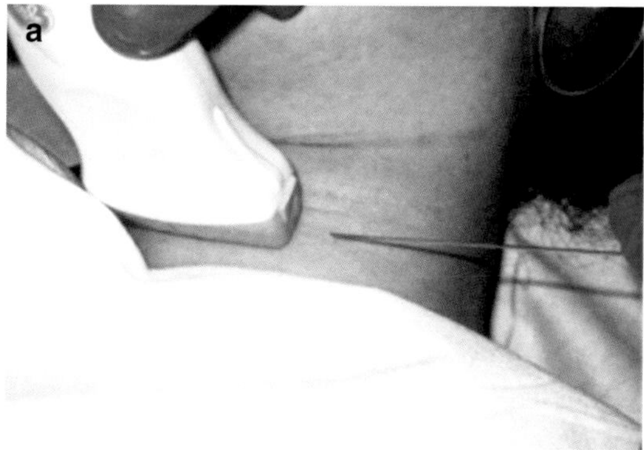

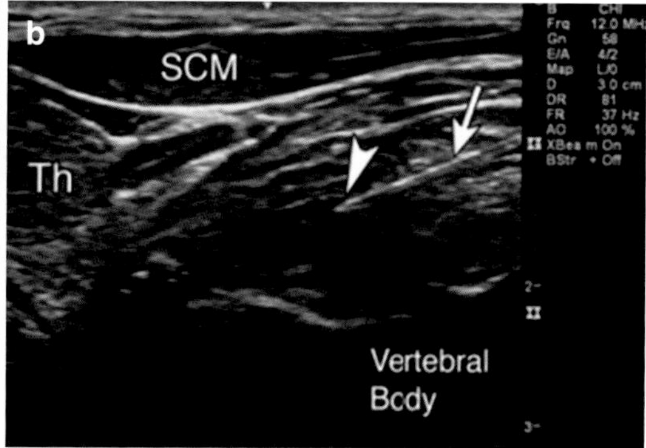

Fig. 18.8 (**a**) Example of axial probe position over stellate ganglion at the level of C6 with in-plane injection technique. (**b**) *Arrowhead* indicates needle tip in the prevertebral fascia; *white arrow* indicates needle; *SCM* sternocleidomastoid, *Th* thyroid; vertebral body labeled

- Probe positioning: Start by placing the probe at C7 in the axial plane. As you scan cephalad, the anterior tubercle of C6 comes into view. Now at the level of C6, visualize the anterior tubercle of C6, longus colli muscle and prevertebral fascia, carotid artery, and thyroid gland.
- Markings: There are a number of significant anatomical structures to mark and note in this region. Identify the esophagus, trachea, carotid artery, internal jugular vein, and inferior thyroidal artery.
- Needle position: The needle is inserted in-plane from lateral to medial aiming at the prevertebral fascia just anterior to the longus colli muscle. Plan out the course of the needle to avoid puncturing important structures. If the needle path can cause injury to these structures, adjust the probe position or insert the needle with a more oblique trajectory.
- Safety considerations: Avoid the esophagus and trachea medially and the carotid artery, internal jugular vein, inferior thyroid, and vertebral arteries laterally. A phrenic nerve block can occur and cause diaphragmatic paresis.

Pearls

- The stellate ganglion lies medial to the scalene muscles.
- Stellate ganglion is formed by the fusion of the inferior cervical and first thoracic ganglion.
- A nerve stimulator can help to identify the phrenic nerve and avoid inadvertent diaphragmatic paresis.

Equipment Needed

- High-frequency linear array transducer
- 25G 1.5–3.5″ needle
- 1–3 mL of short-acting anesthetic for local anesthesia
- 10–20 mL of long-acting anesthetic for the block (Fig. 18.8).

Greater Occipital Nerve

Indications

Greater occipital nerve (GON) blocks are indicated for the treatment of occipital neuralgia and have been used for a variety of headache disorders including cluster and cervicogenic, acute and chronic migraines, post-dural puncture, and even a case report for spontaneous intracranial hypotension headache [3, 7, 55, 56, 62, 75]. The originally described procedure uses palpation of the occipital artery at the level of the superior nuchal ridge and injecting just medial [29]. The challenge with this method, however, is that palpation of the occipital artery can be difficult and there can be variability in the course of both the occipital artery and GON. In most cases, the GON arises from the C2 dorsal ramus and courses around the inferior aspect of the inferior oblique muscle (IOM) and ultimately between the IOM and the semispinalis capitis (SSC) muscle [53]. The GON can become irritated and entrapped at a number of locations including where the GON emerges from the C2 dorsal ramus between C1 and C2, where the nerve courses between the IOM and SSC muscles, where the nerve pierces the belly of the SSC, and as the nerve exits from the tendinous aponeurosis of the trapezius [46, 60].

Scanning Technique and Important Anatomy

The patient should lie prone with slight cervical flexion to expose the suboccipital region. The ultrasound transducer should be placed over the bifid C2 spinous process and moved one level cephalad to C1. The IOM is located just superficial to C1 and the SSC just superficial to the IOM. The GON is a hyperechoic round or elliptical structure that lies within the plane between the IOM and SSC before it pierces superficially through the SSC [10]. Doppler should be utilized to visualize and avoid the occipital artery (Fig. 18.9).

Injection Technique

- Patient positioning: Lay the patient prone with the neck in slight flexion. A pillow can be placed under the chest.
- Probe positioning: Start by placing the transducer transverse (axial) over the bifid spinous process of C2. The posterior arch of C1 will appear smooth. The inferior obliquus capitis muscle attaches to the spinous process of C2 and transverse process of C1. Follow the inferior obliquus capitis in-plane as it moves laterally and cranially. The GON sits in the fascial plane between the inferior obliquus capitis and semispinalis capitis muscle.
- Markings: Use Doppler to identify any branches of the occipital artery to avoid inadvertent puncture.
- Needle position: The needle is inserted in-plane from lateral to medial. Advance until the needle is close to the nerve sheath. If the nerve cannot be clearly visualized, then place medication in the fascial plane between IOM and SSC.
- Safety considerations: Prior to placing the needle, Doppler may help to identify the occipital vessels.

Pearls

- The C2 spinous process is bifid which distinguishes it from the smooth posterior arch of C1.
- Placing the neck in slight flexion will help to clear room for the ultrasound transducer.
- Rotate the probe slightly (lateral end more cranial than medial end) to help bring the inferior obliquus capitis muscle parallel to the probe.

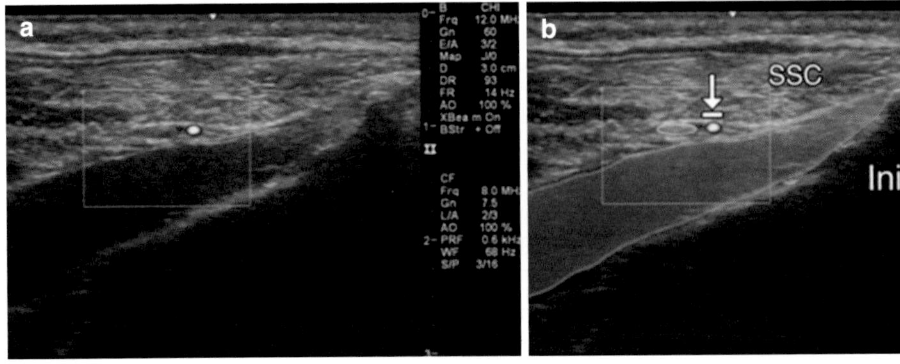

Fig. 18.9 (**a**) Axial view of the GON with Doppler. (**b**) *Orange* indicates IOM, *SSC* and inion labeled; *arrow with stop* indicates occipital artery; *yellow* indicates GON

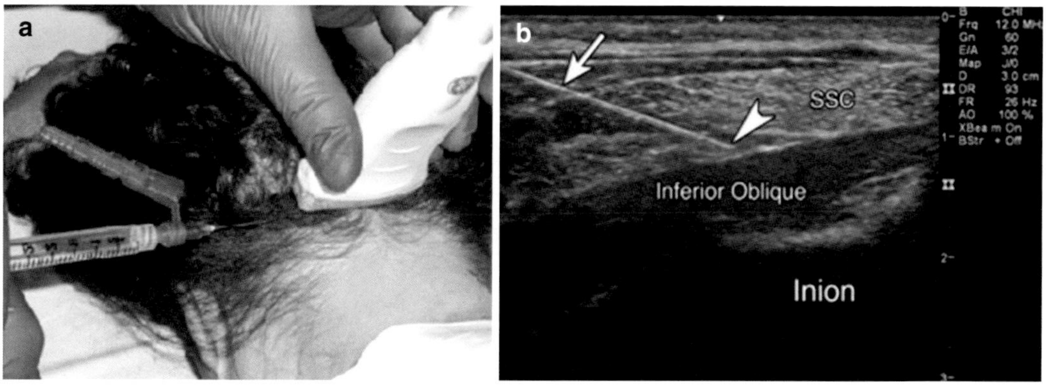

Fig. 18.10 (**a**) Example of axial probe position over GON with in-plane injection technique. (**b**) *Arrowhead* indicates needle tip adjacent to GON; *white arrow* indicates needle; *SSC*, inion, and inferior oblique labeled

Equipment Needed

- High-frequency linear array transducer
- 25G 1.5″ needle
- 0.5–1 mL of steroid preparation
- 1–3 mL of local anesthetic (Fig. 18.10).

Lumbar Medial Branch Blocks and Zygapophyseal Joint

Indications

Facet-mediated low back pain is very common and accounts for up to 45% of axial lumbar pain [8, 52]. The zygapophyseal or facet joints are diarthrodial and formed by the superior and inferior articular processes (SAP and IAP). In the lumbar spine, these joints are innervated by the medial branches of the dorsal rami of the level involved and the level above. For example, the L4–5 facet joint is innervated by the L3 and L4 medial branches. It is important to note that the L5 dorsal ramus does not have a medial branch, so the dorsal ramus itself is targeted [12, 14]. Lumbar facet-mediated pain is usually described as dull/achy in nature and typically localized to the axial lower back, but can occasionally radiate into the buttocks and proximal thigh [8]. Loading the facet joint with oblique extension may reproduce symptoms; however, the gold standard is image-guided comparative anesthetic medial branch blocks [14, 54]. The use of ultrasound guidance for performing diagnostic medial blocks compared to fluoroscopic guidance provides the advantage of avoiding radiation exposure while being just as accurate [28, 32, 37, 41].

Scanning Technique and Important Anatomy

The patient should be placed in the prone position. The transducer should be placed longitudinally to identify the correct level and then rotated axially to obtain the "crown sign." Alternatively, it can be placed axially over the upper aspect of the sacrum to start and then translated cephalad as the hyperechoic midline spinous processes are counted until the desired level is reached. Move the transducer laterally and center it over the junction of the SAP and transverse process (TP) (Fig. 18.11).

Injection Technique

- Patient positioning: Lay the patient prone with a pillow under the pelvis.
- Probe positioning: Start by finding your desired level as above. Keep the probe in an axial view and identify the "crown" sign, transverse process deep, z-jt in the middle, and spinous process superficial, all in the same view. Center the probe over the z-jt.
- Markings: Mark the spinal levels beginning at the sacrum as you scan cephalad. This can be

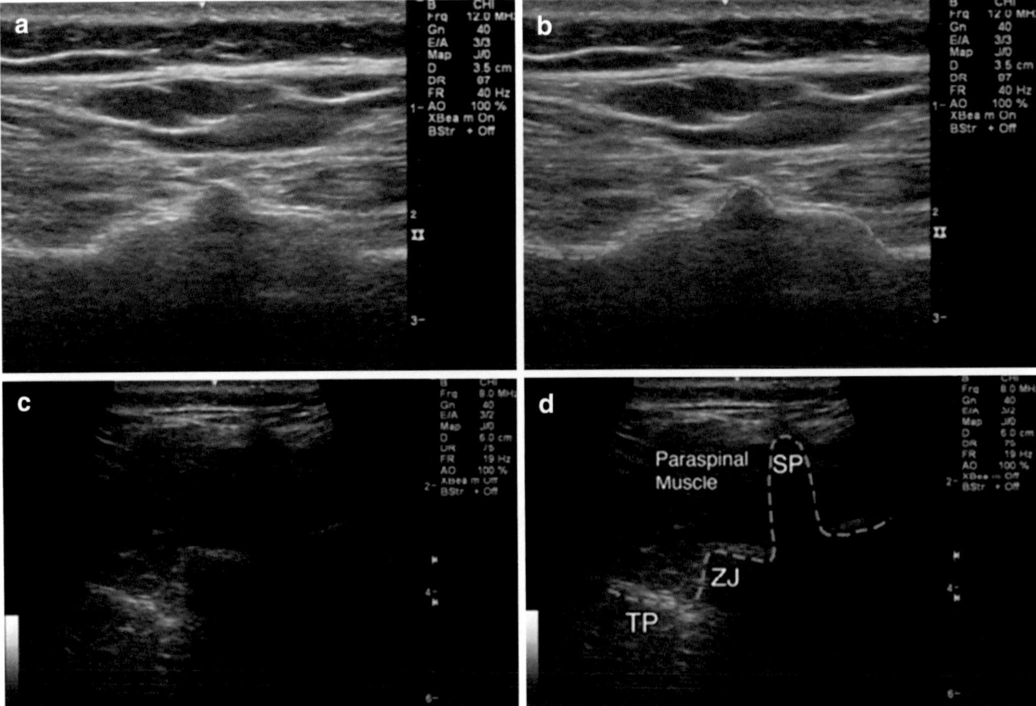

Fig. 18.11 (**a**) Axial view over sacrum. (**b**) Dashed orange line outlines dorsal sacrum. (**c**) Axial view over L5 vertebrae. (**d**) *Dashed orange line* outlines L5 posterior elements; *SP* spinous process, *ZJ* zygapophyseal joint, *TP* transverse process; paraspinal muscle labeled

done by scanning axially or sagittally from the midline using the sacrum as a landmark.

- Needle position: The needle is inserted in-plane from lateral to medial toward the base of the SAP and the transverse process for the medial branches and toward the cleft formed by the IAP and SAP for the z-jt.
- Safety considerations: Prior to placing the needle, Doppler may help to identify any vessels. If the needle is too caudal or cephalad, it may enter the epidural space.

Pearls

- Fine-tuning or toggling the probe once it is in position over the facet joint in the axial plane will help to visualize the joint opening.
- After the target is reached, turn the probe sagittally to view the needle tip on the upper part of the transverse process to confirm it is in proper position for the medial branch block.

Equipment Needed

- Curvilinear transducer or a wide-footprint linear transducer with a low-mid frequency
- Spinal needle 22–25G 3.5–5″
- 0.5–1 mL of steroid preparation per level
- 0.5–1 mL of local anesthetic per level (Fig. 18.12).

Caudal

Indications

Caudal epidural injection is one of the oldest interventional procedures for treating pain due to lumbar spinal stenosis or disc herniation. This approach may be preferred for patients who have undergone previous surgery or have difficult anatomy whereby lumbar transforaminal access is difficult. It also has a lower risk of inadvertent

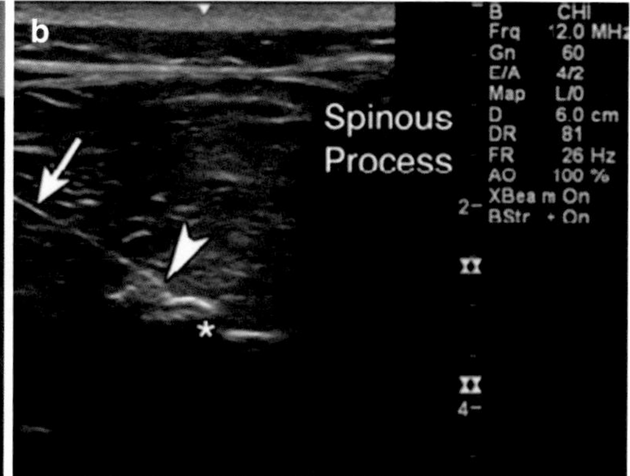

Fig. 18.12 (**a**) Example of axial probe position over L5 z-jt joint with in-plane injection technique. (**b**) *Arrowhead* indicates needle tip at z-jt, *arrow* indicates needle tip, and *asterisk* indicates z-jt; spinous process labeled

intrathecal injection [42]. Caudal injections are typically performed under fluoroscopic guidance and can be performed with either a shallow or steep angle approach depending on the patient's specific anatomy [72]. Even under image guidance, there can be inadvertent needle placement 25.9% of the time [74]. Ultrasound-guided needle placement provides a reasonable alternative to fluoroscopy with 96% accuracy [67]. Use of Doppler to avoid vasculature has shown very high accuracy rates as well [77]. It has also been shown that there is no statistically significant difference in terms of pain or disability between fluoroscopic and ultrasound-guided caudal injections [66].

Scanning Technique and Important Anatomy

With the patient in a prone position, palpate the sacral hiatus with a sterile gloved hand. Place the transducer axially across the sacrum, midline and proximal to the sacral hiatus. Scan distally until the sacral cornua appear as an inverted U-shape structure and the sacrococcygeal ligament is seen as a horizontal hyperechoic line just deep to them. Rotate the transducer 90 degrees to obtain a long-axis view to visualize the sacrum and sacral canal [9] (Fig. 18.13).

Injection Technique

- Patient positioning: Lay the patient prone comfortably on the table.
- Probe positioning: Start by placing the transducer short axis (transverse) to the midsacrum and scan caudad until the sacral cornua appear. Rotate the probe 90° to give a sagittal and longitudinal picture, and center the sacral hiatus on the screen.
- Markings: Mark the placement of the probe and needle entry site once the ideal position is found so that the area can be sterilized and found quickly again. You can also mark the distance between S2 and S4 so you know the distance to the thecal sac.
- Needle position: The needle is inserted in-plane from caudal to cephalad aiming at the sacral hiatus. The needle should be inserted deep to the dorsal aspect of the sacrum. Some resistance by the sacrococcygeal ligament and a "pop" may be appreciated.
- Safety considerations: Carefully aspirate to ensure no blood or cerebrospinal fluid is returned.

Pearls

- Once the needle advances through the sacrococcygeal ligament, begin aspiration and injection. Do not advance the needle too far as the dural sac typically ends at S2 and the nee-

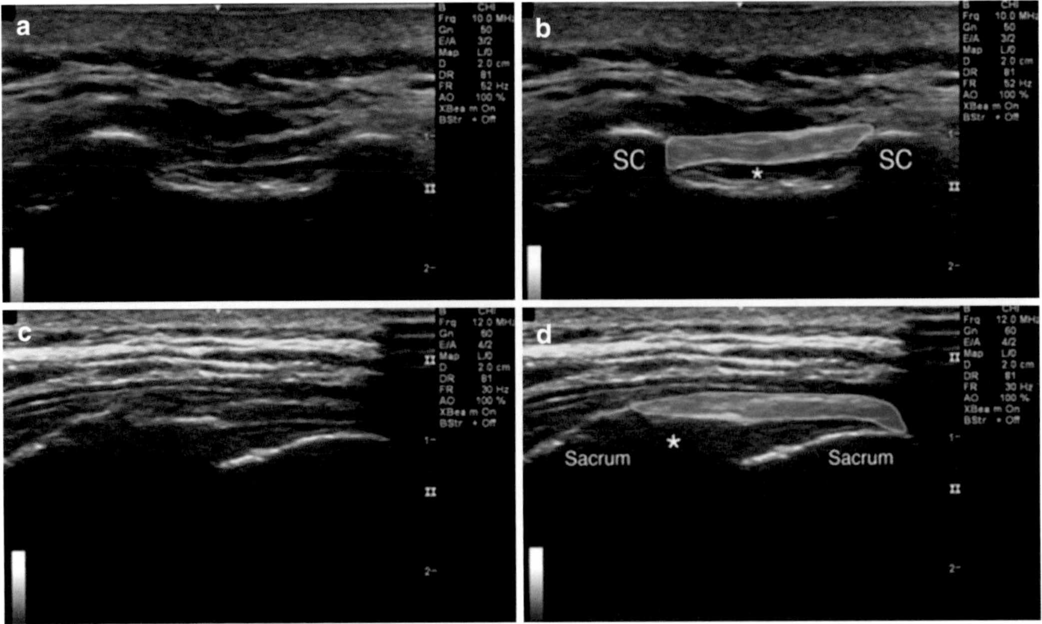

Fig. 18.13 (**a**) Axial view over sacral cornua. (**b**) *Green* indicates sacrococcygeal ligament; *SC* sacral cornua; *asterisk* indicates sacral hiatus. (**c**) Sagittal view of sacral hiatus. (**d**) Dorsal sacrum (left); *green* indicates sacrococcygeal ligament; *asterisk* indicates sacral hiatus

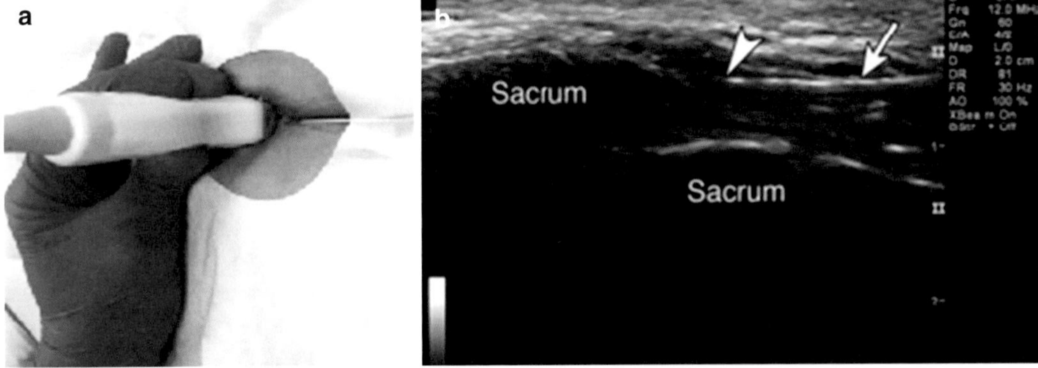

Fig. 18.14 (**a**) Example of sagittal probe position over sacrum with in-plane injection technique. (**b**) *Arrowhead* indicates needle tip traversing toward sacral hiatus; *arrow* indicates needle

dle cannot be visualized anterior to the dorsal bony aspect of the sacrum.

- Injection volume of 20 mL can reach S1 100%, L5 89%, L4 84%, and L3 19% of the time.

Equipment Needed

- High-frequency linear array transducer
- 22 or 25G 3.5″ spinal needle
- 2 mL of steroid preparation
- 0–4 mL of local anesthetic
- 0–6 mL of normal saline (Fig. 18.14).

Sacroiliac Joint

Indications

The diagnosis of sacroiliac joint (SIJ)-mediated pain is based on a combination of history of low back/buttock pain and physical exam; however, there are no reliable imaging studies or specific physical exam maneuvers to accurately diagnose SIJ dysfunction. SIJ injections provide both diagnostic and therapeutic value and can confirm the SIJ as the pain generator [5, 21, 49, 76]. The precise innervation of the SIJ is complex and not fully understood. Some authors argue a combination of anterior and posterior innervation, whereas others suggest innervation entirely posterior from the lateral branches of the dorsal rami [13, 19, 20, 30].

Scanning Technique and Important Anatomy

The patient should be placed in the prone position with the transducer placed transversely over the posterior superior iliac spine (PSIS) and translated medially to identify the S1 foramen. Translate the transducer caudally to identify the inferior SIJ recess/capsule, located lateral to the S2 foramen (Fig. 18.15).

Injection Technique

- Patient positioning: Lay the patient in the prone position with a pillow under the pelvis.
- Probe positioning: Start by placing the transducer short axis (transverse) to the sacrum at the level of the sacral hiatus. Move the probe lateral and cephalad until the cleft between the sacrum and ilium is centered on the screen. The probe should be positioned 1 cm above the lower end of the joint.
- Markings: No significant vascular or neural structures need to be marked.
- Needle position: The needle should be inserted in-plane from medial to lateral parallel to the transducer for optimal needle visualization.
- Safety considerations: Prior to placing the needle, Doppler may help to identify any vessels. Take care in osteoporotic individuals to not advance the needle through bone.

Pearls

- The injection can be performed in the lower third of the SIJ which is synovial, while the upper portion is fibrous and not a true joint.
- Target the most inferior portion of the joint.
- Push the needle through the posterior ligament, and feel a pop to help confirm joint entry rather than a periarticular injection.

Equipment Needed

- Curvilinear or linear array 6–10 mHz transducer
- 22G 3.5″ spinal needle
- 1–2 mL of steroid preparation
- 1–2 mL of local anesthetic (Fig. 18.16).

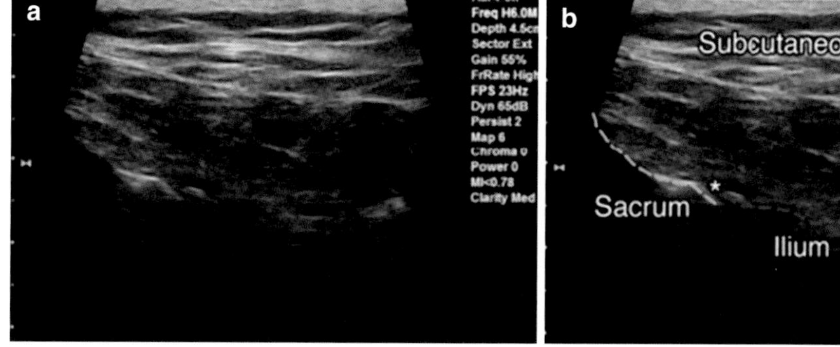

Fig. 18.15 (**a**) Axial view of the SIJ. (**b**) *Dashed orange line* outlines the sacrum, *dashed purple* line outlines the ilium, and *asterisk* indicates joint space; subcutaneous fat labeled

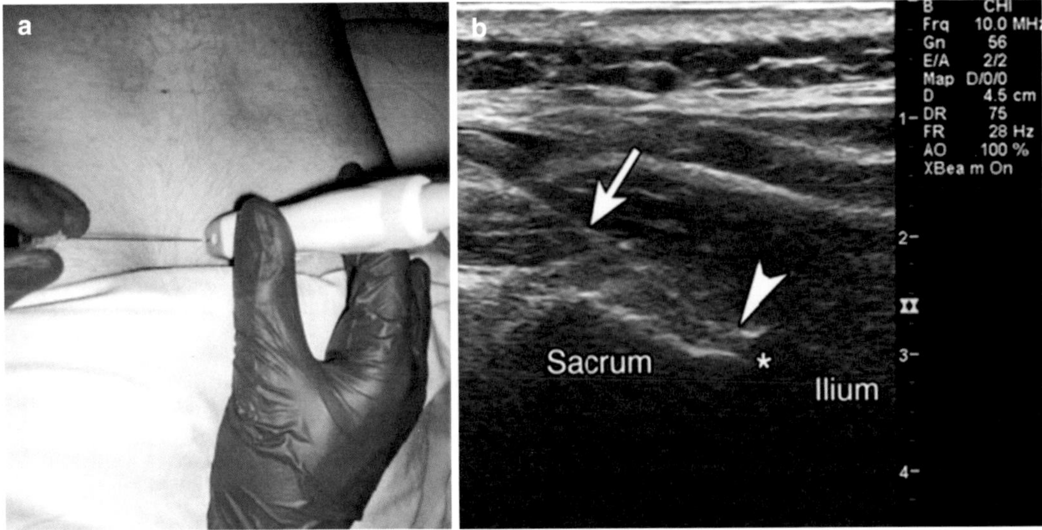

Fig. 18.16 (**a**) Example of axial probe position over SIJ with in-plane injection technique. (**b**) *Arrowhead* indicates needle tip entering SIJ, *arrow* indicates needle, and *asterisk* indicates joint space; sacrum and ilium labeled

References

1. Abdi S, Zhou Y, Patel N, Saini B, Nelson J. A new and easy technique to block the stellate ganglion. Pain Physician. 2004;7(3):327–31.
2. Aeschbach A, Mekhail NA. Common nerve blocks in chronic pain management. Anesthesiol Clin North Am. 2000;18(2):429–59, viii.
3. Allen SM, Mookadam F, Cha SS, Freeman JA, Starling AJ, Mookadam M. Greater occipital nerve block for acute treatment of migraine headache: a large retrospective cohort study. J Am Board Fam Med. 2018;31(2):211–8.
4. Barnsley L, Bogduk N. Medial branch blocks are specific for the diagnosis of cervical zygapophyseal joint pain. Reg Anesth. 1993;18(6):343–50.
5. Berthelot J-M, Labat J-J, Le Goff B, Gouin F, Maugars Y. Provocative sacroiliac joint maneuvers and sacroiliac joint block are unreliable for diagnosing sacroiliac joint pain. Joint Bone Spine. 2006;73(1):17–23.
6. Boswell MV, Colson JD, Sehgal N, Dunbar EE, Epter R. A systematic review of therapeutic facet joint interventions in chronic spinal pain. Pain Physician. 2007;10(1):229–53.
7. Bovim G, Sand T. Cervicogenic headache, migraine without aura and tension-type headache. Diagnostic blockade of greater occipital and supra-orbital nerves. Pain. 1992;51(1):43–8.
8. Bykowski JL, Wong WHW. Role of facet joints in spine pain and image-guided treatment: a review. AJNR Am J Neuroradiol. 2012;33(8):1419–26.
9. Chen CP, Wong AM, Hsu C-C, Tsai W-C, Chang C-N, Lin S-C, et al. Ultrasound as a screening tool for proceeding with caudal epidural injections. Arch Phys Med Rehabil. 2010;91(3):358–63.
10. Cho JC-S, Haun DW, Kettner NW. Sonographic evaluation of the greater occipital nerve in unilateral occipital neuralgia. J Ultrasound Med. 2012;31(1):37–42.
11. Cohen SP, Huang JHY, Brummett C. Facet joint pain--advances in patient selection and treatment. Nat Rev Rheumatol. 2013;9(2):101–16.
12. Cohen SP, Raja SN. Pathogenesis, diagnosis, and treatment of lumbar zygapophysial (facet) joint pain. Anesthesiology. 2007;106(3):591–614.
13. Dreyfuss P, Henning T, Malladi N, Goldstein B, Bogduk N. The ability of multi-site, multi-depth sacral lateral branch blocks to anesthetize the sacroiliac joint complex. Pain Med. 2009;10(4):679–88.
14. Dreyfuss P, Schwarzer AC, Lau P, Bogduk N. Specificity of lumbar medial branch and L5 dorsal ramus blocks. A computed tomography study. Spine. 1997;22(8):895–902.
15. Dwyer A, Aprill C, Bogduk N. Cervical zygapophyseal joint pain patterns. I: a study in normal volunteers. Spine. 1990;15(6):453–7.
16. Eichenberger U, Greher M, Kapral S, Marhofer P, Wiest R, Remonda L, et al. Sonographic visualization and ultrasound-guided block of the third occipital nerve [Internet]. Anesthesiology. 2006:303–8. Available from: https://doi.org/10.1097/00000542-200602000-00016.
17. Finlayson RJ, Etheridge J-PB, Vieira L, Gupta G, Tran DQH. A randomized comparison between ultrasound- and fluoroscopy-guided third occipital nerve block [Internet]. Regional Anesthesia Pain Med. 2013:212–7. Available from: https://doi.org/10.1097/aap.0b013e31828b25bc.

18. Finlayson RJ, Thonnagith A, Elgueta MF, Perez J, Etheridge J-PB, Tran DQH. Ultrasound-guided cervical medial branch radiofrequency Neurotomy: can multitined deployment Cannulae be the solution? Reg. Anesth Pain Med. 2017;42(1):45–51.
19. Fortin JD, Dwyer AP, West S, Pier J. Sacroiliac joint: pain referral maps upon applying a new injection/arthrography technique. Part I: Asymptomatic volunteers. Spine. 1994;19(13):1475–82.
20. Fortin JD, Kissling RO, O'Connor BL, Vilensky JA. Sacroiliac joint innervation and pain. Am J Orthop. 1999a;28(12):687–90.
21. Fortin JD, Washington WJ, Falco FJ. Three pathways between the sacroiliac joint and neural structures. AJNR Am J Neuroradiol. 1999b;20(8):1429–34.
22. Freire V, Grabs D, Lepage-Saucier M, Moser TP. Ultrasound-guided cervical facet joint injections: a viable substitution for fluoroscopy-guided injections? J Ultrasound Med. 2016;35(6):1253–8.
23. Frey C, Yeh PC, Jayaram P. Effects of antiplatelet and nonsteroidal anti-inflammatory medications on platelet-rich plasma: a systematic review. Orthop J Sports Med. 2020;8(4):2325967120912841.
24. Galiano K, Obwegeser A, Bale R, Harlander C, Schatzer R, Schocke M, et al. Ultrasound-guided and CT-navigation-assisted periradicular and facet joint injections in the lumbar and cervical spine: a new teaching tool to recognize the sonoanatomic pattern [Internet]. Regional Anesthesia Pain Med. 2007:254–7. Available from: https://doi.org/10.1016/j.rapm.2007.02.008.
25. Garvican ER, Cree S, Bull L, Smith RK, Dudhia J. Viability of equine mesenchymal stem cells during transport and implantation. Stem Cell Res Ther. 2014;5(4):94.
26. Ghai A, Kaushik T, Wadhera R, Wadhera S. Stellate ganglion blockade-techniques and modalities. Acta Anaesthesiol Belg. 2016;67(1):1–5.
27. Graziani F, Ivanovski S, Cei S, Ducci F, Tonetti M, Gabriele M. The in vitro effect of different PRP concentrations on osteoblasts and fibroblasts. Clin Oral Implants Res. 2006;17(2):212–9.
28. Greher M, Kirchmair L, Enna B, Kovacs P, Gustorff B, Kapral S, et al. Ultrasound-guided lumbar facet nerve block: accuracy of a new technique confirmed by computed tomography. Anesthesiology. 2004;101(5):1195–200.
29. Greher M, Moriggl B, Curatolo M, Kirchmair L, Eichenberger U. Sonographic visualization and ultrasound-guided blockade of the greater occipital nerve: a comparison of two selective techniques confirmed by anatomical dissection [Internet]. Br J Anaesthesia. 2010:637–42. Available from: https://doi.org/10.1093/bja/aeq052.
30. Grob KR, Neuhuber WL, Kissling RO. Innervation of the sacroiliac joint of the human. Z Rheumatol. 1995;54(2):117–22.
31. Guttuso T Jr. Stellate ganglion block for treating hot flashes: a viable treatment option or sham procedure? Maturitas. 2013;76(3):221–4.
32. Han SH, Park KD, Cho KR, Park Y. Ultrasound versus fluoroscopy-guided medial branch block for the treatment of lower lumbar facet joint pain: a retrospective comparative study. Medicine. 2017;96(16):e6655.
33. Hayase J, Patel J, Narayan SM, Krummen DE. Percutaneous stellate ganglion block suppressing VT and VF in a patient refractory to VT ablation. J Cardiovasc Electrophysiol. 2013;24(8):926–8.
34. Hoeft MA, Rathmell JP, Monsey RD, Fonda BJ. Cervical transforaminal injection and the radicular artery: variation in anatomical location within the cervical intervertebral foramina. Reg Anesth Pain Med. 2006;31(3):270–4.
35. Hogan QH, Erickson SJ. MR imaging of the stellate ganglion: normal appearance. AJR Am J Roentgenol. 1992;158(3):655–9.
36. Huntoon MA. Anatomy of the cervical intervertebral foramina: vulnerable arteries and ischemic neurologic injuries after transforaminal epidural injections. Pain. 2005;117(1–2):104–11.
37. Hurdle M-FB. Ultrasound-guided spinal procedures for pain: a review. Phys Med Rehabil Clin N Am. 2016;27(3):673–86.
38. Jayaram P, Yeh PC, Cianca J. Platelet-rich plasma protocols can potentiate vascular emboli: contraindications to platelet-rich plasma. The Journal of the International Society [Internet] jisprmorg; 2019a. Available from: http://www.jisprm.org/article.asp?issn=2349-7904;year=2019;volume=2;issue=2;spage=104;epage=106;aulast=Jayaram.
39. Jayaram P, Yeh P, Patel SJ, Cela R, Shybut TB, Grol MW, et al. Effects of aspirin on growth factor release from freshly isolated leukocyte-rich platelet-rich plasma in healthy men: a prospective fixed-sequence controlled laboratory study. Am J Sports Med SAGE Publications Sage CA: Los Angeles, CA. 2019b;47(5):1223–9.
40. Jee H, Lee JH, Kim J, Park KD, Lee WY, Park Y. Ultrasound-guided selective nerve root block versus fluoroscopy-guided transforaminal block for the treatment of radicular pain in the lower cervical spine: a randomized, blinded, controlled study. Skelet Radiol. 2013;42(1):69–78.
41. Jung H, Jeon S, Ahn S, Kim M, Choi Y. The validation of ultrasound-guided lumbar facet nerve blocks as confirmed by fluoroscopy. Asian Spine J. 2012;6(3):163–7.
42. Kao S-C, Lin C-S. Caudal epidural block: an updated review of anatomy and techniques. Biomed Res Int. 2017;26(2017):9217145.
43. Lee S-H, Kang CH, Lee S-H, Derby R, Yang SN, Lee JE, et al. Ultrasound-guided radiofrequency neurotomy in cervical spine: sonoanatomic study of a new technique in cadavers. Clin Radiol. 2008;63(11):1205–12.
44. Leriche R, Fontaine R, Others. De l'infiltration stellaire dans les embolies cérébrales, dans les spasmes vasculaires postopératoires de l'encéphale et chez les hémiplégiques. Rev Chir Paris. 1936;74:755–8.

45. Lipov E, Ritchie EC. A review of the use of stellate ganglion block in the treatment of PTSD. Curr Psychiatry Rep. 2015;17(8):63.
46. Loukas M, El-Sedfy A, Tubbs RS, Louis RG Jr, Wartmann CHT, Curry B, et al. Identification of greater occipital nerve landmarks for the treatment of occipital neuralgia. Folia Morphol (Warsz). 2006;65(4):337–42.
47. Makharita MY, Amr YM, El-Bayoumy Y. Effect of early stellate ganglion blockade for facial pain from acute herpes zoster and incidence of postherpetic neuralgia. Pain Physician. 2012;15(6):467–74.
48. Malhotra G, Abbasi A, Rhee M. Complications of transforaminal cervical epidural steroid injections. Spine (Phila Pa 1976). 2009;34(7):731–9.
49. Manchikanti L, Staats PS, Singh V, Schultz DM, Vilims BD, Jasper JF, et al. Evidence-based practice guidelines for interventional techniques in the management of chronic spinal pain. Pain Physician. 2003;6(1):3–81.
50. Martinoli C, Bianchi S, Santacroce E, Pugliese F, Graif M, Derchi LE. Brachial plexus sonography: a technique for assessing the root level. AJR Am J Roentgenol. 2002;179(3):699–702.
51. Matula C, Trattnig S, Tschabitscher M, Day JD, Koos WT. The course of the prevertebral segment of the vertebral artery: anatomy and clinical significance. Surg Neurol. 1997;48(2):125–31.
52. Mooney V, Robertson J. The facet syndrome. Clin Orthop Relat Res. 1976;115:149–56.
53. Mosser SW, Guyuron B, Janis JE, Rohrich RJ. The anatomy of the greater occipital nerve: implications for the etiology of migraine headaches [Internet]. Plastic Reconstructive Surg. 2004:693–7. Available from: https://doi.org/10.1097/01.prs.0000101502.22727.5d.
54. Nadler SF, Malanga GA. Introduction: an evidence-based approach to the musculoskeletal physical examination [Internet]. Musculoskeletal Physical Examinat. 2006:1–5. Available from: https://doi.org/10.1016/b978-1-56053-591-1.50008-1.
55. Nair AS, Kodisharapu PK, Anne P, Saifuddin MS, Asiel C, Rayani BK. Efficacy of bilateral greater occipital nerve block in postdural puncture headache: a narrative review. Korean J Pain. 2018;31(2):80–6.
56. Naja ZM, El-Rajab M, Al-Tannir MA, Ziade FM, Tawfik OM. Occipital nerve blockade for cervicogenic headache: a double-blind randomized controlled clinical trial. Pain Pract Wiley OnlineLibrary. 2006;6(2):89–95.
57. Narouze SN. Ultrasound-guided interventional procedures in pain management: evidence-based medicine. Reg Anesth Pain Med. 2010;35(2 Suppl):S55–8.
58. Narouze S, Vydyanathan A. Ultrasound-guided cervical transforaminal injection and selective nerve root block. Tech Reg Anesth Pain Manag. 2009;13(3):137–41.
59. Narouze S, Vydyanathan A, Patel N. Ultrasound-guided stellate ganglion block successfully prevented esophageal puncture. Pain Physician. 2007;10(6):747–52.
60. Natsis K, Baraliakos X, Appell HJ, Tsikaras P, Gigis I, Koebke J. The course of the greater occipital nerve in the suboccipital region: a proposal for setting landmarks for local anesthesia in patients with occipital neuralgia. Clin Anat. 2006;19(4):332–6.
61. Navani A, Manchikanti L, Albers SL, Latchaw RE, Sanapati J, Kaye AD, et al. Responsible, safe, and effective use of biologics in the Management of low Back Pain: American Society of Interventional Pain Physicians (ASIPP) guidelines. Pain Physician. 2019;22(1S):S1–74.
62. Niraj G, Critchley P, Kodivalasa M, Dorgham M. Greater occipital nerve treatment in the Management of Spontaneous Intracranial Hypotension Headache: a case report. Headache. 2017;57(6):952–5.
63. Obernauer J, Galiano K, Gruber H, Bale R, Obwegeser AA, Schatzer R, et al. Ultrasound-guided versus computed tomography-controlled facet joint injections in the middle and lower cervical spine: a prospective randomized clinical trial. Med Ultrason. 2013;15(1):10–5.
64. O'Connell NE, Wand BM, Gibson W, Carr DB, Birklein F, Stanton TR. Local anaesthetic sympathetic blockade for complex regional pain syndrome. Cochrane Database Syst Rev. 2016;7:CD004598.
65. Pal GP, Routal RV, Saggu SK. The orientation of the articular facets of the zygapophyseal joints at the cervical and upper thoracic region. J Anat. 2001;198(Pt 4):431–41.
66. Park Y, Lee JH, Park KD, Ahn JK, Park J, Jee H. Ultrasound-guided vs. fluoroscopy-guided caudal epidural steroid injection for the treatment of unilateral lower lumbar radicular pain: a prospective, randomized, single-blind clinical study. Am J Phys Med Rehabil. 2013;92(7):575.
67. Peng PWH, Narouze S. Ultrasound-guided interventional procedures in pain medicine: a review of anatomy, sonoanatomy, and procedures: part I: nonaxial structures. Reg Anesth Pain Med. 2009;34(5):458–74.
68. Radhakrishnan K, Litchy WJ, O'Fallon WM, Kurland LT. Epidemiology of cervical radiculopathy. A population-based study from Rochester, Minnesota, 1976 through 1990. Brain. 1994;117(Pt 2):325–35.
69. Rong X, Liu Z, Wang B, Chen H, Liu H. The facet orientation of the subaxial cervical spine and the implications for cervical movements and clinical conditions. Spine. 2017;42(6):E320–5.
70. Schneider BJ, Maybin S, Sturos E. Safety and complications of cervical epidural steroid injections. Phys Med Rehabil Clin N Am. 2018;29(1):155–69.
71. Sehgal N, Dunbar EE, Shah RV, Colson J. Systematic review of diagnostic utility of facet (zygapophysial) joint injections in chronic spinal pain: an update. Pain Physician. 2007;10(1):213–28.
72. Sekiguchi M, Yabuki S, Satoh K, Kikuchi S. An anatomic study of the sacral hiatus: a basis for successful caudal epidural block. Clin J Pain. 2004;20(1):51–4.
73. Siegenthaler A, Schliessbach J, Curatolo M, Eichenberger U. Ultrasound anatomy of the nerves

supplying the cervical zygapophyseal joints: an exploratory study. Reg Anesth Pain Med. 2011;36(6):606–10.
74. Stitz MY, Sommer HM. Accuracy of blind versus fluoroscopically guided caudal epidural injection. Spine. 1999;24(13):1371–6.
75. Terzi T, Karakurum B, Üçler S, İnan LE, Tulunay C. Greater occipital nerve blockade in migraine, tension-type headache and cervicogenic headache [Internet]. J Headache Pain. 2002:137–41. Available from: https://doi.org/10.1007/s101940200031.
76. van der Wurff P, Buijs EJ, Groen GJ. A multitest regimen of pain provocation tests as an aid to reduce unnecessary minimally invasive sacroiliac joint procedures. Arch Phys Med Rehabil. 2006;87(1):10–4.
77. Yoon JS, Sim KH, Kim SJ, Kim WS, Koh SB, Kim B-J. The feasibility of color Doppler ultrasonography for caudal epidural steroid injection [Internet]. Pain. 2005:210–4. Available from: https://doi.org/10.1016/j.pain.2005.08.014.
78. Zhang X, Shi H, Zhou J, Xu Y, Pu S, Lv Y, et al. The effectiveness of ultrasound-guided cervical transforaminal epidural steroid injections in cervical radiculopathy: a prospective pilot study. J Pain Res. 2019;12:171–7.

19 Musculoskeletal Ultrasound-Guided Regenerative Medicine

Angela N. Cortez
and Rhoel James Timothy O. Dejano

The History of Ultrasound and Physiatry

Physiatry was one of the first fields to take on the ultrasound in its scope of practice, starting with the founding of the American Institute for Ultrasound in Medicine (AIUM) among a group physiatrists in 1951 [1]. Its use in the field has evolved as ultrasound technology has evolved, starting initially with therapeutic ultrasound as a heating modality [2]. By 1958, Dr. Karl Dussik published the first report on musculoskeletal ultrasonography, heralding a movement in musculoskeletal applications in physiatry that has escalated in the twenty-first century [2–4]. Physiatrists' role in the history of ultrasound has uniquely positioned the field in guiding its applications and evolution [5].

The American Academy of Physical Medicine and Rehabilitation describe physiatrists as physicians who are "muscle and bone experts who treat injuries or illnesses that affect how you move." Specifically, goals of the field involve diagnosing and treating pain and restoring maximum function lost through injury illness or disabling conditions [6]. The physiatrist's understanding of functional anatomy and biomechanics lends itself to wanting accurate information in the patient room, in real time, to guide clinical decision-making and management. By 1999, Primack demonstrated musculoskeletal ultrasound as an extension of the clinical exam, an idea that largely gained momentum among physiatrists in the twenty-first century with improvements in technology [7]. Just as electrodiagnostic testing has long been thought of as an extension of the clinical exam in the physiatrist, the ultrasound has taken arguably equal importance with the physiatrist as a diagnostic tool.

The Ultrasound as an Extension of the Physiatrist

The musculoskeletal ultrasound has now been coined the "stethoscope" of the physiatrist, as its many current advantages (e.g., convenience, portability, high resolution, dynamic real-time properties) facilitate prompt diagnosis, functional information, and interactive imaging of musculoskeletal conditions [8]. Nearly half of the publications on musculoskeletal ultrasound were in the field of physical medicine and rehabilitation over a 25-year period, and its integration into physiatric education has been seen globally [2,

A. N. Cortez (✉)
Department of Physical Medicine & Rehabilitation, University of California at Davis, Sacramento, CA, USA

R. J. T. O. Dejano
Department of Internal Medicine, University of Cebu Medical Center, Cebu City, Philippines

Y. El Miedany (ed.), *Musculoskeletal Ultrasound-Guided Regenerative Medicine*,
https://doi.org/10.1007/978-3-030-98256-0_19

9]. Simultaneously, the evolution of musculoskeletal ultrasound has produced alongside it the development of interventional ultrasound in physiatry. Insomuch as a trained practitioner can now both identify pathology in real-time and accurately provide an ultrasound-guided intervention, its use in physiatry is expansive.

Ultrasound in Physiatric Musculoskeletal Medicine

Joint Injections

Musculoskeletal-related conditions are a primary source of worldwide disability, with osteoarthritis one of the leading causes [10]. Hip and knee osteoarthritis account for 17 million years lived with disability globally [11]. Physiatrists use a multitude of interventions to decrease pain and improve function due to joint pain, and ultrasound-guided interventions allow for accurate and convenient in-office treatment options. For osteoarthritis, several studies have confirmed the accuracy of ultrasound-guided interventions to various joints, and intervention accuracy can maximize the efficacy of the desired injectate, such as PRP, prolotherapy, hyaluronic acid, or corticosteroids [12–14].

Commonly performed joint injections include hip joint injections, glenohumeral joint injections, and subtalar joint injections. Deeper joints and small joints are particularly useful under ultrasound guidance. The accuracy of ultrasound-guided interventions allows for therapeutic options to diminish pain, in addition to diagnostic options via anesthetic infiltration to differentiate pain generators from nearby structures (e.g., hip joint and iliopsoas tendon). Joint effusions and Baker's cysts are quickly visualized and fully aspirated to improve mobility via ultrasound.

Tendon and Bursa Injections

Tendinopathies have seen increasing prevalence with an increase in recreational sports [15]. Individuals over age 35 experience higher risk of overuse tendinopathies, and tendinopathies are the most common cause of chronic shoulder pain in the general population [15, 16]. Optimizing function and improving performance can be difficult in the context of chronic tendinopathies, as treatment is often protracted and requires careful adherence from the patient. Physiatrists are optimized at assessing biomechanical abnormalities that predispose their patients to tendinopathy and at developing a realistic rehabilitation program [15]. Identifying calcific tendinopathies especially of the supraspinatus, enthesophytes, tendon thickening indicative of tendinopathy, and dynamic assessment of snapping tendons are within the capabilities of musculoskeletal ultrasound [17]. Within this framework, musculoskeletal ultrasound allows for direct visual participation of the patient and in-office reassurance of their diagnosis and treatment plan [18].

The ability to directly visualize tendon structures increases accuracy of established procedures and has also allowed for interventional procedures not previously available 10 to 15 years ago [14]. Subacromial and greater trochanteric hip injections have been mainstays for the treatment of common musculoskeletal pathologies, but direct visualization of the tendon has allowed for the development of procedures such as needle tenotomy of the gluteus medius and minimus tendons for chronic tendinopathy. Other interventional examples include high-volume injection of the paratenon to disrupt neovessel abnormalities in Achilles tendinopathy and barbotage of a calcific rotator cuff tendon [19].

Injections in Soft Tissue

Within the scope of the physiatrist are peripheral nerve disorders, including carpal tunnel syndrome and Morton neuromas. Available studies have shown ultrasound-guided Morton neuroma injections to be highly accurate and comparable to MRI in diagnostic accuracy [14, 20]. Carpal tunnel syndrome, a common disorder among adults, can be treated with corticosteroid injection as an alternative to splinting. A critical review of the literature has found ultrasound-guided carpal tunnel injections to be less painful and more efficacious than landmark-based injections [14]. Given those findings, the physiatrist, armed with electrodiagnostic machine and an ultrasound as "stethoscopes," can be a patient's single point of contact from diagnosis to treatment of various compressive focal mononeuropathies.

Ultrasound in Rehabilitation

Musculoskeletal injuries are a prominent focus for physiatrists in musculoskeletal ultrasound, but its use can be conveniently applied in rehabilitation settings, within the backdrop of brain injury, spinal cord injury, and amputation [21].

Post-stroke Shoulder Pain

Stroke is a common syndrome and the second most common cause of disability worldwide. In spastic hemiparesis, post-stroke shoulder pain is a frequent complication with likely multiple pathologies, including shoulder subluxation, shoulder impingement, adhesive capsulitis, and rotator cuff and biceps tendinopathies [21, 22]. Hemiparesis in stroke begins with a flaccid stage, which is the most common period for the emergence shoulder subluxation [23]. It is characterized by the inferior displacement of the humeral head due to impaired muscle tone, which can predispose the shoulder to other disorders including tendinopathy. Ultrasound has been found useful in the measurement of post-stroke shoulder subluxation and can easily be performed bedside for those with mobility impairments [23]. In the same manner, ultrasound-guided diagnostic and therapeutic interventions for rotator cuff and biceps pathologies in post-stroke shoulder pain can be performed with good specificity and accuracy to the benefit of the patient [14, 21].

Spinal Cord Injury Considerations

In patients with spinal cord injury, rehabilitation can include the use a manual wheelchair to regain independent mobility. Increased loads into the upper limb from manual wheelchair use have been associated with a high prevalence of shoulder and wrist pain in this population due to overuse [24]. Correspondingly, treating upper limb pain can be critical for those who rely on their upper limbs for independent mobility and activities of daily living [24, 25]. Pathologies include rotator cuff tendinopathy, shoulder impingement, biceps tendinopathy, ulnar neuropathy at the elbow, and carpal tunnel syndrome [21, 26].

Heterotopic ossification is another common complication after spinal cord injury with incidence ranges of 10–53% and approximately 20–30% of these patients with clinically significant disease [27]. Symptoms include decreased joint range of motion, swelling, and pain. Bisphosphonates have been found effective at halting the progression of heterotopic ossification, though the medication was found most effective when used prior to positive findings on radiographs which can take 4 to 6 weeks [28–30]. Triple-phase bone scan is currently the mainstay for early diagnosis, though its low specificity can be problematic at differentiating the disease from other potential sources such as deep venous thrombosis, infection, and tumors [27]. Ultrasound has long demonstrated to be superior to plain radiographs at the early detection of heterotopic bone formation [29, 30]. In contrast to triple-phase bone scan, ultrasound is more specific and highly sensitive for the early detection and intervention of heterotopic ossification, with increased portability to allow for bedside applications [27, 29, 30].

Botulinum Toxic Injections

Common to both stroke and spinal cord injury is spasticity, which is velocity-dependent muscle tone that has the potential to limit function in patients. Botulinum toxin injections are commonly used for targeted treatment of spasticity and can be guided via electromyography, electrical stimulation, and ultrasound [21]. Injection accuracy is crucial for treatment efficacy and avoidance of neurovascular structures, which makes ultrasound well-suited for this role. Electromyography, although widely available, requires the patient to activate muscle, a task that can be limited in those with stroke or spinal cord injury, and both electromyography and electrical stimulation can be painful for the patient [31]. Musculoskeletal ultrasound, in contrast, allows for precise localization of the targeted muscle, avoidance of neurovascular structures, and arguably improved efficacy and safety [31].

Amputee Limb Complications

Limb amputation is a potentially disabling event that can achieve generally good functional outcomes. Chronic amputation-related pain, however, has been reported in up to 95% of amputees [32]. Stump neuromas, bony pressure points, prosthetic-induced soft tissue inflammation, and heterotopic ossification are all potential sources of pain that can be easily evaluated with ultrasound. Phantom limb syndrome is another common source of pain, though best diagnosed once other causes are excluded [33]. Similar to ultrasound guidance in Morton neuroma injections, stump neuromas can be accurately injected using ultrasound guidance, thereby reducing the need for surgery [33, 34]. “Sonopalpation” or the use of ultrasound-guided palpation to identify painful structures can aid the identification of a neuroma or a bony pressure point as a source of stump pain [21, 35]. Lastly, soft tissue inflammation from uneven stump loading can result in stump bursitis or fluid collection that is readily seen with ultrasound and can provide data to assist with prosthetic modification [21, 33, 36]. Ultrasound-guided aspiration of fluid collections can also differentiate bursitis from infection [36].

Conclusion

Musculoskeletal ultrasound has seen substantial growth among physiatrists over several decades to aid both the diagnostic evaluation and the interventional treatment of various disorders. The musculoskeletal ultrasound can be thought of as an extension of physiatrist. Applications in physical medicine and rehabilitation are immense and only briefly surveyed in this chapter. Physiatrists should anticipate continued development in musculoskeletal ultrasound applications within their practice as the technology advances.

References

1. Valente C. History of the American Institute of Ultrasound in Medicine. J Ultrasound Med. 2005;14:131–42.
2. Finnoff J, Smith J, Nutz D, et al. A musculoskeletal ultrasound course for physical medicine and rehabilitation residents. Am J Phys Med Rehabil. 2010;89(1):56–69.
3. Primack S. Past, present, and future considerations for musculoskeletal ultrasound. Phys Med Rehabil Clin N Am. 2016;27(3):749–52.
4. Kane D, Grassi W, Sturrock R, et al. A brief history of musculoskeletal ultrasound: 'From bats and ships to babies and hips'. Rheumatology. 2004;43(7):931–3.
5. Smith J, Finnoff J. Diagnostic and interventional musculoskeletal ultrasound: part 2. Clinical applications. PMR. 2009;1(2):162–77.
6. Lexell J. What’s on the horizon: defining physiatry through rehabilitation methodology. PMR. 2012;4(5):331–4.
7. Primack S. Musculoskeletal ultrasound: the clinician's perspective. Radiol Clin N Am. 1999;37(4):617–22.
8. Akkaya N, Ulaşlı AM, Özçakar L. Use of musculoskeletal ultrasound in clinical studies in physiatry: the "stethoscope" is also becoming the “pen”. J Rehabil Med. 2013;45(7):701–2.
9. Özçakar L, Tok F, Murat Ulaşli A, et al. What actually changed after the use of musculoskeletal ultrasound? An international survey study in PRM. Eur J Phys Rehabil Med. 2014;50(4):469–7.
10. Neogi T. The epidemiology and impact of pain in osteoarthritis. Osteoarthr Cartil. 2013;21(9):1145–53.
11. O'Neill T, McCabe P, McBeth J. Update on the epidemiology, risk factors and disease outcomes of osteoarthritis. Best Pract Res Clin Rheumatol. 2018;32(2):312–26.

12. Sofka C, Saboeiro G, Adler R. Ultrasound-guided adult hip injections. J Vasc Interv Radiol. 2005;16(8):1121–3.
13. Smith J, Hurdle M, Weingarten T. Accuracy of Sonographically guided intra-articular injections in the native adult hip. J Ultrasound Med. 2009;28(3):329–3.
14. Finnoff J, Hall M, Adams E, et al. American medical Society for Sports Medicine position statement: interventional musculoskeletal ultrasound in sports medicine. Clin J Sport Med. 2015;25(1):6–22.
15. Maffulli N, Wong J, Almekinders L. Types and epidemiology of tendinopathy. Clin Sports Med. 2003;22(4):675–92.
16. Silverstein B, Viikari-Juntura E, Fan Z, et al. Natural course of nontraumatic rotator cuff tendinitis and shoulder symptoms in a working population. Scand J Work Environ Health. 2006;32(2):99–108.
17. Ozçakar L, Tok F, De Muynck M, et al. Musculoskeletal ultrasonography in physical and rehabilitation medicine. J Rehabil Med. 2012;44(4):310–8.
18. Özçakar L, Kara M, Chang K, et al. Nineteen reasons why physiatrists should do musculoskeletal ultrasound: EURO-MUSCULUS/USPRM recommendations. Am J Phys Med Rehabil. 2015;94(6):e45–9.
19. De Muynck M, Parlevliet T, Cock D, et al. Musculoskeletal ultrasound for interventional physiatry. Eur J Phys Rehabil Med. 2012;48(4):675–87.
20. Xu Z, Duan X, Yu X, et al. The accuracy of ultrasonography and magnetic resonance imaging for the diagnosis of Morton's neuroma: a systematic review. Clin Radiol. 2015;70(4):351–8.
21. Ozçakar L, Carli A, Tok F, et al. The utility of musculoskeletal ultrasound in rehabilitation settings. Am J Phys Med Rehabil. 2013;92(9):805–17.
22. Van Ouwenaller C, Laplace P, Chantraine A. Painful shoulder in hemiplegia. Arch Phys Med Rehabil. 1986;67(1):23–6.
23. Park G, Kim J, Sohn S, et al. Ultrasonographic measurement of shoulder subluxation in patients with post-stroke hemiplegia. J Rehabil Med. 2007;39(7):526–30.
24. Subbarao J, Klopfstein J, Turpin R. Prevalence and impact of wrist and shoulder pain in patients with spinal cord injury. J Spinal Cord Med. 1995;18(1):9–13.
25. Mercer J, Boninger M, Koontz A, et al. Shoulder joint kinetics and pathology in manual wheelchair users. Clin Biomech. 2006;21(8):781–9.
26. Gellman H, Chandler D, Petrasek J, et al. Carpal tunnel syndrome in paraplegic patients. J Bone Joint Surg Am. 1988;70(4):517–9.
27. Van Kuijk A, Geurts A, Van Kuppevelt H. Neurogenic heterotopic ossification in spinal cord injury. Spinal Cord. 2002;40(7):313–26.
28. Teasell R, Mehta S, Aubut J, et al. Systematic review of the therapeutic interventions for heterotopic ossification after spinal cord injury. Spinal Cord. 2010;48(7):512–21.
29. Cassar-Pullicino V, McClelland M, Badwan D, et al. Sonographic diagnosis of heterotopic bone formation in spinal injury patients. Paraplegia. 1993;31(1):40–50.
30. Thomas E, Cassar-Pullicino V, McCall I. The role of ultrasound in the early diagnosis and management of heterotopic bone formation. Clin Radiol. 1991;43(3):190–6.
31. Alter K. High-frequency ultrasound guidance for neurotoxin injections. Phys Med Rehabil Clin N Am. 2010;21(3):607–30.
32. Ephraim P, Wegener S, MacKenzie E, et al. Phantom pain, residual limb pain, and back pain in amputees: results of a national survey. Arch Phys Med Rehabil. 2005;86(10):1910–9.
33. Henrot P, Stines J, Walter F. Imaging of the painful lower limb stump. Radiographics. 2000;20:S219–3.
34. Ernberg L, Adler R, Lane J. Ultrasound in the detection and treatment of a painful stump neuroma. Skelet Radiol. 2003;32(5):306–9.
35. Provost N, Bonaldi V, Sarazin L. Amputation stump neuroma: ultrasound features. J Clin Ultrasound. 1997;25(2):85–9.
36. Foisneau-Lottin A, Martinet N, Henrot P. Bursitis, adventitious bursa, localized soft-tissue inflammation, and bone marrow edema in tibial stumps: the contribution of magnetic resonance imaging to the diagnosis and management of mechanical stress complications. Arch Phys Med Rehabil. 2003;84(5):770–7.

Part VI

Sports Medicine

Ultrasound-Guided Exercises 20

Michael Francis Obispo

History of Ultrasound Use in Exercise

In 1958, Dussik et al. [12, 32] measured the acoustic attenuation of articular and periarticular tissues including the skin, adipose tissue, muscle, tendon, articular capsule, articular cartilage, and bone, which, thereafter, became the first published article on the use of musculoskeletal ultrasound. The initial publication detailing the application of diagnostic ultrasound scanning for physical rehabilitation was done in 1968 by Ikai and Fukunaga [29], who made a correlation between the size of upper limb muscles on ultrasound and the strength they generate. McDonald and Leopold [38] published one of the earliest uses of ultrasound for the musculoskeletal system in 1972 when they conducted scans to differentiate a Baker's cyst from thrombophlebitis. In 1980, Archie Young [64] made a comparative measurement of atrophy through the use of tape measure and ultrasound scans.

The practice of integrating the use of ultrasound in therapeutic exercises began with a series of papers between 1993 and 2006 which documented core muscle activity of the transversus abdominis, lumbar multifidus, pulmonary diaphragm, and lumbopelvic muscles particularly in patients suffering from low back pain. In particular, Julie Hides [21] was able to detect atrophy of the lumbar multifidus via ultrasound at the spinal level corresponding to the symptoms of acute low back pain. She also noted that there was no immediate recovery of the lumbar multifidus once pain subsided [22] and that specific exercises reduced the frequency of recurrence of low back pain [23]. Also of significance was a paper by Hodges and Moseley [26] which was able to note the altered neuromuscular control and preparatory recruitment of the diaphragm and transversus abdominis muscles in patients with low back pain. In May 2006, the term "rehabilitative ultrasound imaging" or RUSI was coined at a symposium in San Antonio, Texas. The objective of this meeting was to develop the best practice guidelines for the use of ultrasound imaging for the abdominal, pelvic, and posterior spine muscles and to develop an international collaborative research agenda related to the use of ultrasound imaging [53]. The consensus from this meeting illustrated the use of ultrasound not just as a means for assessment but also as an instructional tool in the conduct of therapeutic exercise. It was agreed that RUSI would be defined as a sonographic procedure utilized by physiotherapists to evaluate muscle and other soft tissues, along with their respective functions during exercise and physical tasks, to assist in the formulation of therapeutic interventions aimed at improving neuromuscular function [61].

M. F. Obispo (✉)
Department of Physical and Rehabilitation Medicine, De La Salle Medical and Health Sciences Institute, Dasmariñas, Cavite, Philippines
e-mail: mbobispo@dlshsi.edu.ph

Y. El Miedany (ed.), *Musculoskeletal Ultrasound-Guided Regenerative Medicine*,
https://doi.org/10.1007/978-3-030-98256-0_20

Box 20.1 RUSI Benefit

Jackie Whittaker [60] enumerated the following benefits of using ultrasound for exercise as derived from the 2006 RUSI consensus:

- Ultrasound imaging enhances the observation, palpatory, and instructional skills of a clinician in order to confirm or negate their findings.
- Ultrasound imaging is a tool for teaching which allows a clinician to explain and demonstrate the subtleties of the specific motor control impairment.
- Ultrasound imaging is an invaluable form of biofeedback when attempting to increase or decrease a specific muscle tension or to coordinate activity of muscle groups.

Biofeedback in Exercise

Exercise has long been recognized as a mainstay in facilitating proper physiologic healing of various conditions for more than a century. While various surgical and interventional procedures have progressed in alleviating pain in many neuromusculoskeletal conditions, exercise is consistently included in all long-term rehabilitation planning. A randomized controlled trial by Jielile et al. [30] comparing cast immobilization and early post-operative rehabilitation for the treatment of neglected Achilles tendon rupture showed better clinical outcomes and faster overall tendon healing with early rehabilitation comprising weight bearing exercises. Additionally, a meta-analysis conducted by Hayden et al. [19] showed that exercise therapy reduced average pain and functional limitations in individuals with persistent low back pain.

One of the ways exercises are conducted at a rehabilitation setting is through the use of biofeedback to facilitate adaptive responses for normal or near-normal movement patterns after an injury [52]. But there are times that there is no injury involved and the symptoms are a result of behavior and habits that have formed in a period of time. While it is easy to modify overt activities like shooting a basketball, where an individual's sensory processes are mostly adequate enough to be aware and cognizant of the activity at hand, including any faults in carrying out the action, it is not the same for ambiguous activities like modifying the contraction of trunk muscles. This is a recurring problem among therapists instructing patients and who are challenged to properly visually elucidate how the activity is to be done.

According to Scmidt and Wrisberg [47], an intrinsic feedback is information provided by an individual's sensory system, which is usually adequate to refine a task performance. An extrinsic or augmented feedback information, on the other hand, is provided by an external source (i.e., an instrument or another individual) when sensory responses fail. Intrinsic feedback deficit resulting in altered proprioception and muscle response may come from a disrupted paraspinal muscle spindle input and/or an imprecise central processing leading to an impaired position sense [5]. This may be compensated by extrinsic feedback strategies through the mechanism of (a) central nervous system facilitation to provide an optimal sensory-motor loop; (b) patient awareness, confidence, and volitional control over specific physiological processes; (c) motivation; and (d) reinforcement of repetition of successful action of tasks [44]. Ribiero et al. [44] recommend using extrinsic feedback in therapy at reduced frequency or to avoid constant cueing to avoid dependency and to focus on providing information on general movement patterns with attention to its effect after a number of trials.

Giggins et al. [18] classified the most frequently used biofeedback tools used in physical rehabilitation as either biomechanical or physiological. Biomechanical feedback measures movement, forces, and posture through the use of inertial sensors, force/pressure plates, electrogoniometers, and camera systems. The physiological biofeedback measurements are conducted for the neuromuscular and cardiorespiratory systems in rehabilitation. The neuromuscular biofeedback, which involves the use of electromyography or ultrasound, is of particular interest to this chapter as it is involved in refining movement or action for tasks.

Ultrasound-Guided Lumbar Core Exercise

With a number of researches pertaining to the use of ultrasound to assess the trunk muscles, there has been a renewed interest in applying ultrasound scanning for low back pain especially in the area of training the core muscles. According to Fatoye [16], the prevalence of low back pain in 2019 is at 1.4–20.0% with an incidence ranging from 0.024% to 7.0% in Canada, the USA, Sweden, Belgium, Finland, Israel, and the Netherlands.

The lumbar "core" muscles, which include the diaphragm as the roof, the pelvic floor muscles as the floor, and the abdominal muscles and paraspinals as the cylindrical covering, all serve as a form of muscular corset to stabilize the trunk regardless of movement or position [2, 45]. Maintaining lumbar spinal stability involves (1) a passive support system, which relies on the patency of joints, ligaments, and fascia; (2) an active contraction system, in which lumbar spinal movement and stability are maintained by coordinated co-contraction of the core muscles; and (3) a discerning central nervous system [1]. Porterfield [42] described this mechanism as akin to a tent where the lumbar spine serves as the central pole, the core muscles as the guy wires, and the thoracolumbar and abdominal fascia as the tent canvass. It is the coordinated co-contraction of the core muscles as well as the tensigrity of the surrounding fascia that minimizes lumbosacral instability. As previously mentioned early on this chapter, the trunk muscles in an individual with low back pain exhibit (1) altered neuromuscular control presenting as loss of anticipatory contraction of the deep core muscles (transversus abdominis, deep multifidus, diaphragm, pelvic floor muscles) [26] and (2) deficits in muscle control that do not immediately resolve with resolution of pain and are not addressed with traditional strengthening exercises [23].

The treatment, as proposed by Whittaker [60], is primarily to address motor control by first eliminating any hypertonic activity of the superficial trunk muscles, followed by the isolated and then coordinated co-activation of the deep core muscles to be done cognitively and as independently as possible from the superficial muscles. She adds that ultrasound scanning has a major role in this motor relearning process during the cognitive and associative stages of learning.

The cognitive stage is described as providing real-time information to educate a patient regarding their precise problem, as well as providing the specifics of the task at hand [60]. Ultrasound scanning comes into play when it is used to identify hypertonic or atrophied muscle groups in the resting state, as well as the onset, speed, and duration of the contraction of the muscle on dynamic testing. The goal here is to provide awareness to the patient as to what is happening internally by providing a visual anatomical analogy to augment their proprioceptive and kinesthetic perception of the activity to be carried out.

The associative stage is mainly comprised of the biofeedback function upon which motor control performance can be modified. Ultrasound imaging is invaluable in providing biofeedback in a patient with low back pain through minimizing hypertonicity and/or through facilitating activity of hypotonic muscles. Superficial core muscles like the obliquus abdominis externus, the obliquus abdominis internus, and the superficial multifidus are usually hypertonic in low back pain. Some strategies suggested by Whittaker to help reduce the hypertonicity of these muscles are through positional changes and breathing pattern modifications while monitoring these changes on real-time ultrasound scans [60]. For hypotonic functioning deep core muscles, targeted facilitation strategies like performing abdominal drawing-in maneuvers [20, 54] and modified forms of Kegel's exercise [59, 62] are some of the activities that can be taught to patients first under ultrasound guidance to help refine the proper action before these are integrated to functional tasks.

Ultrasound evaluation for the anterior trunk muscles is done in a supine position with the hips and knees slightly flexed to lessen the tension to the pelvis. For the assessment of the transversus abdominis, external obliques, and internal obliques, the transducer is placed on the lumbar/flank region in a transverse orientation (Fig. 20.1). Preferential activation of the transverse abdominis is performed by instructing the patient to perform an abdominal hollowing or a drawing-in maneuver. The examination of the pelvic floor muscles is also done in supine with hips and knees slightly flexed and with a full bladder to improve visualization of the pelvic floor. The transducer is placed midline and superior to the pubis and is examined at both the sagittal and transverse planes (Figs. 20.2 and 20.3, respectively). Preferential activation of the pelvic floor

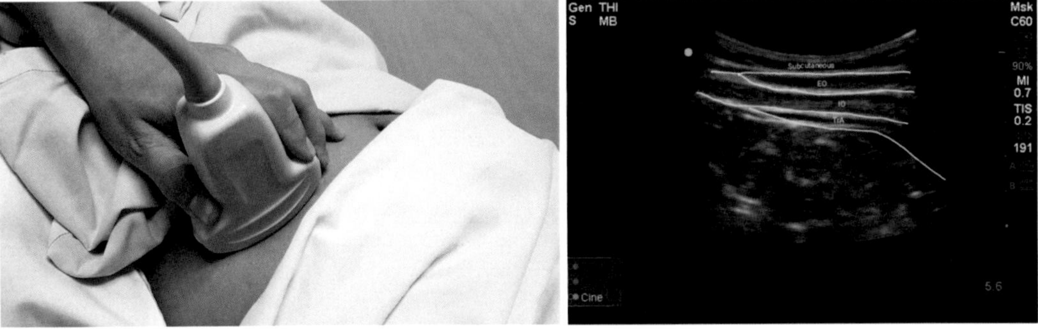

Fig. 20.1 Placement of ultrasound transducer over the anterior abdominal wall for sonographic assessment of the transversus abdominis (TrA), abdominal internal oblique (IO), and abdominal external oblique (EO) [60]

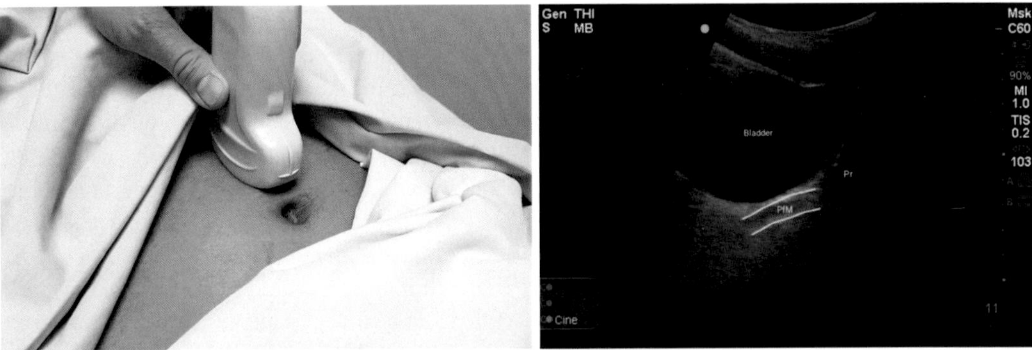

Fig. 20.2 Ultrasound transducer placement for evaluation of pelvic floor muscles (PfM) in longitudinal or long-axis view [60]. Pr prostate

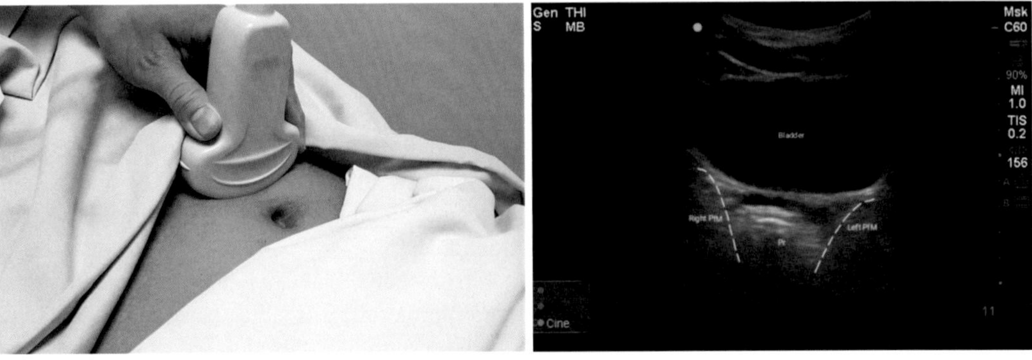

Fig. 20.3 Ultrasound transducer placement for evaluation of pelvic floor muscles (PfM) in transverse or short-axis view [60]. Pr prostate

muscles may be done by providing instructions on how to simulate a Kegel's exercise. For examination of the multifidus muscle at the posterior trunk, the patient is placed either in prone or side-lying. Transverse plane examination of the multifidus is done with the transducer in midline over the vertebra of interest (Fig. 20.4). Sagittal plane examination of the multifidus is performed at the paraspinal region approximately visualizing the area of the lumbar facet joints (Fig. 20.5). Preferential activation of the lumbar multifidus muscle may be carried out through the use of visualization instructional techniques of the action to be performed to induce a near isolated contraction of the muscle at the desired segment [60].

The studies done by Henry [20] and that of Worth [63] were able to note that the use of ultrasound imaging showed better reproducibility in performing abdominal drawing-in maneuvers or abdominal hallowing activities with lesser number of repetitions to perform effectively as compared to just using the verbal and tactile feedback done in most clinics. However, the data on both studies was inconclusive as to the retention of the skill. Teyhen et al. [54] had contrasting findings of no improvement of preferential activation of the transversus abdominis in a 4-day period. A systematic review of 36 articles by Ghamkar et al. [17] revealed that ultrasound imaging had good reliability and validity in differentiating a healthy subject from one suffering from low back pain, as well as in monitoring rehabilitation outcome measures. However, the ability of ultrasound imaging to provide a diagnosis (i.e., spinal stenosis, disc herniation, soft tissue pathology, etc.) of the low back pain based on pathological features on sonoanatomy did not allow for defini-

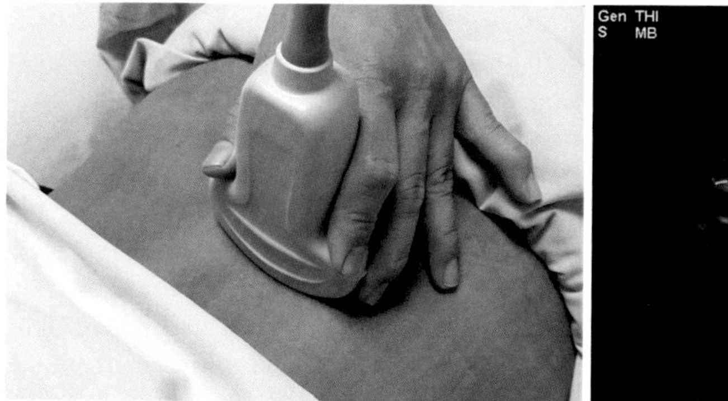
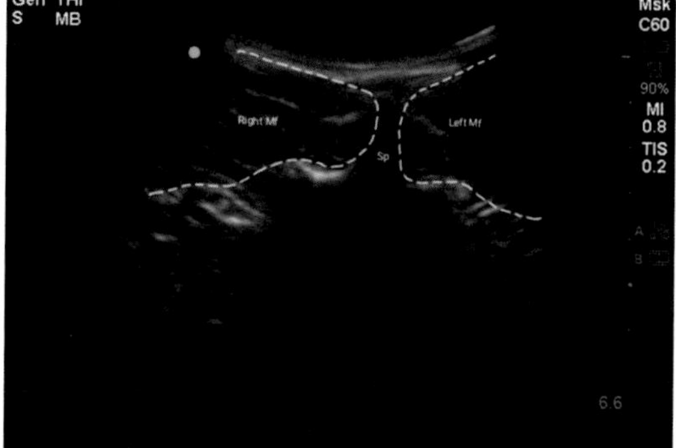

Fig. 20.4 Ultrasound transducer placement for evaluation of the multifidus muscles (Mf) in transverse or short-axis view [60]. Sp lumbar spinous process

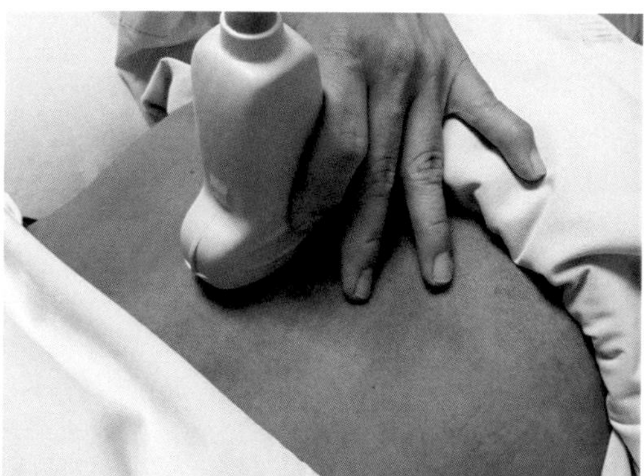
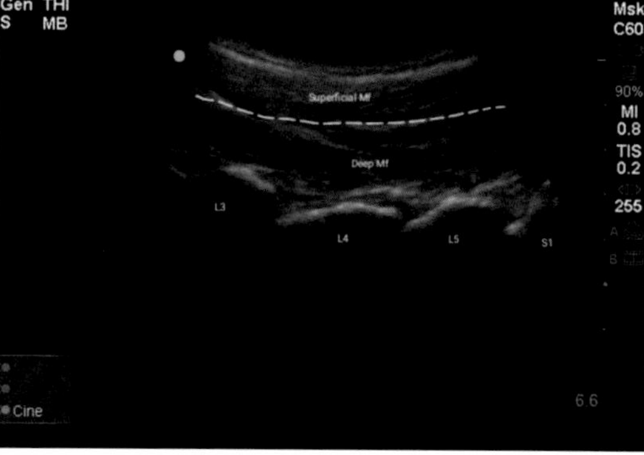

Fig. 20.5 Ultrasound transducer placement for evaluation of the multifidus muscles (Mf) in longitudinal or long-axis view [60]. S1 sacral vertebra, L3–L5 lumbar vertebra levels 3–5

tive conclusion because of the very low diagnostic capability at the spinal area [55]. The varying results on the benefits of ultrasound scanning in patients with low back pain may be attributed to the heterogeneity of sample population as well as the differences in the testing or scanning protocols.

The challenge with engaging on core muscle training is taking into consideration the complex nature of trunk control, stability, and mobility. There may be a paradox involved when a patient is instructed to relax the internal and external abdominal obliques while at the same time trying to contract the transversus abdominis muscle. Also, an individual may also be disoriented if a coordinated contraction of the different muscle groups is required to be done. Eyal Lederman [37] has warned that core exercises may contribute to the development of continuous and abnormal patterns of trunk muscle use resulting in the development of symptoms. There is strong evidence to support that stabilization exercises help in the short-term management of low back pain as compared to regular exercises, but is not particularly beneficial with regard to addressing long-term disability [11, 50, 57]. It should therefore be stressed that core programs should be used judiciously and only as an adjunct to other interventions in addressing a patient with low back pain.

Ultrasound in Neurodynamics

Special tests in physical examination such as the slump test, the straight leg raise test, and even the brachial plexus tension test have pointed to the concept of "neural tension" as a biomechanical source of pain especially during nerve impingement as suggested by David Butler [6]. Ellis and Hing [14] state that it is vital that the nerves are in a position to adapt to mechanical loads by undergoing mechanical processes like elongation, sliding, cross-sectional change, angulation, and compression. Otherwise, the nerves would be susceptible to neural edema, hypoxia, ischemia, and fibrosis in the event of failure of the dynamic protective mechanisms to function.

The treatment of nerve impingement using ultrasound in recent years has mostly been done through nerve hydrodissection or hydrorelease, which is a process of separating the nerve from the surrounding fascia and tissues [8]. Prior to the advent of nerve hydrodissection, physiotherapists have long been employing a similar concept through a series of mobilization and exercise to help relieve the symptoms of nerve impingement in patients who are averse to surgical intervention [4, 35, 36]. Michael Shacklock [49] defines *neurodynamics* as a form of mobilization, exercise, and positional treatment mostly for pain management by addressing the interaction between neural tissue and its surrounding structures by evoking both a mechanical and physiological response that affects neural sensitivity. The mechanical responses include changes in neural movement or sliding, neural tension, intraneural pressure changes, viscoelastic function, and alterations in the cross-sectional shape of the nerve. The physiological responses involve sympathetic activation and alterations in intraneural blood flow, impulse traffic, and axonal transport.

The advent of the use of ultrasound imaging in dynamic, real-time assessment of the nerves has provided a means by which to document the nerve excursion through neurodynamics. A systematic review of 18 studies which was done by Kasehagen et al. [33] revealed moderate reliability in using ultrasound imaging to measure the excursion of the median, sciatic, and tibial nerves; high to very high reliability in measuring the common fibular nerve excursion; and moderate to high reliability for assessing the radial nerve excursion. The clinical implications of this paper show that ultrasound imaging can help assess and document impingement of specific nerves as well as suggest the type of neural mobilization to be undertaken.

Treatment with neurodynamics is initially carried out passively through limb or body positioning and through mobilizations carried out by a therapist. These mobilization techniques have been classified as either "tensioners" or "sliders" [9]. Neural "tensioner" acts to lengthen the nerve bed. It is performed very similarly to the various limb tensioning tests where the sensitivity of the nerve is reproduced by placing both ends of a joint, through which the nerve in question traverses the limb, away from each other in a stretched position. A neural "slider" is performed by placing one joint end into a stretched position, while the other joint end is in a slack position. The alternating stretch-slack of both joint ends going to the same direction would produce an excursion or gliding motion of the nerve which is also called "neural flossing." Moksha et al. [40] conducted a study on 60 patients with nonspecific low back pain who underwent neurodynamic mobilization. It was revealed that neural sliders produced a significant reduction in pain severity and disability scores as compared to performing neural tensioner techniques.

In a meta-analysis conducted by Basson et al. [3] pertaining to the effectiveness of performing neural mobilizations for neuromusculoskeletal conditions, it was found that:

- Slump and straight leg raise techniques for neural mobilization are recommended in improving nerve-related low back pain severity and disability scores (level A evidence).
- Cervical lateral glide techniques for neural mobilization are recommended for improving nerve-related neck and arm pain severity (level A evidence).
- There were no significant positive effects for conducting neural mobilization for patients with carpal tunnel syndrome (level A evidence). It was noted, however, that sliding techniques resulted in the reduction of intraneural edema and improvement in pain and function.
- No definite recommendations could be derived on performing neural mobilization for lateral epicondylalgia, although one study with low risk of bias showed improvement of pain with cervical lateral glide technique.
- Straight leg raise technique for neural mobilization is recommended for tarsal tunnel syndrome and plantar heel pain based on two studies with low risk of bias.

Ultrasound imaging is able to monitor the neural excursion in real time especially when a patient is progressed to actively perform the neural mobilization movements themselves. The imaging is carried out with the transducer placed in a longitudinal or long-axis orientation in relation to the level of interest of the nerve to be examined, and the extremity chain is moved accordingly while monitoring for nerve excursion (Fig. 20.6). A study conducted by Richard Ellis [13] noted that the excursion of the sciatic nerve was greatest toward the mid to late ranges of performance of the neural mobilization. An in vivo cross-sectional study conducted by Coppieters et al. [10] revealed markedly different sciatic nerve excursions for neurodynamic techniques combining movements for the hip and the knee. In another in vivo study to determine if spinal posture had an effect on sciatic nerve excursion, it was found that changes in spinal posture have little effect on sitting-based neural mobilization exercises for the sciatic nerve in healthy

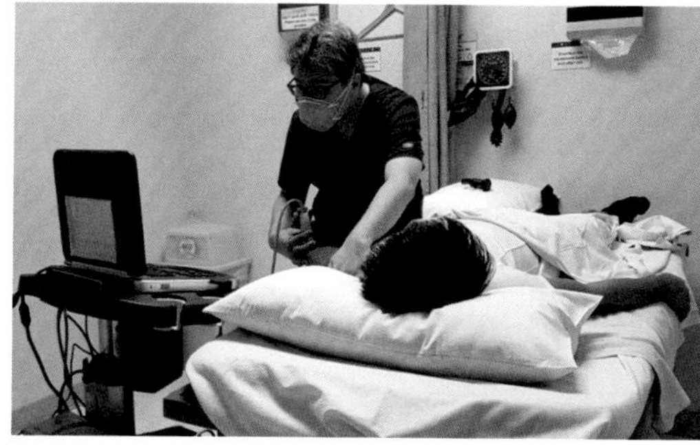

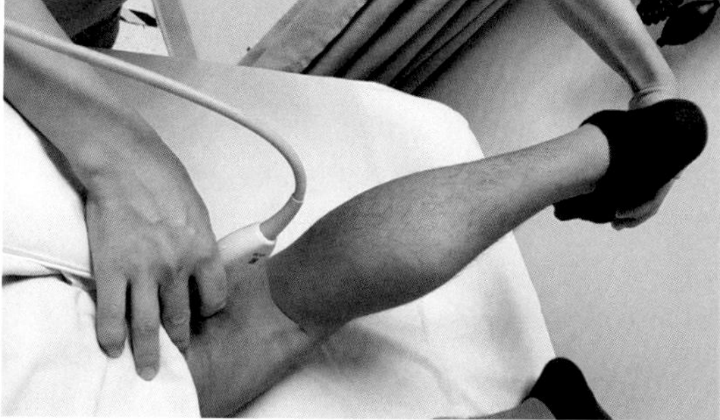

Fig. 20.6 Sonologist positioning and ultrasound probe placement while conducting neural flossing of the median nerve (*left*) and neural mobilization of the sciatic nerve (*right*)

subjects [15]. These are the few studies which provide an insight on ultrasound as an imaging tool in monitoring the treatment of a patient especially when adjusting the manner in which the neural mobilization is to be carried out. However, it is highly advised that further research is required before definitive recommendations on its feedback utilization can be made.

Other Applications of Ultrasound in Exercise

The chapter has mainly focused on ultrasound-guided exercises for the core trunk muscles as well as for its application in neurodynamics due to the growing number of researches in the field. Nevertheless, it must be noted that there are other emerging areas in rehabilitation and physiotherapy where ultrasound imaging is slowly gaining recognition. Jopowicz et al. [31] reviewed some papers addressing scapular dysfunction in shoulder pain through the assessment of the involved scapular muscles. Rosińska et al. [46] proposed a post-operative Achilles tendon rehabilitation through the assessment of tendon gliding and of feedback on gastrocnemius muscle activity. Khoshkhoo et al. [34] conducted sonographic examinations on the effect of strength training to the vastus medialis obliquus (VMO) of the knee. The application in most of these studies is similar to how ultrasound is applied to the core trunk muscles where the characteristic of the muscle contraction is monitored and adjusted accordingly.

The development of shear-wave elastography to grade soft tissue tension or stiffness has recently been gaining popularity in rehabilitation [27]. Elastography not only has the potential to monitor tendon healing, but it may also predict the active and passive forces that a muscle generates as derived from its stiffness [28]. It is no wonder that elastography has already undergone a study to monitor the activity of the transversus abdominis during exercises [24]. One area of focus on research on elastography is on the diagnosis of myofascial pain syndrome, where Quintner et al. [43] argue the validity of the diagnosis as there is still no objective measure to document the so-called myofascial trigger points. The studies of Stecco et al. [51] and of Turo and Otto [56] have started to foray on using elastography to map out muscles where the trigger points may be present. This has the potential to aid in the monitoring and planning for intervention of these muscles which would include tension control as well as relaxation techniques. The use of elastography is not limited to the musculoskeletal system as a systematic review conducted by Wee and Simon [58] showed that peripheral neuropathies have presented with increased stiffness regardless of the etiology. This, in turn, has generated studies on its application to monitor neurodynamic treatments to the median nerve [48] and sciatic nerve [41].

Conclusion

It can be deduced by conventional analysis that the most common symptom for patients who undergo a musculoskeletal ultrasound scan is the symptom of pain. The International Association for the Study of Pain (IASP) defines pain as "an unpleasant sensory and emotional experience associated with actual or potential tissue damage, or described in terms of such damage" [39]. It can be inferred that pain does not necessarily require an injury to precede the occurrence of symptoms. It also means that pain, especially in non-traumatic conditions, is more likely to be multifactorial in origin which, at times, may not be necessarily reflected by imaging procedures like ultrasonography [7]. The fact that pain is also considered a form of "experience," it is paramount that contextual factors around any treatment options to be employed are considered carefully. It is, therefore, in the patient's best interest to carry out an individualized, multi-modal, and biopsychosocial form of treatment in which ultrasound guidance is just one of the options to be considered to provide variation, novelty, and engagement in the performance of exercises, as well as to enhance the therapeutic alliance between the patient and the clinician.

The premise by which ultrasound imaging may improve outcomes in rehabilitation is through its ability to measure neuromuscular dysfunction and as a tool for the provision of feedback [25]. It has shown good reliability in determining changes in neuromuscular morphology and function, as well as fair reliability in determining the presence of pathology in the core trunk muscles and the peripheral nerves [25]. The evidence to date is still inconclusive on the use of musculoskeletal ultrasound to help guide the various therapeutic exercises used in the rehabilitation of a patient. Further research in this area is still highly recommended to refine the manner of its usage. The evidence, at best, suggests that feedback through the use of ultrasound guidance imaging may be employed at the early stages of treatment and only as an adjunct to other high-quality options as recommended by best practice guidelines. For long-term management, its utilization should be limited to the occasional monitoring of treatment especially in refractory cases in order to avoid dependency to the procedure and to improve resilience to the condition at hand.

Acknowledgment Peter Esselbach, BPhty, BSc (Hons), Assoc Dip App Sc (Med US)

Rodiel Kirby Baloy, PT, EdS, DPT, MS

Franklin Domingo, MD, FPARM, RMsk

Paolo Belleza

Capt. Danilo Obispo

Asian Hospital and Medical Center (Department of Physical Medicine and Rehabilitation)

References

1. Akbari A, Khorashadizadeh S, Abdi G. The effect of motor control exercise versus general exercise on lumbar local stabilizing muscles thickness: randomized controlled trial of patients with chronic low back pain. J Back Musculoskelet Rehabil. 2008;21:105–12.
2. Akuthota V, Nadler SF. Core strengthening. Arch Phys Med Rehabil. 2004;85:86–92.
3. Basson A, Olivier B, Ellis R, et al. The effectiveness of neural mobilization for neuromusculoskeletal conditions: a systematic review and meta-analysis. J Orthop Sports Phys Ther. 2017;47(9):593–615.
4. Boyd BS, Nee RJ, Smoot B. Safety of lower extremity neurodynamic exercises in adults with diabetes mellitus: a feasibility study. J Man Manip Ther. 2017;25(1):30–8.
5. Brumagne S, Cordo P, Lysens R, Verschueren S, Swinnen S. The role of paraspinal muscle spindles in lumbosacral position sense in individuals with and without low back pain. Spine. 2000;25(8):989–94.
6. Butler DS. Adverse mechanical tension in the nervous system: a model for assessment and treatment. Aust J Physiother. 1989;35(4):227–38.
7. Cadogan A, McNair PJ, Laslett M, Hing WA. Diagnostic accuracy of clinical examination and imaging findings for identifying subacromial pain. PLoS One. 2016;11(12):e0167738.
8. Cass SP. Ultrasound-guided nerve hydrodissection what is it? A review of the literature. Curr Sports Med Rep. 2016;15(1):20–2.
9. Coppieters MW, Butler DS. Do 'sliders' slide and 'tensioners' tension? An analysis of neurodynamic techniques and considerations regarding their application. Man Ther. 2008;13(3):213–21.
10. Coppieters MW, Andersen LS, Johansen R, et al. Excursion of the sciatic nerve during nerve mobilization exercises: an in vivo cross-sectional study using dynamic ultrasound imaging. J Orthop Sports Phys Ther. 2015;45(10):731–7.
11. Coulombe BJ, Games KE, Neil ER, Eberman LE. Core stability exercise versus general exercise for chronic low back pain. J Athl Train. 2017;52(1):71–2.
12. Dussik KT, Fritch DJ, Kyriazidou M, Sear RS. Measurements of articular tissues with ultrasound. Am J Phys Med. 1958;37:160–5.
13. Ellis RF. Neurodynamic evaluation of the sciatic nerve during neural mobilisation: ultrasound imaging assessment of sciatic nerve movement and the clinical implications for treatment (PhD thesis, Auckland University of Technology, Auckland, New Zealand). 2011. Retrieved from http://hdl.handle.net/10292/3402.
14. Ellis RF, Hing WA. Neural mobilization: a systematic review of randomized controlled trials with an analysis of therapeutic efficacy. J Manual Manipulat Ther. 2008;16(1):8–22.
15. Ellis R, Osborne S, Whitfield J. The effect of spinal position on sciatic nerve excursion during seated neural mobilisation exercises: an in vivo study using ultrasound imaging. J Manual Manipulat Ther. 2017;25(2):98–105.
16. Fatoye F, Gebrye T, Odeyemi I. Real-world incidence and prevalence of low back pain using routinely collected data. Rheumatol Int. 2019;39(4):619–26.
17. Ghamkhar L, Emami M, Mohseni-Bandpei MA, Behtash H. Application of rehabilitative ultrasound in the assessment of low back pain: a literature review. J Bodywork Movement Ther. 2011;15:465–777.
18. Giggins OM, Persson UM, Caulfield B. Biofeedback in rehabilitation. J Neuroeng Rehabil. 2013;10:60.
19. Hayden JA, Wilson MN, Stewart S, et al. Exercise treatment effect modifiers in persistent low back pain: an individual participant data meta-analysis of 3514

participants from 27 randomised controlled trials. Br J Sports Med. 2020;54(21):1277–78.
20. Henry SM, Westervelt KC. The use of real-time ultrasound feedback in teaching abdominal hollowing exercises to healthy subjects. J Orthop Sports Phys Ther. 2005;35:338–45.
21. Hides JA, Stokes MJ, Saide M, Jull GA, Cooper DH. Evidence of lumbar multifidus muscle wasting ipsilateral to symptoms in patients with acute/subacute low back pain. Spine. 1994;19:165–72.
22. Hides JA, Richardson CA, Jull GA. Multifidus muscle recovery is not automatic after resolution of acute, first-episode low back pain. Spine. 1996;21:2763–9.
23. Hides JA, Jull GA, Richardson CA. Long-term effects of specific stabilizing exercises for first-episode low back pain. Spine. 2001;26:E243–8.
24. Hirayama K, Akagi R, Moniwa Y, et al. Transversus abdominis elasticity during various exercises: a shear wave ultrasound elastography study. Int J Sports Phys Ther. 2017;12(4):601–6.
25. Hodges P. Ultrasound imaging in rehabilitation: just a fad? J Orthop Sports Phys Ther. 2005;35(6):333–7.
26. Hodges PW, Moseley GL. Pain and motor control of the lumbopelvic region: effect and possible mechanisms. J Electromyogr Kinesiol. 2003;13:361–70.
27. Hug F. Advancing musculoskeletal rehabilitation using elastography. ASPETAR Sports Med J. 2016;5(1):166–71.
28. Hug F, Tucker K, Gennisson J, et al. Elastography for muscle biomechanics: toward the estimation of individual muscle force. Exerc Sport Sci Rev. 2015;43(3):125–33.
29. Ikai M, Fukunaga T. Calculation of muscle strength per unit cross-sectional area of human muscle by means of ultrasonic measurement. Int Z Angew Physiol Einschl Arbeitsphysiol. 1968;26:26–32.
30. Jielile J, Badalihan A, Qianman B, et al. Clinical outcome of exercise therapy and early post-operative rehabilitation for treatment of neglected Achilles tendon rupture: a randomized study. Knee Surg Sports Traumatol Arthrosc. 2016;24:2148–55.
31. Jopowicz R, Jopowicz M, Czarnocki Ł, et al. Current uses of ultrasound imaging in musculoskeletal rehabilitation. Ortop Traumatol Rehabil. 2017;19(6):503–11.
32. Kane D, Grassi W, Sturrock R, Balint PV. A brief history of musculoskeletal ultrasound: 'From bats and ships to babies and hips'. Rheumatology (Oxford). 2004;43(7):931–3.
33. Kasehagen B, Ellis R, Pope R, et al. Assessing the reliability of ultrasound imaging to examine peripheral nerve excursion: a systematic literature review. Ultrasound Med Biol. 2018;44(1):1–13.
34. Khoshkhoo M, Killingback A, Robertson CJ, Adds PJ. The effect of exercise on vastus medialis oblique muscle architecture: an ultrasound investigation. Clin Anat. 2016;29(6):752–8.
35. Koulidis K, Veremis Y, Anderson C, Heneghan NR. Diagnostic accuracy of upper limb neurodynamic tests for the assessment of peripheral neuropathic pain: a systematic review. Musculoskelet Sci Pract. 2019;40:21–33.
36. Lau YN, Ng J, Lee SY, et al. A brief report on the clinical trial on neural mobilization exercise for joint pain in patients with rheumatoid arthritis. Z Rheumatol. 2019;78(5):474–8.
37. Lederman E. The myth of core stability. J Bodyw Mov Ther. 2010;14:84–98.
38. McDonald D, Leopold G. Ultrasound B-scanning in the differentiation of Baker's cyst and thrombophlebitis. Br J Radiol. 1972;45:729–32.
39. Merskey H, Bogduk N. Classification of chronic pain. In: IASP task force on taxonomy. 2nd ed. Seattle: IASP Press; 1994.
40. Moksha J, Medha D, Swati M. Effectiveness of sliders vs tensioners on pain and disability in nonspecific low back pain with associated lower limb symptoms: a pretest posttest experimental study. Int J Health Sci Res. 2019;9(9):46–52.
41. Neto T, Freitas SR, Andrade RJ, et al. Shear wave elastographic investigation of the immediate effects of slump neurodynamics in people with sciatica. J Ultrasound Med. 2020;39(4):675–81.
42. Porterfield JA, DeRosa C. Mechanical low back pain: perspectives in functional anatomy. 2nd ed. Philadelphia: WB Saunders; 1998.
43. Quintner JL, Bove GM, Cohen ML. A critical evaluation of the trigger point phenomenon. Rheumatology (Oxford). 2015;54(3):392–9.
44. Ribeiro DC, Sole G, Abbott JH, Milosavljevic S. Extrinsic feedback and management of low back pain: a critical review of the literature. Man Ther. 2011;16(3):231–9.
45. Richardson C, Jull G, Hodges P, Hides J. Therapeutic exercise for spinal segmental stabilization in low back pain: scientific basis and clinical approach. Edinburgh: Churchill Livingstone; 1999.
46. Rosińska AB, Ciszkowska-Łysoń B, Śmigielski R. Original algorithm of rehabilitation protocol with use of ultrasound – study based on Achilles tendon reconstruction cases. Orthop J Sports Med. 2014;2(3 Suppl):2325967114S00167.
47. Schmidt RA, Wrisberg CA. Motor learning and performance: a situation-based learning approach. 4th ed. Champaign: Human Kinetics; 2008. p. 395.
48. Schrier VJMM, Lin J, Gregory A, et al. Shear wave elastography of the median nerve: a mechanical study. Muscle Nerve 2020. https://doi.org/10.1002/mus.26863. [Epub ahead of print].
49. Shacklock M. Neurodynamics. Physiotherapy. 1995;81(1):9–16.
50. Smith BE, Littlewood C, May S. An update of stabilisation exercises for low back pain: a systematic review with meta-analysis. BMC Musculoskelet Disord. 2014;15:416.
51. Stecco A, Pirri C, Caro R, Raghavan P. Stiffness and echogenicity: development of a stiffness-echogenicity matrix for clinical problem solving. Eur J Transl Myol. 2019;29(3):8476.

52. Tate JJ, Milner CE. Real-time kinematic, temporospatial, and kinetic biofeedback during gait retraining in patients: a systematic review. Phys Ther. 2010;90(8):1123–34.
53. Teyhen D. Rehabilitative ultrasound imaging symposium San Antonio, TX, May 8-10, 2006. J Orthop Sports Phys Ther. 2006;36:A1–3.
54. Teyhen D, Miltenberger C, Deiters H, et al. The use of ultrasound imaging of the abdominal drawing-in maneuver in subjects with low Back pain. J Orthop Sports Phys Ther. 2005;35:346–55.
55. Todorov P, Nestorova R, Batalov A. Diagnostic value of musculoskeletal ultrasound in patients with low back pain – a review of the literature. Med Ultrason. 2018;20(1):80–7.
56. Turo D, Otto P. Shear wave elastography for characterizing muscle tissue in myofascial pain syndrome. J Acoust Soc Am. 2013;133(5):3358.
57. Wang XQ, Zheng JJ, Yu ZW. A meta-analysis of core stability exercise versus general exercise for chronic low back pain. PLoS One. 2012;7(12):e52082. https://doi.org/10.1371/journal.pone.0052082. Epub 2012 Dec 17.
58. Wee TC, Simon NG. Ultrasound elastography for the evaluation of peripheral nerves: a systematic review. Muscle Nerve. 2019;60(5):501–12.
59. Whittaker J. Abdominal ultrasound imaging of pelvic floor muscle function in individuals with low back pain. J Manual Manipulat Ther. 2004;12(1):44–9.
60. Whittaker J. Ultrasound imaging for rehabilitation of the lumbopelvic region: a clinical approach. Edinburgh: Churchill Livingstone; 2007.
61. Whittaker JL, Teyhen DS, Elliott JM, Cook K, Langevin HM, Dahl HH, et al. Rehabilitative ultrasound imaging: understanding the technology and its applications. J Orthop Sports Phys Ther. 2007;37(8):434–49.
62. Whittaker J, Thompson J, Teyhen D, Hodges P. Rehabilitative ultrasound imaging of pelvic floor muscle function. J Orthop Sports Phys Ther. 2007;37(8):487–98.
63. Worth SA, Henry SM, Bunn JY. Real-time ultrasound feedback and abdominal hollowing exercises for people with low back pain. NZ J Physiother. 2007;35(1):4–11.
64. Young A, Hughes I, Russell P, et al. Measurement of quadriceps muscle wasting by ultrasonography. Rheumatology. 1980;19(3):141–8.

21 Evolution of Sports Ultrasound

Jeffrey Smith, Allison N. Schroeder, Alexander R. Lloyd, and Kentaro Onishi

Introduction

The history of ultrasound (US) in sports medicine dates back to the 1940s when it was first used as a diagnostic imaging modality by Karl Dussik to image brain tumors [1]. That application expanded into musculoskeletal (MSK) evaluation in 1958 when US was used to measure the attenuation of articular and periarticular tissues [2]. The technology and image quality further improved over the following decade, eventually leading to a paper documenting the ability to differentiate a Baker's cyst from thrombophlebitis [3]. From here, the use of US in athletes expanded beyond the MSK system. Echocardiography was first used in the 1970s to measure left ventricular end-diastolic volume and ventricular wall thickness and mass in an effort to diagnose athletic heart syndrome [4].

Ultrasound's progress was eclipsed in the 1970s and 1980s by computed tomography (CT) and magnetic resonance imaging (MRI), both of which became the advanced imaging technologies of choice for the evaluation of MSK and sports medicine conditions. CT was most useful in identifying bony pathology typically missed on plain films including stress fractures and small intra-articular fractures. MRI became popular for its ability to delineate soft tissues better than any existing imaging technique [5–12]. Despite its early promise, the subpar spatial resolution and operator dependency of US during this period relegated it to a few specific applications outside of the MSK system.

However, further technological progress in the 1980s and 1990s led to renewed interest in applying US to the MSK system, particularly for muscle, ligament, and tendon pathology [13–16]. Rheumatologists were the first to widely adopt diagnostic US use and were the first to deploy it for procedural guidance during joint aspiration [17, 18]. Orthopedic surgeons soon recognized the value of US after several papers correlated sonographically identified rotator cuff pathology with arthrography [19] and postoperative function [20]. Subsequent studies documenting the superiority of US compared to standard radiographs in the diagnosis of transient synovitis of the hip in children also strengthened the case for its utility [21, 22].

The publication of the first MSK US textbooks in the 1990s led to broader awareness of the ways US could be used for diagnostic evaluation and interventional procedures in sports medicine and orthopedics [23, 24]. US was subsequently shown

J. Smith · A. R. Lloyd
University of Pittsburgh Medical Center, Department of PM&R, Pittsburgh, PA, USA
e-mail: smithjd7@upmc.edu

A. N. Schroeder
University of Pittsburgh Medical Center, Pittsburgh, PA, USA
e-mail: schroederan2@upmc.edu

K. Onishi (✉)
University of Pittsburgh Medical Center, Department of PM&R and Orthopedic Surgery, Pittsburgh, Pennsylvania, USA

Y. El Miedany (ed.), *Musculoskeletal Ultrasound-Guided Regenerative Medicine*, https://doi.org/10.1007/978-3-030-98256-0_21

to make injections more accurate than similar injections done with landmark guidance for most peripheral joint and soft tissue injections, further boosting its popularity [25]. With increased interest, US imaging evolved in the early twenty-first century as spatial resolution improved and portability increased [26]. Between 2000 and 2009, there was a 316% increase in procedural use of MSK US [27].

Today, the term "sports US" refers to the use of US for both diagnostic and therapeutic indications in sports medicine and includes the diagnostic and interventional use of US for MSK conditions as well as the diagnostic use of US to evaluate non-MSK conditions in athletes [28–32]. The recent development of US-guided procedures indicates the ongoing interest in applying this technology to improve upon current procedural techniques [33–35]. This chapter will describe the current utility of diagnostic and interventional US in sports medicine. It will also review uses of US in procedures and emerging technologies addressing current limitations in US imaging.

Diagnostic Ultrasound in Sports Medicine

Advantages of Diagnostic Ultrasound in Sports Medicine

There are a number of advantages of diagnostic US compared to other imaging modalities such as x-ray, MRI, and CT (see Table 21.1). With increasing portability, US can be brought to the training rooms, injury clinics, or even athletic events to assist in a timely diagnosis and proper triaging for sports injuries from every organ system [36–40]. Advances in telecommunications, such as fifth-generation (5G) wireless, allow ultrasound scanning to be remotely guided by an experienced practitioner and real-time dynamic imaging for faster diagnosis [41, 42].

US also offers high spatial resolution of soft tissue and neurovascular pathology. A 10 Mhz US probe can achieve axial in-plane resolution of approximately 150 μm, significantly more than the resolution of common clinical MRI machines which only reach 450 μm [43]. One study compared MRI and US in detecting peripheral nerve pathology and found better sensitivity with US, while the two were equivalent in specificity [44]. Because of this high resolution, ultrasound has proven to be a cost-effective diagnostic tool for sports injuries, and if utilized for appropriate indications, it has been shown to potentially save billions of dollars [45–49]. Its real-time assessment allows for dynamic imaging of pathology that may be missed using static imaging such as CT or MRI [50, 51]. It has the benefit of providing imaging of the healthy contralateral side providing a control for comparison [52, 53].

Table 21.1 Advantages of diagnostic US

Advantages of diagnostic US
Portable
Superior spatial resolution over MRI for soft tissue and neurovascular imaging
Cost-effective
Real-time, dynamic imaging
Ease of side-to-side comparative study
Less ionization compared to radiographs and CT
Lack of artifact or distortion near metal hardware
Movement artifact does not impede evaluation
Real-time vascular imaging (Doppler, SMI)
Tissue characterization (shear wave elastography, strain elastography, US tissue characterization)

MRI magnetic resonance imaging, *CT* computerized tomography, *SMI* superb microvascular imaging, *US* ultrasound

Chronic musculoskeletal diseases such as knee OA, which are more prevalent in athletes, often require imaging to assess severity of disease [54, 55]. As the association of ionizing radiation exposure and cancer risk has become better understood, the potential for significant radiation exposure over athletes' lifetimes has raised concern [56–58]. Ultrasound can provide equivalent imaging for the assessment of disease progression, such as OA-associated pathology, without any of the risks from ionizing radiation exposure [59–61].

Due to higher prevalence of chronic musculoskeletal diseases, athletes are more prone to joint replacement during their lifetime than in the general population [55, 62, 63]. Evaluation of periprosthetic soft tissue can be difficult using CT or

MRI due to metal artifact obscuring structures [64, 65]. US is effective in detecting periprosthetic infections which are a leading cause of cause for revision of THAs and TKAs [66, 67]. Early identification of these infections to avoid revision due to septic loosening could reduce risk of prolonged postoperative pain due to septic joint replacement [68].

Ultrasound has the advantage of avoiding interference from motion artifact which are noted issues with CT and MRI assessment [69, 70]. It also has superior vascular imaging capability such as color and power Doppler which allow the identification of pathology such as muscle, tendon, and bone injury and permit the identification of vessels during ultrasound-guided procedures to limit complications [71, 72]. Neovascularization has been identified as a key finding in tendinosis, and advances in ultrasound technology such as superb microvascular imaging (SMI) have improved the identification of this pathology compared to color or power Doppler [73–75]. Other advances such as elastography or tissue characterization go beyond standard imaging with B mode and allow for a more thorough assessment of mechanical properties of soft tissues [76, 77].

Broad and Expanding Applicability of US Beyond Traditional MSK Applications

As discussed elsewhere in this book, US can be used to evaluate ligaments, muscles, nerves, tendons, and vessels at the point of care [78–80]. However, the use of US in the diagnosis and treatment of athletes has expanded beyond the MSK system. In a study of ultrasonography at the 2008 Beijing Olympics, US was found to be the imaging modality of choice in the Olympic village polyclinic and was most commonly used to evaluate abdominal complaints (41% of US exams performed) [81]. US's portability, real-time results, and accuracy made it an ideal tool for initial imaging at a large sporting event where transportation to local imaging facilities may be complicated or lead to delayed diagnosis. The use in imaging abdominal complaints highlights the technology's utility beyond evaluation of the MSK system.

US in Sports Medicine: Organ System Evaluation

Significant literature exists regarding the use of US for the evaluation of sports-related injuries. This section will highlight relevant organ systems and diagnoses for which US evaluation can be used in sports medicine and will include a discussion of the ways in which US evaluation can facilitate a more rapid and accurate diagnosis.

HEENT

Ocular Evaluation

Ocular examination with US is routinely used by radiologists, ophthalmologists, and emergency medicine physicians as a rapid, radiation-free, and accurate way to evaluate structures of the eye [82, 83]. Sports-related eye injuries account for approximately 1.5% of all sports injuries with higher rates in baseball, basketball, and racquet sports [84–87]. For some athletes, these injuries can lead to long-term vision loss [88]. US can serve as a triage tool on the sidelines to screen for severe eye injuries after trauma and is not hindered by hyphema or lid edema often present in these injuries.

Frequent pathologies seen in sports settings amenable to US evaluation include retinal detachment, retinal hemorrhage, and lens dislocation or subluxation (Fig. 21.1). Retinal detachment requires rapid diagnosis and referral for intervention and can be readily visualized with US[89]. Untreated, symptomatic retinal detachment can progress to complete detachment within days and can result in complete loss of vision. Given the low incidence of retinal detachment among eye injuries in athletes, US is especially useful for ruling out a detachment in the setting of acute vision changes [90–92]. Research has shown that non-radiology specialists can be trained to reliably use US for the identification of retinal

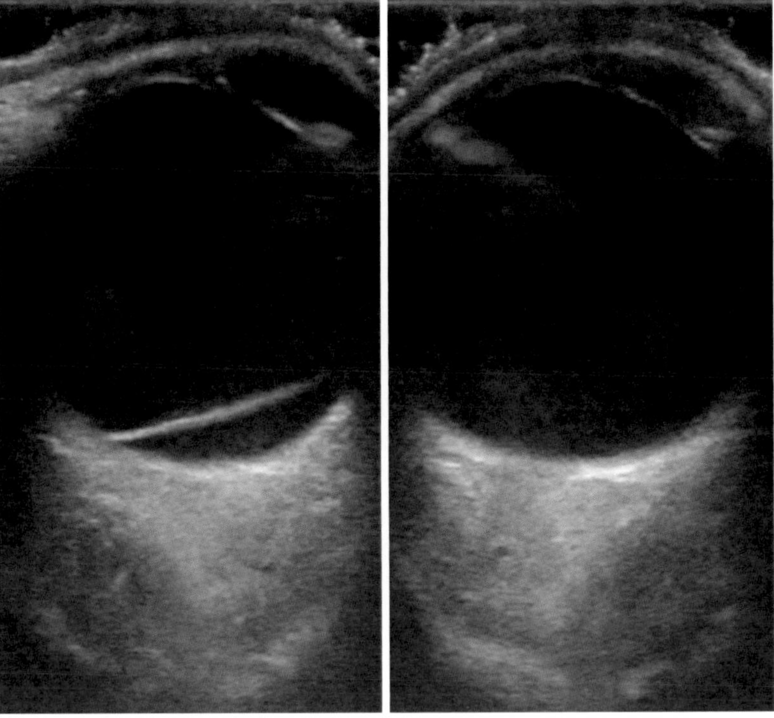

Fig. 21.1 Ocular US: globe on the left reveals a detached retina which is visualized as a hyperechoic line anterior to the posterior wall; the right is normal

detachment with sensitivity ranging from 97 to 100% and specificity from 83 to 100% [89, 93, 94]. Retinal hemorrhage and lens dislocation or subluxation can also be visualized during the same examination, facilitating rapid triage for emergent care and early warning to the emergency department if urgent ophthalmologic evaluation is needed [82].

Ocular US can also be used for an assessment of elevated intracranial pressure (ICP) after head trauma. The optic nerve sheath is contiguous with the dura mater and expands when ICP is elevated. This expansion can be seen on US [95, 96]. A meta-analysis reviewing studies that compared optic nerve sheath diameters on US to CTs with findings suggestive of intracranial compression suggested a cutoff of sheath diameter of 5mm in adults was 95.6% sensitive and 92.3% specific for elevated ICP [97].

Exercise-Induced Laryngeal Obstruction

Exercise-induced laryngeal obstruction (EILO), often referred to as vocal fold dysfunction, is an uncommon and likely underrecognized cause of breathing complaints in sport [98, 99]. The precise etiology is not well understood and is believed to have multiple independent causes that result in partial obstruction of the airway during exercise [99–101]. The presenting symptoms of EILO are very similar to those of exercise-induced asthma, resulting in frequent misdiagnosis [99, 101]. These symptoms include difficulty breathing, chest discomfort, wheezing, dry cough, and a feeling of throat constriction that doesn't respond to standard asthma treatment [102]. Fiber-optic video laryngoscopy is the gold standard for diagnosis, but requires specialized clinical space and equipment, which is often not available to sports medicine physicians, especially when symptoms are occurring [101]. Since symptoms may be context dependent and are transient, US offers the possibility of sideline evaluation and possible diagnosis while the athlete is symptomatic. One study demonstrated the ability to differentiate paradoxical vocal fold motion from normal vocal fold motion with US, but additional research is needed for confirmation [101].

Chest

Echocardiography

While rare, the most common cause of death in sport is sudden cardiac death [103]. These deaths are often preventable with adequate screening, but the type of screening and population to screen is debated [104, 105]. The history and physical exam (H&P) with or without electrocardiogram (EKG) are typically used as screening tools in the preparticipation evaluation (PPE) of athletes, but their effectiveness in disease identification is questioned [106]. A comprehensive review by Harmon et al. found that the pooled sensitivity for the history was 20% (range 7–44%) and 9% for the physical exam (range 3–24%). Both were more specific at 94% and 97%, respectively, but sole use of the H&P will likely omit athletes potentially at risk [106]. While EKG is both sensitive and specific at 94% (79–98%) and 93% (90–96%), respectively, it lacks portability and comes at a monetary cost [106]. Additionally, EKG may have a high false-positive rate, partly as a result of physiologic cardiac changes that occur in athletes and the variability in criteria used to define pathology in those settings [106, 107]. These false positives can exclude healthy athletes from play while subjecting them to prolonged and expensive workups [108, 109].

US has a long history of use in cardiology settings. While current data is insufficient to report well-defined sensitivity and specificity, some research has shown that echocardiography combined with EKG might decrease the false-positive rate and reduce the need for subsequent cardiology referrals [110–112]. One study of 3100 male soccer players who were screened with echocardiography found several cardiac anomalies missed by H&P and EKG, although most were mild valvular abnormalities with unclear clinical significance [113]. Severe abnormalities were rare in the study, and all that were present had an abnormal EKG [113].

The Early Screening for Cardiac Abnormalities with Preparticipation Echocardiography (ESCAPE) protocol was developed specifically to screen for the most concerning cardiac anomalies in athletes using US. It examines the end-diastolic interventricular septal thickness, left ventricular diameter, left ventricular wall thickness, and aortic root diameter [110, 114, 115]. Initial studies on this protocol have shown similar rates for the detection of anomalies between cardiologists and non-cardiologists [110, 116]. The role of screening echocardiography is still being debated and should not replace the H&P or EKG until more comprehensive and systematic research has been performed.

Rib Fracture and Pneumothorax

The etiology of chest pain after trauma can be difficult to determine acutely. Blunt trauma to the thorax can result in rib fracture, which is conventionally diagnosed with radiographs. However, US has been shown to be equivalent or superior to radiographs for rib fracture diagnosis, and its portability allows for rapid evaluation on the sideline or in the training room [117, 118]. On US evaluation, fracture is seen as a discontinuity in the usually smooth, hyperechoic contour of the rib [117].

Pneumothorax is a common sequelae of rib fractures and can be evaluated and diagnosed with US using several techniques [119]. The absence of lung sliding, absence of B lines, and presence of A lines indicate pneumothorax [119–121] (US findings described in Table 21.2) (Fig. 21.2). The absence of lung sliding and presence of A lines have a sensitivity and specificity of 94 and 95%, respectively, for the diagnosis of pneumothorax [119]. Evaluation can be per-

Table 21.2 US findings in the lung exam for pneumothorax. US, ultrasound

US in the lung exam for pneumothorax	
US findings	Description of finding
A lines	Repetitive reverberation artifact of the pleural line
B lines	Wide bands of hyperechoic artifact that originate at the pleural line and traverse the entire US screen in vertical orientation
Comet tail artifact	Short hyperechoic artifacts that originate at the pleural line and only traverse a portion of the screen in vertical orientation
Lung sliding	Parietal pleura sliding against visceral pleura with breathing

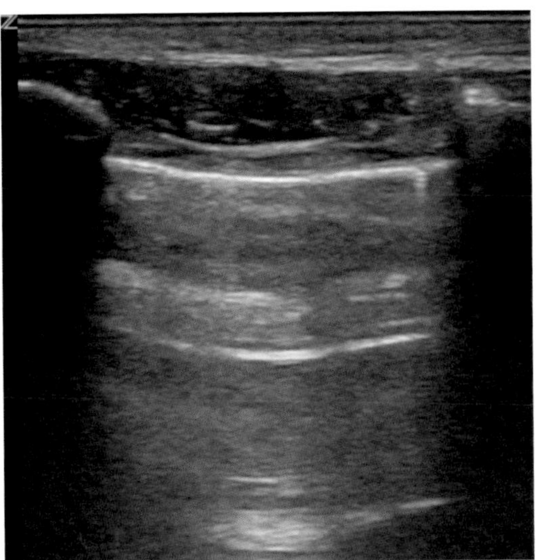

Fig. 21.2 Lung US: comet tail artifact in the upper right extending downward from the pleura; A lines are notable throughout the image; no B lines are present

formed by non-radiologists where x-ray equipment may not be readily available or ambient noise may be too loud to permit auscultation [121–123]. The diagnostic sensitivity and specificity of US evaluation are superior to upright anterior to posterior chest x-ray and similar to CT scan of the chest, which is the gold standard for the diagnosis of pneumothorax [90, 124]. The portability of US allows for point-of-care pneumothorax evaluation and rapid referral for care if present.

Abdomen

Extended FAST (eFAST)

The Focused Assessment with Sonography in Trauma (FAST) was developed in the 1990s to identify abnormal intraabdominal fluid or solid organ injury in the setting of blunt thoracoabdominal trauma [125, 126]. It includes evaluation for hemoperitoneum, liver injury, hemopericardium, pericardial or cardiac injury, and splenic or renal injury and should take the operator 5 minutes or less to perform [125, 127, 128]. The FAST examination was expanded to include the evaluation for pneumothorax and hemothorax and termed the extended FAST (or eFAST) examination. These exams can be performed rapidly, help to triage athletes, do not increase the time to intervention in the emergency department, and may decrease the number of missed life-threatening injuries [127]. However, further research is needed to support its use in sports-specific environments [29].

Splenomegaly Monitoring in Mononucleosis

Infectious mononucleosis is the clinical manifestation of Epstein-Barr viral infection. While common symptoms include fatigue and malaise, transient splenomegaly is the most concerning effect of mononucleosis for athletes [129, 130]. Splenic rupture is a rare, but potentially fatal, complication of return to sport in the setting of splenomegaly [130]. While contact sports are most commonly associated with reports of splenic rupture, rupture can rarely occur with significant Valsalva in non-contact sports [130]. As a result, athletes are often prevented from returning to play for 3 to 4 weeks after disease onset to ensure resolution of their transient splenomegaly [130].

US evaluation of the spleen has been proposed as a possible method to monitor splenomegaly and determine timing for safe return to play. However, there is significant interindividual sonographic variability of spleen size, making normal values difficult to establish [130, 131]. Without consistent baseline measurements, true splenomegaly is difficult to define and cannot guide return-to-play decisions as a result. It is possible that baseline measurements followed by serial scans would prove useful, but this is resource-intensive and likely impractical in many settings. More research is needed to determine the role of US in the evaluation of splenomegaly.

Abdominal Muscle Evaluation

Abdominal muscle pathology can often be visualized with US. Pathology can include herniation of abdominal musculature through its fascial plane or injury to the musculature itself with a resulting defect and herniation of fat or abdominal contents. Spigelian hernias are rare, occur at the edge of the rectus abdominis along the linea semilunaris, and may be difficult to identify with static imaging modalities [132, 133]. These hernias commonly contain fat, but can contain bowel and are seen on US protruding ventrally through the linea semilunaris with Valsalva [133]. Epigastric, umbilical, and incisional hernias can all be visualized as an outright defect in the abdominal wall or with ventral protrusion of abdominal contents with Valsalva [134]. Care should be taken to apply light transducer pressure when attempting to visualize herniation in these areas since it may be prevented or reduced with heavy pressure [135].

Injury to the abdominal musculature can also be visualized with US, including injury to the rectus abdominis, internal and external obliques, and transversus abdominis [136–139]. These injuries are often seen in throwers, who generate significant rotational forces in order to properly execute the throw [140]. These injuries appear on US as disruption of the fibrillar architecture of the muscle and areas of hypoechogenicity at the site of pain and are thought to represent hemorrhage, edema, and muscle fiber disruption [137].

Inguinal and Femoral Hernia Evaluation

US evaluation is often used to visualize hernias because they can be dynamically imaged during provocation maneuvers. Hernias may cause diffuse and nonspecific pain in the groin and lower abdomen, making it difficult to differentiate from other pain generators and difficult to diagnose based on physical exam alone [141, 142]. Inguinal hernias are most common in men and can be either indirect or direct [143]. Indirect hernias involve herniation of abdominal contents through the deep inguinal ring and are visualized on dynamic US as tissue extension lateral to the external iliac vessels or inferior epigastric vessels [133, 144]. Direct hernias involve herniation of abdominal contents directly through Hesselbach's triangle in the abdominal wall, and dynamic US evaluation will show abnormal anterior movement of tissue medial to the inferior epigastric vessels [133, 144].

Femoral hernias are the most common type of hernia in women [145]. They occur below the level of the inguinal ligament, and dynamic US evaluation will reveal superior to inferior herniation of abdominal contents into the femoral canal medial to the femoral neurovasculature and ventral to the pectineus muscle [133, 144].

Hernia Mimickers: Groin Pain in the Athlete

Evaluation of groin pain in the athlete should include examination of pain generators in the area, particularly if a true hernia is absent. "Sports hernia" and "athletic pubalgia" are ambiguous terms often used to describe groin pain in athletes and generally do not reflect a hernia of any kind. Instead, they encompass the broad differential of gastrointestinal, MSK, or neurologic pathologies that may cause groin pain, including intraarticular and periarticular hip joint pathology, musculotendinous injuries (including abdominals, hip adductors, and iliopsoas), inflammatory bowel disease, or nerve entrapment syndromes [146, 147]. US can help narrow this broad differential diagnosis through its ability to evaluate the abdominal wall musculature (as described above), the rectus abdominis/adductor plate, and the adductor tendon origin dynamically at high resolution [141, 146] [148]. Additionally, the iliopsoas can be scanned dynamically to evaluate for snapping iliopsoas tendon [149, 150]. Nerves that can contribute to groin pain, including genitofemoral nerve, obturator nerve, or medial femoral cutaneous nerve, can also be evaluated [151–153].

MSK

US evaluation of the MSK system is covered in extensive detail in Chaps. 5, 6, 7, 8, 9, 10, and 11 of this book. US is effective for the evaluation of a wide variety of MSK complaints, including major joints, muscles, tendons, and ligaments in the extremities [28].

Peripheral Nerve Injuries

Peripheral nerve injuries are believed to be rare in athletes but may just be underrecognized by clinicians [154]. Peripheral nerve injuries can contribute to significant pain and inability to return to play [155, 156]. While electrodiagnostic testing (EDX) is the most common method to localize and determine the nature of these lesions, diagnosis is often delayed by the one to several weeks it takes for EDX to be positive [157]. During this time, athletes may be symptomatic and unable to return to play without an accurate diagnosis to guide effective treatment. While US is not a substitute for EDX, it can assist in localizing nerve injury and facilitate diagnosis and early management [158, 159]. The development of high-resolution US (HRUS), typically defined as 12 MHz or greater depending on the depth of evaluation, allows for the evaluation of nerve or fascicle enlargement indicating compression or irritation and visualization of small nerves that would be difficult or impossible to evaluate with EDX and that may not be adequately visualized on MRI [158, 160–164]. US examination is also less painful than EDX testing and may be better tolerated than EDX. Finally, US can supplement EDX since EDX is a physiologic test that evaluates the strength and speed of nerve conductions, while US evaluates other characteristics such as morphology of the nerve and nerve fascicles or nerves' relationship to surrounding structures that might contribute to nerve irritation [165–172].

Characteristics of nerve injury seen on US include increased nerve or fascicle cross-sectional area due to edema, increased connective tissue formation from scarring, thickened and hyperechoic epineurium, or a hypoechoic internal appearance [169, 173, 174]. A study of nerve characteristics in peripheral nerve compression found increased transverse cross-sectional area (CSA) was most reliable for the diagnosis of nerve injury [175]. Several neuropathies that can be identified on US are described below, but this is not a comprehensive list, and research on peripheral nerve evaluation with US is ongoing.

Median Nerve

Carpal tunnel syndrome (CTS) is the most common mononeuropathy in the general population and is also common among wheelchair athletes [176, 177]. US has been used in the diagnosis of CTS and has shown sensitivity and specificity similar to EDX in several studies while also allowing immediate therapeutic injection or US-guided transverse carpal ligament release [178–183]. CSA of the median nerve at the inlet of the carpal tunnel has been found to be most sensitive and specific in diagnosing CTS [184]. While normal nerve size can vary and exact cutoffs are still debated, median nerve CSA between 9.0 and 12.6mm^2 measured at the inlet has been shown to have sensitivity of 81% and specificity of 84% [184]. The color Doppler, power Doppler sonography, and contrast-enhanced ultrasonography can be used to identify median nerve hyperemia in the acute stage of CTS [185–187]. Superb microvascular imaging (SMI) is a novel technology which allows improved visualization of flow of both small and large vessels without requiring contrast enhancement and may be more sensitive to detecting blood flow changes due to CTS [188, 189].

Ulnar Nerve

The second most common upper extremity neuropathy is ulnar entrapment, often at the ulnar groove of the cubital tunnel, less frequently caused by the humeroulnar arcade [190]. This occurs with compression or recurrent subluxation of the nerve. While entrapment at the elbow occurs most commonly in baseball players, it can occur at the hand or wrist, especially in Guyon's canal between the pisiform and the hook of hamate in wheelchair athletes, cyclists, and skiers [191, 192]. While EDX remains the gold standard for the localization of ulnar neuropathy, diagnostic accuracy improves when US is performed concomitantly [193, 194]. The normal ulnar nerve size varies between individuals and anatomic location, but some suggest a cutoff of 10 mm^2 or greater as a diagnostic of cubital tunnel syndrome [195]. One study of patients in whom EDX was unsuccessful in localization found all injury locations were identifiable with HRUS [196].

Sciatic Nerve Branches

The common fibular nerve is frequently injured through direct trauma in football, hockey, and soccer players as it is superficial and prone to trauma at the lateral knee near the fibular head [197]. It is also susceptible to repetitive stress in runners [198, 199]. The tibial nerve can be injured in combination with the fibular nerve in acute ligamentous knee injuries, dislocations, fractures, or entrapment in tarsal tunnel syndrome at the medial ankle [200]. Both nerves can be visualized at the posterior distal thigh and can be traced to determine if and where injury occurred, providing diagnostic value comparable to that of MRI [201–205].

Lateral Femoral Cutaneous Nerve

Meralgia paresthetica, or neuropathy of the lateral femoral cutaneous nerve, is another commonly discussed focal mononeuropathy described in gymnasts, baseball players, and soccer players [206–210]. Diagnosis of this injury with EDX is possible, but can be technically difficult and may be significantly limited by body habitus [211]. Multiple reports have demonstrated HRUS is useful in identifying nerve entrapment at the lateral end of the inguinal ligament and for performing guidance diagnostic blocks and pain relief [212, 213].

Brachial Plexus

The brachial plexus is a common area for neuropathic injury in sports, especially those involving blunt trauma [214]. While most brachial plexus injuries are "stingers" that cause transient motor and sensory symptoms, others like neurogenic thoracic outlet syndrome (nTOS) result can also result in injuries to brachial plexus structures [215]. nTOS is the most common type of thoracic outlet syndrome comprising more than 95% of cases and can result from cervical trauma or from repetitive overhead activities that result in relative hypertrophy of muscles such as the pectoralis minor that can compress the brachial plexus and cause symptoms consistent with lower trunk brachial plexopathy [216]. While still under debate, US may be useful in identifying anomalous fibromuscular bands, sometimes referred to as "Roos ligaments," compressing the lower trunk of the brachial plexus and causing nTOS [217]. It can also be useful in evaluating pectoral muscles for compression and tension placed upon the medial and lateral cord [218, 219]. Nerve compression between the clavicle, first rib, and scalene muscles due to muscle hypertrophy can cause brachial plexus compression and occurs more frequently among overhead athletes compared to the general population [220]. Ultrasound can identify the entrapment and guide anesthetic injection to the anterior scalene muscle to promote relaxation which correlates with good surgical outcomes [221, 222]. EDX can identify lesions that result in prolonged symptoms, but abnormalities will only appear after several weeks of persistent symptoms. US is capable of immediately visualizing nerve roots from the vertebral foramina through the trunks, divisions, cords, and branches to the axillary region, potentially providing earlier visualization of significant pathology and more rapid subsequent intervention although the clavicle can interrupt visualization from the supraclavicular area to the subpectoral area [223].

Vascular Injuries

While vascular injuries are uncommon in sports, they can cause significant symptoms in all extremities and should be considered when claudication symptoms are present. Vascular causes of exertional lower leg pain include external iliac artery endofibrosis and popliteal artery entrapment syndrome. External iliac artery endofibrosis results from intimal fibrosis of the arterial wall resulting in progressive stenosis and subsequent ischemic pain during exercise [224]. It is typically seen in endurance athletes such as cyclists and marathon runners [225]. Untreated, endofibrosis can lead to arterial dissection or thrombosis [226, 227]. US can be used to identify endofibrotic lesions, which appear as a segmental thickening of the intimal arterial wall with increased echogenicity of the arterial wall [228]. Doppler studies are normal at rest but show a decreased ankle brachial index (ABI) following exercise [229].

Popliteal artery entrapment occurs due to the compression of the artery by the anatomy of the gastrocnemius or popliteus muscles or dynamic compression by the soleus and can cause claudication symptoms [230, 231]. If undiagnosed, it can progress functional occlusion during activity, aneurysm, or thrombosis [232]. According to a meta-analysis, US Doppler ABI has a sensitivity of 90%, but specificity data is limited and may result in a high number of false-positive sonographic findings as a result [233]. This is supported by a study that found arterial occlusion induced with knee extension and subsequent plantarflexion and dorsiflexion in up to 50% of asymptomatic individuals [234].

Overhead athletes can also incur vascular injuries, especially aneurysms of the axillary artery and its branches including the posterior circumflex humeral artery (PCHA). This can lead to thrombosis or emboli causing subsequent digital ischemia [235–237]. Both symptomatic and asymptomatic volleyball players have been found to have PCHA aneurysms with a high prevalence of symptoms of digital ischemia thought to be secondary to microemboli [238, 239]. US has shown promise in the recognition of a PCHA aneurysm, which appears as a segmental vessel dilatation of greater than 50% compared to the closest normal-appearing vessel segment [240].

Overhead athletes are also susceptible to vasculogenic thoracic outlet syndrome, which can be of two forms: arterial thoracic outlet syndrome (aTOS) due to compression of the subclavian artery and venous thoracic outlet syndrome (vTOS) due to compression of the subclavian vein [241]. vTOS presents with fatigue or numbness that worsens when the arm is abducted and externally rotated [242, 243]. US has proven to have a role in diagnosis as episodes of occlusion have been identified by Doppler US, especially while observing during provocative maneuvers of the extremity [244, 245].

US in Sports Medicine: Physiologic Measures

US has been used experimentally to monitor physiologic parameters in an attempt to optimize training regimens and improve sports performance.

Muscle Glycogen

Evaluation of muscle glycogen content, an important source of energy for athletes, may help athletes evaluate their body's response to training stimuli and assist with nutrition decisions. This might subsequently help prevent fatigue and overtraining syndrome while helping athletes and coaches optimize competition, training, recovery, and nutrition strategies [246–248]. Currently, muscle biopsy is the gold standard for determining glycogen quantity, but this is an invasive and uncomfortable procedure that is unrealistic for use during training. An application called MuscleSound (MuscleSound LLC, Denver, CO) has been developed using US to quantify and correlate the water content of muscles with glycogen content. Two studies funded by MuscleSound LLC have shown a strong correlation between muscle biopsy and MuscleSound measured glycogen content [249, 250]. An independently funded study found poor correlation between glycogen quantity measured by MuscleSound when compared to muscle biopsy [251]. More research is needed on the validity of this technology before the utility of noninvasive measure of muscle glycogen content can be established.

Body Composition

Many athletes, especially those in weight-sensitive sports, monitor and attempt to modulate body composition to improve performance [252]. US has been identified as a tool to assist in determining body fat measurements by measuring the thickness of adipose tissue [253]. This could replace the traditional use of fat calipers, which lack accuracy due to tissue compression during measurement [254, 255]. US was shown to have a better inter-rater reliability than the use of calipers for measuring body fat composition, but US scanning protocols for body composition are still under development [256].

Tendon Stiffness

Prior muscle or tendon injury has been identified as one of the major risk factors in the recurrence of injury and thus has been examined as a factor in determining return to play. Identifying weakened tissue is important in both diagnosing injury and determining timing for safe return to play without risking reinjury. Elastography estimates tissue hardness and can be used to estimate the mechanical properties of tissues. This may, in turn, help with early identification of at-risk individuals, outcome tracking, and treatment monitoring [257]. There are three types of elastography: acoustic radiation force impulse elastography, compression (strain) elastography, and shear wave elastography. Unfortunately, technical issues such as a lack of standardization and insufficient data on the characteristics of normal versus diseased tissues still limit the wide use of elastography [257]. The types of elastography and their respective utility in sports medicine are highlighted below.

Acoustic radiation force impulse (ARFI) elastography uses focused acoustic beams to convert acoustic compression waves to shear waves by absorbing acoustic energy [258]. The reaction of tissue to this process is monitored within the range of excitation, and images are generated from sequential data collection with lateral movement at given positions. The speed of shear wave propagation outside the range of excitation is used to estimate the tissue shear modulus [259]. While ARFI elastography has been used extensively in hepatic imaging, it has only recently received investigation in musculoskeletal evaluation [258, 260, 261].

SE uses US imaging to measure the amount of deformation following manual compression. Software then converts tissue hardness into a color map on the US machine. It has been used to evaluate tendon pathology including Achilles tendon [262–264], patellar tendon [264], epicondylar tendons of the elbow [265–270], rotator cuff tendons [268, 271–274], and biceps tendon [275]. Most studies have found that pathologic tendons are softer than normal tendon, with only one study finding that pathologic Achilles tendons are stiffer than normal tendons [276]. Additionally, SE has been used to show that healing Achilles tendons postoperatively are stiffer than normal tendons [277, 278]. Further studies are needed to validate the inter- and intra-rater reliability of SE and determine its role in the diagnosis of tendon injury and its use for monitoring recovery [279].

SWE uses an acoustic radiation force pulse to generate shear waves that propagate perpendicular to the US beam and can be converted to a measure of density using Young's modulus [280]. SWE produces a more objective and quantitative assessment compared to strain elastography since the operator is not involved in stressing the tissues. Shear wave has been used to evaluate muscle, ligaments, and tendons [281, 282]. Findings have largely paralleled those seen with SE including softening of tendinopathic tendons [283, 284] and stiffening of post-surgical tendons [285]. SWE has also been used to monitor gastrocnemius, soleus, and Achilles tendon injuries and may be useful in guide return to play [286, 287]. As with SE, further studies on SWE are needed to validate inter- and intra-rater reliability and determine its role in the diagnosis of tendon injury, ability to monitor recovery, and usefulness in guiding return to play.

US tissue characterization (UTC) was developed to provide a standard assessment of tissue stiffness [77]. UTC utilizes a motorized device that guarantees a fixed US transducer position that obtains 600 contiguous transverse images in 45 seconds at intervals of 0.2 millimeters over a 12 centimeter distance to render a 3D block of US images [288]. After images are obtained, a complex algorithm characterizes each area of tendon into one of four echotypes based on pixel stability which is correlated to stiffness [288]. UTC has primarily been used for large tendons and ligaments, such as the Achilles tendon and patellar ligament [289–293]. Of note, the device used for standardized image acquisition in UTC has to be built specifically for each tendon. Similar to strain elastography (SE) and shear wave elastography (SWE), the role of UTC in the diagnosis of pathologic conditions and guiding return to play is yet to be determined, but shows promise in its ability to monitor the effect of load or treatment on tendon structure [77].

US in Sports Medicine: Guiding Return to Play

As discussed above, the improving portability of US and the ability to perform serial examinations make US an ideal imaging modality for guiding return-to-play decisions. Many physicians utilize

US both to immediately assess ability to return to play on the field (i.e., triage) and to help determine when an athlete is sufficiently healed to resume play. However, imaging criteria and published guidelines are lacking, and clinicians generally rely on a combination of clinical examination and functional performance measures correlated with imaging findings when returning athletes to sport. A few studies on muscle injuries in athletes have shown that evidence of disorganized fibrous tissue, intramuscular hematoma, intermuscular hematoma, and power Doppler signal on US examination predict longer time to return to play [294–296].

Interventional Use of Ultrasound for Procedural Guidance

Advantages of Interventional US in Sports Medicine

Ultrasound also has multiple advantages when used to assist with sports medicine procedures (see Table 21.3). If an interventional treatment is determined to be needed following diagnostic US, it can often be performed immediately after evaluation without the additional time delay required when obtaining an MRI or CT for diagnosis [80]. Injection accuracy is improved with the utilization of ultrasound for needle guidance for most structural targets [297, 298]. Doppler US can also be used to visualize blood vessels to evaluate vascular malformations as well as vascularity of soft tissue masses which can contribute to diagnosis [299–301]. The use of US guidance is even more important for advanced procedures such as barbotage and percutaneous fasciotomy and tenotomy (described in more detail below), which could not be performed accurately without US guidance [302–304]. Some US-guided interventions have additionally shown shorter recovery times with less post-procedural pain than open surgical procedures with similar clinical outcomes [305, 306]. Many peripheral nerve procedures exist and can relieve pain; however, they all require perineural needle placement which increases risk of nerve injury through intraneural injection or nerve penetration [307, 308].

Table 21.3 Advantages of interventional US

Advantages of interventional US
Immediate intervention following diagnosis
Improved accuracy of most injection procedures
Visualization of nearby vascular and neural structures to avoid inadvertent injuries
Conversion to less invasive interventions for traditionally operative interventions

The American Medical Society for Sports Medicine (AMSSM) has suggested that US-guided procedures can be divided into three different generations [309]. First-generation techniques are those that apply US guidance to improve accuracy of established procedures. Second-generation techniques are those that have been developed primarily as a result of US guidance and utilize commonly available needles. Examples include needle tenotomy for chronic or calcific tendinosis, neovessel ablation and tendon scraping, fenestration of the transverse carpal ligament, A1 pulley fenestration, and nerve hydrodissection. Third-generation techniques utilize specially designed surgical tools or devices to duplicate well-established surgical procedures under US guidance. These include A1 pulley release using a hook knife, carpal tunnel release using Guo wires or specially designed devices, and tenotomy or fasciotomy using meniscotomes, Guo wires, or hook knives [25].

First-Generation Procedures

Since the initial use of US by Karl Dussik to evaluate the MSK system, US's ability to visualize both soft tissue and neurovascular structures has made it popular for procedural guidance. The use of US for diagnosis affords an easy transition to performance of US-guided procedures with superior accuracy to palpation guidance [302]. In a position statement on US-guided procedures, the AMSSM concluded that there is high-quality evidence that US-guided injections are more accurate than landmark-guided injections in large joints (accuracy 91–100% for US-guided and 64–81% for landmark-guided), intermediate joints (approximately 95% for US-guided and

78% for landmark-guided), small joints (accuracy 94–100% for US-guided and 0–96% for landmark-guided), and tendon sheaths (accuracy 87–100% for US-guided and 27–60% for landmark-guided), though the difference in efficacy and cost has not yet been determined [309]. Individual joint procedures are discussed in more detail in Chaps. 5, 6, 7, 8, 9, 10, and 11.

Historically, corticosteroid injection near the target structure was believed to be sufficient to provide therapeutic benefit. The local and systemic effects of corticosteroid allowed for therapeutic benefit even if the injection was not precisely placed. As corticosteroid use has fallen out of favor due to its toxic effects on tendon and cartilage, newer agents have arisen that are thought to require precise placement at the site of injury for maximum efficacy. These include autologous blood products, bone marrow, adipose tissue, allogenic amniotic membrane, or dextrose solutions [309]. As a result, it is recommended to perform these injections under US guidance to achieve the highest injection accuracy and best outcomes [309]. Further information on and discussion of regenerative medicine injectates can be found in Chaps. 1, 2, and 3, and procedures are reviewed in Chaps. 12 and 13.

Second-Generation Procedures

Greater spatial resolution has made it possible to perform procedures that require detailed needle visualization beyond mere guidance to a target. This includes using needles to fenestrate or cut a pathologic calcification, ligament, tendon, or retinaculum.

Calcific Barbotage

Calcific barbotage is used for the treatment of calcific tendinopathy [310, 311] and is most effective for intratendinous calcification rather than osseous extension [312]. The goal of the procedure is to break up the painful calcifications within the tendon. This involves lavage of the calcific particles using injection of normal saline and a needle (commonly 18-gauge) to repeatedly inject and aspirate the calcification under direct US guidance [313]. Soft and middle-sized calcifications generally respond best to this treatment [314]. Repeat barbotage may be required to fully address some calcific lesions [315] and may be combined with subacromial corticosteroid injection for greater relief [316]. Several reviews and meta-analyses describe calcific barbotage as safe and effective for the treatment of calcific rotator cuff tendinosis [313, 316–318]. Compiled results show up to 55% improvement in pain and indicate that it can be used as a first-line treatment [313, 316–318]. Calcific barbotage may also be used to treat calcific tendinopathy of the gluteal tendons [319] and the common extensor tendon at the elbow [320].

Neovessel Ablation

Neovessel ablation procedures include tendon scraping and high-volume image-guided injection (HVIGI) that can be performed together or in isolation under US guidance. The goal of these procedures is to disrupt the neovessels and neonerves that grow from fat pads like Hoffa's or Kager's fat pad that lie deep to large tendons. These neonerves and neovessels are thought to contribute to pain associated with patellar [321] and Achilles [322] tendinopathy. US with color Doppler allows for the visualization and targeting of these neovessels pre-procedurally with the hope of subsequently disrupting the accompanying neonerves. A significant advantage of these extra-tendinous procedures is that the integrity of the tendon is not compromised. This results in a more rapid return to activity after the procedure than what is recommended for intra-tendinous procedures.

The tendon scraping procedure can be performed entirely under US guidance through an 11-blade stab incision with an 18-gauge needle or meniscotome inserted perpendicular to the tendon under US guidance. This is then passed back and forth in a sweeping motion deep to the tendon at the area of neovascularization. While the utility of open and mini-open surgical tendon scraping to treat Achilles tendinosis is well documented, only one study has examined percutaneous Achilles tendon scraping under US guidance. In that study, percutaneous scraping of 19 tendons showed similar efficacy to an open procedure [322]. One case has been published on the use of tendon scraping to treat patellar tendinopathy that resulted in complete resolution of symptoms and full return to play at 4 weeks with no recurrence at 11-month follow-up[321].

HVIGI typically consists of a 40–50mL injection of normal saline and aims to separate the tendon from the deep fat pad while disrupting neovessels and neonerves [323–331]. HVIGI has been shown to improve pain and physical function in multiple case reports, case series, one randomized controlled trial (RCT), and a retrospective cohort study, but rates of return to sport varied [323, 325–330, 332]. When compared to PRP or eccentric exercises alone, HVIGI had better results at 6 weeks than PRP and eccentric exercises alone, and both PRP and HVIGI were superior to eccentric exercises alone at 24 weeks [324]. HVIGI to treat greater trochanteric pain syndrome [333] and shoulder impingement [331] have been studied by one author, but found either no benefit or only short-term benefit, respectively.

Third-Generation Procedures

More recently, specific tools have been developed to perform procedures under US guidance that were historically performed by open or arthroscopic surgery. US-guided procedures allow for smaller incision sites that are associated with reduced post-procedure pain and improved function with a more rapid return to baseline activity. These procedures are also likely less costly with lower complication rates and increased patient satisfaction [334–336]. However, if these procedures are performed by practitioners with inadequate anatomical and procedural competence, they carry significantly higher risk for injury to surrounding structures. Correct identification of the anatomy and pathology is central to any US-guided procedure, and most third-generation procedures should be practiced on cadavers prior to use in patients. Use of cutting devices without adequate experience could lead to severe and irreversible injury to critical structures. Therefore, these procedures are best performed by experienced sonographers and proceduralists.

Ligament or Retinaculum Release

Ligament or retinaculum release can now be performed under US guidance through a very small incision. This has been demonstrated with release of the transverse carpal ligament (TCL) in carpal tunnel syndrome, release of the A1 pulley in trigger finger, release of the flexor retinaculum in tarsal tunnel syndrome, and release of the first dorsal compartment of the wrist to treat de Quervain's tenosynovitis.

Release of the TCL under US guidance to treat carpal tunnel syndrome has evolved from a procedure done with US assistance to one done completely under US guidance through needle fenestration [337–339], use of a wire to cut the TCL [340–342], use of a hook knife to cut the TCL [305, 343–347], or use of commercially available devices such as the SX-ONE device [348–351]. US guidance allows for the direct visualization of pertinent anatomy that must be avoided during the procedure. This includes the transverse safe zone (bordered radially by the median nerve and ulnarly by the hook of the hamate or ulnar artery), palmar cutaneous branch of the median nerve, Berrettini branch, recurrent motor branch of the median nerve, and other neurovascular anomalies [352]. Overall, studies on US-guided carpal tunnel release with the SX-ONE device report successful release of the TCL in over 600 wrists with minimal complications and a 95% success rate [348].

Trigger finger release with a needle can be performed under US guidance with improved cosmesis and fewer days absent from work than open surgical release [306, 353, 354]. This is commonly performed after failure of a corticosteroid injection. Trigger finger release under US guidance can also be accomplished with use of a hook knife or wire to cut in a retrograde direction (intra or extra sheath) or use of a needle or needle knife (Nokor needle) to cut in an anterograde direction [355]. Cadaveric and clinical data have shown a higher complete pulley release rate when using a hook knife instead of a needle [355–358]. When compared to surgery, US-guided trigger finger release has a shorter procedure time, lower cost, and more rapid return to normal activities [306, 359].

US-guided tarsal tunnel release with a hook knife [360] and first dorsal compartment release with a needle have also been described. These procedures theoretically afford less pain, are lower cost, and have a more rapid recovery than their respective surgical procedures, but more research is needed [361].

Tendon, Muscle, or Fascial Release

Tendon, muscle, and fascial release can be performed under US guidance and is most beneficial for those who are poor surgical candidates or need a more rapid return to activities than that afforded by surgery. To date, several cadaveric and a few patient studies of these techniques have been published. Current limitations to these procedures include operator skill and lack of procedure-specific tools. The procedures are highlighted below, although a full description of these techniques is beyond the scope of this chapter.

Biceps tendon release using different devices (hook knife, scalpel, banana blade, retractable blade, serrated blade) with retrograde cutting of the biceps tendon at various locations (rotator interval, bicipital anchor, and bicipital groove) have been described [362–364]. Cases performed in the bicipital groove using a scalpel or hook knife were most successful in releasing the long head of the biceps in cadavers.

Plantaris tendon release using a hook knife [365] and adductor release using a Guo cutting wire [366] in a retrograde direction under US guidance have been described in cadavers and are thought to be safe.

Plantar fascia release under US guidance using a hook knife to cut in a retrograde medial to lateral direction [367] in cadavers or a beaver blade to cut in a deep to superficial direction in patients [368] have been found to be successful.

Fasciotomy of the anterior and lateral compartments of the lower leg for treatment of chronic exertional compartment syndrome has also been successfully performed on cadavers under US guidance using a meniscotome and anterograde release [34].

Although many of these procedures are still in development, the use of US to guide procedures offers a promising method to minimize the invasiveness of surgical procedures, decrease recovery time, and decrease cost. However, additional research is needed to develop specific tools to improve the ease of US-guided procedures and to directly compare outcomes between surgical and non-surgical procedures. The next step in the development of US-guided procedures is to determine if repair of tissues performed under US guidance has similar outcomes to open or arthroscopic surgical procedures and what differences in complications and rehabilitation protocols and timeline are noted. A protocol outlining US-guided repair of the lateral ligament complex of the ankle has been published and shows promise [369].

US in Orthopedics: Use of US in Preoperative Planning and in the Operating Room

In addition to assisting with diagnosis, US can be used to assist orthopedic surgeons during preoperative planning and intraoperatively to augment visualization of relevant structures. Several studies have shown that preoperative sonographic measurements of the patellar tendon [370], quadriceps tendon [371], and gracilis and semitendinosus tendons [372–374] predict ACL graft size. Preoperative US mapping of peripheral nerves targeted for surgical intervention has also been used to speed identification and access to the target, minimize tissue destruction, and decrease operating time [375]. US can also be utilized preoperatively to tag nerves commonly injured during certain procedures that are difficult to localize intraoperatively. This includes avoiding sensitive structures during Achilles tendon repair [376], plantar fascia repair [377], and medial elbow arthroscopy [378] and localizing the lateral femoral cutaneous nerve for operative decompression [379].

Current Limitations and Future Directions

In spite of the dramatic expansion of US technology over the last several decades, US still has several limitations (Table 21.4). Overcoming these limitations is the topic of ongoing research, and promising methods are discussed below.

While US is often touted as a portable imaging modality, especially compared to x-ray, MRI, and CT, companies continue to push the limits of portability to make US truly "pocket-portable." The first US machine small enough to be used on the battlefield was developed in 1996 [380], and portable US machines have continued to demonstrate utility in field clinics after natural disasters [381]. Transducers that attach to phones and tablets are now commonplace. Transducers the size of a pen are actively in development, but several disadvantages and barriers to production remain for these small devices. Smaller probes and US machines often compromise image resolution, field of view, ability to employ multiple scanning modes (such as Doppler), machine durability, and battery life (although alternative battery sources, such as solar power, are also in development) [382]. In spite of that, technological progress continues to move toward a world where sideline US evaluation could be as simple as pulling out a durable, pocket-sized probe that syncs wirelessly with a mobile device or laptop.

Table 21.4 Limitations of US and research addressing these limitations. US, ultrasound

Limitation	Future direction/research
Lack of high-quality portable images	Technological improvements and improved resolution of small US machines with transducers the size of a pen. Transducers that attach to phones and tablets
Operator dependent	Access to education. Standardization of image acquisition
Inability to visualize deep structures (particularly in obese patients) due to beam attenuation	Tissue harmonic imaging, spatial compound imaging, speckle reduction, and tissue aberration correction
Inability to penetrate bone and visualize inside joints	Development of tools for in-office arthroscopy such as MiEye
Limited field of view	Extended view imaging
Conventional US is in two dimensions	3D US imaging

The "operator dependency" of US is frequently cited as a weakness, but this is likely improving as US training increases. US training is being incorporated into medical school, residency programs, fellowships, and national workshops to improve and standardize operator skill [383, 384]. The number of articles cited in PubMed that utilize US to evaluate MSK conditions has increased exponentially since the 1970s with over 2800 articles published in 2018 alone. Despite this, inter-rater reliability in MSK and nerve evaluation still varies based on the site examined, whether the tissue is healthy or pathologic, and how much training the examiner has received [385–389]. New technology, such as UTC, attempts to standardize US evaluation by removing the human operator, but remains impractical for widespread implementation as described previously.

Additionally, US evaluation is limited by beam attenuation caused by superficial structures that impede deeper visualization. B-mode US relies on high-frequency sound waves to provide sufficient spatial resolution for tissue differentiation, but these high-frequency waves are attenuated when they pass through tissue layers, especially subcutaneous fat. This makes sonographic imaging of obese patients difficult. While deeper penetration can be achieved by using a lower-frequency transducer, this results in decreased resolution [390]. Tissue harmonic imaging (THI) is one attempt to overcome this problem. It utilizes higher-frequency harmonic sound waves produced by the original US wave interacting with nonlinear tissues of deep structures. These higher-frequency waves reflected from deep structures are captured by the probe, allowing for higher-resolution visualization of deep structures that would not be possible with standard B-mode US [391, 392]. In addition to

THI, technological developments such as spatial compound imaging, speckle reduction, and tissue aberration correction are all image processing enhancements that improve image resolution [393–395].

US field of view is limited by the size of the transducer, which traditionally provides a two-dimensional view. As a result, the examiner must formulate a three-dimensional (3D) view in their mind using orthogonal planes and may need to gather multiple images to measure a long structure. To overcome this limitation, extended field of view US was developed in the late 1990s. It uses image registration technology to stitch together a larger field of view and allow for accurate measurement of larger objects including rotator cuff tears, fluid collections, and masses [396, 397]. 3D US has been developed to overcome the 2D nature of current US evaluation. It utilizes processing of data from multiple US images to form a 3D image. Though primarily used outside of the MSK system [398–400], it has also been trialed in the assessment of muscle volume and muscle fascicle length and architecture [48, 401].

Conclusion

US has played a role in MSK evaluation for over 50 years and has several advantages over other imaging modalities. Recent progress has expanded the scope of US in sports medicine to include other organ systems. US is an ideal imaging modality for injury evaluations at sporting events for its portability. Further, new programs enable physiologic and biological assessment of injured tissues to make return-to-play decisions. Its use in procedural guidance has improved the accuracy of existing office-based procedures while also opening the door for US-based micro-invasive surgical interventions. Ongoing research continues to expand the diagnostic and interventional capabilities of US, broadening the indications of US in the hands of skilled sports medicine physicians.

References

1. Dussik KT. Ultraschall-Diagnostik, insbesondere bei Gehirnerkrankungen, mittels Hyperphonographie. Zeitschrift fur physikalische Therapie, Bader- und Klimaheilkunde. 1948;1(9-10):140–5.
2. Dussik KT, Fritch DJ, Kyriazidou M, Sear RS. Measurements of articular tissues with ultrasound. Am J Phys Med. 1958;37(3):160–5.
3. McDonald DG, Leopold GR. Ultrasound B-scanning in the differentiation of Baker's cyst and thrombophlebitis. Br J Radiol. 1972;45(538):729–32.
4. Morganroth J, Maron BJ, Henry WL, Epstein SE. Comparative left ventricular dimensions in trained athletes. Ann Intern Med. 1975;82(4):521–4.
5. Levinsohn EM. Computerized tomography of the musculoskeletal system. JAMA. 1980;244(3):278–80.
6. Sauser DD, Billimoria PE, Rouse GA, Mudge K. CT evaluation of hip trauma. AJR. Am J Roentgenol. 1980;135(2):269–74.
7. Danzig L, Resnick D, Greenway G. Evaluation of unstable shoulders by computed tomography. A preliminary study. Am J Sports Med. 1982;10(3):138–41.
8. Murcia M, Brennan RE, Edeiken J. Computed tomography of stress fracture. Skelet Radiol. 1982;8(3):193–5.
9. Somer K, Meurman KO. Computed tomography of stress fractures. J Comput Assist Tomogr. 1982;6(1):109–15.
10. Mandelbaum BR, Finerman GA, Reicher MA, et al. Magnetic resonance imaging as a tool for evaluation of traumatic knee injuries. Anatomical and pathoanatomical correlations. Am J Sports Med. 1986;14(5):361–70.
11. Verhaven EF, Shahabpour M, Handelberg FW, Vaes PH, Opdecam PJ. The accuracy of three-dimensional magnetic resonance imaging in the diagnosis of ruptures of the lateral ligaments of the ankle. Am J Sports Med. 1991;19(6):583–7.
12. Reinig JW, McDevitt ER, Ove PN. Progression of meniscal degenerative changes in college football players: evaluation with MR imaging. Radiology. 1991;181(1):255–7.
13. Fornage BD, Touche DH, Segal P, Rifkin MD. Ultrasonography in the evaluation of muscular trauma. Journal of Ultrasound in Medicine : Official Journal of the American Institute of Ultrasound in Medicine. 1983;2(12):549–54.
14. Fornage BD. Achilles tendon: US examination. Radiology. 1986;159(3):759–64.
15. Fornage BD, Rifkin MD, Touche DH, Segal PM. Sonography of the patellar tendon: preliminary observations. AJR. Am J Roentgenol. 1984;143(1):179–82.

16. Coral A, van Holsbeeck M, Adler RS. Imaging of meniscal cyst of the knee in three cases. Skelet Radiol. 1989;18(6):451–5.
17. Cooperberg PL, Tsang I, Truelove L, Knickerbocker WJ. Gray scale ultrasound in the evaluation of rheumatoid arthritis of the knee. Radiology. 1978;126(3):759–63.
18. De Flaviis L, Scaglione P, Nessi R, Ventura R, Calori G. Ultrasonography of the hand in rheumatoid arthritis. Acta radiologica (Stockholm, Sweden : 1987). 1988;29(4):457–60.
19. Crass JR, Craig EV, Thompson RC, Feinberg SB. Ultrasonography of the rotator cuff: surgical correlation. J Clin Ultrasound: JCU. 1984;12(8):487–91.
20. Harryman DT 2nd, Mack LA, Wang KY, Jackins SE, Richardson ML, Matsen FA 3rd. Repairs of the rotator cuff. Correlation of functional results with integrity of the cuff. J Bone Joint Surg Am Vol. 1991;73(7):982–9.
21. Marchal GJ, Van Holsbeeck MT, Raes M, et al. Transient synovitis of the hip in children: role of US. Radiology. 1987;162(3):825–8.
22. van Holsbeeck M, van Holsbeeck K, Gevers G, et al. Staging and follow-up of rheumatoid arthritis of the knee. Comparison of sonography, thermography, and clinical assessment. Journal of Ultrasound in Medicine: Official Journal of the American Institute of Ultrasound in Medicine. 1988;7(10):561–6.
23. van Holsbeeck M, Introcaso J. Musculoskeletal Ultrasound. St Louis: Mosby; 1991.
24. Fornage B. Musculoskeletal Ultrasound. New York: Churchill Livingstone; 1995.
25. Finnoff JT, Hall MM, Adams E, et al. American Medical Society for Sports Medicine (AMSSM) position statement: interventional musculoskeletal ultrasound in sports medicine. Br J Sports Med. 2015;49(3):145–50.
26. Jacobson JA. Musculoskeletal ultrasound and MRI: which do I choose? Semin Musculoskelet Radiol. 2005;9(2):135–49.
27. Sharpe RE, Nazarian LN, Parker L, Rao VM, Levin DC. Dramatically increased musculoskeletal ultrasound utilization from 2000 to 2009, especially by podiatrists in private offices. J Am Coll Radiol: JACR. 2012;9(2):141–6.
28. Finnoff JT. The evolution of diagnostic and interventional ultrasound in sports medicine. PM & R: The Journal of Injury, Function, and Rehabilitation. 2016;8(3 Suppl):S133–8.
29. Finnoff JT, Ray J, Corrado G, Kerkhof D, Hill J. Sports ultrasound: applications beyond the musculoskeletal system. Sports Health. 2016;8(5):412–7.
30. Blaivas M. Bedside emergency department ultrasonography in the evaluation of ocular pathology. Acad Emerg Med Off J Soc Acad Emerg Med. 2000;7(8):947–50.
31. Staub LJ, Biscaro RRM, Kaszubowski E, Maurici R. Chest ultrasonography for the emergency diagnosis of traumatic pneumothorax and haemothorax: a systematic review and meta-analysis. Injury. 2018;49(3):457–66.
32. Venckunas T, Mazutaitiene B. The role of echocardiography in the differential diagnosis between training induced myocardial hypertrophy versus cardiomyopathy. J Sports Sci Med. 2007;6(2):166–71.
33. Peck E, Jelsing E, Onishi K. Advanced ultrasound-guided interventions for tendinopathy. Phys Med Rehabil Clin N Am. 2016;27(3):733–48.
34. Lueders DR, Sellon JL, Smith J, Finnoff JT. Ultrasound-guided fasciotomy for chronic exertional compartment syndrome: a cadaveric investigation. PM & R: The Journal of Injury, Function, and Rehabilitation. 2017;9(7):683–90.
35. Smith J, Alfredson H, Masci L, Sellon JL, Woods CD. Sonographically guided plantaris tendon release: a cadaveric validation study. PM & R: The Journal of Injury, Function, and Rehabilitation. 2019;11(1):56–63.
36. Ojaghihaghighi S, Lombardi KM, Davis S, Vahdati SS, Sorkhabi R, Pourmand A. Diagnosis of traumatic eye injuries with point-of-care ocular ultrasonography in the emergency department. Ann Emerg Med. 2019;74(3):365–71.
37. Daniel MC, Restori M, Acheson J, Dahlmann-Noor A. Ocular ultrasound to detect raised intracranial pressure. Pediatr Emerg Care. 2017;33(3):e4.
38. Scharonow M, Weilbach C. Prehospital point-of-care emergency ultrasound: a cohort study. Scandinavian J Trauma Resuscitat Emerg Med. 2018;26(1):49.
39. Saranteas T, Mavrogenis AF, Mandila C, Poularas J, Panou F. Ultrasound in cardiac trauma. J Crit Care. 2017;38:144–51.
40. Miele V, Piccolo CL, Trinci M, Galluzzo M, Ianniello S, Brunese L. Diagnostic imaging of blunt abdominal trauma in pediatric patients. La Radiologia medica. 2016;121(5):409–30.
41. Editorial: 5G-based mhealth bringing healthcare convergence to reality. IEEE Rev Biomed Eng. 2019;12:2–3.
42. Nicholls M. Ultrasound scanning via a 5G network. 2019.; https://healthcare-in-europe.com/en/news/ultrasound-scanning-via-a-5g-network.html. Accessed 8 Aug, 2020.
43. Ali ZS, Pisapia JM, Ma TS, Zager EL, Heuer GG, Khoury V. Ultrasonographic evaluation of peripheral nerves. World neurosurgery. 2016;85:333–9.
44. Zaidman CM, Seelig MJ, Baker JC, Mackinnon SE, Pestronk A. Detection of peripheral nerve pathology: comparison of ultrasound and MRI. Neurology. 2013;80(18):1634–40.
45. Bureau NJ, Ziegler D. Economics of Musculoskeletal Ultrasound. Current Radiology Reports. 2016;4:44.
46. Mandeville R, Wali A, Park C, Groessl E, Walker FO, Cartwright MS. Cost-effectiveness of neuromuscular ultrasound in focal neuropathies. Neurology. 2019;92(23):e2674–8.
47. Parker L, Nazarian LN, Carrino JA, et al. Musculoskeletal imaging: medicare use, costs, and

potential for cost substitution. J Am Coll Radiol: JACR. 2008;5(3):182–8.
48. Weide G, van der Zwaard S, Huijing PA, Jaspers RT, Harlaar J. 3D ultrasound imaging: fast and cost-effective morphometry of musculoskeletal tissue. J Visualized Experiments: JoVE. 2017;129
49. Guillin R, Botchu R, Bianchi S. Sonography of orthopedic hardware impingement of the extremities. Journal of Ultrasound in Medicine: Official Journal of the American Institute of Ultrasound in Medicine. 2012;31(9):1457–63.
50. Draghi F, Bortolotto C, Draghi AG, Gitto S. Intrasheath instability of the peroneal tendons: dynamic ultrasound imaging. Journal of Ultrasound in Medicine: Official Journal of the American Institute of Ultrasound in Medicine. 2018;37(12):2753–8.
51. Fisher CL, Rabbani T, Johnson K, Reeves R, Wood A. Diagnostic capability of dynamic ultrasound evaluation of supination-external rotation ankle injuries: a cadaveric study. BMC Musculoskelet Disord. 2019;20(1):502.
52. Rossi F, Zaottini F, Picasso R, Martinoli C, Tagliafico AS. Ankle and foot ultrasound: reliability of side-to-side comparison of small anatomic structures. J Ultrasound Med. 2019;38(8):2143–53.
53. Tagliafico A, Martinoli C. Reliability of side-to-side sonographic cross-sectional area measurements of upper extremity nerves in healthy volunteers. J Ultrasound Med. 2013;32(3):457–62.
54. Kellgren JH, Lawrence JS. Radiological assessment of osteo-arthrosis. Ann Rheum Dis. 1957;16(4):494–502.
55. Tveit M, Rosengren BE, Nilsson J, Karlsson MK. Former male elite athletes have a higher prevalence of osteoarthritis and arthroplasty in the hip and knee than expected. Am J Sports Med. 2012;40(3):527–33.
56. Cross TM, Smart RC, Thomson JE. Exposure to diagnostic ionizing radiation in sports medicine: assessing and monitoring the risk. Clinical Journal of Sport Medicine: Official Journal of the Canadian Academy of Sport Medicine. 2003;13(3):164–70.
57. Pearce MS, Salotti JA, Little MP, et al. Radiation exposure from CT scans in childhood and subsequent risk of leukaemia and brain tumours: a retrospective cohort study. Lancet (London, England). 2012;380(9840):499–505.
58. Pijpe A, Andrieu N, Easton DF, et al. Exposure to diagnostic radiation and risk of breast cancer among carriers of BRCA1/2 mutations: retrospective cohort study (GENE-RAD-RISK). BMJ : British Medical Journal. 2012;345:e5660.
59. Adams JG, McAlindon T, Dimasi M, Carey J, Eustace S. Contribution of meniscal extrusion and cartilage loss to joint space narrowing in osteoarthritis. Clin Radiol. 1999;54(8):502–6.
60. Fife RS, Brandt KD, Braunstein EM, et al. Relationship between arthroscopic evidence of cartilage damage and radiographic evidence of joint space narrowing in early osteoarthritis of the knee. Arthritis Rheum. 1991;34(4):377–82.
61. Podlipská J, Guermazi A, Lehenkari P, et al. Comparison of diagnostic performance of semi-quantitative knee ultrasound and knee radiography with MRI: oulu knee osteoarthritis study. Sci Rep. 2016;6:22365.
62. Davies MAM, Kerr ZY, DeFreese JD, et al. Prevalence of and risk factors for total hip and knee replacement in retired national football league athletes. Am J Sports Med. 2019;47(12):2863–70.
63. Volpi P, Quaglia A, Carimati G, Petrillo S, Bisciotti GN. High incidence of hip and knee arthroplasty in former professional, male football players. J Sports Med Phys Fitness. 2019;59(9):1558–63.
64. Chun KA, Cho KH. Postoperative ultrasonography of the musculoskeletal system. Ultrasonography (Seoul, Korea). 2015;34(3):195–205.
65. Jacobson JA, Lax MJ. Musculoskeletal sonography of the postoperative orthopedic patient. Semin Musculoskelet Radiol. 2002;6(1):67–77.
66. Bureau NJ, Ali SS, Chhem RK, Cardinal E. Ultrasound of musculoskeletal infections. Semin Musculoskelet Radiol. 1998;2(3):299–306.
67. Bozic KJ, Kamath AF, Ong K, et al. Comparative epidemiology of revision arthroplasty: failed THA poses greater clinical and economic burdens than failed TKA. Clin Orthop Relat Res. 2015;473(6):2131–8.
68. van Kempen RW, Schimmel JJ, van Hellemondt GG, Vandenneucker H, Wymenga AB. Reason for revision TKA predicts clinical outcome: prospective evaluation of 150 consecutive patients with 2-years follow-up. Clin Orthop Relat Res. 2013;471(7):2296–302.
69. Barrett JF, Keat N. Artifacts in CT: recognition and avoidance. Radiographics: A Review Publication of the Radiological Society of North America, Inc. 2004;24(6):1679–91.
70. Singh DR, Chin MS, Peh WC. Artifacts in musculoskeletal MR imaging. Semin Musculoskelet Radiol. 2014;18(1):12–22.
71. Boesen MI, Boesen M, Langberg H, et al. Musculoskeletal colour/power Doppler in sports medicine: image parameters, artefacts, image interpretation and therapy. Clin Exp Rheumatol. 2010;28(1):103–13.
72. Lambros V. Use of doppler ultrasound to avoid injection complications. Plastic Reconstruct Surg. 2019;144(4):724e.
73. Alfredson H, Ohberg L. Neovascularisation in chronic painful patellar tendinosis--promising results after sclerosing neovessels outside the tendon challenge the need for surgery. Knee Surgery, Sports Traumatology, Arthroscopy: Official Journal of the ESSKA. 2005;13(2):74–80.
74. Hoksrud A, Ohberg L, Alfredson H, Bahr R. Color Doppler ultrasound findings in patellar tendinopathy (jumper's knee). Am J Sports Med. 2008;36(9):1813–20.

75. Arslan S, Karahan AY, Oncu F, Bakdik S, Durmaz MS, Tolu I. Diagnostic performance of superb microvascular imaging and other sonographic modalities in the assessment of lateral epicondylosis. Journal of Ultrasound in Medicine: Official Journal of the American Institute of Ultrasound in Medicine. 2018;37(3):585–93.
76. Domenichini R, Pialat JB, Podda A, Aubry S. Ultrasound elastography in tendon pathology: state of the art. Skelet Radiol. 2017;46(12):1643–55.
77. Rabello LM, Dams OC, van den Akker-Scheek I, Zwerver J, O'Neill S. Substantiating the use of ultrasound tissue characterization in the analysis of tendon structure: a systematic review. Clin J Sport Med. 2019;
78. Hootman JM, Dick R, Agel J. Epidemiology of collegiate injuries for 15 sports: summary and recommendations for injury prevention initiatives. J Athl Train. 2007;42(2):311–9.
79. Patel DR, Yamasaki A, Brown K. Epidemiology of sports-related musculoskeletal injuries in young athletes in United States. Transl Pediatrics. 2017;6(3):160–6.
80. Smith J, Finnoff JT. Diagnostic and interventional musculoskeletal ultrasound: part 2. Clinical applications. PM & R: The Journal of Injury, Function, and Rehabilitation. 2009;1(2):162–77.
81. He W, Xiang DY, Dai JP. Sonography in the 29th olympic and paralympic games: a retrospective analysis. Clin Imaging. 2011;35(2):143–7.
82. Kilker BA, Holst JM, Hoffmann B. Bedside ocular ultrasound in the emergency department. European Journal of Emergency Medicine: Official Journal of the European Society for Emergency Medicine. 2014;21(4):246–53.
83. Kendall CJ, Prager TC, Cheng H, Gombos D, Tang RA, Schiffman JS. Diagnostic ophthalmic ultrasound for radiologists. Neuroimaging Clin N Am. 2015;25(3):327–65.
84. Jones NP. One year of severe eye injuries in sport. Eye (London, England). 1988;2(Pt 5):484–7.
85. Haring RS, Sheffield ID, Canner JK, Schneider EB. Epidemiology of sports-related eye injuries in the United States. JAMA ophthalmology. 2016;134(12):1382–90.
86. Miller KN, Collins CL, Chounthirath T, Smith GA. Pediatric sports- and recreation-related eye injuries treated in US emergency departments. Pediatrics. 2018;141(2).
87. Micieli JA, Easterbrook M. Eye and Orbital Injuries in Sports. Clin Sports Med. 2017;36(2):299–314.
88. Leivo T, Haavisto AK, Sahraravand A. Sports-related eye injuries: the current picture. Acta Ophthalmol. 2015;93(3):224–31.
89. Vrablik ME, Snead GR, Minnigan HJ, Kirschner JM, Emmett TW, Seupaul RA. The diagnostic accuracy of bedside ocular ultrasonography for the diagnosis of retinal detachment: a systematic review and meta-analysis. Annals Emerg Med. 2015;65(2):199–203.e191.
90. MacEwen CJ. Sport associated eye injury: a casualty department survey. Br J Ophthalmol. 1987;71(9):701.
91. Filipe JA, Barros H, Castro-Correia J. Sports-related ocular injuries. A three-year follow-up study. Ophthalmology. 1997;104(2):313–8.
92. Barr A, Baines PS, Desai P, MacEwen CJ. Ocular sports injuries: the current picture. Br J Sports Med. 2000;34(6):456.
93. Baker N, Amini R, Situ-LaCasse EH, et al. Can emergency physicians accurately distinguish retinal detachment from posterior vitreous detachment with point-of-care ocular ultrasound? Am J Emerg Med. 2018;36(5):774–6.
94. Shinar Z, Chan L, Orlinsky M. Use of ocular ultrasound for the evaluation of retinal detachment. J Emergency Med. 2011;40(1):53–7.
95. Major R, Girling S, Boyle A. Ultrasound measurement of optic nerve sheath diameter in patients with a clinical suspicion of raised intracranial pressure. Emergency medicine journal : EMJ. 2011;28(8):679–81.
96. Tayal VS, Neulander M, Norton HJ, Foster T, Saunders T, Blaivas M. Emergency department sonographic measurement of optic nerve sheath diameter to detect findings of increased intracranial pressure in adult head injury patients. Ann Emerg Med. 2007;49(4):508–14.
97. Ohle R, McIsaac SM, Woo MY, Perry JJ. Sonography of the optic nerve sheath diameter for Detection of Raised Intracranial Pressure Compared to Computed tomography: a systematic review and meta-analysis. Journal of Ultrasound in Medicine: Official Journal of the American Institute of Ultrasound in Medicine. 2015;34(7):1285–94.
98. Halvorsen T, Walsted ES, Bucca C, et al. Inducible laryngeal obstruction: an official joint European Respiratory Society and European Laryngological Society statement. The European Respiratory Journal. 2017;50(3).
99. Christensen PM, Thomsen SF, Rasmussen N, Backer V. Exercise-induced laryngeal obstructions: prevalence and symptoms in the general public. European Archives of Oto-Rhino-Laryngology: Official Journal of the European Federation of Oto-Rhino-Laryngological Societies (EUFOS): Affiliated with the German Society for Oto-Rhino-Laryngology - Head and Neck Surgery. 2011;268(9):1313–9.
100. Wilson JJ, Wilson EM. Practical management: vocal cord dysfunction in athletes. Clinical Journal of Sport Medicine : Official Journal of the Canadian Academy of Sport Medicine. 2006;16(4):357–60.
101. Finnoff JT, Orbelo DM, Ekbom DC. Can ultrasound identify paradoxical vocal fold movement? a pilot study. Clinical Journal of Sport Medicine : Official Journal of the Canadian Academy of Sport Medicine. 2018;
102. Griffin SA, Walsted ES, Hull JH. Infographic. The breathless athlete: EILO. Br J Sports Med. 2019;53(10):616–7.

103. Harmon KG, Drezner JA, Wilson MG, Sharma S. Incidence of sudden cardiac death in athletes: a state-of-the-art review. Br J Sports Med. 2014;48(15):1185–92.
104. Boden BP, Breit I, Beachler JA, Williams A, Mueller FO. Fatalities in high school and college football players. Am J Sports Med. 2013;41(5):1108–16.
105. Corrado D, Pelliccia A, Bjornstad HH, et al. Cardiovascular pre-participation screening of young competitive athletes for prevention of sudden death: proposal for a common European protocol. Consensus Statement of the Study Group of Sport Cardiology of the Working Group of Cardiac Rehabilitation and Exercise Physiology and the Working Group of Myocardial and Pericardial Diseases of the European Society of Cardiology. Eur Heart J. 2005;26(5):516–24.
106. Harmon KG, Zigman M, Drezner JA. The effectiveness of screening history, physical exam, and ECG to detect potentially lethal cardiac disorders in athletes: a systematic review/meta-analysis. J Electrocardiol. 2015;48(3):329–38.
107. Drezner JA, Sharma S, Baggish A, et al. International criteria for electrocardiographic interpretation in athletes: Consensus statement. Br J Sports Med. 2017;51(9):704–31.
108. Maron BJ, Friedman RA, Kligfield P, et al. Assessment of the 12-lead ECG as a screening test for detection of cardiovascular disease in healthy general populations of young people (12-25 Years of Age): a scientific statement from the American Heart Association and the American College of Cardiology. Circulation. 2014;130(15):1303–34.
109. Malhotra R, West JJ, Dent J, et al. Cost and yield of adding electrocardiography to history and physical in screening Division I intercollegiate athletes: a 5-year experience. Heart Rhythm. 2011;8(5):721–7.
110. Yim ES, Basilico F, Corrado G. Early screening for cardiovascular abnormalities with preparticipation echocardiography: utility of focused physician-operated echocardiography in preparticipation screening of athletes. Journal of Ultrasound in Medicine: Official Journal of the American Institute of Ultrasound in Medicine. 2014;33(2):307–13.
111. Gleason CN, Kerkhof DL, Cilia EA, et al. Early screening for cardiovascular abnormalities with preparticipation echocardiography: feasibility study. Clinical Journal of Sport Medicine: Official Journal of the Canadian Academy of Sport Medicine. 2017;27(5):423–9.
112. Lucas C, Kerkhof DL, Briggs JE, Corrado GD. The use of echocardiograms in preparticipation examinations. Curr Sports Med Rep. 2017;16(2):77–83.
113. Rizzo M, Spataro A, Cecchetelli C, et al. Structural cardiac disease diagnosed by echocardiography in asymptomatic young male soccer players: implications for pre-participation screening. Br J Sports Med. 2012;46(5):371–3.
114. Kerkhof DL, Gleason CN, Basilico FC, Corrado GD. Is there a role for limited echocardiography during the preparticipation physical examination? PM & R: The Journal of Injury, Function, and Rehabilitation. 2016;8(3 Suppl):S36–44.
115. Yim ES, Kao D, Gillis EF, Basilico FC, Corrado GD. Focused physician-performed echocardiography in sports medicine: a potential screening tool for detecting aortic root dilatation in athletes. Journal of Ultrasound in Medicine: Official Journal of the American Institute of Ultrasound in Medicine. 2013;32(12):2101–6.
116. Yim ES, Gillis EF, Ojala K, MacDonald J, Basilico FC, Corrado GD. Focused transthoracic echocardiography by sports medicine physicians: measurements relevant to hypertrophic cardiomyopathy. Journal of Ultrasound in Medicine: Official Journal of the American Institute of Ultrasound in Medicine. 2013;32(2):333–8.
117. Griffith JF, Rainer TH, Ching AS, Law KL, Cocks RA, Metreweli C. Sonography compared with radiography in revealing acute rib fracture. AJR. Am J Roentgenol. 1999;173(6):1603–9.
118. Battle C, Hayward S, Eggert S, Evans PA. Comparison of the use of lung ultrasound and chest radiography in the diagnosis of rib fractures: a systematic review. Emergency Med J: EMJ. 2019;36(3):185–90.
119. Lichtenstein DA, Meziere G, Lascols N, et al. Ultrasound diagnosis of occult pneumothorax. Crit Care Med. 2005;33(6):1231–8.
120. Lichtenstein D, Meziere G, Biderman P, Gepner A. The comet-tail artifact: an ultrasound sign ruling out pneumothorax. Intensive Care Med. 1999;25(4):383–8.
121. Berkoff DJ, English J, Theodoro D. Sports medicine ultrasound (US) beyond the musculoskeletal system: use in the abdomen, solid organs, lung, heart and eye. Br J Sports Med. 2015;49(3):161–5.
122. Lichtenstein DA, Menu Y. A bedside ultrasound sign ruling out pneumothorax in the critically ill. Lung sliding Chest. 1995;108(5):1345–8.
123. Lyon M, Walton P, Bhalla V, Shiver SA. Ultrasound detection of the sliding lung sign by prehospital critical care providers. Am J Emerg Med. 2012;30(3):485–8.
124. Soldati G, Testa A, Sher S, Pignataro G, La Sala M, Silveri NG. Occult traumatic pneumothorax: diagnostic accuracy of lung ultrasonography in the emergency department. Chest. 2008;133(1):204–11.
125. Rozycki GS, Ochsner MG, Schmidt JA, et al. A prospective study of surgeon-performed ultrasound as the primary adjuvant modality for injured patient assessment. J Trauma. 1995;39(3):492–8; discussion 498-500.
126. Kirkpatrick AW, Sirois M, Laupland KB, et al. Hand-held thoracic sonography for detecting post-traumatic pneumothoraces: the Extended Focused Assessment with Sonography for Trauma (EFAST). J Trauma. 2004;57(2):288–95.

127. Brun PM, Bessereau J, Chenaitia H, et al. Stay and play eFAST or scoop and run eFAST? That is the question! Am J Emerg Med. 2014;32(2):166–70.
128. Bloom BA, Gibbons RC. Focused Assessment with Sonography for Trauma (FAST). StatPearls. Treasure Island (FL): StatPearls Publishing LLC; 2019.
129. Ceraulo AS, Bytomski JR. Infectious mononucleosis management in athletes. Clin Sports Med. 2019;38(4):555–61.
130. Putukian M, O'Connor FG, Stricker P, et al. Mononucleosis and athletic participation: an evidence-based subject review. Clinical Journal of Sport Medicine: Official Journal of the Canadian Academy of Sport Medicine. 2008;18(4):309–15.
131. Hosey RG, Mattacola CG, Kriss V, Armsey T, Quarles JD, Jagger J. Ultrasound assessment of spleen size in collegiate athletes. Br J Sports Med. 2006;40(3):251–4; discussion 251-254.
132. Smereczynski A, Kolaczyk K, Lubinski J, Bojko S, Galdynska M, Bernatowicz E. Sonographic imaging of Spigelian hernias. J Ultrasonography. 2012;12(50):269–75.
133. Jacobson JA. Fundamentals of musculoskeletal ultrasound. 3rd ed. Philadelphia, PA: Elsevier; 2018.
134. Bradley MJ, Cosgrove DO. Chapter 41 - The abdominal wall, peritoneum and retroperitoneum. In: Allan PL, Baxter GM, Weston MJ, editors. Clinical ultrasound. 3rd ed. Edinburgh: Churchill Livingstone; 2011. p. 798–827.
135. Gokhale S. Three-dimensional sonography of muscle hernias. J Ultrasound Med. 2007;26(2):239–42.
136. Connell D, Ali K, Javid M, Bell P, Batt M, Kemp S. Sonography and MRI of rectus abdominis muscle strain in elite tennis players. AJR. Am J Roentgenol. 2006;187(6):1457–61.
137. Obaid H, Nealon A, Connell D. Sonographic appearance of side strain injury. AJR. Am J Roentgenol. 2008;191(6):W264–7.
138. Stevens KJ, Crain JM, Akizuki KH, Beaulieu CF. Imaging and ultrasound-guided steroid injection of internal oblique muscle strains in baseball pitchers. Am J Sports Med. 2010;38(3):581–5.
139. Minardi J, Shaver E, Monseau A, Pratt A, Layman SM. Right lower quadrant pain in a young female: ultrasound diagnosis of rectus abdominis tear. J Emergency Med. 2015;49(5):623–6.
140. Nealon AR, Kountouris A, Cook JL. Side strain in sport: a narrative review of pathomechanics, diagnosis, imaging and management for the clinician. J Sci Med Sport. 2017;20(3):261–6.
141. Thorborg K, Reiman MP, Weir A, et al. Clinical examination, diagnostic imaging, and testing of athletes with groin pain: an evidence-based approach to effective management. J Orthopaedic Sports Phys Therapy. 2018;48(4):239–49.
142. Niebuhr H, Konig A, Pawlak M, Sailer M, Kockerling F, Reinpold W. Groin hernia diagnostics: dynamic inguinal ultrasound (DIUS). Langenbeck's Arch Surg. 2017;402(7):1039–45.
143. Jenkins JT, O'Dwyer PJ. Inguinal hernias. BMJ. 2008;336(7638):269–72.
144. Vasileff WK, Nekhline M, Kolowich PA, Talpos GB, Eyler WR, van Holsbeeck M. Inguinal hernia in athletes: role of dynamic ultrasound. Sports health. 2017;9(5):414–21.
145. HerniaSurge G. International guidelines for groin hernia management. Hernia. 2018;22(1):1–165.
146. Weir A, Brukner P, Delahunt E, et al. Doha agreement meeting on terminology and definitions in groin pain in athletes. Br J Sports Med. 2015;49(12):768–74.
147. Omar IM, Zoga AC, Kavanagh EC, et al. Athletic pubalgia and "sports hernia": optimal MR imaging technique and findings. Radiographics: A Review Publication of the Radiological Society of North America, Inc. 2008;28(5):1415–38.
148. Brandon CJ, Jacobson JA, Fessell D, et al. Groin pain beyond the hip: how anatomy predisposes to injury as visualized by musculoskeletal ultrasound and MRI. AJR. Am J Roentgenol. 2011;197(5):1190–7.
149. Tagliafico A, Bignotti B, Rossi F, Sconfienza LM, Messina C, Martinoli C. Ultrasound of the hip joint, soft tissues, and nerves. Semin Musculoskelet Radiol. 2017;21(05):582–8.
150. Jacobson JA, Khoury V, Brandon CJ. Ultrasound of the groin: techniques, pathology, and pitfalls. Am J Roentgenol. 2015;205(3):513–23.
151. Tagliafico A, Bignotti B, Cadoni A, Perez MM, Martinoli C. Anatomical study of the iliohypogastric, ilioinguinal, and genitofemoral nerves using high-resolution ultrasound. Muscle Nerve. 2015;51(1):42–8.
152. Martinoli C, Miguel-Perez M, Padua L, Gandolfo N, Zicca A, Tagliafico A. Imaging of neuropathies about the hip. Eur J Radiol. 2013;82(1):17–26.
153. Pivec C, Bodner G, Mayer JA, et al. Novel demonstration of the anterior femoral cutaneous nerves using ultrasound. Ultraschall Med, 2018. https://doi.org/10.1055/s-0043-121628.
154. Zuckerman SL, Kerr ZY, Pierpoint L, Kirby P, Than KD, Wilson TJ. An 11-year analysis of peripheral nerve injuries in high school sports. Physician Sports Med. 2019;47(2):167–73.
155. Takazawa H, Sudo N, Akoi K. Statistical observation of nerve injuries in athletes. Brain Nerve Injuries. 1971;3:11–7.
156. Lorei MP, Hershman EB. Peripheral nerve injuries in athletes. Treatment and prevention. Sports Med (Auckland, N.Z.). 1993;16(2):130–47.
157. Robinson LR. Traumatic injury to peripheral nerves. Muscle Nerve. 2000;23(6):863–73.
158. Smith JK, Miller ME, Carroll CG, et al. High-resolution ultrasound in combat-related peripheral nerve injuries. Muscle Nerve. 2016;54(6):1139–44.
159. Padua L, Di Pasquale A, Liotta G, et al. Ultrasound as a useful tool in the diagnosis and management of traumatic nerve lesions. Clinical Neurophysiology: Official Journal of the International Federation of Clinical Neurophysiology. 2013;124(6):1237–43.

160. Moritz T, Prosch H, Pivec CH, et al. High-resolution ultrasound visualization of the subcutaneous nerves of the forearm: a feasibility study in anatomic specimens. Muscle Nerve. 2014;49(5):676–9.
161. Bianchi S, Becciolini M, Urigo C. Ultrasound imaging of disorders of small nerves of the extremities: less recognized locations. Journal of Ultrasound in Medicine: Official Journal of the American Institute of Ultrasound in Medicine. 2019;38(11):2821–42.
162. Mifune Y, Inui A, Sakata R, et al. High-resolution ultrasound in the diagnosis of trigger finger and evaluation of response to steroid injection. Skelet Radiol. 2016;45(12):1661–7.
163. Riegler G, Brugger PC, Gruber GM, Pivec C, Jengojan S, Bodner G. High-resolution ultrasound visualization of pacinian corpuscles. Ultrasound Med Biol. 2018;44(12):2596–601.
164. Riegler G, Lieba-Samal D, Brugger PC, et al. High-resolution ultrasound visualization of the deep branch of the ulnar nerve. Muscle Nerve. 2017;56(6):1101–7.
165. De Maeseneer M, Brigido MK, Antic M, et al. Ultrasound of the elbow with emphasis on detailed assessment of ligaments, tendons, and nerves. Eur J Radiol. 2015;84(4):671–81.
166. Deimel GW, Hurst RW, Sorenson EJ, Boon AJ. Utility of ultrasound-guided near-nerve needle recording for lateral femoral cutaneous sensory nerve conduction study: does it increase reliability compared with surface recording? Muscle Nerve. 2013;47(2):274–6.
167. Gans P, Van Alfen N. Nerve ultrasound showing Martin–Gruber anastomosis. Muscle Nerve. 2017;56(5):E46–7.
168. Lucchetta M, Liotta GA, Briani C, et al. Ultrasound diagnosis of peroneal nerve variant in a child with compressive mononeuropathy. J Pediatr Surg. 2011;46(2):405–7.
169. van Alfen N, Mah JK. Neuromuscular ultrasound: a new tool in your toolbox. Canadian Journal of Neurological Sciences / Journal Canadien des Sciences Neurologiques. 2018;45(5):504–15.
170. Baute V, Strakowski JA, Reynolds JW, et al. Neuromuscular ultrasound of the brachial plexus: a standardized approach. Muscle Nerve. 2018;58(5):618–24.
171. Bignotti B, Cadoni A, Assini A, Martinoli C, Tagliafico A. Fascicular involvement in common fibular neuropathy: evaluation with ultrasound. Muscle Nerve. 2016;53(4):532–7.
172. Jelsing EJ, Presley JC, Maida E, Hangiandreou NJ, Smith J. The effect of magnification on sonographically measured nerve cross-sectional area. Muscle Nerve. 2015;51(1):30–4.
173. Kalia V, Jacobson JA. Imaging of peripheral nerves of the upper extremity. Radiol Clin N Am. 2019;57(5):1063–71.
174. Silvestri E, Martinoli C, Derchi LE, Bertolotto M, Chiaramondia M, Rosenberg I. Echotexture of peripheral nerves: correlation between US and histologic findings and criteria to differentiate tendons. Radiology. 1995;197(1):291–6.
175. Azman D, Hrabac P, Demarin V. Use of multiple ultrasonographic parameters in confirmation of carpal tunnel syndrome. Journal of Ultrasound in Medicine: Official Journal of the American Institute of Ultrasound in Medicine. 2018;37(4):879–89.
176. Boninger ML, Robertson RN, Wolff M, Cooper RA. Upper limb nerve entrapments in elite wheelchair racers. Am J Phys Med Rehabil. 1996;75(3):170–6.
177. Burnham RS, Steadward RD. Upper extremity peripheral nerve entrapments among wheelchair athletes: prevalence, location, and risk factors. Arch Phys Med Rehabil. 1994;75(5):519–24.
178. Duncan I, Sullivan P, Lomas F. Sonography in the diagnosis of carpal tunnel syndrome. AJR. Am J Roentgenol. 1999;173(3):681–4.
179. El Miedany YM, Aty SA, Ashour S. Ultrasonography versus nerve conduction study in patients with carpal tunnel syndrome: substantive or complementary tests? Rheumatology (Oxford, England). 2004;43(7):887–95.
180. Lee D, van Holsbeeck MT, Janevski PK, Ganos DL, Ditmars DM, Darian VB. Diagnosis of carpal tunnel syndrome. Ultrasound versus electromyography. Radiol Clin N Am. 1999;37(4):859–72. x
181. Visser LH, Smidt MH, Lee ML. High-resolution sonography versus EMG in the diagnosis of carpal tunnel syndrome. J Neurol Neurosurg Psychiatry. 2008;79(1):63–7.
182. Wiesler ER, Chloros GD, Cartwright MS, Smith BP, Rushing J, Walker FO. The use of diagnostic ultrasound in carpal tunnel syndrome. J Hand Surg. 2006;31(5):726–32.
183. Yesildag A, Kutluhan S, Sengul N, et al. The role of ultrasonographic measurements of the median nerve in the diagnosis of carpal tunnel syndrome. Clin Radiol. 2004;59(10):910–5.
184. Torres-Costoso A, Martinez-Vizcaino V, Alvarez-Bueno C, Ferri-Morales A, Cavero-Redondo I. Accuracy of ultrasonography for the diagnosis of carpal tunnel syndrome: a systematic review and meta-analysis. Arch Phys Med Rehab. 2018;99(4):758–65.e710.
185. Rahmani M, Ghasemi Esfe AR, Vaziri-Bozorg SM, Mazloumi M, Khalilzadeh O, Kahnouji H. The ultrasonographic correlates of carpal tunnel syndrome in patients with normal electrodiagnostic tests. La Radiologia medica. 2011;116(3):489–96.
186. Vanderschueren GA, Meys VE, Beekman R. Doppler sonography for the diagnosis of carpal tunnel syndrome: a critical review. Muscle Nerve. 2014;50(2):159–63.
187. Volz KR, Evans KD, Kanner CD, Dickerson JA. Detection of intraneural median nerve microvascularity using contrast-enhanced sonography: a pilot study. Journal of Ultrasound in Medicine : Official Journal of the American Institute of Ultrasound in Medicine. 2016;35(6):1309–16.

188. Chen J, Chen L, Wu L, et al. Value of superb microvascular imaging ultrasonography in the diagnosis of carpal tunnel syndrome: compared with color Doppler and power Doppler. Medicine. 2017;96(21):e6862.
189. Karahan AY, Arslan S, Ordahan B, Bakdik S, Ekiz T. Superb microvascular imaging of the median nerve in carpal tunnel syndrome: an electrodiagnostic and ultrasonographic study. Journal of Ultrasound in Medicine: Official Journal of the American Institute of Ultrasound in Medicine. 2018;37(12):2855–61.
190. Campbell WW. Ulnar neuropathy at the elbow. Muscle Nerve. 2000;23(4):450–2.
191. Olivo R, Tsao B. Peripheral nerve injuries in sport. Neurol Clin. 2017;35(3):559–72.
192. Łasecki M, Olchowy C, Pawluś A, Zaleska-Dorobisz U. The Snapping elbow syndrome as a reason for chronic elbow neuralgia in a tennis player - MR, US and sonoelastography evaluation. Pol J Radiol. 2014;79:467–71.
193. Ellegaard HR, Fuglsang-Frederiksen A, Hess A, Johnsen B, Qerama E. High-resolution ultrasound in ulnar neuropathy at the elbow: a prospective study. Muscle Nerve. 2015;52(5):759–66.
194. Schertz M, Mutschler C, Masmejean E, Silvera J. High-resolution ultrasound in etiological evaluation of ulnar neuropathy at the elbow. Eur J Radiol. 2017;95:111–7.
195. Chang KV, Wu WT, Han DS, Özçakar L. Ulnar nerve cross-sectional area for the diagnosis of cubital tunnel syndrome: a meta-analysis of ultrasonographic measurements. Arch Phys Med Rehabil. 2018;99(4):743–57.
196. Alrajeh M, Preston DC. Neuromuscular ultrasound in electrically non-localizable ulnar neuropathy. Muscle Nerve. 2018;58(5):655–9.
197. Peer S, Kovacs P, Harpf C, Bodner G. High-resolution sonography of lower extremity peripheral nerves: anatomic correlation and spectrum of disease. Journal of Ultrasound in Medicine: Official Journal of the American Institute of Ultrasound in Med. 2002;21(3):315–22.
198. Masakado Y, Kawakami M, Suzuki K, Abe L, Ota T, Kimura A. Clinical neurophysiology in the diagnosis of peroneal nerve palsy. Keio J Med. 2008;57(2):84–9.
199. Hainline BW. Peripheral nerve injury in sports. Continuum (Minneapolis, Minn.). 2014;20(6 Sports Neurology):1605–28.
200. Krivickas LS, Wilbourn AJ. Peripheral nerve injuries in athletes: a case series of over 200 injuries. Semin Neurol. 2000;20(2):225–32.
201. Bucklan JN, Morren JA, Shook SJ. Ultrasound in the diagnosis and management of fibular mononeuropathy. Muscle Nerve. 2019;60(5):544–8.
202. Bignotti B, Assini A, Signori A, Martinoli C, Tagliafico A. Ultrasound versus MRI in common fibular neuropathy. Muscle Nerve. 2017;55(6):849–57.
203. Fantino O. Role of ultrasound in posteromedial tarsal tunnel syndrome: 81 cases. J Ultrasound. 2014;17(2):99–112.
204. Tsukamoto H, Granata G, Coraci D, Paolasso I, Padua L. Ultrasound and neurophysiological correlation in common fibular nerve conduction block at fibular head. Clinical Neurophysiology: Official Journal of the International Federation of Clinical Neurophysiology. 2014;125(7):1491–5.
205. Wu WT, Chang KV, Özçakar L. Ultrasound facilitates the diagnosis of tarsal tunnel syndrome: intraneural ganglion cyst of the tibial nerve. J Ultrasound. 2019;22(1):95–8.
206. Kho KH, Blijham PJ, Zwarts MJ. Meralgia paresthetica after strenuous exercise. Muscle Nerve. 2005;31(6):761–3.
207. Macgregor J, Moncur JA. Meralgia paraesthetica--a sports lesion in girl gymnasts. Br J Sports Med. 1977;11(1):16–9.
208. Otoshi K, Itoh Y, Tsujino A, Kikuchi S. Case report: meralgia paresthetica in a baseball pitcher. Clin Orthop Relat Res. 2008;466(9):2268–70.
209. Ulkar B, Yildiz Y, Kunduracioglu B. Meralgia paresthetica: a long-standing performance-limiting cause of anterior thigh pain in a soccer player. Am J Sports Med. 2003;31(5):787–9.
210. Esser S, Thurston M, Nalluri K, Muzaurieta A. "Numb-Leg" in a crossfit athlete: a case presentation. PM & R: The Journal of Injury, Function, and Rehabilitation. 2017;9(8):834–6.
211. Seror P. Somatosensory evoked potentials for the electrodiagnosis of meralgia paresthetica. Muscle Nerve. 2004;29(2):309–12.
212. Aravindakannan T, Wilder-Smith EP. High-resolution ultrasonography in the assessment of meralgia paresthetica. Muscle Nerve. 2012;45(3):434–5.
213. Tagliafico A, Serafini G, Lacelli F, Perrone N, Valsania V, Martinoli C. Ultrasound-guided treatment of meralgia paresthetica (lateral femoral cutaneous neuropathy): technical description and results of treatment in 20 consecutive patients. Journal of Ultrasound in Medicine: Official Journal of the American Institute of Ultrasound in Medicine. 2011;30(10):1341–6.
214. Cunnane M, Pratten M, Loughna S. A retrospective study looking at the incidence of 'stinger' injuries in professional rugby union players. Br J Sports Med 2011;45(15):A19.
215. Safran MR. Nerve injury about the shoulder in athletes, part 2: long thoracic nerve, spinal accessory nerve, burners/stingers, thoracic outlet syndrome. Am J Sports Med. 2004;32(4):1063–76.
216. Stewman C, Vitanzo PC Jr, Harwood MI. Neurologic thoracic outlet syndrome: summarizing a complex history and evolution. Curr Sports Med Rep. 2014;13(2):100–6.
217. Arányi Z, Csillik A, Böhm J, Schelle T. Ultrasonographic identification of fibromuscular

bands associated with neurogenic thoracic outlet syndrome: the "wedge-sickle" sign. Ultrasound Med Biol. 2016;42(10):2357–66.
218. Pesser N, Teijink JAW, Vervaart K, et al. Value of ultrasound in the diagnosis of neurogenic thoracic outlet syndrome. European Journal of Vascular and Endovascular Surgery: The Official Journal of the European Society for Vascular Surgery. 2020;59(5):852–3.
219. Sucher BM. Thoracic outlet syndrome-postural type: ultrasound imaging of pectoralis minor and brachial plexus abnormalities. PM & R: The Journal of Injury, Function, and Rehabilitation. 2012;4(1):65–72.
220. Shutze W, Richardson B, Shutze R, et al. Midterm and long-term follow-up in competitive athletes undergoing thoracic outlet decompression for neurogenic thoracic outlet syndrome. J Vasc Surg. 2017;66(6):1798–805.
221. Jordan SE, Ahn SS, Gelabert HA. Combining ultrasonography and electromyography for botulinum chemodenervation treatment of thoracic outlet syndrome: comparison with fluoroscopy and electromyography guidance. Pain physician. 2007;10(4):541–6.
222. Torriani M, Gupta R, Donahue DM. Sonographically guided anesthetic injection of anterior scalene muscle for investigation of neurogenic thoracic outlet syndrome. Skelet Radiol. 2009;38(11):1083–7.
223. Graif M, Martinoli C, Rochkind S, et al. Sonographic evaluation of brachial plexus pathology. Eur Radiol. 2004;14(2):193–200.
224. Abraham P, Saumet JL, Chevalier JM. External iliac artery endofibrosis in athletes. Sports Med (Auckland, N.Z.). 1997;24(4):221–6.
225. Menon D, Onida S, Davies AH. Overview of arterial pathology related to repetitive trauma in athletes. J Vasc Surg. 2019;70(2):641–50.
226. Nakamura KM, Skeik N, Shepherd RF, Wennberg PW. External iliac vein thrombosis in an athletic cyclist with a history of external iliac artery endofibrosis and thrombosis. Vasc Endovasc Surg. 2011;45(8):761–4.
227. Willson TD, Revesz E, Podbielski FJ, Blecha MJ. External iliac artery dissection secondary to endofibrosis in a cyclist. J Vasc Surg. 2010;52(1):219–21.
228. Abraham P, Leftheriotis G, Bourre Y, Chevalier JM, Saumet JL. Echography of external iliac artery endofibrosis in cyclists. Am J Sports Med. 1993;21(6):861–3.
229. Fernandez-Garcia B, Alvarez Fernandez J, Vega Garcia F, et al. Diagnosing external iliac endofibrosis by postexercise ankle to arm index in cyclists. Med Sci Sports Exerc. 2002;34(2):222–7.
230. Joy SM, Raudales R. Popliteal artery entrapment syndrome. Curr Sports Med Reports. 2015;14(5):364–7.
231. Cho KJ, Kang S, Ko S, Baek J, Kim Y, Park NK. Neurovascular compression caused by popliteus muscle enlargement without discrete trauma. Ann Rehabil Med. 2016;40(3):545–50.
232. Levien LJ, Veller MG. Popliteal artery entrapment syndrome: more common than previously recognized. J Vasc Surg. 1999;30(4):587–98.
233. Sinha S, Houghton J, Holt PJ, Thompson MM, Loftus IM, Hinchliffe RJ. Popliteal entrapment syndrome. J Vascular Surg. 2012;55(1):252–62. e230.
234. Erdoes LS, Devine JJ, Bernhard VM, Baker MR, Berman SS, Hunter GC. Popliteal vascular compression in a normal population. J Vasc Surg. 1994;20(6):978–86.
235. Jackson MR. Upper extremity arterial injuries in athletes. Semin Vasc Surg. 2003;16(3):232–9.
236. Rohrer MJ, Cardullo PA, Pappas AM, Phillips DA, Wheeler HB. Axillary artery compression and thrombosis in throwing athletes. J Vasc Surg. 1990;11(6):761–8; discussion 768-769.
237. Schneider K, Kasparyan NG, Altchek DW, Fantini GA, Weiland AJ. An aneurysm involving the axillary artery and its branch vessels in a major league baseball pitcher. A case report and review of the literature. Am J Sports Med. 1999;27(3):370–5.
238. van de Pol D, Kuijer PP, Langenhorst T, Maas M. High prevalence of self-reported symptoms of digital ischemia in elite male volleyball players in the Netherlands: a cross-sectional national survey. Am J Sports Med. 2012;40(10):2296–302.
239. van de Pol D, Maas M, Terpstra A, et al. Ultrasound assessment of the posterior circumflex humeral artery in elite volleyball players: aneurysm prevalence, anatomy, branching pattern and vessel characteristics. Eur Radiol. 2017;27(3):889–98.
240. van de Pol D, Maas M, Terpstra A, Pannekoek-Hekman M, Kuijer PP, Planken RN. B-Mode sonographic assessment of the posterior circumflex humeral artery: the SPI-US Protocol-A technical procedure in 4 steps. Journal of Ultrasound in Medicine: Official Journal of the American Institute of Ultrasound in Medicine. 2016;35(5):1015–20.
241. Nichols AW. Diagnosis and management of thoracic outlet syndrome. Curr Sports Med Rep. 2009;8(5):240–9.
242. Daniels B, Michaud L, Sease F Jr, Cassas KJ, Gray BH. Arterial thoracic outlet syndrome. Curr Sports Med Rep. 2014;13(2):75–80.
243. Farrar TA, Rankin G, Chatfield M. Venous thoracic outlet syndrome: approach to diagnosis and treatment with focus on affected athletes. Curr Sports Med Reports. 2014;13(2):81–5.
244. Demondion X, Vidal C, Herbinet P, Gautier C, Duquesnoy B, Cotten A. Ultrasonographic assessment of arterial cross-sectional area in the thoracic outlet on postural maneuvers measured with power Doppler ultrasonography in both asymptomatic and symptomatic populations. Journal of Ultrasound in Medicine: Official Journal of the American Institute of Ultrasound in Medicine. 2006;25(2):217–24.
245. Longley DG, Yedlicka JW, Molina EJ, Schwabacher S, Hunter DW, Letourneau JG. Thoracic outlet syndrome: evaluation of the subclavian vessels by

color duplex sonography. AJR. Am J Roentgenol. 1992;158(3):623–30.
246. Coggan AR, Coyle EF. Reversal of fatigue during prolonged exercise by carbohydrate infusion or ingestion. J Appl Physiol (Bethesda, Md. : 1985). 1987;63(6):2388–95.
247. Coggan AR, Coyle EF. Carbohydrate ingestion during prolonged exercise: effects on metabolism and performance. Exerc Sport Sci Rev. 1991;19:1–40.
248. Coyle EF, Coggan AR, Hemmert MK, Ivy JL. Muscle glycogen utilization during prolonged strenuous exercise when fed carbohydrate. J Appl Physiol (Bethesda, Md. : 1985). 1986;61(1):165–72.
249. Hill JC, Millan IS. Validation of musculoskeletal ultrasound to assess and quantify muscle glycogen content. A novel approach. Phys Sportsmed. 2014;42(3):45–52.
250. Nieman DC, Shanely RA, Zwetsloot KA, Meaney MP, Farris GE. Ultrasonic assessment of exercise-induced change in skeletal muscle glycogen content. BMC Sports Sci Med Rehab. 2015;7:9.
251. Bone JL, Ross ML, Tomcik KA, Jeacocke NA, Hawley JA, Burke LM. Ultrasound technology fails to provide indirect estimate of muscle glycogen concentration: 1891 Board #43 June 2, 2: 00 PM - 3: 30 PM. Med Sci Sports Exercise. 2016;48(5S).
252. Fogelholm M. Effects of bodyweight reduction on sports performance. Sports Medicine (Auckland, N.Z.). 1994;18(4):249–67.
253. Ramirez ME. Measurement of subcutaneous adipose tissue using ultrasound images. Am J Phys Anthropol. 1992;89(3):347–57.
254. Muller W, Lohman TG, Stewart AD, et al. Subcutaneous fat patterning in athletes: selection of appropriate sites and standardisation of a novel ultrasound measurement technique: ad hoc working group on body composition, health and performance, under the auspices of the IOC Medical Commission. Br J Sports Med. 2016;50(1):45–54.
255. Storchle P, Muller W, Sengeis M, et al. Standardized ultrasound measurement of subcutaneous fat patterning: high reliability and accuracy in groups ranging from lean to obese. Ultrasound Med Biol. 2017;43(2):427–38.
256. Müller W, Horn M, Fürhapter-Rieger A, et al. Body composition in sport: a comparison of a novel ultrasound imaging technique to measure subcutaneous fat tissue compared with skinfold measurement. Br J Sports Med. 2013;47(16):1028.
257. Prado-Costa R, Rebelo J, Monteiro-Barroso J, Preto AS. Ultrasound elastography: compression elastography and shear-wave elastography in the assessment of tendon injury. Insights Into Imaging. 2018;9(5):791–814.
258. Karatekin YS, Karaismailoglu B, Kaynak G, et al. Does elasticity of Achilles tendon change after suture applications? Evaluation of repair area by acoustic radiation force impulse elastography. J Orthop Surg Res. 2018;13(1):45.
259. Nightingale K. Acoustic Radiation Force Impulse (ARFI) imaging: a review. Curr Med Imaging Rev. 2011;7(4):328–39.
260. Cho SH, Lee JY, Han JK, Choi BI. Acoustic radiation force impulse elastography for the evaluation of focal solid hepatic lesions: preliminary findings. Ultrasound Med Biol. 2010;36(2):202–8.
261. Kural Rahatli F, Turnaoglu H, Haberal KM, et al. Acoustic radiation force impulse elastography findings of achilles tendons in patients on chronic hemodialysis and in renal transplant patients. Experimental and Clinical Transplantation: Official Journal of the Middle East Society for Organ Transplantation. 2018;
262. De Zordo T, Chhem R, Smekal V, et al. Real-time sonoelastography: findings in patients with symptomatic achilles tendons and comparison to healthy volunteers. Ultraschall in der Medizin (Stuttgart, Germany: 1980). 2010;31(4):394–400.
263. Klauser AS, Miyamoto H, Tamegger M, et al. Achilles tendon assessed with sonoelastography: histologic agreement. Radiology. 2013;267(3):837–42.
264. Ooi CC, Richards PJ, Maffulli N, et al. A soft patellar tendon on ultrasound elastography is associated with pain and functional deficit in volleyball players. J Sci Med Sport. 2016;19(5):373–8.
265. De Zordo T, Lill SR, Fink C, et al. Real-time sonoelastography of lateral epicondylitis: comparison of findings between patients and healthy volunteers. AJR. Am J Roentgenol. 2009;193(1):180–5.
266. Ahn KS, Kang CH, Hong SJ, Jeong WK. Ultrasound elastography of lateral epicondylosis: clinical feasibility of quantitative elastographic measurements. AJR. Am J Roentgenol. 2014;202(5):1094–9.
267. Park G, Kwon D, Park J. Diagnostic confidence of sonoelastography as adjunct to greyscale ultrasonography in lateral elbow tendinopathy. Chin Med J. 2014;127(17):3110–5.
268. Kocyigit F, Kuyucu E, Kocyigit A, Herek DT, Savkin R, Aslan UB. Investigation of biomechanical characteristics of intact supraspinatus tendons in subacromial impingement syndrome: a cross-sectional study with real-time sonoelastography. Am J Phys Med Rehabil. 2016;95(8):588–96.
269. Klauser AS, Pamminger M, Halpern EJ, et al. Extensor tendinopathy of the elbow assessed with sonoelastography: histologic correlation. Eur Radiol. 2017;27(8):3460–6.
270. Klauser AS, Pamminger MJ, Halpern EJ, et al. Sonoelastography of the common flexor tendon of the elbow with histologic agreement: a cadaveric study. Radiology. 2017;283(2):486–91.
271. Seo JB, Yoo JS, Ryu JW. The accuracy of sonoelastography in fatty degeneration of the supraspinatus: a comparison of magnetic resonance imaging and conventional ultrasonography. J Ultrasound. 2014;17(4):279–85.
272. Seo JB, Yoo JS, Ryu JW. Sonoelastography findings of supraspinatus tendon in rotator cuff tendinopathy without tear: comparison with magnetic reso-

nance images and conventional ultrasonography. J Ultrasound. 2015;18(2):143–9.
273. Tudisco C, Bisicchia S, Stefanini M, Antonicoli M, Masala S, Simonetti G. Tendon quality in small unilateral supraspinatus tendon tears. Real-time sonoelastography correlates with clinical findings. Knee Surgery, Sports Traumatology, Arthroscopy : Official Journal of the ESSKA. 2015;23(2):393–8.
274. Lee SU, Joo SY, Kim SK, Lee SH, Park SR, Jeong C. Real-time sonoelastography in the diagnosis of rotator cuff tendinopathy. J Shoulder Elb Surg. 2016;25(5):723–9.
275. Seo JB, Yoo JS, Ryu JW. Sonoelastography findings of biceps tendinitis and tendinosis. J Ultrasound. 2014;17(4):271–7.
276. Sconfienza LM, Silvestri E, Cimmino MA. Sonoelastography in the evaluation of painful Achilles tendon in amateur athletes. Clin Exp Rheumatol. 2010;28(3):373–8.
277. Tan S, Kudas S, Ozcan AS, et al. Real-time sonoelastography of the Achilles tendon: pattern description in healthy subjects and patients with surgically repaired complete ruptures. Skelet Radiol. 2012;41(9):1067–72.
278. Busilacchi A, Olivieri M, Ulisse S, et al. Real-time sonoelastography as novel follow-up method in Achilles tendon surgery. Knee Surgery, Sports Traumatology, Arthroscopy: Official Journal of the ESSKA. 2016;24(7):2124–32.
279. Brage K, Hjarbaek J, Kjaer P, Ingwersen KG, Juul-Kristensen B. Ultrasonic strain elastography for detecting abnormalities in the supraspinatus tendon: an intra- and inter-rater reliability study. BMJ Open. 2019;9(5):e027725.
280. Gennisson JL, Deffieux T, Fink M, Tanter M. Ultrasound elastography: principles and techniques. Dia Intervent Imaging. 2013;94(5):487–95.
281. Dirrichs T, Quack V, Gatz M, Tingart M, Kuhl CK, Schrading S. Shear Wave Elastography (SWE) for the evaluation of patients with tendinopathies. Acad Radiol. 2016;23(10):1204–13.
282. Coombes BK, Tucker K, Vicenzino B, et al. Achilles and patellar tendinopathy display opposite changes in elastic properties: A shear wave elastography study. Scand J Med Sci Sports. 2018;28(3):1201–8.
283. Aubry S, Nueffer JP, Tanter M, Becce F, Vidal C, Michel F. Viscoelasticity in Achilles tendonopathy: quantitative assessment by using real-time shear-wave elastography. Radiology. 2015;274(3):821–9.
284. Chen XM, Cui LG, He P, Shen WW, Qian YJ, Wang JR. Shear wave elastographic characterization of normal and torn achilles tendons: a pilot study. Journal of Ultrasound in Medicine : Official Journal of the American Institute of Ultrasound in Medicine. 2013;32(3):449–55.
285. Zhang LN, Wan WB, Wang YX, et al. Evaluation of elastic stiffness in healing achilles tendon after surgical repair of a tendon rupture using in vivo ultrasound shear wave elastography. Medical Science Monitor: International Medical Journal of Experimental and Clinical Research. 2016;22:1186–91.
286. Yoshida K, Itoigawa Y, Maruyama Y, Kaneko K. Healing Process of Gastrocnemius Muscle Injury on Ultrasonography Using B-Mode Imaging, Power Doppler Imaging, and Shear Wave Elastography. Journal of Ultrasound in Medicine : Official Journal of the American Institute of Ultrasound in Medicine. 2019;38(12):3239–46.
287. Washburn N, Onishi K, Wang JH. Ultrasound elastography and ultrasound tissue characterisation for tendon evaluation. J Orthopaedic Transl. 2018;15:9–20.
288. van Schie HT, Bakker EM, Jonker AM, van Weeren PR. Efficacy of computerized discrimination between structure-related and non-structure-related echoes in ultrasonographic images for the quantitative evaluation of the structural integrity of superficial digital flexor tendons in horses. Am J Vet Res. 2001;62(7):1159–66.
289. Docking SI, Cook J. Pathological tendons maintain sufficient aligned fibrillar structure on ultrasound tissue characterization (UTC). Scand J Med Sci Sports. 2016;26(6):675–83.
290. Rosengarten SD, Cook JL, Bryant AL, Cordy JT, Daffy J, Docking SI. Australian football players' Achilles tendons respond to game loads within 2 days: an ultrasound tissue characterisation (UTC) study. Br J Sports Med. 2015;49(3):183–7.
291. Docking SI, Rosengarten SD, Cook J. Achilles tendon structure improves on UTC imaging over a 5-month pre-season in elite Australian football players. Scand J Med Sci Sports. 2016;26(5):557–63.
292. van Ark M, Rio E, Cook J, et al. Clinical improvements are not explained by changes in tendon structure on ultrasound tissue characterization after an exercise program for patellar tendinopathy. Am J Phys Med Rehabil. 2018;97(10):708–14.
293. Pereira CS, Santos RCG, Whiteley R, Finni T. Reliability and methodology of quantitative assessment of harvested and unharvested patellar tendons of ACL injured athletes using ultrasound tissue characterization. BMC Sports Science, Medicine & Rehabilitation. 2019;11:12.
294. Torres RJL, Hattori S, Kato Y, Yamada S, Ohuchi H. Ultrasonography and return to play of the different clinical grading of quadriceps contusions: a case series. J Med Ultrasonics (2001). 2018;45(2):375–80.
295. Guillodo Y, Bouttier R, Saraux A. Value of sonography combined with clinical assessment to evaluate muscle injury severity in athletes. J Athl Train. 2011;46(5):500–4.
296. Yoshida K, Itoigawa Y, Maruyama Y, Kaneko K. Healing process of gastrocnemius muscle injury on ultrasonography using B-mode imaging, power doppler imaging, and shear wave elastography. Journal of Ultrasound in Medicine: Official Journal of the American Institute of Ultrasound in Medicine. 2019;

297. Lee JH, Lee JU, Yoo SW. Accuracy and efficacy of ultrasound-guided pes anserinus bursa injection. J Clin Ultrasound: JCU. 2019;47(2):77–82.
298. Hashiuchi T, Sakurai G, Morimoto M, Komei T, Takakura Y, Tanaka Y. Accuracy of the biceps tendon sheath injection: ultrasound-guided or unguided injection? A randomized controlled trial. J Shoulder Elb Surg. 2011;20(7):1069–73.
299. Brull R, Perlas A, Cheng PH, Chan VW. Minimizing the risk of intravascular injection during ultrasound-guided peripheral nerve blockade. Anesthesiology. 2008;109(6):1142; author reply 1144, 1144-1145.
300. Zhang M, Pessina MA, Higgs JB, Kissin EY. A vascular obstacle in ultrasound-guided hip joint injection. J Med Ultrasound. 2018;26(2):77–80.
301. Carra BJ, Bui-Mansfield LT, O'Brien SD, Chen DC. Sonography of musculoskeletal soft-tissue masses: techniques, pearls, and pitfalls. Am J Roentgenol. 2014;202(6):1281–90.
302. Lento PH, Strakowski JA. The use of ultrasound in guiding musculoskeletal interventional procedures. Phys Med Rehabil Clin N Am. 2010;21(3):559–83.
303. Jacobson JA, Kim SM, Brigido MK. Ultrasound-guided percutaneous tenotomy. Semin Musculoskelet Radiol. 2016;20(5):414–21.
304. Koh JS, Mohan PC, Howe TS, et al. Fasciotomy and surgical tenotomy for recalcitrant lateral elbow tendinopathy: early clinical experience with a novel device for minimally invasive percutaneous microresection. Am J Sports Med. 2013;41(3):636–44.
305. Rojo-Manaute JM, Capa-Grasa A, Chana-Rodríguez F, et al. Ultra-minimally invasive ultrasound-guided carpal tunnel release: a randomized clinical trial. Journal of Ultrasound in Medicine: Official Journal of the American Institute of Ultrasound in Medicine. 2016;35(6):1149–57.
306. Nikolaou VS, Malahias MA, Kaseta MK, Sourlas I, Babis GC. Comparative clinical study of ultrasound-guided A1 pulley release vs open surgical intervention in the treatment of trigger finger. World J Orthopedics. 2017;8(2):163–9.
307. Strakowski JA. Ultrasound-guided peripheral nerve procedures. Phys Med Rehabil Clin N Am. 2016;27(3):687–715.
308. Brull R, Hadzic A, Reina MA, Barrington MJ. Pathophysiology and etiology of nerve injury following peripheral nerve blockade. Reg Anesth Pain Med. 2015;40(5):479–90.
309. Finnoff JT, Hall MM, Adams E, et al. American medical society for sports medicine position statement: interventional musculoskeletal ultrasound in sports medicine. Clinical Journal of Sport Medicine: Official Journal of the Canadian Academy of Sport Medicine. 2015;25(1):6–22.
310. de Witte PB, Kolk A, Overes F, Nelissen R, Reijnierse M. Rotator cuff calcific tendinitis: ultrasound-guided needling and lavage versus subacromial corticosteroids: five-year outcomes of a randomized controlled trial. Am J Sports Med. 2017;45(14):3305–14.
311. de Witte PB, Selten JW, Navas A, et al. Calcific tendinitis of the rotator cuff: a randomized controlled trial of ultrasound-guided needling and lavage versus subacromial corticosteroids. Am J Sports Med. 2013;41(7):1665–73.
312. Klontzas ME, Vassalou EE, Karantanas AH. Calcific tendinopathy of the shoulder with intraosseous extension: outcomes of ultrasound-guided percutaneous irrigation. Skelet Radiol. 2017;46(2):201–8.
313. Lanza E, Banfi G, Serafini G, et al. Ultrasound-guided percutaneous irrigation in rotator cuff calcific tendinopathy: what is the evidence? A systematic review with proposals for future reporting. Eur Radiol. 2015;25(7):2176–83.
314. Bazzocchi A, Pelotti P, Serraino S, et al. Ultrasound imaging-guided percutaneous treatment of rotator cuff calcific tendinitis: success in short-term outcome. Br J Radiol. 2016;89(1057):20150407.
315. Oudelaar BW, Schepers-Bok R, Ooms EM. Huis In 't Veld R, Vochteloo AJ. Needle aspiration of calcific deposits (NACD) for calcific tendinitis is safe and effective: Six months follow-up of clinical results and complications in a series of 431 patients. Eur J Radiol. 2016;85(4):689–94.
316. Arirachakaran A, Boonard M, Yamaphai S, Prommahachai A, Kesprayura S, Kongtharvonskul J. Extracorporeal shock wave therapy, ultrasound-guided percutaneous lavage, corticosteroid injection and combined treatment for the treatment of rotator cuff calcific tendinopathy: a network meta-analysis of RCTs. European Journal of Orthopaedic Surgery & Traumatology: Orthopedie Traumatologie. 2017;27(3):381–90.
317. Gatt DL, Charalambous CP. Ultrasound-guided barbotage for calcific tendonitis of the shoulder: a systematic review including 908 patients. Arthroscopy. 2014;30(9):1166–72.
318. Wu YC, Tsai WC, Tu YK, Yu TY. Comparative effectiveness of nonoperative treatments for chronic calcific tendinitis of the shoulder: a systematic review and network meta-analysis of randomized controlled trials. Arch Physical Med Rehab. 2017;98(8):1678–92.e1676.
319. Jo H, Kim G, Baek S, Park HW. Calcific tendinopathy of the gluteus medius mimicking lumbar radicular pain successfully treated with barbotage: a case report. Ann Rehabil Med. 2016;40(2):368–72.
320. Abate M, Salini V, Schiavone C. Ultrasound-guided percutaneous lavage in the treatment of calcific tendinopathy of elbow extensor tendons: a case report. Malaysian Orthopaedic J. 2016;10(2):53–5.
321. Hall MM, Rajasekaran S. Ultrasound-guided scraping for chronic patellar tendinopathy: a case presentation. PM & R: the Journal of Injury, Function, and Rehabilitation. 2016;8(6):593–6.

322. Alfredson H. Ultrasound and Doppler-guided mini-surgery to treat midportion Achilles tendinosis: results of a large material and a randomised study comparing two scraping techniques. Br J Sports Med. 2011;45(5):407–10.
323. Humphrey J, Chan O, Crisp T, et al. The short-term effects of high volume image guided injections in resistant non-insertional Achilles tendinopathy. J Sci Med Sport. 2010;13(3):295–8.
324. Boesen AP, Hansen R, Boesen MI, Malliaras P, Langberg H. Effect of high-volume injection, platelet-rich plasma, and sham treatment in chronic midportion achilles tendinopathy: a randomized double-blinded prospective study. Am J Sports Med. 2017;45(9):2034–43.
325. Chan O, O'Dowd D, Padhiar N, et al. High volume image guided injections in chronic Achilles tendinopathy. Disabil Rehabil. 2008;30(20-22):1697–708.
326. Maffulli N, Spiezia F, Longo UG, Denaro V, Maffulli GD. High volume image guided injections for the management of chronic tendinopathy of the main body of the Achilles tendon. Physical Therapy in Sport: Official Journal of the Association of Chartered Physiotherapists in Sports Medicine. 2013;14(3):163–7.
327. Abate M, Di Carlo L, Verna S, Di Gregorio P, Schiavone C, Salini V. Synergistic activity of platelet rich plasma and high volume image guided injection for patellar tendinopathy. Knee Surgery, Sports Traumatology, Arthroscopy: Official Journal of the ESSKA. 2018;26(12):3645–51.
328. Crisp T, Khan F, Padhiar N, et al. High volume ultrasound guided injections at the interface between the patellar tendon and Hoffa's body are effective in chronic patellar tendinopathy: a pilot study. Disabil Rehabil. 2008;30(20-22):1625–34.
329. Maffulli N, Del Buono A, Oliva F, Testa V, Capasso G, Maffulli G. High-volume image-guided injection for recalcitrant patellar tendinopathy in athletes. Clinical Journal of Sport Medicine: Official Journal of the Canadian Academy of Sport Medicine. 2016;26(1):12–6.
330. Morton S, Chan O, King J, et al. High volume image-guided Injections for patellar tendinopathy: a combined retrospective and prospective case series. Muscles Ligaments Tendons J. 2014;4(2):214–9.
331. Morton S, Chan O, Ghozlan A, Price J, Perry J, Morrissey D. High volume image guided injections and structured rehabilitation in shoulder impingement syndrome: a retrospective study. Muscles Ligaments Tendons J. 2015;5(3):195–9.
332. Wheeler PC, Mahadevan D, Bhatt R, Bhatia M. A comparison of two different high-volume image-guided injection procedures for patients with chronic noninsertional achilles tendinopathy: a pragmatic retrospective cohort study. J Foot Ankle Surg. 2016;55(5):976–9.
333. Morton S, Chan O, Price J, et al. High volume image-guided injections and structured rehabilitation improve greater trochanter pain syndrome in the short and medium term: a combined retrospective and prospective case series. Muscles Ligaments Tendons J. 2015;5(2):73–87.
334. Gilberts EC, Beekman WH, Stevens HJ, Wereldsma JC. Prospective randomized trial of open versus percutaneous surgery for trigger digits. J Hand Surg. 2001;26(3):497–500.
335. Nakamichi K, Tachibana S. Ultrasonographically assisted carpal tunnel release. J Hand Surg. 1997;22(5):853–62.
336. Nakamichi K, Tachibana S, Yamamoto S, Ida M. Percutaneous carpal tunnel release compared with mini-open release using ultrasonographic guidance for both techniques. J Hand Surg. 2010;35(3):437–45.
337. McShane JM, Slaff S, Gold JE, Nazarian LN. Sonographically guided percutaneous needle release of the carpal tunnel for treatment of carpal tunnel syndrome: preliminary report. Journal of Ultrasound in Medicine: Official Journal of the American Institute of Ultrasound in Medicine. 2012;31(9):1341–9.
338. Guo XY, Xiong MX, Lu M, et al. Ultrasound-guided needle release of the transverse carpal ligament with and without corticosteroid injection for the treatment of carpal tunnel syndrome. J Orthop Surg Res. 2018;13(1):69.
339. Guo XY, Xiong MX, Zhao Y, et al. Comparison of the clinical effectiveness of ultrasound-guided corticosteroid injection with and without needle release of the transverse carpal ligament in carpal tunnel syndrome. Eur Neurol. 2017;78(1-2):33–40.
340. Guo D, Guo D, Guo J, Malone DG, Wei N, McCool LC. A cadaveric study for the improvement of thread carpal tunnel release. J Hand Surg. 2016;41(10):e351–7.
341. Guo D, Guo D, Guo J, Schmidt SC, Lytie RM. A clinical study of the modified thread carpal tunnel release. Hand (New York, N.Y.). 2017;12(5):453–60.
342. Burnham R, Playfair L, Loh E, Roberts S, Agur A. Evaluation of the effectiveness and safety of ultrasound-guided percutaneous carpal tunnel release: a cadaveric study. Am J Phys Med Rehabil. 2017;96(7):457–63.
343. Capa-Grasa A, Rojo-Manaute JM, Rodriguez FC, Martin JV. Ultra minimally invasive sonographically guided carpal tunnel release: an external pilot study. Orthopaedics & Traumatology, Surgery & Research: OTSR. 2014;100(3):287–92.
344. Rojo-Manaute JM, Capa-Grasa A, Rodriguez-Maruri GE, Moran LM, Martinez MV, Martin JV. Ultra-minimally invasive sonographically guided carpal tunnel release: anatomic study of a new tech-

nique. Journal of Ultrasound in Medicine: Official Journal of the American Institute of Ultrasound in Medicine. 2013;32(1):131–42.

345. Chern TC, Kuo LC, Shao CJ, Wu TT, Wu KC, Jou IM. Ultrasonographically guided percutaneous carpal tunnel release: early clinical experiences and outcomes. Arthroscopy: The Journal of Arthroscopic & Related Surgery : Official Publication of the Arthroscopy Association of North America and the International Arthroscopy Association. 2015;31(12):2400–10.
346. Petrover D, Hakime A, Silvera J, Richette P, Nizard R. Ultrasound-guided surgery for carpal tunnel syndrome: a new interventional procedure. Semin Interv Radiol. 2018;35(4):248–54.
347. Petrover D, Silvera J, De Baere T, Vigan M, Hakime A. Percutaneous ultrasound-guided carpal tunnel release: study upon clinical efficacy and safety. Cardiovasc Intervent Radiol. 2017;40(4):568–75.
348. Henning PT, Yang L, Awan T, Lueders D, Pourcho AM. Minimally invasive ultrasound-guided carpal tunnel release: preliminary clinical results. Journal of Ultrasound in Medicine: Official Journal of the American Institute of Ultrasound in Medicine. 2018;37(11):2699–706.
349. Henning T, Lueders D, Chang K, Yang L. Ultrasound-Guided carpal tunnel release using dynamic expansion of the transverse safe zone in a patient with postpolio syndrome: a case report. PM & R: The Journal of Injury, Function, and Rehabilitation. 2018;10(10):1115–8.
350. Latzka EW, Henning PT, Pourcho AM. Sonographic changes after ultrasound-guided release of the transverse carpal ligament: a case report. PM & R: The Journal of Injury, Function, and Rehabilitation. 2018;10(10):1125–9.
351. Beckman JP, Sellon JL, Lachman N, Smith J. Sonographically detected transligamentous median nerve branch. Am J Phys Med Rehabil. 2018;97(9):e87–8.
352. Sytsma TT, Ryan HS, Lachman N, Kakar S, Smith J. Anatomic relationship between the hook of the hamate and the distal transverse carpal ligament: implications for ultrasound-guided carpal tunnel release. Am J Phys Med Rehabil. 2018;97(7):482–7.
353. Rajeswaran G, Healy JC, Lee JC. Percutaneous release procedures: trigger finger and carpal tunnel. Semin Musculoskelet Radiol. 2016;20(5):432–40.
354. Rajeswaran G, Lee JC, Eckersley R, Katsarma E, Healy JC. Ultrasound-guided percutaneous release of the annular pulley in trigger digit. Eur Radiol. 2009;19(9):2232–7.
355. Smith J, Rizzo M, Lai JK. Sonographically guided percutaneous first annular pulley release: cadaveric safety study of needle and knife techniques. J Ultrasound Med. 2010;29(11):1531–42.
356. Rojo-Manaute JM, Rodriguez-Maruri G, Capa-Grasa A, Chana-Rodriguez F, Soto Mdel V, Martin JV. Sonographically guided intrasheath percutaneous release of the first annular pulley for trigger digits, part 1: clinical efficacy and safety. Journal of Ultrasound in Medicine : Official Journal of the American Institute of Ultrasound in Medicine. 2012;31(3):417–24.
357. Guo D, Guo D, Guo J, McCool LC, Tonkin B. A cadaveric study of the thread trigger finger release: the first annular pulley transection through thread transecting technique. Hand (New York, N.Y.). 2018;13(2):170–5.
358. Pan M, Sheng S, Fan Z, et al. Ultrasound-guided percutaneous release of A1 pulley by using a needle knife: a prospective study of 41 cases. Front Pharmacol. 2019;10:267.
359. Rojo-Manaute JM, Capa-Grasa A, Del Cerro-Gutierrez M, Martinez MV, Chana-Rodriguez F, Martin JV. Sonographically guided intrasheath percutaneous release of the first annular pulley for trigger digits, part 2: randomized comparative study of the economic impact of 3 surgical models. Journal of Ultrasound in Medicine : Official Journal of the American Institute of Ultrasound in Medicine. 2012;31(3):427–38.
360. Marcos AI, Villanueva-Martinez M, Barrett SL, Rodriguez-Collazo ER, Sanz-Ruiz P. Ultrasound-guided release of the tibial nerve and its distal branches: a cadaveric study. J Ultrasound Med. 2018;
361. Lapegue F, Andre A, Pasquier Bernachot E, et al. US-guided percutaneous release of the first extensor tendon compartment using a 21-gauge needle in de Quervain's disease: a prospective study of 35 cases. Eur Radiol. 2018;28(9):3977–85.
362. Levy B, Ducat A, Gaudin P, et al. Ultrasound-guided percutaneous tenotomy of the long head of the biceps tendon: a non-reliable technique. Knee Surgery, Sports Traumatology, Arthroscopy: Official Journal of the ESSKA. 2012;20(6):1027–30.
363. Aly AR, Rajasekaran S, Mohamed A, Beavis C, Obaid H. Feasibility of ultrasound-guided percutaneous tenotomy of the long head of the biceps tendon--A pilot cadaveric study. J Clin Ultrasound: JCU. 2015;43(6):361–6.
364. Sconfienza LM, Mauri G, Messina C, et al. Ultrasound-guided percutaneous tenotomy of biceps tendon: technical feasibility on cadavers. Ultrasound Med Biol. 2016;42(10):2513–7.
365. Smith J, Alfredson H, Masci L, Sellon JL, Woods CD. Sonographically guided plantaris tendon release: a cadaveric validation study. PM & R: The Journal of Injury, Function, and Rehabilitation. 2018.
366. Boettcher BJ, Hollman JH, Stuart MJ, Finnoff JT. Ultrasound-guided cutting wire release of the proximal adductor longus tendon: a feasibility study. Orthopaedic J Sports Med. 2019;7(8):2325967119866010.

367. Vohra PK, Japour CJ. Ultrasound-guided plantar fascia release technique: a retrospective study of 46 feet. J Am Podiatr Med Assoc. 2009;99(3):183–90.
368. Debrule MB. Ultrasound-guided weil percutaneous plantar fasciotomy. J Am Podiatr Med Assoc. 2010;100(2):146–8.
369. Hattori S, Alvarez CAD, Canton S, Hogan MV, Onishi K. Ultrasound-guided ankle lateral ligament stabilization. Curr Rev Musculoskel Med. 2019;12(4):497–508.
370. Seijas R, Rius M, Barastegui D, Ares O, Rivera E, Alvarez-Diaz P. Sonographic measurement of the patellar tendon should predict autograft Bone Patellar Tendon Bone (BPTB) size: comparison of anatomical and clinical findings. Journal of Investigative Surgery: The Official Journal of the Academy of Surgical Research. 2019:1–6.
371. Takeuchi S, Rothrauff B, Taguchi M, Fu F, Onishi K. Prediction of quadriceps tendon autograft diameter with preoperative ultrasonography for individualized anterior cruciate ligament reconstruction. Paper presented at: Orthopaedic Research Society2020; Phoenix, Arizona.
372. Takenaga T, Yoshida M, Albers M, et al. Preoperative sonographic measurement can accurately predict quadrupled hamstring tendon graft diameter for ACL reconstruction. Knee Surgery, Sports Traumatology, Arthroscopy: Official Journal of the ESSKA. 2019;27(3):797–804.
373. Rodriguez-Mendez LM, Martinez-Ruiz JJ, Perez-Manzo R, Corona-Hernandez JL, Alcala-Zermeno JL, Sanchez-Enriquez S. Preoperative ultrasonographic prediction of hamstring tendon diameter for anterior cruciate ligament repair. J Knee Surg. 2017;30(6):544–8.
374. Sumanont S, Mahaweerawat C, Boonrod A, Thammaroj P, Boonrod A. Preoperative ultrasound evaluation of the semitendinosus tendon for anterior cruciate ligament reconstruction. Orthopaedic J Sports Med. 2019;7(1):2325967118822318.
375. Gofeld M, Bristow SJ, Chiu S, Kliot M. Preoperative ultrasound-guided mapping of peripheral nerves. J Neurosurg. 2013;119(3):709–13.
376. Chavez J, Hattori S, Kato Y, Takazawa S, Yamada S, Ohuchi H. The use of ultrasonography during minimally invasive Achilles tendon repair to avoid sural nerve injury. J Med Ultrasonics (2001). 2019;46(4):513–4.
377. Ohuchi H, Ichikawa K, Shinga K, Hattori S, Yamada S, Takahashi K. Ultrasound-assisted endoscopic partial plantar fascia release. Arthroscopy Tech. 2013;2(3):e227–30.
378. Ohuchi H, Torres RJL, Shinga K, et al. Ultrasound-assisted posteromedial portal placement of the elbow joint to prevent ulnar nerve injury. Arthroscopy Tech. 2017;6(4):e1087–91.
379. Hanna AS, Ehlers ME, Lee KS. Preoperative ultrasound-guided wire localization of the lateral femoral cutaneous nerve. Operative Neurosurgery (Hagerstown, Md.). 2017;13(3):402–8.
380. Hwang J-J, Quistgaard J, Souquet J, Crum LA. Portable ultrasound device for battlefield trauma. Paper presented at: 1998 IEEE Ultrasonics Symposium. Proceedings (Cat. No. 98CH36102)1998.
381. Shorter M, Macias DJ. Portable handheld ultrasound in austere environments: use in the Haiti disaster. Prehospital Disaster Med. 2012;27(2):172–7.
382. Nolting L, Baker D, Hardy Z, Kushinka M, Brown HA. Solar-powered point-of-care sonography: our himalayan experience. Journal of Ultrasound in Medicine: Official Journal of the American Institute of Ultrasound in Medicine. 2019;38(9):2477–84.
383. Berko NS, Goldberg-Stein S, Thornhill BA, Koenigsberg M. Survey of current trends in postgraduate musculoskeletal ultrasound education in the United States. Skelet Radiol. 2016;45(4):475–82.
384. Wu WT, Chang KV, Han DS, Ozcakar L. Musculoskeletal ultrasound workshops in postgraduate physician training: a pre- and post-workshop survey of 156 participants. BMC Med Education. 2019;19(1):362.
385. Drolet P, Martineau A, Lacroix R, Roy JS. Reliability of ultrasound evaluation of the long head of the biceps tendon. J Rehabil Med. 2016;48(6):554–8.
386. Fowler JR, Hirsch D, Kruse K. The reliability of ultrasound measurements of the median nerve at the carpal tunnel inlet. J Hand Surg. 2015;40(10):1992–5.
387. Garcia-Santibanez R, Dietz AR, Bucelli RC, Zaidman CM. Nerve ultrasound reliability of upper limbs: Effects of examiner training. Muscle Nerve. 2018;57(2):189–92.
388. Ishida H, Suehiro T, Suzuki K, Watanabe S. Muscle thickness and echo intensity measurements of the rectus femoris muscle of healthy subjects: Intra and interrater reliability of transducer tilt during ultrasound. J Bodyw Mov Ther. 2018;22(3):657–60.
389. Tamborrini G, Marx C, Micheroli R. Inter-rater reliability in the classification of supraspinatus tendon tears using 3D ultrasound - a question of experience? J Ultrasonography. 2016;16(66):252–9.
390. Modica MJ, Kanal KM, Gunn ML. The obese emergency patient: imaging challenges and solutions. Radiographics: A Review Publication of the Radiological Society of North America, Inc. 2011;31(3):811–23.
391. Averkiou MA, Roundhill DN, Powers JE. A new imaging technique based on the nonlinear properties of tissues. Paper presented at. 1997 IEEE Ultrasonics Symposium Proceedings. An International Symposium (Cat. No.97CH36118); 5-8 Oct. 1997, 1997.
392. Ward B, Baker AC, Humphrey VF. Nonlinear propagation applied to the improvement of resolution in diagnostic medical ultrasound. J Acoustical Soc Am. 1997;101(1):143–54.

393. Meuwly JY, Thiran JP, Gudinchet F. Application of adaptive image processing technique to real-time spatial compound ultrasound imaging improves image quality. Investig Radiol. 2003;38(5):257–62.
394. Barr RG, Maldonado RL, Georgian-Smith D. Comparison of conventional, compounding, computer enhancement, and compounding with computer enhancement in ultrasound imaging of the breast. Ultrasound Quarterly. 2009;25(3):129–34.
395. McLaughlin GW. Practical aberration correction methods. Ultrasound. 2007;15(2):99–104.
396. Weng L, Tirumalai AP, Lowery CM, et al. US extended-field-of-view imaging technology. Radiology. 1997;203(3):877–80.
397. Lin EC, Middleton WD, Teefey SA. Extended field of view sonography in musculoskeletal imaging. J Ultrasound Med. 1999;18(2):147–52.
398. Lang RM, Addetia K, Narang A, Mor-Avi V. 3-dimensional echocardiography: latest developments and future directions. J Am Coll Cardiol Img. 2018;11(12):1854–78.
399. Merz E, Abramowicz JS. 3D/4D ultrasound in prenatal diagnosis: is it time for routine use? Clin Obstet Gynecol. 2012;55(1):336–51.
400. Fenster A, Blake C, Gyacskov I, Landry A, Spence JD. 3D ultrasound analysis of carotid plaque volume and surface morphology. Ultrasonics. 2006;44(Suppl 1):e153–7.
401. Rana M, Wakeling JM. In-vivo determination of 3D muscle architecture of human muscle using free hand ultrasound. J Biomech. 2011;44(11):2129–35.

Use of Musculoskeletal Ultrasound and Regenerative Therapies in Sports

22

Jeimylo C. de Castro

Musculoskeletal Ultrasound in Sports

Musculoskeletal ultrasound has significantly improved over the years as a primary tool for diagnosing musculoskeletal injuries in the sports activity. As technology improves coupled with its unique dynamic feature of looking at tissues, the ability to provide real-time information is enhanced. High-quality diagnostic ultrasound, however, cannot be done without an accurate clinical history of the injury, knowledge of gender-specific injuries, and an understanding of the mechanism of injuries especially in diagnosing defects and determining appropriate treatment among amateur and professional athletes alike [1]. Several technological features were added in the ultrasound such as higher resolution linear array probes, tissue harmonic imaging, extended field of view, two-dimensional matrix probe technology, power Doppler sonography, and elastography. All these features make it easier for the sonologist to detect and characterize a variety of musculoskeletal pathologies [2]. With all the challenges in the healthcare industry, the use of ultrasound provides a less costly alternative to MRI scan, with one notable drawback, which is its operator-dependency [2]. A well-trained and competent sonologist is needed for consistent and reliable imaging studies.

With regard to sports injuries, there is always the question of which comes first – the need for precision and diagnostic sensitivity of the machine to be able to deliver the appropriate treatment or the upgrading of the machine itself to get the advantage of the market? In professional sports, one feature in ultrasound, for instance, that stands out is tissue harmonic imaging (THI). This provides greater contrast in resolution for tendons and muscles with similar impedance [3]. For instance, the use of THI at 7.5 MHz will collect the information at 14 MHz, thus enabling the image to be shown at greater resolution even at deeper structures. Further, it reduces most of the artifacts such as reverberation, and improves the signal-to-noise ratio [3]. Some studies show that this feature is best for diagnosing shoulder lesions, especially subscapular tendons [4, 5]. Another feature that enhances visualization of the image is an extended field of view technique or panoramic view. With this, large lesions can be viewed easily, especially those involving the knees and thigh muscles [3]. To improve the lateral resolution of the image, and improve the images of deeper planes, a real-time compound ultrasound system can be used

J. C. de Castro (✉)
Chair, Physical Medicine and Rehabilitation Department, The Medical City-South Luzon, Sta. Rosa, Laguna, Philippines

Medical Director/CEO, SMARTMD Center for Non-Surgical Pain Interventions, Makati City, Philippines

Y. El Miedany (ed.), *Musculoskeletal Ultrasound-Guided Regenerative Medicine*, https://doi.org/10.1007/978-3-030-98256-0_22

[6]. Also, the use of power Doppler enables images to be obtained in painful tendinopathies and inflammatory conditions which correlate well with MRI scans [3]. Recently, Afandi and Astawa did a 10-year systematic review of athletes suffering from tendinopathies using elastography ultrasound (EUS) between 2009 and 2019 using 59 articles. The study showed that both strain and shear-wave elastographies are reliable techniques in musculoskeletal ultrasound and have shown higher sensitivity, specificity, and accuracy in diagnosing early tendon pathologies than the B-mode conventional ultrasound. EUS is also used as a tool to evaluate and guide ongoing treatments in post-op rehabilitation monitoring and to predict a return to play especially in high-level professional athletes. Various tendons are amenable to this technique such as rotator cuff and rotator cuff tendons, common extensor tendons of the elbow, patellar tendons, Achilles tendon, and the plantar fascia [7]. Of particular interest and unique feature of ultrasound also is dynamic imaging. Dynamic ultrasound is affected, however, by the field of view, which is typically 40–60 mm wide, and the frame rate. The field of view can be improved by using either an extended field of view feature or probes with a larger field of view. The frame rate refers to the number of images the ultrasound can acquire in 1 second [8]. In one study, dynamic ultrasound of a lateral ankle injury involving calcaneofibular ligament (CFL) showed that ultrasound has a sensitivity of 90% and a specificity of 100%, with a positive predictive value (PPV) of 100% and a negative predictive value of 91.7% as compared to MRI [9]. Dynamic imaging in ultrasound can be used to evaluate multidirectional laxity of a structure, assess tendon subluxation, and support the clinical decision of a referral [10, 11]. It can also be used for ultrasound-guided interventional procedures to aid the practitioner in optimal needle placement [12]. Contrast-enhanced ultrasound (CEUS) is another feature in ultrasound which is used to visualize other organs in the body, but recently it has been found useful for visualizing musculoskeletal injuries. In a study by Kunz and colleagues, CEUS was used to predict the outcome of previously large supraspinatus (SSP) tear sustaining retear after surgical repair. In the past, MRI-based parameters like tear size, fatty infiltration, and tendon retraction are measured pre-operatively together with the demographic data of the patient. Similarly, the postoperative morphologic changes seen in the MRI scan can hardly be used to predict outcomes, and thus has weak to moderate predictive strength. This was observed in a number of patients at risk for poor functional outcome or failed tendon healing because of the inability of the lesion to be detected by MRI imaging. In this study, muscle perfusion assessment by CEUS is used postoperatively reflecting the regenerative potential of the SSP muscle/tendon system rather than the morphologic parameters in MRI. Results showed that preoperative CEUS-based assessment of SSP perfusion significantly correlated with early postoperative shoulder function and tendon retear after surgical repair. Therefore, it helps identify patients who are at low or high risk for tendon retear by assessing microcirculation as a surrogate parameter for tissue vitality and metabolism [13].

Wengert and colleagues compared the use of high-resolution ultrasound and magnetic resonance arthrography (MRA) in sports-related shoulder injuries. Usually, MRA is used to assess intraarticular abnormities and rotator cuff injuries by application of contrast agent with better visualization of intraarticular shoulder injuries as compared to conventional MRI scan. This study has shown that high-frequency ultrasound is a reliable modality for the rotator cuff, long head biceps (LHB) tendon, and acromioclavicular joint over MRA based on its diagnostic accuracy, comfortability, cost-effectiveness, and availability. However, for other structures, MRA remains the gold standard of diagnosis [14]. It is also recommended that in any sports injury, musculoskeletal ultrasound should be used as an initial study for patients with acute and chronic shoulder pain [15, 16]. Conventional radiographs should always be used as a baseline imaging modality for any shoulder injuries [14].

The use of musculoskeletal ultrasound will be much simple with the advent of capacitive micromachined transducer (CMUT). It is a breakthrough in ultrasound technology where a single probe instead of various probes for different ultrasound examinations can be applicable. In contrast to conventional ultrasound, CMUT does not utilize crystals. Instead, it makes use of the new generation silicon wafer technology composed of innumerable tiny vibration drum cells formed in the micrometer scale. These cells are arranged in a matrix array that improves spatial resolution where the frequency bandwidth is in the range of 2–22 MHz. Its e-focusing feature allows better penetration with less focus-dependency. It has the ability to image all or most of the image fields during each transmission by its fast parallel beam-forming ability. CMUT delivers one probe for all ultrasound examinations. Moreover, with all its fancy development, there is a need to improve in terms of the resolution of the superficial tissues and Doppler signal to validate its claim over the lead-based piezoelectric linear probes [17].

An emerging development in the diagnosis of sports injury is the fusion of MRI-US technology. Although it technically requires fusion imaging hardware, it is a good choice for sports-related injuries such as partial- or full-thickness tendon tears, nerve entrapments, muscle strains, ligamental sprains, joint effusions, and other soft-tissue injuries. This is usually done by using previously acquired MRI scans and is then fused with real-time US. The linkage is made possible by the fusion imaging hardware whereby an electromagnetic sensor attached to the US probe sends positional data to the fusion US machine. By selecting two or more recognizable landmarks, locking a plane, and then registering the images on each of the two studies, this linkage is done. US fusion technology allows simultaneous viewing of the MRI which corresponds with real-time US images on the US monitor on any plane. This combination of imaging techniques can lead to a more accurate diagnosis and better clinical decisions during a sports injury. While the US provides imaging studies for the more superficial structures, MRI provides better imaging with deeper structures like muscle injuries [18].

Musculoskeletal Ultrasound/Regenerative Therapies in Upper Extremity Sports Injuries

Shoulder

The shoulder is one of the most affected areas in swimming and water sports. This is by far the most frequent chronic injury in swimmers representing about 40–90% of limiting shoulder pain among swimmers [19]. Generally, the symptoms are caused by overuse injuries and affect the subacromial region, rotator cuff, long head of the biceps, subcoracoid and subacromial-subdeltoid bursae, which are best diagnosed by ultrasound [1, 20, 21]. Lengthy swimming careers may lead to a reduction in the mechanical properties of the supraspinatus muscle and tendon with an increased likelihood of rotator cuff pathology over the years [22]. Surprisingly, the pathological changes that lead to pain among elite swimmers are not known, although ultrasound findings suggest overuse tendinopathy and glenohumeral ligamentous laxity [19]. In water polo sports, a complex combination of shoulder pathologies is seen in the early asymptomatic stage. As a result, the use of ultrasound is useful in the quick management of and regular follow-up of shoulder modifications in regular practice in sports medicine [23].

Generally, the patient with rotator cuff tears (Fig. 22.1) usually presents with pain and weakness of the lateral deltoid. Pain is usually felt at night when the patient sleeps on that side affected. The most effective examination tests are the active painful arc test, drop arm test, and weakness on external rotation [24]. A study by Wengert and colleagues, comparing US to MRA to assess shoulder pathology, showed that US is superior to MRA in assessing rotator cuff, long head of the biceps, posterior labrum, and the AC joint with the additional feature of dynamic examination of US in conjunction with clinical examination [14]. Also, muscle degeneration as the consequence of

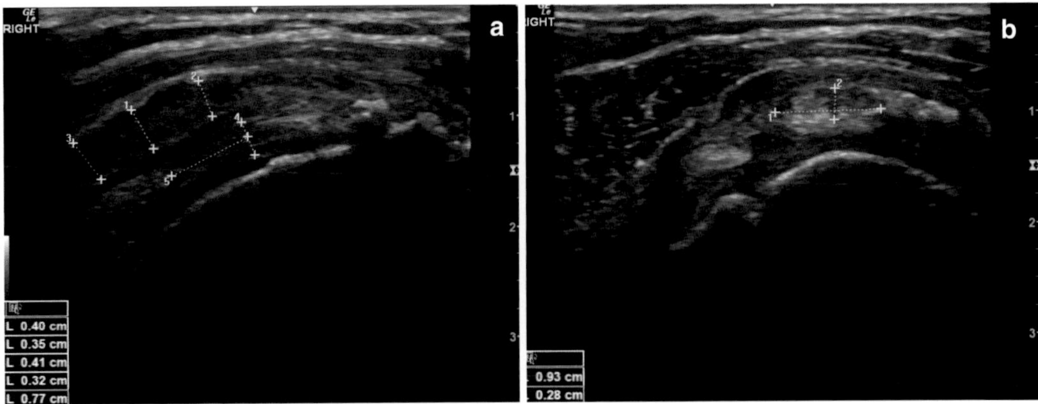

Fig. 22.1 (**a**) A longitudinal view of the supraspinatus tendon showing full-thickness tear with hypoechoic swelling of the subdeltoid bursa. Note the cortical irregularity of the greater tuberosity of the humerus which serves as the attachment of the supraspinatus tendon. (**b**) Short-axis view of the supraspinatus tendon full-thickness tear with some hyperechoic changes indicative of calcium deposits

supraspinatus tendon tear could be best visualized by contrast-enhanced ultrasound (CEUS) examination rather than by MRI scan. CEUS assesses muscular vitality by assessing microvascular perfusion of the muscle tissue after rotator cuff repair and thus serves as a quantitative method to evaluate rotator cuff muscles [25, 26].

Asymptomatic rotator cuff tears are common among overhead and throwing athletes, and with particular interest are the baseball pitchers [26]. The increased risk of tendinopathy occurred during the late cocking phase of throwing causing an internal shoulder impingement [28]. Most of these asymptomatic patients surprisingly do not develop symptoms of pain even up to 5 years follow-up of ongoing, competitive play [29, 30]. Most of them showed articular-sided tears of the supraspinatus and infraspinatus muscles without any symptoms at all [30]. In fact, some of them in a repeat MRI scan may show resolution of the tendinopathy or partial tears of the rotator cuff, years after retirement from sports activity, and does not progress to full tears [31]. So, the question is what is the cause of the shoulder pain? Among non-athletes, Yamaguchi sonographically found that enlargement of the tears in 50% of patients may be the cause of pain [31], while other ultrasound studies showed that shoulder pain with partial- and/or full-thickness tears is associated with increasing age [32, 33]. The presence of pain in the shoulder among athletes do not correlate with the presence of shoulder pathologies such as tendinopathies or tendon tears as these findings may be present in asymptomatic individuals [26]. Moreover, among baseball pitchers experiencing shoulder pain, an ultrasound study detected an increase in width of the infraspinatus and long head of biceps tendon as early as 50 pitches as a response to overload experience with no associated decrease in echogenicity [27]. In a study by Takenaga and colleagues on healthy college baseball players with a career length of at least 10 years, shear-wave ultrasound elastography was used to measure elasticity. The study showed that the posterior and postero-inferior capsules of the shoulder were stiffer and thicker in the throwing shoulder than in the non-throwing shoulder. Further, posterior capsule elasticity has greater effect on glenohumeral internal rotation deficit (GIRD) than did posterior capsule thickness, and thus this non-invasive procedure will help identify players who are at risk for shoulder injuries [34]. Moreover, pitchers with GIRD usually show dominant humeral retro torsion [35]. Humeral retro torsion is also seen as an adaptive change among young healthy baseball athletes (8–14 years old) during throwing activities and could influence shoulder motion at a young age [36].

Shoulder injuries might in some way affect the brachial plexus nerves. In a systematic review by Chin and colleagues on traumatic brachial plexus injury studies up to July 2016, covering seven studies, the use of ultrasound as a diagnostic tool was most sensitive in lesions in the upper and middle (C5-C7) than in the lower spinal nerves (C8, T1). However, the window for ultrasound examination in these studies was up to about a 27-month period. Identifying surgical candidates is most needed within the 3- to 6-month period and as such the question of whether the US is sensitive enough to diagnose cases in the acute stage is raised. The value of the US as a first-line diagnostic tool for traumatic brachial plexus injuries needs further standardized studies. However, this does not preclude the fact that this tool has a great potential for such cases [37]. Unless there is an indication of a peripheral nerve injury, the use of ultrasound as a screening modality for athletes with suspected peripheral nerve entrapment due to atrophy of supra- and infraspinatus muscles with or without pain is not warranted [38].

Pectoralis muscle injuries occur when the athlete is eccentrically contracted, with the shoulder extended, abducted, and externally rotated. Patients often complain of pain, swelling, and weakness [39, 40]. While this is rare, this is common among weightlifters and occurred during the eccentric phase of bench press [39]. Ultrasound is a valuable modality for assessment but has its limitations. MRI scan remains the diagnostic imaging of choice. Surgical intervention is recommended for complete tears of pectoralis muscles with a return to play at about 6 months [41].

Ultrasound can also be used to evaluate whether a certain exercise modality provides the promised effect on a particular muscle being trained. Sachdeva and colleagues assessed different strength training for the supraspinatus muscle. Their study showed that strength training using prone horizontal abduction was effective for maintaining fiber bundle length (FBL) and facilitating increases in strength in multiple modes allowing the muscle to produce greater forces over a larger range of motion of the shoulder joint. Thus, this is a more effective exercise for supraspinatus strengthening [42].

The use of ultrasound to diagnose shoulder conditions in sports medicine could not be overemphasized. In undifferentiated shoulder pain, a bedside ultrasound showed a change in diagnosis in 53% of cases and a change in management in 60% of cases. It also resulted in a new order of MRI in 28% of cases and an elimination of an MRI order in 21% of patients [43]. Arthroscopic techniques remain the gold standard for treating most rotator cuff tears providing similar functional results to open and mini-open surgery with an additional advantage of lesser postoperative complications [44]. Pain in post-arthroscopic surgery, however, was more significant in smaller tears than in larger tears because of more vigorous healing in smaller tears from 6 weeks to 6 months after surgery [45]. Regenerative injection therapies are becoming popular as an alternative treatment to surgery due to their potential to provide healing and shorter recovery as in the case of platelet-rich plasma (PRP) (Fig. 22.2). The use of PRP therapy in rotator cuff conditions did not show any improvement when used in an interstitial supraspinatus tear as compared with saline injections [46]. Ultrasound-guided peritendinous subacromial hyaluronic acid (HA) injection over the supraspinatus tendon combined with physical therapy showed high efficacy in the treatment of supraspinatus tendinopathy resulting in an earlier return to play and with lesser rehabilitation sessions [47]. Cai and colleagues did a study combining PRP and sodium hyaluronate (SH) to treat partial-thickness rotator cuff tear and compared the results with either PRP alone or SH alone. A study showed that the combination of PRP + SH as compared with either PRP alone or SH alone yielded a better clinical outcome in terms of healing and showing a cumulative effect after repeated injections. This combination treatment enhanced the recovery of small- to medium-sized bursal-sided tears by alleviating pain and decreasing tear size over a 12-month period (pretreatment AP size = 7.38 ± 1.06; 1-year post-treatment AP size = 1.52 ± 0.62) [48]. PRP was also used as an adjunct treatment for post-arthroscopic supraspinatus repair. A midterm evaluation was done to see any effect of PRP on the healing tissues. This

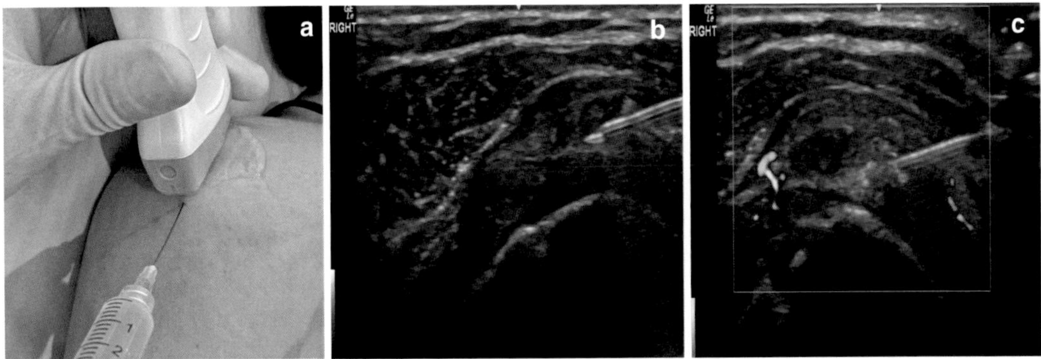

Fig. 22.2 (**a**) Ultrasound-guided LR-PRP injection of the supraspinatus tendon. (**b**, **c**) Short axis ultrasound approach to the torn supraspinatus tendon using LR-PRP using both B-mode and power Doppler to ensure that no vital structures are hit during the approach

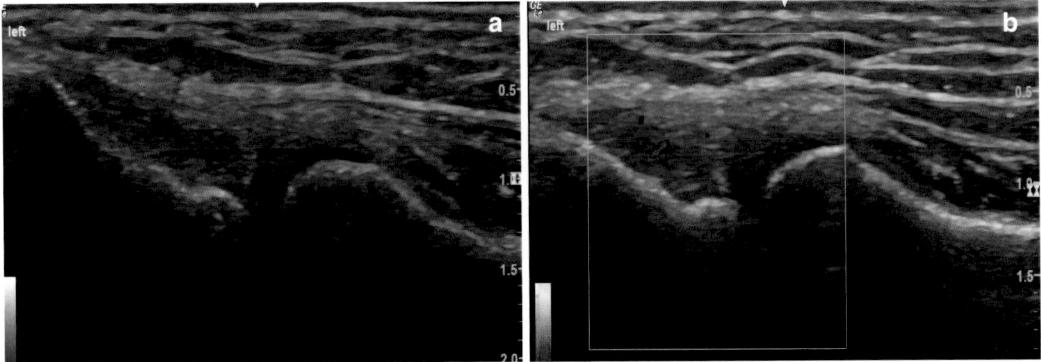

Fig. 22.3 (**a**) A 51-year-old female complaining of lateral elbow pain for more than 6 months with prior history of repetitive wrist extension activities showed the following ultrasound findings. Note the hypoechoic lesion over the inner layer of the common wrist extensor tendon with the absence of a distinct fibrillar pattern of the tendon consistent with tendinosis. (**b**) Ultrasound image with power Doppler showed mild inflammatory reaction over the inner layer of the common wrist extensor tendon with possible involvement of the lateral ulnar collateral ligament. Also note the thickening of the common wrist extensor tendon

study showed that there is significant pain-free abduction strength on the shoulder treated with PRP but no difference in terms of tendon repair and durability and resistance to tendon reinjuries as compared to the control group [49]. An ultrasound-guided PRP injection post-arthroscopically also does not improve early tendon-bone healing or functional recovery [50].

Elbow

Elbow ultrasound is a very useful modality both for diagnosis and for guided procedures. The use of unique and novel features in ultrasound machines will help establish a clinical diagnosis and at the same time guide practitioners to find the most appropriate medical and surgical management. Lateral elbow pain has an incidence of 1–2% and is due to an overuse injury of the common wrist extensor origin of the lateral epicondyle of the elbow [51]. Lateral elbow tendinopathy (Fig. 22.3) is one of the most common pathologies affecting the elbow both in sports and occupational settings. Pain in this area is usually exacerbated by wrist extension as this is the origin of common wrist extensor tendons. For lack of inflammatory findings, this is often referred to as tendinosis. Ultrasound findings are characterized by structural changes such as tendon thickening, hypo echogenicity, intrasubstance tears, and neovascularity [52]. Of these features, the most significant clinical findings relating to a poor prognosis are the presence of lateral collateral ligament (LCL) tear and the size of the largest intrasubstance tears which may require either surgical intervention or regenerative therapies [52]. Early tendon pathology can be assessed by elastography to avoid further degeneration of tendons which otherwise cannot be seen when using conventional ultrasound [7]. Moreover, sonopalpation to induced tenderness over the lateral epicondyle in an ultrasound examination showed that maximum tenderness corresponds to the exact site of pathology, rules out other differential diagnoses, and guides ultrasound-guided intralesional injections [53]. In one study, recalcitrant lateral elbow tendinopathy responds favorably with ultrasound-guided percutaneous tenotomy which was followed up after 3 years [54]. Ultrasound-guided tenotomy has the benefits of pain relief, improved physical function, and high patient satisfaction [55]. In a randomized controlled trial study, the use of platelet-rich plasma for chronic lateral epicondylitis led to pain relief earlier than autologous whole blood [56].

Among young professional baseball pitchers, one of the first changes sonographically in the medial elbow is the increase in ulnar collateral ligament (UCL) thickness, which increases over time professionally [57] but is not seen among young high school pitchers [58]. It is measured at the midportion of the UCL without stress at the elbow [57]. As you can see, injury to the UCL can be a career-threatening defect for elite overhead-throwing athletes causing pain, decreased control, and velocity to the pitcher [57, 59]. And as such, assessing this structure can provide essential guidance as to the best possible training and treatment. In a cadaveric study, the release of the anterior bundle of UCL results in the greatest increase in joint gapping as measured by medial elbow stress ultrasound (SUS), which is measured by the greatest distance of the ulnohumeral valgus joint gapping (difference of 90° elbow flexion valgus stress minus resting elbow). The anterior bundle of the UCL is the primary stabilizer of the medial elbow against valgus stress [59]. A recent study by Park and colleagues showed that stress ultrasound can be used to diagnose complete medial UCL tears in athletes when joint gapping is greater than 0.5 mm at 30° of elbow flexion and greater than 1 mm at 90° of elbow flexion [60]. It was also found out that increasing the pitch velocity by 10 km/hour would increase the risk of medial epicondyle abnormality and medial elbow pain by three times, together with the number of practices per week [61]. Thus, valgus stress stabilization exercises involving the flexor digitorum superficialis (FDS), especially of the middle and index fingers, provide medial elbow support for UCL [62]. In fact, hand gripping reduces medial elbow joint gapping compared with rest as shown in elastography measurements [63]. For partial UCL tears, ultrasound-guided PRP injection is an effective treatment [64] with an added benefit of early return to play [65].

Among adolescents, repetitive throwing activities in sports may put a strain over the immature capitellum of the elbow and may cause capitellar osteochondritis dessicans (COCD) [66]. This condition may cause fragmentation of the osteochondral bone that may be unstable and may cause pains. The evaluation of the stability of the lesion is important so that practitioners can decide between operative and nonoperative options. Stable lesions tend to heal with simple elbow rest, but unstable lesions require surgery [67]. In the past, preoperative MRI scans play an important role in the diagnosis, with a sensitivity of 84% and specificity of 70% [68]. In this study, ultrasound was a useful tool in evaluating fragment instability in COCD. It is superior to MRI with a sensitivity of 92% and a specificity of 100% [67].

Wrist and Hand

Approximately 25% of all sports-related injuries involve the wrist and hand [69]. With its intricate structural makeup, The unique demand of sports upon the hands and wrists of athletes makes this area very susceptible to injuries. The mechanism of injury

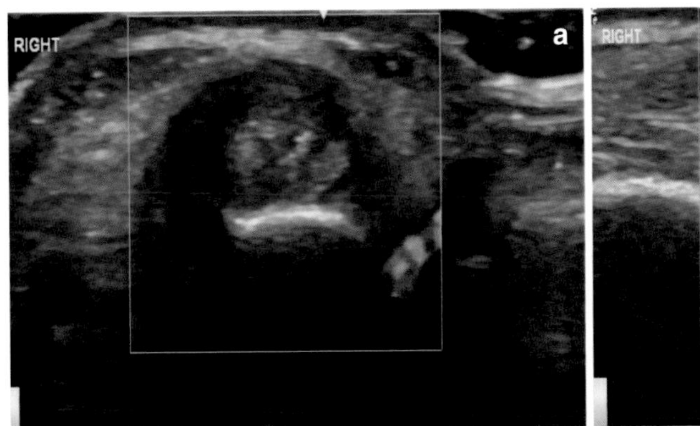

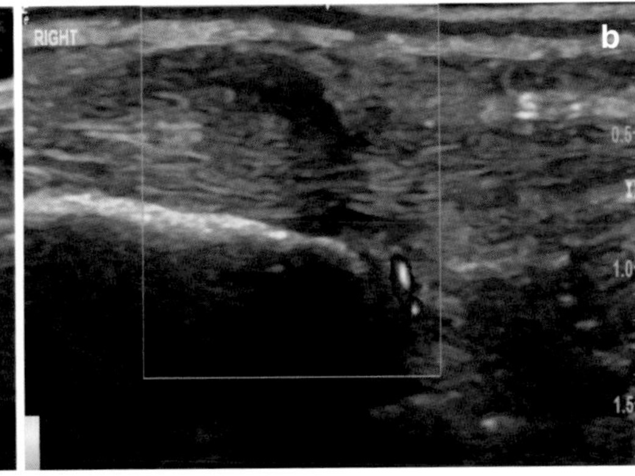

Fig. 22.4 (**a**) Short-axis view of the first dorsal compartment of the wrist with abductor pollicis longus (APL) and extensor pollicis brevis (EPB), with a relatively swollen sheath and mild effusion of a 51-year-old female complaining of radial wrist pain for 10 months. (**b**) The long-axis view showed the extent of swelling of the sheath of the first dorsal compartment of the wrist with an active inflammatory process

and an ideal, quick, available, and reliable diagnostic imaging tool are important factors for decision-making in the management of these injuries.

The most common tendinopathy affecting the wrist and hand is De Quervain's tenosynovitis [70]. This is brought about by repetitive thumb extension and abduction with thickening of the abductor pollicis longus (APL) and extensor pollicis brevis (EPB) tendons under the first dorsal compartment of the wrist (Fig. 22.4).

A positive Finkelstein test confirms the site of the problem [71]. Ultrasound findings showed marked hypoechogenic thickening along the tendon of EPB due to thickened extensor retinaculum with associated hypervascularity and effusion by power Doppler signal [72, 73]. Intersection syndrome or Oarsman's wrist is a friction between the first dorsal compartment tendons passing over the tendons of the second dorsal compartment of the dorsal wrist which sometimes could be mistaken for De Quervain's tenosynovitis. The site of the pain and tenderness are more proximal with intersection syndrome [74]. It is usually located 4–8 cm proximal to the Lister's tubercle where these groups of tendons intersect. A distal intersection syndrome also exists where the third dorsal wrist compartment intersects with the second dorsal wrist compartment but not as common. Ultrasound findings showed effusion within the sheath by power Doppler and with peritendinous edema within the tendon sheaths at the intersection [75, 76]. Given its low prevalence rate of 0.20%, ultrasound is useful for patients who are refractory to conservative therapy, and planning for surgical intervention is an option. Ultrasound imaging is also needed to identify anatomical variants and guide interventional procedures [76]. Among volleyball and water polo players, repetitive wrist flexion or overstretching of the wrist can cause tendenitis of the flexor carpi radialis (FCR) tendon. Pain develops as this tendon thickens which run right adjacent to the flexor retinaculum of the carpal tunnel [77]. FCR tenosynovitis is characterized sonographically by effusion and/or thickening of the synovial membrane surrounding the FCR tendon. Tenosynovitis of mechanical origin is characterized by effusion prevails [78]. In contrast, tenosynovitis associated with RA or chronic inflammatory disorders and thickening of the synovial membrane (pannus) prevail [79]. Tendinopathy, on the other hand, is characterized as tendon thickening and heterogeneous hypoechogenicity with or without superficial tearing [78].

Extensor carpi ulnaris (ECU) injuries are usually seen among players in golf, baseball, hockey, tennis, and other racquet sports. The mechanism of injury is characterized by repetitive microtrauma or a sudden traumatic event during wrist flexion, supination, and ulnar deviation as seen in tennis or in the leading hand in the downward phase of a golf stroke [71]. There is typically tenderness over the ECU groove and pain is initiated during resisted wrist extension and ulnar deviation. Supination with ulnar deviation of the wrist might uncover subluxation of the ECU [71]. There is about an 8.9% incidence of a wrist injury which may affect ECU. The common features of injury that might affect ECU are a combination of forces such as wrist flexion during supination and ulnar deviation or sudden lateral force applied when the tendon is engaged in strong isometric contraction such as in tennis, golf, or rugby sports. In tennis, it usually occurs in double-handed backhand stroke. In golf, it usually affects the leading wrist, which is the wrist that faces the target. In traumatic ECU subluxation, the leading wrist moves from radial deviation to a neutral position at impact. Subsequently, the momentum puts the leading wrist toward ulnar deviation, with the ECU contracting isometrically to counteract the ulnar deviation, which then brings the club through the end of the golf swing with an impact. This reaction together with the body's reaction can result in the failure of the subsheath with ECU subluxation. In rugby, the attempt of player to clutch the ball on the chest with the forearm in maximal supination, with the wrist in flexion and ulnar deviation, and his/her attempt to increase the isometric contraction of the ECU may tear the subsheath and thus ECU tendon subluxation [80]. ECU synergy test has been shown to be specific for ECU tendinosis [81]. Ultrasound findings for tenosynovitis showed anechoic, easily compressible fluid surrounding the tendon with minimal or absent vascularity on power Doppler [80]. However, for tendinopathy, tendon thickening may be subtle during the early stages and so it is important to do a side-to-side comparison. Over time, as the disease progresses, tendon thickening will be more pronounced with neovascularization on power Doppler [80, 82].

Sports injury over the ulnar side of the wrist can involve the triangular fibrocartilage complex (TFCC) (Fig. 22.5) such as in athletes who rotate and grip baseball bats, racquets, and golf clubs. As you know TFCC is a soft tissue complex that supports and stabilizes the distal radioulnar and ulnocarpal joints [83]. In an acute injury of the wrist, TFCC may be injured because of hyperextension and pronation of the axially loaded ulnar-deviated wrist. Patient will usually complain of deep aching pain or pain with gripping associated with clicking during pronation and supination of the wrist [71]. Although attempts to diagnose TFCC lesions using high-resolution ultrasound have been proposed, no agreement has yet been made as to the lesions in TFCC [84]. The sensitivity, specificity, and accuracy of MRI and USG

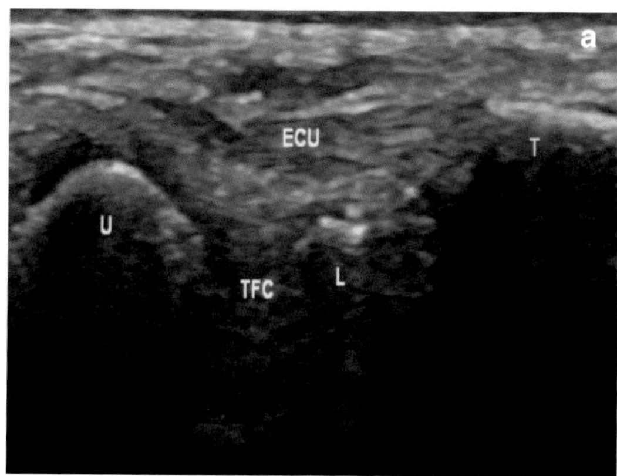

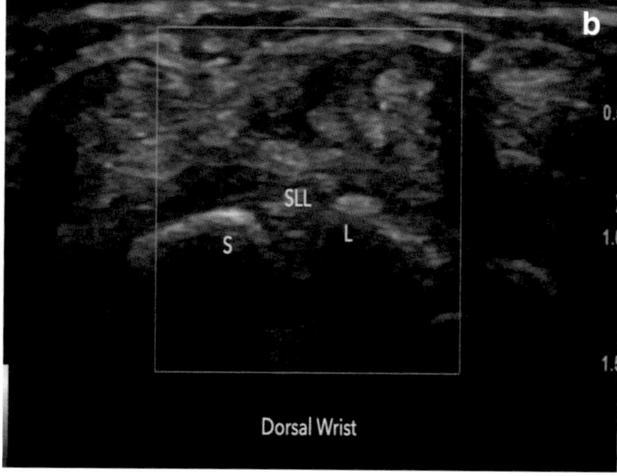

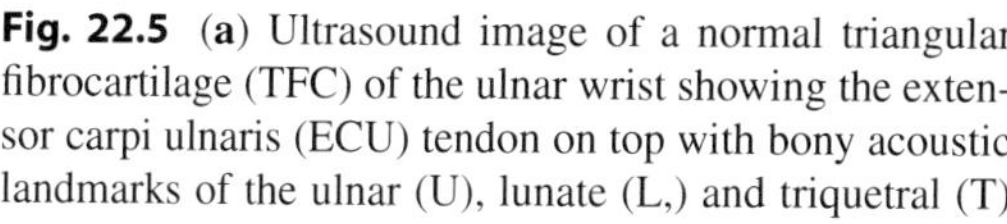
Fig. 22.5 (**a**) Ultrasound image of a normal triangular fibrocartilage (TFC) of the ulnar wrist showing the extensor carpi ulnaris (ECU) tendon on top with bony acoustic landmarks of the ulnar (U), lunate (L,) and triquetral (T) bones with the TFC between the ulna and lunate bones. (**b**) Ultrasound image of the dorsal scapholunate ligament (SLL) with the bony acoustic landmark of the scaphoid (S) and lunate (L) bones

for TFCC tear were 75%, 100%, 87.5% and 0%, 50% and 50%, respectively [85].

Scapulolunate (SL) ligament (Fig. 22.5) tears can occur following a position of impact in contact sports such as football and rugby. The mechanism of injury is wrist hyperextension, ulnar deviation, and supination [71]. Tenderness is induced between the third and fourth dorsal extensor wrist compartments. A radiographic PA clenched fist view may show greater than 5 mm widening between the scaphoid and lunate (Terry Thomas sign), which is diagnostic of a complete tear of the SL ligament [86]. Ultrasound scanning begins at the Lister's tubercle of the dorsal wrist in the transverse plane and then slowly advances distally with the proximal pole of the scaphoid bone in view distal to the radiocarpal joint space. Adjust the probe to visualize both the scaphoid and the lunate and avoid anisotropy. The SL ligament fibers which connect the scaphoid and lunate are characterized by a triangular echogenic structure with a compact and fibrillar hyperechoic echotexture [87]. The dorsal portion of this ligament is visualized up to 78% of normal wrists [88]. Tears in the SL ligament are interpreted as a loss of the normal echogenic appearance, disruption or absence of the normal ligament, or presence of concurrent fluid or an associated ganglion [89]. Dynamic ultrasound examination for SL ligament instability assessment has a high specificity and accuracy but a low sensitivity. Thus, other diagnostic modalities may be used in conjunction with ultrasound to establish a diagnosis [90].

The injury to the ulnar collateral ligament (UCL) of the thumb is quite common and is often seen in skiing, basketball, and football [91]. Injury to the UCL happened in an abducted thumb as in a fall of an outstretched hand at the thumb metacarpophalangeal joint (MCPJ) [71]. An acute injury is what is referred to as a skier's thumb [92] in contrast to a chronic attritional insufficiency injury of the same structure which is referred to as a gamekeeper's thumb [93]. The thumb UCL has two portions: the proper which is more dorsally located and the accessory which is volarly located. A Stener lesion occurs when the adductor pollicis aponeurosis is interposed between the torn-off UCL and the proximal phalanx insertion [71]. The adductor pollicis aponeurosis normally lies superficial to the UCL [94]. Ultrasound imaging of the UCL is done orthogonally in the coronal plane relative to the metacarpal bone. Correct transducer placement consists of finding the shallow groove or concavity at the ulnar aspect of the distal first metacarpal between the apex of the lateral tubercle and articular surface, and a similar but smaller groove in the ulnar aspect of the proximal phalanx near the phalangeal collateral tubercle where the UCL is attached [95–97]. A displaced UCL is characterized by the absence of UCL fibers spanning the first MCP joint and well-defined heterogeneous mass-like abnormality proximal to the apex to the metacarpal lateral tubercle [95]. A displaced full-thickness tear of the UCL is characterized by retraction of the proximal UCL to the proximal edge of the adductor aponeurosis which is referred to as the Stener lesion [98]. To ensure correct imaging, passive flexion of the first IP joint causes isolated movement of the adductor aponeurosis but not the UCL (Martinolli technique) [95]. For complete tears, reconstruction surgery is needed. For partial tears, hand-based thumb spica is recommended [71].

Sagittal band ruptures (Boxer's knuckles) represent zone 5 extensor tendon injuries [99]. As the primary lateral stabilizer of the tendon over the MCP joint, the sagittal band attaches to the extensor hood and runs to the volar part of the finger to insert at the volar plate [100]. The injury occurs when there is a direct force toward a flexed digit with the wrist in flexion and ulnar deviation [101]. A typical radial-sided sagittal band rupture occurs resulting in pain and swelling with ulnar subluxation of the extensor tendon with MCP flexion [99]. The index and middle fingers are commonly affected among professionals with the ring and little fingers among amateurs. Overall, the middle finger is affected in 48% of sagittal band injuries [102]. Rayan and Murray proposed a classification for closed sagittal band injuries depending on the degree of structural abnormality [103]. Dynamic ultrasound is extremely useful in assessing the extent of the injury with subluxation of the extensor tendons seen during

MCP joint flexion [104, 105]. A transverse scan of the dorsal finger is done with finger extension and 30° MCP flexion. The sagittal band appears as a hypoechoic band on both sides of the common extensor tendon. The transverse and oblique bands are not visible by ultrasound. A sagittal band rupture is shown as a discontinuity in the alignment of the sagittal band. Dynamic scanning will help in evaluating the stability of the extensor tendon with ulnar deviation in the index, middle, and ring fingers but not with the little finger even if the fingers are stressed in flexion [106]. Splinting in full finger extension with PIP joint-free is done if there is no subluxation or dislocation. Operative treatment is done for a ruptured sagittal band with dislocation or subluxation [71].

Among basketball and volleyball players, boutonniere deformity may occur because of volar dislocation or forced flexion of the PIP joint with rupture of the triangular ligament at the distal end of the central slip. Boutonniere deformity is described as PIP joint flexion and hyperextension of the DIP joint with the lateral bands migrating volarly [71]. The patient is tested by flexing the PIP to 90° and asking the patient to actively extend the DIP in this position. A patient with disrupted central slip will demonstrate rigid DIP hyperextension or a positive Elson test. Isolated central slip will not result in Boutonniere deformity and may appear innocuous if not carefully assessed [99]. High-frequency ultrasound can be used to assess central slip injuries.

Rock climbing is becoming common nowadays and it does not go without injury. The pressure imposed upon the finger pulley system during frequent climbing causes ruptures at the A2 and A4 pulley systems usually at the middle and ring fingers [71]. Such lesions result from overuse injuries with anterior displacement of the flexor tendons (bowstringing) and reduced digital performance. High-frequency ultrasound shows a gap detected between the bone and flexor tendons in the injured area and can be elicited by active forced flexion. There is also an associated effusion inside the sheath of the flexor tendon [107]. Annular pulleys are usually hyperechoic relative to the tendons with fibrillar appearance but with a tendency to anisotropy [108]. High-frequency ultrasound provides the diagnostic ability for A2 and A4 ruptures. The threshold value was determined to evaluate the optimal tendon-bone distance for pulley rupture diagnosis in an ultrasound cadaveric study. For A2 pulley rupture, the threshold distance is 1.9 mm and 1.85 mm for A4 pulley rupture [109]. Bodner and colleagues in a comparative study between high-frequency ultrasound and MRI found that a complete ruptured pulley showed a distance of 3 mm between tendon and bone in an extended finger, and a distance of 5 mm during finger flexion confirmed the diagnosis [110]. The sensitivity of ultrasound for depiction of pulley injuries is about 98% with 100% specificity [111].

Finger injuries represent 38% of all upper extremity injuries [112]. Jersey finger or sweater finger is an avulsion of the flexor digitorum profundus tendon at the volar aspect of the distal phalanx due to forced hyperextension of the DIP joint while the finger is actively flexed. The FDP of the ring finger is more commonly involved. It is commonly seen during football and rugby sports [113]. Physical examination showed loss of active DIP joint flexion of the involved digit with the inability to make a full fist [113]. A related condition where there is loss of terminal extension function of the DIP joint of the fingers is referred to as mallet finger. A jamming force at the fingertip while the DIP joint is in active extension results in avulsion of the extensor tendon. Mallet fingers can occur in softball, baseball, football, basketball, or soccer. The patient usually presents with an inability to fully extend the DIP joint [113]. A high-frequency ultrasound is placed at the volar area of the distal phalanx of the involved finger in long-axis view. In Jersey finger, ultrasound shows an irregular hyperechoic fragment located at the proximal metaphysis of the middle phalanx just distal to A3 pulley of the flexor tendons. The common synovial tendon sheath contained a small hypoechoic effusion [114]. In partial tears, ultrasound demonstrates hypoechoic, fusiform swelling of the tendon and focal discontinuity of the internal fibrillar pattern. For complete tears, the ruptured tendon cannot be seen at the injury site, and the distal, retracted tendon presents as a hypoechoic and irregular lesion with posterior acoustic shadowing [115]. The accuracy of ultrasound is noted when it is done after 1 day but within 7 days of injury as the immediate hematoma of the area might obliterate the structures being imaged. If done after 1 day, the accuracy of ultrasound is 100%, 88% if done on the same day of the injury, and 85.7% when done after 7 days. Overall, the sensitivity of diagnostic ultrasound is 96% and specificity is 95% [116]. In the surgical management of Jersey finger, the use of ultrasound helps in identifying the proximal end of the ruptured tendon in 72% of cases and to decide as to whether to do a direct repair or not [116]. Return to play is expected between 8 and 12 weeks post-treatment [113]. Mallet finger appears on the ultrasound as an irregular, hypoechoic soft tissue lesion at the distal shaft of the middle phalanx, after it has retracted. When an avulsion fracture accompanies the mallet finger, a retracted bone accompanies the retracted tendon [115]. Splinting for both conditions may serve as conservative interventions for these athletes for 6 weeks [71].

Scaphoid fractures are the most injured carpal bones seen among college football players [117] representing about 10.6–29 per 100,000 per year or 2% of all fractures [118, 119]. It also represents 60% of carpal fractures and 11% of hand fractures [120]. This is a hyperextension injury that occurred in a pronated and radially deviated hand. Pain is felt at the radial side of the wrist (snuffbox), especially during pincer grasp and axial loading of the thumb [71]. An early correct diagnosis is important to avoid "overtreatment" with unnecessary immobilization or "undertreatment" which carries the risk of nonunion, delayed union or osteonecrosis, carpal instability, and osteoarthritis [121, 122]. Ultrasound assessment is considered positive when one of the four of the following criteria is seen: a fracture line, a subperiosteal or subcapsular hematoma, a ridge or a contour crossing the cortex of the scaphoid, and displacement of the deep branch of the radial artery from the radial cortex of the scaphoid [123]. In a previous study, Munk and colleagues (2000) showed that the accuracy of ultrasound was 84%, sensitivity 50%, specificity 91%, PPV 56%, and NPV 90%, and thus ultrasound is not recommended for early diagnosis based on their studies [123]. Recently, Kwee and Kwee (2018) in their systematic search found that radiographically occult scaphoid fracture using ultrasound has a sensitivity of 77.8–100% and a specificity of 71.4–100%, adding the presence of cortical disruption as the sole diagnostic criterion, which might be the reason for the high sensitivity and specificity. Most of the fractures in the scaphoid bone are seen in the scaphoid waist and thus are very accessible to ultrasound imaging [122]. In cases where an ultrasound confirmed the presence of scaphoid fractures, additional CT or MRI is requested to identify the location and extent of the fracture [122]. In another study, Malahias and colleagues in 2019 showed that ultrasound has a sensitivity of 90% and a specificity of 85.7% in diagnosing occult scaphoid fractures and has noted that ultrasound can be used only under strict circumstances for early diagnosis of occult scaphoid fracture. Moreover, the presence of subperiosteal hematoma and cortical discontinuity confirmed its presence. Further, if the ultrasound is negative and symptoms persist, MRI or CT scan is required for definitive diagnosis [124]. In contrast, CT and MRI have a sensitivity of 72% and 88%, respectively [125].

Scaphoid fracture is a very critical condition that needs timely and appropriate treatment where the aim of the treatment is the union of scaphoid fracture [119]. In Sweden, the risk of diagnosed nonunion after a diagnosed scaphoid fracture was 2.4% [126] with serious consequences after prolonged immobilization referred to as scaphoid nonunion advanced collapse (SNAC) wrist [127]. As previously mentioned, there is a need to avoid "overtreatment" or "undertreatment" as both cases carry sequelae of risk. In a recent study by Commandeur and colleagues, a graduated and guarded immobilization using below elbow cast where the thumb is not immobilized and the wrist is in a slightly extended position is suggested. A 6-week period of immobilization is done with intermittent clinical and radiological evaluation. If no consolidation occurs, immobilization is extended with 2 weekly evaluations, with no agreed extent of immobilization period. There is no evidence that other conservative treatments like electromagnetic field therapy or pulsed low-intensity ultrasound therapy work [128]. In Europe, cast immobilization is reported to have 90–95% healing [119], and CT before and CT after the immobilization are recommended to ensure optimal results [129]. CT investigation is needed to determine whether fractures are displaced or non-displaced. Conservative treatment usually has been reported to result in a nonunion rate of 10–14% for non-displaced fractures and 50% for displaced fractures. Persistent pain, however, may indicate incomplete or delayed union or may be associated with other injuries [120, 130]. Proximal scaphoid fractures with their tenuous blood supply should be treated operatively to maximize union rates [131], while distal pole scaphoid fractures should be treated nonoperatively with predictably high union rates [132] due to its well-vascularized region. A minimally displaced or non-displaced waist scaphoid fracture will heal successfully (90%) after conservative management at 6 weeks, while unstable and severely displaced fracture must be treated operatively [120]. Return to work is assessed by CT scan when the scaphoid fracture is united with more than 50% trabecular bridging across the fracture site, and wrist range and grip strength should be within 20–40% of the contralateral side [120, 133]. An ultrasound-guided PRP treatment was reported on a nonunion scaphoid fracture with complete healing after doing an MRI and CT scan [134].

Peripheral Nerve Injury Secondary to Sports in the Upper Extremity

Sports injury affecting the peripheral nerves is usually secondary to compression, traction, ischemia, and laceration [135]. Unlike the musculoskeletal system, peripheral nerve injuries may develop in an insidious manner with subtle clinical signs and symptoms. Pain is not always present and gross muscle atrophy may be seen over time as nerve injury progresses. Muscle strength testing may not be reliable during the acute stage as athletes may compensate for the movement by using muscle substitution. Referred pain may complicate the presentation of the problem and as such a comprehensive neurologic test must always be performed to identify the specific nerve involved. Electromyographic tests can aid in the diagnosis of neuropathies. However, it takes 2–3 weeks before the nerve injury before fibrillation potentials and positive sharp waves can be observed. With Wallerian degeneration, significant motor amplitudes change may only be detected after a week. For the sensory amplitudes, the change may be significant after 10 days of injury [135]. Following trauma, high-frequency ultrasound can determine the type of injury, localize the proximal and distal nerve stumps, and differentiate between acute and chronic peripheral nerve injuries. Compared to MRI, high-frequency ultrasound provides quick, reliable, dynamic, and cost-effective diagnostic imaging devices [136]. Kullmer and colleagues in tracking down the changes after muscle denervation found out that there is a decrease in muscle diameter and an increase in overall echogenicity on ultrasound by day 14 after denervation, while MRI showed a decrease in muscle diameter with associated increased signal intensity indicating its first sign of denervation by day 21. Then, 28 days post-denervation, the ultrasound findings of muscle atrophy because of denervation are detectable on day 28 and are characterized by an increase in echogenicity, while the same atrophic changes in the muscle as a result of denervation are detectable on MRI on day 35. EMG showed spontaneous activity more than 11 days after denervation [137]. This study recommends the use of ultrasound and EMG for complete functional and anatomical assessment of the sequelae of early denervation [137]. In another study focusing on detecting focal peripheral nerve pathology, ultrasound is more sensitive than MRI (93% vs 67%), has equivalent specificity (86%), and better identifies multifocal lesions than MRI [138]. High-resolution ultrasound shows good diagnostic utility and management of peripheral nerve lesions [139]. Ultrasound has been found to aid in the decision-making regarding conservative or surgical treatment and is an ideal diagnostic complement to clinical electrophysiological testing for peripheral neuropathies [140].

Jacobson and colleagues noted the earliest sign of nerve entrapment as decreased echogenicity of the connective tissue layers of a nerve trunk, with the nerve appearing globally hypoechoic. Later, it will show a hypoechoic enlargement. Sonopalpation can also be done to elicit pain over the site of nerve distribution. Denervation changes as described above will be noted in the muscle being innervated characterized by abnormally increased echogenicity. Muscle atrophy will be shown over time as significant evidence of peripheral nerve injury [141]. Overall, high-frequency ultrasound is a useful complementary tool for assessing peripheral nerve lesions in the context of finding the exact location, course, continuity, and extent of traumatic nerve lesions and for assessing nerve entrapment and tumors if there is any [142]. High-frequency ultrasound can also identify different degrees of peripheral nerve injury from mild hypoechoic swelling, continuity of epineurium, the absence and/or swelling of the fascicles, and whether there is continuity in the epineurium in the case of neurotmesis. It cannot, however, show the myelin sheath and axons; thus, current damages to this structure are indistinguishable [143]. While EMG provides the physiological status of the nerve, the concurrent use of US can complement it by providing morphological information [143].

Brachial Plexus Injury or "Stingers"

Brachial plexus injury (BPI) is common among athletes who play football or other collision sports. It is sometimes referred to as "stingers." Stinger is referred to as a transient episode of shooting or electric pain with acute onset after an impact to the head and/or shoulder [144]. The most affected nerve is the brachial plexus followed by radial and ulnar nerve, and then by the axillary nerve in that order of frequency [145]. This type of injury affects about 49–65% of college football players and with a recurrence rate of about 87% [146, 147]. The mildest and most common form of brachial plexus injury is referred to as neuropraxia. It is characterized by a loss of sensation and motor function due to focal demyelination which could last for 6 weeks without any treatment followed by spontaneous recovery. A damaged axon with associated Wallerian degeneration is an injury referred to as axonotmesis. It commonly involves C5 and C6 levels. With an intact epineurium, it could slowly recover but longer than neuropraxia for several months. There is pain, burning, or tingling sensation, such that it is referred to as "burner" or "stinger." Muscle weakness is seen over the deltoid, supraspinatus, and coracobrachialis muscles [146]. Electrodiagnostic studies, MRI scans, and high-frequency ultrasound are useful to localize the lesion, define an appropriate treatment, and monitor functional prognosis [148]. Chin and colleagues in a systematic review on the value of ultrasound for traumatic BPI noted that high-frequency ultrasound is an effective diagnostic tool for traumatic adult BPI. The sensitivity of lesion detection is higher in the upper and middle levels (C5 is 93%; C6 is 94%; C7 is 95%) than in the lower spinal nerves (C8 is 71%; T1 is 56%) with an overall ultrasound sensitivity of 87%, while MRI has an overall sensitivity of 81% [37]. High-frequency ultrasound (Fig. 22.6) can very well visualize the cords of the brachial plexus and the level of the root avulsion, and, if there is any rupture of the cord, it can detect any disruption of the nerves [149].

Spinal Accessory Nerve

Spinal accessory nerve (SAN) injury occurs secondary to blunt trauma of the posterior triangle of the neck or a traction injury when a blow depresses the shoulder while the head moves in the opposite direction [150]. This is commonly seen in football, lacrosse, and hockey. The trapezius muscle is paralyzed but the sternocleidomastoid is spared since the injury happened distal to its innervation [150]. The location of the SAN in this area is very superficial and covered only by the skin and subcutaneous fascia. There is an obvious drooping of the shoulder, loss of shoulder elevation, and pain [151]. High-frequency ultrasound showed the nerves at the posterolateral border of the SCM (Fig. 22.6) and the anterior border of the trapezius [152]. However, actual transection of the nerve may not be seen by ultrasound. That is why it is important to evaluate

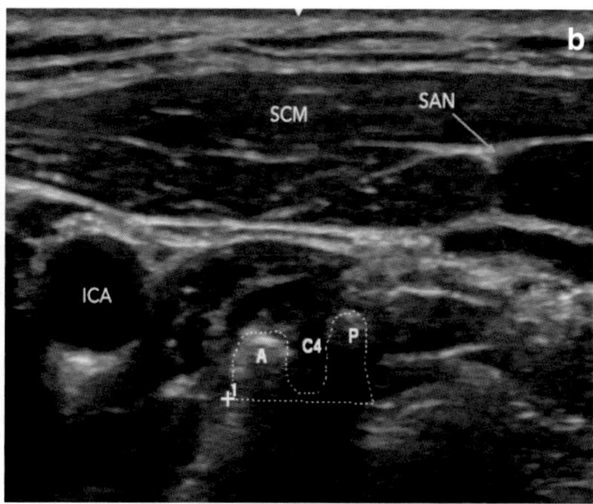

Fig. 22.6 (**a**) The brachial plexus nerves are found in between the anterior scalene (AS) and middle (MS) muscles as shown here in this ultrasound image. (**b**) The spinal accessory nerve (SAN) is found in the fascial sheath in the middle of the sternocleidomastoid muscle (SCM) when scanned proximally in the neck. Also shown here is the fourth cervical nerve (C4) root in between the anterior (A) and posterior (P) tubercle and the internal carotid artery (ICA)

the status of the trapezius to check for fatty infiltration or echogenicity which confirms denervation of the muscle [153].

Long Thoracic Nerve

Sports-related injuries affecting the long thoracic nerve (LTN) are usually associated with extreme hyperabduction movements such as what is seen in archery, wrestling, soccer, boxing, tennis, bowling, hockey, gymnastics, and weightlifting. When serratus anterior muscle undergoes winging, it is minimal in resting position and is only accentuated during forward flexion and while pushing with arms extended forward [154]. Serratus anterior basically serves as the primary stabilizer of the scapula. Inman noted that serratus anterior is important in sustaining primary scapulohumeral function [155]. Patients with long thoracic nerve impingements usually present with pain, paresthesia, and weakness of the serratus anterior [156]. Only with severe cases will it present with medial winging and medial translation or rotation of the scapula, or projection of the medial scapular border may concurrently take place [157]. It is not unusual however to see long thoracic nerve entrapment not associated with trauma and this is usually due to anatomical variations, especially within the scalene musculature, and not all patients with anatomical entrapment will present with symptoms. Also, in this same study, only 86.5% pierced the middle scalene muscles [156]. Since there is no cutaneous distribution coming from the long thoracic nerve to explain the sensation of pain, the pain could arise from the increased sensitization of the nerve fibers resulting from nerve trunk injuries referring to pain into the neck or from the thoracic posterior rami with its cutaneous branches because of stretching from scapular winging referred to as interscapular pain [156]. High-frequency ultrasound will show at least four areas to scan the long thoracic nerve: at the cervical region, at the supraclavicular level, at the infraclavicular level, and at the midaxillary line beside the lateral thoracic artery [158].

Suprascapular Nerve

Suprascapular nerve (Fig. 22.7) injury could be injured in sports with compression at the level of the suprascapular notch associated with backpackers, volleyball players, weightlifters, and baseball pitchers [135]. It is considered the most injured brachial plexus peripheral nerve branch among athletes [159]. The nerve arises from the upper trunk or sometimes directly from C5 nerve root. It provides motor branches to the supraspi-

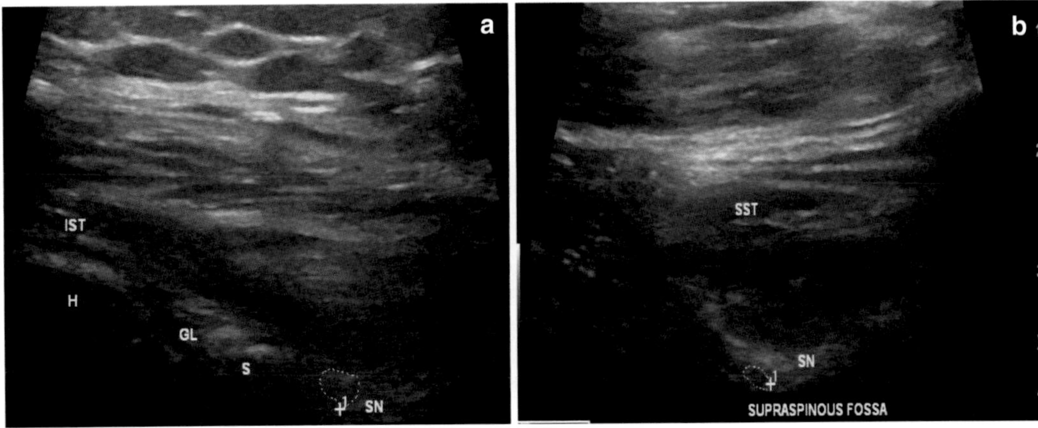

Fig. 22.7 (**a**) Ultrasound image of the suprascapular nerve (SN) at the level of the spinoglenoid notch at the posterior shoulder. (**b**) Ultrasound image of the suprascapular nerve (SN) at the level of the supraspinous fossa at the superior portion of the shoulder underneath the supraspinatus tendon. IST Infraspinatus tendon, H humerus, GL glenoid labrum, S scapula

natus and infraspinatus muscles. The sensory branch innervates the acromioclavicular joint, glenohumeral joint, and subacromial bursa. The most frequent site of injury is at the suprascapular notch where the nerve travels under the superior transverse scapular ligament. It does not injure the nerve at the spinoglenoid notch except in sports involving overhead activities [160]. Contemori and Biscarini reported the higher shoulder position during overhead activities where the hitting shoulder incurred isolated infraspinatus atrophy due to injury of the suprascapular nerve at the spinoglenoid notch [161]. In fact, it was reported that up to 20–45% of volleyball players had evidence of isolated infraspinatus muscle impairment [162, 163]. There is also a subsequent reduction of position sense in the affected shoulder suggesting an impairment of the shoulder sensorimotor control system resulting from reduced afferent proprioceptive information. Overall, this results in reduced shoulder functional stability and increased risk of injury. This study highlights the fact that the proprioceptive system serves a very important role in the preservation of functional joint stability. Athletes with this type of isolated nerve injury can benefit from a specific proprioceptive and neuromuscular preventive training program [161]. In other studies, it was also reported that the lesion at the spinoglenoid notch affecting the suprascapular nerve is usually incomplete showing some function of the muscle and thus most athletes are asymptomatic with teres minor compensating for the infraspinatus dysfunction [162]. High-frequency ultrasound can demonstrate the suprascapular nerve at the suprascapular notch appearing as a thin, hypoechoic structure lying over the echogenic bony floor of the groove, especially for lean individuals. However, in cases where it is not visualized due to the thick musculature, a color Doppler may provide a clue to the location of the nerve as it visualizes its neighboring vascular bundle. In 96%, the superior transverse suprascapular ligament could be visualized and in 86% the vascular bundle which is the suprascapular artery can be shown demonstrating the location of the suprascapular nerve [164].

Axillary Nerve

The axillary nerve is commonly injured in wrestling, weightlifting, rugby, hockey, and football players. It is the most injured peripheral nerve in 9–18% of anterior shoulder dislocations. The mechanism of injury is usually a direct blow to the lateral deltoid usually seen during hockey collisions or in football or rugby [135, 165]. Its nerve fibers originate from the upper trunk and C5 and C6 cervical roots. Before innervating the deltoid and teres minor muscles, it courses posteriorly through the quadrangular space [135]. Neurological complications following shoulder dislocation occur more often in patients aged more than 40 or 50 years, with an associated increased risk if it remains dislocated more than 12 hours. The axillary nerve is susceptible to stretch injury after a shoulder dislocation due to its numerous attachments with the deltoid muscle and thus more often associated with infraclavicular brachial plexus injury [165]. Moreover, most of the axillary nerve injuries are part of the combined brachial plexus injury and only 0.3–6% are isolated axillary nerve injuries [162]. Athletes with axillary nerve injury may be asymptomatic, regardless of whether it is complete or incomplete lesions. Only when they exercise will they show easy fatigabilities such as when they do an overhead activity or heavy lifting. These present with reduced abduction strength or inability to raise the arms. There is a sensory deficit at the lateral arm. Sometimes, it is possible to have intact sensation with complete deltoid muscle weakness. In the later stage, there is atrophy of the deltoid and teres minor, unless the lesion is beyond the quadrilateral space, in which case, these two muscles are spared [162]. A unique syndrome referred to as quadrilateral space (Fig. 22.8) syndrome is a chronic compression syndrome of the axillary nerve in athletes whose sports require repetitive throwing motions. Fibrous bands developed at the inferior border of the teres minor eventually compress the posterior humeral circumflex artery and axillary nerve with subsequent complete denervation of the deltoid and teres minor. Compression of the structures is more severe in shoulder abduction and externally rotated positions [166]. High-frequency ultrasound can image the quadrilateral space (Fig. 22.8). The probe is positioned in the long axis of the humerus 2 cm below the posterolateral border of the acromion at the dorsal aspect of the arm. With the aid of the color Doppler, the posterior humeral circumflex artery could be detected, and the axillary nerve is right next to it. Also, note any sign of denervation and atrophy of the deltoid [167]. Ultrasound is also preferred as a first-line diagnostic modality for axillary nerve trauma [168].

Musculocutaneous Nerve

The musculocutaneous nerves may be injured by a stretch with anterior shoulder dislocations or compressed with hypertrophied coracobrachialis in weightlifters [135]. The musculocutaneous nerve arises from the lateral cord together with

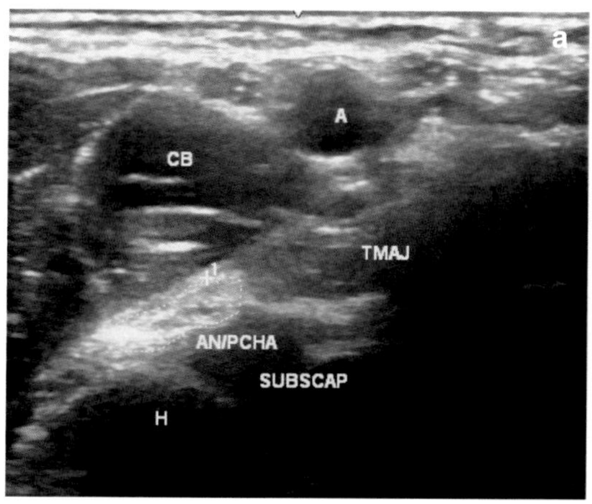

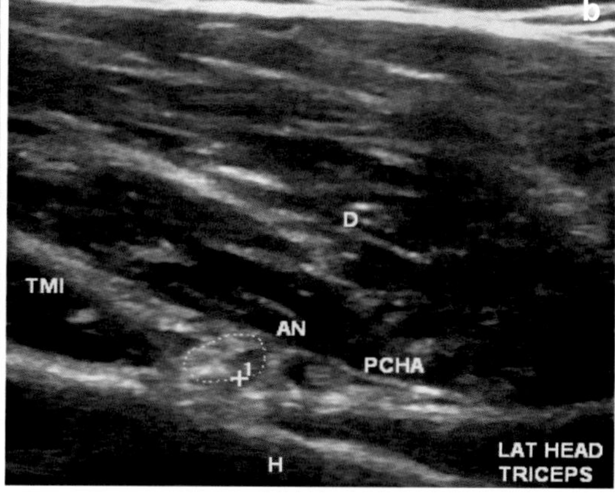

Fig. 22.8 (**a**) Ultrasound image of the axillary nerve (AN) at the axillary shown beside the posterior circumflex humeral artery (PCHA). This is otherwise known as an anterior view of the axillary nerve. (**b**) The posterior view of the axillary nerve (AN) together with the posterior circumflex humeral artery (PCHA) seen in between teres minor (TMI), lateral head of the triceps muscle and the deltoid (D) muscle, and the humeral bone as a bony acoustic landmark or otherwise referred to as quadrilateral space. CB coracobrachialis, TMAJ teres major, Subscap subscapularis

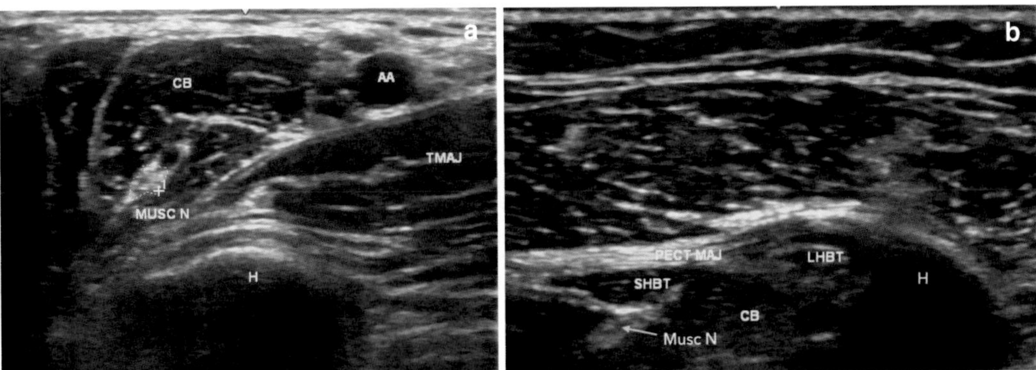

Fig. 22.9 (**a**) Ultrasound image of the musculocutaneous nerve (Musc N) at the level of the axillary fossa using the axillary artery (AA) as the reference in short-axis view. The musculocutaneous nerve perforates through the coracobrachialis muscle (CB). (**b**) Ultrasound image of the musculocutaneous nerve (Musc N) at the level of the pectoralis major (PECT MAJ) tendon attachment to the mid-humeral (H) bone. Also seen are the tendons of the short head (SHBT) and long head of the biceps tendon (LHBT). TMAJ teres major

the median nerve and lateral pectoral nerve. They come from C5, C6, and C7 spinal nerve roots. It pierces the coracobrachialis at the level of the axilla and then descends in between the biceps brachii and brachialis muscles. In a unique way, the coracobrachialis muscle is supplied by this nerve before it enters the muscle, while the biceps and brachialis are supplied after it enters the muscle. In the elbow, the nerve perforates the fascia lateral to the biceps tendon and continues to the forearm as the lateral antebrachial cutaneous nerve [169]. Among weightlifters, the most common injury is the injury to musculocutaneous nerve at the level of the coracobrachialis (Fig. 22.9) as well as in between the biceps brachii and brachialis leading to ischemic injury of the nerve with focal demyelination and variable axonal degeneration [170]. Traction mechanism can also injure this nerve when the elbow is in full extension as in the case of skydiving where the arms are in abduction, extension, and externally rotated position [171]. The second mechanism of musculocutaneous nerve injury involves the distal branch at the level of the superficial antebrachial fascia and the biceps tendon. In about 10% of such injury is iatrogenic in nature and is induced by the the displacement of the humeral shaft fracture when using Russell-Taylor splints. It usually affects the lateral antebrachial cutaneous branch of the musculocutaneous nerve [172]. Clinically, a proximal lesion will present with a mixed motor and sensory deficit, with associated weakness of the elbow flexors and sensory deficit at the lateral forearm, while the distal lesion is a purely sensory deficit with accentuation of symptoms during elbow extension and forearm pronation [169, 173]. Ultrasound is a useful tool for diagnosing traumatic injury of the musculocutaneous nerve complementing MRI and EMG tests. Two positions are suggested in imaging this nerve: one is tracing the nerve while the arms is at the side of the trunk. The musculocutaneous nerve is at the anatomical position but located deep in the muscle. The other position is when the hand is placed behind the head and in this way the musculocutaneous nerve becomes more superficial [174]. High-resolution ultrasound shows a fusiform stretching neuroma located between the long head and the short head of the biceps brachii or between the biceps and coracobrachialis muscles. Color Doppler did not show any increased flow on the site of the neuroma [174].

Median Nerve

The median nerve injury can occur in different segments of the upper extremity. The median nerve arises from the lateral cord (C5-C7 roots) and from medial contributions (C8-T1 roots) [135]. Repetitive movements of the elbow and forearm can cause impingement of the median nerve at the level of the pronator teres muscle.

The median nerve is entrapped in between the two heads of the pronator teres muscle or under the proximal edge of the flexor digitorum superficialis arch or at the lacertus fibrosus of the elbow. Resisted elbow flexion with the forearm supinated can be used to test if the entrapment occurred in the lacertus fibrosus [175]. This is common among baseball players, archers, pitchers, tennis players, and weightlifters. There is usually associated pain in the volar forearm and numbness of the first three fingers including the radial half of the fourth digit much like the carpal tunnel syndrome but with peculiar numbness of the thenar eminence without nocturnal pains. Pain is elicited during pronation and supination motion. Resisting the pronation motion could reproduce the symptoms [150, 176]. The second entrapment takes place at the forearm affecting the motor branch of the median nerve, referred to as anterior interosseous nerve syndrome (syndrome of Nevin and Kiloh). Entrapment of this nerve occurs superior to the elbow at the ligament of Struther where it forms part of the median nerve. It may also be entrapped at the site where the median pierces the two heads of the pronator teres. The anterior interosseous nerve (motor) passes deep to the tendinous bridge connecting the humeroulnar and radial heads of the flexor digitorum superficialis muscles (sublimis bridge) [177]. The anterior interosseous nerve (AIN) innervates the pronator quadratus, FPL, and FDP of the second and third digit [178]. The AIN is deep to the flexor pollicis longus, flexor digitorum profundus of the second and third digits, and pronator quadratus in the forearm. Or it can also be compressed at the FCR, FDS origin deep into the pronator teres head, or by an accessory head of the FPL (Gantzer muscle). There is an inability to make an "OK" sign (weakness of the FPL and FDP of the second digit) with no sensory deficit [176, 179]. Carpal tunnel syndrome is a common entrapment of the median nerve at the volar wrist especially seen among wheelchair users representing about 8% among disabled athletes [180]. Recently, with the advent of gaming in electronic sports or e-sports, there is a growing incidence of symptoms related to carpal tunnel syndrome. A competing athlete in e-sports would regularly spend 12–15 hours a day practicing dynamic and repetitive movements using a mouse and a keyboard [181]. Among long-distance cyclists, numbness over the palmar hand was reported, and although in most cases, the deep branch of the ulnar nerve to the first dorsal interossei was affected, the median nerve is also compressed especially exacerbating symptoms of carpal tunnel syndrome [182]. High-frequency ultrasound is an effective tool for diagnosing median nerve entrapment syndromes in the upper extremity. Although EMG/NCS is a common test to confirm carpal tunnel syndrome, the sensitivity of NCS has only a range of 49–84% and the specificity is more than 95% [183]. In fact, 25% of clinical CTS revealed a normal NCS study [184, 185]. An ultrasound diagnostic test (Fig. 22.10) has a sensitivity of 77.6% and a specificity of 86.8% for

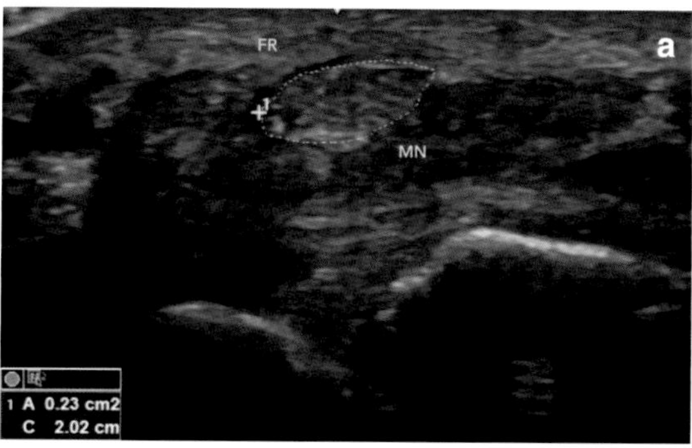

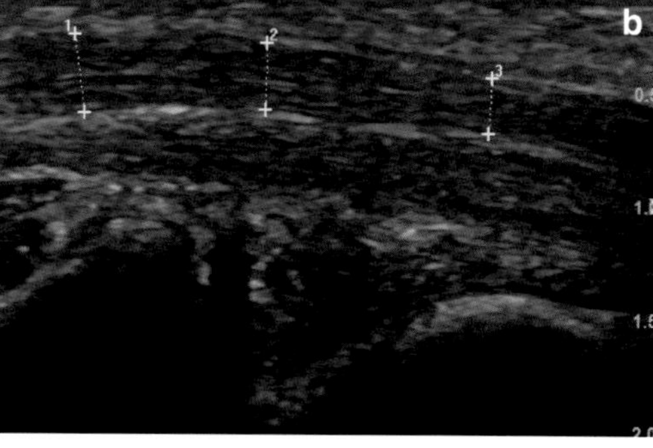

Fig. 22.10 (**a**, **b**) Ultrasound images of the short and longitudinal views of the median nerve (MN) at the level of the wrist of a 62-year-old male patient who is complaining of numbness for more than 6 months duration. It showed a swollen median nerve with associated minimal loss of fascicular pattern. FR, flexor retinaculum

CTS and can be useful in clinical CTS which might reveal a normal CTS [186]. Although ultrasound can provide morphologic abnormality in CTS, it cannot provide information about axonal loss or coexisting neuromuscular conditions which the electrodiagnostic test can do [187]. The work of Cartwright and colleagues will significantly alter the way peripheral nerve injuries can be diagnosed when using an ultra-high frequency ultrasound such as in a median nerve by counting the number of fascicles in the nerve [188]. In the pronator teres median nerve entrapment, a high-frequency ultrasound study showed that a CSA of 4.9–12.9 mm^2 is considered normal and is suggested when the normal side-to-side comparison is not available. However, an upper limit of side-to-side difference of >3.0 mm^2 is considered abnormal [189]. Ultrasound of the AIN is inconclusive due to its deep location in the forearm and its size unless there is a mass [177]. Transverse high-resolution ultrasound can visualize the anterior interosseous nerve by assessing the echogenicity of the innervated muscles such as the FPL, FDP of the second and third digit, and pronator quadratus [190]. In a systematic review, Malahias and colleagues reported that PRP treatment is recommended for mild to moderate CTS but not in severe CTS patients [191].

Ulnar Nerve

Ulnar nerve injury at the elbow is the second most common injury in the upper extremity seen in throwing athletes after "burner" or "stinger." Valgus instability which causes traction on the ulnar nerve at the medial elbow makes it very susceptible to injury and pain [192]. The strain of overhead throwing on the medial elbow of the baseball pitcher occurs at the acceleration phase where the large rotational moments of the elbow produce a large amount of force in all parts of elbow articulations [192]. In fact, Andrews called this combination of forces in the elbow causing a spectrum of disorders as valgus extension overload syndrome (VEO) [193]. The repetitive nature of this activity may drive the tissue to eventually absorb the stress. As a result, the anterior bundle of the UCL may eventually fail. Subsequently, it will injure the ulnar nerve causing neuritis. The subtle laxity and stretching of the medial elbow structures due to VEO syndrome may also injure the ulnar nerve [192]. In a cadaveric study by Mihata and colleagues, the greatest strain in the UCL and ulnar elongation at the medial elbow occurs during 60° and 90° of elbow flexion, thus causing cubital tunnel syndrome [194]. It is important though to determine whether the injuries primarily affect the UCL without the presence of ulnar neuritis or whether the ulnar neuritis is secondary to a deficient or lax UCL [192]. The first stage of ulnar neuritis includes medial elbow pain and muscle weakness without numbness [195]. The clinical diagnostic criteria for ulnar neuritis include the following: medial elbow pain or numbness at the ulnar side, tenderness or Tinel sign at the site of the ulnar nerve around the elbow, and weakness of the intrinsic muscle strength of the abductor digiti minimi, adductor pollicis, or positive elbow flexion test. All three criteria must be satisfied to come up with the diagnosis [195]. Other entrapment sites of the ulnar nerve are found at the Arcade of Struthers in the arm. This thin aponeurotic band extends from the medial head of the triceps to the intermuscular septum. This area is a confluence of structures made up of the medial head of the triceps, medial intermuscular septum, and the internal brachial ligament. It is approximately 6–8 cm proximal to the medial epicondyle of the elbow and the ulnar nerve passes underneath the arcade in about 70–80% of individuals. The second entrapment is what is described above, the cubital tunnel. Compression of the ulnar nerve by the Osborne ligament may diminish the gliding of the ulnar nerve during elbow flexion and extension [192, 196]. When Osborne's ligament has a pathologic fusion of the layers, it can reduce the cross-sectional area of the cubital tunnel by as much as 40% during elbow flexion [197]. The third entrapment site for the ulnar nerve occurs as the nerve enters the two heads of the flexor carpi ulnaris at the deep fascia of the anterior forearm. Lastly, ulnar nerve entrapment can occur at the confluence of fascia from the flexor digitorum superficialis to the ring finger [192]. Hand numbness on the ulnar side, ulnar nerve subluxation, and UCL injury are strong predictors of poor outcome after a period of conservative treatment, and surgery provides an excellent result [195]. Described as the "cyclists' palsy" or "handlebar palsy," this ulnar neuropathy is quite common among bicyclists. It is characterized by a gradual onset of numbness and tingling sensation at the little and ring fingers and/or weakness of the ulnar-innervated muscles of the hand and fingers. Recently, cyclists' palsy usually occurs as an isolated deep motor branch lesion. At the Guyon's canal in the palmar wrist, the ulnar nerve can be entrapped anywhere along the course of the nerve in which case the signs and symptoms vary as to whether it is a mixed sensory and motor (proximal), a pure sensory (middle), or a pure motor (distal) ulnar neuropathy. The floor of this canal is formed by the piso-hamate ligament and transverse carpal ligament, the roof by volar carpal ligament, the radial wall by the abductor digiti minimi and hook of the hamate, and the ulnar wall by the pisiform bone. In the hand, the ulnar nerve divides into a superficial sensory branch that supplies the palmar surface of the little finger and the ulnar half of the ring finger and the deep motor branch which supplies all the small muscles of the hand except the radial two lumbricals and the median innervated thenar muscles, except the deep head of the FPB [198, 199]. The superficial sensory branch divides into two branches after it gives off a branch to the palmaris brevis. These two branches consist of the common digital branch to the fourth web space at the lateral and an ulnar (medial) proper digital nerve to the medial side of the finger [200]. A rare ulnar nerve injury may occur at the thumb among bowlers referred to as bowler's thumb. Patients with this condition will usually complain of a painful nodule found at the volar surface of the hand between the first and second web space. It is described as a posttraumatic neuroma of the thumb due to a repetitive friction affecting the thumb ulnar digital nerve [201].

At the level of Arcade of Struthers, which is about 8 cm proximal to the medial epicondyle, an ulnar nerve entrapment in this area shows a hypoechoic enlargement of the ulnar nerve with evidence of fascial thickening. Normally, the ulnar nerve will appear normal distal to the FCU during an entrapment in this site [196]. High-frequency ultrasound is a reliable tool for evaluation of the ulnar nerve at the elbow and its related structures around the elbow and to diagnose any pathological conditions [202]. The main ultrasound finding at the medial elbow is an increase in the cross-sectional area (CSA) diameter at the affected side (Fig. 22.11). This method is the most accepted means of diagnosing entrapment neuropathies of the ulnar nerve. Ultrasound showed a sensitivity of 93.1% and a specificity of 50% using nerve conduction studies as reference [203]. Thickening of the epineurium was observed with patients with dislocating nerves at

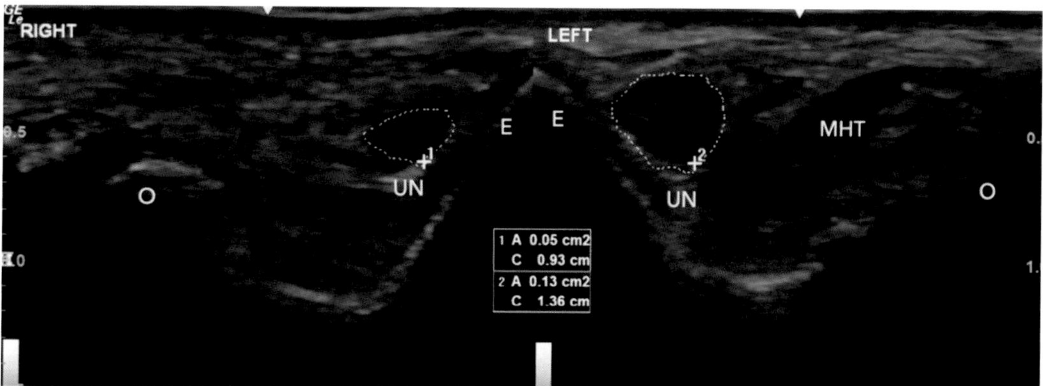

Fig. 22.11 Side-to-side comparison of the ultrasound images of the ulnar nerve (UN) where the left elbow showed an abnormal hypoechoic swelling at the level of the cubital tunnel. Note the medial head of the triceps (MHT) seen at the medial side of the elbow. Some patients may experience instability of the ulnar nerve while being pushed by the MHT during a dynamic flexion-extension motion. E epicondyle, O olecranon

the medial elbow which is a similar finding among leprosy patients. Among baseball pitchers, for instance, there is a significant increase in the distance of the ulnar nerve from the elbow as it approaches 120° flexion in the throwing arm as compared to the non-throwing arm, thus an increased tendency for nerve subluxation and nerve irritation [204]. Interestingly, Scheidl and colleagues have found that ultrasound can distinguish between axonal loss and demyelination. In their study of the ulnar neuropathy at the elbow (UNE), diagnosed by electrodiagnostic studies, a larger CSA of ulnar nerve at the medial epicondyle correlates with axonal loss, as opposed to demyelinating lesions (mean CSA 10.1 mm^2 in demyelinating versus 15.2 mm^2 in axonal loss) [205].

High-frequency ultrasound of the ulnar digital nerve of the thumb in bowler's thumb is placed at the level of the MCP in long-axis view. It shows a gradual hypoechoic enlargement of the ulnar digital nerve with enlarged hypoechoic fascicles with hyperechoic epineural thickening [201]. In the cyclists' palsy, where the ulnar nerve is injured at the area around Guyon's canal, the nerve appears thickened in a high-resolution ultrasound in the proximal side of the lesion. For the deep branch of the ulnar nerve, two sites can cause ulnar nerve entrapment. The first one is between the fibro-osseous tunnel formed by the tendon origin of the hypothenar muscles (roof) and the pisohamate ligament (floor). The other one is between the tendinous arch of the transverse and adductor heads of the adductor pollicis muscle [206]. Other studies identified five areas of ulnar nerve entrapment in the palmar wrist and hand among the cyclists [199].

Radial Nerve

The radial nerve arises from the posterior cord at C5-T1 spinal nerve roots. It usually runs posterior to the axillary artery at the axilla and then courses through the long and medial heads of the biceps brachii muscles to go posterior up to the level of the humeral groove, (Fig. 22.12a) which is a common entrapment site for the radial nerve. The radial nerve then perforates through the intermuscular septum laterally and then it enters the anterior compartment of the arm distally. Before it goes beyond the elbow, it innervates the following muscles: extensor carpi radialis longus and brevis, triceps, and brachioradialis muscles. From the elbow, it gives off two branches: superficial radial nerve (sensory) and posterior interosseous nerve (motor), which is the branch that goes beneath the supinator mus-

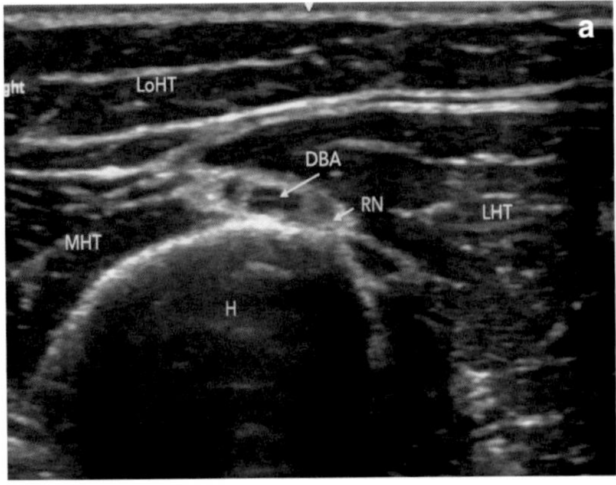

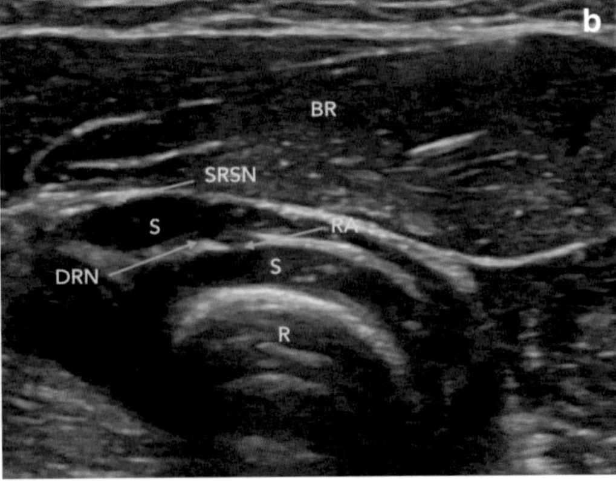

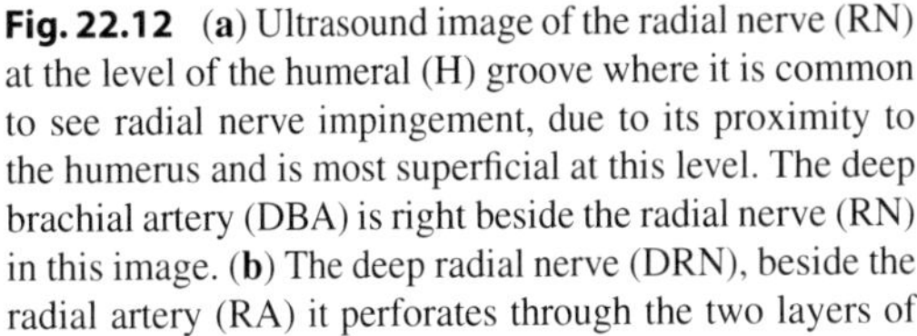

Fig. 22.12 (**a**) Ultrasound image of the radial nerve (RN) at the level of the humeral (H) groove where it is common to see radial nerve impingement, due to its proximity to the humerus and is most superficial at this level. The deep brachial artery (DBA) is right beside the radial nerve (RN) in this image. (**b**) The deep radial nerve (DRN), beside the radial artery (RA) it perforates through the two layers of the supinator muscles at the level of the proximal elbow, which is on top of the radius (R). The superficial radial sensory nerve (SRSN) splits from the main radial nerve branch at this level. LoHT long head triceps muscle, LHT lateral head triceps muscle, MHT medial head triceps muscle, BR brachioradialis (BR) muscle

cle at the Arcade of Frohse (Fig. 22.12b) and is thickened in 30% of individuals. This is the most common site of entrapment of the radial nerve in the radial tunnel. The other area of entrapment of the posterior interosseous nerve is the fascial bands connecting the brachioradialis and brachialis muscles, the leash of Henry, an arcade of anastomosing branches of the radial recurrent artery, and the tendinous edge of extensor carpi radialis brevis muscle. The superficial radial nerve runs over the posterolateral aspect of the forearm, to the wrist and the hand to innervate the first, second, third, and radial half of the fourth digits except the distal phalanx, which is a median-innervated area. The posterior interosseous nerve runs distally to innervate the muscles namely the extensor pollicis longus and brevis, extensor carpi ulnaris, and finger extensors [207]. Radial tunnel syndrome is commonly observed in tennis and Frisbee players, weightlifters, and rowers. It is usually due to hyperextension injuries of the elbow, or repetitive pronation and supination of the forearm, or direct compression of the nerve [207–209]. This is characterized by pain mimicking a tennis elbow in contrast with a posterior interosseous nerve (PIN) syndrome (supinator syndrome) which is characterized by weakness of the extensor muscles of the forearm without pain. The boundary of the radial tunnel includes the humeroulnar joint and deep layer of the supinator muscle posteriorly; the fibrous attachments between brachialis and brachioradialis, and ECRB laterally; the superficial layer of the supinator muscle anteriorly; and the biceps brachii medially [209]. Ultrasound of the radial nerve inside the tunnel shows a hypoechoic swelling of the deep branch of the radial nerve with the Arcade of Frohse being the most common site of entrapment [177, 209]. In fact, ultrasound confirms 83% of abnormal electrodiagnostic findings of the posterior interosseous nerve with additional information such as PIN enlargement nerve continuity or laceration in trauma [210]. In a sports injury involving the arm, the radial nerve is the most injured peripheral nerve occurring in 9.5% of humeral fractures. Also, an avulsion fracture of the distal humerus at the origin of the brachioradialis muscle has sustained an associated superficial radial nerve injury in a lacrosse player in this case report [211]. Ultrasound over the humeral groove shows hypoechoic swelling of the radial nerve with loss of fascicular pattern. In the presence of fracture, the radial nerve may be displaced at the edge of fracture fragments or be pinched in between them [177]. Radial nerve entrapment can also occur at the radial side of the wrist just above the first dorsal compartment of the wrist. As the superficial radial nerve courses forward from the proximal forearm, it runs beneath the brachioradialis and perforates through the antebrachial fascia of the distal forearm. It moves superficially over the APL and EPB tendons of the radial wrist [212]. High-frequency ultrasound can visualize the nerve in this area as in the case of Wartenberg Syndrome (or cheiralgia paresthetica). Patients complain of pain and paresthesia along the distal forearm, thumb, and index finger, much like a De Quervain's tenosynovitis [213].

Musculoskeletal Ultrasound/Regenerative Therapies in Lower Extremity Sports Injuries

Lower extremity sports injuries are becoming common regardless of the status of an individual. In the past, some sports activities are only played by the upper-class people, but recently with sports activity becoming an exercise activity or lifestyle, it has become accessible to all people. And so, it goes with sports injuries. In a study by Brant and colleagues among US high school athletes, they described the epidemiology of lower extremity sports injuries over a 10-year period from 2005 to 2016. The study showed that the highest injury rate among both genders was seen in soccer, followed by basketball, cross-country, track and field, volleyball, softball/baseball with the lowest injury seen in tennis, swimming, and diving. In each individual sport, girls have a higher rate of lower extremity injuries as seen in soccer. Regardless of sports activity, the highest injury was an ankle sprain, with the anterior talofibular ligament being the most strained ligament for both genders [214]. Moreover, the most common ligament injured among boys is the patellar tendon, and for girls, it is the anterior cruciate ligament [214]. In another study, it was reported that athletes with moderate to high sport specialization or those athletes specializing in a single sport have a higher risk of lower extremity injuries [215].

Hip

Groin pain is such a broad term that initially has caused many physicians to describe this condition to refer to non-specific sports injury affecting the hip. It was not until 2015 that an impressive group of leaders in this field met in Doha during the First World Conference on Groin Pain in Athletes and subsequently published their consensus report. The result of this meeting provided four new subcategories of groin pain: adductor-related, pubic-related, inguinal-related, and iliopsoas-related groin pain [216]. Sports hip injuries account for about 6% of all sports injuries and counting. It is usually seen in athletes who require pivoting and cutting associated with rapid acceleration and deceleration. These injuries consist of adductor strains, osteitis pubis, and athletic pubalgia, or core muscle injury previously described as "sports hip triad" [217]. There is also an associated range of motion limitation due to femoroacetabular impingement [217]. This categorization of sports hip injury, however, could be outdated, although many sports physicians still use this. To our discussion, we will describe this as objectively as possible referring to a particular and specific condition. The "core" also was coined by exercise and fitness experts to refer to the entire body from the chest to the midthigh. And this is also further subdivided into four categories namely muscular, hip, back, and everything else. Thus, a core muscle injury is an injury of any structure from the chest to the midthigh [216].

Hip flexor strain was the most common diagnosis with intraarticular injuries taking a toll on days lost in competition (94.2 days) [216]. In a study by Epstein and colleagues, it was reported that these injuries made up 10.6% of all hip and groin injuries [218]. Among professional basketball players like the NBA, groin pulls and sports hernias are the most common hip and groin pains, but this condition responds well with conservative treatments. However, a third of them continue to experience hip pain after retirement and 16.7% of them may soon require total hip arthroplasty [219]. This rate is higher than that found in the population older than 50 years, which is 15% [220]. Among soccer players, they have reported that a decreased hip range of motion (HROM) is associated with more hip and groin-related symptoms independent of a cam hip deformity [221]. Serner and colleagues characterized athletes with groin injuries in the hip flexor muscles using an MRI study among 156 athletes with groin injuries. The study showed that athletes with hip flexor injuries predominantly involve rectus femoris and iliacus but rarely in combination. Moreover, rectus femoris injuries are usually secondary to kicking and then sprinting, whereas iliacus injuries took place during a change in direction. Also, the indirect tendon is usually involved in most proximal rectus femoris injuries while a distinct iliacus and psoas major injuries occurred at the muscle-tendon junction [222].

Anterior/Medial Hip

In adductor strains, the adductor longus is the usual source of symptoms and pathology in athletes, commonly seen among soccer players and ice hockey players and representing 23% of all muscle injuries. There is a reinjury rate of 18% with a mean time lost in the play of about 2 weeks [217, 223]. Reinjuries are higher in professional ice hockey with a recurrence rate of 23.5% [223]. Usually, the reinjuries take a longer time to recover as compared to the original injury which is why it is important that appropriate and timely rehabilitation must be performed. Athletes usually report medial thigh pain aggravated by resisted adduction and passive stretching of adductors. Injuries over the myotendinous area are usually located more distally [217]. Surprisingly, the mechanism of injury of adductor tears is non-contact in 77% of cases followed by overuse injury which has a rate of 12.8%.

Such injury resulted in a time loss of 7–13 days. However, surgery is not required for such injury [224]. Moreover, it was reported by Ralston and colleagues among NCAA Women's Soccer Players that the most common tears are found in adductor and iliopsoas/sartorius muscles with a rate of about 81.5%. These injuries occurred during practice and were sustained during the preseason [224].

Core muscle injury, sometimes referred to as athletic pubalgia or "sports hernia," is an injury about the chest and the mid-thigh. The muscles attaching through the fibrocartilage covering the pubic bone stabilize the pelvis and thus form a harness that allows the trunk to move with the legs. The following muscles are important in stabilizing the core: rectus abdominis, the three adductors such as the pectineus, adductor longus, and adductor brevis, which serve a primary role. Other muscles such as the iliopsoas and rectus femoris may secondarily get involved [216]. The rectus abdominis, adductor longus, and brevis muscles and pectineus muscles are attached to the fibrocartilaginous plate at the anterior pelvis close to the pubic symphysis and pubic tubercles [216, 225]. This injury is seen in sports that require pivoting and cutting as in the case of ice hockey, soccer, or American football [217]. A classic symptom is pain over the pubis, abdominal obliques, rectus abdominis, adductor longus insertion at the pubis. Resisted sit-ups cause pain over the distal rectus abdominis and with resisted adduction [226]. Core injuries can be unilateral, bilateral, or midline in location [225]. Ultrasound can be an inexpensive and effective first step in diagnosing this injury. The presence of edema around the pubic bone or evidence of laxity or atrophy of the abdominal musculature is an indication that an MRI is needed to confirm the pathology [216]. MRI showed cleft sign over the rectus abdominis/adductor aponeurosis at the anterior pelvis [227]. A poor MRI image, however, might show diffuse haziness around the pubic bone which may be interpreted as a pubic bone stress fracture and the patient might unnecessarily be told to rest and be non-weight-bearing for months. Moreover, if this injury is related to muscle detachment in the case of core muscle injury, then the pain will return when resuming athletic activities [216]. Depending on the MRI findings, the plate detachment because of the injury could be found in the midline, right, or left lateral or there may be a posterior extension of the injuries of the fibrocartilage plate from the pubis. Chronic plate detachment may occur in a long-standing injury without any treatment, where spicules of granulation tissue occupy between the fibrocartilaginous plates and the pubic bone. Degenerative detachments may occur because of repetitive motion simulating a chronic plate detachments with a lytic appearance. Peripubic and bone marrow edema may signify a plate detachment [216]. The patient responds well with conservative therapies like rest and physical therapy, although the pain can recur once athletic activity resumes. Steroids are prescribed by some to relieve pain. Platelet-rich plasma is also prescribed by other practitioners, but with an increased incidence of heterotopic ossification at the site of injection, caution is needed in considering such treatment. The definitive treatment for core muscle injuries is surgical repair. The presence of an indirect hernia must be fixed as well, as this can contribute to the imbalance of forces of the abdominal musculature and the hip joint. Treating this laxity contributes to the complete restoration of the muscle acting on the pubic bone and hip [216, 228]. In fact, except for core endurance, the core strength, core proprioception, and neuromuscular control of the core contribute to lower extremity injuries if not addressed appropriately [229].

There are lots of debate on the nomenclature as to whether osteitis pubis is part of the "sports hernia" injuries or could be an altogether separate entity. The incidence is about 0.5–8% with a higher incidence with distance runners or those athletes involved in kicking such as in male soccer players [230]. In fact, in another study, it was reported that 86% of patients suffering from groin pain, treated for osteitis pubis and/or sports hernia, had radiographic evidence of femoroacetabular impingement (FAI) [231]. In contrast, there is a prevalence rate of about 1.8–2.6% of symphysis pubis abnormality in patients with FAIs [232]. As part of the groin pain in sports injury of the anterior pelvis, there is evidence to say that athletes could suffer from this condition. This is described as a painful overuse injury of the symphysis pubis causing lower abdominal pain and/or groin pain [217]. The pubic symphysis acting as a fulcrum balances the forces coming from two antagonists muscles: the rectus abdominis acting to elevate the pelvis and the three adductors (pectineus, adductor longus, and brevis) acting to depress it during core rotation and extension. When these muscles are imbalanced which may be subsequently injured, the symphyseal biomechanics are altered with subsequent injury to the pubic bone and later degeneration of the cartilage in the symphysis pubis [217]. This is where an overlap of signs and symptoms is observed between osteitis pubis and athletic pubalgia. The one distinguishing mark is pain elicited by palpation over the pubic symphysis or pain on resisted sit-ups (positive spring test) at the lateral edge of the rectus abdominis [217]. The bilateral adductor test also has been found to be a sensitive test for this condition [230]. As this is a chronic condition, the radiographic findings may show lytic changes over the pubic symphysis, sclerosis, and widening of the symphysis pubis [217]. A "flamingo view" where the patient stands on one leg on an AP view will show the instability of the pelvis where a vertical subluxation of more than 2 mm or a widening of more than 7 mm of the pubic symphysis is pathognomonic for this condition [230]. In contrast, MRI shows subchondral bone edema with bilateral involvement, although it is more visible on the affected side [217]. There is a hyperintense signal on the T2-weighted images around the pubic symphysis on cases with less than 6 month duration of symptoms. For patients with a longer duration of symptoms, there is usually subchondral sclerosis, subchondral resorption, with bony irregularity, pubic beak-like appearance [230].

This condition is usually self-limited and may respond to conservative treatments such as rest, ice, inflammatory conditions, and physical rehabilitation with the goal of correcting muscle imbalance around the pubic symphysis, stretching, and strengthening of pelvic musculature [233]. Ultrasound imaging can show tendon, muscle, and aponeurosis abnormalities around the pubic symphysis together with cortical irregularities, but MRI can show deep and intraosseous abnormalities [234]. MRI is the preferred imaging modality, but ultrasound provides a dynamic assessment of soft tissue abnormality and guided intervention. When used for guided intervention, it is placed sagittally over the pubis and the needle is introduced superior to inferior approach. It has a limited role in the diagnosis of symphysial dysfunction and in osteitis pubis [235].

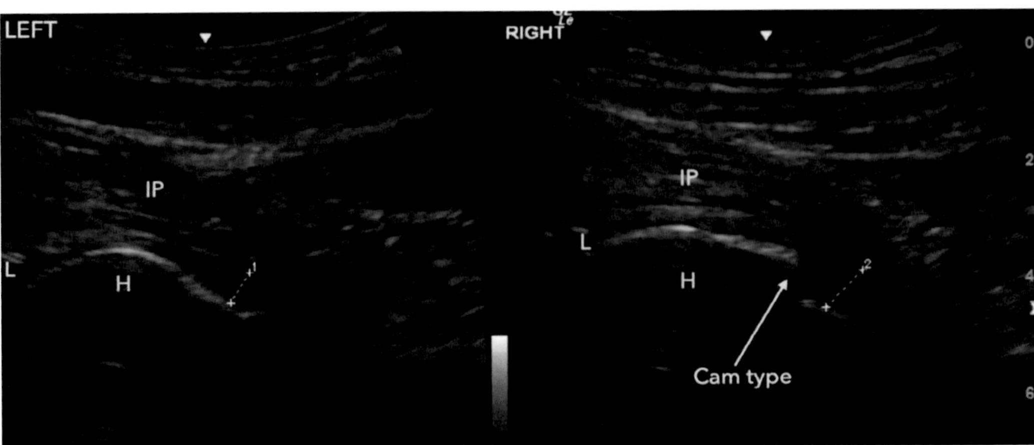

Fig. 22.13 Side-to-side comparison of the anterior hip joint of a 50-year-old male patient complaining of anterior right hip pain, the left being asymptomatic and the right hip showing pains during >60° of hip flexion. Ultrasound showed a cortical step-off sign over the anterior femoral head, typical of the cam type femoroacetabular impingement with associated hypoechoic swelling of the anterior recess. IP iliopsoas, L labrum, H femoral head

Labral tears of the anterior hip are quite common among athletes manifested as a dull anterior hip or groin pain with signs of clicking and buckling [236]. It is often the result of trauma or injury which subsequently causes subluxation or dislocation of the femoral head and is associated with chondral injuries either at the acetabular or at the femoral side [237]. Femoroacetabular impingement (FAI) (Fig. 22.13) is the most common cause of labral tear [238]. It is estimated that there is a prevalence rate of 38% of labral tears in young asymptomatic athletes and 56% in professional and adult collegiate athletes. Most of the labral tears (84%) are found in the anterosuperior portion of the hip [236]. Rankin and colleagues reported a higher prevalence rate of FAI in men (45%) and labral tears among women (47.7%) [239]. It has three basic types:, the cam-type, where there is a bony protrusion at the anterolateral head-neck junction and therefore this collides with the acetabular rim during motion disrupting the chondrolabral conjunction and eventually delaminating the articular cartilage and labrum; the pincer type, where the acetabulum creates an over coverage of the femoral head causing a breakdown of the cartilage and labrum during motion; and the mixed type [240]. It was reported that 83.7% had a cam deformity and 28% had a pincer deformity and the average alpha angle was 66.7° [231]. Aiba and colleagues use multiplanar reconstruction computed tomography (mCT) for the detection of subclinical coincidence of hip OA and FAI with a labral tear. They reported the 2-mm rule narrow joint space which was previously used radiographically and applied it using mCT to detect poor outcomes of hip arthroscopy in favor of hip arthroplasty surgery [240]. Patients with FAI complain of gradually developing anterior hip pain (Fig. 22.13) radiating to the knee and in most cases occurring at night and can be aggravated by walking, pivoting, running, and prolonged sitting. An anterior hip impingement test where the hip and the knee are flexed to 90° and then adducted and internally rotated confirms that the labral tear is anterior. For posterior hip impingement test, the patient lies prone with hip and knee extended. The hip and knee are then extended, adducted, and externally rotated indicating a posterior labral tear when pain is present during the maneuver [241]. Interestingly, Fukushima and colleagues reported the severity of synovitis and chondral injury to be more important pathologies for the origin of hip pain than labral tears or instability. Moreover, the pain is due to inflammatory cytokines such as TNF-α and IL-6 [242]. There is an increase of fibronectin-aggrecan complex (FAC) and COMP (cartilage oligomeric matrix protein) in FAI and is seen among young athletes. Thus, FAI instead of the aging process causes hip OA. There is also a consistent increase of IL-6 in hip OA but with varied results in TNF-α and IL-1 [243].

Ultrasound of the anterior hip around an abnormal labral morphology usually showed a hypoechoic labral cleft with a detachment of the labrum from the acetabular rim confirming a labral tear [236]. Usually the presence of paralabral cyst by ultrasound is an indication of a labral tear. Filling a labral cleft with fluid in the case of a hip effusion improves the detection of the labral tear [244]. MRA arthrography however has better sensitivity than ultrasound for the detection of labral tears [245]. Labral tears can initially be treated using rest, ice, NSAIDs, activity modification, and physical rehabilitation [236]. In a prospective study, the use of ultrasound-guided platelet-rich plasma injection showed a significant effect in terms of pain and function for hip labral tear treatment in patients who are refractory to conservative treatments for an 8-week period follow-up [246].

The rectus femoris is the most common injury of the anterior hip and comes second after hamstring injuries among athletes [247]. The injuries could be attributed to their biarticular nature, the predominance of fast-twitch muscle types, and powerful eccentric and concentric contractions. Athletes sustain these injuries with the hip in extension and knee in flexion such as in football and rugby [236] during kicking and sprinting [222]. The indirect head is the most common site of injury affecting the central aponeurosis of the musculotendinous part of the structure. The injury has an insidious onset with athletes complaining of only mild pain and spasms at the anterior thigh [222, 236]. Acutely injured indirect head of the rectus femoris appears in the ultrasound as ill-defined, thickened, and heterogeneous central tendon with a bull's eye pattern on transverse view due to its edema formation [248]. Chronic injuries of the indirect head appear in ultrasound as a thickened hypoechoic form with loss of fibrillar pattern and a posterior acoustic shadowing due to scar formation. Acute, high-grade strains of the indirect head of the rectus femoris appear in ultrasound as a complete disruption with bizarre tendon retraction mimicking a soft tissue mass. Myofascial injuries are a distinct abnormality in the muscle tissue which is better visualized by MR imaging [236].

Iliopsoas muscle strain and tendon tears were commonly seen secondary to a sports injury especially among men although they were rarely found in the normal population (prevalence of 0.66%) [236]. The injury is usually associated with age and gender rather than with specific activity. Patients with a mean age of 53 years were seen suffering from partial tendon tears of the iliopsoas and patients under 65 years were more often found to have only muscle strains and partial tears. Those beyond 65 years usually present with complete iliopsoas tendon tear with associated hip flexion weakness [249]. Iliopsoas disorders are shown to be the cause of chronic groin pain in about 12–36% of athletes and in 25–30% of acute groin pain [250]. Trauma in the psoas is associated with team sports and canoeing. It was also associated with sports involving kicking and jumping such as football, basketball, and gymnastics [236]. This may lead to any of the three distinct lesions in the iliopsoas, such as the fleshy part of the muscle, the myotendinous junction (small), and the lower part of the tendon insertions in the lesser trochanter. Of the three lesions, this is the most disabling and is associated with hip flexion weakness [251]. Iliopsoas tendinopathy was reported after acute and overuse injuries. It has also been found to be associated with internal hip snapping, osteophyte formation, and post-arthroplasty impingement. This is shown in ultrasound as the hypoechoic heterogeneous appearance of the tendon with loss of fibrillar pattern, hypertrophic changes of the iliopsoas tendon, and neoangiogenesis by power Doppler ultrasound. Partial-thickness musculotendinous tears appear as focal discontinuity of the fibrillar patterns with associated anechoic focal fluid on transverse view, while full-thickness tears appear as full discontinuity of the fibers, with a fluid-filled gap with its distal fibers retracted [236, 252].

Internal snapping hip syndrome was once described as a snapping of the iliopsoas tendon over the iliopectineal eminence or the lesser trochanter [253]. This condition is reported among ballet dancers and football players. Moreover, this is observed in patients when climbing stairs or when one gets out of the car or stands up from a chair [254]. Tatu and colleagues have found out that the most medial fibers of the iliacus muscle merged with the psoas muscle as an accessory tendon making up the iliopsoas tendon, while the most lateral fibers of the iliacus muscle ended up without any tendon on the anterior portion of the lesser trochanter and infratrochanteric region. The most inferior fibers of the iliacus muscle joined the main iliopsoas tendon from the arcuate line. Another muscle overlying on its anterolateral surface reached the anterior aspect of the lesser trochanter and infratrochanteric area without a tendon, called an ilio-infratrochanteric muscle [255]. Guillin and colleagues, deriving their knowledge from the cadaveric studies of Tatu, made the first attempt to study the dynamic movement of the iliopsoas muscle and tendon by sonographic examination. Under ultrasound imaging, in a dynamic movement of hip flexion, abduction, and external rotation (frog-leg position), the psoas major tendon (PMT) moved laterally and followed an externally oriented rotational course around the medial fibers of the iliacus (MFI) (Fig. 22.14B). The rotating movement was clockwise on the left hip and counterclockwise on the right hip. None of the tendon glides on the superior pubic ramus without any muscular interposition of the PMT and MFI. Thus, as the PMT glides around the MFI, the MFI was then entrapped between the PMT and the superior pubic ramus. The snap created occurred during the last phase of external rotation at the vicinity of the anterior inferior iliac spine. When the hip is brought back to extension, the

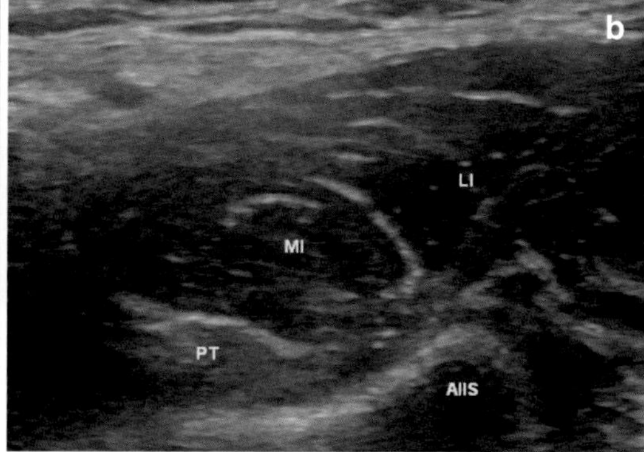

Fig. 22.14 (**a**) Ultrasound image of the greater trochanter in short axis view showing the bony apex (*), serving as the key landmark between the lateral (L) and anterior (A) facets. The gluteus minimus (Gmin) is seen attaching to the anterior facet and the gluteus medius (Gmed) attaching to the lateral facet. Also shown are the gluteus max (Gmax) and the iliotibial tract (ITT). Usually, the subgluteus maximus or trochanteric bursa is seen way posterior between the gluteus maximus and posterior facet. (**b**) Ultrasound image of the anterior hip in short-axis view at the level of the anterior inferior iliac spine (AIIS) shows the psoas tendon (PT), medial iliacus (MI), and lateral iliacus (LI)

PMT and MFI followed a reverse course until the initial position is reached. Moreover, the MFI was distinguished from the lateral fibers of the iliacus (LFI) by a thin echoic interface named "intramuscular fascia of the iliacus muscle" [256]. In another study, Deslandes and colleagues have debunked the snapping of the iliopsoas tendon against the iliopubic eminence. The sudden tendon snap, therefore, is created between the psoas tendon and the medial iliacus as described by Guillin [256, 257]. This dynamic maneuver as observed in ultrasound is present in up to 40% of normal subjects where even the athletes with this physiological phenomenon may not be aware [256]. The repetitive snapping may then cause inflammation with subsequent pain [257]. The other causes of painful snapping hip were between the two components of the bifid psoas major tendon at the level of the anterior inferior iliac spine while in the frog-leg position [257], at the postoperative period of total hip arthroplasty where there is an overlap of the prosthetic cup at the anterior acetabular rim [258]. The ultrasound procedure is done by putting the probe in a transverse oblique plane between the anterior inferior iliac spine and superior pubic ramus with the iliopsoas complex at the middle of the image. The patient is asked to perform hip flexion-abduction-external rotation motions followed by extension and adduction. The probe is adjusted more laterally during the initial motion and moves a little medially toward the later part of the rotation of the hip to visualize the presence of a snap [258]. Interestingly, Audenaert and colleagues refuse to fully agree with Guillin and Deslandes that the snapping exclusively does not involve the iliopectineal eminence but further added his observation in the increase in tendon excursion with a decreasing ischiofemoral distance, the presence of femoral malrotation, and its association with female sex [259].

Snapping of the hip is usually classified as intra-articular or extra-articular depending on the appropriate location. Intra-articular snapping hip is caused by any impingement occurring at the hip joint such as due to labral tears, synovial chondromatosis, ligamentum teres tears, fracture fragments, or any loose bodies inside the joint space. Extra-articular hip snapping is the most common form and is further subdivided into internal or external snapping hip [260]. Additionally, a posterior snapping caused by the proximal hamstring origin may also occur [261]. The previous one was just described above lengthily. In the external form of snapping, the thickened posterior portion of the iliotibial band

(ITB) or the thickened anterior edge of the gluteus maximus muscle.

Posterior portion of the iliotiband band (ITB) or the thickened anterior edge of gluteus maximus muscle snaps over the greater trochanter during flexion and extension of the hip or by mere walking producing a "click" or a snap-on motion (Fig. 22.14A). Moreover, snapping cannot be induced when a patient walks with the leg in external rotation since the thickened band moves anterior to the greater trochanter. With the repetitive motion of the hip like running and ballet, it may cause inflammation and pain. Women are often more affected than men. To some patients, the snapping may not cause any pain at all [260, 262, 263]. The prevalence of this condition in both symptomatic and asymptomatic cases are unknown [264]. Clinically, the snapping can be elicited when the patient lies on the side with the affected leg passively extended or flexed in a neutral position [265]. The ITB lies posterior to the greater trochanter when the hip is extended, and it moves anteriorly when the knee and hip are flexed. Thus, when the posterior part of the thickened portion of the proximal ITB moves forward on a flexed knee in an abrupt motion, the snapping occurs [264]. In some cases, it is also possible that the distal gluteus maximus muscle may snap during hip flexion over the greater trochanter [260]. MRI is the standard imaging diagnostic tool, but ultrasound imaging can help also in the assessment. Ultrasound usually showed an increased thickness of the iliotibial tract/band with heterogeneous echogenicity indicating tendinopathy. Dynamic imaging will demonstrate the translation of the IT tract over the gluteus medius tendon which is connected anteriorly with tensor fascia lata and posteriorly by the gluteus maximus muscle/tendon while the hip is being extended and then flexed [260]. Treatment for this condition includes rest, NSAIDs, physical therapy, and stretching of the iliotibial band. Patients who are refractory to this treatment may undergo injection with steroid, platelet-rich plasma, or local anesthetic with steroids providing short-term relief. Platelet-rich plasma as a possible treatment has not been thoroughly investigated for external hip snapping, although it has been used for recalcitrant trochanteric tendinopathies [266, 267]. Surgical lengthening of the ITB by Z-plasty or endoscopic IT tract release is reserved for those unresponsive for any treatment mentioned above [260, 268]. The open IT release showed a recurrence rate of 11% compared to an arthroscopic IT release with very minimal complication [269].

Posterior Hip

Hamstring injuries are one of the most common injuries involving athletes. Their prevalence among professional baseball players is 12–15% [270] The spectrum of these injuries can be as simple as a hamstring strain to severe ruptures, occurring either proximally, at the mid-substance, or distally [271]. Acute hamstring strain is the most common muscle strain with a high rate of recurrence, with some studies reporting that one in three hamstring strains will recur within the first 2 weeks of return to sports [272–274]. The most common hamstring injuries affect the proximal tendons following a history of forceful hip flexion and knee extension. It is characterized by sudden and acute onset of pain with ecchymosis over the posterior thigh distal to the ischial tuberosity [275]. It is usually measured 2.3 cm distal to the ischial tuberosity [276] and there is an associated difficulty in sitting and weight-bearing. The ecchymosis can after a few days extend to the distal posterior thigh and posterior leg. To some extent, the posterior cutaneous branch of the sciatic nerve could impinge because of the hematoma and the retracted tendon can cause numbness and neuropathic pains. In the early phase of injury, walking and running could be very challenging [271]. Proximal hamstring strains and avulsions are more common with the long head of the biceps femoris most often injured, and the musculotendinous tendinous junction is a possible location. Moreover, the injury involving the long head of the biceps femoris tendon occurs during high-speed running, especially during the late swing and early stance phases of gait [277] and semimembranosus being the next commonly injured muscle happens during extensive stretching [278]. Proximal hamstring avulsions occur predominantly in the middle-aged patient and rarely in patients below

30 years of age with older female affected during activities of daily living [279]. Regardless of whether the hamstring injury is distal or proximal, the patient usually presents with a feeling of snap at the posterior thigh and knee flexion weakness with associated pain and stiffness, making weight-bearing a difficult task. In an isolated biceps femoris rupture, pain can be felt at the lateral or posterolateral aspect of the thigh [271]. Recent biomechanical studies also revealed that hamstring muscle-tendon complex has a significant role in the rotational stability of the knee. In fact, hamstring is an ACL agonist and thus it protects the ACL from an added injury [280]. MRI and ultrasound are the modalities of choice for hamstring injuries with MRI showing better sensitivity for proximal hamstring tendinopathy. Ultrasound findings of tendinopathy showed hypoechoic thickening of the tendon with associated peritendinous fluid. There is also an echogenic focus of calcific tendinopathy with cortical irregularity and tender on sonopalpation [281]. Partial-thickness tears are better visualized by MRI than ultrasound especially if there are subtle lesions involving the semimembranosus muscle. For complete hamstring avulsion, an initial radiographic study is needed to rule out any bony avulsion injury. Ultrasound is useful in this type of injury to identify complete avulsion injury especially in a setting where MRI is not practical to use. But once surgery is being considered, MRI is useful to characterize the details of the injury including the extent of muscle retraction and the number of tendons involved [282]. Most hamstring strains, tendinopathy, or partial-thickness tears can be treated conservatively but proximal hamstring avulsions or injury of the entire hamstring muscle complex requires surgery. Moreover, surgical treatment may be indicated for partial thickness tear after a failure of conservative treatment, involving two tendons with a retraction of >2 cm or complete with three tendon injuries [282–284]. Conservative treatment may include physiotherapy, extracorporeal shock wave therapy, and PRP injections [284]. There are no significant results to recommend the use of PRP in recent studies [285, 286] for hamstring injuries, although one study reported a shorter return to play in those athletes with grade 2 hamstring injuries [287]. As mentioned earlier, sciatic nerve impingement whose main symptom is pain may be secondarily affected in proximal hamstring avulsion injuries but is underrecognized. However, Wilson and colleagues have reported that with surgery, these symptoms are likely to improve and thus should be taken into consideration when discussing the risks and benefits of operative repair [288]. Subbu and colleagues in their study found that the meantime of 22 days post-injury provides the best timing for surgery with a quicker return to preinjury level of play to about 16 weeks. The greater the delay to surgery, the wider the retraction of the proximal hamstring complex [289]. Surgical treatment of proximal hamstring tendon avulsions results in good clinical outcomes with early return to sports. Furthermore, surgical repair of partial and complete tears provides similar clinical outcomes but with higher complication with complete avulsions [290]. Return to play (RTP) is usually based on any of these three grading systems derived from the MRI findings. It includes the Modified Peetrons, Chan Grading, or the BAMIC Classification of hamstring injury [291], the Chan [292] or the BAMIC Classification [293] of hamstring injury. Wangensteen and colleagues did a prospective study of these different classification systems to assess their ability to predict time to return to sports. Their study concluded that these MRI classification systems cannot be used alone to predict return to sports after hamstring injuries. Instead, the specific MRI system must be specified to avoid misinterpretation when using it [294]. Eggleston and colleagues in their study among Australian Football Players reported a longer RTP in intramuscular injuries >5 cm of the longitudinal length of intramuscular disruption or 50% of intramuscular cross-sectional area based on MRI findings. Furthermore, the intramuscular injuries of the proximal long head of the biceps femoris with concomitant injuries of the biceps femoris/semitendinosus muscles had the longest RTP [295]. There are mixed results in the recoveries among athletes with hamstring injuries as shown in this study when using PRP treatment as compared to physical rehabilitation

alone [286] with one study saying that PRP with physical rehabilitation showing good growth factor concentration with early return to play to pre-injury level in 21 days for grade 2 hamstring tear than physical rehabilitation alone [296]. Reinjuries post-PRP, however, are common and are usually reported within the first 4 weeks and 100 days in 53% and 70% of cases, respectively, after return to play. Based on the MRI findings, the site for reinjuries is located where the initial injury happened [297]. It was reported that reinjuries remain high at 12–63% [280]. Exercise-based interventions decreased hamstring injury risk with no added benefits on load progression and frequencies in preventing further injury [298]. Flexibility and strength though remain an important clinical parameter during rehabilitation in ensuring a decrease in acute hamstring injuries as depicted by MRI scans. Moreover, flexibility testing by means of passive straight leg raise test instead of active knee extension test was independently associated with recovery times after hamstring injuries [299]. Also, medical staff like physicians and physiotherapists were consulted for deciding on the return to play (RTP), instead of the sports science staffs, coaches, and players as they are the gatekeepers of the RTP decision [300].

Knee

Anterior Cruciate Ligament

Sports injury involving the knee remains the most common injuries among athletes. In a 10-year study by Gage and colleagues assessing different knee impairments in the emergency room, about 50% of knee injuries are due to sporting or recreational activities with soft tissue injuries accounting for most cases [301]. Around 90% of those seeking medical help end up undergoing ACL reconstruction [302]. One of the most injured ligaments in the knee is the anterior cruciate ligament (ACL). It usually arises from the medial margin of the lateral femoral condyle. It is composed of two bundles which are the longer anteromedial bundle and a shorter posterolateral bundle, and each is functionally distinct. The anteromedial bundle is functionally taut on flexion and is the primary restraint to anterior tibial translation during flexion, while the posterolateral bundle is taut in extension and is restraint during anterior tibial translation in extension and it assists in rotatory control [303, 304]. These bundles originate from the medial aspect of the lateral femoral condyle within the intercondylar notch and course its way anteriorly to insert into the anterior aspect of the intercondylar eminence of the tibia [304]. With its distinct attachment, ACL can stabilize the knee in different angles. For instance, the anteromedial bundle stabilizes the knee when it is flexed to >30° knee flexion. But when the knee is in <30° flexion including knee extension, the posterolateral bundle of ACL assumes the role of stabilizing it. Interestingly, both bundles exhibit identical loads when the knee absorbs valgus stress and internal tibial torques while flexed to 15° (pivot shift test) [304]. Non-contact injuries involving the ACL happen when there is an anterior tibial translation coupled with either varus or valgus loading in a planted foot (pivot shift injuries) which usually occur in a soccer game due to abrupt changes in direction. This makes up most ACL injuries [305]. Whereas contact injuries affecting the ACL happen whereby a valgus force is applied on a partially flexed knee or in a hyperextended knee. This injury could simultaneously involve the medial meniscus and medial collateral ligament as it is bound together structurally [303]. ACL tears present with a large hemarthrosis in about 41–75% of acute knee injuries [306]. Among the tests used for evaluating ACL injuries, the following tests have better sensitivity – Lachman's, anterior drawers, and pivot shift tests [307]. For definite diagnostic purposes, MRI is still the imaging of choice [304]. Recently, a systematic review on the use of ultrasound was reported by Lee and Yun which showed that ultrasound is an excellent tool for diagnosing ACL with a sensitivity of 88% and a specificity of 96% provided it is performed by experienced musculoskeletal radiologists [308]. One caveat to note here is the presence of fats. The extent of ACL can be seen in patients with a low proportion of fat around the knee, adding that the femoral attachment of the ACL is only partially visualized [309] (Fig. 22.15). Anteriorly, the patient's knee is

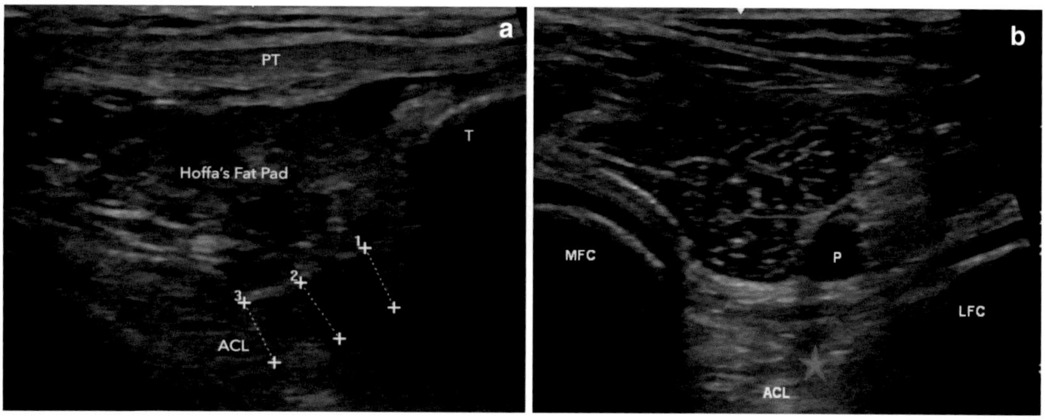

Fig. 22.15 (**a**) Ultrasound image of the anterior knee in 90° knee flexion showed the anterior cruciate ligament (ACL). Also shown are the patellar tendon (PT) and Hoffa's fat pad. (**b**) Ultrasound image of the posterior knee in short-axis view with medial femoral condyle (MFC) and lateral femoral condyle (LFC) as bony landmarks to locate for the anterior cruciate ligament seen at the lateral aspect (*) of the intercondylar notch. P popliteal artery

flexed to 90° and the probe (7–10 MHz) is positioned parallel to the tibia in the sagittal plane just below the inferior pole of the patella. The probe is moved to 30° counterclockwise so that the probe is parallel to the ACL fibers. Posteriorly, in a prone position, the probe is positioned in a posterior intercondylar view (transverse view with lateral and medial femoral in view) to assess the ACL attachment (Fig. 22.15). The normal appearance of ACL is a small oval-shaped, hypoechoic structure. A tear appears as a hypoechoic collection along the lateral wall of the femoral intercondylar notch (femoral notch sign), representing hematoma at the proximal attachment of the ACL, where most tears appear.

Furthermore, these findings were confirmed by MRI and arthroscopy. It is not clear when hematoma can resolve, but it can last for as long as 10 weeks post-injury [310]. Other indirect signs by ultrasound include PCL wave sign and capsular protrusion sign [311]. Moreover, to enhance better diagnosis, the patient must be scanned in prone, rather than in supine, position and must be compared to the contralateral knee all the time [308]. Mautner and colleagues found out that the PCL wave sign had the highest sensitivity at 84.9% and the femoral notch sign had the highest specificity at 93.8%, but a sensitivity of 56.6%. If 2 or 3 of the signs were positive, the sensitivity was at 86.8% and the specificity was at 87.5%. In addition, a thickened PCL compared to the normal side is considered a positive sign for ACL rupture. Partial midsubstance tears can be missed using this indirect sign [312]. Most ACL tears can be proximal at the femoral attachment (43%) or midsubstance (52%) of the ligament [314]. Surgical treatment is the preferred mode of treatment for young, active individuals and athletes with high physical demands and those patients who remain symptomatic after a trial of conservative treatments with physical rehabilitation [313]. A return to pre-injury sports after a unilateral ACL injury post-reconstruction procedure is about 53–83% and return to pivoting sports is about 83% [315, 316]. Return to pre-injury sports is about 40% in bilateral ACL post-reconstruction procedure. Interestingly, fear of reinjury was cited as the most common cause for failure to return to sport after the second reconstruction [315, 317], which is why it is important to make a psychological readiness assessment of athletes regarding treatment plans and physical rehabilitation process to prepare them for their return to sports activity [318, 319]. In another study, the rate of return to sports is 50% after a year post-reconstruction and about 67% 2 years after that, with rates of second ACL injury affecting younger athletes up to 35% [320]. This same study however showed that 23% of athletes passed the return-to-play test batteries which provided a 60% decrease in the risk of graft rupture but with a surprisingly 235% risk for contralateral ACL injury. Thus, it would be difficult to apply these data clinically [320]. In a recent review, an isokinetic strength protocol with concentric tests at 60°/s was found out to be the most reliable assessment method for return to sports [321]. In another study, return to sports in an ACL-deficient knee treated with conservative therapy consisting of quadriceps strengthening and dynamic stability training and not reconstructive surgery showed that 89% of them led an active sporting life with one-third of them returning to pivoting sports [322]. However, it is also observed that there is a high rate of OA-related changes in MRI among young adults during the first 1–5 years post-ACL reconstruction with two-thirds showing some joint deterioration. There is also an accelerated degenerative change observed among older and overweight patients especially affecting the patellofemoral cartilage [323]. In fact, ACL injury alone, regardless of age, was observed to increase the inflammatory markers which subsequently led to the development of osteoarthritis, and ACL reconstruction did not reverse this process. However, ACL reconstruction can improve knee kinematics and reduce secondary damages to the cartilage and meniscus [324]. Wellsandt and colleagues compared the existence of osteoarthritis between those treated operatively and those treated non-operatively under a progressive criterion-based rehabilitation 5 years after an ACL injury. Results showed that 5% of those treated non-operatively had tibiofemoral osteoarthritis in contrast to 23% of those treated operatively. These findings are not statistically significant [325]. Smith and colleagues showed similar results 10 years after an ACL injury was treated non-operatively versus operative treatment, although the post-ACL reconstruction knees have a higher likelihood of developing degenerative processes [326]. One study though reported a reduction of post-traumatic osteoarthritis following ACL reconstruction, for anatomic ACL reconstruction versus non-anatomic techniques. Anatomic ACL reconstruction is defined as AARSC (Anatomic ACL Reconstruction Scoring Checklist) score of ≥8 and is associated with a lower prevalence of OA in long-term follow-up [327]. Maximal medical improvement is no longer detectable 1 year after ACL reconstruction [328]. Several studies show that the use of PRP as a treatment for ligament healing did not show any significant effect [329, 330]. In fact, increasing PRP concentration negatively affected ligament strength and histological characteristics [329].

Posterior Cruciate Ligament

The posterior cruciate ligament is the largest intra-articular ligament. It originates from the medial femoral condyle within the intercondylar notch and inserts in between the two tibial plateau posterior to the tibial spine at the posterior intercondyloid fossa [331]. Posterior cruciate ligament injuries of the knee represent about 38–44% [332] of acute knee trauma with hemarthrosis with isolated tears representing about 1–5% [306, 333]. The most common mechanism of injury is a posteriorly directed force against the tibia or knee hyperflexion with a plantarflex foot, but without the "pop" that you commonly encounter in ACL injury. This is what commonly occurred in a "dashboard injury" where an individual seated on the front seat of a car in an accident had been hit by a dashboard with the proximal tibia absorbing the posteriorly directed force. In sports injury, it may occur when the athletes fall on the knee in a plantarflex foot [334]. With this given mechanism of injury, it can also involve other structures such as the posterolateral corner (PLC), of which 60% of PCL cases are found which includes the lateral collateral ligament and the medial collateral ligament following a high energy trauma or accident. The medial peripheral lesion is more common among biking and skiing accidents [335]. Other structures of the PLC that may be involved includes coronary ligament, popliteofibular ligament, popliteus tendon, and arcuate ligament [336]. The PCL usually prevents the posterior translation of the tibia while the PLC is the most important restraint in varus stress and is acting as a secondary restraint against posterior tibial translation on the lateral tibiofemoral compartment, but both are restraints to external rotation of the tibia [337, 338]. Both PCL and PLC restrain the knee in high flexion angles while PLC is the main restraint in low flexion angles [338]. Posterior cruciate ligament may also be injured because of multiligament injuries of the knee such as what occurred in an ACL type of injury with hyperextension or hyperflexion of the knee with a rotational component and varus/valgus stress [339]. Thus, combined injuries are more common than isolated PCL injuries [335] and sports is the most common cause for surgically treated PCL injuries except handball [340].

Physical examination for patient with suspected PCL injuries includes posterior drawer test. For isolated PCL injuries, posterior tibial translation will be decreased with internal tibial rotation due to the restraints exerted by the superficial medial collateral ligament and posterior oblique ligament. With the amount of posterior tibial translation during the posterior drawer test, a grading system is used for determining severity of PCL injuries. Grade I injuries are defined when the amount of posterior tibial translation is about 0–5 mm as compared to the contralateral knee. Grade III injuries are defined as those with more than 10 mm posterior tibial translation and grade II injuries are the ones in between. For complete PCL tear, a quadriceps active test can be used. Patient is placed in supine position while the knee is flexed to 90°. The patient is asked to contract the quadriceps isometrically while the examiner stabilizes the foot. In a complete PCL tear, the quadriceps contraction will reduce the posteriorly subluxed tibia [341]. Hematoma from the back of the knee confirms the presence of PCL tear [334]. A dimple sign in the medial knee is pathognomonic of a non-reducible knee dislocation [342].

MRI remains the gold standard for the diagnosis of a suspected PCL injury with 100% specificity and sensitivity but needs to be correlated with the history and physical examination especially in acute cases [334]. In chronic PCL cases, however, the sensitivity is only up to 62.5%. So, to increase diagnostic sensitivity in diagnosing chronic PCL tear, a 2.0 mm posteromedial tibial translation is performed to increase the sensitivity of MRI to 80% and the specificity to 89%. For revision cases, MRI has a sensitivity of 18.1%, but with 3.66 mm of posterior tibial translation (PTT) in the medial compartment, it shows a sensitivity of 92% and a specificity of 72% [343]. As mentioned previously, combined injuries are more common than isolated PCL injuries. In an isolated PCL injury, 25% shows an associated

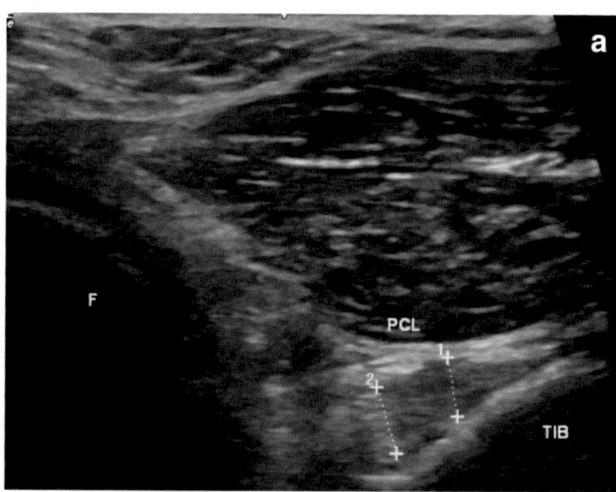

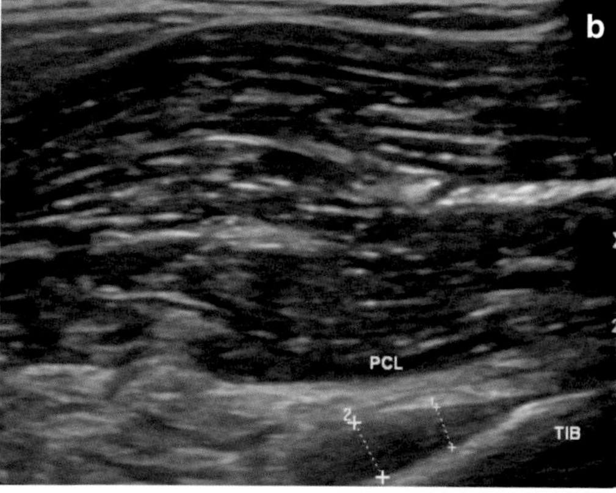

Fig. 22.16 (**a**, **b**) Sagittal ultrasound imaging over the posterior medial knee shows the anechoic structure of the posterior cruciate ligament (PCL) as it attaches at the posterior tibia. The posterior cruciate ligament is hypoechoic as a result of anisotropy. Thickness is usually <1 cm

meniscal injury. Usually, 69% of the isolated PCL injury may occur in the midsubstance with 27% occurring proximally and can be partial or complete tear [344]. Another modality for diagnosis is the use of ultrasound. A 2D ultrasound technique with sonoelastography introduced by Wang and colleagues hold promise in the diagnosis of PCL injuries. The transducer is placed longitudinally at the inferomedial aspect of the popliteal fossa at the posterior intercondylar area of the proximal tibia. The PCL attachment is measured 2 cm proximal to the tibial insertion (Fig. 22.16). A sprain is identified when there is a hypoechoic swelling as compared to the contralateral knee. A partial tear is defined as a hypoechoic gap with preserved partial continuity and a complete disruption is defined as a complete discontinuity of the ligament. It was reported in that study that a minimum thickness of PCL to ≥6.5 mm yielded a sensitivity of 90.6% and a specificity of 86.7% in the diagnosis of PCL strain injury. Thus, hypoechoic swelling (increased thickness) and softening (by elastography) are compatible with PCL injury and can be used as a screening tool for diagnosis [309, 345]. A torn PCL appears in ultrasound as heterogeneously hypoechoic with an indistinct and wavy posterior margin [309] or a focal disruption of the ligament [346]. Lee and Yun in their study reported that knee ultrasound in the diagnosis of PCL has a sensitivity and specificity of 99% provided the examiner performs side to side comparison of the images, and dynamic ultrasound is performed by a competent and experienced musculoskeletal radiologist [308] (Fig. 22.16). Ultrasound can image the PCL using a posterior longitudinal approach to the knee. A ruptured PCL in ultrasound is characterized by an interruptions close to its insertion into the intercondylar fossa [347]. Dynamic ultrasound stress test was also shown to have a sensitivity of 83% and a specificity of 100% for injury of the lateral collateral ligament and posterolateral corner structures and thus can predict the need for surgery in 100% of patients who required posterolateral repair or reconstruction [348].

The initial approach in the management of PCL injuries is by determining whether it is an acute or chronic injury. An acute and isolated but uncommon PCL tear can be managed by conservative treatment, while a chronic PCL tear with knee instability will usually require surgical intervention [334]. An acute PCL tear has good intrinsic healing capability when treated conservatively, although it heals in an elongated and attenuated condition with 62–75% of cases showing good continuity by MRI findings [349–351]. The MRI is evaluated between 2 months and 17 months after a PCL injury showing good continuity [350, 351]. However, another study suggests surgery for those with grade II or grade III PCL injuries [352]. Under usual clinical conditions, it is reported that more than 50% of PCL is seen by clinicians after more than a year of injury [343]. If it is part of the multi-ligament injuries, prompt treatment and management are very important [334]. Conservative treatment may for a time provide certain relief, but there is a high rate of arthrosis in the medial and patellofemoral compartments due to altered kinematics and loads. These arthritic findings can also be used to determine the chronicity of the knee injury. Recent findings showed that avoiding posterior tibial translation forms part of the conservative management of patients with PCL injury to optimize ligament healing. It includes also strengthening of the quadriceps and core musculature with a progressive range of motion exercises. At 12 weeks, interval training may commence followed by agility work and sports-specific exercises to prepare athletes for return to sports. This protocol has a high rate of return to sport [341]. Chronic PCL injuries with less than 8 mm posterior tibial subluxation have the potential to heal with ligament fiber restoration as shown in MRI findings [353]. For proximal or distal avulsion type PCL tears, it is recommended that arthroscopic primary repair may be performed in which the ligament can be reattached to its original insertions and origins. The advantage of this procedure is faster rehabilitation and preservation of the native tissue with a return to their pre-injury competitive level and with a full range of motion [354]. There is no evidence that PRP works for PCL injuries [329].

Lateral (Fibular) Collateral Ligament Injury

A blow to the medial side of the knee or hyperextension stress across the knee in non-contact injury can injure the lateral collateral ligament (LCL). Sports like gymnastics and tennis contribute to the increased incidence of lateral knee trauma. In a study of more than 200,000 knee injuries from different sporting events, isolated LCL pathology is represented by <2% [355]. As a primary varus stabilizer of the knee, failure to recognize its pathology in a multiligamentous trauma can result in instability and unsatisfactory outcome after a cruciate ligament reconstruction [356]. The lateral collateral ligament also acts as a secondary restraint to external rotation together with the popliteofibular ligament (PFL). The LCL, PFL, arcuate ligament, and fabellofibular ligament are the static stabilizers of the posterolateral corner (PLC), and together, they resist posterior displacement of the tibia, varus instability, and external tibial rotation [357, 358]. Furthermore, it also provides stability to the PLC of the knee, together with the popliteus muscle-tendon unit and the PFL [359]. An angle of 30° knee flexion is observed to have the highest degree of varus laxity and thus is important in the clinical assessment of LCL laxity [360]. As the knee is further flexed, the control of the LCL on the knee is increasingly less and, therefore, the LCL is loaded at the early range of the knee flexion [356]. Varus laxity in an extended knee can otherwise provide clues to an associated injury of either or both cruciate ligaments [361]. Claes and colleagues [362] proposed a term called lateral collateral ligament complex (LLC) to include LCL and anterolateral ligament (ALL) which is commonly observed to be specific in Brazilian jiu-jitsu (BJJ) injuries occurring in about 25.9% of athletes [363]. The mechanism of injury in BJJ is described as a varus injury on a flexed knee with varying degrees of external rotation [364]. Care should also be noted in patients with LCL injury presenting with radiographic signs of avulsion injury of the fibular head otherwise referred to as arcuate sign or arcuate fracture. This could point to the possibility of posterolateral corner injury. Undiagnosed PLC injury could give rise to recurrent instability, failed anterior cruciate ligament reconstruction, and early onset of osteoarthritis [365]. Shekari and colleagues have found an association between LCL injuries and ALL injuries [366].

The assessment of varus laxity regarding the LCL knee injury is done with the knee at 30° flexion. A varus opening of ≤5 mm indicates a low-grade injury and >10 mm a high-grade injury. Anything in between is a moderate grade varus injury. Athletes with high-grade injuries should be assessed further for possible multiligamentous injuries [356]. Warren has noted an

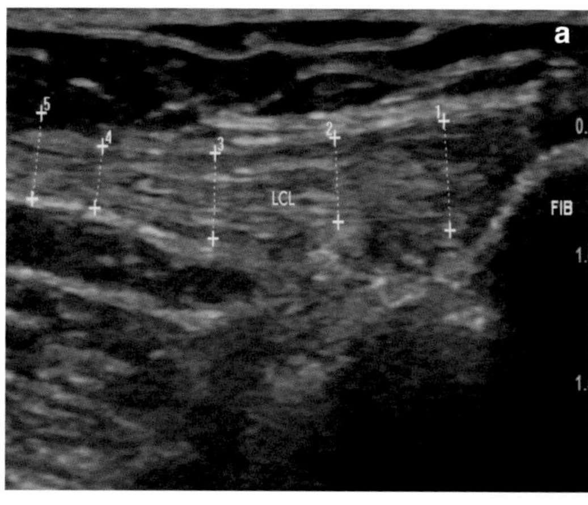

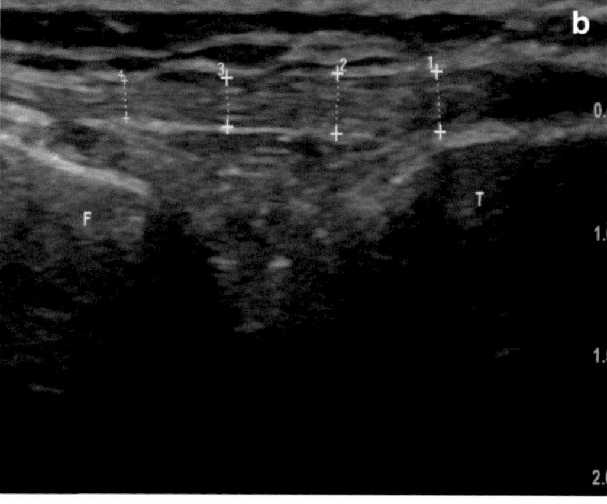

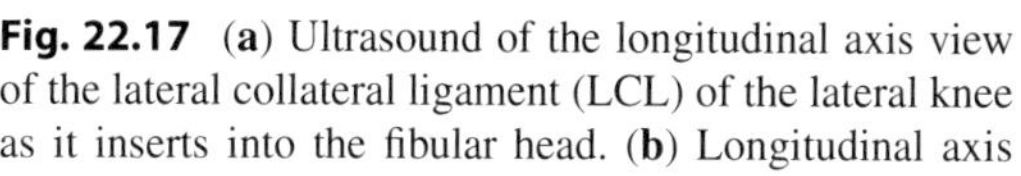

Fig. 22.17 (**a**) Ultrasound of the longitudinal axis view of the lateral collateral ligament (LCL) of the lateral knee as it inserts into the fibular head. (**b**) Longitudinal axis view of the iliotibial band as it inserts into the Gerdy's tubercle of the tibia. Fib fibula, F femur, T tibia

increase in varus opening to about 5–9° for combined LCL-popliteus injury which was confirmed arthroscopically to an opening of 9–10 mm [367]. MRI remains the imaging of choice for LCL injury with a sensitivity of about 58% [368]. Grade I is the least severe characterized by subcutaneous fluid around the midsubstance or in any of the insertions. Grade II indicates partial tears in the LCL in any part of the ligament with associated edema formation. Grade III is a complete tear of the LCL with edema formation [369]. Ultrasound of the lateral knee is a useful modality for both static and dynamic imaging (Fig. 22.17a). Sekiya and colleagues reported that static ultrasound of the LCL has a sensitivity of about 92%, specificity of 75%, and accuracy of 88%; popliteus has a sensitivity of 33%, specificity of 100%, and an accuracy of 50%; and popliteofibular ligament has a sensitivity of 67%, specificity of 75%, and an accuracy of 69%. Dynamic ultrasound stress imaging is used to measure the lateral joint space width which is normally <10.5 mm. The need for posterolateral corner surgery is based on a value >10.5 mm. This dynamic stress testing has a sensitivity of 83% and a specificity of 100% for injuries of the LCL and PLC. This has a positive predictive value of 100%, a negative predictive value of 75%, and an accuracy of 88% [348]. Anterolateral ligament (ALL) is found in 97% of cadaveric studies [362] such that it shares a common origin with LCL of the lateral femoral condyle and then runs deep and oblique to the ITB and finally inserts 2 cm posterior to the ITB insertions. By flexing the knee to 90 degrees, a better view of ALL is visible by ultrasound [370].

Conservative treatments for LCL injuries are reserved for grade I or II injuries. Surgical repair and interventions are done for grade III midsubstance tears and in chronic lateral instability due to LCL injury [371]. The same holds true for PLC injuries where grades I and II are treated conservatively with good responses to treatment. High suspicion of PLC injuries must be made in the presence of arcuate fractures involving the fibular head and such condition is best diagnosed by MRI and treated during the first 3 weeks post-injury with improved outcomes [365]. Thus, PLC grade III injuries have good outcomes with surgical intervention. Semitendinosus graft for grade III LCL injuries is reported to have good subjective and objective results [356]. There are limited studies regarding the use of PRP in ligament injuries. No evidence of its effects on healing was observed on ligaments [372] except in decreasing pain in both the short and long terms [373].

Medial Knee Ligaments

Medial collateral ligament (MCL) injuries result from a valgus force from a direct force to the lateral knee in a planted foot associated with sudden pain and a popping sound [374] usually seen in sports like hockey, football, and skiing. About 43% to 52% accounts for this injury which is considered the most injured ligament of the knee occurring more among contact than non-contact sports activities [375]. The medial knee is made up of static and dynamic structural stabilizers. Among the static stabilizers, it includes the superficial and deep MCL or medial capsular ligament and posterior oblique ligament. The dynamic medial knee stabilizers include the musculotendinous unit of semimembranosus, quadriceps, and pes anserinus [376]. There are three layers of the MCL, namely the superficial sartorial fascia layer, the middle superficial MCL with the posterior oblique ligament (POL), and the deep MCL with the knee capsule [377]. A bursa exists between the middle superficial and deep MCL which is not seen unless there is a fluid collection in between [378]. Although rare, medial knee pain can be due to MCL bursitis due to the osteophytes of knee OA [379]. The superficial MCL originates from the medial femoral condyle and inserts underneath the pes anserine 4–5 cm from the medial joint line. Its anterior fibers are taut in flexion and lax in full extension (Fig. 22.18). The deep portion of the MCL is made of different confluence of ligaments namely the meniscofemoral, meniscocapsular, and meniscotibial. Posterior to the MCL is the posteromedial corner (PMC) called posterior oblique ligament (POL), which is a condensation of the capsule, together with semimembranosus and medial meniscus. This complex is tight in extension [376]. As a primary restraint to valgus stress,

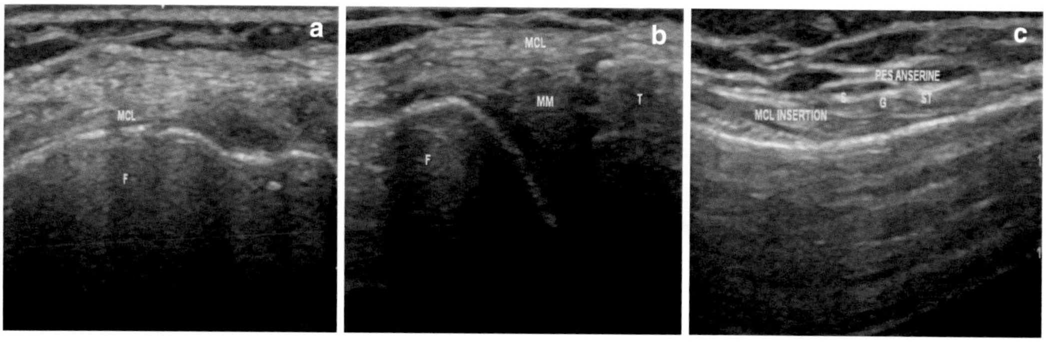

Fig. 22.18 (**a**) Ultrasound image of the longitudinal view of the medial collateral ligament (MCL) as it inserts from the femoral condyle (F). (**b**) Ultrasound image of the medial collateral ligament (MCL) in relation to the medial meniscus (MM), where the inner fiber of the medial collateral ligament (MCL) is attached to the medial meniscus (MM) and the superficial layer is free. (**c**) Ultrasound image of the distal insertion of the medial collateral ligament (MCL) in longitudinal view deep to the pes anserine structures made up of sartorius (S), gracilis (G), and semitendinosus (ST) in the tibia (T)

MCL exerts 78% of resistance at 25° knee flexion. In full extension, the PMC with ACL contributes to valgus stress with MCL still restraining 57% of the force. Thus, valgus laxity in flexion is highlighted with an isolated MCL injury but with an additional laxity in knee extension when PMC and ACL are injured. Moreover, in full extension, the greatest strain is at the posterior part of the MCL, while strain at the anterior fibers is constant in all flexion angles [380]. Recently, the study of Kramer and colleagues confirmed prior research by Gardiner regarding injuries affecting the proximal portion of the MCL in its posterior origin when the knee is in full extension among pediatric and adolescent athletes [381]. Moreover, Wierer and colleagues reported that the superficial MCL capsuloligamentous structure is the most important restraint in anteromedial instability with the deep MCL and POL playing minor roles. Thus, the superficial MCL is the key medial restraint to valgus rotation, anteromedial translation, and external tibial torsion [382].

The mechanism of injury is either a direct blow to the lateral knee on a planted foot or pivoting activity that produces a valgus moment in the knee [377]. Although most athletes are injured by direct contact, they will typically complain of pain with weight-bearing characterized by wobbling gait and instability due to pain. Local swelling is usually seen at the femoral origin (most common) of the MCL. The presence of an effusion is a warning sign of an intraarticular injury [383]. Three different grading systems are used for MCL injuries based on MRI findings and clinical findings. Grade I injury refers to an intact fiber with surrounding edema, grade II injury shows partial disruption, and grade III injury shows complete fiber disruption and avulsion [384]. Stress testing of the MCL is done with the knee in 0-30 degrees flexion while applying valgus force at the medial joint line. The grading is based on AMA and is as follows: grade I, 0–5 mm opening with painful/firm endpoint, grade III, with >10 mm opening with soft or absent endpoint, and grade II, in between with firm endpoint [385]. Although rare, distal superficial MCL lesion could occur and appear in the MRI as a "wavy" lesion, described as fibers with a serpentine morphology. Also, when the proximal stump of the superficial MCL is located superficial to the pes anserine and sartorius fascia, it is referred to as Stener-like lesion (SLL). Further, a distal lesion of the superficial MCL is characterized as an injury inferior to the medial joint line [386]. This type of lesion is always accompanied by other structural injuries. Boutin and colleagues reported a concomitant tear of ACL at 82%, PCL tear of 22%, deep MCL tear of 61%, and lateral compartment osseous injury of 94% with or without SLL-associated findings [387]. Injury of the PMC and oblique popliteal ligament gave rise to pain, functional genu recurvatum instability, and failed ACL reconstruction [388]. Ultrasound of the MCL of the knee is an acceptable modality in showing the anatomical detail of the superficial structures of the knee which may be difficult when using other diagnostic modalities. Skill and experience though define the best results for diagnosing an MCL injury [388].

An isolated MCL injury, whether sprains or tears (grades I and II), is treated conservatively with good functional outcomes. However, when a grade III or complete MCL injury with concomitant major ligament tears is diagnosed, surgical intervention is always indicated. Moreover, the rare distal superficial MCL injury at or near the distal tibial attachment is always an indication for surgery because of poor anatomic ligament healing and chronic valgus instability with any conservative interventions [387].

The use of platelet-rich growth factors in MCL injuries is beneficial for early return to athletic activities as shown in one study [389]. Three case studies were reported showing recovery of the damaged MCL, indicating that PRP hastened the healing process of ruptured ligaments of both superficial and deep layers of the MCL [390].

Iliotibial Band Injuries

The iliotibial band (ITB) is a vital structure in the knee that provides restraint in internal rotation together with the anterolateral ligament. The distal insertion of the ITB at the Gerdy's tubercle of the proximal tibia (Fig. 22.17b) may appear simple at first, except for the fact that the cadaveric study of Godin and colleagues provides us a complex and comprehensive understanding of how it is attached both at the distal femur and proximal tibia. Two separate bundles at the distal femur were identified referred to as Kaplan fibers. The proximal deep bundle (proximal Kaplan fibers) arises from the undersurface of the ITB and attach to the proximal ridge of the proximal femoral diaphysis, 53.6 mm proximal to the lateral epicondyle, while the distal deep bundle (distal Kaplan fibers) goes from lateral to distal and then medial and inserts at the supracondylar flare of the distal femur 31.4 mm proximal to the lateral epicondyle. The superficial lateral geniculate artery can serve as the reference as it is found just distal to the distal Kaplan fibers with the capsulo-osseous layer of the ITB attached proximally to the lateral gastrocnemius tubercle [391]. Capsulo-osseous layer is also sometimes referred to as the ALL and other different names were made to refer to it like short lateral ligament, mid-third lateral capsular ligament, and lateral capsular ligament [392]. Recently, Landreau and colleagues [392] identified another distinct structure after doing a cadaver dissection via a posterior approach, but a previous study by Terry and colleagues used anterior approach [393]. This structure was identified as "condylar strap" of the ITB, and this is attached to the deep ITB and the femoral epicondylar area, which plays a role in anterolateral knee rotatory stability [392]. The Kaplan fibers earlier described by Godin and colleagues [391] could very much be seen in a routine MRI scan in an ACL-intact knee. With its important role as a secondary stabilizer in the ACL-deficient knee, its identification plays an important role in the non-pathologic state. Moreover, it is suggested that the best plane to identify the Kaplan fibers in both normal and pathologic states is in the sagittal plane with the coronal plane being the worst. The identification of the superior geniculate artery, lateral gastrocnemius origin, and lateral joint line has a good correlation with cadaver studies and thus are appropriate references for MRI identification of such structures [394]. In a related study, Batty and colleagues reported a rate of 23.7% in diagnosing Kaplan injuries by MRI when done before 90 days as compared to the 6.4% rate when performed after 90 days. Moreover, there is an increase in associated injury by radiological findings involving lateral meniscal injury, posteromedial tibial bone marrow edema, and injury to the lateral and medial collateral ligament in a Kaplan fiber injury. Due to its role in providing anterolateral rotatory knee stability, its injury implies a high energy level of injury to the lateral knee. It is, however, reported that only about 18.6% of patients with an ACL injury show injuries involving the Kaplan fibers [395]. Herbst and colleagues, however, noted that the rotatory knee stability is provided by the anterolateral complex of the knee which is composed of the three Seebacher layers and capsule-osseous layer of the ITB and the anterolateral joint capsule (ALC) [396]. Getgood and colleagues with the ALC Consensus Group Meeting included the anterolateral ligament (ALL) as part of the ALC [397].

Iliotibial band syndrome (ITBS) is an inflammation of the distal part of the ITB and is second only to patellofemoral pain as the most common chronic pathologies of the knee among runners, with females twice as much as males being affected. Aside from runners, it also affects cyclists and field hockey, basketball, and soccer players [398]. Sinclair and colleagues have reported that the peak ITB strain and strain velocity alongside the impingement duration are highest during the run and cut movements compared to the hop and that the medial and off the shelf orthosis attenuates the mechanism linked to the cause among female runners [398].

Ultrasound of the knee provides excellent visualization of the structures of the knee including ITB. Under normal conditions, it appears as a linear fibrillar structure from the lateral femoral condyle to the Gerdy's tubercle of the tibia. A dynamic imaging technique can be done over the femoral condyle during flexion and extension of the knee to detect any snapping [399]. Iliotibial band syndrome in ultrasound shows soft tissue edematous swelling, discrete fluid collection between the iliotibial bands, and lateral femoral condyle suggestive of adventitial bursitis with thickening of the iliotibial band at the Gerdy's tubercle as an inconsistent finding [399]. Sometimes, cortical irregularity may be seen at the lateral femoral condyle. Note the presence of the fluid effusion at the lateral recess of the suprapatellar bursa which may be confused for the fluid deep to the ITB [399]. It is possible that the fluid collection deep to the ITB can be due to fat pad compression and not to the actual ITB itself during running [400]. The use of PRP in the treatment of the iliotibial band has not been studied lengthily, although ultrasound-guided injection of related structures including the iliotibial band shows an effect with a return to dancing within 6 months of therapy [401].

Patellar Tendon Sports Injuries

Patellar tendinopathy otherwise referred to as "jumper's knee" is an overuse injury of the patella associated with sports such as running, jumping, and kicking due to its repetitive and explosive activities. It is found in 55% of male basketball players. The pathology in the tendon is usually characterized by microinjury to the tendon fibers, local mucoid degeneration, necrosis, and loss of transitional fibrocartilaginous tissue at its insertion site to the bone but often with no sign of inflammation [402]. This problem could take a toll on the athlete's performance, especially with continuous sports activity, and develop into partial patellar tendon tears (PPTT). This can eventually lead to prolonging recovery time, reduced performance, and increased time off from sports and with a foreseeable unnecessary retirement from their sports. Golman and colleagues reported that PPTT usually occurred at the posterior and posteromedial portion of the patellar tendon in 91% of cases which could be explained by its poor vascularity in that region [402]. The cadaveric findings of Pang and colleagues have reported that the anterior patella is supplied by three blood vessels namely inferolateral geniculate, anterior tibial recurrent, and inferomedial geniculate while the posterior patellar tendon receives its blood supply from the smaller arteries of the retropatellar anastomotic arch in the Hoffa's fat pad [403]. In fact, the collagen content and turnover of the entire patella are the same in all its length, although the glycosaminoglycans (GAG) content is higher in the insertion and distal regions [404]. The patellar tendon thickness as measured by axial MRI scans of >8.8 mm has a high correlation of tear of the patellar tendon. In fact, athletes with >11.5 mm thickness or >50% tear thickness were less likely to improve with conservative interventions [402]. On the other hand, patellar tendinopathy may be either symptomatic or asymptomatic. These observations are important in predicting which

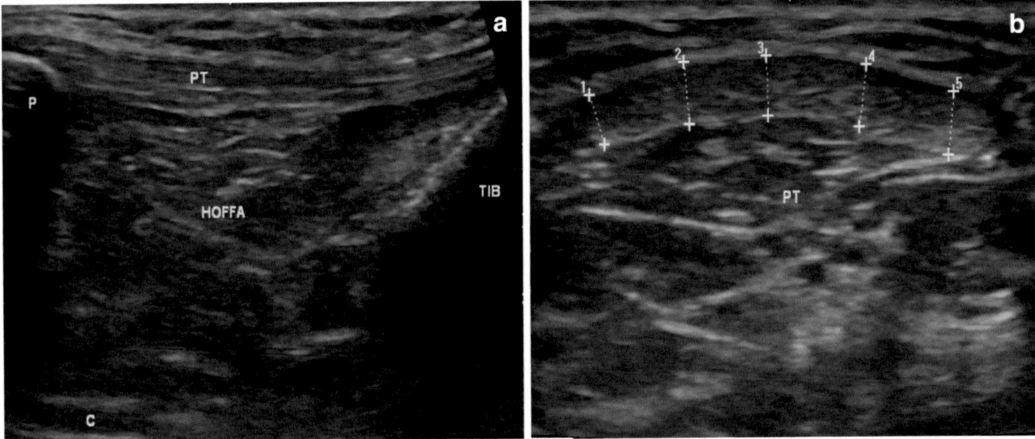

Fig. 22.19 (**a**) Ultrasound image of the longitudinal axis view of the fibrillar pattern of the patellar tendon (PT) from its attachment in the patella (P) and inserts distally at the tibia (TIB). Deep to the patellar tendon is the Hoffa's fat pad and the hypoechoic hyaline cartilage (C). (**b**) Short-axis view of the proximal portion of the patellar tendon (PT) where most of the pathology can be seen

athletes are at risk for tendon pain, which is found in 45% in volleyball and 32% in basketball players [405]. Ultrasound imaging is a useful tool in determining which athletes will develop tendon pain or not in asymptomatic athletes. For instance, if an asymptomatic athlete does not show evidence of structural changes such as thickening, hypoechogenicity, and neovascularization, asymptomatic athletes are at low risk for developing any patellar tendon pain. In fact, an athlete can continue competitive sports activity even up to 3 years without any problem. Of those ultrasound characteristics providing the highest association to pain, neovascularization followed by hypoechogenicity emerges as consistent findings [26] (Fig. 22.19).

Platelet-rich plasma therapy reported good results for patellar tendinopathies by Di Matteo and colleagues in a systematic review, although there are limited studies available to recommend its use for such patients. It is therefore recommended as a second line of treatment when other conservative measures fail [406]. Le and colleagues recommend the use of LR-PRP for patellar tendinopathy showing good results in 6-month and 12-month follow-up [407].

Meniscal Injuries

Meniscal injuries are common among athletes and are usually caused by a combination of axial loading and rotational forces that is translated on the meniscus. It could be injured in isolation or in a combination of other related structures such as the ligaments and articular cartilages. One of the symptoms felt by an injured athlete is characterized by pain, swelling, and a peculiar locking, buckling, and catching sensation [408]. Medial meniscal tears are more common than lateral tears with males more commonly affected than females with a ratio of 2:1–4:1 [409]. Moreover, meniscal root tears were reported to occur in association with multi-ligament knee injuries (less than 2%) because of compressive forces, with valgus injury patterns seen associated with lateral root tears and varus injury patterns seen in medial root tears. Meniscal root injuries are associated with rapid extrusion of the meniscus and rapid deterioration of the articular cartilage which when left untreated leads to poor function and subsequent surgery [410].

In a recent study by Vaishya and colleagues, elite athletes of Indian and Brazilian origin showed that a quarter of them undergo surgery such as partial arthroscopic meniscectomies with lateral meniscectomy showing poorer prognosis

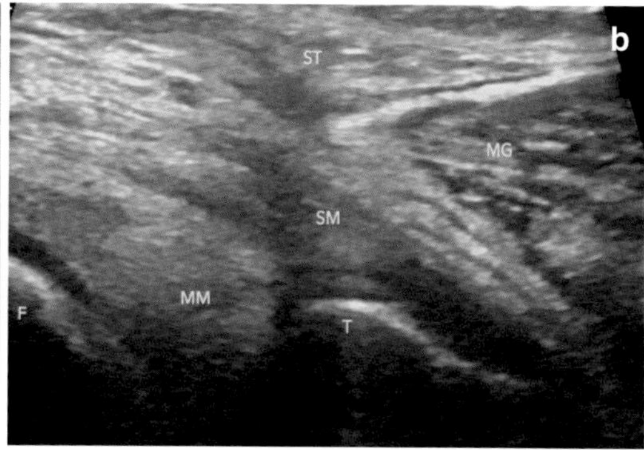

Fig. 22.20 (**a**) Ultrasound image of a 51-year-old male complaining of medial knee pain showed a bulging medial meniscus (MM) deep to the medial collateral ligament (MCL). (**b**) Ultrasound image of a 52-year-old female complaining of a posterior knee pain showing a bulging and degenerated medial meniscus (MM) deep to the semimembranosus tendon (SM). Also seen are the medial gastrocnemius (MG) muscle and semitendinosus (ST) tendon. F femur, T tibia

than the medial side. The poor prognosis is associated with a return to the previous level of play, longer recovery, more problems post-surgery, and a need for further arthroscopy [411]. In addition, a peculiar observation is seen among side midfielders showing the shortest recovery period with the goalkeepers showing the longest recovery period reflecting the dynamic activity assigned to these players. Football has the highest knee injury during the summer Olympics while Alpine skiing showed the greatest knee injuries during winter [411]. MRI remained as the imaging of choice for meniscal tears. It has a sensitivity and specificity of 93% and 88% for medial meniscal tears and 79% and 95% for lateral tears, respectively. The low sensitivity of lateral meniscal tears can however be complemented by a confirmatory arthroscopic finding [408]. Similarly, ultrasound as a diagnostic tool (Fig. 22.20) was sensitive and specific and comparable to MRI in diagnosing meniscal injuries as reported by Xia and colleagues, and its use for routine examination of meniscal injuries of the knee is recommended [412]. Although MRI remains to be the imaging of choice for meniscal knee injuries, ultrasound can be used to diagnose meniscal injuries in acute knee injuries as confirmed by an arthroscopuc examination in acute knees [413]. Of special note, however, is the ability of rigorous physical examination by experienced clinicians using tests such as Thessaly's, McMurray's, and Apley's to make a correct diagnosis of meniscal injuries equal or even better than MRI [414].

Up until the present, arthroscopic partial meniscectomy (APM) remains very popular among orthopedic surgeons for the treatment of meniscal injuries. However, recent studies reported that meniscal repair is a more viable and more effective alternative for such conditions. This procedure aims to achieve meniscal healing while avoiding the early onset of degenerative change of partial meniscectomy, especially among young and active athletes. Moreover, this procedure does not come without a long-term failure rate of less than 10% at a 2-year follow-up and a long-term failure rate (5 years) of 30%. Thus, there is a need to look for other alternative procedures such as meniscal allografting which shows an 89.2% 10-year follow-up survival rate [415]. The technique of meniscal allograft transplantation is becoming the standard of care for total meniscal insufficiency. Further, artificial scaffold-based meniscal substitution although still evolving for the treatment of irreparable partial meniscal injuries is becoming a feasible procedure in improving outcomes, especially for patients with post-meniscectomy syndrome. This progress in treatment is due to more comprehensive tissue engineering [416]. A recent systematic review by

Belk and colleagues reported that an additional PRP treatment after meniscal repair did not show any difference in outcomes at midterm follow-up [417].

Ankle and Lower Leg

Ankle and lower leg injuries remain one of the most common sites of sports injuries. In a recent study by Lucasti and colleagues among professional baseball players, covering 2011–2016, the most common injuries included leg contusions, anterior talofibular ligament sprains, unspecified ankle sprains, ankle contusions, and gastrocnemius strains. A review of the epidemiological data showed that ligamentous sprains (37%) followed by muscle strains (13%), bone problems (6%), and tendon injuries (6%) were noted [418]. Of this, the ankle lateral collateral ligament (LCL) complex takes precedence as one of the most injured areas in the ankle. This complex includes anterior talofibular ligament (ATFL), calcaneofibular ligament (CFL), posterior talofibular ligament (PTFL), and anterior tibiofibular ligament (injured in high ankle sprain) [419].

Ankle Inversion Sprain

Ankle sprain used to be the most common injury among athletes [420]. In the past, 10–36% of professional football players have suffered from ankle sprain [421]. However, with an improved preventive rehabilitation strategies and stricter games rules, the incidence rate decreased to 10–15% [422]. It has now become the fourth most common injury in sports. In one study, half of those with acute injuries may lead to chronic ankle sprain in their lifetime. Most often, an inversion ankle injury may affect the lateral ankle ligament (ATF ligament), with 30% to 40% progressing into chronic ankle injury because of non-healing. Recent findings point to the injury of the intra-articular superior fascicle of the anterior talofibular ligament which is commonly affected during an inversion ankle injury (Fig. 22.21). The intra-articular location of the superior fascicle could be the reason for its impaired healing [423]. The inferior fascicle of the ATFL is attached to the calcaneofibular ligament (CFL) through the arciform fibers. Together, they form what is referred to as the lateral fibulotalocalcaneal ligament (LFTCL) complex, which is present in 100% of cases studied by Vega and colleagues. Moreover, the inferior fascicle of the ATFL and the anterior border of the CFL are attached to the subtalar joint capsule [424]. Injury to the superior fascicle of ATFL leads to ankle microinstability and is a subtle form of a lateral

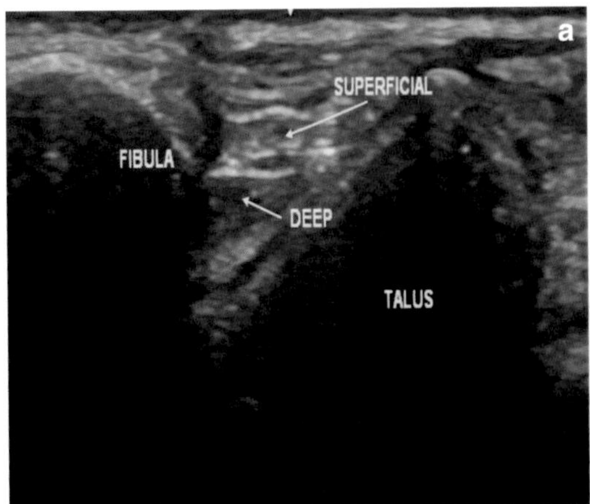

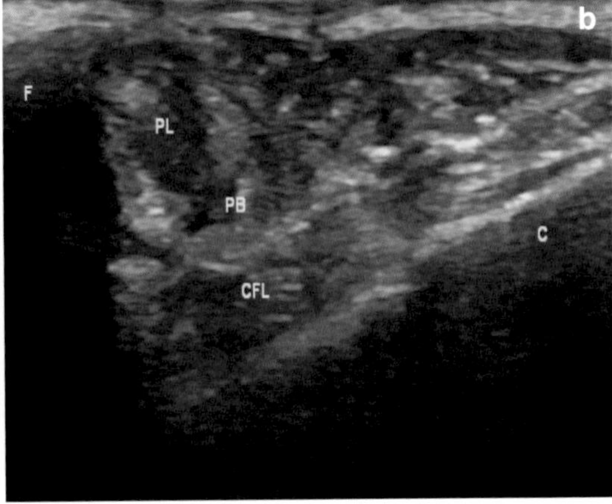

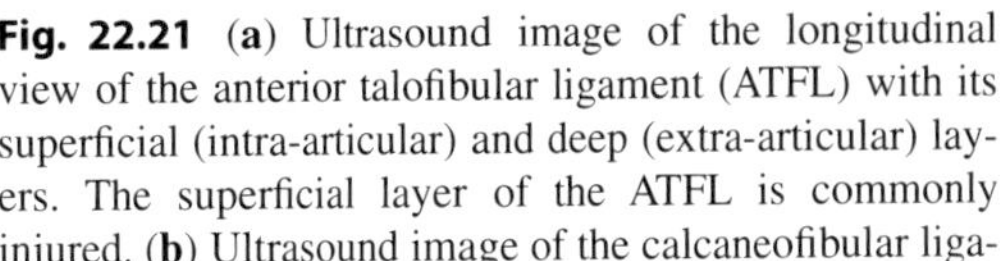

Fig. 22.21 (**a**) Ultrasound image of the longitudinal view of the anterior talofibular ligament (ATFL) with its superficial (intra-articular) and deep (extra-articular) layers. The superficial layer of the ATFL is commonly injured. (**b**) Ultrasound image of the calcaneofibular ligament (CFL) deep to the peroneus longus (PL) and peroneus brevis (PB) tendons. Typically, the deep layers of ATFL are attached to the anterior border of the CFL through the arciform fibers which form a complex referred to as lateral fibulotalocalcaneal ligament (LFTCL)

ankle injury. The LFTCL complex is an extra-articular structure and as such can heal when injured. This is the main lateral ankle joint stabilizer and is an isometric structure. Injury to this ligament complex could lead to classical lateral ankle instability [423]. Injury to the inferior and superior ATFL however will result in chronic ankle instability [424]. Presently, no studies can confirm whether an intra-articular lateral ankle injury or its hidden pathology could be the reason for its instability and chronic involvement. Other residual symptoms include chronic pain and muscular weakness. A study has shown that previous history of ankle sprains increases the chance of incurring a recurrent ankle sprain up to 2 to 5 times compared to those with no history of ankle injury regardless of the severity [420].

In a typical ankle inversion sprain, the superior fascicle of ATFL being the weakest absorbed the initial brunt of the injury and became the first to be affected (Fig. 22.21). With an additional force during an ankle inversion injury, the inferior fascicle together with the CFL is impaired. Finally, an added and continuous force will eventually damage the posterior talofibular (PTFL) ligament that could possibly lead to lateral ankle dislocation [424].

MRI remains the modality of choice for diagnosing ligamental injuries with a sensitivity of 92–100% and a specificity of 100% for ATFL injuries. In comparison with arthroscopy, however, MRI can correctly identify the injured part of the ATFL in 93% of cases in contrast to ultrasound at 63% [420]. In a meta-analysis reported by Seok and colleagues, the diagnostic capability of ultrasound has a sensitivity of 99% and a specificity of 92% for ATFL injuries. It has a sensitivity and specificity of 95% and 99%, respectively, for CFL injuries. In subgroup analysis, ultrasound has a sensitivity and specificity of 95% and 82% for complete ATFL tears and a sensitivity and specificity of 90% and 82% for partial ATFL tears, respectively, and thus is recommended as the first line of diagnostic modality replacing stress radiography [419]. This data was concurred by the systematic review studies on ultrasound of the ankle done by Lee and colleagues, which are recently published in 2020 [425]. Surgery and arthroscopy are said to be the highest quality standard of reference. Chen and colleagues have shown that ultrasound has a 93.8% sensitivity and 90.9% specificity for chronic lateral injuries involving CFL with intraoperative surgical findings as the standard of reference [426].

The initial focus of treatment and rehabilitation with ankle sprain includes reducing pain while at the same time effort should be made to restore the range of motion and strength of the patient. Persistent pain and instability even in the absence of fracture may be an indication for surgery. The use of orthobiologics however showed promise in this case, although no large-scale studies have been reported. There are reported cases of a faster return to play and greater functional improvement with platelet-rich plasma injections, especially in high ankle sprains [427]. However, for a lateral ankle sprain, there is no significant difference in effect using an LR-PRP for acute ankle injury [407].

Return to play for a lateral ankle injury is a more challenging task with several variables to be considered in the process. These variables include clinical, functional, sport-specific, psychosocial, and decision-modifying. In a recent study, it was advised not to include a time-contingent approach as each variable can change as the patient moves to its return to sports processes [428].

High Ankle Sprain

High ankle sprain or otherwise called syndesmotic sprains are not as common as ankle inversion sprains but is three to four times more severe than lateral ankle sprains. It is usually seen in men's football, ice hockey, and wrestling. It usually affects the syndesmosis of the distal tibiofibular joint causing significant chronic pain and ankle instability. A recent systematic review reported by Prakash showed that sporting population especially during the second or third decade of life are more prone to this injury with the highest risk during the competition [429]. Traumas involving this joint may injure the anterior inferior tibiofibular ligament (AITFL), posterior inferior tibiofibular ligament (PITFL), and

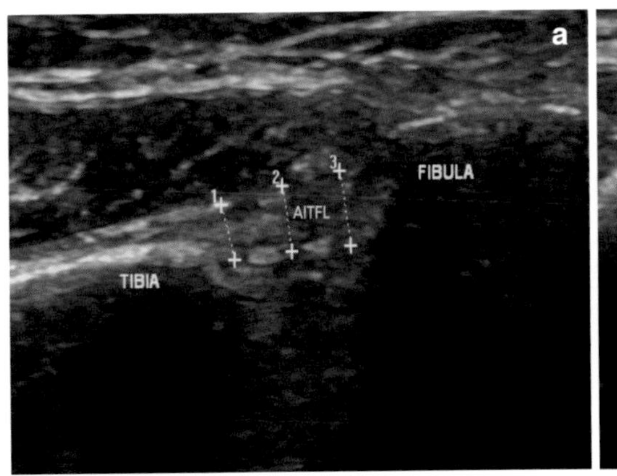

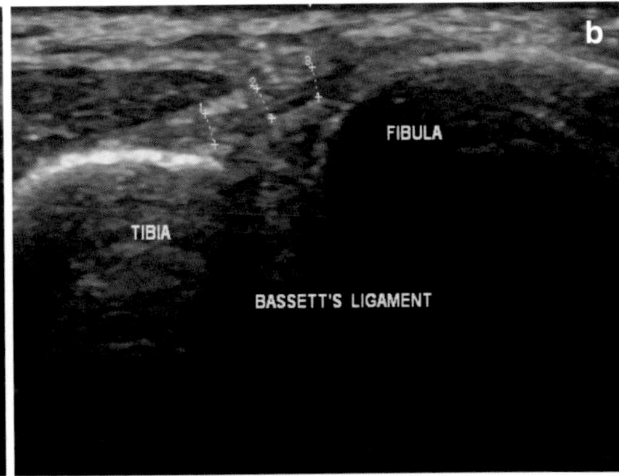

Fig. 22.22 (**a**) Ultrasound image of the anterior inferior tibiofibular ligament (AITFL) which is commonly injured in a high ankle sprain or what is referred to as AITFL proper. (**b**) Ultrasound image of the distal component of AITFL referred to as Bassett's ligament. This structure can also cause anterior ankle impingement

the interosseous ligament. The AITFL has two components: the AITFL proper and the distal Bassett's ligament which can cause anterior ankle impingement (Fig. 22.22). The most stable ligament, PITFL, is also made up of two components: superficial and deep, which is also referred to as transverse ligament. The interosseous ligament is contiguous with the proximal interosseous membrane [430].

Syndesmotic injuries are usually caused by excessive rapid-pivoting ankle rotation or combined ankle dorsiflexion in a pronated foot with a forceful external rotation of calcaneo-talar-fibular complex on a fixed forefoot [431]. The ligaments of the ankle are injured in this order of frequency from the most to the least common: AITFL, interosseous ligament, and rarely the PITFL [430]. The deep deltoid ligament may also be consequentially affected by this injury. Recent biomechanical studies reveal a multidirectional instability with anteroposterior translational and rotational instability of the distal fibula relative to the tibia. What eventually separates the distal tibia and fibula is the rotation of the talus in the mortise, with the fibula rotating externally and moving posteriorly and laterally [431]. In a related study, this injury when accompanied with tibial periosteal stripping by the avulsion of extra-osseous vasculature may lead to osteonecrosis in about 3–4 weeks following the initial injury [432].

Misdiagnosed syndesmosis injury is a usual source of disability and delayed return to sport. Although MRI is considered the imaging of choice for a suspected high ankle sprain, it has a lower chance of diagnosing it correctly after 6 weeks post-injury, with 12 weeks post-injury showing a normal MRI scan despite the ankle instability. In fact, posterior malleolar edema is the only sign of a complete syndesmosis injury with a surprisingly normal appearance of PITFL [433]. In a recent study, Calder and colleagues identified in MRI scans, a subcircumferential edema, 4–6 cm above the ankle joint in patients with syndesmosis injury which they coined as broken "ring of fire." It has a specificity of 97% and a sensitivity of 49%. This finding is seen when there is substantial trauma to disrupt part of the interosseous membrane leading to bleeding around that area [434]. Ultrasound can provide excellent visualization of the syndesmotic ligaments of the ankle and differentiate the pathology of each ligament (Fig. 22.22). It can provide stress maneuvers and dynamic evaluation to ensure whether a particular ligament is partially or completely torn [435]. In fact, ultrasound has a sensitivity of 66% and a specificity of 91% for detecting AITFL pathology using a 13 MHz probe as compared to MRI [436]. Recent studies, however, showed 100% sensitivity and specificity for AITFL pathologies using dynamic stress ultrasonography, but this study had a very small sample size [437]. Moreover, Fisher and colleagues noted that a supination external rotation (SER) stress ultrasonography test with 25% of AITFL fibers intact will be able to sustain the force and will have a tibiofibular space widening of up to about 5.4 mm and thus can be treated conservatively. However, in complete tears, stress ultrasonography was reported to show a tibiofibular space widening of 6 mm (normal is 4.5 mm). Therefore, dynamic stress ultrasonography is a useful evaluation of the extent of AITFL injuries [438]. Becciolini and colleagues recently published a paper detailing the technique for imaging the PITFL using ultrasound where both the superficial and deep components are visualized [430]. In another recent study, a sagittal translation was done in ankle syndesmotic injury using ultrasound with significant and reliable results [439].

There are several approaches for treating these injuries which include physical rehabilitation, bracing, neuromuscular training, use of nonsteroidal anti-inflammatory drugs, manual therapy, and surgery. Orthobiologics treatment was reported in two studies [427], with one study using a single injection of platelet-rich plasma in syndesmosis injuries of the ankle involving the AITFL and tibiofibular joint showing a faster return to play [440]. Samra and colleagues in a related study showed similar results [441]. The only limitation for both studies is the small sample sizes [427].

Poor outcomes for acute ankle sprains are affected by several factors. However, none of them seemed to be consistent. Of these factors, early surgical intervention is suggested for the following group of athletes/patients: high level/high demand athletes, severe injuries which include bone bruise, multi-ligament involvement, persistent pain, and sprain recurrence, and lastly, the presence of associated injuries like bony avulsion or cartilage injury [442].

Medial Ankle Sprains

Unlike lateral ankle sprains, medial ankle sprains have more severe pathomechanism of injury. It is associated with comorbidities, requiring longer treatment and recovery times. Understanding the injury mechanism is the key to effective rehabilitation and prevention protocols. In a kinematic analysis, Wade and colleagues have reported that a combination of ankle dorsiflexion during heel strike followed by a rapid eversion is associated with a non-contact ankle eversion sprain [443]. Medial ankle sprains represent 15% of all ankle sprains. The incidence of this injury increases in the presence of associated trauma such as lateral ligament injuries, malleolar fractures, or syndesmotic disruptions [444]. In fact, in an arthroscopic study reported by Hintermann and colleagues, 40% of patients with chronic ankle instability revealed a different type of injury involving the deltoid ligament [445].

The deltoid ligament is made up of three consistent ligaments (tibiospring ligament, tibionavicular ligament, and deep posterior tibiotalar ligament) and three variable ligaments (superficial posterior tibiotalar ligament, tibiocalcaneal ligament, and deep anterior tibiotalar ligament). These ligaments are recognized as an important stabilizer of the medial tibiotalar joint [444]. Furthermore, the ankle ligaments can be divided into superficial and deep structures. The deep ligaments of the deltoid are the deep posterior tibiotalar ligament (major ligament) and deep anterior tibiotalar ligament. The rest of the ligaments on the medial side of the ankle comprising the deltoid ligament are superficial in location [446]. The rich vascularity of the deltoid ligament is one reason why injury to this structure heals with conservative treatment; otherwise, any disruption to the blood supply during an ankle trauma may predispose it to delayed or inadequate ligament healing [444]. Moreover, when the injury to the ligaments involves the superficial ligaments, and the deep ligaments are intact, the medial clear space (MCS) of the medial ankle is not altered, and thus conservative management can be used to treat such patients. However, when a combination of superficial and deep ligaments is injured, the medial clear space is significantly altered and thus this type of injury requires a surgical approach for treatment, regardless of whether there is a bony fracture or not [446].

Magnetic resonance imaging (MRI) scans remain as the gold standard imaging modality to diagnose deltoid ligament injuries including other associated abnormalities like bone edema, intra-articular lesions, and joint effusions. However, it cannot provide any assessment on ankle stability due to its static images. An arthroscopic examination may show the integrity of the medial ankle. However, it is an invasive procedure. Ultrasound proves to be a potential imaging modality that can assess for ankle stability due to its dynamic capability, portability, and non-invasiveness. Rosa and colleagues have reported using ultrasonography that an intact deltoid ligament (DL) had a medial clear space (MCS) of 2.7 +/− 0.5 mm, a partial DL tear had an MCS of 5.2 +/− 2.4 mm, and a complete DL tear had an MCS of 9.9 +/− 5.8 mm. Those with superficial DL tear had a mean MCS of 4.2 +/− 0.3 mm, those with deep tears had a mean MCS of 4.5 +/− 0.6 mm, and those with tears in the two layers had a MCS of 6.2 +/− 3.6 mm [447]. Thus, ultrasound showed 100% sensitivity and 90% specificity in this study. Arthroscopic examination using gravity stress views, an MCS greater than 5 mm had complete ruptures, those with less than 5 mm, but greater than 4 mm MCS is either intact or partial DL tear [446]. As fracture is commonly associated with deltoid ligament injuries, there is always a need to surgically repair the ruptured ligament and its associated fracture or dislocation. Failure to surgically repair the deltoid ligament tears may lead to early osteoarthritis due to malalignment during weight-bearing. There is a relatively safe zone for surgical repair in the medial ankle without injuring the saphenous nerve or vein in the ankle [447]. Salameh and colleagues have confirmed that a surgical repair of tibial fractures with the concurrent repair of the deltoid ligament has shown a better anatomical reduction of the ankle with reduced MCS, lower pain scores, and lower complication rate [448]. No studies about orthobiologic treatment for deltoid ligament were reported at present.

Achilles Tendon Injuries

Achilles tendon pathologies are very common among athletes and their involvement from any trauma in sports is debilitating. Chronic tendinosis is often seen in overuse injuries and usually responds with conservative treatments. When no improvement is seen in 6 months trial of conservative treatment, surgical debridement is considered. Acute Achilles tendon ruptures are observed to be increasing due to a more active older population engaging in exercise and sports activities. Thus, the pathology of the Achilles tendon can be acute or chronic or could be a spectrum of tendinosis to actual tears, affecting both athletes and nonathletes alike [449].

Being the largest and strongest tendon in the human body, the Achilles tendon is a confluence of the gastrocnemius and soleus muscles inserted into the posterior calcaneal bone. From its origin, it spans three joints and is therefore actively involved in knee flexion, ankle dorsiflexion, and hindfoot inversion. The etiology of Achilles tendon injuries can be due to any of the two possible theories, namely, the chronic and degenerative changes that come by age, or can be secondary to medications such as fluoroquinolones or corticosteroids or due to acute healthy traumatic injuries. Other factors that could possibly predispose injury include biomechanical malalignment such as hyper-pronation or inappropriate footwear [450]. This hyper-pronation causes the rotation of the tendon to be accentuated which consequently decreases the blood flow to the Achilles tendon, a phenomenon referred to as “whipping action” [451]. Arner and colleagues [452] have postulated that the tendon that has undergone degenerative changes could be coming from an aging process and thus deprived itself of a normal blood flow which leads to hypoxia and altered metabolism. This represents about 25% of Achilles tendon injuries [453]. In fact, this injury is difficult to diagnose and is more demanding in terms of treatment and management. It is more challenging to diagnose it in the early stage [453]. Moreover, Achilles tendon rupture is not always preceded by tendinous degeneration and is common among patients with non-sports-related injuries and those with low sports activity [450]. However, Barfred and colleagues have observed in a rat model, that what occurs among healthy subjects happened in a push-off type activity where an obliquely loaded tendon at a short ini-

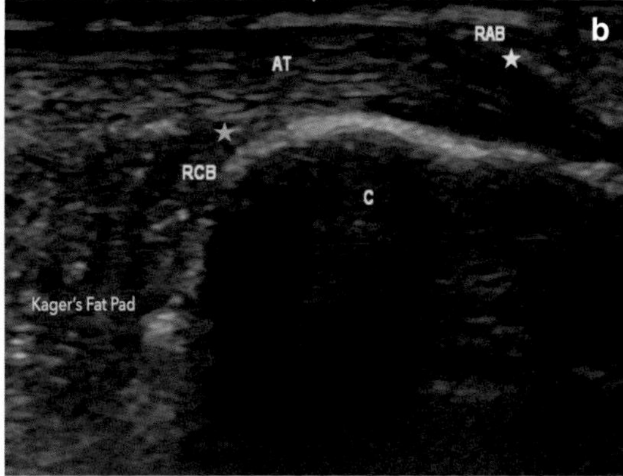

Fig. 22.23 (**a**, **b**) Ultrasound images of the Achilles tendon in longitudinal views show the Achilles tendon fiber as it inserts into the posterior calcaneal (**c**) bone. Deep to the Achilles tendon is shown the retrocalcaneal bursa (RCB) and superficial to it is the retroachilles bursa (RAB). The Kager's fat pad is shown anterior to the Achilles tendon

tial length is under a maximum muscle contraction. This asynchrony is common among athletes who do not train consistently before engaging in a challenging sports activity [454]. Most tears occur about 3–6 cm proximal to the insertion at the calcaneus and usually this is because of a paucity of vascularity by the posterior tibial artery and this decreases over time and age [455] (Fig. 22.23). The ruptures usually occur between 30 and 50 years, with older ones taking more time for healing after any intervention is done [455]. Among the different types of sports, basketball takes the lead for acute Achilles tendon rupture, followed by soccer and tennis [456].

There are systematic ways to identify an Achilles tendon tear in a patient. A typical patient will report a pop at the time of injury, with immediate pain and an inability to plantarflex the ankle or bear weight [455]. During a physical examination, a defect can be palpable along the length of the Achilles tendon. The most widely used test is Thompson's or Simmond's test. It has a sensitivity of 96% and a specificity of 93% [457]. Diagnostic modalities can further confirm your diagnosis by using either MRI or ultrasound. MRI is the gold standard for a suspected Achilles tendon tear. It has a sensitivity of 94%, a specificity of 81%, and an overall accuracy of 89% [458]. However, diagnostic ultrasound is a readily available modality because of its portability. It has the capability of diagnosing tear, partial or complete, tendinosis, type, and level of the rupture and can monitor the changes during the healing process. Because of its dynamic capability, an ultrasound-guided Thompson test has a sensitivity of 86% and a specificity of 91% when compared with static ultrasound imaging alone [459]. It is, however, user-dependent and requires a great deal of familiarity and training to be able to make an accurate diagnosis [455]. Ultrasound changes, however, maybe also seen in asymptomatic patients and may be worth mentioning especially since these are athletes who are engaged in active sports, such as among runners and soccer players. The presence of neovascularization followed by focal hypoechogenicity had a direct correlation with the development of tendon pain. Caution however must be observed when interpreting such findings [26]. Moreover, elastography ultrasound is another feature in ultrasound that can make an early diagnosis for tendon pathologies such as in Achilles tendon where tendon stiffness is being assessed as well as monitoring post-op rehabilitation to evaluate and guide on-going treatments [7].

There are varied techniques of treatment in an Achilles tendon rupture with competing results of interventions, with each intervention showing its own benefits and disadvantages. In the past, it is common to have an immediate surgical intervention for an Achilles tendon rupture. However, there are issues that come with operative interventions such as infections, and devastating wound complications [455, 460]. Presently, nonoperative treatment finds its way among clinicians which consists of early mobilization and functional rehabilitation with significantly good outcomes such as reduced re-rupture rate. However, this approach may take several weeks of intensive physiotherapy to achieve optimal results [455]. Aufwerber and colleagues underscored the importance of accelerated postoperative protocol with immediate loading and ankle motion in 6 months in Achilles tendon rupture [461]. From the surgical standpoint, the more conventional operative care appears to be evolving where most surgeons prefer the less invasive surgical technique such as minimally invasive and percutaneous surgical technique over the open technique with the advantages of lesser risk for wound complications and infections but carry with it a more challenging learning curve for surgeons [460, 462, 463].

Orthobiologic interventions such as platelet-rich plasma (PRP) therapy have shown significant benefits in an Achilles tendon injury. Neph and colleagues have recently noted that PRP injection can be further potentiated for tendon regeneration when mechanical loading rehabilitation protocols are incorporated in Achilles tendinopathy [464]. For Achilles tendon rupture (ATR), however, Boesen and colleagues in a recently published randomized, double-blinded prospective study have not shown tendon healing or improved patient-reported outcomes and functional and clinical outcomes in the first 12 months after an ATR by using PRP [465].

Athletes sustaining an ATR faced a challenging year ahead with 30.6% of them unable to return to play. In fact, functional deficits are not evident until after a year post-operatively. Moreover, the level of play akin to their previous performance can only be achieved 2 years post-operatively [466].

New Features in Ultrasonography

Musculoskeletal ultrasound is a very useful tool as a quick and convenient way to diagnose neuromusculoskeletal conditions. Aside from its unique feature of dynamic imaging, it has several features that are now being included like ultrasound elastography, ultrasound tissue characterization (UTC), and contrast-enhanced ultrasound (CEUS). Ultrasound elastography is very useful for identifying at-risk tendons among athletes. In a study of asymptomatic foot players, preseason softening of the Achilles tendon on strain elastography (SE) has a direct correlation for the development of symptoms postseason [467]. Moreover, shear wave elastography (SWE) or otherwise called dynamic elastography quantifies the stiffness of the tendons. It however requires a depth of at least 0.4 cm for the SWE to be generated. A depth of 9 cm from the surface of the skin cannot be assessed properly due to pulse attenuation [467]. To bypass the depth limitation, especially for shallow structures, applying a 5-mm layer of coupling gel may serve as a stand-off [468]. It also has limited capability in assessing fluid-filled structures and soft tissue embedded in harder and incompressible tissues [467]. SWE has shown great utility in rotator cuff conditions as they correlate with functional scores. In one study, it was shown that long years of participation in sports revealed a decrease in stiffness of the supraspinatus tendon which corresponds to increased thickness in ultrasound and a self-reported decline in function [469]. Compared to SE, SWE is more objective, quantitative, and reproducible. This ultrasound feature can also be used to monitor the progress of the rehabilitation program. For instance, a postoperative Achilles tendon shows a progressive increase in stiffness in SWE after completing a rehabilitation program indicating an improved functional score. The increase in stiffness can be due to the physiological healing process which shows a disorganized collagen fiber. The same holds true with eccentric loading in an Achilles tendon which shows an increased tendon stiffness in SWE [467]. In general, SWE showed that tendinopathic tendons and fasciae were heterogeneous and had reduced stiff patterns or are softer than normal tendons and tissue elasticity decreased [470]. Thus, ultrasound elastography is an important technique to promote an early diagnosis long before a conventional ultrasound shows any changes, to identify the risk of injury, and to evaluate rehabilitation interventions [471]. In fact, the combination of elastography and conventional ultrasound is more powerful than power Doppler and conventional ultrasound. Thus, it is recommended that before further evaluation with MRI, ultrasound elastography can make a difference in diagnosing early tendon pathology both among athletes and non-athletes alike such that it can predict an ongoing pathology in what otherwise may appear as normal in a conventional ultrasound and preclude further injury [7]. It has also been reported to have very good applicability in nerve entrapments. In fact, the loss of elasticity of either the nerve itself or the carpal tunnel in the case of carpal tunnel syndrome or both can precede any change in conventional neural cross-sectional measurements. And that is why with all these advancements in ultrasound techniques, new guidelines might emerge as to the current diagnostic practice [472].

Ultrasound tissue characterization (UTC) is used both in research and in clinical practice to quantify the structure specifically of the tendons. A conventional ultrasound has limited capability to detect minimal intratendinous changes and to quantify tendon structure and as such is simply using gross description like hypoechogenic zone or tendon diameter and cross-sectional area. UTC, therefore, converts a tendon structure into a three-dimensional data block and then calculates the stability of the brightness of the pixels over contiguous transverse images [473]. Wezenbeck and colleagues did a study [474] on the Achilles tendon of 70 physiotherapy students, with 26 males and 44 females with no history of Achilles tendon injury. By using UTC, the study reported that normal, healthy individuals showed a predominance of echo type I in males and echo type II among female counterparts at both the insertion and midportion, which could be due to the estrogen hormone in the females. Moreover, there is a predominance of echo type I at the midportion and a predominance of echo type II at the insertion site of the Achilles tendon. Echo types II, III, and IV represent alterations in tendon bundles, with echo type IV showing the most alterations in tendon architecture. The predominance of echo type II does not necessarily mean an abnormality but instead is a necessary morphological, histological, and functional requirement with an increased level of glycosaminoglycans (GAG) in the region. This finding showed that UTC can quantify subtle differences in tendon structure that may precede the development of symptoms in an abnormal tendon [474].

Contrast-enhanced ultrasound (CEUS) is a technique using micro-bubble-based intravenous contrast agents that can enhance the vascular flow of a particular structure being imaged and allow the assessment of microcirculation during ultrasound imaging. It can show microvascularity and blood perfusion in real time and can detect neovascularization at the capillary level [475]. In this case, a second-generation contrast agent used is sulfur hexafluoride (Sonovue®, Bracco Imaging, Milan, Italy), and this solution has shown a good safety profile with no reported fatalities so far. In fact, it was reported to have a better safety profile than the MRI contrast agent gadolinium [476]. Other contrast agents used in the past include Levovist and Sonazoid. The 2017 guidelines of the European Federation of Societies for Ultrasound in Medicine and Biology (EFSUMB) introduced CEUS for non-hepatic applications. It was initially intended for inflammatory joint diseases and eventually was applied for microperfusion assessment for bone and muscle tissue [475]. CEUS, however, has a specific window of time that corresponds to the phase of contrast for ideal ultrasound scanning [475].

Other advanced ultrasound techniques include microvascular imaging or superb microvascular imaging (SMI) wherein an extremely subtle blood flow detects inflammation and malignancy without the use of contrast agents and any invasive procedures. In traditional color and power Doppler technologies, the clutter is removed by suppressing low-velocity components, with loss of visibility and data. The SMI works by suppressing low-flow signals and separating these low-flow signals from overlaying the artifacts of tissue motion while at the same time preserving the low-flow components and enhancing detail and definition. It was reported to be better than power Doppler ultrasound in assessing hypervascularity in median nerve neuropathy such as in

CTS. It can also identify neovascularization associated with tendinopathies [475]. It is however available in selected high-resolution ultrasound machines like the Aplio 500 US system by Toshiba (Toshiba Medical Systems, Tokyo, Japan) and Xario 200 Platinum Series by Canon Medical Systems, USA.

With all these exciting developments, it can be assured that musculoskeletal ultrasound can emerge further as an indispensable tool for musculoskeletal sports diagnosis, a guide to prevent further injuries in a seemingly asymptomatic patient, and an instrument to assist in rehabilitation and interventional procedures and provide objective ways to return to play.

The use of ultrasound to improve the accuracy of regenerative interventions is a vital addition in any interventional procedure. Its optimal use by a trained and experienced physician will enable quick and prompt diagnosis of an injury and provide a precision-guided ultrasound interventional procedure, either in the clinic, hospital, or even during an actual sports event. It is important, however, to recognize its limitations and to understand and decide when to consider other available diagnostic modalities that can provide better sensitive and specific imaging when necessary.

> Study to shew thyself approved unto God. 2 Timothy 2:15 (KJV)

Acknowledgment Special thanks to the Almighty God for providing me the inspiration and guidance in preparing this chapter and to my wife Kyna and my two kids: Rafael Bennett de Castro and Zarah Francine de Castro.

References

1. Robotti G, Draghi F, Bortolotto C, Canepa M. Ultrasound of sports injuries of the musculoskeletal system: gender differences. J Ultrasound. 2020;23:279–85.
2. Healy J. The value of ultrasound in sports medicine. Hosp Med. 2002;63(10):593–7.
3. Jiménez Díaz J, Alvarez Rey G, Balius Matas R, Berral De La Rosa F, Padilla E, Villa Vicente J. New technologies applied to ultrasound diagnosis of sports injuries. Adv Ther. 2008;25(12):1315–30.
4. Strobel K, Zanetti M, Nagy L, Hodler J. Suspected rotator cuff lesions: tissue harmonic imaging versus conventional US of the shoulder. Radiology. 2004;230:243–9.
5. Oktar SO, Yucel C, Ozdemir H, Uluturk A, Isik S. Comparison of conventional sonography, real-time compound sonography, tissue harmonic sonography, and tissue harmonic compound sonography of abdominal and pelvic lesions. Am J Roentgenol. 2003;181:1341–7.
6. Weng L, Tirumalai AP. Method and apparatus for generating large compound ultrasound images. U.S. Patent 5575286; 1996. Available at: www.freepatentsonline.com/5575286.html.
7. Afandi R, Astawa P. The use of elastography-ultrasound in diagnosing tendinopathy related sport injury: a 10 years trend systematic review. Orthop J Sports Med. 2019;7(11_suppl6):1.
8. Van Hooren B, Teratsias P, Hodson-Tole E. Ultrasound imaging to assess skeletal muscle architecture during movements: a systematic review of methods, reliability, and challenges. J Appl Physiol. 2020;128(4):978–99.
9. Alvarez C, Hattori S, Kato Y, Takazawa S, Adachi T, Yamada S, Ohuchi H. Dynamic high-resolution ultrasound in the diagnosis of calcaneofibular ligament injury in chronic lateral ankle injury: a comparison with three-dimensional magnetic resonance imaging. J Med Ultrason. 2020;47(2):313–7.
10. Angelopoulou K, McReynolds K. Use of dynamic ultrasound imaging for assessment of the fibular collateral ligament of the knee. J Orthop Sports Phys Ther. 2020;49(3):210.
11. Martin K, Wake J, Van Buren JP. Ultrasound evaluation of the peroneal tendons in an asymptomatic elite military population: a prospective cohort study. Mil Med. 2020;185(Supplement_1):420–2.
12. Murray T, Roberts D, Rattan B, Murphy D, Cresswell M. Dynamic ultrasound-guided trochanteric bursal injection. Skeletal Radiol. 2020;49:1155–8.
13. Kunz P, Mick P, Gross S, Schmidmaier G, Zeifang F, Weber M, Fischer C. Contrast-Enhanced Ultrasound (CEUS) as predictor for early retear and functional outcome after supraspinatus tendon repair. J Orthop Res. 2020;38(5):1150–8.
14. Wengert G, Schmutzer M, Bickel H, Sora M, Polanec S, Weber M, Schueller-Weidekamm C. Reliability of high-resolution ultrasound and magnetic resonance arthrography of the shoulder in patients with sports-related shoulder injuries. PLoS One. 2019;14(9):1–12.
15. Ottenheim RP, Cals JW, Weijers R, Vanderdood K, de Bie RA, Dinant GJ. Ultrasound imaging for tailored treatment of patients with acute shoulder pain. Ann Fam Med. 2015;13(1):53–5.
16. Chauhan NS, Ahluwalia A, Sharma YP, Thakur L. A prospective comparative study of high- resolution ultrasound and MRI in the diagnosis of rotator cuff tears in a tertiary hospital of North India. Pol J Radiol. 2016;81:491–7.
17. Draghi F, Lomoro P, Bortolotto C, Mastrogirolamo L, Calliada F. Comparison between a new ultrasound

probe with a capacitive micromachined transducer (CMUT) and a traditional one in musculoskeletal pathology. Acta Radiol. 2020;1:1–7.
18. Wong-On M, Til-Pérez L, Balius R. Evaluation of MRI-US fusion technology in sports-related musculoskeletal injuries. Adv Ther. 2015;32(6):580–94.
19. Rodeo S, Nguyen J, Cavanaugh J, Patel Y, Adler R. Clinical and ultrasonographic evaluations of the shoulders of elite swimmers. Am J Sports Med. 2016;44(12):3214–21.
20. Draghi F, Scudeller L, Draghi AG, Bortolotto C. Prevalence of subacromial-subdeltoid bursitis in shoulder pain: an ultrasonographic study. J Ultrasound. 2015;18:151–8.
21. Kennedy JC, Hawkins RJ. Swimmer's shoulder. Phys Sportsmed. 1974;2:34–8.
22. Dischler J, Baumer T, Finkelstein E, Siegal D, Bey M. Association between years of competition and shoulder function in collegiate swimmers. Sports Health. 2017;10(2):113–8.
23. Galluccio F, Bellucci E, Porta F, Tofani L, De Paulis A, Bianchedi D, Barskova T, Matucci-Cerinic M. The waterpolo shoulder paradigm: results of ultrasound surveillance at poolside. BMJ Open Sport Exerc Med. 2017;3(1):1–4.
24. AKT answer relating to shoulder injuries. InnovAiT. 2020;13(1):e12–2.
25. Fischer C, Gross S, Zeifang F, Schmidmaier G, Weber M, Kunz P. Contrast-enhanced ultrasound determines supraspinatus muscle atrophy after cuff repair and correlates to functional shoulder outcome. Am J Sports Med. 2018;46(11):2735–42.
26. Splittgerber LE, Ihm JM. Significance of asymptomatic tendon pathology in athletes. Curr Sports Med Rep. 2019;18(6):192–200.
27. Popchak A, Hogaboom N, Vyas D, Abt J, Delitto A, Irrgang J, Boninger M. Acute response of the infraspinatus and biceps tendons to pitching in youth baseball. Med Sci Sports Exerc. 2017;49(6):1168–75.
28. Corpus KT, Camp CL, Dines DM, et al. Evaluation and treatment of internal impingement of the shoulder in overhead athletes. World J Orthop. 2016;7:776–84.
29. Connor PM, Banks DM, Tyson AB, et al. Magnetic resonance imaging of the asymptomatic shoulder of overhead athletes: a 5- year follow-up study. Am J Sports Med. 2003;31:724–7.
30. Lesniak BP, Baraga MG, Jose J, et al. Glenohumeral findings on magnetic resonance imaging correlate with innings pitched in asymptomatic pitchers. Am J Sports Med. 2013;41:2022–7.
31. Schar MO, Dellenbach S, Pfirrmann CW, et al. Many shoulder MRI findings in elite professional throwing athletes resolve after retirement: a clinical and radiographic study. Clin Orthop Relat Res. 2018;476:620–31.
32. Yamaguchi K, Tetro AM, Blam O, et al. Natural history of asymptomatic rotator cuff tears: a longitudinal analysis of asymptomatic tears detected sonographically. J Shoulder Elb Surg. 2001;10:199–203.
33. Yamaguchi K, Ditsios K, Middleton WD, et al. The demographic and morphological features of rotator cuff disease. A comparison of asymptomatic and symptomatic shoulders. J Bone Joint Surg Am. 2006;88:1699–704.
34. Takenaga T, Sugimoto K, Goto H, Nozaki M, Fukuyoshi M, Tsuchiya A, Murase A, Ono T, Otsuka T. Posterior shoulder capsules are thicker and stiffer in the throwing shoulders of healthy college baseball players. Am J Sports Med. 2015;43(12):2935–42.
35. Noonan T, Shanley E, Bailey L, Wyland D, Kissenberth M, Hawkins R, Thigpen C. Professional pitchers with Glenohumeral Internal Rotation Deficit (GIRD) display greater humeral retrotorsion than pitchers without GIRD. Am J Sports Med. 2015;43(6):1448–54.
36. Greenberg E, Lawrence J, Fernandez-Fernandez A, McClure P. Humeral retrotorsion and glenohumeral motion in youth baseball players compared with age-matched nonthrowing athletes. Am J Sports Med. 2017;45(2):454–61.
37. Chin B, Ramji M, Farrokhyar F, Bain JR. Efficient imaging: examining the value of ultrasound in the diagnosis of traumatic adult brachial plexus injuries, a systematic review. Neurosurgery. 2018;83(3):323–32. https://doi.org/10.1093/neuros/nyx483.
38. Igielska-Bela B, Baczkowski B, Flisikowski K. Shoulder ultrasound in the diagnosis of the suprascapular neuropathy in athletes. Open Med (Wars). 2020;15(1):147–51.
39. Provencher CDRMT, Handfield K, Boniquit MT, Reiff SN, Sekiya JK, Romeo AA. Injuries to the pectoralis major muscle: diagnosis and management. Am J Sports Med. 2010;38(8):1693–705.
40. Doods SD, Wolfe SW. Injuries to the pectoralis major. Sports Med. 2002;32(14):945–52.
41. Liem B, Olafsen N. Pectoralis major injuries: return to play potential. Curr Phys Med Rehabil Rep. 2017;5(2):91–7.
42. Sachdeva R, Farthing J, Kim S. Evaluation of supraspinatus strengthening exercises based on fiber bundle architectural changes. Scand J Med Sci Sports. 2017;27(7):736–45.
43. Goodman M, Schmitt R, Petron D, Gee C, Mallin M. The effect of bedside ultrasound on diagnosis and management of patients presenting to a sports medicine clinic with undifferentiated shoulder pain. J Diagn Med Sonogr. 2015;31(2):82–5.
44. Randelli P, Menon A, Nocerino E, Aliprandi A, Feroldi F, Mazzoleni M, Boveri S, Ambrogi F, Cucchi D. Long-term results of arthroscopic rotator cuff repair: initial tear size matters: a prospective study on clinical and radiological results at a minimum follow-up of 10 years. Am J Sports Med. 2019;47(11):2659–69.
45. Yeo D, Walton J, Lam P, Murrell G. The relationship between intraoperative tear dimensions and postoperative pain in 1624 consecutive arthroscopic rotator cuff repairs. Am J Sports Med. 2017;45(4):788–93.

46. Schwitzguebel A, Kolo F, Tirefort J, Kourhani A, Nowak A, Gremeaux V, Saffarini M, Lädermann A. Efficacy of platelet-rich plasma for the treatment of interstitial supraspinatus tears: a double-blinded, randomized controlled trial. Am J Sports Med. 2019;47(8):1885–92.
47. Flores C, Balius R, Álvarez G, Buil M, Varela L, Cano C, Casariego J. Efficacy and tolerability of peritendinous hyaluronic acid in patients with supraspinatus tendinopathy: a multicenter, randomized, controlled trial. Sports Med Open. 2017;3(1):1–8.
48. Cai Y, Sun Z, Liao B, Song Z, Xiao T, Zhu P. Sodium hyaluronate and platelet-rich plasma for partial-thickness rotator cuff tears. Med Sci Sports Exerc. 2019;51(2):227–33.
49. Ebert J, Wang A, Smith A, Nairn R, Breidahl W, Zheng M, Ackland T. A midterm evaluation of postoperative platelet-rich plasma injections on arthroscopic supraspinatus repair: a randomized controlled trial. Am J Sports Med. 2017;45(13):2965–74.
50. Wang A, McCann P, Colliver J, Koh E, Ackland T, Joss B, Zheng M, Breidahl B. Do postoperative platelet-rich plasma injections accelerate early tendon healing and functional recovery after arthroscopic supraspinatus repair? Am J Sports Med. 2015;43(6):1430–7.
51. Shiri R, Viikari-Juntura E, Varonen H, Heliovaara M. Prevalence and determinants of lateral and medial epicondylitis: a population study. Am J Epidemiol. 2006;154(11):1065–74.
52. Clarke A, Ahmad M, Curtis M, Connell D. Lateral elbow tendinopathy. Am J Sports Med. 2010;38(6):1209–14.
53. Noh K, Moon Y, Jacir A, Kim K, Gorthi V. Sonographic probe induced tenderness for lateral epicondylitis: an accurate technique to confirm the location of the lesion. Knee Surg Sports Traumatol Arthrosc. 2010;18(6):836–9.
54. Seng C, Mohan P, Koh S, Howe T, Lim Y, Lee B, Morrey B. Ultrasonic percutaneous tenotomy for recalcitrant lateral elbow tendinopathy. Am J Sports Med. 2016;44(2):504–10.
55. Stover D, Fick B, Chimenti RL, Hall MM. Ultrasound-guided tenotomy improves physical function and decreases pain for tendinopathies of the elbow: a retrospective review. J Shoulder Elb Surg. 2019;28(12):2386–93.
56. Thanasas C, Papadimitriou G, Charalambidis C, Paraskevopoulos I, Papanikolaou A. Platelet-rich plasma versus autologous whole blood for the treatment of chronic lateral elbow epicondylitis. Am J Sports Med. 2011;39(10):2130–4.
57. Atanda A, Buckley P, Hammoud S, Cohen S, Nazarian L, Ciccotti M. Early anatomic changes of the ulnar collateral ligament identified by stress ultrasound of the elbow in young professional baseball pitchers. Am J Sports Med. 2015;43(12):2943–9.
58. Marshall N, Keller R, Van Holsbeeck M, Moutzouros V. Ulnar collateral ligament and elbow adaptations in high school baseball pitchers. Sports Health. 2015;7(6):484–8.
59. Ciccotti M, Hammoud S, Dodson C, Cohen S, Nazarian L, Ciccotti M. Stress ultrasound evaluation of medial elbow instability in a cadaveric model. Am J Sports Med. 2014;42(10):2463–9.
60. Park JY, Kim H, Lee JH, Heo T, Park H, Chung SW, Oh KS. Valgus stress ultrasound for medial ulnar collateral ligament injuries in athletes: is ultrasound alone enough for diagnosis? J Shoulder Elb Surg. 2020;29(3):578–86.
61. Kurokawa D, Muraki T, Ishikawa H, Shinagawa K, Nagamoto H, Takahashi H, Yamamoto N, Tanaka M, Itoi E. The influence of pitch velocity on medial elbow pain and medial epicondyle abnormality among youth baseball players. Am J Sports Med. 2020:48(7): 1601–07
62. Hoshika S, Nimura A, Takahashi N, Sugaya H, Akita K. Valgus stability is enhanced by flexor digitorum superficialis muscle contraction of the index and middle fingers. J Orthop Surg Res. 2020;15(1):121.
63. Hattori H, Akasaka A, Otsudo T, Hall T, Amemiya K, Mori Y, Sakaguchi K, Tachibana Y. Changes in medial elbow elasticity and joint space gapping during maximal gripping: reliability and validity in evaluation of the medial elbow joint using ultrasound elastography. J Shoulder Elbow Surg. 2020. https://doi.org/10.1016/j.jse.2019.11.005.
64. Podesta L, Crow S, Volkmer D, Bert T, Yocum L. Treatment of partial ulnar collateral ligament tears in the elbow with platelet-rich plasma. Am J Sports Med. 2013;41(7):1689–94.
65. Gordon A, De Luigi A. Adolescent pitcher recovery from partial ulnar collateral ligament tear after platelet-rich plasma. Curr Sports Med Rep. 2018;17(12):407–9.
66. Matsuura T, Suzue N, Iwame T, et al. Prevalence of osteochondritis dessicans of the capitellum in young baseball players: results based on ultrasonographic findings. Orthop J Sports Med. 2014;2(8):1.
67. Yoshizuka M, Sunagawa T, Nakashima Y, Shinomiya R, Masuda T, Makitsubo M, Adachi N. Comparison of sonography and MRI in the evaluation of stability of capitellar osteochondritis dissecans. J Clin Ultrasound. 2018;46(4):247–52.
68. Satake H, Takahara M, Harada M, et al. Preoperative imaging criteria for unstable osteochondritis dessicans of the capitellum. Clin Orthop Relat Res. 2013;471(4):1137.
69. Rettig AC. Athletic injuries of the wrist and hand. Part 1. Traumatic injuries of the wrist. Am J Sports Med. 2003;31:1038–48.
70. Rumball JS, Lebrun CM, Di Ciacca SR, Orlando K. Rowing injuries. Sports Med. 2005;35(6):537–55.
71. Avery DM, Rodner CM, Edgar CM. Sports-related wrist and hand injuries: a review. J Orthop Surg Res. 2016;11:99. https://doi.org/10.1186/s13018-016-0432-8.
72. Karthik K, Carter-Esdale CW, Vijayanathan S, Kochhar T. Extensor pollicis brevis tendon dam-

age presenting as De Quervain's disease following kettleball training. BMC Sports Sci Med Rehabil. 2013;5:13. https://doi.org/10.1186/2052-1847-5-13.
73. Knobloch K, Gohritz A, Spies M, et al. Neovascularisation in de Quervain's disease of the wrist: novel combined therapy using sclerosing therapy with polidocanol and eccentric training of the forearms and wrists—a pilot report. Knee Surg Sports Traumatol Arthr. 2008;16:803–5. https://doi.org/10.1007/s00167-008-0555-5.
74. Hanlon DP, Luellen JR. Intersection syndrome: a case report and review of literature. J Emerg Med. 1999;17(6):969–71.
75. Montechiarello S, Miozzi F, D'Ambrosio I, Giovagnorio F. The intersection syndrome: ultrasound findings and their diagnostic value. J Ultrasound. 2010;13(2):70–3.
76. Draghi F, Bortolotto C. Intersection syndrome: ultrasound imaging. Skeletal Radiol. 2014;43(3):283–7.
77. Brink PR, Franssen BB, Disseldorp DJ. A simple blind tenolysis for flexor carpi radialis tendinopathy. Hand (NY). 2015;10(2):323–7.
78. Luong D, Smith J, Bianchi S. Flexor carpi radialis tendon ultrasound pictorial essay. Skeletal Radiolog. 2014;43(6):745–60.
79. Naredo E, D'Agostino MA, Wakefield RJ, Moller I, Ballint PV, Filippucci E, et al. Reliability of a consensus-based ultrasound score for tenosynovitis in rheumatoid arthritis. Ann Rheuma Dis. 2013; 72(8): http://dx.doi.org/10.1136/annrheumdis-2012-202092.
80. Campbell D, Campbell R, O'Connor P, Hawkes R. Sports-related extensor carpi ulnaris pathology: a review of functional anatomy, sports injury and management. Br J Sports Med. 2013;47:1105–11.
81. Ruland RT, Hogan CJ. The ECU synergy test: an aid to diagnose ECU tendonitis. J Hand Surg [Am]. 2008;33:1777–82.
82. Bianchi S, Martinoli C, editors. Ultrasound of the musculoskeletal system. Berlin, Heidelberg: Springer; 2007. p. 425–94.
83. Palmer AK. Triangular fibrocartilage complex lesions: a classification. J Hand Surg. 1989;14:594–606.
84. Wu WT, Chang KV, Mezian K, Naňka O, Yang YC, Hsu YC, Hsu PC, Özçakar L. Ulnar wrist pain revisited: ultrasound diagnosis and guided injection for triangular fibrocartilage complex injuries. J Clin Med. 2019;8(10):1540.
85. El-Deek AMF, Dawood EMAEH, Mohammed AAM. Role of ultrasound versus magnetic resonance imaging in evaluation of non-osseous disorders causing wrist pain. Egypt J Radiol Nucl Med. 2019;50(8) https://doi.org/10.1186/s43055-019-0008-9.
86. Elsaftawy A. Radial wrist extensors as a dynamic stabilizers of scapholunate complex. Pol Przegl Chir. 2013;85(8):452–9.
87. Jacobson JA, Oh E, Propeck T, Jebson PJL, Jamadar JA, Hayes CW. Sonography of the scapulolunate ligament in four cadaveric wrists: correlation with MR arthrography and anatomy. Am J Roentgenol. 2002;179(2):523–7.
88. Griffith J, Chan D, Ho P, Zhao L, Hung L, Metreweli C. Sonography of the normal scapholunate ligament and scapholunate joint space. J Clin Ultrasound. 2001;29:223–9.
89. Finlay K, Lee R, Friedman L. Ultrasound of intrinsic wrist ligament and triangular fibrocartilage injuries. Skeletal Radiol. 2004;33(2):85–90.
90. Dao KD, Solomon DJ, Shin AY, Puckett ML. The efficacy of ultrasound in the evaluation of dynamic scapholunate ligamentous instability. JBJS. 2004;86(7):1473–8.
91. Rhee PC, Jones DB, Kakar S. Management of thumb metacarpophalangeal ulnar collateral ligament injuries. J Bone Joint Surg Am. 2012;94(21):2005–12.
92. Gerber C, Senn F, Matter P. Skier's thumb. Surgical treatment of recent injuries to the ulnar collateral ligament of the thumb's metacarpophalangeal joint. a. J Sports Med. 1981;9(3):171–7.
93. Campbell CS. Gamekeeper's thumb. J Bone Joint Surg Br. 1955;37-B(1):148–9.
94. Melville DM, Jacobson JA, Fessell DP. Ultrasound of the ulnar collateral ligament: technique and pathology. Am J Roentgenol. 2014;202(2):W168.
95. Melville D, Jacobson J, Haase S, Brandon C, Brigido M, Fessell D. Ultrasound of displaced ulnar collateral ligament tears of the thumb: the Stener lesion revisited. Skeletal Radiol. 2013;42(5):667–73.
96. Canella Moraes Carmo C, Cruz GP, Trudell D, Hughes T, Chung C, Resnick D. Anatomical features of metacarpal heads that simulate bone erosions: cadaveric study using computed tomography scanning and sectional radiography. J Comput Assist Tomogr. 2009;33:573–8.
97. Kataoka T, Moritomo H, Miyake J, Murase T, Yoshikawa H, Sugamoto K. Changes in shape and length of the collateral and accessory collateral ligaments of the metacarpophalangeal joint during flexion. J Bone Joint Surg Am. 2011;93:1318–25.
98. Shinohara T, Horii E, Majima M, et al. Sonographic diagnosis of acute injuries of the ulnar collateral ligament of the metacarpophalangeal joint of the thumb. J Clin Ultrasound. 2007;35:73–7.
99. Grandizio L, Klena J. Sagittal band, boutonniere, and pulley injuries in the athlete. Curr Rev Musculoskelet Med. 2017;10(1):17–22.
100. Wheeldon FT. Recurrent dislocation of extensor tendons in the hand. J Bone Joint Surg Br. 1954;36B:612–7.
101. Boyes J. Bunnell's surgery of the hand. 4th ed. Boyes J, editor. Philadelphia: Lippincott; 1984.
102. Shinohara T, Nakamura R, Suzuki M, Maeda N. Extensor mechanism laxity at the metacarpophalangeal joint as identified by a new provocative test: predisposition to dislocation. J Hand Surg. 2005;30:79–82.

103. Rayan GM, Murray D. Classification and treatment of closed sagittal band injuries. J Hand Surg. 1994;19:590–4.
104. Lopez-Ben R, Lee DH, Nicolodi DJ. Boxer knuckle (injury of the extensor hood with extensor tendon subluxation): diagnosis with dynamic US. Report of three cases. Radiology. 2003;228:642–6.
105. Karsandas A, Self A, Tuckett J, Sinha R, Hide G. The boxer's knuckle—injury to the sagittal band. A review of the anatomy with ultrasound and MRI correlation. ESSR 2016/P-0050. https://doi.org/10.1594/essr2016/P-0050.
106. Kichouh M, Vanhoenacker F, Jager T, Roy P, Pouders C, Marcelis S, Hedent E, Mey J. Functional anatomy of the dorsal hood or the hand: correlation of ultrasound and MR findings with cadaveric dissection. Eur Radiol. 2009;19(8):1849–56.
107. Martinoli C, Bianchi S, Nebiolo M, Derchi LE, Garcia JF. Sonographic evaluation of digital annular pulley tears. Skeletal Radiol. 2000;29:387–91.
108. Boutry N, Titecat M, Demondion X, Glaudy E, Fontaine C, Cotten A. High frequency ultrasonographic examination of the finger pulley system. J Ultrasound Med. 2005;24(10):1333–9.
109. Schoffl I, Hugel A, Schoffl V, Rascher W, Jungert J. Diagnosis of complex pulley ruptures using ultrasound cadaver models. Ultrasound Med Biol. 2017;43(3):662–9.
110. Bodner G, Rudisch A, Gabl M, Judmaier W, Springer P, Klauser A. Diagnosis of digital flexor tendon annular pulley disruption: comparison of high frequency ultrasound and MRI. Ultraschall Med. 1999;20(4):131–6.
111. Klauser A, Frauscher F, Bodner G, Halpern EJ, Schocke MF, Springer P, et al. Finger pulley injuries in extreme rock climbers: depiction with dynamic ultrasound. Radiology. 2002;222(3):755. https://doi.org/10.1148/radiol.2223010752.
112. Ootes D, Lambers KT, Ring DC. The epidemiology of upper extremity injuries presenting to the emergency department in the United States. Hand (NY). 2012;7:18–22.
113. Bachoura A, Ferikes A, Lubahn J. A review of mallet finger and jersey finger injuries in the athlete. Curr Rev Musculoskelet Med. 2017;10(1):1–9.
114. de Gautard G, de Gautard R, Celi J, Jacquemoud G, Bianchi S. Sonography of Jersey finger. J Ultrasound Med. 2009;28(3):389–92.
115. Bianchi S, Martinolli C. Ultrasound of the musculoskeletal system. Ney York: Springer; 2007.
116. Gilleard O, Silver D, Ahmad Z, Devaraj V. The accuracy of ultrasound in evaluating closed flexor tendon ruptures. Eur J Plast Surg. 2010;33(2):71–4.
117. Sendher R, Ladd AL. The scaphoid. Orthop Clin North Am. 2013;44(1):107–20.
118. Garala K, Taub NA, Dias JJ. The epidemiology of fractures of the scaphoid: impact of age, gender, deprivation and seasonality. Bone Joint J. 2016;98-B(5):654–9.
119. Dias J, Kantharuban S. Treatment of scaphoid fractures: European approaches. Hand Clin. 2018;33(3):501–9.
120. Clementson M, Björkman A, Thomsen N. Acute scaphoid fractures: guidelines for diagnosis and treatment. EFORT Open Rev. 2020;5(2):96–103.
121. Mack GR, Bosse MJ, Gelberman RH, Yu E. The natural history of scaphoid nonunion. J Bone Joint Surg. 1984;66A:504–9.
122. Kwee R, Kwee T. Ultrasound for diagnosing radiographically occult scaphoid fracture. Skeletal Radiol. 2018;47(9):1205–12.
123. Munk B, Bolvig L, Kroner K, Christiansen T, Borris L, Boe S. Ultrasound for diagnosis of scaphoid fractures. J Hand Surg. 2000;25(4):369–71.
124. Malahias M, Nikolaou V, Chytas D, Kaseta M, Babis G. Accuracy and interobserver and intraobserver reliability of ultrasound in the early diagnosis of occult scaphoid fractures: diagnostic criteria and a way of interpretation. J Surg Orthop Adv. 2019;28(1):1–9.
125. Mallee WH, Wang J, Poolman RW, Kloen P, Maas M, de Vet HC, Doornberg JN. Computed tomography versus magnetic resonance imaging versus bone scintigraphy for clinical suspected scaphoid fractures in patients with negative plain radiographs. Cochrane Database Syst Rev. 2015;6:CD010023.
126. Swärd E, Schriever T, Franko M, Björkman A, Wilcke M. The epidemiology of scaphoid fractures in Sweden: a nationwide registry study. J Hand Surg (Eur Vol). 2019;44(7):697–701.
127. Ram AN, Chung KC. Evidence-based management of acute non-displaced scaphoid waist fractures. J Hand Surg Am. 2009;34:735–8.
128. Commandeur J, Rhemrev S, Buijze G, Beeres F. Conservative treatment of scaphoid fractures. Ned Tijdschr Geneeskd. 2020;2020(163):1.
129. Suh N, Grewal R. Controversies and best practices for acute scaphoid fracture management. J Hand Surg (Eur Vol). 2018;43(1):4–12.
130. Grewal R, Lutz K, MacDermid JC, Suh N. Proximal pole scaphoid fractures: a computed tomographic assessment of outcomes. J Hand Surg Am. 2016;41:54–8.
131. Saltzman EB, Rancy SK, Lee SK, Wolfe SW. Acute management of proximal pole scaphoid fractures. In: Buijze ZE, Jupiter JB, editors. Scaphoid fractures: evidence-based management. Philadelphia: Elsevier; 2017.
132. Clementson M, Thomsen N, Beskajov J, Jorgsholm P, Bjorkman A. Long term outcomes after distal scaphoid fractures: a 10-year follow up. J Hand Surg Am. 2017;42(11):927.e1–7.
133. Fowler JR, Hughes TB. Scaphoid fractures. Clin Sports Med. 2015;34:37–50.
134. Mekaouche M, Merabet M, Koriche H. Platelet rich plasma therapy for scaphoid fracture nonunion. Med. 2018.
135. Feinberg J, Nadler S, Krivickas L. Peripheral nerve injuries in the athlete. Sports Med. 2012;24(6):385–408.

136. Toros T, Karabay N, Ozaksar T, Sugun S, Kayalar M, Bal E. Evaluation of the peripheral nerves of the upper limb with ultrasonography. A comparison of ultrasonographic examination and the intra-operative findings. J Bone Joint Surg Br. 2009;91-B(6):762. https://doi.org/10.1302/0301-620X.91B6.22284.
137. Küllmer K, Sievers K, Reimers C, Rompe J, Müller-Felber W, Nägele M, Harland U. Changes of sonographic, magnetic resonance tomographic, electromyographic, and histopathologic findings within a 2-month period of examinations after experimental muscle denervation. Arch Orthop Trauma Surg. 1998;117(5):228–34.
138. Zaidman CM, Seelig MJ, Baker JC, Mackinnon SE, Pestronk A. Detection of peripheral nerve pathology. Comparison of ultrasound and MRI. Neurology. 2013;80(18) https://doi.org/10.1212/WNL.0b013e3182904f3f.
139. Lee FC, Singh H, Nazarian LN, Ratliff JK. High resolution ultrasonography in the diagnosis of intra-operative management of peripheral nerve lesions. J Neurosurg. 2011. https://doi.org/10.3171/2010.2.JNS091324.
140. Martinolli C, Tagliafico A, Bianchi S, Bodner G, Padua L, Schenone A, Graif M. Peripheral nerve abnormalities. Ultrasound Clin. 2007;2(4):655–67.
141. Jacobson JA, Wilson TJ, Yang LJS. Sonography of common peripheral nerve disorders with clinical correlation. J Ultrasound Med. 2016;35(4):683–93.
142. Koenig RW, Pedro MT, Heinen CP, Schmidt T, Richter HP, Antoniadis G, Kretschmer T. High resolution ultrasonography in evaluating peripheral nerve entrapment and trauma. Neurosurg Focus. 2009;26:E13.
143. Zhu J, Liu F, Li D, Shao J, Hu B. Preliminary study of the types of traumatic peripheral nerve injuries by ultrasound. Eur Radiol. 2010;21(5):1097–101.
144. Kawasaki T, Ota C, Yoneda T, Maki N, Urayama S, Nagao M, Nagayama M, Kaketa T, Takazawa Y, Kaneko K. Incidence of stingers in young Rugby players. Am J Sports Med. 2015;43(11):2809–15.
145. Chan JS, Ip JW. Upper limb nerve injuries in sport. In: Luchetti R, Pegoli L, Bain G, editors. Hand and wrist injuries in combat sports. Cham: Springer; 2018. p. 297–303.
146. Chao S, Pacella M, Torg J. The pathomechanics, pathophysiology and prevention of cervical spinal cord and brachial plexus injuries in athletics. Sports Med. 2012;40(1):59–75.
147. Robertson WC, Eichman PL, Clancy WG. Upper trunk brachial plexopathy in football players. JAMA. 1979;241:1480–2.
148. Belviso I, Palermi S, Sacco AM, Romano V, Corrado B, Zappia M, Sirico F. Brachial plexus injuries in sports medicine: clinical evaluation, diagnostic approaches, treatment options and rehabilitative interventions. J Funct Morphol Kinesiol. 2020;5(2):22. https://doi.org/10.3390/jfmk5020022.
149. Srivastava PK. High resolution ultrasound of brachial plexus. Ultrasound Med Biol. 2017;43(suppl1):S242.
150. Lorei M, Hershman E. Peripheral nerve injuries in athletes. Sports Med. 2012;16(2):130–47.
151. Lu J, Haman SP, Ebraheim NA. Vulnerability of the spinal accessory nerve in the posterior triangle of the neck: a cadaveric study. Healio Orthop. 2002;25(1):71–4.
152. Canella C, Demondion X, Abreu E, Marchiori E, Cotten H, Cotton A. Anatomical study of spinal accessory nerve using ultrasonography. Eur J Radiol. 2013;82(1):56–61.
153. Bodner G, Harpf C, Gardetto A, Kovacs P, Gruber H, Peer S, Mallhoui A. Ultrasonography of the accessory nerve: normal and pathologic findings in cadavers and patients with iatrogenic accessory nerve palsy. J Ultrasound Med. 2002;21(10):1159–63.
154. Üstün ÖS. Isolated long thoracic nerve injury case presentation: a sports injury. Acta Neurol Belg. 2020;120(1):199–200.
155. Inman VT, Saunders JB, Abbott LC. Observations on the function of the shoulder joint. J Bone Joint Surg. 1944;26:1–30.
156. Williams A, Smith H. Anatomical entrapment of the dorsal scapular and long thoracic nerves, secondary to brachial plexus piercing variation. Anat Sci Int. 2019;95(1):67–75.
157. Wiater JM, Flatow EL. Long thoracic nerve injury. Clin Orthop Relat Res. 1999;368:17–27.
158. Chang KV, Wu WT, Mezian K, Nanka O, Ozcakar L. Sonoanatomy revisited: long thoracic nerve. Med Ultrason. 2019;21(3):349–52.
159. Nuber GW, McCarthy WJ. Neurovascular disorders: clinical assessment and treatment. In: Jobe FW, editor. Operative techniques in upper extremity sports injuries. St Louis: Mosby; 1996. p. 373–87.
160. Cummins C, Bowen M, Anderson K, Messer T. Suprascapular nerve entrapment at the spinoglenoid notch in a professional baseball pitcher. Am J Sports Med. 1999;27(6):810–2.
161. Contemori S, Biscarini A. Shoulder position sense in volleyball players with infraspinatus atrophy secondary to suprascapular nerve neuropathy. Scand J Med Sci Sports. 2018;28(1):267–75.
162. Safran M. Nerve injury about the shoulder in athletes, part 1. Am J Sports Med. 2004;32(3):803–19.
163. Becker J. Infraspinatus atrophy in a volleyball player a case of a Bennett lesion causing nerve impingement. Curr Sports Med Rep. 2014;13(6):358–60.
164. Yücesoy C, Akkaya T, Özel O, Cömert A, Tüccar E, Bedirli N, Ünlü E, Hekimoğlu B, Gümüş H. Ultrasonographic evaluation and morphometric measurements of the suprascapular notch. Surg Radiol Anat. 2009;31(6):409–14.
165. Perlmutter G, Apruzzese W. Axillary nerve injuries in contact sports. Sports Med. 2012;26(5):351–61.
166. Lee S, Saetia K, Saha S, Kline DG, Kim DH. Axillary nerve injury associated with sports. J Neurosurg. 2011;31(5):E10. https://doi.org/10.3171/2011.8.FOCUS11183.

167. Feng S, Hsiao M, Wu C, Özçakar L. Ultrasound-guided diagnosis and management for quadrilateral spsce Syndrome. Pain Med. 2017;18(1):184–6.
168. Gruber H, Peer S, Loescher W, Bauer T, Loizides A. Ultrasound imaging of the axillary nerve and its role in the diagnosis of traumatic impairment. Ultraschall Med. 2014;35(4):332–8.
169. Guerri-Guttenberg R, Ingolotti M. Classifying musculocutaneous nerve variations. Clin Anat. 2009;22(6):671–83.
170. Papanikolaou A, Maris J, Tsampazis K. Isolated musculocutaneous nerve palsy after heavy physical activity. Injury Extra. 2005;36:486–8.
171. Mautner K, Keel JC. Musculocutaneous nerve injury after simulated free fall in a vertical wind-tunnel: a case report. Arch Phys Med Rehabil. 2007;88:391–3.
172. Blyth MJ, Macleod CM, Asante DK, Kinninmonth AW. Iatrogenic nerve injury with the Russell-Taylor humeral nail. Injury. 2003;34:227–8.
173. Gillingham BL, Mack GR. Compression of the lateral antebrachial cutaneous nerve by the biceps tendon. J Shoulder Elb Surg. 1996;5:330–2.
174. Tagliafico A, Michaud J, Marchetti A, Garello I, Padua L, Martinoli C. US imaging of the musculocutaneous nerve. Skeletal Radiol. 2011;40(5):609–16.
175. Lee MJ, LaStayo PC. Pronator syndrome and other nerve compressions that mimic carpal tunnel syndrome. J Orthop Sports Phys Ther. 2004;34(10):601–9.
176. Cass S. Upper extremity nerve entrapment syndromes in sports: an update. Curr Sports Med Rep. 2014;13(1):16–21.
177. Martinoli C, Bianchi S, Pugliese F, Bacigalupo L, Gauglio C, Valle M, Derchi L. Sonography of entrapment neuropathies in the upper limb (wrist excluded). J Clin Ultrasound. 2004;32(9):438–50.
178. Youngner J, Matsuo K, Grant T, Garg A, Samet J, Omar I. Sonographic evaluation of uncommonly assessed upper extremity peripheral nerves: anatomy, technique, and clinical syndromes. Skeletal Radiol. 2018;48(1):57–74.
179. Andrea C, PierLuigi B, Guglielmo L. Median nerve disorders at the elbow. In: Bain G, Eygendaal D, van Riet R, editors. Surgical techniques for trauma and sports related injuries of the elbow. Springer, Berlin, Heidelberg: Berlin, Heidelberg; 2019. p. 751–5.
180. Meirelles LM, Fernandes CH, Ejnisman B, Cohen M, Gomes dos Santos JB, Albertoni WM. The prevalence of carpal tunnel syndrome in adapted sports athletes based on clinical diagnostic. Orthop Traumatol Surg Res. 2020. https://doi.org/10.1016/j.otsr.2020.02.004.
181. Geoghegan L, Wormald J. Sport-related hand injury: a new perspective of e-sports. J Hand Surg (Eur Vol). 2019;44(2):219–20.
182. Akuthota V, Plastaras C, Lindberg K, Tobey J, Press J, Garvan C. The effect of long-distance bicycling on ulnar and median nerves. Am J Sports Med. 2005;33(8):1224–30.
183. Mousavi AA, Saied AR. Comparison of sonography and electrodiagnostic tests in diagnosis and treatment of carpal tunnel syndrome. World Appl Sci J. 2011;15:490–5.
184. Taylor-Gjevre RM, Gjevre JA, Nair B. Suspected carpal tunnel syndrome: do nerve conduction study results and symptoms match? Can Fam Phys. 2010;56:250–4.
185. Werner RA, Andary M. Electrodiagnostic evaluation of carpal tunnel syndrome. Muscle Nerve. 2011;44:597–607.
186. Aktürk S, Büyükavcı R, Ersoy Y. Median nerve ultrasound in carpal tunnel syndrome with normal electrodiagnostic tests. Acta Neurol Belg. 2020;120(1):43–7.
187. Mhoon J, Juel V, Hobson-Webb L. Median nerve ultrasound as a screening tool in carpal tunnel syndrome: correlation of cross-sectional area measures with electrodiagnostic abnormality. Muscle Nerve. 2012;46(6):861–70.
188. Cartwright M, Baute V, Caress J, Walker F. Ultrahigh-frequency ultrasound of fascicles in the median nerve at the wrist. Muscle Nerve. 2017;56(4):819–22.
189. Babaei-Ghazani A, Roomizadeh P, Nouri E, Raeisi G, Yousefi N, Asilian-mahabadi M, Moeini M. Ultrasonographic reference values for the median nerve at the level of pronator teres muscle. Surg Radiol Anat. 2018;40(9):1019–24.
190. Hide I, Grainger A, Naisby G, Campbell R. Sonographic findings in the anterior interosseous nerve syndrome. J Clin Ultrasound. 1999;27(8):459–64.
191. Malahias M, Chytas D, Mavrogenis A, Nikolaou V, Johnson E, Babis G. Platelet-rich plasma injections for carpal tunnel syndrome: a systematic and comprehensive review. Eur J Orthop Surg Traumatol. 2018;29(1):1–8.
192. Dowdle S, Chalmers P. Management of the Ulnar Nerve in throwing athletes. Curr Rev Musculoskelet Med. 2020;13:449–56.
193. Andrews JR. Bony injuries about the elbow in the throwing athletes. Instr Course Lect. 1985;34:323–31.
194. Mihata T, Akeda M, Kunzler M, McGarry MH, Neo M, Lee TQ. Ulnar collateral ligament insufficiency affects cubital tunnel syndrome during throwing motion: a cadaveric biomechanical study. J Shoulder Elb Surg. 2019;28(9):1758–63.
195. Maruyama M, Satake H, Takahara M, Harada M, Uno T, Mura N, Takagi M. Treatment for ulnar neuritis around the elbow in adolescent baseball players: factors associated with poor outcome. Am J Sports Med. 2017;45(4):803–9.
196. Sivak W, Hagerty S, Huyhn L, Jordan A, Munin M, Spiess A. Diagnosis of ulnar nerve entrapment at the arcade of struthers with electromyography and ultrasound. Plastic Reconstr Surg Global Open. 2016;4(3):e648.
197. Tubbs RS, Deep A, Shoja MM, Mortazavi MM, Loukas M, Cohen-Gadol AA. The arcade of

Struthers: an anatomical study with potential neurosurgical significance. Surg Neurol Int. 2011;2:184.

198. Elhassan B, Steinmann S. Entrapment neuropathy of the ulnar nerve. J Am Acad Orthop Surg. 2007;15(11):672–81.
199. Akyü MZ. Fit, Cyclist's neuropathy a compression syndrome of the deep motor branch of the ulnar nerve a case report. Neurosurg Q. 2015;25(3):337–40.
200. Doyle JR, Botte MJ. Surgical anatomy of the hand and upper extremity. Philadelphia, London: Lippincott, Williams and Wilkins; 2003. p. 575–81.
201. Wajid H, LeBlanc J, Shapiro D, Delzell P. Bowler's thumb: ultrasound diagnosis of a neuroma of the ulnar digital nerve of the thumb. Skeletal Radiol. 2016;45(11):1589–92.
202. Draghi F, Bortolotto C, Ballerini D, Preda L. Ultrasonography of the ulnar nerve in the elbow: video article. J Ultrasound, OnlineFirst. 2020;23(3):335–36
203. Ellegaard H, Fuglsang-Frederiksen A, Hess A, Johnsen B, Qerama E. High-resolution ultrasound in ulnar neuropathy at the elbow: a prospective study. Muscle Nerve. 2015;52(5):759–66.
204. Aird C, Thoirs K, Maranna S, Massy-Westropp N. Ultrasound measurements and assessments of the ulnar nerve at the elbow and cubital tunnel: a scoping review. J Diagn Med Sonogr. 2019;35(6):474–82.
205. Schneidl E, Bohm J, Farbaky Z, et al. Ultrasonography of ulnar neuropathy at the elbow: axonal involvement leads to greater nerve swelling than demyelinating nerve lesion. Clin Neurophysiol. 2013;124:619–5.
206. Riegler G, Lieba-Samal D, Brugger P, Pivec C, Platzgummer H, Vierhapper M, Muschitz G, Jengojan S, Bodner G. High-resolution ultrasound visualization of the deep branch of the ulnar nerve. Muscle Nerve. 2017;56(6):1101–7.
207. Cavaletti G, Marmiroli P, Alberti G, Michielon G, Tredici G. Sport-related peripheral nerve injuries: part 1. Sport Sci Health. 2004;1(2):55–60.
208. Dickerman RD, Stevens QEJ, Cohen AJ, Jaikumar S. Radial tunnel syndrome in an elite power athlete: a case of direct compressive neuropathy. J Peripher Nerve Sys. 2002;7:229–32.
209. Meng S, Tinhofer I, Weninger W, Grisold W. Ultrasound and anatomical correlation of the radial nerve at the arcade of Frohse. Muscle Nerve. 2015;51(6):853–8.
210. Dietz A, Bucelli R, Pestronk A, Zaidman C. Nerve ultrasound identifies abnormalities in the posterior interosseous nerve in patients with proximal radial neuropathies. Muscle Nerve. 2016;53(3):379–83.
211. Marchant MH, Gambardella RA, Podesta L. Superficial radial nerve injury after avulsion fracture of the brachioradialis muscle origin in a professional lacrosse player: a case report. J Shoulder Elb Surg. 2009;18(6):E9–E12.
212. Chang K, Hung C, Özçakar L. Snapping thumb and superficial radial nerve entrapment in De Quervain disease: ultrasound imaging/guidance revisited. Pain Med. 2015;16(11):2214–5.
213. Miller TT, Reinus WR. Nerve entrapment syndromes of the elbow, forearm and wrist. Am J Roentgenol. 2010;195(3):585–94.
214. Brant J, Johnson B, Brou L, Comstock R, Vu T. Rates and patterns of lower extremity sports injuries in all gender-comparable US high school sports. Orthop J Sports Med. 2019;7(10):1–7.
215. McGuine T, Bell D, Brooks M, Hetzel S, Pfaller A, Post E. The effect of sport specialization on lower extremity injury rates in high school athletes. Orthop J Sports Med. 2017;5(7_suppl6):1.
216. Poor A, Roedl J, Zoga A, Meyers W. Core muscle injuries in athletes. Curr Sports Med Rep. 2018;17(2):54–8.
217. Lynch T, Bedi A, Larson C. Athletic hip injuries. J Am Acad Orthop Surg. 2017;25(4):269–79.
218. Epstein DM, Mchugh M, Yorio M, Neri B. Intraarticular hip injuries in national hockey league players: a descriptive epidemiological study. Am J Sports Med. 2013;41(2):343–8.
219. Ekhtiari S, Khan M, Burrus T, Madden K, Gagnier J, Rogowski J, Maerz T, Bedi A. Hip and groin injuries in professional basketball players: impact on playing career and quality of life after retirement. Sports Health. 2019;11(3):218–22.
220. Maradit Kremers H, Larson DR, Crowson CS, et al. Prevalence of total hip and knee replacement in the United States. J Bone Joint Surg Am. 2015;97:1386–97.
221. Tak I, Glasgow P, Langhout R, Weir A, Kerkhoffs G, Agricola R. Hip range of motion is lower in professional soccer players with hip and groin symptoms or previous injuries, independent of cam deformities. Am J Sports Med. 2016;44(3):682–8.
222. Serner A, Weir A, Tol J, Thorborg K, Roemer F, Guermazi A, Yamashiro E, Hölmich P. Characteristics of acute groin injuries in the hip flexor muscles — a detailed MRI study in athletes. Scand J Med Sci Sports. 2018;28(2):677–85.
223. Eckard T, Padua D, Dompier T, Dalton S, Thorborg K, Kerr Z. Epidemiology of hip flexor and hip adductor strains in National Collegiate Athletic Association Athletes, 2009/2010-2014/2015. Am J Sports Med. 2017;45(12):2713–22.
224. Ralston B, Arthur J, Makovicka J, Hassebrock J, Tummala S, Deckey D, Patel K, Chhabra A, Hartigan D. Hip and groin injuries in National Collegiate Athletic Association Women's soccer players. Orthop J Sports Med. 2020;8(1):1–6.
225. Palisch A, Zoga AC, Meyers WC. Imaging of athletic pubalgia and core muscle injuries: clinical and therapeutic correlations. Clin Sports Med. 2013;32(3):427–47.
226. Meyers WC, Foley DP, Garrett WE, Lohnes JH, Mandlebaum BR. PAIN (Performing Athletes with Abdominal or Inguinal Neuromuscular Pain Study Group): management of severe lower abdominal or

inguinal pain in high-performance athletes. Am J Sports Med. 2000;28(1):2–8.
227. Zoga AC, Kavanagh EC, Omar IM, et al. Athletic pubalgia and "sports hernia": MR imaging findings. Radiology. 2008;247(3):797–807.
228. Kopelman D, Kaplan U, Hatoum OA, et al. The management of sportsman's groin hernia in professional and amateur soccer players: a revised concept. Hernia. 2016;20:69–75.
229. De Blaiser C, Roosen P, Willems T, Danneels L, Bossche LV, De Ridder R. Is care stability a risk factor for lower extremity injuries in an athletic population? A systematic review. Phys Ther Sport. 2018;30:48–56.
230. Via A, Frizziero A, Finotti P, Oliva F, Randelli F, Maffulli N. Management of osteitis pubis in athletes: rehabilitation and return to training – a review of the most recent literature. Open Access J Sports Med. 2018;10:1–10.
231. Economopoulos KJ, Milewski MD, Hanks JB, Hart JM, Diduch DR. Radiographic evidence of femoroacetabular impingement in athletes with athletic pubalgia. Sports Health. 2014;6(2):171–7.
232. Krishnamoorthy V, Kunze K, Beck E, Cancienne J, O'Keefe L, Ayeni O, Nho S. Radiographic prevalence of symphysis pubis abnormalities and clinical outcomes in patients with femoroacetabular impingement syndrome. Am J Sports Med. 2019;47(6):1467–72.
233. Frizziero A, Vittadini F, Pignataro F, et al. Conservative management of tendinopathies around hip. Muscles Ligaments Tendons J. 2016;6(3):281–92.
234. Brandon CJ, Jacobson JA, Fessell D, Dong Q, Morag Y, Girish G, Jamadar D. Groin pain beyond the hip: how anatomy predisposes to injury as visualized by musculoskeletal ultrasound and MRI. Am J Roentgenol. 2011;197(5):1190–7.
235. Campbell R. Ultrasound of the athletic groin. Semin Musculoskelet Radiol. 2013;17(1):34–42.
236. Lungu E, Michaud J, Bureau N. US assessment of sports-related hip injuries. Radiographics. 2018;38(3):867–89.
237. Kelly B, Weiland D, Schenker M, Philippon MJ. Arthroscopic labral repair in the hip: surgical technique and review of the literature. Arthroscopy. 2005;21:1496–504.
238. Wenger D, Kendell K, Miner M, Trousdale RT. Acetabular labral tears rarely occur in the absence of bony abnormalities. Clin Orthop Relat Res. 2004;426:145–50.
239. Rankin A, Bleakley C, Cullen M. Hip joint pathology as a leading cause of groin pain in the sporting population. Am J Sports Med. 2015;43(7):1698–703.
240. Aiba H, Watanabe N, Fukuoka M, Wada I, Murakami H. Radiographic analysis of subclinical appearances of the hip joint among patients with labral tears. J Orthop Surg Res. 2019;14(1):1–6.
241. Su T, Chen GX, Yang L. Diagnosis and treatment of labral tear. Chin Med J. 2019;132(2):211–9.
242. Fukushima K, Inoue G, Fujimaki H, Uchida K, Miyagi M, Nagura N, Uchiyama K, Takahira N, Takaso M. The cytokine expression in synovial membrane and the relationship with pain and pathological findings at hip arthroscopy. J Exp Orthop. 2017;4(1):1–7.
243. Lynch T, O'Connor M, Minkara A, Westermann R, Rosneck J. Biomarkers for femoroacetabular impingement and hip osteoarthritis: a systematic review and meta-analysis. Am J Sports Med. 2019;47(9):2242–50.
244. Mervak BM, Morag Y, Marcantonio D, Jacobson J, Brandon C, Fessell D. Paralabral cysts of the hip: sonographic evaluation with magnetic resonance arthrographic correlation. J Ultrasound Med. 2012;31(3):495–500.
245. Jin W, Kim KI, Rhyu KH, et al. Sonographic evaluation of the anterosuperior hip labral tears with magnetic resonance arthrographic correlation. J Ultrasound Med. 2012;31(3):439–47.
246. De Luigi A, Blatz D, Karam C, Gustin Z, Gordon A. Use of platelet-rich plasma for the treatment of acetabular labral tear of the hip. Am J Phys Med Rehabil. 2019;98(11):1010–7.
247. Kassarjian A, Rodrigo RM, Santisteban JM. Intrasmuscular degloving injuries to the rectus femoris: findings at MRI. Am J Roentgenol. 2014;202(5):W475–80.
248. Lutterbach-Penna RA, Kalume-Brigido M, Morag Y, Boon T, Jacobson JA, Fessell DP. Ultrasound of the thigh: focal, compartmental, or comprehensive examination? Am J Roentgenol. 2014;203(5):1085–92.
249. Bui K, Ilaslan H, Recht M, Sundaram M. Iliopsoas injury: an MRI study of patterns and prevalence correlated with clinical findings. Skeletal Radiol. 2008;37(3):245–9.
250. Anderson CN. Iliopsoas: pathology, diagnosis and treatment. Clin Sports Med. 2016;35(3):419–33.
251. Bouvard M, Roger B, Laffond J, Lippa A, Tassery F. Iliopsoas muscle injuries. In: Roger B, Guermazi A, Skaf A, editors. Muscle injuries in sport athletes. Sports and traumatology. Cham: Springer; 2017. p. 245–59.
252. Blankenbaker DG, Tuite MJ. Iliopsoas musculotendinous unit. Semin Musculoskelet Radiol. 2008;12(1):13–27.
253. Lyons JC, Peterson LF. The snapping iliopsoas tendon. Mayo Clin Proc. 1984;59:327–9.
254. Lee KS, Rosas HG, Phancao JP. Snapping hip: imaging and treatment. Semin Musculoskelet Radiol. 2013;17(3):286–94.
255. Tatu L, Parratte B, Vuillier F, Diop M, Monnier G. Descriptive anatomy of the femoral portion of the iliopsoas muscle. Anatomical basis of anterior snapping of the hip. Surg Radiol Anat. 2001;23:371–4.
256. Guillin R, Cardinal E, Bureau N. Sonographic anatomy and dynamic study of the normal iliopsoas musculotendinous junction. Eur Radiol. 2008;19(4):995–1001.
257. Deslandes M, Guillin R, Cardinal E, Hobden R, Bureau NJ. The snapping iliopsoas tendon; new

mechanisms using dynamic sonography. Am J Roentgenol. 2008;190:576–81.
258. Bureau NJ. Sonographic evaluation of the snapping hip syndrome. J Ultrasound Med. 2013;32(6):895–900.
259. Audenaert EA, Khanduja V, Claes P, Malviya A, Steenackers G. Mechanics of psoas tendon snapping. A virtual population study. Front Bioeng Biotechnol. 2020;8:264.
260. Flato R, Passanante G, Skalski M, Patel D, White E, Matcuk G. The iliotibial tract: imaging, anatomy, injuries, and other pathology. Skeletal Radiol. 2017;46(5):605–22.
261. Scillia A, Choo A, Milman E, et al. Snapping of the proximal hamstring origin: a rare cause of coxa saltans: a case report. J Bone Joint Surg Am. 2011;93:e1251–3.
262. Yen Y, Lewis CL, Kim Y. Understanding and treating the snapping hip. Sports Med Arthrosc Rev. 2015;23(4):194–9.
263. Pelsser V, Cardinal E, Hobden R, et al. Extra-articular snapping hip: sonographic findings. Am J Roentgenol. 2001;176:67–73.
264. Potalivo G, Bugiantella W. Snapping hip syndrome: systematic review of surgical treatment. Hip Int. 2017;27(2):111–21.
265. Krishnamurthy G, Connolly B, Narayanan U, Babyn P. Imaging findings in external snapping hip syndrome. Pediatr Radiol. 2007;37(12):1272–4.
266. Via AG, Fioruzzi A, Randelli F. Diagnosis and management of snapping hip syndrome: a comprehensive review of literature. Rheumatol Curr Res. 2017;17(4):1–7.
267. Walker-Santiago R, Wojnowski NM, Lall AC, Maldonado DR, Rabe SM, Domb BG. Platelet-rich plasma versus surgery for the management of recalcitrant greater trochanteric pain syndrome: a systematic review. Arthroscopy. 2020;36(3):875–88.
268. Lewis CL. Extra-articular snapping hip: a literature review. Sports Health. 2010;2(3):186–90.
269. Pierce T, Kurowicki J, Issa K, Festa A, Scillia A, McInerney V. External snapping hip: a systematic review of outcomes following surgical intervention: external snapping hip systematic review. Hip Int. 2018;28(5):468–72.
270. Ekstrand J, Hagglund M, Walden M. Injury incidence and injury patterns in professional football: the UEFA injury study. Br J Sports Med. 2011;45(7):553–8.
271. Alzahrani M, Aldebeyan S, Abduljabbar F, Martineau P. Hamstring injuries in athletes: diagnosis and treatment. JBJS Rev. 2015;3(6):11.
272. Chu S, Rho M. Hamstring injuries in the athlete: diagnosis, treatment, and return to play. Curr Sports Med Rep. 2016;15(3):184–90.
273. Orchard J, Best TM, Verrall GM. Return to play following muscle strains. Clin J Sport Med. 2005;15:436–41.
274. Heiderscheit BC, Sherry MA, Silder A, et al. Hamstring strain injuries: recommendations for diagnosis, rehabilitation and injury prevention. J Orthop Sports Phys Ther. 2010;40:67–81.
275. van der Made A, Tol J, Reurink G, Peters R, Kerkhoffs G. Potential hamstring injury blind spot: we need to raise awareness of proximal hamstring tendon avulsion injuries. Br J Sports Med. 2019;53(7):390–2.
276. Askling CM, Tengvar M, Saartok T, Thorstensson A. Acute first-time hamstring strains during slow-speed stretching: clinical, magnetic resonance imaging and recovery characteristics. Am J Sports Med. 2007;35(10):1716–24.
277. Kenneally-Dabrowski C, Brown N, Lai A, Perriman D, Spratford W, Serpell B. Late swing or early stance? A narrative review of hamstring injury mechanisms during high-speed running. Scand J Med Sci Sports. 2019;29(8):1083–91.
278. Made A, Wieldraaijer T, Kerkhoffs G, Kleipool R, Engebretsen L, Dijk C, Golanó P. The hamstring muscle complex. Knee Surg Sports Traumatol Arthrosc. 2015;23(7):2115–22.
279. Irger M, Willinger L, Lacheta L, Pogorzelski J, Imhoff A, Feucht M. Proximal hamstring tendon avulsion injuries occur predominately in middle-aged patients with distinct gender differences: epidemiologic analysis of 263 surgically treated cases. Knee Surg Sports Traumatol Arthrosc. 2020;28(4):1221–9.
280. Stępień K, Śmigielski R, Mouton C, Ciszek B, Engelhardt M, Seil R. Anatomy of proximal attachment, course, and innervation of hamstring muscles: a pictorial essay. Knee Surg Sports Traumatol Arthrosc. 2018;27(3):673–84.
281. Beatty N, Félix I, Hettler J, Moley P, Wyss J. Rehabilitation and prevention of proximal hamstring tendinopathy. Curr Sports Med Rep. 2017;16(3):162–71.
282. Degen R. Proximal hamstring injuries: management of tendinopathy and avulsion injuries. Curr Rev Musculoskelet Med. 2019;12(2):138–46.
283. Brucker PU, Imhoff AB. Functional assessment after acute and chronic ruptures of the proximal hamstring tendons. Knee Surg Sports Traumatol Arthrosc. 2005;13(5):411–8.
284. Cohen SB, Rangavajjula A, Vyas D, Bradley JP. Functional results and outcomes after repair of proximal hamstring avulsions. Am J Sports Med. 2012;40(9):2092–8.
285. Seow D, Shimozono Y, Tengku Yusof T, Yasui Y, Massey A, Kennedy J. Platelet-rich plasma injection for the treatment of hamstring injuries: a systematic review and meta-analysis with best-worst case analysis. Am J Sports Med. 2020;1:1–9.
286. Manduca M, Straub S. Effectiveness of PRP injection in reducing recovery time of acute hamstring injury: a critically appraised topic. J Sport Rehabil. 2018;27(5):480–4.
287. Bradley J, Lawyer T, Ruef S, Towers J, Arner J. Platelet-rich plasma shortens return to play in National Football League Players with acute hamstring injuries. Orthop J Sports Med. 2020;8(4):1–5.

288. Wilson T, Spinner R, Mohan R, Gibbs C, Krych A. Sciatic nerve injury after proximal hamstring avulsion and repair. Orthop J Sports Med. 2017;5(7):1–8.
289. Subbu R, Benjamin-Laing H, Haddad F. Timing of surgery for complete proximal hamstring avulsion injuries. Am J Sports Med. 2015;43(2):385–91.
290. Willinger L, Siebenlist S, Lacheta L, Wurm M, Irger M, Feucht M, Imhoff A, Forkel P. Excellent clinical outcome and low complication rate after proximal hamstring tendon repair at mid-term follow up. Knee Surg Sports Traumatol Arthrosc. 2020;28(4):1230–5.
291. Ekstrand J, Healy JC, Walden M, et al. Hamstring muscle injuries in professional football: the correlation of MRI findings with return to play. Br J Sports Med. 2012;46:112–7.
292. Chan O, Del Buono A, Best TM, Maffuli N. Acute muscle strain injuries: a proposed new classification system. Knee Surg Sports Traumatol Athrosc. 2012;20:2356–62.
293. Pollock N, James SLJ, Lee JC, Chakraverty R. British athletics muscle injury classification: a new grading system. Br J Sports Med. 2014;48:1347–51.
294. Wangensteen A, Guermazi A, Tol J, Roemer F, Hamilton B, Alonso J, Whiteley R, Bahr R. New MRI muscle classification systems and associations with return to sport after acute hamstring injuries: a prospective study. Eur Radiol. 2018;28(8):3532–41.
295. Eggleston L, McMeniman M, Engstrom C. High-grade intramuscular tendon disruption in acute hamstring injury and return to play in Australian Football players. Scand J Med Sci Sports. 2020;30(6):1073–82.
296. Gaballah A, Elgeidi A, Bressel E, Shakrah N, Abd-Alghany A. Rehabilitation of hamstring strains: does a single injection of platelet-rich plasma improve outcomes? (clinical study). Sport Sci Health. 2018;14(2):439–47.
297. Wangensteen A, Tol J, Witvrouw E, Van Linschoten R, Almusa E, Hamilton B, Bahr R. Hamstring Reinjuries occur at the same location and early after return to sport. Am J Sports Med. 2016;44(8):2112–21.
298. Vatovec R, Kozinc Z, Šarabon N. Exercise interventions to prevent hamstring injuries in athletes: a systematic review and meta-analysis. Eur J Sport Sci. 2021;20(7):992–04
299. Crema M, Guermazi A, Reurink G, Roemer F, Maas M, Weir A, Moen M, Goudswaard G, Tol J. Can a clinical examination demonstrate intramuscular tendon involvement in acute hamstring injuries? Orthop J Sports Med. 2017;5(10):1–8.
300. Dunlop G, Ardern C, Andersen T, Lewin C, Dupont G, Ashworth B, O'Driscoll G, Rolls A, Brown S, McCall A. Return-to-play practices following hamstring injury: a worldwide survey of 131 premier league football teams. Sports Med. 2020;50(4):829–40.
301. Gage BE, McIlvain NM, Collins CL, Fields SK, Comstock RD. Epidemiology of 6.6 million knee injuries presenting to United States emergency departments from 1999 through 2008. Acad Emerg Med. 2012;19(4):378–85.
302. Bien DP, Dubuque TJ. Considerations for late stage ACL rehabilitation and return to sport to limit re-injury risk and maximize athletic performance. Int J Sports Phys Ther. 2015;10:256–71.
303. Naraghi A, White L. Imaging of athletic injuries of knee ligaments and menisci: sports imaging series. Radiology. 2016;281(1):23–40.
304. Elkin J, Zamora E, Gallo R. Combined anterior cruciate ligament and medial collateral ligament knee injuries: anatomy, diagnosis, management recommendations, and return to sport. Curr Rev in Musculoskelet Med. 2019;12(2):239–44.
305. MacMahon PJ, Palmer WE. A biomechanical approach to MRI of acute knee injuries. Am J Roentgenol. 2011;197(3):568–77.
306. LaPrade RF, Wentorf FA, Fritts H, Gundry C, Hightower CD. A prospective magnetic resonance imaging study of the incidence of posterolateral and multiple ligament injuries in acute knee injuries presenting with a hemarthrosis. Arthroscopy. 2007;23(12):1341–7.
307. Benjaminse A, Gokeler A, van der Schans CP. Clinical diagnosis of an anterior cruciate ligament rupture: a meta-analysis. J Orthop Sports Phys Ther. 2006;36:267–88.
308. Lee S, Yun S. Efficiency of knee ultrasound for diagnosing anterior cruciate ligament and posterior cruciate ligament injuries: a systematic review and meta-analysis. Skeletal Radiol. 2019;48(10):1599–610.
309. Tsai WH, Chiang YP, Lew RJ. Sonographic examination of knee ligaments. Am J Phys Med Rehabil. 2015;94(8):e77–9.
310. Ptasznik R, Feller J, Bartlett J, Fitt G, Mitchell A, Hennessey O. The value of sonography in the diagnosis of traumatic rupture of the anterior cruciate ligament of the knee. Am J Roentgenol. 1995;164:1461–3.
311. Chylarecki C, Hierholzer G, Tabertshofer H. Ultrasound criteria of fresh rupture of the anterior cruciate ligament (in German). Unfallchirurgie. 1995;21:109–17.
312. Mautner K, Sussman WI, Nanos K, Blazuk J, Brigham C, Sarros E. Validity of indirect ultrasound findings in acute anterior cruciate ligament ruptures. J Ultrasound Med. 2019;38:1685–92.
313. Alazzawi S, Sukeik M, Ibrahim M, Haddad F. Management of anterior cruciate ligament injury: pathophysiology and treatment. Br J Hosp Med. 2016;77(4):222–5.
314. Van der List JP, Mintz DN, DiFelice GS. The location of anterior cruciate ligament tears: a prevalence study using magnetic resonance imaging. Orthop J Sports Med. 2017;5:2325967117709966.
315. Webster K, Feller J, Kimp A, Whitehead T. Low rates of return to preinjury sport after bilateral anterior cruciate ligament reconstruction. Am J Sports Med. 2019;47(2):334–8.

316. Lindanger L, Strand T, Mølster A, Solheim E, Inderhaug E. Return to play and long-term participation in pivoting sports after anterior cruciate ligament reconstruction. Am J Sports Med. 2019;47(14):3339–46.
317. Clifford A, Buckley E, O'Farrell D, Louw Q, Moloney C. Fear of movement in patients after anterior cruciate ligament reconstruction. Physiother Pract Res. 2017;38(2):113–20.
318. Faleide A, Inderhaug E, Vervaat W, Breivik K, Bogen B, Mo I, Trøan I, Strand T, Magnussen L. Anterior cruciate ligament—return to sport after injury scale: validation of the Norwegian language version. Knee Surg Sports Traumatol Arthrosc. 2020;OnlineFirst:1–10.
319. Hirohata K, Aizawa J, Furuya H, Mitomo S, Ohmi T, Ohji S, Ohara T, Koga H, Yagishita K, Webster K. The Japanese version of the anterior cruciate ligament-return to sport after injury (ACL-RSI) scale has acceptable validity and reliability. Knee Surg Sports Traumatol Arthrosc. 2020;OnlineFirst:1–7.
320. Webster K, Hewett T. What is the evidence for and validity of return-to-sport testing after anterior cruciate ligament reconstruction surgery? A systematic review and meta-analysis. Sports Med. 2019;49(6):917–29.
321. Undheim MB, Cosgrave C, King E, et al. Isokinetic muscle strength and readiness to return to sport following anterior cruciate ligament reconstruction: is there an association? A systematic review and a protocol recommendation. Br J Sports Med. 2015;49:1305–10.
322. Keays S, Newcombe P, Keays A. Nearly 90% participation in sports activity 12years after non-surgical management for anterior cruciate ligament injury relates to physical outcome measures. Knee Surg Sports Traumatol Arthrosc. 2018;27(8):2511–9.
323. Patterson B, Culvenor A, Barton C, Guermazi A, Stefanik J, Morris H, Whitehead T, Crossley K. Worsening knee osteoarthritis features on magnetic resonance imaging 1 to 5 years after anterior cruciate ligament reconstruction. Am J Sports Med. 2018;46(12):2873–83.
324. Cheung E, DiLallo M, Feeley B, Lansdown D. Osteoarthritis and ACL reconstruction—myths and risks. Curr Rev Musculoskelet Med. 2020;13(1):115–22.
325. Wellsandt E, Failla M, Axe M, Snyder-Mackler L. Does anterior cruciate ligament reconstruction improve functional and radiographic outcomes over nonoperative management 5 years after injury? Am J Sports Med. 2018;46(9):2103–12.
326. Smith TO, Postle K, Penny F, McNamara I, Mann CJV. Is reconstruction the best management strategy for anterior cruciate ligament rupture? A systematic review and meta-analysis comparing anterior cruciate ligament reconstruction versus non-operative treatment. Knee. 2014;21:462–70.
327. Rothrauff B, Jorge A, de Sa D, Kay J, Fu F, Musahl V. Anatomic ACL reconstruction reduces risk of post-traumatic osteoarthritis: a systematic review with minimum 10-year follow-up. Knee Surg Sports Traumatol Arthrosc. 2020;28(4):1072–84.
328. Agarwalla A, Puzzitiello R, Liu J, Cvetanovich G, Gowd A, Verma N, Cole B, Forsythe B. Timeline for maximal subjective outcome improvement after anterior cruciate ligament reconstruction. Am J Sports Med. 2019;47(10):2501–9.
329. LaPrade R, Goodrich L, Phillips J, Dornan G, Turnbull T, Hawes M, Dahl K, Coggins A, Kisiday J, Frisbie D, Chahla J. Use of platelet-rich plasma immediately after an injury did not improve ligament healing, and increasing platelet concentrations was detrimental in an in vivo animal model. Am J Sports Med. 2018;46(3):702–12.
330. Wang D, Rodeo SA. Platelet-rich plasma in orthopaedic surgery: a critical analysis review. JBJS Rev. 2017;5(9):1–10.
331. Arthur J, Haglin J, Makovicka J, Chhabra A. Anatomy and biomechanics of the posterior cruciate ligament and their surgical implications. Sports Med Arthrosc Rev. 2020;28(1):e1–e10.
332. Fanelli GC, Edson CJ. Posterior cruciate ligament injuries in trauma patients: part II. Arthroscopy. 1995;11:526–9.
333. Petrigliano FA, McAllister DR. Isolated posterior cruciate ligament injuries of the knee. Sports Med Arthrosc Rev. 2006;14:206–12.
334. Verhulst F, MacDonald P. Diagnosing PCL injuries: history, physical examination, imaging studies, arthroscopic evaluation. Sports Med Arthrosc Rev. 2020;28(1):2–7.
335. Schlumberger M, Schuster P, Eichinger M, Mayer P, Mayr R, Immendörfer M, Richter J. Posterior cruciate ligament lesions are mainly present as combined lesions even in sports injuries. Knee Surg Sports Traumatol Arthrosc. 2020;OnlineFirst:1–8.
336. Sekiya JK, Haemmerle MJ, Stabile KJ, et al. Biomechanical analysis of a combined double-bundle posterior cruciate ligament and posterolateral corner reconstruction. Am J Sports Med. 2005;33:360–9.
337. Apsingi S, Nguyen T, Bull AM, et al. The role of PCL reconstruction in knees with combined PCL and posterolateral corner deficiency. Knee Surg Sports Traumatol Arthrosc. 2008;16:104–11.
338. Petrillo S, Volpi P, Papalia R, Maffulli N, Denaro V. Management of combined injuries of the posterior cruciate ligament and posterolateral corner of the knee: a systematic review. Br Med Bull. 2017;123(1):47–57.
339. Kannus P, Bergfeld J, Jarvinen M, et al. Injuries to the posterior cruciate ligament of the knee. Sports Med. 1991;12:110–31.
340. Owesen C, Sandven-Thrane S, Lind M, Forssblad M, Granan LP, Aroen A. Epidemiology of surgically treated posterior cruciate ligament injuries in

Scandinavia. Knee Surg Sports Traumatol Arthrosc. 2017;25:2384–91.
341. Wang D, Graziano J, Williams R, Jones K. Nonoperative treatment of PCL injuries: goals of rehabilitation and the natural history of conservative care. Curr Rev Musculoskelet Med. 2018;11(2):290–7.
342. Xu B, Xu H, Tu J, et al. Initial assessment and implications for surgery: the missed diagnosis of irreducible knee dislocation. J Knee Surg. 2018;31:254–63.
343. DePhillipo N, Cinque M, Godin J, Moatshe G, Chahla J, LaPrade R. Posterior tibial translation measurements on magnetic resonance imaging improve diagnostic sensitivity for chronic posterior cruciate ligament injuries and graft tears. Am J Sports Med. 2018;46(2):341–7.
344. Ringler MD, Shotts EE, Collins MS, et al. Intra-articular pathology associated with isolated posterior cruciate ligament injury on MRI. Skeletal Radiol. 2016;45:1695–703.
345. Wang L, Yang T, Huang Y, Chou W, Huang C, Wang C. Evaluating posterior cruciate ligament injury by using two-dimensional ultrasonography and sonoelastography. Knee Surg Sports Traumatol Arthrosc. 2016;25(10):3108–15.
346. Miller T. Sonography of injury of the posterior cruciate ligament of the knee. Skeletal Radiol. 2002;31(3):149–54.
347. Suzuki S, Kasahara K, Futami T, Iwasaki R, Ueo T, Yamamuro T. Ultrasound diagnosis of pathology of the anterior and posterior cruciate ligaments of the knee joint. Arch Orthop Trauma Surg. 2004;110(4):200–3.
348. Sekiya JK, Swaringen JC, Wojtys EM, Jacobson JA. Diagnostic ultrasound evaluation of posterolateral corner knee injuries. Arthroscopy. 2010;26(4):494–9.
349. Shelbourne KD, Davis TJ, Patel DV. The natural history of acute, isolated, nonoperatively treated posterior cruciate ligament injuries: a prospective study. Am J Sports Med. 1999;27(3):276–83.
350. Akisue T, Kurosaka M, Yoshiya S, Kuroda R, Mizuno K. Evaluation of healing of the injured posterior cruciate ligament: analysis of instability and magnetic resonance imaging. Arthroscopy. 2001;17(3):264–9.
351. Rodriguez W Jr, Vinson EN, Helms CA, Toth AP. MRI appearance of posterior cruciate ligament tears. Am J Roentgenol. 2008;191(4):1031.
352. Chan TW, Kong CC, del Buono A, et al. Acute augmentation for interstitial insufficiency of the posterior cruciate ligament. A two to five year clinical and radiographic study. Muscles Ligaments Tendon J. 2016;6:58–63.
353. Mariani PP, Margheritini F, Christel P, Bellelli A. Evaluation of posterior cruciate ligament healing: a study using magnetic resonance imaging and stress radiography. Arthroscopy. 2005;21(11):1354–61.
354. Vermeijden H, van der List J, DiFelice G. Arthroscopic posterior cruciate ligament primary repair. Sports Med Arthrosc Rev. 2020;28(1):23–9.
355. Bushnell BD, Bitting SS, Crain JM, Boublik M, Schlegel TF. Treatment of magnetic resonance imaging-documented isolated grade III lateral collateral ligament injuries in National Football League athletes. Am J Sports Med. 2010;38(1):86–91.
356. Grawe B, Schroeder AJ, Kakazu R, Messer MS. Lateral collateral ligament injury about the knee: anatomy, evaluation, and management. J Am Acad Orthop Surg. 2018;26(6):e120–7.
357. Wilson WT, Deakin AH, Payne AP, Picard F, Wearing SC. Comparative analysis of the structural properties of the collateral ligaments of the human knee. J Orthop Sports Phys Ther. 2012;42(4):345–51.
358. Buzzi R, Aglietti P, Vena LM, Giron F. Lateral collateral ligament reconstruction using a semitendinous graft. Knee Surg Sports Traumatol Arthrosc. 2004;12(1):36–42.
359. Lim HC, Bae JH, Bae TS, Moon BC, Shyam AK, Wang JH. Relative role changing of lateral collateral ligament on the posterolateral rotatory instability according to the knee flexion angles: a biomechanical comparative study of role of lateral collateral ligament and popliteofibular ligament. Arch Orthop Trauma Surg. 2012;132(11):1631–6.
360. Coobs BR, LaPrade RF, Griffith CJ, Nelson BJ. Biomechanical analysis of an isolated fibular (lateral) collateral ligament reconstruction using an autogenous semitendinosus graft. Am J Sports Med. 2007;35(9):1521–7.
361. Devitt BM, Whelan DB. Physical examination and imaging of the lateral collateral ligament and posterolateral corner of the knee. Sports Med Arthrosc. 2015;23(1):10–6.
362. Claes S, Vereecke E, Maes M, Victor J, Verdonk P, Bellemans J. Anatomy of the anterolateral ligament of the knee. J Anat. 2013;223(4):321–8.
363. Temponi E, Saithna A, de Carvalho L, Teixeira B, Sonnery-Cottet B. Nonoperative treatment for partial ruptures of the lateral collateral ligament occurring in combination with complete ruptures of the anterolateral ligament: a common injury pattern in Brazilian Jiu-Jitsu athletes with acute knee injury. Orthop J Sports Med. 2019;7(1):1–7.
364. Davis BA, Hiller LP, Imbesi SG, Chang EY. Isolated lateral collateral ligament complex injury in rock climbing and Brazilian jiu-jitsu. Skeletal Radiol. 2015;44(8):1175–9.
365. Rosas H. Unraveling the posterolateral corner of the knee. Radiographics. 2016;36(6):1776–91.
366. Shekari I, Shekarchi B, Abbasian M, Minator Sajjadi M, Momeni Moghaddam A, Kazemi S. Predictive factors associated with anterolateral ligament injury in the patients with anterior cruciate ligament tear. Indian J Orthop. 2020;OnlineFirst:1–10.
367. Warren R. Editorial commentary: knee lateral collateral ligament injury is more common than we thought. Arthroscopy. 2019;33(12):2182–3.
368. Bonadio MB, Helito CP, Gury LA, Demange MK, Pecora JR, Angelini FJ. Correlation between mag-

netic resonance imaging and physical exam in assessment of injuries to posterolateral corner of the knee. Acta Ortop Bras. 2014;22(3):124–6.
369. Mirowitz SA, Shu HH. MR imaging evaluation of knee collateral ligaments and related injuries: comparison of T1-weighted, T2-weighted, and fat-saturated T2-weighted sequences. Correlation with clinical findings. J Magn Reson Imaging. 1994;4(5):725–32.
370. Cianca J, John J, Pandit S, Chiou-Tan FY. Musculoskeletal ultrasound imaging of the recently described anterolateral ligament of the knee. Am J Phys Med Rehabil. 2014;93(2):186.
371. Moulton S, Matheny L, James E, LaPrade R. Outcomes following anatomic fibular (lateral) collateral ligament reconstruction. Knee Surg Sports Traumatol Arthrosc. 2015;23(10):2960–6.
372. Silva A, Sampaio R. Anatomic ACL reconstruction: does the platelet-rich plasma accelerate tendon healing? Knee Surg Sports Traumatol Arthrosc. 2009;17(6):676–82.
373. Chen X, Jones I, Park C, Vangsness C. The efficacy of platelet-rich plasma on tendon and ligament healing: a systematic review and meta-analysis with bias assessment. Am J Sports Med. 2018;46(8):2020–32.
374. Reider B. Medial collateral ligament injuries in athletes. Sports Med. 2012;21(2):147–56.
375. Motamedi A, Gowd A, Nazemi A, Gardner S, Behrend C. Incidence, positional distribution, severity, and time missed in medial collateral ligament injuries of the knee in NCAA division I football athletes. J Am Acad Orthop Surg Global Res Rev. 2017;1(5):1–4.
376. Chen L, Kim P, Ahmad C, Levine W. Medial collateral ligament injuries of the knee: current treatment concepts. Curr Rev Musculoskelet Med. 2007;1(2):108–13.
377. Warren LF, Marshall JL. The supporting structures and layers on the medial side of the knee: an anatomical analysis. J Bone Joint Surg Am. 1979;61:56–62.
378. De Maeseneer M, Van Roy F, Lenchik L, Barbaix E, De Ridder F, Osteaux M. Medial capsular and supporting structures of the knee: MR imaging-anatomic correlation. Radiographics. 2000;20:83–9.
379. Nur H, Aytekin A, Gilgil E. Medial collateral ligament bursitis in a patient with knee osteoarthritis. J Back Musculoskelet Rehabil. 2018;31(4):589–91.
380. Gardiner JC, Weiss JA, Rosenberg TD. Strain in the human medial collateral ligament during valgus loading of the knee. Clin Orthop Relat Res. 2001;391:266–74.
381. Kramer D, Miller P, Berrahou I, Yen Y, Heyworth B. Collateral ligament knee injuries in pediatric and adolescent athletes. J Pediatr Orthop. 2020;40(2):71–7.
382. Wierer G, Milinkovic D, Robinson J, Raschke M, Weiler A, Fink C, Herbort M, Kittl C. The superficial medial collateral ligament is the major restraint to anteromedial instability of the knee. Knee Surg Sports Traumatol Arthrosc. 2020;OnlineFirst:1–12.
383. Craft J, Kurzweil P. Physical examination and imaging of medial collateral ligament and posteromedial corner of the knee. Sports Med Arthrosc Rev. 2015;23(2):e1–6.
384. Sanders TG, Miller MD. A systematic approach to magnetic resonance imaging interpretation of sports medicine injuries of the knee. Am J Sports Med. 2005;33:131–48.
385. Injuries, American Medical Association. Committee on the Medical Aspects of Sports, Subcommittee on Classification of Sports Injuries in Standard Nomenclature for Athletic Injuries. 1966. A.M.A. 99–100.
386. Taketomi S, Uchiyama E, Nakagawa T, et al. Clinical features and injury patterns of medial collateral ligament tibial side avulsions: "wave sign" on magnetic resonance imaging is essential for diagnosis. Knee. 2014;21(6):1151–5.
387. Boutin R, Fritz R, Walker R, Pathria M, Marder R, Yao L. Tears in the distal superficial medial collateral ligament: the wave sign and other associated MRI findings. Skeletal Radiol. 2020;49(5):747–56.
388. Maeseneer M, Marcelis S, Boulet C, Kichouh M, Shahabpour M, Mey J, Cattrysse E. Ultrasound of the knee with emphasis on the detailed anatomy of anterior, medial, and lateral structures. Skeletal Radiol. 2014;43(8):1025–39.
389. Yoshioka T, Akihiro K, Toshikatsu W, Katsuya A, Kenta U, Masataka S, Naoyuki O. The effects of plasma rich in growth factors (PRGF-Endoret) on healing of medial collateral ligament of the knee. Knee Surg Sports Traumatol Arthrosc. 2013;21(8):1763–9.
390. Yoshida M, Marumo K. An autologous leukocyte-reduced platelet-rich plasma therapy for chronic injury of the medial collateral ligament in the knee: a report of 3 successful cases. Clin J Sport Med. 2019;29(1):e4–6.
391. Godin J, Chahla J, Moatshe G, Kruckeberg B, Muckenhirn K, Vap A, Geeslin A, LaPrade R. A comprehensive reanalysis of the distal iliotibial band: quantitative anatomy, radiographic markers, and biomechanical properties. Am J Sports Med. 2017;45(11):2595–603.
392. Landreau P, Catteeuw A, Hamie F, Saithna A, Sonnery-Cottet B, Smigielski R. Anatomic study and reanalysis of the nomenclature of the anterolateral complex of the knee focusing on the distal iliotibial band: identification and description of the condylar strap. Orthop J Sports Med. 2019;7(1):1–9.
393. Terry GC, Hughston JC, Norwood LA. The anatomy of iliopatellar band and iliotibial tract. Am J Sports Med. 1986;14(1):39–45.
394. Batty L, Murgier J, O'Sullivan R, Webster K, Feller J, Devitt B. The Kaplan Fibers of the iliotibial band can be identified on routine knee magnetic resonance imaging. Am J Sports Med. 2019;47(12):2895–903.
395. Batty L, Murgier J, Feller J, O'Sullivan R, Webster K, Devitt B. Radiological identification of injury to the Kaplan Fibers of the iliotibial band in association

with anterior cruciate ligament injury. Am J Sports Med. 2020;48(9):2213–20.
396. Herbst E, Albers M, Burnham J, Shaikh H, Naendrup J, Fu F, Musahl V. The anterolateral complex of the knee: a pictorial essay. Knee Surg Sports Traumatol Arthrosc. 2017;25(4):1009–14.
397. Getgood A, Brown C, Lording T, Amis A, Claes S, Geeslin A, Musahl V. The anterolateral complex of the knee: results from the international ALC consensus group meeting. Knee Surg Sports Traumatol Arthrosc. 2018;27(1):166–76.
398. Sinclair J, Ingram J, Butters B, Brooks D, Stainton P, Taylor P. A three-experiment examination of iliotibial band strain characteristics during different conditions using musculoskeletal simulation. Sport Sci Health. 2020;16(4):727–36
399. Jiménez Díaz F, Gitto S, Sconfienza L, Draghi F. Ultrasound of iliotibial band syndrome. J Ultrasound. 2020;23:379–85.
400. Abdelshahed D, Neuman S, Oh-Park M. Dynamic change in ultrasonographic findings in iliotibial band syndrome after running. Am J Phys Med Rehabil. 2018;97(2):e13.
401. Jain N, Bauman P, Hamilton WG, Merkle A, Adler RS. Can elite dancers return to dance after ultrasound-guided platelet-rich plasma injections? J Dance Med Sci. 2018;22(4):225–32.
402. Golman M, Wright M, Wong T, Lynch T, Ahmad C, Thomopoulos S, Popkin C. Rethinking patellar tendinopathy and partial patellar tendon tears: a novel classification system. Am J Sports Med. 2020;48(2):359–69.
403. Pang J, Shen S, Pan WR, Jones IR, Rosen WM, Taylor GI. The arterial supply of the patellar tendon: anatomical study with clinical implications for knee surgery. Clin Anat. 2009;22(3):371–6.
404. Zhang C, Couppé C, Scheijen J, Schalkwijk C, Kjaer M, Magnusson S, Svensson R. Regional collagen turnover and composition of the human patellar tendon. J Appl Physiol. 2020;128(4):884–91.
405. Liam OB, Engebretsen L, Bahr R. Prevalence of jumper's knee among elite athletes from different sports: a cross-sectional study. Am J Sports Med. 2005;33:561–7.
406. Di Matteo B, Filardo G, Kon E, Marcacci M. Platelet-rich plasma: evidence for the treatment of patellar and Achilles tendinopathy—a systematic review. Musculoskelet Surg. 2014;99(1):1–9.
407. Le A, Enweze L, DeBaun M, Dragoo J. Current clinical recommendations for use of platelet-rich plasma. Curr Rev Musculoskelet Med. 2018;11(4):624–34.
408. Blake M, Lattermann C, Johnson D. MRI and arthroscopic evaluation of meniscal injuries. Sports Med Arthros Rev. 2017;25(4):219–26.
409. Clayton RA, Court-Brown CM. The epidemiology of musculoskeletal tendinous and ligamentous injuries. Injury. 2008;39:1338–44.
410. Kosy J, Matteliano L, Rastogi A, Pearce D, Whelan D. Meniscal root tears occur frequently in multi-ligament knee injury and can be predicted by associated MRI injury patterns. Knee Surg Sports Traumatol Arthrosc. 2018;26(12):3731–7.
411. Vaishya R, Kambhampati S, Vaish A. Meniscal injuries in the Olympic and elite athletes. Indian J Orthop. 2020;54(3):281–93.
412. Xia X, Chen H, Zhou B. Ultrasonography for meniscal injuries in knee joint: a systematic review and meta-analysis. J Sports Med Phys Fitness. 2017;56(10):1179–87.
413. Cook JL, Cook CR, Stannard JP, Vaughn G, et al. MRI versus ultrasonography to assess meniscal abnormalities in acute knees. J Knee Surg. 2014;27:319–24.
414. Hashemi S, Ranjbar M, Tahami M, Shahriarirad R, Erfani A. Comparison of accuracy in expert clinical examination versus magnetic resonance imaging and arthroscopic exam in diagnosis of meniscal tear. Adv Orthop. 2020;2020:1895852.
415. Bhan K. Meniscal tears: current understanding, diagnosis, and management. Cureus. 2020;12(6):1–8.
416. Winkler P, Rothrauff B, Buerba R, Shah N, Zaffagnini S, Alexander P, Musahl V. Meniscal substitution, a developing and long-awaited demand. J Exp Orthop. 2020;7(1):1–15.
417. Belk J, Kraeutler M, Thon S, Littlefield C, Smith J, McCarty E. Augmentation of meniscal repair with platelet-rich plasma: a systematic review of comparative studies. Orthop J Sports Med. 2020;8(6):1–9.
418. Lucasti C, Dworkin M, Warrender W, Winters B, Cohen S, Ciccotti M, Pedowitz D. Ankle and lower leg injuries in professional baseball players. Am J Sports Med. 2020;48(4):908–15.
419. Seok H, Lee S, Yun S. Diagnostic performance of ankle ultrasound for diagnosing anterior talofibular and calcaneofibular ligament injuries: a meta-analysis. Acta Radiol. 2020;61(5):651–61.
420. D'Hooghe P, Cruz F, Alkhelaifi K. Return to play after a lateral ligament ankle sprain. Curr Rev Musculoskelet Med. 2020;13(3):281–8.
421. Anderson RL, Engebretsen L, Kennedy N, LaPrade R, Wegner AM, Giza E. Epidemiology and mechanisms and ankle pathology in football. In: The ankle in football. Paris: Springer; 2014. p. 31–59.
422. Ekstrand J, Hagglund M, Walden M. Injury incidence and injury patterns in professional football: the UEFA injury study. Br J Sports. 2011;45(7):553–8.
423. Vega J, Karlsson J, Kerkhoffs G, Dalmau-Pastor M. Ankle arthroscopy: the wave that's coming. Knee Surg Sports Traumatol Arthrosc. 2020;28(1):5–7.
424. Vega J, Malagelada F, Manzanares Céspedes M, Dalmau-Pastor M. The lateral fibulotalocalcaneal ligament complex: an ankle stabilizing isometric structure. Knee Surg Sports Traumatol Arthrosc. 2020;28(1):8–17.
425. Lee S, Yun S. Ankle ultrasound for detecting anterior talofibular ligament tear using operative finding as reference standard: a systematic review

and meta-analysis. Eur J Trauma Emerg Surg. 2020;46(1):73–81.

426. Chen Y, Cai Y, Wang Y. Value of ultrasonography for detecting chronic injury of the lateral ligaments compared with ultrasonography findings. Br J Radiol. 2014;87(1033):20130406

427. Chen E, McInnis K, Borg-Stein J. Ankle sprains: evaluation, rehabilitation, and prevention. Curr Sports Med Rep. 2019;18(6):217–23.

428. Tassignon B, Verschueren J, Delahunt E, Smith M, Vicenzino B, Verhagen E, Meeusen R. Criteria-based return to sport decision-making following lateral ankle sprain injury: a systematic review and narrative synthesis. Sports Med. 2019;49(4):601–19.

429. Prakash A. Epidemiology of high ankle sprains: a systematic review. Foot Ankle Spec. 2020;13(5):420–30.

430. Becciolini M, Bonacchi G, Stella S, Galletti S, Ricci V. High ankle sprain: sonographic demonstration of a posterior inferior tibiofibular ligament avulsion. J Ultrasound. 2020;23(3):431–3.

431. Tampere T, D'Hooghe P. The ankle syndesmosis pivot shift "Are we reviving the ACL story?". Knee Surg Sports Traumatol Arthrosc. 2020;OnlineFirst:1–4.

432. Baldassarre R, Pathria M, Huang B, Dwek J, Fliszar E. Periosteal stripping in high ankle sprains: an association with osteonecrosis. Clin Imaging. 2020;67:237–45.

433. Randell M, Marsland D, Ballard E, Forster B, Lutz M. MRI for high ankle sprains with an unstable syndesmosis: posterior malleolus bone oedema is common and time to scan matters. Knee Surg Sports Traumatol Arthrosc. 2019;27(9):2890–7.

434. Calder J, Mitchell A, Lomax A, Ballal M, Grice J, van Dijk N, Lee J. The broken "Ring of Fire": a new radiological sign as predictor of syndesmosis injury? Orthop J Sports Med. 2017;5(3):2325967117695064.

435. Park J, Lee S, Choo H, Kim S, Gwak H, Lee S. Ultrasonography of the ankle joint. Ultrasonography. 2017;36(4):321–35.

436. Milz P, Milz S, Steenborn M, et al. Lateral ankle ligament and tibiofibular syndesmosis: 13 MHz frequency sonography and MRI compared in 20 patients. Act Orthop Scand. 1998;69:51–5.

437. Mei-Dan O, Kots E, Barchilon V, Massarwe S, Nyska M, Mann G. A dynamic ultrasound examination for the diagnosis of ankle syndesmotic injury in professional athletes: a preliminary study. Am J Sports Med. 2009;37(5):1009–16.

438. Fisher C, Rabbani T, Johnson K, Reeves R, Wood A. Diagnostic capability of dynamic ultrasound evaluation of supination-external rotation ankle injuries: a cadaveric study. BMC Musculoskelet Disord. 2019;20(1):1–7.

439. Hagemeijer N, Chang S, Saengsin J, Waryasz G, Kerkhoffs G, DiGiovanni C, Guss D. Reproducibility and reliability of dynamic ultrasound for evaluating tibiofibular translation in the sagittal plane. Foot Ankle Orthop. 2019;4(4):1.

440. Laver L, Carmont MR, McConkey MO, et al. Plasma rich in growth factors (PRGF) as a treatment for high ankle sprain in elite athletes: a randomized controlled trial. Knee Surg Sport Traumatol Arthrosc. 2015;23:3383–92.

441. Samra DJ, Sman AD, Rae K, et al. Effectiveness of a single platelet-rich plasma injection to promote recovery in rugby players with ankle syndesmosis injury. BMJ Open Sport Exerc Med. 2017;3:1–7.

442. Ferreira J, Vide J, Mendes D, Protásio J, Viegas R, Sousa M. Prognostic factors in ankle sprains: a review. EFORT Open Rev. 2020;5(6):334–8.

443. Wade F, Mok K, Fong D. Kinematic analysis of a televised medial ankle sprain. Asia Pac J Sports Med Arthrosc Rehabil Technol. 2018;2018(12):12–6.

444. Haynes J, Gosselin M, Cusworth B, McCormick J, Johnson J, Klein S. The arterial anatomy of the deltoid ligament: a cadaveric study. Foot Ankle Int. 2017;38(7):785–90.

445. Hintermann B, Boss A, Schafer D. Arthroscopic findings in patients with chronic ankle instability. Am J Sports Med. 2002;30(3):402–9.

446. Rosa I, Rodeia J, Fernandes P, Teixeira R, Saldanha T, Consciência J. Ultrasonographic assessment of deltoid ligament integrity in ankle fractures. Foot Ankle Int. 2020;41(2):147–53.

447. Acevedo J, Kreulen C, Cedeno A, Baumfeld D, Nery C, Mangone P. Technique for arthroscopic deltoid ligament repair with description of safe zones. Foot Ankle Int. 2020;41(5):605–11.

448. Salameh M, Alhammoud A, Alkhatib N, Attia A, Mekhaimar M, D'Hooghe P, Mahmoud K. Outcome of primary deltoid ligament repair in acute ankle fractures: a meta-analysis of comparative studies. Int Orthop. 2020;44(2):341–7.

449. Egger A, Berkowitz M. Achilles tendon injuries. Curr Rev Musculoskelet Med. 2017;10(1):72–80.

450. Park Y, Kim T, Choi G, Kim H. Achilles tendinosis does not always precede Achilles tendon rupture. Knee Surg Sports Traumatol Arthrosc. 2018;27(10):3297–303.

451. Wezenbeek E, Willems T, Mahieu N, Van Caekenberghe I, Witvrouw E, De Clercq D. Is Achilles tendon blood flow related to foot pronation? Scand J Med Sci Sports. 2017;27(12):1970–7.

452. Arner O, Lindholm A, Orell SR. Histologic changes in subcutaneous rupture of the Achilles tendon: a study of 74 cases. Acta Chir Scand. 1959;116(5-6):484–90.

453. Maffulli N, Via A, Oliva F. Chronic Achilles tendon rupture. Open Orthop J. 2017;11:660–9.

454. Barfred T. Achilles tendon rupture: etiology and pathogenesis of subcutaneous rupture on the basis of the literature and rupture experiments in rats. Acta Orthop Scand. 1973;44(suppl152):1–126.

455. Binkley HM, Douglass D, Phillips K, Wise SL. Rehabilitation and return to sport after nonsur-

gical treatment of Achilles tendon rupture. Strength Cond J. 2020;42(3):90–9.
456. Caldwell J, Lightsey H, Trofa D, Swindell H, Greisberg J, Vosseller J. Seasonal variation of Achilles tendon injury. JAAOS Global Res Rev. 2018;2(8):1–6.
457. Schwieterman B, Haas D, Columber K, Knupp D, Cook C. Diagnostic accuracy of physical examination tests of the ankle/foot complex: a systematic review. Int J Sports Phys Ther. 2013;8:416–26.
458. Bleakney RR, White LM, Maffuli N. Imaging of the Achilles tendon. Foot Ankle Clin. 2005;10:239–54.
459. Griffin MJ, Olson K, Heckmann N, Charlton TP. Realtime Achilles ultrasound Thompson (RAUT) test for the evaluation and diagnosis of acute achilles tendon rupture. Foot Ankle Int. 2017;38:36–40.
460. Meulenkamp B, Stacey D, Fergusson D, Hutton B, Mlis R, Graham I. Protocol for treatment of Achilles tendon ruptures; a systematic review with network meta-analysis. Syst Rev. 2018;7:247.
461. Aufwerber S, Heijne A, Edman G, Silbernagel K, Ackermann P. Does early functional mobilization affect long-term outcomes after an Achilles tendon rupture? A randomized clinical trial. Orthop J Sports Med. 2020;8(3):1–9.
462. Carpenter D, Dederer K, Weinhold P, Tennant J. Endoscopically assisted percutaneous Achilles tendon repair: a biomechanical and clinical pilot. Foot Ankle Orthop. 2019;4(4):1.
463. Lima M, Patel M, Kadakia A. Percutaneous treatment of Achilles tendon rupture: a patient report outcome study. Foot Ankle Orthop. 2019;4(4):1.
464. Neph A, Schroeder A, Enseki K, Everts P, Wang J, Onishi K. Role of mechanical loading for platelet-rich plasma-treated Achilles tendinopathy. Curr Sports Med Rep. 2020;19(6):209–16.
465. Boesen A, Boesen M, Hansen R, Barfod K, Lenskjold A, Malliaras P, Langberg H. Effect of platelet-rich plasma on nonsurgically treated acute Achilles tendon ruptures: a randomized, double-blinded prospective study. Am J Sports Med. 2020;48(9):2268–76.
466. Trofa D, Miller J, Jang E, Woode D, Greisberg J, Vosseller J. Professional athletes' return to play and performance after operative repair of an Achilles tendon rupture. Am J Sports Med. 2017;45(12):2864–71.
467. Washburn N, Onishi K, Wang J. Ultrasound elastography and ultrasound tissue characterisation for tendon evaluation. J Orthop Translat. 2018;15:9–20.
468. Taljanovic M, Gimber L, Becker G, Latt L, Klauser A, Melville D, Gao L, Witte R. Shear-wave elastography: basic physics and musculoskeletal applications. Radiographics. 2017;37(3):855–70.
469. Dischler JD, Baumer TG, Finkelstein E, Siegal DS, Bey MJ. Association between years of competition and shoulder function in collegiate swimmers. Sports Health. 2018;10(2):113–8.
470. Hackett L, Aveledo R, Lam P, Murrell G. Reliability of shear wave elastography ultrasound to assess the supraspinatus tendon: an intra and inter-rater in vivo study. Shoulder Elbow. 2020;12(1):18–23.
471. Prado-Costa R, Rebelo J, Monteiro-Barroso J, Preto A. Ultrasound elastography: compression elastography and shear-wave elastography in the assessment of tendon injury. Insights Imaging. 2018;9(5):791–814.
472. Gruber L, van Holsbeeck MT, Khoury V, Deml C, Gabl MF, Jaschke W, Klauser AS. Compliance assessment and flip-angle measurement of the median nerve: sonographic tools for carpal tunnel syndrome assessment? Eur Radiol. 2019;29:588–98.
473. van Ark M, Rabello L, Hoevenaars D, Meijerink J, van Gelderen N, Zwerver J, van den Akker-Scheek I. Inter- and intra-rater reliability of ultrasound tissue characterization (UTC) in patellar tendons. Scand J Med Sci Sports. 2019;29(8):1205–11.
474. Wezenbeek E, Mahieu N, Willems T, Van Tiggelen D, De Muynck M, De Clercq D, Witvrouw E. What does normal tendon structure look like? New insights into tissue characterization in the Achilles tendon. Scand J Med Sci Sports. 2017;27(7):746–53.
475. Van Holsbeeck MT, Soliman S, van Kerkhove F, Craig J. Advance musculoskeletal ultrasound techniques: what are the applications? Am J Roentgenol. 2020. https://doi.org/10.2214/AJR.20.22840.
476. Fischer C, Kunz P, Strauch M, Weber M, Doll J. Safety profile of musculoskeletal contrast-enhanced ultrasound with sulfur hexafluoride contrast agent. Ther Clin Risk Manag. 2020;16:269–80.

Part VII

Future of Regenerative Medicine

Regenerative Medicine: Challenges and Opportunities

23

Susan Plummer and Yasser El Miedany

Introduction

Regenerative medicine encompasses innovative interdisciplinary strategies which principally involves both cell and gene therapies, tissue engineering and non-biologic constructs and aims at tissue repair and regeneration. With its potential to create living and functional cells, the created living tissues can be used to replace or repair those which have sustained potentially irreparable damage due to disease, injury, trauma, age or attained through genetic and congenital defects [1]. Broadly, regenerative medical approaches include harnessing, guiding, stimulating or replacing endogenous repair or developmental processes. With the potential facility to produce life-saving therapies for some genetic diseases affecting skin or blood, regenerative medicine represents a substantial hope for managing obstinate disorders.

So far regenerative medicine has only proved itself and shown efficacy in just a few specific clinical conditions such as haematopoietic and dermatology conditions. Consequently the enthusiasm about regenerative medicine and its wide-ranging potential of disease management created a gap between anticipations and the authenticities of transforming technology into standard clinical practice [2]. In mid-2020, the European Academies' Science Advisory Council (EASAC) and the Federation of European Academies of Medicine (FEAM) published their report on 'Challenges and Potential in Regenerative Medicine' [3] to highlight the challenges and opportunities of regenerative medicine for the scientific community, health services, regulating authorities, as well as policy-makers, and to deliver recommendations on the principles and options for change to inform the EU strategy.

For several years tissue engineering therapy was mostly confined to bone marrow transplantation for epidermis transplantation for large burns as well as haematological disorders. On their path to clinical translation, stem cell and gene therapies were confronted by enormous challenges—a status that started to change by the end of the 1990s. The past two decades have witnessed an exponential progress in experimental therapies as tissue engineering therapy started to enter the clinical arena. However, the outcomes of these clinical studies varied from unequivocal clinical efficacy for formerly intractable and incurable conditions to (more often) a modest or null effect. Elaboration of the underlying causes of such broad variation in the studies' outcomes

S. Plummer (✉)
Faculty of Medicine, Health and Social Care, Canterbury Christ Church University, Canterbury, Kent, UK
e-mail: susan.plummer@canterbury.ac.uk

Y. El Miedany
Institute of Medical Sciences, Canterbury Christ Church University, Canterbury, Kent, UK

Y. El Miedany (ed.), *Musculoskeletal Ultrasound-Guided Regenerative Medicine*,
https://doi.org/10.1007/978-3-030-98256-0_23

has further highlighted the challenges facing regenerative medicine.

This chapter will address some critical scientific issues for evidence-based implementation and regulation of regenerative medicine. It will start by addressing the challenges facing regenerative medicine, followed by the available opportunities and how to respond to these challenges. The chapter will conclude by a trial to answer the question: is there a bright future for regenerative medicine?

Challenges

Clinical

The Evidence Crisis

There is a main hurdle in the regenerative medicine field in that stem cell-based protocols are often applied to patients with very weak experimental base or understanding of the pathophysiology. Furthermore, the fact that the cells lack a precisely identifiable molecular and chemical structure makes its comparison to chemical compounds unapplicable. This has led to the conclusion that it is very difficult to standardise the research methodology [4]. This is further complicated by the finding that medicinal products used in regenerative research may vary when prepared in the variable research centres and even within the same centre if prepared at different times [5].

This data reflected on the smart trial designs and uniformity in reporting in regenerative medicine research. Whilst randomised control trials (RCTs) are considered the most commonly recognised as showing the most reliable evidence when assessing the safety and efficacy of a new therapeutic intervention and for gaining regulatory body sanctions [6], in the year 2019, only half of the 12 approved advanced therapy medicinal products (ATMPs) in Europe were tested in RCTs, and many of these used small sample sizes (ranging from 99 to 512). The other half were carried out only in single-arm studies (this is according to the European public assessment reports (EPAR) on the European Medicines Agency (EMA) website) [7].

But although it is tempting to insist that all new therapeutics should be evaluated in rigorous RCTs, this may not actually be possible for rare diseases that have few or no effective treatment options available [8]. It is therefore important to consider other measures that can help to improve the strength of evidence for cell and gene therapies [9]. For example, systematic reviews and meta-analyses pool data from multiple studies and registries and can be used to provide more precise estimates of effect or risk, particularly when results from individual trials are inconclusive.

Fortunately there are emerging methods of evidence synthesis designed to support decision-makers facing heterogeneous data. Evidence mapping is one such method which systematically depicts a broad (often heterogeneous) evidence body in order to identify knowledge gaps and opportunities for future research. In contrast to traditional systematic reviews and meta-analyses, whose results are typically presented in the form of dense tables and figures, evidence maps are most often designed to be user-friendly and interactive [10].

The considerably limited supporting clinical evidence for long-term safety and efficacy make it impossible to distinguish between 'good' and 'bad' clinical activity [1]. Furthermore, the absence of reliable clinical knowledge from trials makes it very difficult for both health-care professionals and patients who cannot be informed adequately of the risks and benefits of a certain treatment approach. Therefore more comprehensive reporting might be the clue to facilitate the development of rapid and reliable evidence and to promote valid pooling of data. In addition in a trial to tackle such challenge, innovative tools such as interactive and dynamic evidence maps could be used to track the evidence in real time and allow the field to make better sense of the heterogeneity across the total evidence landscape. In fact, combining these approaches would represent a significant step forward increasing confidence in the existing evidence and paving the way to a smooth integration of these innovative treatments into mainstream clinical practice [7].

Augmented Access

Another challenge results from the premature marketing approval and commercialisation of expensive approaches, facilitated by regulatory authority initiatives for accelerated access [5]. There is concern that schemes for conditional marketing approval lead to medicinal products with limited evidence of clinical benefit.

Distinguishing between the 'good' and the 'bad' clinical activity can be difficult. The biomedical companies might start working based on a rational hypothesis, gather some evidence and publish in reputable journals, but data can be inflated and inadequately replicated, whilst risk and benefit are inadequately ascertained [6]. Furthermore, granting conditional (accelerated) access transfers financial costs and the burdens of medical uncertainty from drug developers to health-care systems and consequently from trial participants (who should be required to undergo a rigorous informed consent process) to health-care consumers (who are not) [4].

One partial solution could be the adoption of novel regulatory models such as limited approval with intensive collection of new clinical evidence before a drug becomes universally available. As a further step, drugs that have not yet shown clinical outcome benefit could be made available at just the cost of production, or most profits could be kept in escrow, until adequate trials are completed [8, 9].

The EASAC-FEAM report [3] advises that in an era of international competitiveness when some regulatory frameworks have become increasingly permissive, it is essential that the EU does not lower its regulatory threshold without assessing the consequences for patient safety, health-care budgets and public trust in science [10, 11].

Commercial Clinics

Several new ATMPs face challenges particularly regarding manufacturing know-how, reimbursement and prices as well as having access to the market. This reflects the difficulties such companies face to make the leap from laboratory sense to commercial reality. Therefore many of these companies working in this field are trying hard to find approaches to unlock these products' potential [9].

Another challenge that remains unabated is the unregulated products and services which are offered in the commercial clinics, bringing high hopes of a broad range of positive outcomes but use poorly recognised therapies; ambiguous scientific rationale, with poor or low effectiveness evidence; and potential concerns regarding its safety concerns. This is presented in association with the primary intention of making financial profits [12]. In a trial to combat these issues, some principles have been suggested by the EASAC-FEAM who endorsed vibrant and available clinical efficacy evidence and to keep the patients who are contemplating such therapies fully informed. A vital criterion that should be highlighted, particularly for the patients making their decision whether to share in a novel clinical trial, is that they should not be expected to pay for clinical research [3].

Ethical and Governance Crisis

On engaging with the public, contacting the press and decision-making bodies in the variable national health systems, scientists face many ethical and governance issues. Political agendas may not match the public expectations. In some centres, a novel therapy authorisation might be a politically hot issue, even when effectiveness is unverified, and the cost to taxpayers means other patients may get deprived of effective and established treatments. Furthermore, there is evidence that some national regulatory systems have become too permissive, and there are examples (such as in Asia) where regulatory review pathways have been amended specifically to encourage approval of regenerative medicine [11, 13]. In other instances the regulatory authority allowed stem cells, if minimally manipulated and homologous, not to be subject to the same regulatory mechanism as drugs [14]. In addition it has been observed in the context of the recent controversy about synthetic trachea transplantation that part of the World Medical Association's Helsinki Declaration might be misinterpreted and merits revision to provide better safeguards against experimentation at the physician's own discretion [15].

The controversy about synthetic trachea transplantation is a very good example of the ethical and governance crisis that is worth mentioning to learn from. In January 2016 a documentary was aired on the public Swedish television [16, 17], telling the story of a thoracic surgeon (PM) at the Karolinska Institute in Stockholm and his trials to develop an innovative approach to replace parts of the trachea by growing stem cells on a synthetic scaffold, which was then implanted into a patient. The first operation, carried out in 2011 at the Karolinska University Hospital, was broadcasted as a groundbreaking attainment, published in prestigious medical journals and hailed by the press. Five years later a different picture was drawn. A 3-hour documentary called The Experiments (Experimenten) was aired on the Swedish public television (SVT) [18] and presented follow-up of surgeries performed implanting the synthetic trachea in both Sweden and similar surgeries in Russia. The documentary showed interviews with the patients' close relatives who believed that the operations contributed to the patients' premature deaths. In addition the documentary shared data revealing that the surgeries lacked proper scientific support and regulatory approval [19]. The magnitude of the crisis can be illustrated by the reaction of the Royal Swedish Academy of Science as reported in *The Lancet* [20]. Several inquiries on issues ranging from research fraud to criminal misconduct were commenced following the airing of the documentary [19] (Karolinska Institute 2016: Karolinska Institute (2016) 'ACTREM' <http://ki.se/en/clintec/actrem> (the site was removed in late March 2016). Four members of the Nobel Prize committee in physiology or medicine resigned. The vice-chancellor of the Karolinska Institute, Professor Hamsten, resigned after formerly defending the thoracic surgeon PM. In April 2016, *The Lancet* published an expression of concern, noting the 'ongoing uncertainty about the integrity of the work reported in this paper; while reserving a final decision for when current investigations are completed' [19].

Ethical problems are raised by conflicting values and by interests that pull in different directions. If and when interests or values clash (when certain values or interests can only be achieved at the expense of others), principles are available that can guide the decision-making [2]. The Lancet commission published in 2018 [1] highlighted the different ways in which stem cell therapy can be accessed: 'Patients can access stem cell and regenerative therapies in four ways. First, and most straightforwardly, when a therapy has been tested and received marketing approval for the indication for which the clinical team intends to use it. Second, in the context of a clinical trial. Third, through permitted non-research access to a treatment that does not have marketing approval for that indication—including hospital exemption within the EU, and also off-label or compassionate use. Fourth and more crucially, through direct recruitment (usually through the internet) from commercial entities whose activity is not scrutinised or approved by any regulatory body'.

Though such challenges can be difficult to address and solve, a strategy to tackle such hurdle can rely on coordinated approach based on four main pillars: better science, better governance better funding models and better public and patient engagement. Together with warranting regulatory procedures which are transparent, robust and evidence-based and the expectation to be speedy and accurate, there is much else to be done. The academies' consensus has highlighted specific priorities including reinvigoration of EU research infrastructure, particularly for translational and clinical research [20], support for new models of partnership between academia and industry whilst ensuring ethical development [14], inserting regenerative medicine in curricula for medical education and professional training [21], alerting against non-peer-reviewed 'predatory' journals [22], developing health services' institutional readiness in relation to regenerative medicine research and engaging with the public and patients to counter misinformation [2].

Demand

The global stem cell therapy market is projected to reach USD 401 million by 2026 from USD 187 million in 2021, at a compound annual growth rate (CAGR) of 16.5% during the forecast period. Growth in this market is majorly driven by the increasing investment in stem cell research and the rising number of GMP-certified stem cell manufacturing plants. The stem cell therapy market is segmented into North America, Europe and Asia Pacific, followed by rest of the world. The stem cell therapy market in the Asia Pacific region is expected to grow at the highest CAGR during the forecast period. Factors such as the growing adoption of stem cell-based treatment in the region and the growing approval and commercialisation of stem cell-based products for degenerative disorders drive the growth of the stem cell therapy market in the region [23].

One of the key factors boosting the growth of this market is the limitations of traditional organ transplantation such as the risk of infection, rejection and immunosuppression risk. Another drawback of conventional organ transplantation is that doctors have to depend on organ donors completely. All these issues can be eliminated by the application of stem cell therapy. Another factor which is helping the growth in this market is the growing pipeline and development of drugs for emerging applications. Increased research studies aiming to widen the scope of stem cell will also fuel the growth of the market. Scientists are constantly engaged in trying to find out novel methods for creating human stem cells in response to the growing demand for stem cell production to be used for disease management. This has been supported by the results of research studies revealing successful translation of stem cell therapies to patients that have augmented the hope that such regenerative strategies may one day become a treatment for a wide range of vexing diseases (2). This is of particular interest for those patients who have no other therapeutic option but to resort to stem cell clinics or products given conditional marketing status on the basis of inadequate evidence.

Over the past 2 years during the COVID-19 epidemic, an escalating demand for stem cell research products has been reported. This has been attributed to several factors including (1) the use of stem cells in the treatment of COVID-19 complications, such as immune and respiratory complications; (2) promise of mesenchymal cells (MSCs) for ameliorating COVID-induced respiratory distress, such as ARDS; (3) accelerated pathways for regulatory approvals during COVID-19; (4) surging funding for stem cell research due to support from BARDA, CIRM, NIAID and other groups; (5) increased interest among pharmaceutical companies in stem cell R&D programs related to COVID-19; and (6) potential for stem cells to support the management of the global COVID-19 pandemic [24].

Such growing demand on stem cell therapy and its potential to change the future of medicine represents a major challenge particularly to ensure patients' safety. The general public must be cautious of clinics that exploit people's desperation for a cure. On the other hand, whilst researchers are working to use stem cells to improve health care, they have to make sure that it is carried out safely with some form of oversight.

Finance

Research into biomedical innovations has the potential to yield economic and health benefits. However, noteworthy financial investment is mandatory to bring these innovations from 'bench to bedside' [1, 2]. As such it is no surprise that several funding agencies as well as governments considered that fostering commercialisation is vital to make the economic and medical potential of biomedical research a reality and to deliver on promised targets and benefits [25–28].

Commercialisation is defined as 'links between both publicly funded researchers and industry; and efforts to turn university - based research into marketable products and services' [29, 30].

The field of stem cell research has been subject to significant commercialisation pressure. Scientists are facing pressure to develop stem cell therapies that will reach the clinic within a short period, from both the funding agencies as well as the public [22, 31, 32]. To date, there has been only limited progress in translating stem cell research into clinical therapies, but this has not lowered the expectations or enthusiasm for the field, as the phenomenon of 'stem cell tourism' attests [32]. The commercialisation pressures facing stem cell researchers are likely to continue into the foreseeable future.

A major challenge comes to the surface on evolving the financial models. For some novel approaches, limited experimental evidence may be existing based on a rational starting research hypothesis, published in reputable journals and involving expert scientists. But the data are then endorsed in an unbalanced way by company sources with the consequence that the distinction between validated and replicated or premature and unsubstantiated therapeutic claims may become harder. That is, instead of the initial simple scenario where 'good' and 'bad' clinical centres could easily be contrasted, there is now a continuum from one extreme to the other without clear boundaries. Lack of published information may indicate a more general lack of evidence, for example, on cell characteristics and clinical effects, and an intention to claim beneficial properties in multiple indications [3].

Such financial challenges highlight the need for regulatory authorities to build good scientific links with the companies and their regulatory advisory committees to ensure the presence of an appropriately robust evidence base, even when encouraging early access to innovation by patients who may have few or no other options. There are also related issues for what should be allowed in terms of promotional medical claims on company websites when no marketing authorisation has yet been granted and the use by companies of selected patient results when other information is not supportive [33].

Media

Public views can significantly influence governmental policy and consequently can have a large impact on regenerative medicine and stem cell research. Therefore it is vastly important for the public to be informed of scientific advancements and what they mean. Additionally it is vital that researchers are in tune with how the public perceives regenerative medicine research. In general, news media is the primary way the public learns about scientific and medical breakthroughs. However, several questions have been raised and await answers. These include the following: How does the media portray regenerative medicine and stem cell research? Do the articles available in the media promote unrealistic expectations? And what topics about regenerative medicine research does the media focus on?

In their study [34], Kalina Kamenova and Timothy Caulfield tried to answer these questions. Of the 307 newspaper articles analysed, 37.1% focused on clinical translation, and 22.8% discussed new scientific discoveries. Only 1.6% of the articles focused on the ethical issues of regenerative medicine and stem cells. The majority (57.7%) of all newspaper articles between 2009 and 2014 presented the future of regenerative medicine and stem cell research in a positive and optimistic tone.

Responding to the Challenges: The Opportunities

In spite of the fact that research in regenerative medicine next generation cell and gene therapies has been going on for years and the hype around stem cell therapies, tissue engineering and its potential value, it has only recently started to become commercially available, and relatively few patients have benefited to date. Worldwide, 64 ATMPs have been reported including 34 cell therapies, 20 gene therapies and 10 tissue engineering products. Whilst not a relatively small figure, it is far eclipsed by the number of products that have entered clinical development and stalled there [3].

The path to the market is rather complex, expensive, time-consuming and highly regulated. Even for those products that are successful, not that many of them have the potential to become blockbusters. In February 2021, one of the biotech companies 'Humacyte' broadcasted its decision to go public, inaugurating its move from a clinical-stage company to a commercial one. The company, which develops regenerative human tissues that can be implanted in any patient without the need for immunosuppressive drugs, is expected to hit the market with a value of $1.1bn [34].

Endorsing the conversion of science to clinical application necessitates strong ethical review and commitment of the sponsors of research. Clinical research is not cheap, and EU-level funding mechanisms are warranted, in particular to advance from limited phase research to academic investigator-led, clinically based studies, including clinical trials (and active comparator designs). Funding provided by professional organisations such as EU can help to coordinate and build initial critical mass in clinical research [35].

Participation of the patients in the study design and follow-up can be beneficial particularly for the new models of regenerative medicine translation [20]. There is also scope for public investment, at the EU level, in evolving platform technologies which can be implemented in multiple applications, e.g. gene therapy vectors. Furthermore, there is also an opportunity for a closer relationship between the clinical and social sciences and humanities. This would enable researchers to get better understanding of the social and ethical implications and public expectations of regenerative medicine [36]. This will also enable social scientists to better understand about the clinical trials' practicalities.

Building new links between academia and industry in regenerative medicine is vital to make such partnership a reality [37]. Such partnership paves the way for several potential roles, for generating tools, promoting applications and clinical translation. It may also help in bridging the financial gaps in early product development. Sustained funding provided by either professional authority such as EU as well as national organisations is also central to indorse networks able to bring together multiple regenerative medicine disciplines (e.g. EuroStemCell). This will not only help to explore the clinical potential but also to set up the fundamental research base that provides the initial resource for any future pipeline in regenerative medicine [38].

Tackling the gaps in health-care education on regenerative medicine is also vital to endorse such innovative development. Unfortunately so far in most medical schools at either undergraduate or postgraduate level, little mention is made about regenerative medicine although there are some cases of good practice represented by courses on haematological stem cell approaches [21]. Efforts to progress medical education need to consider two main factors: first, tackling the gaps in training on ethical, legal and societal issues in regenerative medicine, including how to involve other stakeholders, especially patients, in research design and review [39] and second, training for primary care professionals to advise patients on how to access and assess good evidence. This was supported by the findings of a recent research which highlighted the need to improve information for these professionals about regenerative medicine [40].

Tackling the publication practices is vital to ensure the integrity of the published research. The development of guidelines/recommendations for clinical trial registration/study design, data analysis and reproducibility, as well as reporting, is important to ensure that the outcomes of failed trials are documented, particularly as most journals give priority to successful trials or trials claimed as such. Furthermore, there should be strategies supporting the open accessibility of negative data to enable independent analysis as part of strong and comprehensive procedures to track and coordinate evidence development [3]. On another front, the scientific community should carefully consider the issue of appraising the quality of journal publications. The launch of predatory, non-peer-reviewed open access journals and the paucity of expert reviewers for the increasing manuscript numbers represent a major challenge that require tackling in the publication practices issue. Therefore there is a role for medical research charity patient groups to provide resources, whereby patients can seek advice.

Is There a Bright Future for Regenerative Medicine?

Since the birth of the biotechnology industry in the late 1970s, many transformational technologies and new therapies have been announced improving medical care and benefitting patients. Further, in many areas of medicine exciting progress continues. However, there are many areas where standard of care is fundamentally limited and significant challenges highlighted. So, it is natural to ask: What advances will the next decade bring? How will the landscape evolve in light of key health-care and technology trends? And is there a bright future for regenerative medicine? This will be stratified and discussed briefly below as the main pillars of modern regenerative medicine.

Driver: Availability of Funding for Stem Cell Research

The need for newer and better therapies for the treatment of autoimmune, neurological and cardiovascular diseases has resulted in an overall increase in research activities and the availability of funding for cell-based research. In November 2019, the Australian government released a 10-year roadmap for stem cell research in Australia—The Stem Cell Therapies Mission.

Restraints: Ethical Concerns Related to Embryonic Stem Cells

Several ethical issues are associated with the use of stem cells. Ethical problems are raised by conflicting standards and by interests that pull in variable directions. To move forward, decisions can be taken and even changed as the scientific evidence and value landscape change. These include (1) importance of objective (the targets, whether theoretical or practical, should be of significant value), (2) relevance of means (the means should achieve or at least help to achieve the target), (3) most favourable option (there is no other less risky or controversial means to achieve the target(s)) and (4) non-excessiveness (the means used should not be excessive in relation to the intended target) [3].

Opportunity: Emergence of iPSCs as an Alternative to ESCs

Induced pluripotent stem cells (iPSCs) are adult stem cells that have been genetically reprogrammed back to an embryonic stem cell-like state. iPSCs function similarly to embryonic stem cells (ESCs), having the ability to differentiate into specialised tissue cells according to the gene expression; this makes iPSCs an effective alternative to ESCs. As ESCs are derived from early-stage embryos, they are associated with socio-ethical issues and laws related to contraception, abortion and in vitro fertilisation. The use of iPSCs bypasses the need for human embryos, thus avoiding socio-ethical objections.

The Allogeneic Stem Cell Therapy Segment Dominated the Stem Cell Therapy Market in 2020

Based on type, the global stem cell therapy market is broadly segmented into allogeneic stem cell therapy and autologous stem cell therapy. In 2020, the allogeneic segment accounted for the largest share of the stem cell therapy market. The growth of the allogeneic segment is attributed to the ease of manufacturing and production processes and the increasing availability of novel stem cell products across major geographies.

The Inflammatory and Autoimmune Disease Segment Will Witness the Highest Growth During the Forecast Period

Based on therapeutic application, the global stem cell therapy market is segmented into musculoskeletal disorders, wounds and injuries, cardiovascular diseases, surgeries, inflammatory and autoimmune diseases, neurological disorders and other therapeutic applications (which include ocular diseases, fat loss and peripheral arterial diseases). The neurological disorder segment is expected to grow at the highest CAGR during the forecast period owing to the increasing prevalence of neurological disorders and the high cost of therapy [41].

Conclusion

In conclusion, many areas of clinical medicine could be transformed by advances in regenerative medicine. A mixture of poor-quality science, blurred funding models, unrealistic expectations and unprincipled private clinics threatens regenerative medicine's social licence to function. Tackling these challenges can be the light at the end of the tunnel. If regenerative medicine is to shift from mostly limited bespoke investigational interventions into routine clinical practice, together with ensuring high quality of publication, significant rethinking of the social perception that supports such research and clinical practice in the public arena will take place. Limitations in standard of care and unmet clinical needs, as well as the corresponding anticipation for better outcomes and enhanced quality of life by patients and their families, will continue to drive medical innovation. Such improvements are possible only if investment fuels the innovation and sensible policies are applied to help enable the efficient development of new medicines.

References

1. Cossu G, Birchall M, Brown T, et al. Lancet Commission: stem cells and regenerative medicine. Lancet. 2018;391:883–910.
2. Cossu G, Fears R, Griffin G, Ter Meulen V. Regenerative medicine: challenges and opportunities. Lancet. 2020;395(10239):1746–7.
3. EASAC, FEAM. Challenges and potential in regenerative medicine: a joint report from EASAC and FEAM. Halle (Saale): German National Academy of Sciences Leopoldina. 2020. https://easac.eu/fileadmin/PDF_s/reports_statements/Regenerative_Medicine/EASAC_Regenerative_Medicine_Web_10_September_2020.pdf. Accessed 5th Dec 2021.
4. MacPherson A, Kimmelman J. Ethical development of stem cell-based interventions. Nat Med. 2019;2019(25):1037–44.
5. Lindstrom-Gommers L, Mullin T. International conference on harmonization: recent reforms as a driver of global regulatory harmonization and innovation in medical products. Clin Pharmacol Ther. 2018;2018(105):926–31.
6. Clinical trial evidence supporting FDA approval of novel therapeutic agents, 2005–2012. JAMA. 2014;311:368.
7. Abou-El-Enein M, Hey SP. Cell and gene therapy trials: are we facing an 'evidence crisis'? Lancet. 2019;7:13–4.
8. Djurisic S, Rath A, Gaber S, Garattini S, Bertele V, Ngwabyt SN, Hivert V, Neugebauer EAM, Laville M, Hiesmayr M, Demotes-Mainard J, Kubiak C, Jakobsen JC, Gluud C. Barriers to the conduct of randomised clinical trials within all disease areas. Trials. 2017;18(1):360.
9. Abou-El-Enein M, Grainger DW, Kili S. Registry contributions to strengthen cell and gene therapeutic evidence. Mol Ther. 2018;26(5):1172–6.
10. Miake-Lye IM, Hempel S, Shanman R, Shekelle PG. What is an evidence map? A systematic review of published evidence maps and their definitions, methods, and products. Syst Rev. 2016;5:28.
11. Sipp D, Sleeboom-Faulkner M. Downgrading of regulation in regenerative medicine. Science. 2019;365:644–6.
12. Fu W, Smith C, Turner L, et al. Characteristics and scope of training of clinicians participating in the US direct-to-consumer marketplace for unproven stem cell interventions. JAMA. 2019;321:2463–4.
13. Cyranoski D. The potent effects of Japan's stem-cell policies. Nature. 2019;573:482–5.
14. MacPherson A, Kimmelman J. Ethical development of stem-cell-based therapies. Nat Med. 2019;25:1037–44.

15. Asplund K, Hermerén G. The need to revise the Helsinki Declaration. Lancet. 2017;389:1190–1.
16. Lindquist B. Experimenten [television documentary in three parts]. Stockholm: SVT (in Swedish); 2016.
17. McKelvey M, Saemundsson RJ, Zaring O. A recent crisis in regenerative medicine: analyzing governance in order to identify public policy issues. Sci Public Policy. 2018;45(5):608–20.
18. Horton R. Offline: Paolo Macchiarini - science in conflict. Lancet. 2016;387:732.
19. The Lancet. Expression of concern-tracheobronchial transplantation with a stem-cell-seeded bioartificial nanocomposite: a proof-of-concept study. Lancet. 2016;387:1359.
20. Toure SB, Kleiderman E, Knoppers BM. Bridging stem cell research and medicine: a learning health system. Regen Med. 2018;13:741–52.
21. Wyles SP, Hayden RE, Meyer FB, Terzic A. Regenerative medicine curriculum for next-generation physicians. NPJ Regen Med. 2019;4:3.
22. Dobush L, Heimstädt M, Mayer K, Ross-Hellauer T. Defining predatory journals: no peer review, no point. Nature. 2020;580:29.
23. Global Stem Cell Therapy Market (2021 to 2026) - Growing Demand for Cell & Gene Therapies Presents Opportunities. Research and Markets 2021. https://www.globenewswire.com/en/news-release/2021/05/13/2228889/28124/en/Global-Stem-Cell-Therapy-Market-2021-to-2026-Growing-Demand-for-Cell-Gene-Therapies--Presents-Opportunities.html. Accessed on 12th Dec 2021.
24. Hildreth C. Escalating demand for stem cell research products during COVID-19. Bioinformant. 2020. https://bioinformant.com/stem-cell-research-report/. Accessed on 12th Dec 2021.
25. Pucéat M, Ballis A. Embryonic stem cells: from bench to bedside. Clin Pharmacol Ther. 2007;82:337–9.
26. Henderson GE, Cadigan RJ, Edwards TP, et al. Characterizing biobank organizations in the U.S.: results from a national survey. Genome Med. 2013;5:3.
27. Caulfield T. Sustainability and the balancing of the health care and innovation agendas: the commercialization of genetic research. Sask L Rev. 2003;66:629–46.
28. Mason C. ISSCR 2009 industry panel session: promoting translation and commercialization. Cell Stem Cell. 2009;5:379–84.
29. Caulfield T. Patents or commercialization pressure? A (speculative) search for the right target. J Law Info Sci. 2012;22:122.
30. Caulfield T, Harmon SHE, Joly Y. Open science versus commercialization: a modern research conflict? Genome Med. 2012;4:17.
31. Caulfield T. Stem cell research and economic promises. J Law Med Ethics. 2010;38:303–13.
32. Bubela T, Li MD, Hafez M, Bieber M, Atkins H. Is belief larger than fact: expectations, optimism and reality for translational stem cell research. BMC. 2012;Med 10:133.
33. Murdoch CJ, Caulfield T. Commercialization, patenting and genomics: researcher perspectives. Genome Med. 2009;1:22.
34. Millar A. Regenerative medicine: ready for the big leagues? https://www.pharmaceutical-technology.com/features/regenerative-medicine-ready-for-big-leagues/. Accessed on 26th Dec 2021.
35. Barker RA, Farrell K, Guzman NV, et al. Designing stem-cell based dopamine cell replacement trials for Parkinson's disease. Nat Med. 2019;25:1045–53.
36. Edwards J, Thomas R, Guilliatt R. Regenerative medicine: from the laboratory looking out. Palgrave Communications. 2017;3:27.
37. Corbett MS, Webster A, Hawkins R, Woolacott N. Innovative regenerative medicines in the EU: a better future in evidence? BMC Med. 2017;15:49.
38. de Haan G, de Crom R, Dzierzak E, Mummery C. Regenerative medicine funding policies in Europe and the Netherlands. NPJ Regen Med. 2017;2:1.
39. Illes J, Sipp D, Kleiderman E. A blueprint for the next generation of ELSI research, training and outreach in regenerative medicine. NPJ Regen Med. 2017;2:21.
40. Sola M, Sanchez-Quevedo C, Martin-Piedra MA, et al. Evaluation of the awareness of novel advanced therapies among family medicine residents in Spain. PLoS One. 2019;14:e0214950.
41. Stem Cell Therapy Market by Type (Allogeneic, Autologous), Therapeutic Application (Musculoskeletal, Wound & Injury, CVD, Autoimmune & Inflammatory), Cell Source (Adipose tissue, Bone Marrow, Placenta/Umbilical Cord) - Global Forecasts to 2026. https://www.marketsandmarkets.com/Market-Reports/stem-cell-technologies-and-global-market-48.html. Accessed on 12th Dec 2021.

Index

Y. El Miedany (ed.), *Musculoskeletal Ultrasound-Guided Regenerative Medicine*,
https://doi.org/10.1007/978-3-030-98256-0

K

L

M

N

O